HEMATOLOGIC VALUES *(Continued)*

DETERMINATION	REFERENCE RANGE		NOTES
	Conventional	SI*	
HEMATOLOGY *(continued)*			
Leukocyte count	Newborn: 9000–30,000/μl 1 week: 5000–21,000/μl 1 month: 5000–19,500/μl 6–12 months: 6000–17,500/μl 2 years of age: 6200–17,000μl Child/adult: 4800–10,800/μl	$9.0–30.0 \times 10^9$/liter $5.0–21.0 \times 10^9$/liter $5.0–19.5 \times 10^9$/liter $6.0–17.5 \times 10^9$/liter $6.2–17.0 \times 10^9$/liter $4.8–10.8 \times 10^9$/liter	Hemacytometer
Erythrocyte count	Newborn: 4.4–5.8 million/μl Infant/child: 3.8–5.5 million/μl Adult male: 4.7–6.1 million/μl Adult female: 4.2–5.4 million/μl	$4.4–5.8 \times 10^{12}$/liter $3.8–5.5 \times 10^{12}$/liter $4.7–6.1 \times 10^{12}$/liter $4.2–5.4 \times 10^{12}$/liter	Hemacytometer
Eosinophil count	50–400/μl		Hemacytometer
Reticulocyte count	Newborn (0–2 weeks): 2.5–6.0% Adult: 0.5–2.0% red cells		New methylene blue
Absolute reticulocyte count	60,000/μl		

Erythrocyte sedimentation rate
  (ESR)
	Male: 0–15 mm/hr
	Female: 0–20 mm/hr
			Use EDTA as anticoagulant;
			  Westergren Method

Osmotic fragility of erythrocytes	Initial hemolysis: 0.45% Complete hemolysis: 0.30–0.35%		Use heparin as anticoagulant

Acidified serum test (Ham test)
  for paroxysmal nocturnal
  hemoglobinuria (PNH)
	No hemolysis		

Sugar water test for PNH	Less than 5% red cell hemolysis		

Autohemolysis test	Lysis at 48 hrs: without added
	  dexrose: 0.2%, with added
	  dextrose: 0–0.9%, with added
	  ATP: 0–0.8%		

Heinz body induction test	1 Heinz body per RBC		

Erythrocyte enzymes:
  Glucose—6-phosphate
  dehydrogenase
	5–15 U/g Hb	5–15 U/g	Use special anticoagulant
			  (ACD solution)

Pyruvate kinase	13–17 U/g Hb	13–17 U/g	Use special anticoagulant (ACD solution)
Ferritin (serum)			
Iron deficiency	0–12 ng/ml 13–20 borderline	0–4.8 nmol/liter 5.2–8 nmol/liter borderline	
Iron excess	>400 ng/liter	>160 nmol/liter	
Folic acid			
Normal	>3.3 ng/liter	>7.3 nmol/liter	
Borderline	2.5–3.2 ng/ml	5.75–7.39 nmol/liter	
Haptoglobin	40–336 mg/100 ml	0.4–3.6 g/liter	

*SI—System of International Units.

CLINICAL HEMATOLOGY
AND FUNDAMENTALS
OF HEMOSTASIS

CLINICAL HEMATOLOGY AND FUNDAMENTALS OF HEMOSTASIS

THIRD EDITION

**Denise M. Harmening, PhD,
MT(ASCP), CLS(NCA)**
Editor
Chair and Professor
Department of Medical and Research Technology
University of Maryland School of Medicine
University of Maryland at Baltimore
Baltimore, Maryland

 F. A. DAVIS COMPANY • Philadelphia

F. A. Davis Company
1915 Arch Street
Philadelphia, PA 19103

Printed in the United States of America

Last digit indicates print number: 10 9 8 7 6 5 4 3 2

Publisher: Jean-François Vilain
Developmental Editor: Ralph Zickgraf, Marianne Fithian
Production Editor: Jessica Howie Martin
Cover Designer: Louis J. Forgione

As new scientific information becomes available through basic and clinical research, recommended treatments and drug therapies undergo changes. The author and publisher have done everything possible to make this book accurate, up to date, and in accord with accepted standards at the time of publication. The author, editors, and publisher are not responsible for errors or omissions or for consequences from application of the book, and make no warranty, expressed or implied, in regard to the contents of the book. Any practice described in this book should be applied by the reader in accordance with professional standards of care used in regard to the unique circumstances that may apply in each situation. The reader is advised always to check product information (package inserts) for changes and new information regarding dose and contraindications before administering any drug. Caution is especially urged when using new or infrequently ordered drugs.

Library of Congress Cataloging-in-Publication Data
Clinical hematology and fundamentals of hemostasis / Denise M.
  Harmening, editor.—3rd ed.
     p. cm.
  Includes bibliographical references and index.
  ISBN 0-8036-0135-2 (hardcover)
  1. Hematology. 2. Blood—Diseases. 3. Homeostasis.
I. Harmening, Denise.
  [DNLM: 1. Hematologic Diseases. 2. Hemostasis. 3. Blood Cells—
physiology. 4. Hematopoiesis. WH 100 C6413 1997]
RB145.536 1997
616.1'5—dc20
DNLM/DLC
for Library of Congress   96-29337
                                                                    CIP

To all students, full-time, part-time, past, present, and future, who have touched and will continue to touch the lives of so many educators . . .

It is to you this book is dedicated in the hope of inspiring an unquenchable thirst for knowledge and love of mankind.

PREFACE

The third edition of this text has been designed as a thorough and concise guide to clinical hematology and fundamentals of hemostasis. The textbook is unique in its five-part format, featuring an introduction to clinical hematology and sections on the anemias, white blood cell disorders, hemostasis/thrombosis, and laboratory methods, allowing easy incorporation into block curricula. New chapters on the use of flow cytometry, the molecular diagnostic techniques in hematopathology, and an introduction to thrombosis and anticoagulant therapy are highlights of this edition.

Full color has been incorporated throughout the entire text. The photographs from the 260-color-plate atlas, a prominent feature of previous editions, have been incorporated into the relevant chapters. These color figures, demonstrating peripheral smears, bone marrow aspirates, gross morphology, and clinical manifestations, enhance the text as a foundation for the practice of clinical laboratory science. In addition, the third edition includes more than 300 figures (line drawings and black-and-white photographs) and 400 tables.

The first five chapters (Part I) focus on hematopoiesis, bone marrow examination, red cell metabolism, the pathogenesis of anemia, and the evaluation of red cell morphology. The next ten chapters (Part II) are devoted to anemias, presenting the disease processes leading to abnormal red blood cell morphology. Part III contains nine chapters that focus on white blood cell disorders, including both benign and malignant states. Included are reviews of the leukemias, myelodysplastic syndromes, myeloproliferative disorders, plasma cell dyscrasias, lymphomas, and lipid storage disease. The new chapter introducing flow cytometry is also in this section. Part IV focuses on hemostasis, with chapters devoted to platelet structure and function, vascular and platelet disorders, defects of plasma clotting factors, and the interaction of the fibrinolytic, coagulation, and kinin systems. A final chapter introducing thrombosis and anticoagulant therapy concludes the hemostasis section.

The laboratory methods chapter of the second edition has been expanded into five chapters, which make up the final segment of the text (Part V). This expanded format provides a more comprehensive guide to procedures routinely performed in the clinical hematology and hemostasis laboratory, including routine hematology methods, principles of automated differential analysis, special stains, and coagulation. New in this edition is a chapter on molecular diagnostic techniques in hematopathology.

The text has retained the popular listing of normal hematologic values on the inside covers for quick reference. Chapter outlines, educational objectives, case studies, and study guide questions accompany each chapter. An innovative instructor's guide emphasizing competency-based assessment accompanies the text, and an interactive test-generating system, CyberTest™, is also available. Slides of the 260 color photographs are a new offering.

This new edition, like the first and second, is a culmination of dedicated efforts of a group of prominent professionals. They committed themselves to this project by donating their time and expertise out of concern for a common goal: improving patient care by providing a high-quality practical and usable textbook. To all of these contributors, thank you and congratulations on a wonderful book.

My sincere appreciation is also extended to the following educators and clinicians for their thorough and thoughtful review of the manuscript:

- Joanne Cuomo
  North Shore University Hospital
  Manhasset, New York
- Jane Elder, MS, MT(ASCP)SBB
  Program Director/Instructor
  MLT-AD Program
  Hinds Community College
  Jackson, Mississippi

- Juanita Gurubatham, MA, MT(ASCP)HT
  Assistant Professor and Program Director, Clinical Laboratory Science
  Columbia Union College
  Takoma Park, Maryland
- Virginia C. Hughes, BSMT(ASCP)
  Instructor, Anne Arundel Community College
  Arnold, Maryland
- Karen M. Kiser, MT(ASCP)
  Associate Professor/Education Coordinator
  Department of Clinical Laboratory Technology and Phlebotomy
  St. Louis Community College
  St. Louis, Missouri
- Janice G. LaReau, MS, MT(ASCP)SH
  Assistant Professor and Clinical Laboratory Science Program Director
  Indiana University Northwest
  Gary, Indiana
- Cynthia A. Martine, MEd, MT(ASCP)
  Assistant Professor, Department of Medical Technology
  University of Texas Medical Branch
  Galveston, Texas
- Mary R. McCole, MT(ASCP)SC
  Program Director, Department of Pathology and Laboratory Medicine
  Veterans Administration School of Medical Technology
  Overton Brooks Veterans Medical Center
  Shreveport, Louisiana
- Phyllis Muellenberg, MA, MT(ASCP)
  Program Director, Department of Medical Technology
  University of Nebraska Medical Center
  Omaha, Nebraska
- Mary A. Nelson, MT(ASCP)
  Instructor/Clinical Coordinator
  Medical Laboratory Technician Department
  Madison Area Technical College
  Madison, Wisconsin
- Joseph K. Semak, EdD, MT(ASCP)
  Director Medical Laboratory Technician Program
  Cleveland State Community College
  Cleveland, Tennessee

A very special acknowledgment must be given to Virginia Hughes, my graduate student and technologist, who works at Anne Arundel Hospital. Her many hours of dedicated and meticulous review have ensured a more accurate and usable text.

Finally, I would like to acknowledge the contributions, throughout the book's preparation, of my dedicated coworkers and friends at the Department of Medical and Research Technology, particularly Joanne Manning, Cynthia Stambach, William Haythorn, and Audrey Ford.

In summary, this book has been designed to inspire an unquenchable thirst for knowledge in every medical technologist, hematologist, and practitioner whose knowledge, skills, and ongoing education provide the public with excellence in health care.

D. M. Harmening, PhD, MT(ASCP), CLS(NCA)

CONTRIBUTORS

Ann Bell, MS, SH(ASCP), CLSpH(NCA)
Emeritus Assistant Professor, Medicine
Emeritus Assistant Professor of Clinical Laboratory Sciences
Department of Medicine
Division of Hematology/Oncology
University of Tennessee, Memphis
Health Science Center
Memphis, Tennessee

Rita M. Braziel, MD
Associate Professor, Pathology
Director of Hematopathology, Flow Cytometry, and Molecular Diagnostics
Oregon Health Sciences University
Director of Hematology, Cellular and Molecular Diagnostics
Legacy Laboratory Services
Legacy Health System
Portland, Oregon

Barbara S. Caldwell, MT(ASCP)SH
Clinical Instructor
Department of Medical and Research Technology
University of Maryland School of Medicine
Baltimore, Maryland

Michel M. Canton, PharmD
Director of Clinical and Business Development
American Bioproducts Company
Parsippany, New Jersey

Carol C. Caruana, H(ASCP)SH
Department of Laboratories
North Shore University Hospital
New York University School of Medicine
Manhasset, New York

Betty E. Ciesla, MS, MT(ASCP)SH
School Assistant Professor
Department of Medical and Research Technology
University of Maryland School of Medicine
Baltimore, Maryland

Theresa L. Coetzer, PhD
South African Institute for Medical Research
University of the Witwatersrand
Department of Haematology
Johannesburg, South Africa

Giovanni D'Angelo, FCSLT
Laboratory Director
Department of Hematology
Maisonneuve–Rosemont Hospital
Professor of Hematology
University of Montreal, Faculty of Pharmacy
Montreal, Quebec, Canada

Deirdre E. DeSantis, MS, MT(ASCP)SBB
School Assistant Professor
Department of Medical and Research Technology
University of Maryland School of Medicine
Baltimore, Maryland

Gordon E. Ens, MT(ASCP)
Laboratory Director
Colorado Coagulation Consultants
Associate Editor
Clinical Hemostasis Review
Denver, Colorado

Armand B. Glassman, MD
Olla S. Stribling Chair for Cancer Research
Professor, Head and Chairman
Division and Department of Laboratory Medicine
The University of Texas M.D. Anderson Cancer Center
Houston, Texas

Ralph Green, BAppSci(MLS), FAIMS
Associate Professor in
Immunohematology
Acting Head
Department of Medical Laboratory
Science
Faculty of Biomedical and Health
Sciences
Royal Melbourne Institute of
Technology University
Melbourne, Victoria, Australia

Kathryn A. Grenier, MT(ASCP), CLT(CA)
Director, Clinical Research
Clinical Pathways
Morgan Hill, California

Margaret L. Gulley, MD
Director of Molecular Diagnostics
Department of Pathology
The University of Texas Health
Science Center at San Antonio
and
Audie Murphy Veteran's Hospital
San Antonio, Texas

Sandra Gwaltney-Krause, MA, MT(ASCP)
Former Instructor
Department of Medical Technology
University of South Alabama
Mobile, Alabama

Martin Gyger, MD, FRCP(C)
Professor of Medicine
University of Montreal
Cytogenetics Laboratory Director
Department of Hematology
Maisonneuve–Rosemont Hospital
Montreal, Quebec, Canada

Denise M. Harmening, PhD, MT(ASCP), CLS(NCA)
Chair and Professor
Department of Medical and Research
Technology
University of Maryland School of
Medicine
University of Maryland at Baltimore
Baltimore, Maryland

Chantal Ricaud Harrison, MD
Professor of Pathology
Medical Director/Blood Bank
Department of Pathology
The University of Texas Health
Science Center at San Antonio
San Antonio, Texas

Laurel D. Holmer, MEd, MT(ASCP)SH
Clinical Laboratory Science Program
University of Nevada School of
Medicine
Reno, Nevada

Ellen Hope, MS, SH(ASCP)H
Professor of Clinical Sciences
Department of Clinical Sciences
School of Health
California State University,
Dominguez Hills
Carson, California

Virginia Hughes, BS, MT(ASCP)
Instructor
Department of Allied Health Sciences
Anne Arundel Community College
Arnold, Maryland

Dan M. Hyder, MD
Department of Pathology and
Laboratory Medicine
Southwest Washington Medical
Center
Vancouver, Washington

Bette Jamieson, MEd, SH(ASCP)
Hematology Supervisor
Department of Hematology
Children's Hospital
Denver, Colorado

Carmen J. Julius, MD
Department of Pathology and
Laboratory Medicine
The Ohio State University
Columbus, Ohio

Joette Kizer, MT(ASCP)
Manager, Hematology/Flow
Cytometry and Cytogenetics Sections
Department of Pathology and
Laboratory Medicine
Medical University of South Carolina
Charleston, South Carolina

John Lazarchick, MD
Professor and Director
Hematology/Hemostasis
Department of Pathology and Clinical
Medicine
Medical University of South Carolina
Charleston, South Carolina

Susan J. Leclair, MS, CLS(NCA)
Department of Medical Laboratory
Science
University of Massachusetts
Dartmouth
North Dartmouth, Massachusetts

Linda D. Lemery, MBA, MT(ASCP)DLM
Instructor
Medical Laboratory
Technology Department
Alamance Community College
Graham, North Carolina

James M. Long, MD, LtCol(sel), USAF
Department of Hematology and Oncology
David Grant Medical Center/SGOMO
Travis Air Force Base
Vacaville, California

Joe Marty, MS, MT(ASCP)
Assistant Professor (Clinical)
Department of Pathology
University of Utah Health Sciences
Center
Salt Lake City, Utah

Sara McCarron, MD
Department of Laboratory Medicine
The University of Texas
M. D. Anderson Cancer Center
Houston, Texas

Milka M. Montiel, MD
Professor, Department of Pathology
Director, Hematology Laboratory
Deputy Chair, Clinical Services
The University of Texas Health
Science Center at San Antonio
San Antonio, Texas

Suzy L. Nicol, MT(ASCP)SBB
Department of Transfusion Medicine
The Johns Hopkins Hospital
Baltimore, Maryland

J. Michael Odell, MD
Department of Pathology
Legacy Laboratory Services
Legacy Health System
Portland, Oregon

Elinor J. B. Peerschke, PhD
Professor of Pathology
Director, Clinical Hematology
Laboratory
Cornell University School of Medicine
New York, New York

Mary Loring Perkins, MS, MT(ASCP)SH
System Manager, Hematology,
Cellular and Molecular Diagnostics
Legacy Laboratory Services
Legacy Health System
Portland, Oregon

Sherrie L. Perkins, MD, PhD
Department of Pathology
University of Utah Health Sciences
Center
Salt Lake City, Utah

Sharon L. Schwartz, MT(ASCP)
Department of Laboratories
North Shore University Hospital
New York University School of
Medicine
Manhasset, New York

Sue J. Sim, MD
Department of Laboratory Medicine
The University of Texas
M.D. Anderson Cancer Center
Houston, Texas

Catherine M. Spier, MD
Associate Professor
University of Arizona
Department of Pathology
Health Science Center
Tucson, Arizona

Ronald G. Strauss, MD
Medical Director, DeGowin Blood
Center
Professor of Pathology and Pediatrics
University of Iowa Hospitals and
Clinics
Iowa City, Iowa

Mitra Taghizadeh, MS, MT(ASCP), CLS(NCA)
Clinical Assistant Professor
Department of Medical and Research
Technology
University of Maryland School of
Medicine
Baltimore, Maryland

Janis Wyrick-Glatzel, MS, MT(ASCP)
Associate Professor of Clinical
Laboratory Science
Program in Clinical Laboratory
Science
University of Nevada at Las Vegas
Las Vegas, Nevada

Stan Zail, MB, BCh, MD, FRCPath (London)
South African Institute for Medical
Research
University of the Witwatersrand
Department of Haematology
Johannesburg, South Africa

CONTENTS

Part I

INTRODUCTION TO CLINICAL HEMATOLOGY

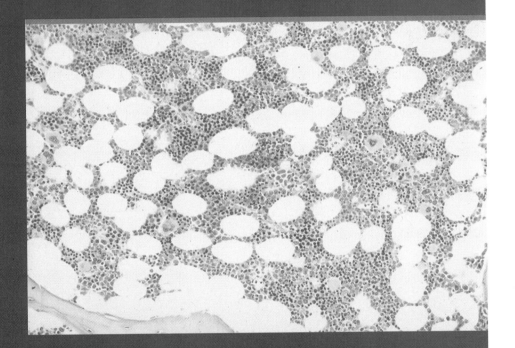

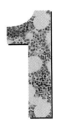

1

Hematopoiesis: Morphology of Human Blood and Marrow Cells

Ann Bell, MS, SH(ASCP), CLSpH(NCA)
Virginia Hughes, BS, MT(ASCP)

Objectives

At the end of this chapter, the learner should be able to:

BASIC MORPHOLOGY AND BASIC CONCEPTS

1. Define *hematopoiesis.*
2. Name the organs that are responsible for hematopoiesis in the fetus.
3. List the proper cell maturation sequence of the erythroid series.
4. Give two or more morphological characteristics of each nucleated red cell in the erythrocytic series.
5. List the proper cell sequence for granulocytopoiesis.
6. Differentiate the morphologic features of the myeloblast, progranulocyte, neutrophilic myelocyte, neutrophilic metamyelocyte, and neutrophilic band.
7. Describe the two main differences between a neutrophilic band and neutrophilic segmented cell.
8. Describe morphological features that are helpful in identifying monocytes and lymphocytes.
9. Describe the morphology of reactive lymphocytes.
10. Describe the difference between osteoblasts and osteoclasts.

MOLECULAR HEMATOLOGY AND ADVANCED CONCEPTS

11. Describe the function of colony-stimulating factors and define the acronyms CFU-GEMM and GM–CSF.
12. Define "cluster designation" in the CD nomenclature.

BASIC MORPHOLOGY AND BASIC CONCEPTS

Hematopoiesis

Definition

Hematopoiesis, the dynamic process of blood cell production and development, is characterized by a constant turnover of cells. The hematopoietic system continuously maintains a cell population of leukocytes, erythrocytes, and platelets through a complex network of tissues, organs, stem cells, and regulatory factors.[1,2] This network is responsible for the maturation and division of undifferentiated cells, which are cells that cannot be identified morphologically and are not yet committed to a specific cell lineage, into operational cell lines. Lymphocytes perform immune functions; granulocytes fight infections; red cells transport oxygen and excrete carbon dioxide; and platelets maintain hemostasis, a process in which the formation of blood clots and bleeding are halted (Table 1–1).

Hematopoietic cells, including lymphocytes, are derived from a pool of pluripotential stem cells (cells with the ability to develop into several cell lines). The pluripotential stem cell has the capacity for continuous self-replication and proliferation and the ability to differentiate into progenitor cells for each cell line. Under the influence of cytokines (growth factors) such as colony-stimulating factors and interleukins, progenitors divide and differentiate to form the mature cellular elements of the blood.[2] The hematopoietic system consists of the bone marrow, liver, spleen, lymph nodes, and thymus. These tissues and organs are involved in the production, maturation, and destruction of blood cells. The entire hematopoietic process evolves around the stem cells that support hematopoiesis, the progenitor cells that are committed to particular lineages, and the regulatory factors (growth factors) to which the hematopoietic system responds. These features enable the hematopoietic system to respond to such stimuli as infection, bleeding, or hypoxia by increasing hematopoiesis, with emphasis on the cell type needed.[1-3]

Ontogeny (Origin) of Hematopoiesis

During the first weeks of embryonic life, hematopoiesis begins in the mesoderm of the yolk sac, with mesenchymal stem cells forming large primitive nucleated erythroid cells (Fig. 1–1). Yolk sac production of these nucleated erythroid cells begins to decline in about 6 weeks and ends in about 2 months.[1-7]

The fetal liver assumes responsibility for hematopoiesis about the second month, with the yolk sac nucleated red blood cells migrating to the liver and re-

maining there until the seventh month.[1,2] From the third to the sixth month, splenic hematopoiesis also occurs. At approximately 7 months of fetal life, the responsibility for hematopoiesis shifts from the liver to the bone marrow, which then becomes the major site of blood cell development in the fetus.[1] Production of hematopoietic cells in the bone marrow is termed *medullary hematopoiesis*.[2,7] Fetal marrow becomes filled with red blood cells during hematopoiesis. Bones of the toes, fingers, vertebrae, ribs, and pelvis, along with the long bones and cranium, are filled with erythroid cells; early lymphocytic cells also may be formed during fetal life. A few megakaryocytes (precursors to platelets) first appear at approximately 3 months of fetal life, and granulocytes are observed at about 5 months.[6]

At birth, the liver and spleen have ceased hematopoietic cell development and the active sites of hematopoiesis are in bone cavities (red marrow). Bone seems to provide a microenvironment that is appropriate for proliferation and maturation of cells.[1] Hematopoiesis occurs in the extravascular part of the red marrow, with a single layer of epithelial cells separating the extravascular marrow compartment from the intravascular compartment (venous sinuses). When new blood cells produced in the marrow are almost mature and ready to circulate in the peripheral blood, the migrating cells leave the marrow parenchyma by squeezing through cytoplasmic fenestrations in sinus endothelial lining cells and emerging into venous sinuses[1-4,7] (see Chap. 2).

During infancy and early childhood, hematopoiesis takes place in the entire medullary space, with the volume of marrow in the newborn infant almost equaling the hematopoietic marrow space of adults.

Hematopoiesis gradually decreases in the shaft of the long bones, and after age 4 fat cells begin to appear in the long bones.[1] Around age 18 to 20, hematopoietic marrow is found exclusively in the sternum, ribs, pelvis, vertebrae, and skull. Other bones contain primarily fat (yellow marrow). After age 40, marrow in the sternum, ribs, pelvis, and vertebrae is composed of equal amounts of hematopoietic tissue and fat.[1] Generally, hematopoiesis is sustained in a steady state, with production of mature cells equaling blood cell removal. When demand for blood cells is increased, active hematopoiesis may again be found in the spleen, liver, and other tissues as a compensatory mechanism known as *extramedullary hematopoiesis*.[1,2,7]

Hematopoiesis can be divided into activity in the bone marrow by division of cells into two separate pools: the stem cell pool and the bone marrow pool, with eventual release of mature cells into the peripheral blood (Fig. 1–2). It is assumed that in the bone marrow microenvironment a stem cell pool exists where morphologically unidentifiable multipotential stem cells (MSCs) and unipotential committed colony-forming units (CFUs) reside. In addition, there is a bone marrow pool that can be divided into two cell pools: cells that are proliferating and maturing and cells that are stored for later release into the peripheral blood. In the peripheral blood, two pools of cells can also be considered: those that are functional with circulation and those that exist in a storage form. For example, in the granulocytic cell line in the bone marrow pool, there is a component for proliferation and mat-

TABLE 1–1	**Hematopoietic Cell Function**
Cell	**Function**
Granulocytes	Fight infection
Lymphocytes	Cellular and humoral immunity
Erythrocytes (red cells)	Transport oxygen and excrete carbon dioxide
Platelets	Maintain hemostasis

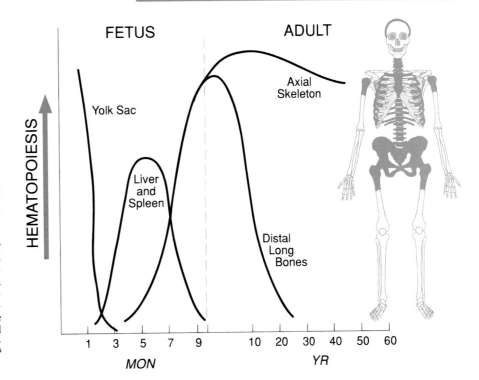

FIGURE 1-1 Location of active marrow growth in the fetus and adult. During fetal development, hematopoiesis is first established in the yolk sac mesenchyme, later moves to the liver and spleen, and finally is limited to the body skeleton. From infancy to adulthood, there is a progressive restriction of productive marrow to the axial skeleton and proximal ends of the long bones, shown as the shaded areas on the drawing of the skeleton. (From Hillman and Finch,[5] with permission.)

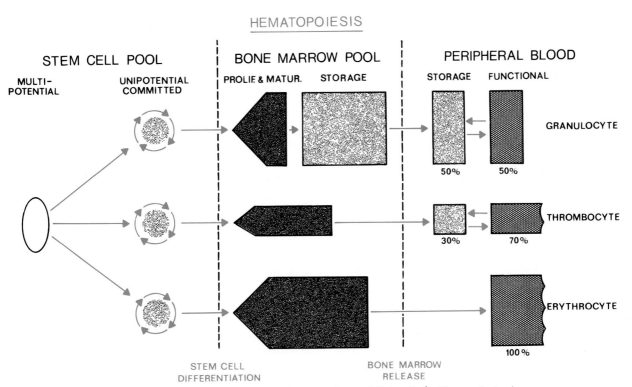

FIGURE 1-2   Hematopoiesis. (From Erslev and Gabuzda,[4] with permission.)

uration, and a storage component. As seen in Figure 1–2, the granulocytic cells in the peripheral blood also contain 50% of circulating cells and 50% of storage cells. Those cells stored around the walls of the blood vessels are sometimes referred to as the marginating storage pool.[2]

For platelets (also known as thrombocytes), the peripheral blood contains 70% in circulation and 30% in storage in the spleen. As shown in Figure 1–2, the bone marrow pool consists of only proliferating and maturing platelet precursor cells.

Red cells, known as erythrocytes, are 100% circulating in peripheral blood in a functional state. In the bone marrow pool, these cells comprise a large component of proliferating and maturing red cell precursors.

Morphology of Human Blood and Marrow Cells

Residing in the bone marrow is a pool of hematopoietic stem cells that, through cell kinetics, stimulation by growth factors, and influence by the microenvironment, differentiate and become committed to production of one cell line.[2] The progenitor cells develop into morphologically recognizable cell lines with distinctive features. Each cell in the maturation process has particular recognizable characteristics. In this chapter, erythropoiesis, granulopoiesis, monopoiesis, megakaryopoiesis, and lymphopoiesis will be discussed. The morphology of other closely related marrow cells, namely, osteoblasts, osteoclasts, and the tissue granulocytes, is also presented for completeness.

Identification of cells in peripheral blood and marrow smears depends on smears made properly and stained satisfactorily with Wright's stain. The preparation of blood smears is described in Chapter 31.

Erythropoiesis

The Erythron

The erythron is the total population of mature erythrocytes and their precursors in blood and bone marrow and other sites. The use of this term indicates that the widely distributed red blood cells function as a unit.[1] The term *erythropoiesis* identifies the entire process by which the erythrocytes are produced in the bone marrow.[2]

In response to erythropoietin, a growth factor that stimulates the erythroid precursors, erythropoiesis occurs in the central sinus beds of medullary marrow over a period of about 5 days through at least three successive reductions or divisions: from rubriblast to prorubricyte to rubricyte, and finally to metarubricyte (orthochromatic normoblast) (Fig. 1–3, middle column). With each successive developmental stage, there is a reduction in cell volume, condensation of chromatin, loss of nucleoli, decrease in ribonucleic acid (RNA) in the cytoplasm, decrease in mitochondria, and gradual increase in synthesis of hemoglobin. The nucleus of the metarubricyte is eventually extruded, leaving a nonnucleated polychromatophilic (diffusely basophilic) erythrocyte that is released into the circu-

lating blood to mature in 1 to 2 days. From 14 to 16 erythrocytes are produced from one rubriblast.[1]

Rubriblast (Pronormoblast, Proerythroblast)

The rubriblast, the earliest recognizable cell of the erythrocytic series, has a round, primitive nucleus with visible nucleoli and chromatin strands that are indistinct and dispersed (Figs. 1–4 through 1–8). There is no evidence of clumped chromatin. The nucleus stains reddish blue with Wright's stain. The cytoplasm stains royal blue because of the presence of RNA. The nuclear-to-cytoplasmic ratio in a rubriblast is 4:1.

Rubriblasts range in size from 14 to 19 μm. A rubriblast differs little from a myeloblast. Usually a rubriblast is slightly larger than a myeloblast and has more cytoplasm, which stains a deeper blue.

Rubriblasts constitute 1% or less of the cells observed in normal bone marrow (Table 1–2). Rubriblasts usually divide within 12 hours to make two daughter cells (prorubricytes).[1,8]

Prorubricyte (Basophilic Normoblast, Basophilic Erythroblast)

Prorubricytes, the daughter cells of rubriblasts, require about 20 hours to develop (Figs. 1–9 through 1–12). Normal bone marrow contains about four times as many prorubricytes as rubriblasts.[1,8] The prorubricyte is differentiated from the rubriblast by the coarsening of the chromatin pattern, and the nucleoli are ill-defined or not visible under light microscopy. As the prorubricyte matures, it accumulates more RNA and hemoglobin. The predominant color of the cytoplasm is blue because of the staining of RNA, but there may be a pinkish tinge reflecting the presence of varying amounts of hemoglobin.[8] The nuclear-to-cytoplasmic ratio in the prorubricyte is the same as its precursor (4:1). A prorubricyte is normally somewhat smaller than a rubriblast. Normal marrow contains from 1 to 4% prorubricytes (Table 1–2). The division of the prorubricyte forms cells (rubricytes) that are smaller than prorubricytes but have twice the amount of hemoglobin.[8]

Rubricyte (Polychromatic Normoblast, Polychromatic Erythroblast)

Rubricytes are smaller than prorubricytes (12 to 15 μm) (Figs. 1–13 and 1–14). Rubricytes have relatively more cytoplasm and a smaller nucleus than a prorubricyte. The cytoplasm contains varying mixtures of the pink of hemoglobin and the blue of RNA; in the late rubricytes, the pinkish color is usually predominant.[1,8]

Nuclear chromatin is thickened and irregularly condensed in the rubricyte. Light-staining parachromatin areas are visible among the dark-blue-staining, irregular pyknotic masses. Nucleoli are no longer visible.[8] The nuclear-to-cytoplasmic ratio in a rubricyte is 4:1.

The transit time for rubricytes is about 30 hours, and there are approximately three times as many rubricytes as prorubricytes in marrow. Marrow in a normal adult contains 10% to 20% rubricytes (Table 1–2). Rubricytes are not present in the normal peripheral

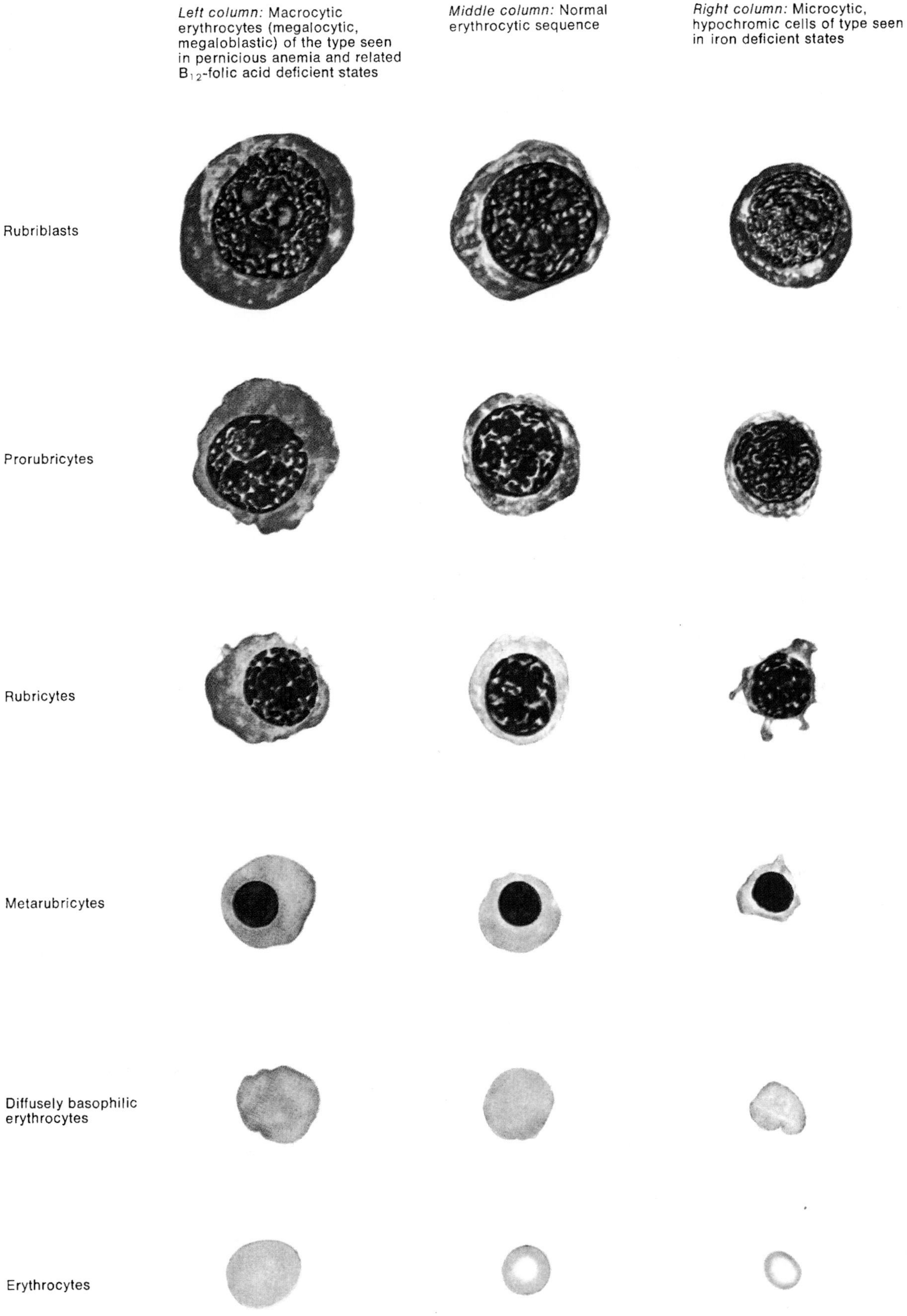

Left column: Macrocytic erythrocytes (megalocytic, megaloblastic) of the type seen in pernicious anemia and related B_{12}-folic acid deficient states

Middle column: Normal erythrocytic sequence

Right column: Microcytic, hypochromic cells of type seen in iron deficient states

Rubriblasts

Prorubricytes

Rubricytes

Metarubricytes

Diffusely basophilic erythrocytes

Erythrocytes

FIGURE 1–3   Erythrocytic system. Normal erythrocytic sequence. (From Diggs, Sturm, and Bell,[8] with permission.)

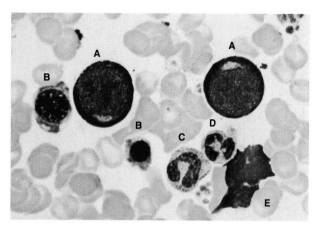

FIGURE 1-4 *A.* Two rubriblasts (note the perinuclear halo). *B.* Two rubricytes. *C.* N. band. *D.* N. segmented. *E.* Smudge cell.

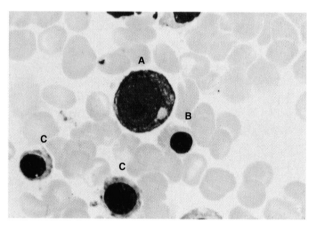

FIGURE 1-5 *A.* Rubriblast. *B.* Metarubricyte. *C.* Two rubricytes.

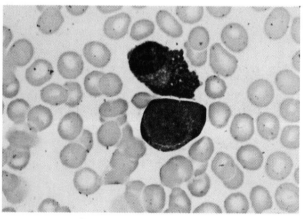

FIGURE 1-6 Center: rubriblast; upper center: plasmacyte.

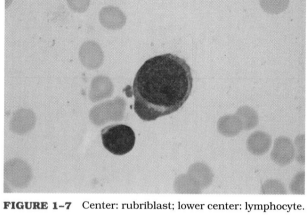

FIGURE 1-7 Center: rubriblast; lower center: lymphocyte.

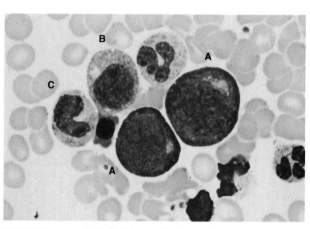

FIGURE 1-8 *A.* Rubriblasts. *B.* N. myelocyte. *C.* N. metamyelocyte.

TABLE 1-2 **Bone Marrow Cells: Normal Adult Values**	
Cell	**Percent**
Stem cell	0–0.01
Myeloblast	0–1
Promyelocyte	1–5
N. myelocyte	2–10
N. metamyelocyte	5–15
N. band	10–40
N. segmented	10–30
Eosinophil	0–3
Basophil	0–1
Lymphocyte	5–15
Plasmacyte	0–1
Monocyte	0–2
Other cells	0–1
Megakaryocyte	0.1–0.5
Rubriblast	0–1
Prorubricyte	1–4
Rubricyte	10–20
Metarubricyte	5–10
WBC: Nucleated RBC Ratio = 4:1	

Source: From Diggs, Sturm, and Bell,[8] with permission.

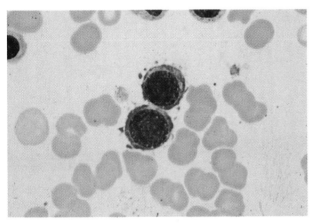

FIGURE 1-9   Prorubricytes.

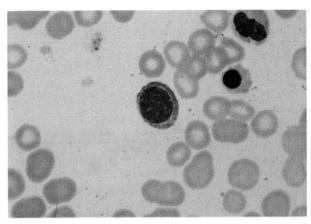

FIGURE 1-12   Center: prorubricyte; right: metarubricyte.

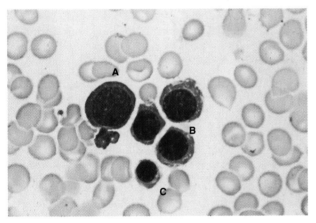

FIGURE 1-10   *A.* Prorubricyte. *B.* Three rubricytes. *C.* Metarubricyte.

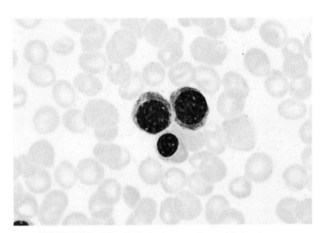

FIGURE 1-13   Rubricytes: early and late stages.

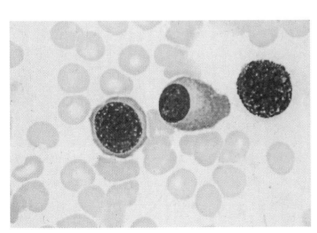

FIGURE 1-11   Left: prorubricyte; center: plasmacyte.

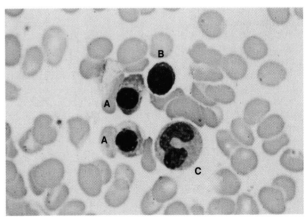

FIGURE 1-14   *A.* Rubricytes. *B.* Lymphocyte. *C.* N. segmented.

blood of adults, but may appear in the peripheral blood of normal newborn infants.[1,8]

Metarubricyte (Orthochromatic Normoblast, Orthochromatic Erythroblast)

Metarubricytes are formed from rubricytes and are recognized by a solid blue-black degenerated nucleus with a nonlinear clumped chromatin pattern (see Fig. 1–10*C* and Fig. 1–12, *right*). The metarubricyte nucleus is incapable of further DNA synthesis. The degenerated nucleus of the metarubricyte is destined to be extruded and will be phagocytized.[8] The nuclear-to-cytoplasmic ratio in a metarubricyte is 1:1.

The cytoplasm is predominantly pinkish (or reddish) because of increasing hemoglobin synthesis, but minimal amounts of blue cytoplasm may remain because of RNA. Mitochondria are no longer evident.[8]

The transit time for metarubricytes is 48 hours.[2] The number of metarubricytes in normal marrow varies between 5% and 10% (Table 1–2). Metarubricytes are not observed in normal adult peripheral blood but can be found in the blood of normal newborn infants.[1,8] The metarubricyte is the smallest of the nucleated erythrocyte precursors (8 to 12 μm).[2]

Diffusely Basophilic Erythrocyte (Polychromatophilic Erythrocyte)

The condensed, pyknotic nucleus of a metarubricyte is extruded, leaving a diffusely basophilic or polychromatophilic cell (Fig. 1–15, cell labeled F). The membrane of the erythrocyte reseals itself. Some of the bluish staining color remains because of the presence of RNA. The erythrocyte contains approximately two thirds of its total hemoglobin content by the time the nucleus is lost. There are decreases in RNA content and mitochondria.[1,8]

A diffusely basophilic erythrocyte is larger than a mature red cell (7 to 10 μm). It is released in 2 to 3 days from the marrow and circulates for 1 or 2 days before maturing into an erythrocyte. Only rarely are diffusely basophilic erythrocytes found in the blood of normal adults; however, polychromatophilic cells are frequently seen in the blood of normal newborn infants.[1,8]

When stained with new methylene blue, diffusely basophilic cells reveal ribosomes in a granulofilamentous arrangement (or network of strands and granules) and are classified as reticulocytes (Fig. 1–16). As ribosomes disappear, the diffusely basophilic cell changes into a mature erythrocyte.[8]

With anemia or hypoxia, erythropoietin stimulates marrow erythroid precursors to proliferate and increase the number of early erythroid cells. An increased number of polychromatophilic cells is delivered early from the marrow, and therefore the reticulocyte count is increased.[1,8]

Erythrocyte (Discocyte, Mature Red Blood Cell)

A normal mature erythrocyte is a biconcave disc that is 7 to 8 μm in mean diameter and 1.5 to 2.5 μm thick; it has a mean volume of 90 femtoliters (fL). After the smear is stained with Wright's stain, an erythrocyte appears as a circular cell with distinct and smooth

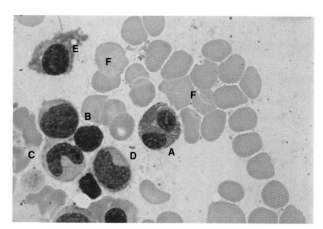

FIGURE 1–15 *A.* E. segmented. *B.* Lymphocyte. *C.* N. band. *D.* N. metamyelocyte. *E.* Plasmacyte. *F.* Two diffusely basophilic red cells.

margins. In the central portion of the erythrocyte, where the cell is thinnest, the intensity of the stain is less than at the marginal area, creating an area of central pallor. Red blood cells are flattened out, lack central pallor, and do not reveal their biconcavity at the feathered end of a bullet-shaped smear.[8]

A mature erythrocyte is not able to synthesize hemoglobin because it is without a nucleus and mitochondria, or ribosomes, but it has a unique, yet limited, metabolism to sustain itself while traversing the microvasculature. The erythrocyte carries oxygen from the lungs to the tissues, where it is exchanged for carbon dioxide. Erythrocytes are pliable or flexible and deformable, making them capable of unusual changes in shape that are necessary for passage through the microcirculation to transport oxygen.[1,8] Refer to Table 1–3 for a summary of the morphological characteristics of each stage of maturation of the red cell.

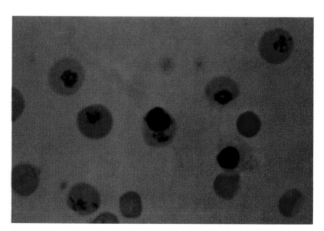

FIGURE 1–16 Reticulocytes. New methylene blue stain of peripheral blood. Note non-nucleated reticulocytes with varying amounts of stained reticulum (RNA). Reticulocytosis is associated with increased erythropoietic activity reflected by polychromasia on the Wright's stain of the peripheral smear. (From Bell, A: Hematology. In Listen, Look, and Learn. Health and Education Resources, Inc., Bethesda, MD, with permission.)

TABLE 1–3   Morphological Characteristics of the Rubricytic (Erythrocytic) Series

	Pronormo-blast (Rubriblast)	Basophilic Normoblast (Prorubricyte)	Polychromato-philic Normoblast (Rubricyte)	Orthochromatic Normoblast (Metarubricyte)	Polychromato-philic Erythrocyte	Mature Erythrocyte
Cell size, μm	14–19	12–17	12–15	8–12	7–10	7–8
N:C ratio	4:1	4:1	4:1	1:1	n/a	n/a
Nuclear shape	Round	Round	Round	Round	n/a; nucleus has been extruded	n/a
Nuclear position	Central	Central	Central	Central	n/a	n/a
Nuclear color/ chromatin	Reddish blue, finely stippled, granular chromatin	Increased, larger granularity of nuclear chromatin	Dark blue, smaller nucleus with parachromatin, increased clumped chromatin	Blue purple, small nucleus with pyknotic degeneration/ condensed chromatin	n/a	n/a
Nucleoli	0–2	Usually none, occasional indistinct nucleolus	None	None	None	None
Color/amount of cytoplasm	Dark or royal blue/slight	Basophilic/slight	Bluish pink/ moderate	Pink/moderate	Clear gray-blue, polychroma-tophilic to pink	Pink
Cytoplasmic granules	None	None	None	None	None	None

Myelopoiesis (Granulocytopoiesis)

Granulocytopoiesis or myelopoiesis is the production of neutrophils, eosinophils, basophils, and monocytes. Mature neutrophils, eosinophils, and basophils have similar patterns of proliferation, differentiation, division, storage in marrow, and delivery to the blood.[2] Maturation and division of the myeloid series in the marrow demonstrate a continuum of development from the blast to the most mature cells (neutrophil segmented), requiring from 7 to 11 days[1,9,10] (Fig. 1–17).

Granulocyte production proceeds after cell line commitment has determined the identity of the maturing cell as a member of the granulocytic series. The system moves cells through passages and compartments where various cellular stages occur in response to various stimuli. The mitotic or proliferative pool contains the committed stem cells, myeloblasts, promyelocytes, and myelocytes (see Fig. 1–2). These cells actively divide and mature, taking 1 to 2 days for each cellular cycle (T_g) (see section on cell cycle kinetics in this chapter). The maturation pool is composed of metamyelocytes and bands and represents the end of DNA synthesis. The transformation of myelocyte to metamyelocyte to band takes about 8 to 9 hours after entry into the maturation pool. The storage pool retains mature cells for release into peripheral circulation.[2] These mature cells leave the marrow by moving through transiently formed pores in endothelial cells that separate marrow parenchyma from venous sinuses; when leaving blood for tissue, cells migrate between endothelial cells (diapedesis).[2] After release, cells become part of the functional pool and reside as circulating cells or as marginated cells, which line blood vessel walls. Cells are released to enter the peripheral blood or vessel walls for a few hours, and then leave the blood to enter tissues and body cavities. Under normal circumstances, the rate at which these cells enter the blood and the rate at which they exit to tissue are in equilibrium.[1,4] As these cells exit the blood for the tissues, they are replaced by other cells from the marrow. Once in the blood, half of the released cells freely circulate while the other half are in a marginating pool on the walls of blood vessels—particularly those in lungs, liver, and spleen.[1,2,7,9] These latter cells leave the peripheral vessels to be directed by chemotactic factors to inflammatory or infectious tissue.[1,7,9–12] After cells enter tissues, they do not reenter the circulation or the marrow.[4,7,9]

Morphological Changes

During maturation, there is a reduction in nuclear volume, condensation of chromatin, change in nuclear shape, appearance and disappearance of primary granules, appearance of secondary granules, color changes in cytoplasm from blue to pinkish, red, and change in size of cells.[1,4,7,9,13]

Maturation of the granulocytic series of cells is characterized by the development of primary blue-staining granules, which are replaced by secondary granules that differ in their affinity for various dyes.[8,11,13] Cells with an affinity for basic dyes are basophils; those that stain reddish orange with the acid dye eosin are eosinophilic; those that do not stain intensely with either acidic or basic dyes are called *neutrophils*. As these motile cells mature, the nucleus undergoes progressive changes from round to multilobular forms.[8,11,12]

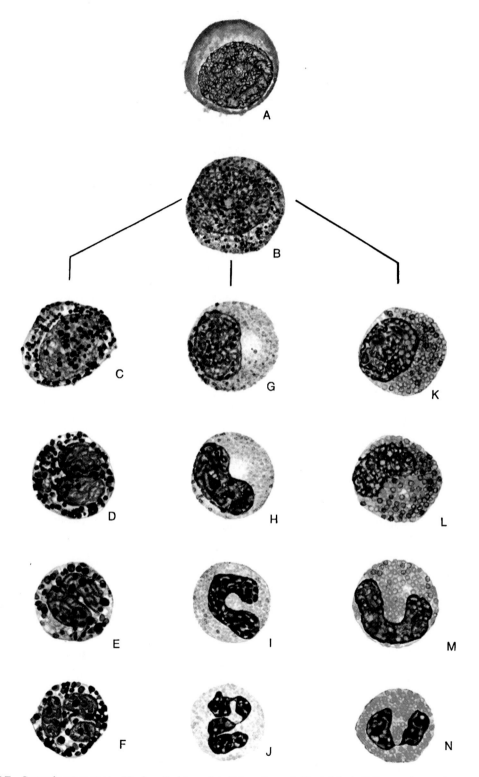

FIGURE 1–17   Granulocytopoiesis: Myelocytic (granulocytic) system. *A.* Myeloblast. *B.* Promyelocyte (progranulocyte. *C.* Basophilic myelocyte. *D.* Basophilic metamyelocyte. *E.* Basophilic band. *F.* Basophilic segmented. *G.* Neutrophilic myelocyte. *H.* Neutrophilic metamyelocyte. *I.* Neutrophilic band. *J.* Neutrophilic segmented. *K.* Eosinophilic myelocyte. *L.* Eosinophilic metamyelocyte. *M.* Eosinophilic band. *N.* Eosinophilic segmented. (From Diggs, Sturm, and Bell,[8] with permission.)

Stages of Differentiation and Maturation

Myeloblast The earliest recognizable cell in the granulocytic series is the myeloblast (Fig. 1–18), which usually has a round nucleus that stains predominantly reddish blue and has a smooth nuclear membrane. The interlaced chromatin strands are delicate, finely dispersed or stippled, and evenly stained, but not clumped. One or more nucleoli of uniform size are usually demonstrable, but occasionally nucleoli may be barely visible.[8] A slight to moderate amount of bluish nongranular cytoplasm stains lighter next to the nucleus than at the periphery of the cell (see Fig. 1–17). The nuclear-to-cytoplasmic ratio in the myeloblast is 4:1. A myeloblast is smaller and has less blue cytoplasm than a rubriblast. After about three to five mitotic divisions, the myeloblast matures into a promyelocyte as primary granules become visible.[1,8] Ultrastructural studies of myeloblasts reveal numerous mitochondria, a Golgi area, and free ribosomes.[1]

Myeloblasts vary in size but are usually about 17 μm.[1] They are not observed in normal peripheral blood. Normal marrow contains 1% or fewer myeloblasts (see Table 1–2). With the appearance of primary granules, the myeloblast has matured into a promyelocyte.[8]

Promyelocyte (Progranulocyte) In the promyelocyte, there are granules that stain dark blue or reddish blue; they may be round or irregular (Figs. 1–19 and 1–20). They appear throughout the cytoplasm and may lie over the nucleus.[8,13] Primary granules are filled with lysosomal granules, which contain myeloperoxidase, acid phosphatase, hydrolytic enzymes, elastase, and β-glucuronidase and other basic proteins, but not alkaline phosphatase.[2,4,7,14]

The nucleus of a promyelocyte is usually round and is large in relation to the cytoplasm. In young promyelocytes, the chromatin is almost as finely granular as it is in a myeloblast. In older cells, the chromatin structure is slightly coarser than that in a myeloblast. Nucleoli may be faintly visible but are not often distinct[8] (see Figs. 1–17, 1–19, and 1–20). The nuclear-to-cytoplasmic ratio in a promyelocyte is 3:1.

The cytoplasm is blue with a relatively light zone ad-

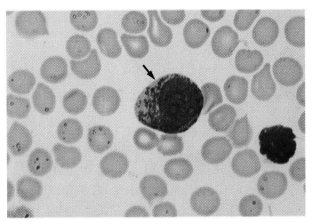

FIGURE 1–19   Center: promyelocyte.

jacent to the nucleus. The periphery of the cytoplasm is smooth and is not indented by neighboring cells.[8]

The size of a promyelocyte can vary depending on the stage of a given cell in the mitotic cycle, but this cell may often be 20 μm and may be larger than a myeloblast. Promyelocytes do not appear in normal peripheral blood. From 1 to 5% of promyelocytes are observed in normal bone marrow[8] (see Table 1–2).

As the promyelocyte matures, nucleoli begin to fade, the chromatin becomes more condensed, and the granules are not as intensely stained. Specific secondary neutrophilic granules begin to appear, and the synthesis of primary granules ceases.[1,8,13] A few primary granules remain through division and maturation and may even appear in segmented neutrophils.[1,8,13]

Neutrophilic Myelocyte When primary granules are no longer synthesized and smaller, less dense secondary neutrophilic granules can be identified, the cell then has matured into a myelocyte[8] (Fig. 1–21, see also Fig. 1–8). The first sign of neutrophilic differentiation has been called the "dawn of neutrophilia" or "beginning neutrophilia," which refers to a relatively light island of ill-defined or barely visible reddish (or pinkish) secondary lysosomal granules that develop adjacent to the nucleus and in proximity to the remaining primary

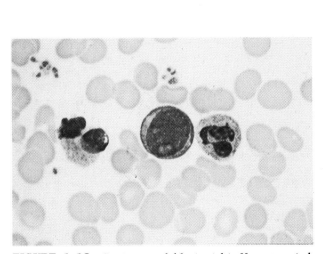

FIGURE 1–18   Center: myeloblast; right: N. segmented; left: disintegrated neutrophil.

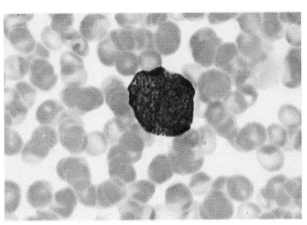

FIGURE 1–20   Promyelocyte.

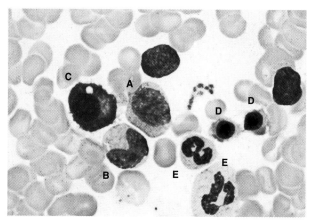

FIGURE 1–21 *A.* N. myelocyte. *B.* N. metamyelocyte. *C.* Plasmocyte. *D.* Metarubricytes. *E.* Segmented neutrophils.

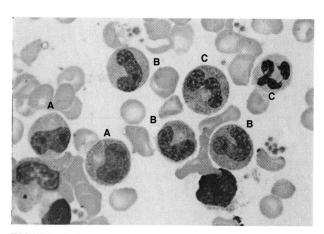

FIGURE 1–22 *A.* Two N. metamyelocytes. *B.* Three N. bands. *C.* Two N. segmented.

granules.[8,13] As myelocytes divide and age, the primary granules become fewer and the secondary (specific) neutrophilic granules predominate. Secondary granules are considered specific granules for neutrophils and contain collagenase, lysozyme, lactoferrin, plasminogen activators, aminopeptidase, and alkaline phosphatase.[1,11,14]

The nuclei of myelocytes can be round, oval, or flattened on one side and usually are not centrally located.[8] Chromatin strands become condensed, partly clumped, and thickened, and are unevenly stained. Nucleoli are absent or indistinct in myelocytes (see Figs. 1–8B, 1–17, and 1–21A). The neutrophilic myelocyte is the last myeloid precursor capable of division.[8]

Neutrophilic myelocytes are often smaller than promyelocytes and have relatively larger amounts of cytoplasm (the ratio of neutrophilic myelocytes to cytoplasm [N:C] is 2:1 or 1:1), which gradually becomes less basophilic and more pinkish. Normal peripheral blood does not contain neutrophilic myelocytes. There are 2% to 10% myelocytes in normal bone marrow[8] (see Table 1–2).

Neutrophilic Metamyelocyte As maturation proceeds, the nucleus becomes slightly indented (bean- or kidney-shaped), which serves to identify the cell as a metamyelocyte[8] (Fig. 1–22; see also Figs. 1–8C and 1–21B). The indentation is less than half the width of the arbitrary round nucleus. There is noticeable condensation with clumping of the chromatin, but the chromatin structure is not as dense as that of the neutrophilic segmented cell. Metamyelocytes do not divide, nor do they have nucleoli.[8] The N:C ratio is now 1:1 and remains so throughout the maturation sequence.

Many small, pinkish secondary granules fill the cytoplasm, and a few primary darker granules may remain (see Fig. 1–17). These maturing cells remain in marrow and form a granulocytic reserve.[2]

Metamyelocytes are minimally smaller than myelocytes (10 to 18 μm) and larger than the neutrophilic band or segmented cell. These cells are rare or absent in normal peripheral blood. There are approximately 5% to 15% metamyelocytes in normal bone marrow[8] (see Table 1–2).

Neutrophilic Band (N. Nonsegmented, N. Nonfilamented) When the stage is reached in which the nuclear indentation is greater than half the width of the nucleus, the cell is identified as a neutrophilic band.[8] The opposite edges of the nucleus become almost parallel for an appreciable distance, giving the appearance of a horseshoe or a curved link of sausage. The nuclear chromatin is clumped and shows degenerative changes, and there is usually a dark pyknotic mass at each pole where the lobe is destined to be.[8] The secondary neutrophilic granules are small and evenly distributed, stain various shades of pink, and contain alkaline phosphatase.[1,8] There may be an occasional dark primary granule (see Fig. 1–17).

Neutrophilic band cells are often slightly smaller than metamyelocytes. Band forms constitute from 2% to 6% of the leukocytes in the peripheral blood of healthy individuals and 10% to 40% of the nucleated cells in bone marrow (Table 1–4; see also Table 1–2).

Neutrophilic Segmented (N. Filamented, N. Polymorphonuclear Leukocyte, PMN) In a neutrophilic segmented cell, the nucleus is normally separated into two to five (usually three) lobes with a narrow filament or strand connecting the lobes (see Figs. 1–21E and 1–22C). Nuclear chromatin is heavily clumped, coarse, or pyknotic and stains purplish red. The cytoplasm in an ideal stain is light pink, and the small, numerous, and evenly distributed secondary granules either stain pink or are neutral.[8] Neutrophil secondary granules are lysosomes that contain alkaline phosphatase.

TABLE 1–4 **Peripheral Blood Cells: Normal Adult Values**		
	Percent	**Per mm^3**
N. band	2–6	100–650
N. segmented	50–70	2400–7500
Eosinophil	0–4	0–450
Basophil	0–2	0–200
Lymphocyte	20–44	1000–4750
Monocyte	2–9	100–1000

Mature neutrophils are approximately twice the size of normal erythrocytes. There are 50% to 70% segmented neutrophils in the peripheral blood of older children and adults and 10% to 30% in normal marrow.[8] Approximately 5% of the neutrophils have one lobe (N. band); 35%, two lobes; 41%, three lobes; 17%, four lobes; and 2%, five lobes.[8] Segmentation of the nucleus enables these motile cells to pass through an opening in endothelial lining cells of capillaries and to "home in on selected prey."[8]

Because there is a gradual transition between the various stages of granulocytes, the division of neutrophils into developmental stages is somewhat arbitrary but is necessary for morphological evaluation. Borderline cells that are difficult to distinguish from each other may be present. The major difficulty arises in differentiating between bands and segmented cells, and in deciding whether the link connecting the lobes is narrow enough to be called a filament or wide enough to be identified as a band. A filamented or segmented cell has a threadlike connection between two lobes, and there is no visible chromatin between the two sides. In a band cell are two distinct margins with nuclear chromatin material visible between the margins.[8] Lobes of nuclei often touch each other or overlap, and it is impossible to see the connecting filaments. If the margin of a lobe can be traced as a definite and continuing line from one side of the nucleus across the isthmus to the other side, then it may be assumed that a filament is present even though it is not visible. In attempting to differentiate between a segmented cell and a band cell, identification should not be made on a single morphological characteristic but rather on

combined features.[8] If there is doubt in identifying a borderline cell, the questionable cell should be placed in the mature category.[8] Table 1-5 summarizes the morphological characteristics of the granulocytic (neutrophilic series).

Tissue Neutrophil Tissue neutrophils are large marrow cells with ample cytoplasm that is irregular with blunt pseudopods, is often multipointed, and has nebulous cytoplasmic streamers (Fig. 1-23). These cells are readily indented by adjacent marrow cells or are squeezed between them. Often there are long and tenuous cytoplasmic extensions that seem to wrap around other cells. These cells are not phagocytic and seldom have vacuoles in the cytoplasm.[8,15]

The cytoplasm stains light blue and has a fine latticelike structure. Granules vary in number and stain various shades of red to blue, but most stain reddish purple. Many of the granules tend to be arranged in chains. The beadlike granular aggregates extend into the cytoplasmic projections.[15]

The large round or oval nucleus has a coarse chromatin structure with a distinct linear pattern. Nucleoli are usually conspicuous and stain light blue.[8,15]

Tissue neutrophils are fixed or semifixed tissue cells that have developed neutrophilic granules. They are immobile end-stage cells that are probably derived from the same progenitor cell as neutrophils.

Tissue neutrophils occur infrequently in normal bone marrow; however, they are found in increased numbers in bone marrow smears of patients having conditions in which there is a proliferation of neutrophilic cells such as myelocytic leukemia, myelocytic-monocytic leukemia and myelofibrosis, as well as in

TABLE 1-5 Morphological Characteristics of the Granulocytic (Neutrophilic) Series

	Myeloblast	Promyelocyte (Progranulocyte)	N. Myelocyte	N. Metamyelocyte	N. Band	N. Segmented
Cell size, μm	10–20	10–20	10–18	10–18	10–16	10–16
N:C ratio	4:1	3:1	2:1 or 1:1	1:1	1:1	1:1
Nuclear shape	Round	Round	Oval or round; slightly indented	Usually indented (kidney-shaped)	Elongated, narrow band (horseshoe) shape of uniform thickness	2–5 distinct nuclear lobes
Nuclear position	Eccentric or central	Eccentric or central	Usually eccentric	Central or eccentric	Central or eccentric	Central or eccentric
Nuclear color/chromatin	Light reddish blue, fine meshwork with no aggregation of material	Light reddish blue, fine meshwork, slight aggregation may be seen at nuclear membrane	Reddish blue, fine chromatin with slightly aggregated or granular pattern	Light blue-purple with basophilic chromatin easily distinguishable	Purplish red, clumped granular chromatin	Purplish red clumped granular chromatin
Nucleoli	1–3	1–2	May or may not have nucleolus	None	None	None
Color/amount of cytoplasm	Basophilic/slight	Basophilic/increased	Bluish pink/moderate	Clear pink/moderate	Pink/abundant	Pink/abundant
Cytoplasmic granules	Absent	Present, fine azurophilic, nonspecific granules	Present, azurophilic, *specific* granules	Present, (specific) granules, neutrophilic	Specific granules, fine violet pink	Specific, fine violet pink

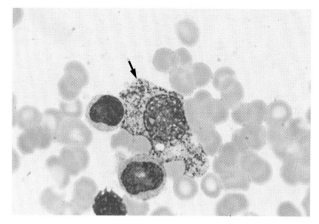

FIGURE 1-23 Tissue neutrophil (large center cell).

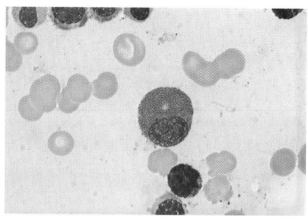

FIGURE 1-25 Center: eosinophilic myelocyte; below: basophil.

neutropenic states in which there is an arrest in the maturation and delivery of cells into the circulating blood.[15]

Eosinophils

Eosinophils are usually easily recognizable because of the large, round, secondary refractile granules that have an affinity for the acid eosin stain[16] (Fig. 1–24; see also Fig. 1–17). With Wright's stain, normal eosinophilic granules become orange to reddish orange. The granules are spherical, uniform in size, and evenly distributed. Because of the size and roundness of the granule, eosinophils can be recognized in unstained moist preparations of blood in light microscopy and in phase microscopy.[8] Eosinophil granules contain an electron-dense crystalloid core when observed with the electron microscope. This crystalloid core is composed mainly of major basic protein (MBP), which binds to acid aniline dyes and may help to explain the staining qualities of the granule.[1,7,14,17] The granules of eosinophils contain various hydrolytic enzymes, including peroxidase, acid phosphatase, aryl sulfatase, β-glucuronidase, phospholipase, cathepsin, and ribonuclease, but lack lysozyme, cationic proteins, and alkaline phosphatase.[1,7,14,16,17]

Eosinophils pass through the same developmental stages as neutrophils: E. myelocyte (Fig. 1–25), E. metamyelocyte (Fig. 1–26A), band (Fig. 1–27A), and segmented stages[1,16] (see Fig. 1–17). The earliest eosinophil (E. myelocyte) has a few dark bluish primary granules intermingled with the few specific reddish-orange granules. During development, the bluish granules become less visible and disappear, and the round specific secondary eosinophil granules fill the cytoplasm.[8]

Eosinophils spend 3 to 6 days in production in marrow before appearing in peripheral blood. Bone marrow provides a storage area for eosinophils so that they can be rapidly mobilized when needed.[1] The factors that regulate production and release of eosinophils into blood are probably different from those of neutrophils. The mean transit time of these cells in the circulatory system of humans has been reported to be about 8 hours, but in some disease states with eosinophilia the time may be longer.[1] Much less is known about the stem cell kinetics of the eosinophils than of the neutrophil.[1] Eosinophils migrate from blood to tissue such as that of the bronchial mucosa, skin, gastrointestinal tract, and vagina, for about 12 days. Eo-

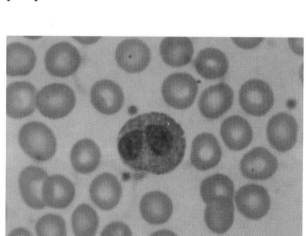

FIGURE 1-24 Eosinophil (segmented).

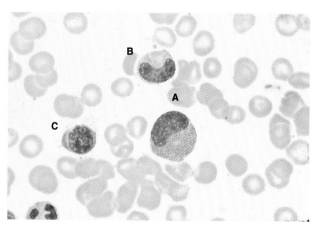

FIGURE 1-26 *A.* E. metamyelocyte. *B.* N. band. *C.* Rubricyte.

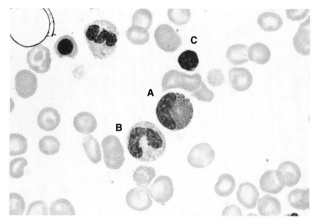

FIGURE 1-27 *A.* E. band. *B.* N. band. *C.* Lymphocyte.

sinophils may migrate from tissue back into blood and marrow.[16] Eosinophils, which are motile, can migrate between endothelial cells into tissue or into an area of inflammation in the same manner as neutrophils.

Normal adult peripheral blood contains 0% to 4% eosinophils, with approximately the same number observed in normal bone marrow (see Tables 1–2 and 1–4). In normal blood, eosinophils are about the size of neutrophils or slightly larger, and have a band or two-lobed nucleus with condensed chromatin; rarely does an eosinophil have three lobes.[8] Eosinophils

show diurnal variation, with increase at night and decrease in the morning. Table 1–6 summarizes the morphological characteristics of the granulocytic (eosinophilic series).

Tissue Eosinophil   In smears of bone marrow, there may occasionally be a large cell with elongated and tapering cytoplasmic extensions, containing typical reddish-orange granules of the type seen in the eosinophils of the circulating blood.[8,15] The nucleus of such cells, instead of being indented or lobulated, is round or oval and has a well-defined reticular chromatin and often nucleoli. Such cells are identified as tissue eosinophils and are thought to be fixed tissue variants of the more motile eosinophils of the circulating blood.[8,15] Tissue eosinophils arise from the same progenitor cell as eosinophils in marrow and blood.

Basophils

Although basophils constitute 0% to 2% of normal blood cells (see Table 1–4), the large abundant violet-blue (or purple-black) granules aid in the immediate recognition of this cell. These granules are visible above the nucleus as well as lateral to the nucleus, and they obscure most of the nucleus. The granules vary in size from 0.2 to 1.0 μm. They are coarse and unevenly distributed; vary in number, shape, and color; and are less numerous than eosinophil granules. These granules have an affinity for blue or basic thiazine dyes. Basophil granules are also water-soluble. In

TABLE 1-6	**Morphological Characterization of the Granulocytic (Eosinophilic) Series**					
	Myeloblast	Promyelocyte (Progranulocyte)	E. Myelocyte	E. Metamyelocyte	E. Band	E. Segmented
Cell size, μm	10–20	10–20	10–18	10–18	10–16	10–16
N:C ratio	4:1	3:1	2:1 or 1:1	1:1	1:1	1:1
Nuclear shape	Round	Round	Oval or round; slightly indented	Usually indented (kidney-shaped)	Elongated, narrow band shape of uniform thickness	2 distinct nuclear lobes
Nuclear position	Eccentric or central	Eccentric or central	Usually eccentric	Central or eccentric	Central or eccentric	Central or eccentric
Nuclear color/ chromatin	Light reddish blue, fine meshwork with no aggregation of material	Light reddish blue, fine meshwork, slight aggregation may be seen at nuclear membrane	Reddish blue fine chromatin with slightly aggregated or granular pattern	Light blue purple with basophilic chromatin easily distinguishable	Deep blue purple, coarsely granular chromatin	Deep blue purple, coarsely granular chromatin
Nucleoli	1–3	1–2	May or may not have nucleolus	None	None	None
Color/amount of cytoplasm	Basophilic/ scanty	Basophilic and increased	Bluish pink/ moderate	Pink/moderate	Pink/moderate	Pink/moderate
Cytoplasmic granules	Absent	Present, fine azurophilic, nonspecific granules	Present, reddish-orange, uniform (*specific*) eosinophilic granules	Present, reddish-orange, uniform (specific) eosinophilic granules	Present, red, uniform (specific) eosinophilic granules	Present, red, uniform (specific) eosinophilic granules

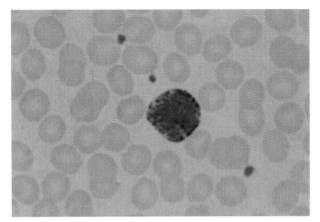

FIGURE 1-28   Center: basophil.

cells that are poorly fixed during staining, the center of the granules may disappear or the entire granule may be washed away, leaving a small, colorless cytoplasmic area.[8]

Based on the shape of their nuclei, basophils are identified as basophilic myelocytes, metamyelocytes, bands, and segmented cells. However, the shape of the nucleus is often masked by the granules[8] (Fig. 1-28; see also Fig. 1-17). The specific violet-blue granules of basophils are formed in the myelocytic stage and continue to be made during the later maturation stages. There are also some smaller granules that do not stain

as darkly as the specific basophil granules but that tend to be more reddish blue.[8,18,19]

Maturation of basophils takes place over 7 days.[1] Mature basophils rarely have more than two segments. Basophils circulate for a few hours in blood, then migrate into skin, mucosa, and other serosal areas.[1]

Basophils in all stages of maturation are smaller than promyelocytes and neutrophil myelocytes; their size approximates that of neutrophils. Basophils show diurnal variation similar to that of eosinophils, increasing at night and decreasing in the morning.[1] Table 1-7 summarizes the morphological characteristics of the granulocytic (basophilic) series.

Tissue Basophil (Mast Cell)

Tissue basophils (mast cells) (Fig. 1-29) and blood basophils are closely related in their functions and biochemical characteristics, but the relationship between them is controversial.[1,8] Both cells participate in a similar manner in acute and delayed allergic reactions. The granules of both cells have similar morphological characteristics and each cell contains histamine and heparin and is water-soluble.[8]

Tissue basophils are derived from the multipotential undifferentiated stem cell and are fixed tissue cells. The cytoplasm of the tissue basophil is filled with large, prominent, intensely stained violet-blue granules. The granules are usually round and about the same size (0.1 to 0.3 μm). They may overlie the margins of the palely stained nucleus or obscure the nucleus com-

TABLE 1-7	**Morphological Characteristics of the Granulocytic (Basophilic) Series**					
	Myeloblast	Promyelocyte (Progranulocyte)	B. Myelocyte	B. Metamyelocyte	B. Band	B. Segmented
Cell size, μm	10–20	10–20	10–18	10–18	10–16	10–16
N:C ratio	4:1	3:1	2:1 or 1:1	1:1	1:1	1:1
Nuclear shape	Round	Round	Oval or round; slightly indented	Usually indented (kidney shaped), oval	Elongated, narrow band shape of uniform thickness	2 distinct nuclear lobes
Nuclear position	Eccentric or neutral	Eccentric or central	Commonly eccentric, may be central	Central or eccentric	Central or eccentric	Central or eccentric
Nuclear color/ chromatin	Light reddish blue, fine meshwork with no aggregation of material	Light reddish blue, fine meshwork, slight aggregation at nuclear rim	Reddish-blue, fine chromatin with slightly aggregated or granular pattern	Light blue purple with basophilic chromatin easily distinguishable	Deep blue purple, coarsely granular chromatin	Deep blue purple, coarsely granular chromatin
Nucleoli	1–3	1–2	May/may not	None	None	None
Color/amount of cytoplasm	Basophilic/Slight	Basophilic/ increased	Bluish pale, moderate	Pale blue, moderate	Pale blue, moderate	Pale blue, moderate
Cytoplasmic granules	Absent	Present, fine azurophilic, nonspecific granules	Present, coarse (*specific*) basophilic, nonuniform	Present, coarse violet blue nonuniform granules	Present coarse violet blue, nonuniform	Present coarse violet blue nonuniform

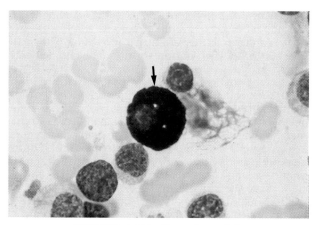

FIGURE 1-29   Tissue basophil.

pletely. The nucleus is small and round or oval and not segmented.[8]

Tissue basophils are widely scattered in connective tissue of various organs, bone marrow, and mucosal areas of serous membranes. In bone marrow, tissue basophils are usually observed in the hypercellular area of a "squashed" smear made from a marrow particle. Some tissue basophils have spindle shapes and jagged margins caused by trauma in the process of aspiration.[8]

Monopoiesis

The mononuclear-phagocyte system is composed of monocytes, macrophages, and their precursors, monoblasts and promonocytes.

Monoblasts and Promonocytes

Monoblasts (Fig. 1–30B) have a large, eccentrically placed nucleus that may be minimally indented, one or two large prominent nucleoli, a fine lacy nuclear

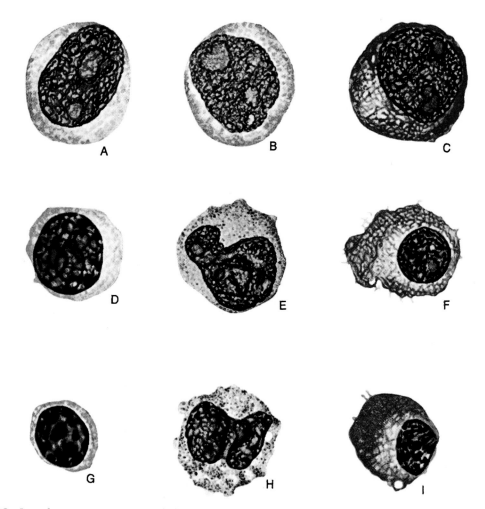

FIGURE 1-30   Lymphocytic, monocytic, and plasmocytic systems. *A.* Lymphoblast. *B.* Monoblast. *C.* Plasmoblast. *D.* Prolymphocyte. *E.* Promonocyte. *F.* Proplasmacyte. *G.* Lymphocyte with clumped chromatin. *H.* Monocyte. *I.* Plasmocyte. (From Diggs, Sturm, and Bell,[8] with permission.)

chromatin, and an agranular cytoplasm that stains a deep blue. The N:C ratio in these cells is 4:1. Monoblasts are nonmotile and nonphagocytic cells. Monoblasts divide and give rise to promonocytes (Fig. 1–31).[8]

Promonocytes (Fig. 1–30E) also are large, have indented or folded nuclei, have fine chromatin and irregular margins, may have a nucleolus, and sometimes contain a few peroxidase-positive granules. The N:C ratio in promonocytes is 3:1 or 2:1. Promonocytes are slightly motile and may infrequently take part in phagocytosis.[8]

Promonocytes and monoblasts are not easily identifiable in bone marrow or peripheral blood smears except in disorders in which there is marked proliferation of monocytic cells. The identification of early monocytic cells is based on slightly indented or folded, large nuclei and on association with more mature cells that have pseudopods and brainlike convolutions in the nucleus.[8]

Monocytes and Macrophages

Monoblasts, which are found in the marrow, divide and develop into promonocytes and then into monocytes. Figure 1–32 shows several different examples. Monocytes enter the circulation for a short time and migrate into tissue to be transformed into tissue macrophages.[1,2]

In thin areas of the peripheral blood smear, the monocyte is about 15 to 18 μm and is larger than the neutrophil. Monocytes have abundant cytoplasm in relation to the nucleus (N:C ratio is 2:1 or 1:1). The scanning electron microscope shows the monocyte to have a ruffled plasma membrane with long, thin microvilli. With Wright's stain, the cytoplasm turns a dull gray-blue, in contrast to the pink cytoplasm of neutrophils.[8] Numerous fine, small, reddish- or purplish-stained, evenly distributed granules in the cytoplasm give the cell a ground-glass appearance. There may be varying numbers of prominent granules in addition to the small granules. Some monocytes may appear nongranular, suggesting rapid turnover. Digestive vacuoles may be observed in the cytoplasm. In disease states, phagocytized erythrocytes, nuclei, cell fragments, bacteria, fungi, and pigment may be present.

The nuclei of monocytes may frequently be kidney-shaped, deeply folded, or indented or occasionally lob-ular. One of the distinctive features of the monocyte is the appearance of brainlike convolutions in the nucleus. Another characteristic is the lacy, often delicate chromatin network of fine strands intermingled with small chromatin clumps.[8]

The shape of the monocyte is variable. Many cells are round; other cells reveal blunt pseudopods that are manifestations of their slow mobility. These ameboid cells continue to move while the blood film is drying and become fixed before the cytoplasmic extensions are retracted. These pseudopods vary in size and number; the outer portion of the outstretched cytoplasm may have a hyaline appearance without granules in contrast to the inner granular cytoplasm.[8]

Three helpful characteristic features of the monocyte are brainlike nuclear convolutions, blunt pseudopods, and dull gray-blue cytoplasm[8] (Figs. 1–33 and 1–34). Kinetic studies have revealed that the half-time clearance of monocytes in the circulation is an average of 8.4 hours.[1,7]

Monocytes account for 2% to 9% or normal blood leukocytes and for less than 2% of normal marrow cells (see Tables 1–2 and 1–4). Monocytes are known to be in the marginating pool of cells. There is not a large reserve pool of monocytes in normal marrow. Monocytes leave the marrow when mature and enter the bloodstream, where they circulate for about 14 hours before entering tissue to transform into macrophages.[1] Macrophages are observed occasionally in normal marrow.

As monocytes grow, they become too large to pass readily through capillaries, and so they move into tissue and convert into macrophages in many organs (e.g., pulmonary alveolar macrophages, peritoneal macrophages, splenic macrophages, Küpffer cells in the liver, and connective tissue macrophages).[1] This transformation involves rapid growth, enlargement, and intensified phagocytic activity. Macrophages do not normally reenter the bloodstream, but may reenter the circulation during inflammation.[1]

Macrophages are large tissue cells (25 to 80 μm) with a round or reniform nucleus and contain one or two nucleoli, clumped chromatin, abundant cytoplasm with vacuoles, numerous azurophilic granules, and irregular shapes.[1] Macrophages are also called *histiocytes* (*histio* = tissue; *cyte* = cell). Table 1–8 summarizes the morphological characteristics of the monocyte-macrophage series.

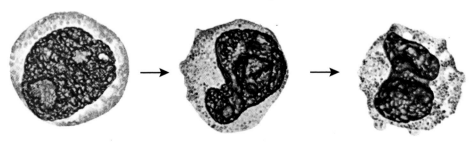

Monoblast   Promonocyte   Monocyte

FIGURE 1–31 The monocytic series.

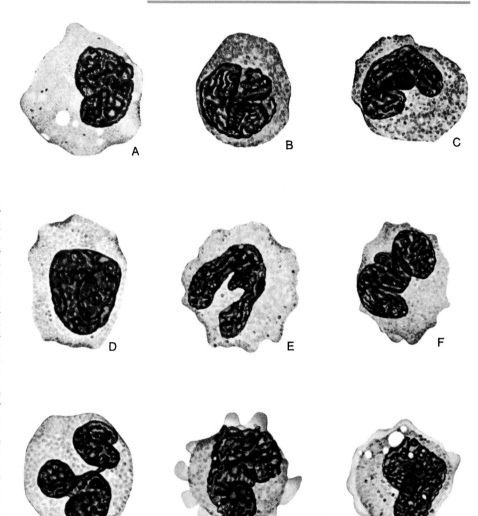

FIGURE 1-32 Monocytes. *A.* Monocyte with "ground-glass" appearance, evenly distributed fine granules, occasional azurophilic granules, and vacuoles in cytoplasm. *B.* Monocyte with opaque cytoplasm and granules and with lobulation of nucleus and linear chromatin. *C.* Monocyte with prominent granules and deeply indented nucleus. *D.* Monocyte without nuclear indentations. *E.* Monocyte with gray-blue color, band type of nucleus, linear chromatin, blunt pseudopods, and granules. *F.* Monocyte with gray-blue color, irregular shape, and multilobulated nucleus. *G.* Monocyte with segmented nucleus. *H.* Monocyte with multiple blunt nongranular pseudopods, nuclear indentations, and folds. *I.* Monocyte with vacuoles and with nongranular ectoplasm and granular endoplasm. (From Diggs, Sturm, and Bell,[8] with permission.)

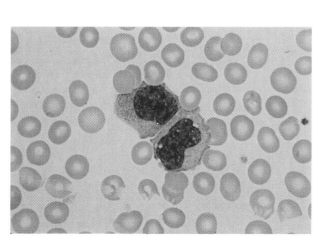

FIGURE 1-33   Monocytes.

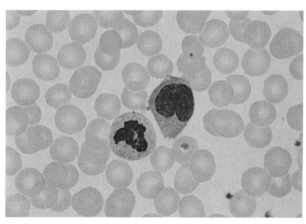

FIGURE 1-34   Right: Monocyte; left: N. segmented.

TABLE 1-8	**Morphological Characteristics of the Monocytic Series**			
	Monoblast	**Promonocyte**	**Mature Monocyte**	**Macrophage**
Cell size, μm	12–20	12–20	15–18	25–80
N:C ratio	4:1	3:1 or 2:1	2:1 or 1:1	1:2 or 1:3
Nuclear shape	Round, oval, or slightly folded	Round with chromatin creases or cerebriform folding, more distinct	Increased folding or elongated	Round or reniform
Nuclear position	Eccentric	Central	Central	Eccentric
Nuclear color/ chromatin	Pale red purple, fine, thready chromatin	Pale red purple, reticular pattern	Blue purple, finer reticular pattern than immature forms	Clumped chromatin
Nucleoli	1–2	0–2	None	1–2
Color/amount of cytoplasm	Basophilic/ moderate	Paler gray-basophilic/ abundant with "bleblike" pseudopodia at border	Pale gray blue/ abundant "bleblike" pseudopodia	Abundant with vacuoles
Cytoplasmic granules	None	May or may not contain fine red dustlike particles	Numerous fine, pale red dustlike particles throughout cytoplasm	Numerous azurophilic granules

Lymphopoiesis

The lymphoid progenitor cell is derived from the multipotential cell. The common lymphoid progenitor cell can differentiate into either T or B cells, depending on the microenvironment (Fig. 1–35). T cells differentiate in the thymus and B cells in adult bone marrow. Null cells, or third-population cells, originate in the bone marrow, although the maturation sequence is unknown.[2] T, B, and null cells cannot be separately identified morphologically but can be distinguished functionally and by immunologic marker studies. (See section on CD nomenclature in this chapter.)

In primary lymphoid organs such as the thymus and bone marrow, lymphocytes differentiate, proliferate, and mature into fully functional immune cells. In secondary lymphoid organs such as lymph nodes, spleen, and mucosal tissues (tonsils, Peyer's patches), lymphocytes communicate and interact with antigen-presenting cells (APCs), phagocytes, and macrophages in an active immune response.[2,7]

Lymphoblasts and Prolymphocytes

The earliest lymphocytes are identified as lymphoblasts and prolymphocytes (see Fig. 1–30A and D), re-spectively. Lymphoblasts contain a large round nucleus with a small or moderate amount of basophilic cytoplasm. The nuclear chromatin strands in lymphoblasts are thin, loose, evenly stained, and not clumped. One or several nucleoli are usually demonstrable.[2] These cells measure 10 to 20 μm in diameter.

Prolymphocytes have an intermediate chromatin pattern that has clumps in some areas of the nucleus but does not appear as clumped as in mature lymphocytes.[8] Parachromatin, which appears reddish purple, may be present in the nucleus. Nucleoli are less distinct than in lymphoblasts. Prolymphocytes are slightly smaller than lymphoblasts (9 to 18 μm). Differences are subtle, and if there is doubt the cell should be called a lymphocyte.[8]

Lymphocytes

Lymphocytes (Fig. 1–36) are the second most numerous cells in the blood; from 20% to 44% of adult blood cells are lymphocytes (see Table 1–4). There are 5% to 15% lymphocytes in bone marrow smears (see Table 1–2). Most lymphocytes are small, varying from 7 to 10 μm compared with monocytes (15 to 18 μm). Large lymphocytes may be 12 to 15 μm or more (Figs. 1–37 and 1–38). Between the small and large lympho-

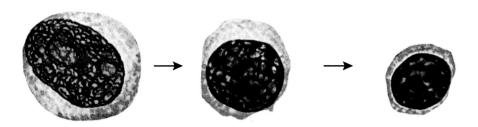

Lymphoblast   Prolymphocyte   Lymphocyte

FIGURE 1–35 The lymphocytic series.

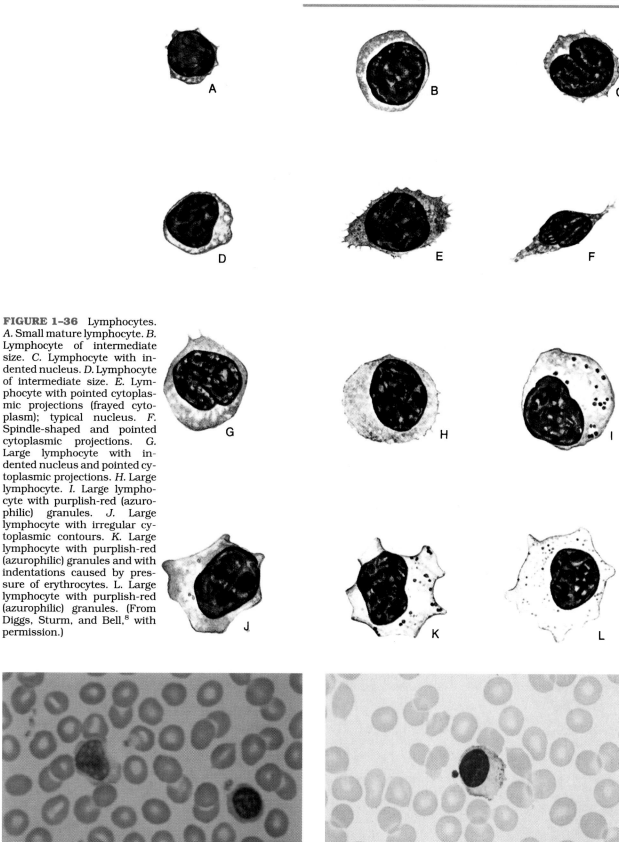

FIGURE 1-36 Lymphocytes. *A.* Small mature lymphocyte. *B.* Lymphocyte of intermediate size. *C.* Lymphocyte with indented nucleus. *D.* Lymphocyte of intermediate size. *E.* Lymphocyte with pointed cytoplasmic projections (frayed cytoplasm); typical nucleus. *F.* Spindle-shaped and pointed cytoplasmic projections. *G.* Large lymphocyte with indented nucleus and pointed cytoplasmic projections. *H.* Large lymphocyte. *I.* Large lymphocyte with purplish-red (azurophilic) granules. *J.* Large lymphocyte with irregular cytoplasmic contours. *K.* Large lymphocyte with purplish-red (azurophilic) granules and with indentations caused by pressure of erythrocytes. L. Large lymphocyte with purplish-red (azurophilic) granules. (From Diggs, Sturm, and Bell,[8] with permission.)

FIGURE 1-37 Lymphocytes. Left: large; right: small.

FIGURE 1-38 Lymphocyte, large.

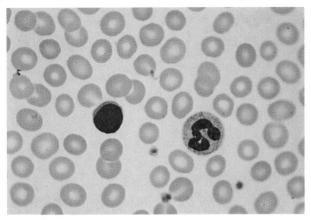

FIGURE 1-39   Left: lymphocyte; right: segmented neutrophil.

cytes are many of intermediate size. Size is not a reliable basis for determining the age or metabolic activity of lymphocytes because the size varies with the thickness of the smear. Lymphocytes tend to become spherical and small in thick areas of the smear; in the thinnest end of the smear, lymphocytes may be spread out and appear large.[8]

Small lymphocytes are usually round with smooth margins (Fig. 1–39). Rarely, a lymphocyte may have a spindle form with an oval nucleus and cytoplasmic filaments extending outward at each end (see Fig. 1–36F). The margin of large lymphocytes frequently is indented by neighboring erythrocytes, causing them to have a serrated (holly-leaf) shape.[8]

With Wright's stain, the color of the cytoplasm is blue, with the intensity of the blue varying from light to dark in different cells. The color is evenly distributed in some cells and uneven in others. The intensity of the blue stain is greater at the periphery of the cell than near the Golgi area adjacent to the nucleus. The cytoplasm of some large lymphocytes that stain a pale sky blue has a structureless appearance; other large cells may reveal fine bluish interlacing fibrils with critical illumination.[8]

Most lymphocytes do not have granules. In some large cells, there may be a few well-defined granules that vary in size, are unevenly distributed, and can be easily counted. These granules are a purplish red and have been called azurophilic; this term is misleading because these granules are predominantly red rather than blue.[8] The diameter of the nucleus of the smallest lymphocyte in peripheral blood is slightly larger than or the same size as a normal erythrocyte in the same microscopic field. The lymphocyte's nucleus, in relation to its cytoplasm, is large (N:C ratio is 4:1), and the nuclei are round or slightly indented. Chromatin structure is lumpy or clumped and stains dark purple with lighter bluish-purple areas between chromatin aggregates.[8]

Nucleoli are present in some lymphocytes but are *not* visible in light microscopy because they are obscured by the darkly stained chromatin masses. The fact that nucleoli may be present in small lymphocytes is evidence that these cells are capable of growth and replication.[8,9] Table 1–9 summarizes the morphological characteristics of the lymphocytic series.

Large Lymphocytes versus Monocytes

A monocyte is often mistaken for a large lymphocyte (Fig. 1–40) because the monocytic cytoplasm may be blue, the granules may be indistinct, the nucleus is round, and blunt pseudopods and digestive vacuoles are missing. To distinguish monocytes from large lymphocytes, the nuclear chromatin structure, character of the cytoplasm, and shape of the cells are useful. The nucleus of a lymphocyte tends to be clumped rather than linear or lacy, as it is in a monocyte. There is a greater tendency for the nuclear chromatin to be condensed at the periphery of the nucleus in the lymphocyte. The brainlike convolutions present in a monocyte are not observed in a lymphocyte.[8]

Large lymphocytes and monocytes may have distinct bluish-red granules. In a monocyte, the large bluish-red granules are interspersed with numerous fine granules in the cytoplasm and cannot be enumerated (see Fig. 1–33). In a lymphocyte, these large granules are prominent and can be counted easily because there are no other granules (Fig. 1–41; see also Fig.

TABLE 1–9	**Characteristics of the Lymphocytic Series**		
	Lymphoblast	**Prolymphocyte**	**Mature Lymphocyte**
Cell size, μm	10–20	9–18	7–10
N:C ratio	4:1	4:1	4:1
Nuclear shape	Round	Round or indented	Round or indented
Nuclear position	Eccentric or central	Eccentric with scanty cytoplasm to one side or round	Eccentric with scanty cytoplasm to one side or round
Nuclear color/chromatin	Undifferentiated red purple/smooth chromatin	Condensed, clumped blue purple chromatin with red purple parachromatin	Homogenous, coarse blue purple nuclear chromatin
Nucleoli	1–2	0–1	None
Color/amount of cytoplasm	Clear basophilic/scanty	Clear basophilic/scanty	Light sky blue/scanty to moderate
Cytoplasmic granules	Absent	Absent	Usually absent, few azurophilic granules seen occasionally

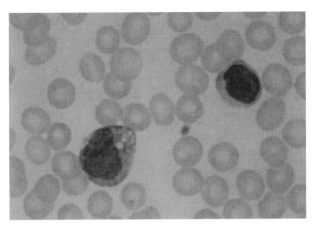

FIGURE 1-40   Left: monocyte; right: lymphocyte.

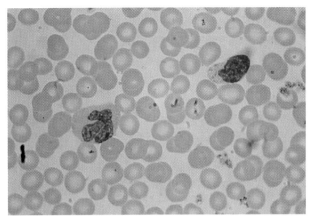

FIGURE 1-41   Left: normal monocyte; right: medium-size lymphocyte.

1-38). Because of the finely granular cytoplasm, the monocyte has a ground-glass appearance, whereas the cytoplasm of the lymphocyte has a relatively clear non-granular background. Large lymphocytes are often deeply indented by neighboring red blood cells. Monocytes tend to project blunt pseudopods between cells or to compress cells, rather than being indented by them.[8] Table 1-10 summarizes and compares the morphological characteristics of large lymphocytes versus monocytes.

Reactive (Activated) Lymphocytes

In reaction to appropriate antigenic stimuli, lymphocytes have been shown to transform into cells that are immunologically competent. The nucleus and cytoplasm of lymphocytes that respond to antigenic stimuli enlarge. The size of activated lymphocytes varies, but usually these cells are large with abundant cytoplasm. The increase in size is due to an increase in DNA in the nucleus and of RNA in the cytoplasm. The nucleus may be oval, indented, or irregularly shaped with an intermediate chromatin pattern, which is less dense than normal small lymphocytes. Some reactive lymphocytes may have a blastlike nucleus with faintly visible nucleoli. Varying degrees of cytoplasmic basophilia may be present; basophilia also may be unevenly distributed. There may be distinctive reddish granules. The cytoplasm may appear bubbly and vacuoles may be

seen.[8] Large reactive lymphocytes may have scalloped margins.

Lymphocytes that respond to antigenic stimuli constitute a wide spectrum of morphological variants. The most striking variants are observed in infectious mononucleosis (see Chap. 17), but reactive lymphocytes are also present, in lesser numbers, in other viral diseases, such as cytomegalovirus (CMV) and human immunodeficiency virus (HIV), infectious hepatitis, and in conditions such as post-transfusion reactions, organ transplants, and serum sickness.[2] Figure 1-42 shows a plasmacytoid reactive lymphocyte. Table 1-11 reviews the morphological characteristics of reactive lymphocytes.

Plasmablasts and Proplasmacytes

Cells designated as plasmablasts are similar to blast cells of other series (see Fig. 1-30C). The nuclei are large in relation to the cytoplasm (N:C ratio is 4:1); appear round with fine, linear chromatin strands; and have a clearly visible nucleolus. Figure 1-43 shows the plasmacytic series. Plasmablasts are identified primarily in the presence of proplasmacytes and plasmacytes but cannot be differentiated easily from other blasts.[8] The plasmablast appears slightly larger than the more mature plasmacyte (16 to 25 μm).

Proplasmacytes and plasmacytes differ from plas-

TABLE 1-10 **Morphological Comparison of Large Lymphocytes and Monocytes**		
	Large Lymphocyte	**Monocyte**
Size, μm	12-15	15-18
Nucleus	Clumped, condensed at periphery	Lacy, brainlike convolutions
Cytoplasmic granules	Bluish red, prominent granules, easily enumerated if present	Bluish red, interdispersed with other granules, not easily enumerated
Cytoplasm	Clear, nongranular background	"Ground-glass" appearance
Cell interactions	Indented by erythrocytes	Projection of blunt pseudopodia

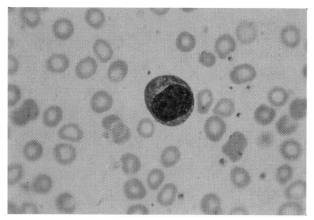

FIGURE 1–42   Plasmacytoid reactive lymphocyte in a drug reaction.

TABLE 1–11	**Morphological Characteristics of Reactive (Activated) Lymphocytes**
Size	Generally larger than mature lymphocytes
Cytoplasm	Usually more abundant than mature lymphocyte, may exhibit striking basophilia; vacuoles may be seen
Cytoplasmic granules	Often distinct reddish granules
Nuclei	Oval-indented nuclei; intermediate chromatin pattern (blastlike)
Nucleoli	Occasionally visible

mablasts in that the color of the cytoplasm is dark blue, the juxtanuclear light areas are prominent, and the nuclei are eccentric. The chromatin structure of the nuclei in proplasmacytes is intermediate between that of plasmablasts and plasmacytes. In proplasmacytes, the nucleolus may be ill-defined or absent.[8] The N:C ratio in proplasmacytes in 3:1.

Plasmablasts and proplasmacytes, although not observed in normal bone marrow, are seen in diseases associated with abnormal immunoglobulin production, especially multiple myeloma.[8]

Plasmacytes (Plasma Cells)

Plasmacytes represent the end stage of B-lymphocyte lineage. They are not observed in peripheral blood smears of normal individuals, but constitute about 1% of the nucleated cells in normal marrow (see Table 1–2). Mature plasmacytes range in size from 10 to 18 μm.[1] They may be round or oval with slightly irregular margins (Figs. 1–44 and 1–45). The cytoplasm is nongranular and usually stains a deep or vibrant blue that has been described as "cornflower" or "larkspur" blue. The cytoplasm adjacent to the nucleus is pale with a perinuclear clear zone containing the Golgi apparatus, and at the cell periphery there are secretory vesicles. Fibrillar structures that stain blue may be demonstrable in the cytoplasm. One or several small vacuoles

may be observed. There is no evidence of phagocytosis of visible particles.[8]

The nucleus of a plasmacyte is relatively small, round, or oval and eccentrically placed in the cell. The nuclear chromatin is clumped or coarse and lumpy, similar to that of a lymphocyte.[8]

Plasmacytes in bone marrow are semifixed cells that are torn in the process of aspiration and appear in marrow smears with irregular spiculate margins. Plasmacytes may cluster around large nongranular or finely granular tissue cells. This contact of plasmacytes with tissue cells is probably a manifestation of the immune response in which antigenic material, processed by macrophages, is transferred to the plasmacytes, which in turn will manufacture immune globulins.[8]

Immune globulins manufactured by plasmacytes produce unusual morphological variants. The proteinaceous material is in the form of round globules that may be red, pink, blue, or almost colorless and are called Russell bodies. The globules may fill the cytoplasm, giving the appearance of a bunch of grapes (berry, grape, or morula cells).[8]

In some cells, the globules are so numerous and so tightly packed that they assume a honeycomb configuration. In other cells, the redness has a diffuse distribution, producing cells called flame cells,[8] which are observed particularly in association with IgA (see Chap. 22, Fig. 22–15). The red-staining proteinaceous material may appear as granules or as pools at the margins; it also may crystallize and produce elongated

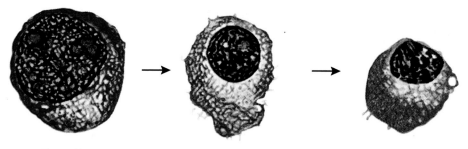

Plasmablast   Proplasmacyte   Plasma Cell

FIGURE 1–43   The plasmacytic series.

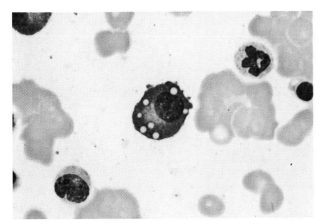

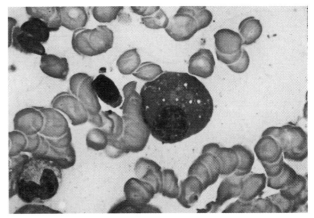

FIGURE 1–44   Center: plasmacyte; upper right: N. segmented, lower left: resting monocyte.

FIGURE 1–45   Center: plasmacyte; left center: small lymphocyte.

crystalline structures that stain reddish.[8] Table 1–12 summarizes the morphological characteristics of the plasmacytic series.

Megakaryocytopoiesis

The megakaryocyte is the largest hematopoietic cell in the bone marrow and descends from the same multipotential stem cell as do the other blood cells. The role of megakaryocytes is to proliferate and then fragment their cytoplasm into platelets, when needed, to maintain a normal number of platelets. The maturation of the megakaryocyte (Fig. 1–46) involves endoreduplication (or endomitosis), which is a process whereby the nuclear material reduplicates but the nucleus does not divide. The result of endoreduplication is a polyploid nucleus. Each nuclear division causes a doubling of the nuclear material. The cytoplasm increases in amount and in number of granules, but does not divide.[1,2] Megakaryoblasts are moderately sized cells in the range of 20 to 45 μm, with a single, round (or slightly oval) primitive nucleus; one or two nucleoli; and basophilic protrusions that stain blue and contain chromophobic globules.[1,2] The scanty cy-

toplasm is nongranular and basophilic. The N:C cytoplasmic ratio is 4:1.

Pathologic alterations in megakaryoblasts are observed in myeloproliferative diseases. The presence of micromegakaryoblasts is typical of acute megakaryocytic leukemia (classified as M7 in the French-American-British [FAB] classification of acute leukemia). They may also be found in the blast crisis of chronic granulocytic leukemia and other acute leukemias. Such cells are small and difficult to distinguish from myeloblasts, but cytoplasmic blebs or budding (suggesting early platelet formation) help to identify micromegakaryoblasts.[7,8]

As the megakaryoblast matures into a promegakaryocyte, it increases both the amount of nuclear material and the amount of cytoplasm itself (N:C ratio is 4:1 to 1:1) (Figs. 1–47 and 1–48). A promegakaryocyte not only increases the size of the nucleus but also becomes lobed, with each lobe having a 2n complement of DNA. The size of the promegakaryocyte ranges from 20 to 80 μm. Reddish granules appear in the enlarging bluish cytoplasm. Electron micrographs reveal that demarcation membranes are beginning to develop as invaginations from the plasma membrane of the megakary-

TABLE 1–12	**Morphological Characteristics of the Plasmacytic Series**		
	Plasmablast	**Proplasmacyte**	**Mature Plasma Cell**
Cell size, μm	16–25	15–20	10–18
N:C ratio	4:1	3:1	2:1 or 1:1
Nuclear shape	Round	Round or oval	Round or oval
Nuclear position	Central	Eccentric	Usually eccentric
Nuclear color/chromatin	Pale red purple, fine stippled chromatin	Red purple, increased granularity of chromatin	Blue purple, dense chromatin with large clumps near nuclear margin
Nucleoli	1–3	0–1	None
Color/amount of cytoplasm	Pale blue/scanty to moderate, frequent perinuclear clear zone	Dark blue/moderate	Dark blue/moderate cytoplasm with perinuclear clear zone, may contain vacuoles
Cytoplasmic granules	None	None	None

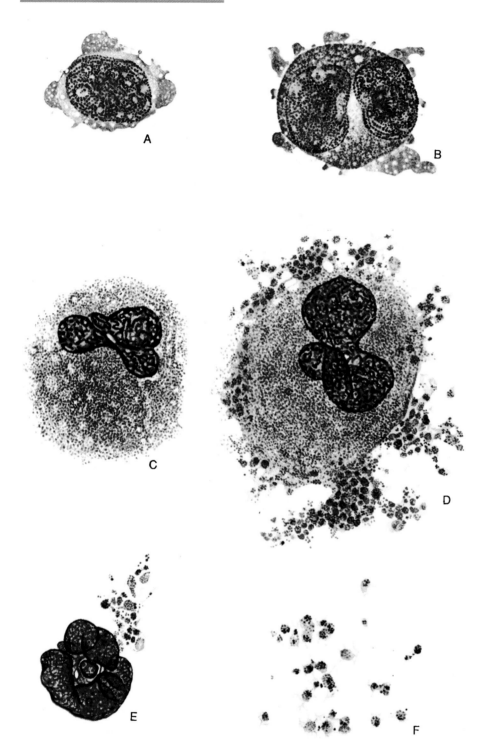

FIGURE 1-46 Megakaryocytic system. *A.* Megakaryoblast with single oval nucleus, nucleoli, and bluish foamy marginal cytoplasmic structures. *B.* Promegakaryocyte with two nuclei, granular blue cytoplasm, and marginal bubbly cytoplasmic structures: *C.* Megakaryocyte with granular cytoplasm and without discrete thrombocytes (platelets). *D.* Metamegakaryocyte with multiple nuclei and with thrombocytes (platelets). *E.* Metamegakaryocyte nucleus with attached thrombocytes. *F.* Thrombocytes (platelets). (From Diggs, Sturm, and Bell,[8] with permission.)

ocyte. The demarcation membrane system establishes an outer limit of each platelet, which arises as a cytoplasmic fragment.[1,2,7]

As endomitosis and DNA synthesis cease and maximum nuclear number (ploidy) is attained, the megakaryocyte has increased in volume with an abundant amount of pinkish cytoplasm and a multilobulated nucleus (Figs. 1–49 and 1–50). The size of the megakaryocyte ranges from 30 to 100 μm. Most of the cells are of the $8n$, $16n$, and $32n$ ploidy classes ($16n$ average ploidy represents eight lobes).[1,7] The chromatin is linear and coarse. Numerous small, uniformly distributed, dense granules that stain reddish blue are present. The demarcation membrane system is uniform

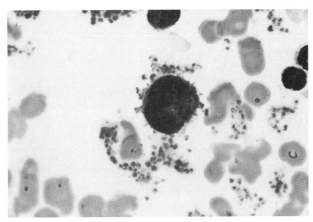

FIGURE 1-47 Center: early megakaryocyte.

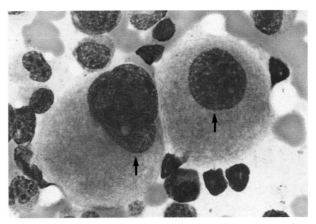

FIGURE 1-49 Megakaryocytes without platelets.

and its lumen open; the cytoplasm is divided into partitions that define platelet limits.[1,7] The N:C ratio at the megakaryocyte stage of development ranges from 1:1 to 1:12.

After maturation is completed, the megakaryocyte membrane ruptures, the entire megakaryocyte cytoplasm fragments, and thrombopoiesis occurs. The polyploid naked nucleus (Fig. 1–51) is soon to be engulfed by a macrophage.[1]

In addition, some mature megakaryocytes are located adjacent to marrow sinuses and extend portions of their cytoplasm through the basement membrane and between endothelial cells of the marrow sinusoids in order to put platelets into the sinus. Membrane-bound platelets are released and swept into the flowing bloodstream from these cytoplasmic projections. Further fragmentation to form individual platelets occurs after release into the sinus. One megakaryocyte can release several thousand platelets.[1,7]

In the past, megakaryocytes were believed to shed platelets from their outer surface. However, transmission electron micrographs demonstrate that mature megakaryocytes have a well-defined marginal zone and that there are only a few channels of the demar-

cation membrane system in which platelets could be shed from the surface. Therefore, during thrombocytopoiesis, the entire megakaryocyte cytoplasm fragments to form platelets.[1,7]

Ultrastructural features and marker studies on megakaryocytes aid in their identification at all stages. Ultrastructural features are the demarcation membrane, alpha granules, and platelet peroxidase activity.[1] Monoclonal antibodies for platelet glycoproteins Ib, IIb, IIIa, factor VIII antigen, beta thromboglobulin, and factor V are markers for all stages of megakaryocytes.[1]

Platelets (or thrombocytes) are cytoplasmic fragments and have no nucleus. In peripheral smears of normal adults, platelets vary in size from 1 to 4 μm. Platelets may be round, oval, or rod-shaped. A variable number of small reddish granules are seen in the hyaline, light-blue cytoplasm. Granules may be concentrated in the center of the platelet, giving the appearance of a nucleus.[2]

Platelets tend to adhere to each other and may form small aggregates in a well-made normal smear. In the thin area of the blood smear where erythrocytes are separated or gently touching each other but not over-

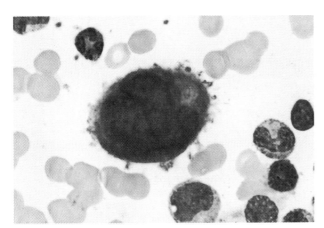

FIGURE 1-48 Center: early megakaryocyte; top left: segmented neutrophil; bottom center: N. metamyelocyte.

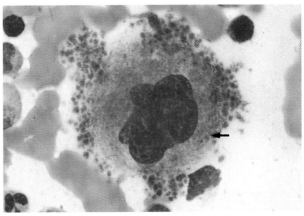

FIGURE 1-50 Megakaryocyte with platelets.

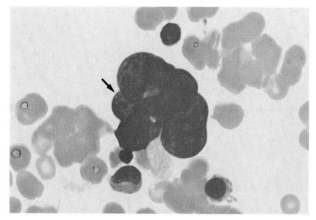

FIGURE 1-51 Naked nuclei, megakaryocyte.

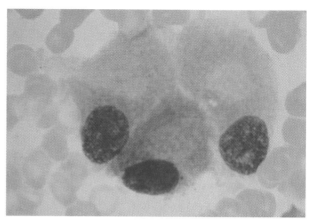

FIGURE 1-52 The osteoblast.

lapping, the number per oil immersion field varies from 7 to 25.[8]

In marrow smears of normal individuals, there are approximately 1 to 4 megakaryocytes per 1000 nucleated cells, and these cells are in the late stage of maturation.[8] Table 1–13 summarizes the morphological characteristics of the megakaryocytic series.

Bone-Derived Cells

The formation of bone marrow cavity results from a complex process in which hematopoietic cells migrate and colonize spaces originally occupied by cartilage and bone. This process occurs both in the long bones of the limbs and in the membranous bones of the skull, which develop directly into bone. Studies have shown that bone formation and hematopoiesis are closely linked, in that the degree of hematopoiesis correlates with the rate of bone turnover.[2,7,20] Two normal, non-hematopoietic cells that exhibit different functions yet play essential roles in the formation of the bone cavity

are the osteoblast and the osteoclast. The hiearchy of cell maturation and bone-derived cells remains unclear.

Osteoblasts

An osteoblast is a large cell that can measure up to 30 μm, with ample cytoplasm and a small, round, eccentrically placed nucleus (Fig. 1–52). These cells may be traumatized in the process of marrow aspiration and smearing and often have irregular shapes and cytoplasmic streamers. The cells may have comet or tadpole shapes. The nucleus may be partially extruded, similar to a small round head on a round body. The nuclear chromatin strands and nuclear margins are well defined and stain purple-red. Usually there is a distinct blue nucleolus.[8]

Throughout the blue cytoplasm are small spherical bodies that are colorless and give a bubbly appearance to the cytoplasm. Within the cytoplasm there is a prominent round or oval chromophobic zone that

TABLE 1-13	**Morphological Characteristics of the Megakaryocytic Series**			
	Megakaryoblast	**Promegakaryocyte**	**Megakaryocyte**	**Thrombocyte**
Cell size, μm	20–45	20–80	30–100	1–4
N:C ratio	4:1	4:1–1:1	1:1–1:12	n/a
Nuclear shape	Usually single round, oval, indented or kidney-shaped	Usually single round, oval indented or kidney-shaped	Lobulated (2 or more lobes)	n/a
Nuclear position	Central or eccentric	Central or eccentric	Central	n/a
Nuclear color/chromatin	Red purple fine chromatin with distinct chromatin	Red purple, increased granularity of nuclear chromatin	Blue purple, granular	n/a
Nucleoli	1–2	0–1, usually less than megakaryoblast	None	n/a
Color/amount of cytoplasm	Basophilic, pseudopodia frequent/scanty	Basophilic/abundant with pseudopodia	Pale blue with pink cast/abundant	Light blue, fragment of megakaryocyte cytoplasm
Cytoplasmic granules	Nongranular	Fine azurophilic granules	Numerous fine azurophilic granules	Reddish-blue, fine, evenly dispersed

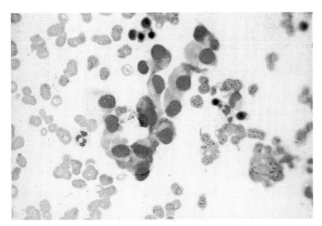

FIGURE 1-53 Group of osteoblasts (center) aspirated from the marrow of a child. (Magnification ×400)

stains lighter than the rest of the cytoplasm. This area is usually away from the nucleus but may be adjacent to it.[8]

Osteoblasts, most often seen in marrow from young children (Fig. 1–53), are responsible for the formation, calcification, and maintenance of trabeculae and cancellous bone.[8] Osteoblasts secrete large amounts of collagen and proteoglycans, contributing to structure of the bone and stromal matrix.[2]

Osteoblasts morphologically resemble plasmacytes, both having irregular shapes, cytoplasmic protrusions, blue cytoplasm, eccentric nuclei, spherical bodies within the cytoplasm, chromophobic areas, cytoplasmic fibrils, and vacuoles.[8] The relatively unstained zone of the plasmacytes is adjacent to the nucleus and partially surrounds the nucleus like a collar, whereas the chromophobic zone of the osteoblast is often distinctly separate from the nuclear margin and, when adjacent to the nucleus, does not surround or enclose the nucleus.[8]

The protein secretions of the plasmacytes impart a reddish background color to the cells that is not de-

monstrable in osteoblasts.[8] Osteoblasts occurring in clusters or aggregates may be misinterpreted as malignant cells. Malignant cells in a cluster are crowded and distorted and their margins are indistinct, rendering it impossible to identify individual cells. The size, shape, structure, and color of malignant cells are variable, whereas osteoblasts are more orderly and uniform. Chromophobic areas in the cytoplasm of osteoblasts are seldom demonstrable in malignant cells.[8]

It is thought that the mature osteoblast arises from the immature preosteoblast exhibiting mitotic activity. Other theories have placed osteoblast formation at the mesenchymal stem cells, which reside in the periosteum. It is probable, however, that many intermediate stages exist in the development of the mature osteoblast, as described by studies using monoclonal antibodies specific for bone phenotypes.[2]

Osteoclasts

Osteoclasts are giant (>100 μm), multinucleated, irregularly shaped marrow phagocytes that are capable of absorption of bone (Fig. 1–54). Osteoclasts have from 2 to 50 nuclei, which are separate, usually round or oval, all about the same size, and haphazardly distributed within the cytoplasm; they have visible nucleoli.[8] Bone-absorbing osteoclasts are formed by fusion of precursor cells derived from the monocyte-macrophage lineage.

The abundant cytoplasm with ragged margin is bluish with numerous reddish lysosomal granules containing acid phosphatase. In thin marrow smears it may be possible to demonstrate a ruffled cytoplasmic fringe consisting of diaphanous veils, fingerlike protrusions, and saccular invaginations.[8]

Osteoclasts and megakaryocytes are sometimes difficult to differentiate because both cells are large with granular cytoplasm, irregular shapes, and multiple nuclei. The nuclei of megakaryocytes are connected by a nuclear strand, have irregular nuclear shapes, and may be superimposed (Fig. 1–55), whereas the nuclei

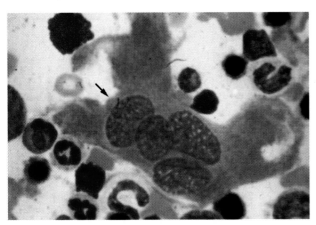

FIGURE 1-54 The osteoclast is usually seen as a single giant cell with multiple and separated nuclei and basophilic granular cytoplasm (center). (Magnification ×640)

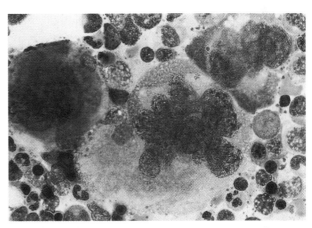

FIGURE 1-55 Megakaryocytes tend to be in small groups with multilobulated single nuclei. Mature megakarocytes have numerous fine cytoplasmic granules, and occasionally platelet units can be seen at their periphery. (Magnification ×640)

TABLE 1–14 **Morphological Characteristics of the Osteoclast and Megakaryocyte**		
	Osteoclast	**Megakaryocyte**
Size, μm	>100	30–100
Shape	Irregular	Irregular
Cytoplasm	Granular	Granular
Nuclei	Multiple, uniform in size, unconnected by nuclear strands	Multiple, connected by nuclear strands, not uniform in size
Number of nuclei	Odd number	Even number

of osteoclasts are separated, uniform in size, and have no visible connections to each other (see Fig. 1–54). The number of nuclei in normal megakaryocytes is even, whereas in osteoclasts it may be uneven.[8] Table 1–14 summarizes and compares the morphological characteristics of the multinucleated osteoclast and the multilobulated megakaryocyte.

Osteoclasts secrete enzymes that aid in dissolution of osteoid tissue and calcific bone. Osteoclastic activating factor (OAF), secreted by plasmacytes in myeloma, is a lymphokine that stimulates osteoclastic activity in the endosteum near groups of myeloma cells. The presence of OAF helps to explain the development of osteolytic bone lesions observed in myeloma.[1,8]

These cells are involved in the degradation (or reabsorption) of bone, which is essential for the formation of the bone marrow cavity and bone remodeling. On the basis of in vivo studies, osteoclasts are thought to originate from hematopoietic stem cells, but a general consensus as to the immediate precursor has not been reached. Theories supporting osteoclasts arising from the monocytic lineage have been well documented; both cells exhibit phagocytic activities and share common antigenic determinants. In vivo and in vitro studies have demonstrated the fusion of monocytes and macrophages into multinucleated cells resembling osteoclasts, in addition to a growth factor acting in the generation of both cell types.[2] Table 1–15 summarizes and compares the morphological characteristics of the osteoblast and the osteoclast.

Introduction to the Cell Cycle

The Generative (G) Cell Cycle Kinetics

When stimulated by hematopoietic growth factors (see section in this chapter on colony-stimulating fac-

tors and interleukins), hematopoietic cells undergo a continuous generative (G) cycle in which the cells divide, differentiate, or remain dormant (Fig. 1–56). The bone marrow contains cell populations in all phases of cell development. The generative cell cycle is divided into five phases: G_0, G_1, S, G_2, and M.[2,7] The cells able to proliferate enter a resting or dormant phase (G_0) after division. From the G_0 state the resting cell enters the G_1 phase, which is the postmitotic rest phase and which directly precedes the deoxyribonucleic acid (DNA) synthesis phase. The cell proceeds into the synthesis (S) phase of active DNA synthesis, where the DNA content is doubled. The next phase is the premitotic rest period (G_2) as the cell prepares to enter the mitotic period (M). During the final, or M, phase, there is cellular division of the chromosomes in the nucleus and the cytoplasm, resulting in two daughter cells.[2,7] T_g is the cycle of one complete mitotic division. After final differentiation, the cell leaves the cycle as a nondividing cell (G_{ND}) (Fig. 1–56).

MOLECULAR HEMATOLOGY AND ADVANCED CONCEPTS

Specific Cell Line Ontogeny

Multipotential Stem Cells—Colony-Forming Units

The morphology of the recognizable stages of peripheral blood and marrow cells has been described. As stated earlier, these cells come from an unrecognizable pluripotential stem cell. The pluripotential stem cell has the capacity for continuous self-replication and also for differentiation into the multipotential stem cell and the lymphoid stem cell without capacity for self-renewal. The multipotential stem cell becomes com-

TABLE 1–15 **Morphological Comparison of Osteoblasts and Osteoclasts**		
	Osteoblast	**Osteoclast**
Size, μm	Up to 30	>100
Nuclei	Round, eccentric, uninuclear	Multinucleated, uniform size
Nucleolus	Present	Present
Cytoplasm	Chromophobic area, usually away from nucleus	Bluish, reddish lysosomal granules, cytoplasmic protrusions
Shape	Resemble plasmacytes	May be confused with megakaryocytes

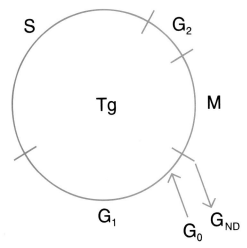

FIGURE 1-56 Cell cycle kinetics. Tg = one complete mitotic division cycle; G_0 = resting or dormant phase; G_1 = postmitotic rest period; S = active DNA synthesis phases; G_2 = premitotic rest period; M = mitotic period; G_{ND} = nondividing cell.

mitted to support progenitor cells for myelopoiesis, erythropoiesis, monopoiesis, and megakaryopoiesis. The lymphoid stem cell line supports lymphopoiesis.[7] The multipotential stem cell was shown to exist in a classic experiment in 1961 by Till and McCullock,[21] who irradiated mice to empty the hematopoietic organs and then injected a suspension of marrow cells intravenously. About a week later, nodules of injected marrow could be observed on the cut surface of the spleen colonies. All cell lines found in normal marrow were generated from the multipotential stem cells in the marrow suspension. The multipotential stem cell giving rise to several cell lines was called the colony-forming unit–granulocyte-erythrocyte-monocyte–macrophage-megakaryocyte (CFU–GEMM).[2,7]

The CFU–GEMM in a colony assay forms a series of progenitor cells (CFU–GM, CFU–Eo, CFU–Bs, CFU–Meg, BFU–E, CFU–E) under appropriate growth conditions. See Table 1–16 for acronyms. CFU–GM makes colonies of granulocytes and monocytes and/or macrophages. CFU–Eo forms colonies of eosinophils. CFU–Bs makes early basophils and mast cells. CFU–Meg

forms megakaryocyte colonies. There are two colonies of erythroid progenitor cells: the early burst-forming unit—erythroid (BFU–E) and the more mature colony-forming unit—erythroid (CFU–E).

The lymphoid stem cell is also derived from the pluripotential stem cell. The lymphoid stem cell has the potential to differentiate into a T or B cell. T cells participate in immune functions of a cellular nature, either directly cytotoxic or in helping or suppressing immune activities through interaction with other immunocompetent cells. B cells differentiate into plasmacytes, which secrete specific immunoglobulins important in the host's defense against infection. Another population of lymphocytes, called null cells, have none of the characteristics of either the T or the B cells. The null cell category includes killer (K) cells, which interact with antibody to cause destruction of antibody-coated targets, and natural killer (NK) cells, which can lyse target cells through direct cytotoxic activity. Their differentiation is uncertain.[1] Table 1–17 lists the different types of lymphocytes and their function.

Colony-Stimulating Factors and Interleukins

Each cell line is dependent on cytokines, which are soluble mediators secreted by cells for the purpose of cell-to-cell communication. Table 1–18 lists the different cell types and the cytokines they produce. Table

TABLE 1-16 Hematopoietic Progenitor Cells

Abbreviation	Full Name
CFU-GEMM	Colony-forming unit—granulocyte, erythrocyte, macrophage-monocyte, megakaryocyte
CFU-GM	Colony-forming unit—granulocyte, macrophage-monocyte
CFU-Eo	Colony-forming unit—eosinophil
CFU-Bas	Colony-forming unit—basophil
CFU-Meg	Colony-forming unit—megakaryocyte
BFU-E	Burst-forming unit—erythrocyte
CFU-E	Colony-forming unit—erythrocyte

TABLE 1-17 Functions of Lymphocytes

Lymphocyte	Function
T cells	Cell mediated immunity
B cells	Humoral immunity
Null cells (killer)	Antibody-dependent cell-mediated lysis
Natural killer (NK) cells	Direct cytotoxic activity

TABLE 1-18 Cellular Cytokine Production

Cell Type	Cytokine*
Endothelial cell	GM-CSF, G-CSF, M-CSF, IL-6
Monocyte-macrophage	GM-CSF, G-CSF, M-CSF, IL-3, IL-6, EPO, SCF
T cell	GM-CSF, IL-2, IL-3, IL-4, IL-5
Fibroblasts	GM-CSF, G-CSF, M-CSF, IL-6, SCF
NK cells	GM-CSF
Osteoblasts	IL-6, GM-CSF
PMN	G-CSF, GM-CSF
B cells	GM-CSF, M-CSF, IL-2, IL-5, IL-6
Marrow stroma	GM-CSF, G-CSF, M-CSF, IL-6, IL-3, SCF, IL-11
Renal parenchyma, liver, and marrow cells	EPO

*mRNA, protein, or specific biologic activity detected at baseline levels or immediately after induction.

TABLE 1–19 **Cytokine Characteristics**
Glycoproteins
Produced by many cell types
Usually act on multiple cell lineages
Interact synergistically with one another
Activate receptors at very low concentrations
Usually act on the neoplastic counterpart of normal target cells
Usually act throughout the maturation hierarchy from stem cell to the terminally differentiated cell

1–19 lists the characteristics of cytokines. Cytokines act on multipotential stem cells to stimulate their proliferation and differentiation to committed cell lines (Fig. 1–57). For a cell to develop from a multipotential cell to a myeloblast, monoblast, erythroblast, or megakaryoblast, cytokines are necessary. Colony-stimulating factors (CSFs) or growth factors and interleukins (ILs) are two types of cytokines. Table 1–20 summarizes the cytokines involved in hematopoietic blood cell development, listing their sources and the target cells that they stimulate.

Colony-stimulating factors and interleukins regulate blood cell development by mediating proliferation, differentiation, and maturation of hematopoietic progenitor cells (see Fig. 1–57).

TRENDS IN THERAPEUTIC MANIPULATION OF HEMATOPOIESIS

Recombinant Cytokines

Many growth factors have been isolated, biochemically characterized, purified, genetically cloned, and produced through recombinant DNA technology.[22–28] During the last 10 years, growth factors G-CSF, GM-CSF, EPO, and the interleukins have been used for preclinical study and for clinical application.[26–28] In vivo, the regulation of hematopoiesis is under control of cytokine production in the basal state, maintaining normal blood counts and the antigen stimulus state, eliciting cytokine stimuli above the basal state to combat infection. CSFs have been used to strengthen patients with cancer and acquired immunodeficiency syndrome (AIDS) and to guard against infection in bone marrow transplant recipients. These factors have also been used to treat patients with anemia caused by either surgery or kidney failure. The blood counts of autologous donors can be raised for donation before surgical procedures. Interleukins are used clinically for wound healing, activating lymphocytes, and assisting in the growth of transplanted or damaged bone marrow.[29–31]

Clinical Trials of Recombinant Cytokines

Clinical trials of recombinant cytokines using biologic substances similar to those in the human body have provided new opportunities for evaluating their clinical usefulness in the treatment of hematologic and oncologic disorders.[29,30] Investigations have shown that recombinant human granulocyte CSF (rHuG-CSF) accelerates recovery from neutropenia induced by myelotoxic chemotherapy for different types of carcinoma.[32] RHuG-CSF has been given to patients receiving myelosuppressive chemotherapy and undergoing autologous bone marrow transplantation to accelerate the rate of neutrophil recovery.[7,33] Clinical trials are being conducted to determine whether rHuG-CSF is effective in correcting severe neutropenia in hematopoietic malignancies, such as hairy-cell leukemia, and also in non-neoplastic hematopoietic diseases, such as aplastic anemia and cyclic neutropenia.[7,29,30]

Recombinant human GM-CSF appears to offer useful therapy with graft failure after bone marrow transplantation.[7,29] Hematopoietic growth factors can be combined with chemotherapy in treating patients with advanced malignancies and bone marrow transplant patients by increasing production of granulocytes and platelets.[23,24] Cytokines can augment mechanisms of host defense in patients with AIDS.[23,24] GM-CSF has been evaluated in HIV-infected (AIDS) patients and has been shown to increase the leukocyte count and to be effective when combined with antiretrieval agents such as AZT (azidothymidine or zidovudine, also Retrovir).[24,25]

IL-3, together with M-CSF, stimulates myelocytes, erythrocytes, and platelet production in aplastic anemia, myelodysplastic syndrome, and prolonged chemotherapy for malignancy.[34]

Chronic anemia caused by renal failure has shown that treatment with recombinant human erythropoietin (rHuEPO) has increased red blood cell (RBC) production and alleviated the anemia in more than 97% of patients.[23,24,31] The rise in hematocrit is dose-dependent and is in proportion to the increase in RBC mass.[7,31] Clinical studies using stem cell factor (SCF) combined with other cytokines are now ongoing in patients with Stage IV breast cancer and non–small cell lung cancer.[35] SCF produced from marrow fibroblasts acts on the hematopoietic stem cells, increasing the proliferation and differentiation to the committed cell lineages. In addition, SCF added to long-term cell culturing extends the growth period of a diverse population of cells.[35]

Clinical trials using other synthesized cytokines are currently in progress to determine activity in controlling hematopoiesis. Each factor needs to be purified and its function determined before the interactions between hematopoietic growth factors in the marrow microenvironment can be completely understood.

The CD Nomenclature

The classification of cell surface antigens on hematopoietic cells has been aided by the development of monoclonal antibody technology. The rapid production of monoclonal antibodies and the development of multiple commercial sources under a variety of trade names and designations led to the development of a standardized nomenclature for human leukocyte dif-

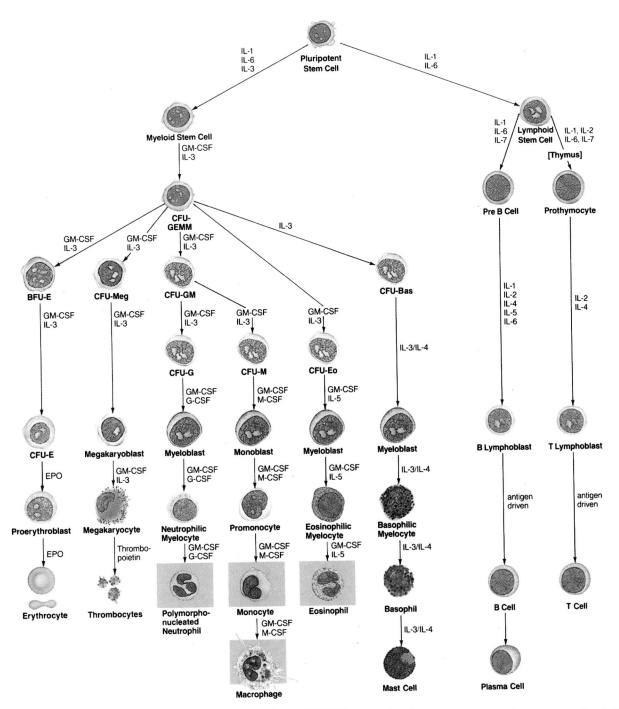

FIGURE 1-57 Regulation of hematopoiesis by cytokines. GM-CSF = granulocyte-monocyte–macrophage–colony stimulating factor; BFU-E = burst-forming unit–unit erythroid; CFU-E = colony forming unit–erythroid; EPO = erythropoietin; G-CSF = granulocyte colony-stimulating factor; M-CSF = monocyte–colony-stimulating factor; CFU-Meg = colony-forming unit–megakaryocyte; CFU-Bas = colony-forming unit–basophil; CFU-GEMM = colony-forming unit–granulocyte, erythroid, monocyte/macrophage, megakaryocyte, CFU-Eo = colony-forming unit–eosinophil; CFU-M = colony-forming unit–monocyte; CFU-G = colony-forming unit–granulocyte; Meg-CSF = megakaryocyte–colony-stimulating factor. (Reprinted from Sandoz Pharmaceuticals Corporation and Schering-Plough, with permission).

TABLE 1–20 **Cytokines Involved in Hematopoietic Blood Cell Development**

	Synonym	Source	Target	Gene Location
GROWTH FACTORS				
Epo	Erythropoietin	Kidney, liver	Erythroid progenitors	7q
G-CSF	Granulocyte colony-stimulating factor	Macrophages, endothelial cells, fibroblasts	Stem cells, neutrophil precursors	17q
GM-CSF	Granulocyte-macrophage colony-stimulating factor	T lymphocytes, macrophages, endothelial cells, fibroblasts	Progenitors for neutrophils, eosinophils, monocytes	5q
M-CSF	CSF-1, Monocyte-macrophage CSF	Endothelial cells, fibroblasts, B cells, monocytes-macrophages, stromal cells	Mononuclear phagocytes	5q
SCF	Stem cell factor, *c-kit ligand*	Fibroblasts	Stem cells	12q
INTERLEUKINS				
IL-1	Hematopoietic-1; response modulator	Macrophages, fibroblasts, endothelial cells	Mononuclear phagocytes progenitor cells	2q
IL-2	T-cell growth factor	T lymphocytes, macrophages	T cells, B cells	4q
IL-3	Multi-CSF	T lymphocytes	Precursors of neutrophils, platelets, monocytes, eosinophils, basophils, stem cells	5q
IL-4	B-cell stimulatory factor I	T lymphocytes	B cells, mast cells, T cells	5q
IL-5	B-cell growth factor II, eosinophil differentiation factor	T lymphocytes	B cells, eosinophils	5q
IL-6	Interferon β hybridoma growth factor	T lymphocytes, macrophages	Stem cells, B cells	7p
IL-7	Lymphopoietin-1	Stromal cells	Pre-B cells, T cells, early granulocytes	8q
IL-8	Granulocyte chemotactic factor	Monocytes, T cells, fibroblasts	Neutrophils, T cells, basophils	4q
IL-9	T-cell growth factor III	T cells	BFU-E, T cells, mast cells	5q
IL-10	Cytokine synthesis inhibitory factor	T cells, macrophages, B cells	B cells, macrophage, T cells, mast cells	1q
IL-11	Adipogenesis inhibitory factor	Stromal, fibroblasts	Megakaryocyte, B cells, mast cells	19q
IL-12	NK cell stimulatory factor	B cells, macrophages	T cells, NK cells	Not reported
IL-13	IL-13	T cells	B cells	5q
IL-14	High-molecular-weight B cell growth factor	T cells	Activated B cells	Not reported

Abbreviations: NK = natural killer cell; BFU-E = burst-forming unit—erythroid

ferentiation antigens termed the CD (cluster designation) nomenclature. In 1989, at a series of International Workshops on human leukocyte differentiation antigens sponsored by the World Health Organization, monoclonal antibodies having similar reactive patterns with tissue, cells, or molecules were assigned to a "cluster" and given a "cluster designation" (CD) number. More than 125 CD antigens have been classified by the Fifth International Workshop on Leukocyte Typing held in Boston in 1993.[7]

With the exception of lymphocytes, the current CD antigens for each cell lineage as determined by the Fifth International Workshop on Leukocyte Typing are given in Table 1–21. Table 1–22 lists the lymphocytic surface markers currently available.

Clinical Applications of Cell Surface Markers

The use of monoclonal antibodies specific to cell surface markers (CDs) allows phenotypic characterization of cells in disease states. By using flow cytometry (see Chap. 24), cells labeled with monoclonal antibodies are sorted and enumerated to identify a specific population of cells.

TABLE 1–21   Surface Markers for the Granulocytic, Monocytic, Megakaryocytic, and Erythrocytic Cell Lines

Myelocytes	Eosinophils	Basophils	Monocytes	Megakaryocytes	Erythrocytes
CD34	CD23	CDw32	CD11a,b,c	CDw41	CD35
CD33	CD33	CD44	CDw12	CDw42	CD55
CD13	CD44	CD45	CD13	CDw12	CD71
CD11b	CD48	CD46	CD14	CDw17	
CD15	CDw50	CD47	CD15	CDw32	
CD16	CDw52	CD48	CDw17	CD36	
CD14	CD53	CDw50	CD31	CD44	
CD10	CD55	CDw52	CDw32	CDw49b	
CDw12	CD11a	CD53	CD35	CD51	
CDw17	CD29	CD11a	CD45RO	CDw60	
CD24	CD18	CD55	CD45RA	CD61	
CD31		CD18	CD45RB	CD63	
CDw32		CD29	CD55	CD62	
CD35		CDw13	CD64		
CD43		CDw17	CD66		
CD44			CD4		
CD45			CD9		
CD45RO			CD36		
CD45RA			CD37		
CD45RB			CD40		
CD46			CD39		
CD47			CD43		
CD48			CD44		
CDw50			CD46		

TABLE 1–22   Lymphocytic Surface Markers

B Cells	T Cells	Natural Killer Cells
CD10	CD2	CD2
CD11a,c/CD18	CD2R*	CD2R
CD19	CD3	CD5
CD20	CD4	CD11a,b,c/CD18
CD21	CD5	CD16
CD22	CD6	CD23*
CD23*	CD7	CD25*
CD24	CD8	CD28
CD25*	CD11a/CD18	CD29
CD29	CD25*	CD56
CD37	CD26*	CD57
CD40	CD27	CD58
CD45	CD28	CD71*
CD58	CD29	
CD71*	CD30*	
CD72	CD45	
CD73	CD48	
CD74	CD56*	
CD77*	CD58	
CD78	CD71*	
	CD73*	

*On activated cells

Certain cell markers have been identified as being present on the cell surface in disease states such as the acute leukemias, autoimmune disease, and thromboembolytic disease. Cell markers have been identified also in the management of renal, cardiac, and bone marrow transplantation.[36] Although diagnosis of disease states is dependent upon clinical presentation, cytochemistry, and examination of morphology, flow-cytometry characterization of cells has added another dimension to disease classification. Monoclonal antibodies are used to characterize cells in the acute leukemias. Such markers allow for the differentiation of myeloblasts, lymphoblasts, monoblasts, megakaryoblasts, and erythroid ontogeny.

REFERENCES

1. Jandl, JH: Blood. In Textbook of Hematology. Little, Brown, Boston, 1987.
2. Lee, GR, Bethell, TC, Foerster, J, et al: Wintrobe's Clinical Hematology, ed 9. Lea & Febiger, Philadelphia, 1993.
3. Beck, WS: Hematology, ed 5. MIT Press, Cambridge, MA, 1991.
4. Erslev, AJ and Gabuzda, TG: Pathophysiology of Blood, ed 3. WB Saunders, Philadelphia, 1985.
5. Hillman, RF and Finch, CA: Red Cell Manual, ed 6. FA Davis, Philadelphia, 1992.
6. Nathan, DG: The beneficence of neonatal hematopoiesis. N Engl J Med 321:1190, 1989.
7. Beutler, E, Lechtman, MA, Coller, BS, and Kepps, TJ. Williams' Hematology, ed 4. McGraw-Hill, New York, 1994.

8. Diggs, LW, Sturm, D, and Bell, A: The Morphology of Human Blood Cells, ed 5. Abbott Laboratories, Abbott Park, IL, 1985.

9. Boggs, DR and Winkelstein, A: White Cell Manual, ed 5. FA Davis, Philadelphia, 1989.

10. Stossell, TP and Cohen, HJ: Neutrophil function normal and abnormal. In Gordon, AS, et al (eds): The Year in Hematology. Plenum Press, New York, 1977.

11. Boggs, DR: Physiology of neutrophil proliferation, maturation, and circulation. Clin Haematol 4:535, 1975.

12. Murphy, P: The Neutrophil. Plenum Press, New York, 1976.

13. Bainton, DF and Farquher, MG: Origin of granules in polymorphonuclear leucocytes; two types derived from opposite faces of the Golgi complex of developing granulocytes. J Cell Biol 28:277, 1966.

14. Zucker-Franklin, D, et al: Atlas of Blood, Function and Pathology, vol 1. Lea & Febiger, Philadelphia, 1988.

15. Diggs, LW and Shibata, S: Ferrata cells—Tissue neutrophils, not artifacts. Lab Med 14:50, 1970.

16. Beeson, PB and Bass, DA: The eosinophil. In Smith, LH (ed): Major Problems in Internal Medicine, vol 14. WB Saunders, Philadelphia, 1977.

17. Zucker-Franklin, D: Eosinophil function and disorders. Adv Intern Med 19:1, 1974.

18. Parwaresch, MR: The Human Blood Basophil. Springer-Verlag, Berlin, 1976.

19. Dvorak, JF and Dvorak, AM: Basophilic leukocytes, structure, function, and role in disease. Clin Haematol, 4(3):658, 1975.

20. Shinar, DM and Roden, GA: Bone and bone marrow relationships and interactions. In Long MW and Wicha MS: The Hematopoietic Microenvironment: The Functional and Structural Basis of Blood Cell Development. The Johns Hopkins Series in Hematology-Oncology. Johns Hopkins University Press, Baltimore, 1993, p 80.

21. Till, TE and McCullock, EA: A direct measurement of the radiation sensitivity of normal mouse bone marrow cells. Radiat Res 14:213, 1961.

22. Ogawa, M: Effects of hematopoietic growth factors on stem cells in vitro. Hematol Oncol Clin North Am 3:453, 1989.

23. Gabrilove, JL: Introduction and overview of hematopoietic growth factors. Semin Hematol 26:1, 1989.

24. Groopman, JE, Molina, JM, and Scaddon, DT: Hematopoietic growth factors. N Engl J Med 321:1449, 1989.

25. Quesenberry, P, Souza, L, and Krantz, S: Growth Factors. American Society of Hematology, Education Program, Atlanta, 1989, pp 98–113.

26. Morstyn, G and Burgess, AW: Hematopoietic growth factors: A review. Cancer Res 48:5624, 1988.

27. Clark, SC and Kamen, R: The human hematopoietic colony-stimulating factors. Science 236:1229, 1987.

28. Griffin, JD: Clinical applications of colony-stimulating factors. Oncology 2:15, 1988.

29. Applebaum, FR: The clinical use of hematopoietic growth factors. Semin Hematol 26(3):7, 1989.

30. Groopman, JE: New directions in hematologic biotherapy. Semin Hematol 26(Suppl):1, 1989.

31. Adamson, JW: The promise of recombinant human erythropoietin. Semin Hematol 26(Suppl):5, 1989.

32. Weisbart, RH, Gasson, JC, and Golde, DW: Physiology of granulocyte and macrophage colony-stimulating factors in host defense. Hematol Oncol Clin North Am 3:401, 1989.

33. Lawson, RA, Sandler, DP, and LeBeau, MM: Acute leukemia: Biology and treatment. American Society of Hematology. Education Program. Nashville, 1994, p 34.

34. Greenberg, PL, deWald, G, and Sawyers, C: Myeloproliferative disorders and myelodysplastic syndromes: Recent therapeutic, cytogenic, and molecular advances.

American Society of Hematology. Education Program, Nashville, 1994, pp 21–33.

35. Morstyn, G, et al: Stem cell factor is a potent synergistic factor in hematopoiesis, Oncology 51:206, 1994.

36. Bauer, KD, Duque, RE, and Shankey, TV: Clinical Flow Cytometry: Principles and Application, Williams & Wilkins, Baltimore, 1993.

QUESTIONS

Basic Morphology

1. Which organ(s) is (are) the primary site(s) for hematopoiesis in the fetus?
   a. Liver
   b. Spleen
   c. Bone marrow
   d. All of the above

2. Which listing represents the proper cell sequence of erythropoiesis?
   a. Rubriblast, prorubricyte, rubricyte, metarubricyte, reticulocyte, erythrocyte
   b. Rubriblast, rubricyte, prorubricyte, metarubricyte, reticulocyte, erythrocyte
   c. Rubriblast, prorubricyte, metarubricyte, rubricyte, reticulocyte, erythrocyte
   d. Rubriblast, reticulocyte, prorubricyte, rubricyte, metarubricyte, erythrocyte

3. What is the best description of a metarubricyte?
   a. Solid, blue-black degenerated nucleus with nonlinear clumped chromatin pattern; no nucleoli; pink cytoplasm
   b. Round nucleus with visible nucleoli; indistinct and dispersed chromatin; blue cytoplasm
   c. Coarse chromatin; ill-defined or absent nucleoli; predominantly blue cytoplasm with pink tinge
   d. Small nucleus; thick and condensed nuclear chromatin; no nucleoli; mixture of pink and blue cytoplasm

4. What is the sequence for the maturation pools of granulocyte production?
   a. Maturation, proliferation, storage, functional (or marginated) pool
   b. Proliferation, maturation, storage, functional (or marginated) pool
   c. Storage, maturation, proliferation, functional (or marginated) pool
   d. Functional (or marginated) pool, storage, proliferation, maturation

5. Which listing represents the proper cell sequence of granulocytopoiesis?
   a. Myeloblast, myelocyte, promyelocyte, metamyelocyte, band, segmented cell
   b. Myeloblast, metamyelocyte, myelocyte, promyelocyte, segmented cell, band
   c. Myeloblast, promyelocyte, myelocyte, metamyelocyte, band, segmented cell
   d. Myeloblast, band, promyelocyte, myelocyte, metamyelocyte, segmented cell

6. Which granulocytic cell has a kidney-shaped nucleus with clumped chromatin and small pink secondary granules with a few primary dark granules?
   a. Band
   b. Myelocyte

c. Promyelocyte
d. Metamyelocyte

7. Which granulocytic cell has large, abundant violet-blue or purple-black granules?
a. Eosinophil
b. Basophil
c. Neutrophil

8. What is the proper cell sequence for the monocyte-macrophage phagocytic system?
a. Monoblast, macrophage, promonocyte, monocyte
b. Monoblast, monocyte, promonocyte, macrophage
c. Monoblast, promonocyte, monocyte, macrophage
d. Monoblast, promonocyte, macrophage, monocyte

9. Which cell classification is described by the following: Second most numerous cell in the blood; usually small and round; intensely blue cytoplasm; and nucleus with clumped dark purple chromatin?
a. Monocyte
b. Lymphocyte
c. Null cell
d. Plasmacyte

Molecular Hematology

10. At what stage of differentiation will cells become committed to one cell line?
a. Pluripotential stem cell
b. Colony-forming unit (CFU)
c. Myeloblast
d. Progranulocyte

ANSWERS

1. **d** (p. 4)
2. **a** (pp. 6, 10)
3. **a** (p. 10)
4. **b** (p. 11)
5. **c** (pp. 13, 14)
6. **d** (p. 14)
7. **b** (p. 17)
8. **c** (pp. 19, 20)
9. **b** (pp. 22, 24)
10. **b** (pp. 32, 33)

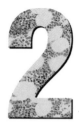# Bone Marrow

Milka M. Montiel, MD

Bone Marrow Structure
Indications for Bone Marrow Studies

Obtaining and Preparing Bone Marrow for Hematologic Studies
Bone Marrow Examination

Objectives

At the end of this chapter, the learner should be able to:
1 Name the bones that participate in active hemopoiesis in adults.
2 List conditions that indicate bone marrow studies.
3 Name the most common skeletal sites for hematologic studies.
4 Explain the role of the technologist during a bone marrow procedure.
5 Describe the preparation of marrow aspirate for laboratory examination.
6 List stains used for dried bone marrow smears.
7 Name some advantages and disadvantages of a bone marrow biopsy.
8 Explain how to calculate the myeloid-to-erythroid (M:E) cell ratio.
9 List conditions for which a bone marrow differential count has diagnostic value.
10 List conditions for which the evaluation of marrow iron stores is essential for diagnosis.

BONE MARROW STRUCTURE

The bone marrow is one of the body's largest organs, representing 3.4% to 4.6% of total body weight and averaging about 1500 g in adults. The hemopoietic marrow is organized around the bone vasculature.[1,2] An artery entering the bone branches out toward the periphery to specialized vascular spaces called *sinuses* (Fig. 2–1). Several sinuses combine in a collecting sinus, which forms a central vein that enters in the systemic circulation. Hemopoietic cords, in which the development of the hemopoietic cells takes place, lie just outside of the sinuses. Following maturation in the cords, the hemopoietic cells cross the walls of the sinuses and enter the blood.[3–5]

Hemopoietic cell colonies are compartmentalized in the cords. Erythropoiesis takes place in distinct anatomic units called *erythropoietic islands*[6] (Fig. 2–2). Each island consists of a macrophage surrounded by a cluster of maturing erythroblasts. Granulopoiesis is less conspicuously oriented toward a distinct reticulum cell, yet may be recognized as a unit[7] (Fig. 2–3).

Early granulocytic precursors are located deep in the cords and about the bone trabeculae. Megakaryopoiesis occurs adjacent to the sinus endothelium. The megakaryocytes protrude small cytoplasmic processes through the vascular wall, delivering platelets directly to the sinusoidal blood.[8] Marrow immunocytes consist of lymphocytes and plasma cells. Lymphocyte production is compartmentalized in lymphocytic follicles, and lymphocytes are randomly dispersed throughout the cords. The lymphocytic follicles are unevenly distributed and tend to influence the variability of the lymphocyte count in aspirated bone marrow samples (Fig. 2–4). Plasma cells are situated along the vascular wall.

The bone marrow is also the source of immune stem cells that on Wright's stain smears are indistinguishable from small lymphocytes. The stem cells of marrow may differentiate to myelopoietic cells or competent immune cells, which carry tissue and humoral immune functions, respectively. Some immune progenitor cells produced in the marrow mature in the thymus as T lymphocytes;[9] others are produced and continue

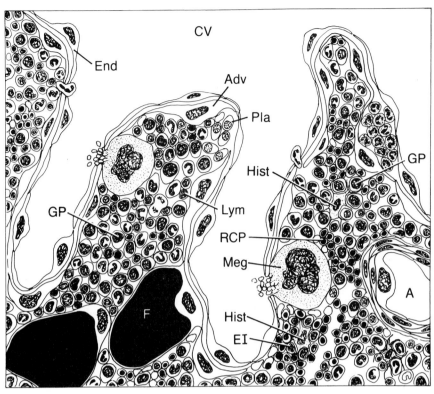

FIGURE 2-1 Graphic presentation of hemopoietic tissue. The vascular compartment consists of arteriole (A) and central sinus (CV). The venous sinusoids are lined by endothelial cells (End), and their wall outside is supported by adventitial-reticulum cells (Adv). Fat tissue (F) is part of the marrow. The compartmentalization of the hemopoiesis is represented by areas of granulopoiesis (GP), areas of erythropoiesis (RCP), and erythropoietic islands (EI) with their nutrient histiocyte (Hist). The megakaryocytes protrude with small cytoplasmic projections through the vascular wall (Meg). Lymphocytes (Lym) are randomly scattered among the hemopoietic cells while plasma cells are usually situated along the vascular wall (Pla.)

their maturation and differentiation in bone marrow as B lymphocytes from the twelfth gestational week throughout life.[10] Therefore, the bone marrow and thymus are primary lymphoid organs of *antigen-independent* progenitor immune cell proliferation and differentiation, which gives rise to new lymphocytes. These new lymphocytes may then populate the secondary lymphoid organs, lymph nodes, spleen, and lymphoid apparatus of the gastrointestinal tract. Under appropriate stimulation the mature lymphocytes of the peripheral lymphoid organs undergo *antigen-dependent*

effector cell proliferation and kinin or antibody production takes place from T and B lymphocytes, respectively (see also Chap. 1).

The meshwork of stromal cells in which the hemopoietic cells are suspended is in a delicate semifluid state and is composed of reticulum cells, histiocytes, fat cells, and endothelial cells. The reticulum cells are associated with fibers that can be visualized after silver staining. They are adjacent to the sinus endothelial cells, forming the outer part of the walls as an adventitial reticulum cell. Their fine cytoplasmic projections

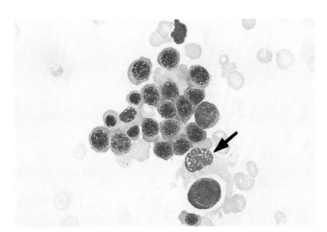

FIGURE 2-2 Erythropoietic island composed mainly of polychromatophilic normoblasts. The nutrient-histiocyte (arrow) is slightly displaced of its central position by smearing of the particle. Its cytoplasmic slender processes envelop a basophilic normoblast, establishing intimate contact with the maturing red cell precursor. (Magnification ×640)

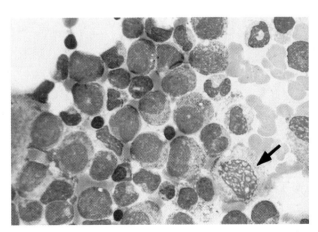

FIGURE 2-3 Compartment of granulopoiesis. A reticulas cell (arrow) with open reticulated chromatin and light blue cytoplasm containing dust-like fine granules is situated among numerous granulocytic precursors, especially myelocytes. (Magnification ×640)

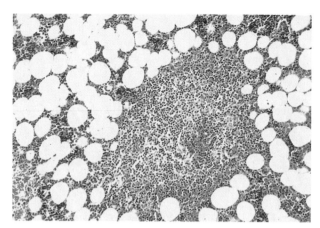

FIGURE 2–4 A lymphocytic nodule (follicle) in bone marrow as shown here may alter very significantly the marrow differential count when aspirated and give a false impression of lymphocytic malignancy. (Magnification ×250)

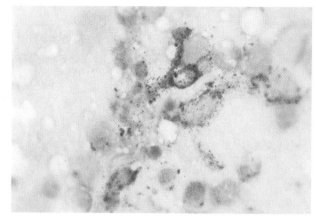

FIGURE 2–6 Two acid phosphatase–positive macrophages in bone marrow of patient treated with chemotherapeutic agents. Macrophages are also scavengers and cleaners of the hemopoietic tissue, so they increase in number during massive destruction of hemopoietic cells. (Magnification ×640)

are extended deep into the cords, making contact with similar projections of other cells. Occasionally, the nuclear region of these cells can be seen deep in the cords surrounded by granulopoiesis. Cytochemically, these cells are alkaline phosphatase–positive (Fig. 2–5). The histiocyte-macrophage is seen as a perisinusoidal cell related to the bone marrow–blood barrier and as a central storage macrophage part of the erythropoietic islands. In the role of storage nutrient cell delivering iron to the growing immature erythroblasts, the storage macrophage sends out long, slender cytoplasmic processes that envelop the erythroid precursors. This extensive and intimate contact with the maturing erythropoietic cells is necessary in transferring iron from the macrophage to the red cell precursors. As phagocytic cells, they also undergo hyperplasia when there is increased destruction of hemopoietic cells. Histochemically, the macrophages are acid phosphatase–positive (Fig. 2–6).

Tissue mast cells (Fig. 2–7), 6 to 12 μm in diameter, are connective tissue cells of mesenchymal origin, nor-

mally present in the bone marrow in varying numbers. They have a round or oval reticular nucleus and abundant blue-purple granules that obscure the nucleus. Their granules contain serotonin and proteolytic enzymes in addition to all other substances that are present in the granules of basophils. Mast cells increase in chronic infections, autoimmune diseases, and especially systemic mastocytosis.

The stromal cells produce an extracellular matrix[11] composed of collagens, glycoproteins, proteoglycans, and other proteins. This extracellular matrix is essential in sustaining normal renewal and differentiation of marrow cells. The fat cells vary in amount according to the age of the individual patient and the skeletal location from which the marrow is obtained. Only a few fat cells are seen in children. These gradually increase after 4 years of age, whereas in adults fat cells average about 50% of the total marrow volume in the vertebras and flat bones of the pelvis. The marrow fat and the extracellular matrix are dynamic tissues, similar to the

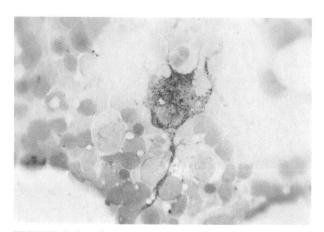

FIGURE 2–5 Alkaline phosphatase-stained reticulum cell extends its slender cytoplasmic projections deep in the hemopoietic cord, maintaining an intimate contact with granulopoiesis. The background cells are stained with neutral red. (Magnification ×640)

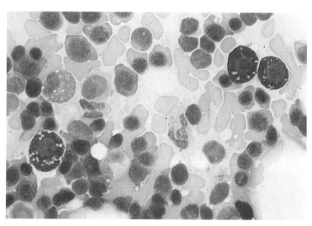

FIGURE 2–7 Three mast cells, known also as tissue basophils, are shown in this marrow aspirate on a background of erythroid hyperplasia. Numerous regular round granules fill their cytoplasm and obscure the nuclear details. (Magnification ×640)

hemopoietic tissue, and they may be altered rapidly in disease.

In marrow aspirates, cells are occasionally seen originating from bone tissue. Osteoblasts are bone matrix–synthesizing cells usually found in groups. They are up to 30 μm in diameter and resemble plasma cells. The osteoblast nucleus has a fine chromatin pattern with a prominent nucleolus. A perinuclear halo, detached from the nuclear membrane with a cytoplasmic bridge, represents the Golgi apparatus area (see Chap. 1, Fig. 1–53). Osteoblasts are alkaline phosphatase-positive. They are characteristically seen in bone marrow aspirates of children and patients with metabolic bone diseases.

Osteoclasts, bone-remodeling cells, are multinucleated giant cells more than 100 μm in diameter that resemble megakaryocytes. The nuclei of the osteoclasts are separated from each other and may have nucleoli (compared with the megakaryocyte nucleus, which is multilobated). Their cytoplasm is well delineated and finely granular (see Chap. 1, Figs. 1–54 and 1–55).

The bone marrow is a highly vascularized tissue from which endothelial cells can occasionally be aspirated. Endothelial cells are more visible in hypoplastic marrows and should not be mistaken for metastatic tumors (Fig. 2–8).

The main function of the marrow is to supply mature hemopoietic cells for the circulating blood in a steady-state condition as well as to respond to increased demands. Self-renewal is maintained by a semidormant pool of pluripotential stem cells, and the mechanism of their commitment to progenitor cells is under intensive investigation. A progenitor is a cell committed to a single line of proliferation and differentiation. Granulocytic, monocytic, eosinophilic, erythroid, and megakaryocyte progenitor cells are influenced in their differentiation by colony-stimulating factors (CSFs).[12–14] (See Chap. 1.) In addition, erythropoiesis is influenced by erythropoietin produced in the kidney.[15,16] In the process of cell egression from the cords to the circulation, a number of releasing factors are

identified. The best characterized of these are granulocyte colony-stimulating factor (G-CSF) and granulocyte-macrophage colony-stimulating factor (GM-CSF), but other factors as components of a complement system, androgenic steroids, and endotoxins may play a role.[17] The endothelial lining of the sinusoids forms a continuous, veil-like wall through which the mature cells migrate from extravascular sites into the circulation.[18] This is accomplished by close contact between mature hemopoietic cells and endothelial cells. A transient migration pore is formed during such contact through which the mature cells pass into the circulation without loss of plasma to the extravascular pool.[19] It is apparent that the bone marrow is subjected to a complex regulation by many cellular and humoral systems of the body and any disease affecting these systems is likely to affect the hemopoiesis.

INDICATIONS FOR BONE MARROW STUDIES

Bone marrow study in the diagnosis of hemopoietic disorders was introduced by Arinkin.[20] Obtaining bone marrow tissue, once a formidable task, has become a standard procedure with current improved techniques. Several techniques have been devised, each having its own merits and limitations. Bone marrow aspiration and bone marrow biopsy are usually performed concurrently.

Although obtaining bone marrow for examination carries little procedural risk for the patient, the procedure is costly and can be painful. For this reason, bone marrow studies should be done only when clearly indicated or whenever the physician expects a beneficial diagnostic result for his or her patient.

Hematologic diseases affecting primarily the bone marrow and causing a decrease or increase of any cellular blood element are among the most common indications. These conditions typically include:

1. Anemias, erythrocytosis, polycythemia
2. Leukopenia and unexplained leukocytosis
3. Appearance of immature or abnormal cells in the circulation
4. Thrombocytopenia and thrombocytosis

It is not rare for more than one blood element to be increased or decreased, as occurs in leukemias and some refractory anemias. In these situations, bone marrow study affords specific information, and usually precedes any other diagnostic procedure.

Systemic diseases may affect the bone marrow secondarily and require bone marrow studies for diagnosis or monitoring patients' conditions. These may include:

1. Solid malignant tumors arising elsewhere in the body, such as lymphomas, carcinomas, and sarcomas, may metastasize to the bone marrow. Patients having any of these solid malignant tumors may undergo bone marrow studies when the initial diagnosis is established for evaluation of the degree of tumor spread and clinical staging of disease. Occasionally the bone marrow study may be the site of first diagnosis of unsuspected disseminated malignant tumor. During the course of malignant disease, additional studies are also

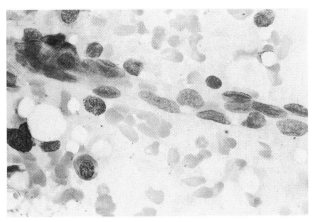

FIGURE 2–8 A string of endothelial cells aspirated from hypocellular marrow. The nuclei are elongated and slightly tapered. The cytoplasm is transparent and barely visible. (Magnification ×640)

performed periodically to monitor the status of tumor spread and its therapeutic response.

2. Infections manifested clinically as "fever of unknown origin" may exhibit granulomas, focal necrosis, or histiocytic proliferation with intracytoplasmic organisms within the marrow. Material for morphological studies and bacterial cultures may be obtained simultaneously during a single procedure. The suspected diagnoses of disseminated tuberculosis, fungal infections (particularly histoplasmosis, cryptococcosis), and some protozoan infections are frequently confirmed through such studies.

3. Hereditary and acquired histiocytoses occasionally involve the bone marrow histiocyte, for example, Gaucher's disease, sea-blue histiocytosis, and hemophagocytic syndrome. A simple procedure such as bone marrow aspiration or biopsy may establish diagnosis.

OBTAINING AND PREPARING BONE MARROW FOR HEMATOLOGIC STUDIES

The most common sites for bone marrow studies in adults are the posterior superior iliac crest, sternum, anterior superior iliac crest, and (very rarely) spinal processes or vertebral bodies (Fig. 2–9). Occasionally, when a localized bone lesion is visualized on a radiograph or computed tomographic (CT) scan, a directed or "open" bone marrow biopsy of the lesion may be done by a radiologist or surgeon in an operating room with the patient under anesthesia. In newborns and infants, marrow for studies can be obtained from the upper end of the tibial bone.

Before performing the procedure, the physician should inform the adult patient or the parent or guardian of a child about the procedure, its risks, and its expected benefits for the diagnostic process. An authorized permission form, the so-called informed consent form, is then signed, allowing the physician to perform the procedure. Signature of the permission form is witnessed by a second person, in many instances the patient's nurse. The actual procedure is performed, often with the assistance of a medical technologist. While the physician performs the procedure and the nurse attends to the patient, the medical technologist gives full attention to processing the specimens. It is the medical technologist's responsibility to see that the samples are adequate. If they are not, the physician is informed immediately so that the procedure can be repeated before the patient is released. Samples are preserved appropriately for histologic, electron microscopic, cytogenetic, immunologic, microbiologic, and other studies as indicated in a particular case.

Equipment

The instrument tray used to perform a bone marrow procedure should contain enough equipment to complete the procedure and to prepare the tissues obtained for the appropriate studies (Table 2–1). A hematology laboratory that routinely assists in performing bone marrow procedures should always

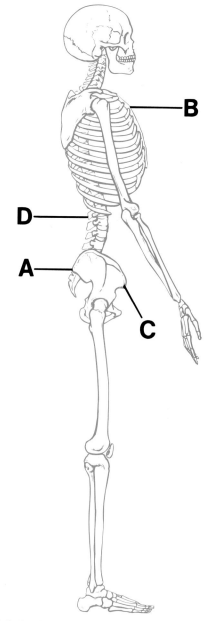

FIGURE 2-9 Common sites for bone marrow studies. *A.* Posterior superior iliac crest. *B.* Sternum. *C.* Anteiror superior iliac crest. *D.* Spinal processes. These indicate the sites of the skeleton in descending order of frequency from which bone marrow tissue is obtained for studies.

have at least two sterile bone marrow trays ready as well as a basic inventory of equipment and reagents to handle aspirated samples and bone biopsies. Complete bone marrow trays are sold as disposable equipment, which may be convenient for some laboratories performing few bone marrow procedures. The disposable tray's convenience is offset by its higher cost and loss of versatility.

Several different styles of aspiration and trephine bone biopsy needles are commonly used (Fig. 2–10). Examples include the University of Illinois sternal needle, with its adjustable guard for aspiration, and var-

TABLE 2–1   Example of a Tray for Bone Marrow Aspiration and Biopsy

Required Materials:
1. 30-mL syringes
2. 20-mL syringes
3. 10-mL syringes
4. 5-mL syringes
5. 2% lidocaine
6. Prepodyne prep
7. Alcohol (70%) or prep
8. 23-gauge needles
9. 21-gauge needles
10. Filter papers
11. Buffered formalin 10% with a pH of about 6.8 or other fixative for histologic processing of bone biopsy and marrow particles
12. Tube containing liquid EDTA anticoagulant
13. One box slides
14. One slide folder
15. One rubber bulb
16. Pasteur pipette
17. Petri dish
18. Sterile blades
19. Gloves (several pairs of different sizes)
20. Sterile gauze and cotton balls
21. Sterile bone marrow aspiration and trephine biopsy needles
22. Applicator sticks
23. Bandage
24. Culture bottles (*not* biphasic) for bacterial culture (Note: Save some bone marrow specimen in syringe for tuberculosis and fungal cultures, when indicated)
25. Pencil to label slides
26. #11 Bard Parker blades

ious modifications of the Vim-Silverman trephine needle for bone biopsy. Examples of such modified trephine needles are the Westerman-Jensen and Jamshidi needles. There are also smaller needles designed for use with infants and children. These original aspiration and trephine needles have been modified by different companies and are manufactured as disposable equipment.

Aspiration

Bone marrow aspiration may be performed as an independent procedure or in conjunction with bone biopsy. It is favored by hematologists in ambulatory and office practice. As a rule, very apprehensive patients and children receive a mild sedative before the procedure. The site selected is shaved if hairy and washed with soap. Then an antiseptic is applied, and the area is draped with sterile towels. A local anesthetic such as 1% to 2% lidocaine (Xylocaine) is infiltrated in the skin, in the intervening tissues between the skin and bone, and in the periosteum of the bone from which the marrow is to be obtained. A cut of about 3 mm is made through the skin with a Bard-Parker blade to facilitate piercing skin and subcutaneous tissue.

The physician penetrates the bone cavity with an aspiration needle, assembled with guard and stylet locked in place. When the marrow cavity is penetrated, the stylet is removed, a syringe is attached to the free end of the needle, and the plunger is quickly pulled, drawing 1.0 to 1.5 mL of marrow particles and sinusoidal blood in the syringe. Because the vacuum created in the syringe is important for rapid and efficient suctioning of cells and particles, the syringe should be

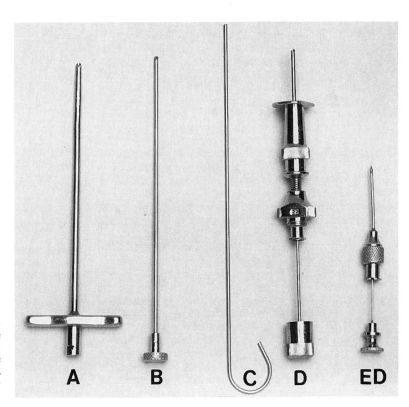

FIGURE 2–10   Trephine biopsy and aspiration needles. *A.* Jamshidi trephine needle biopsy includes a stylet (*B*) and probe (*C*). *D.* University of Illinois sternal aspiration needle with an adjustable guard and stylet. *ED.* A smaller pediatric aspiration needle and trephine biopsy is also shown.

10 mL or larger with a well-fitting plunger. Despite the use of local anesthesia, the patient normally experiences discomfort during the aspiration process (aspiration pain). Accomplishing the aspiration with a quick and continuous pull on the plunger diminishes the patient's discomfort and decreases the chance of clotting the specimen. A clotted specimen is useless for smear preparation because the fibrin threads strip the cytoplasm off the cells and hamper their spreading.

Keeping the volume of the initial aspirate small also prevents dilution of the sample with large amounts of sinusoidal blood while diminishing the quality of the aspirate. This first-aspirated material is used immediately for preparing smears. More aspirate may be obtained in additional syringes if needed for chromosome studies, bacterial cultures, and other tests. Once an adequate aspirate is obtained, the quality of the smear depends entirely on the technologist's skill and speed in preparing the smears and preserving the morphology of the marrow cells. Part of the first aspirate is used for the preparation of direct and marrow particle smears. The other part is placed in an ethylenediaminetetra-acetic acid (EDTA) anticoagulant-containing tube for use later in the laboratory. If some aspirate still remains, it can be left to clot. The clot may be fixed in 10% buffered formalin or other chosen fixative and processed for histologic examination.

Preparation of Bone Marrow Aspirate

All necessary materials, preservatives, and slides should be meticulously clean and in readiness to avoid delay. The aspirate in the first syringe contains mostly blood admixed with fat, marrow cells, and particles of marrow tissue, which should be used for smears. Several direct smears can be prepared immediately, using the technique for blood film preparation. A small drop is placed on a glass slide, and the blood and the particles are dragged behind a spreading slide with a technique similar to that for preparing blood film. Although this method of preparation preserves the cell morphology well, it is inadequate for the evaluation of the cells in relationship to each other and for the estimation of marrow cellularity.

Smears of marrow particles are prepared by pouring a small amount of the aspirate on a glass slide. The marrow tissue is seen as gray particles floating in blood and fat droplets. The particles are aspirated selectively with a plastic dropper or Oxford pipette and transferred to a clean glass slide. These are covered gently with another slide. The two slides are pulled in opposite and parallel directions to smear the particles without crushing the cells. Some techniques recommend using two coverglasses instead.[21] In this process, the marrow particles are squashed between two coverslips, which are then gently pulled apart.

Techniques for preparing particle smears vary from person to person and from laboratory to laboratory. The aspirate may be transferred into a watchglass and the particles collected with a capillary pipette or broken end of a wooden stick applicator. With experience, technologists usually adapt a technique to produce high-quality slides that best suits themselves. The technologist should prepare an adequate number of slides of smeared marrow particles. In cases of newly diagnosed acute leukemias, no fewer than 10 slides should be prepared. These are needed for histochemical stains such as Sudan black, naphthyl AS-D chloracetate esterase, and alpha-naphthyl butyrate esterase (see Chap. 33).

Marrow particle smears are used in the evaluation of cellularity and the relationship of the cells to each other. Well-prepared smears have the added advantage of excellent cell morphology so that subtle changes in cell maturation and cytoplasmic inclusions can be easily recognized.

All direct and particle smears should be labeled with the patient's name, identification number, and date at the bedside and then quickly air-dried.

Measurement of Bone Marrow Aspirate

The EDTA-anticoagulated aspirate can be used for quantitative studies.[21] About 1 mL of marrow aspirate is transferred to a Wintrobe tube and centrifuged at 2800 rpm (at 850 g) for 8 minutes. The fluid is separated into four layers representing fat and perivascular cells, plasma, buffy coat of myeloid-erythroid cells, and erythrocytes (see Fig. 2–11). Each layer is measured and read as a percentage directly from the Wintrobe tube, its volume correlating with a given basic element of the marrow. Smears can be prepared from fat-perivascular and buffy coat layers and used accordingly to study iron and hematopoietic cell and myeloid-to-erythroid (M:E) cell ratio. Such quantitative studies may be useful in estimating cellularity (fat versus buffy coat) when no histologic sections of bone biopsy and marrow particles are available.

Histologic Marrow Particle Preparation

The leftover marrow particles obtained during the aspiration procedure can be processed for histologic examination. The tissue particles, admixed with blood, may be left to clot, then fixed in 10% buffered formalin and processed for histologic sectioning. However, better results are obtained if the blood and particles are transferred to an EDTA-containing tube before clotting sets in. Then the blood is filtered through histowrap filter paper and the concentrated particles enfolded in the paper are fixed in 10% buffered formalin. In the histology laboratory these particles are harvested by scraping the paper and the particles are embedded in agar for further processing.[22]

Bone Biopsy

The bone biopsy is especially indicated when the marrow cannot be aspirated, "dry tap," owing to pathologic alterations encountered in acute leukemias, myelofibrosis, hairy cell leukemia, and other diseases. Trephine bone biopsy is also performed for the diagnosis of neoplastic and granulomatous diseases. For clinical staging of lymphomas and carcinomas, bilateral posterior superior iliac crest biopsies are recommended, which increase the chance to diagnose a focal process. In adults, an 11-gauge Jamshidi biopsy needle is used, whereas in children a 13-gauge needle is preferred. An adequate biopsy is at least 15 mm in

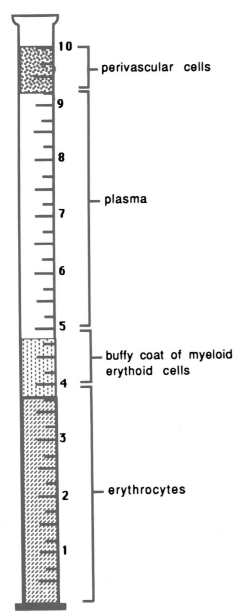

FIGURE 2–11 Quantitative measurement of bone marrow aspirate. Schematic presentation of the four marrow layers formed by centrifugation of aspirate in a Wintrobe tube.

length.[21,23] When a bone biopsy is performed in conjunction with marrow aspirate, it customarily follows the aspirate. This is done by changing the direction of the needle to avoid the aspiration site. It is better yet for the marrow biopsy to be done through a new puncture site in the anesthetized area.

Preparation of Trephine Biopsy

Touch Preparation

The bone core is supported lightly without pressure between the blades of a forceps and touched several times on two or three clean slide surfaces. The biopsy core should not be rubbed on the slide because rub-

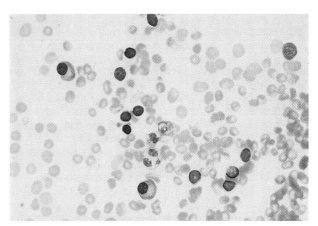

FIGURE 2–12 Wright-stained bone marrow touch preparation. Aspirate was a "dry tap." A few scattered lymphocytes and plasma cells are present. (Magnification ×400)

bing destroys the cells. The slides are air-dried rapidly. The touch preparations are fixed in absolute methanol and stained with Wright-Giemsa stain. In the absence of a good aspirate smear, the touch preparations of the bone marrow biopsy (Fig. 2–12) may be the only source to study cellular details and the maturation sequence of the sample. Sometimes the touch preparations contain enough cells for differential counts and blast evaluation.

Histologic Bone Biopsy Preparation

The biopsy specimen is immersed without delay in B-5 or 10% buffered formalin fixative. Histology laboratories may have a choice of other preferred fixatives such as Zenker's solution or Carnoy's solution.[24,25] After fixation, the biopsy undergoes standard histologic processing of decalcification, dehydration, embedding in paraffin blocks, sectioning of 2- to 3-μm-thick sections, and histologic staining. The advantage of bone marrow biopsy is that it represents a large sample of marrow and bone structures in their natural relationship. A variety of stains can be used to demonstrate marrow iron, reticulum, and collagen. Acid-fast organisms and fungi in granulomatous diseases may be detected quickly with specific stains, offering great advantages in diagnosing these infections. For instance, mycobacterial cultures may require weeks of incubation to show growth of organisms, whereas on tissue sections the histologic and etiologic diagnosis may be made within 10 to 12 hours. At present, when metastatic tumors and lymphomas are found in the bone marrow, monoclonal hybridoma antibodies can be used on histologic material to demonstrate specific tumor markers. Thus, a very precise diagnosis of the origin of a tumor can be made without elaborate, expensive, and invasive techniques.

A disadvantage of the bone biopsy is that fine cellular details are lost in the processing; therefore it is of little value in the diagnosis of leukemias and of some refractory anemias. In these situations, the touch preparation from the biopsy may supply the missing morphologic details. Multiple-touch preparations also offer an opportunity for histochemical stains (Sudan black, naphthyl AS-D chloracetate esterase, alpha-naphthyl butyrate esterase, etc.) that are essential in diagnosis and classification of leukemias.

Trephine bone marrow biopsy may be embedded in methyl methacrylate, synthetic plastic media, and sectioned into 1- to 2-μm-thin sections without decalcification. The morphologic quality of the cells is extremely well preserved, and a differential count can be done on hematoxylin-eosin- or Giemsa-stained slides.[26] However, this technique requires specially trained personnel and equipment and separate handling in the histology laboratory, which increases expenses. The processing time of the tissue also increases, which may not be acceptable for rapid diagnosis. In addition, tissue embedded in plastic media instead of paraffin may not be suitable for immunochemistry studies of bone marrow.

BONE MARROW EXAMINATION

The examination of the bone marrow aspirate smears should start at low magnification with a dry objective of ×10. A scan over the slide permits selection of a suitable area for examination and differential count. "Bare nuclei" caused by destruction of the marrow cells by squashing them or stripping their cytoplasm by fibrin thread should be avoided. An area is selected where the cells are well spread, intact, and not diluted by sinusoidal blood. When marrow particles are examined, such areas are found at the periphery of the particles. At this low magnification, marrow cellularity is also evaluated (Fig. 2–13). The number and distribution of the megakaryocytes are usually noted adjacent to a spicule, about 5 per low magnification field. Nonhematopoietic tumor cells infiltrating the bone marrow could also be seen at this magnification. These are usually larger than the granulocytic or erythropoietic precursors, and are scattered in small groups and clusters (Fig. 2–14).

After the initial scan, immersion oil is applied on the slide and the examination continues on high magnification (oil-immersion objective ×50 or ×100). The high

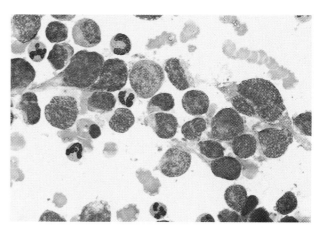

FIGURE 2–14 Metastatic tumor in the bone marrow. The tumor cells are usually pleomorphic and in groups with large nuclear: cytoplasmic ratios, irregular nuclear outlines, and deep blue cytoplasm. (Magnification ×640)

magnification provides details of the nuclear and cytoplasmic maturation process. The iron in histiocytes is visualized as brown-blue granules. Cytoplasmic inclusions of a diagnostic nature can be seen in histiocytes, erythroblasts, and granulocytes. Differential counts of bone marrow are also done with the oil-immersion objective.

Estimation of Bone Marrow Cellularity

The cellularity is reflected in the ratio of nucleated hemopoietic cells to fat cells. Overall marrow cellularity in adults is about 50% (±10%) (Fig. 2–15). The bone biopsy is the most reliable for assessment of cellularity because it offers a large amount of tissue for evaluation. However, the evaluation of the cellularity can also be done on good aspirate smears or marrow particles. The best areas for examination of cellularity in smears are the areas between two uncrushed particles. The ratio of cells to fat is evaluated on low magnification (objective ×10), so that larger areas are included in the field of observation. The empty spaces that result from

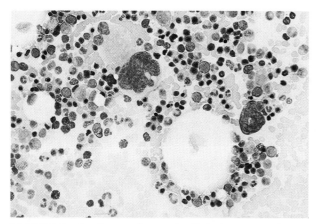

FIGURE 2–13 Smear of normal cellular marrow with normal maturation of erythropoietic, granulocytic, and megakaryocytic cells. (Magnification ×250)

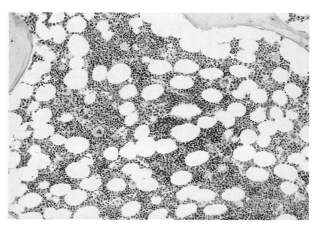

FIGURE 2–15 Normal bone marrow biopsy showing approximately 50% marrow cellularity. Note the megakaryocyte (low power).

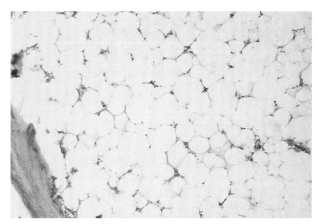

FIGURE 2-16 Markedly hypocellular bone marrow biopsy as commonly seen in severe aplastic anemia (low power).

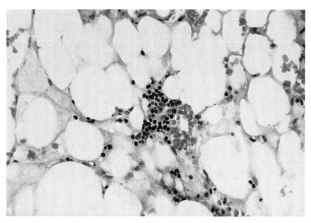

FIGURE 2-18 Bone marrow biopsy showing small lymphoid aggregate or nodule (low power).

the spreading of the cells but are not occupied by fat cells are disregarded and treated as an artifact (see Fig. 2-12). The term *decreased* or *increased* cellularity is applied when less or more than the expected normal number of cells is seen (Figs. 2–16 and 2–17). Precise evaluation can be achieved with experience, and good reproducibility can be attained among several observers. The marrow cellularity can be expressed in percentages, but this is best done on histologic sections of biopsy specimens. Marrow cellularity has diagnostic value when it is related to the M:E ratio, which is calculated after a differential count is performed.

Bone Marrow Differential Count

A bone marrow differential count is an excellent tool for training a novice in bone marrow morphology, and it is widely used in diagnosing and following patients with leukemias, refractory anemias, and myelodysplastic syndromes. Because of the compartmentalization of the hemopoietic cells and high cellularity of marrow, at least 500 to 1000 nucleated cells need to be classified for a representative differential count.[27]

In infants during the first month after birth, dramatic alterations occur in the distribution of the different marrow compartments.[28] At birth there is a predominance of granulocyte precursors, which switches within a month to a predominance of lymphoid elements. In early infancy many lymphocytes have fine chromatin and a high nucleus:cytoplasm ratio, and lack distinct nucleoli. They can be misinterpreted as blasts if the observer is unfamiliar with these characteristics. Suggestion has been made that these lymphoid cells may represent hematogones in the infant marrow.[29,30] In children up to 3 years old, one-third or more of the marrow cellularity is made up of lymphocytes. The lymphocyte number gradually declines to the normal adult level thereafter.

In adult marrow the lymphocytes are distributed both at random among the hemopoietic cells and in lymphocytic follicles (Figs. 2–18 and 2–19). This can introduce significant variation in the differential count from sample to sample in the same patient. The great mass of the adult marrow is composed of granulopoietic and erythropoietic precursors. For the purpose of the differential count, these are enumerated into dif-

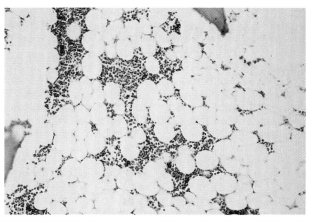

FIGURE 2-17 Bone marrow biopsy showing variable cellularity (low power).

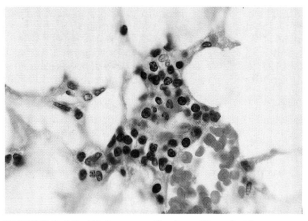

FIGURE 2-19 Higher magnification of lymphoid aggregate depicted in Figure 2-18. (Magnification ×400)

TABLE 2–2   **Differential Cell Count of Bone Marrow in Percent of Total Nucleated Cells***

	At Birth	Up to 1 Month	Children	Adults
Undifferentiated cells	0–2	0–2	0–1	0–1
Myeloblast	0–2	0–2	0–2	0–2
Promyelocyte	0–4	0–4	0–4	0–4
Myelocytes				
Neutrophilic	2–8	2–4	5–15	5–20
Eosinophilic	0–5	0–3	0–6	0–3
Basophilic	0–1	0–1	0–1	0–1
Metamyelocytes and bands				
Neutrophilic	15–25	5–10	5–15	5–35
Eosinophilic	0–5	1–5	1–8	0–5
Basophilic	0–1	0–1	0–1	0–1
Segmented neutrophils	5–15	3–10	5–15	5–15
Pronormoblast	0–3	0–1	0–2	0–1.5
Basophilic normoblast	0–5	0–3	0–5	0–5
Polychromatophilic normoblast	6–20	5–20	5–11	5–30
Orthochromatic normoblast	0–5	0–2	0–8	5–10
Lymphocytes	5–15	5–50	5–35	10–20
Plasma cells	0–2	0–2	0–2	0–2
Monocytes	0–5	0–2	0–4	0–5
M:E ratio based on 500-cell count	3–4.5	3–4.5	1.5–4	2–4

*Normal reference range from the Laboratory Computing Resources of The University of Texas Health Science Center and University Hospital, San Antonio, TX.

ferent categories according to their stage of maturation. (See Chap. 1, Hematopoiesis.) When adequate numbers of cells are tabulated, the percentage of each category is calculated. The ratio between all granulocytes and their precursors and all nucleated red cell precursors represents the M:E ratio.

Some hematologists prefer to exclude the segmented neutrophils from the differential count as being part of the neutrophil storage pool of the marrow. The normal M:E ratio in this case is between 1.5 and 3. However, pathologists and hematologists who interpret the bone marrow histologic sections of particle clot and biopsies in conjunction with marrow smears include the segmented neutrophils in the differential counts because these cannot be excluded in the evaluation of histologic specimens and are part of the marrow cellularity. The normal M:E ratio then is slightly higher and ranges between 2 and 4. The granulopoietic tissue occupies two to four times more marrow space than the erythropoietic precursors, owing to the shorter survival of the granulocytes in the circulation (i.e., neutrophils, 5 to 10 hours versus erythrocytes, 120 days) (see Fig. 2–12). Changes in the survival of granulocytes and erythrocytes are reflected in changes of the M:E ratio.

Megakaryocytes are unevenly distributed, and a differential count is a poor means for their evaluation. Usually 5 to 10 megakaryocytes are seen per microscopic field on low magnification (objective ×10). When clusters of megakaryocytes and promegakaryocytes are seen in every field, it is an indication of megakaryocytic hyperplasia. In a normal cellular marrow, finding fewer than two megakaryocytes per field on screening may indicate megakaryocytic hypoplasia. A marked increase or decrease of the number of megakaryocytes is easy to evaluate, whereas slight to moderate changes are difficult to judge and are better estimated on histologic sections of biopsy and particle specimens.

Table 2–2 represents the data of normal marrow reference ranges used by the computer resources of the University Hospital and University of Texas Health Science Center at San Antonio.

Bone Marrow and Blood Interpretation Based on Cellularity and M:E Ratio Changes

A bone marrow aspirate or biopsy sample represents a minute part of a very large and dynamic organ. Its activity and responses are reflected in blood changes; therefore, evaluation of the bone marrow should always be done in conjunction with evaluation of the peripheral blood. In adult humans with 50% marrow cellularity, about 30% to 40% represents granulopoiesis, and 10% to 15% erythropoiesis with an average M:E ratio of 4:1. When marrow cellularity increases or decreases, preserving the normal M:E ratio, it is indicative of a balanced granulocytic and erythrocytic hyperplasia or hypoplasia, correspondingly. However, if cellularity change occurs simultaneously with M:E ratio change, the interpretation requires a broader understanding of hemopoietic tissue physiology and its reactions during disease.

Cell morphology and the M:E ratio are well represented in random bone marrow specimens. The variations are not significant even when samples are compared from sternal and iliac crest aspirates.[31] However, marrow cellularity is poorly represented in random smears; thus, their interpretation should be considered with some degree of reservation. Even large

TABLE 2–3 Marrow and Blood Interpretation Based on Cellularity and M:E Ratio

Complete Blood Count	Bone Marrow Cellularity	M:E Ratio	Bone Marrow Interpretation
Normal	Increased or decreased*	Normal range	Normal
Neutropenia	Decreased	Decreased	Granulocytic hypoplasia
Neutropenia	Normal or increased	Increased	Decreased neutrophilic survival or ineffective granulopoiesis
Neutrophilia	Normal or increased	Increased	Granulocytic hyperplasia
Anemia	Normal or decreased	Increased	Red cell hypoplasia
Anemia	Normal or increased	Decreased	Erythrocytic hyperplasia or ineffective erythropoiesis†
Erythrocytosis (polycythemia)	Normal or increased	Decreased	Erythrocytic hyperplasia
Pancytopenia	Decreased	Normal range	Marrow hypoplasia
Pancytopenia	Increased	Normal, increased, or decreased	Ineffective myelopoiesis or hypersplenism

*Because of poor presentation of cellularity in random specimen.
†Reticulocyte count is necessary to differentiate between erythrocytic hyperplasia and ineffective erythropoiesis.

biopsy specimens may have a great degree of variation in cellularity.[32] For this reason, in diseases in which marrow cellularity is crucial for the diagnosis (aplastic anemia, marrow hypoplasia), more than one bone biopsy sample may need to be obtained.

Table 2–3 is included to be used only as a simple guide and to give some basic information to the reader; it is not intended to be a diagnostic tool without the patient's clinical history and clinical evaluation of the disease. Also, the variety of problems frequently presented by different patients with the same disease may not fit in such a simple schematic concept.

Bone Marrow Iron Stores

The storage iron of the bone marrow is in the form of hemosiderin. The iron content of hemosiderin is higher than that of ferritin. Other components of hemosiderin are protein, ferritin aggregates, some lipids, and membranes of cellular organelles. Hemosiderin can be seen on unstained smears as golden-yellow granules. On Wright-Giemsa–stained smears, it appears as brownish-blue granules. However, for more precise evaluation, Prussian blue reaction is used to demonstrate the intracytoplasmic iron of histiocytes and red cell precursors. The evaluation of marrow iron stores is essential in the diagnosis of anemias and especially in refractory and dyserythropoietic anemias. When the morphological characteristic of the iron particles in the storage nutrient histiocyte and erythroblastic precursors is an important diagnostic consideration (such as sideroblastic anemias), an iron stain is done on a particle smear. If the overall distribution of the amount of iron is of clinical importance (iron deficiency anemia, anemia of chronic diseases, hemochromatosis and others), then histologic sections of bone marrow biopsy and marrow clotted particles are stained for iron. The

biopsy and the particles are a more reliable source of information because they represent a large sample of hemopoietic tissue. Bone biopsy for iron studies should be decalcified by the EDTA chelating method, which does not affect the storage iron.[24,25] Rapid acid decalcifying solutions extract iron and must not be used in these cases.

Hemosiderin and some ferritin aggregates are seen after staining as bright blue specks and granules. Hemoglobin iron and dispersed ferritin do not stain. Normal marrow iron is seen as fine cytoplasmic granules in histiocytes and 30% to 50% of marrow erythroblasts contain iron specks (sideroblasts). Clumps of iron easily seen on scanning magnification (×10) indicate increased storage, whereas only a few specks of iron found after searching several microscopic fields (×50 or ×100 magnification) indicates decreased iron storage. When no stainable iron is detected on the bone marrow smear or tissue sections, this indicates iron storage depletion or absence.[33] The storage depletion may be reported as "absent," "decreased," "adequate," "moderately increased," and "markedly increased," or it can be given corresponding numerical values from 0 to 4, where 2 represents the normal or adequate iron stored in an adult.

Bone Marrow Report

The bone marrow report usually encompasses the following:

1. The name of the laboratory or physician's office from which the report originates.
2. Patient's addressograph data, including age and relevant clinical summary and/or tentative diagnosis.
3. Description of material received for studies, such as smears of aspirate, marrow particles, and/or bone biopsy(ies).

4. Data of the complete blood count (CBC), white blood cell (WBC) differential count, and a description of the blood smear, preferably from the day on which the bone marrow specimen is obtained. Platelet count should be included, as well as reticulocyte count if available.
5. Bone marrow differential count.
6. Description of cellularity, M:E ratio, granulopoiesis, erythropoiesis, and megakaryopoiesis. Any change of the nonhematopoietic elements of marrow, such as histiocytic hyperplasia, erythrophagocytosis, or metastatic tumor cells, is included in this section of the report. The status of iron stores and special staining procedures performed are reported.
7. Description of histologic sections of marrow particles of bone marrow biopsy, if done.
8. Diagnostic conclusion. It should encompass separate diagnoses of blood and bone marrow, even where the same diagnosis is applicable to both. (Examples: Blood: pancytopenia; Bone marrow left posterior iliac spine aspirate: aplasia; or Blood: acute myelogenous leukemia (FAB-M1) and Bone marrow left posterior iliac crest aspirate: acute myelogenous leukemia, FAB-M1.)

The medical technologist's contribution in this phase is in performing the blood and bone marrow differential count. The examination of the blood and the bone marrow, the correlation with clinical presentation, and the diagnostic conclusions on each specimen are the responsibility of a physician who has adequate training and experience to integrate all available clinical and laboratory information in reaching the correct diagnosis.

REFERENCES

1. Tavassoli, M and Jossey, JM: Bone Marrow, Structure and Function. Alan R Liss, New York, 1978, p 43.
2. Lichtman, MA: The ultrastructure of the hemopoietic environment of the marrow: A review. Exp Hematol 9:391, 1981.
3. Tavassoli, M and Shaklai, M: Absence of tight junctions in endothelium of marrow sinuses: Possible significance for marrow cell egress. Erythropoiesis in bone marrow. Br J Haematol 41:303, 1979.
4. Aoki, M and Tavassoli, M: Dynamics of red cell egress from bone marrow after blood letting. Br J Haematol 49:337, 1981.
5. Aoki, M and Tavassoli, M: Red cell egress from bone marrow in state of transfusion plethora. Exp Hematol 9:231, 1981.
6. Bessis, M: L'ilot érythroblastique, unité fonctionelle de la moelle osseuse. Rev Hematol 13:8, 1958.
7. Western, H and Bainton, DF: Association of alkaline-phosphatase-positive reticulum cells in bone marrow with granulocytic precursors. J Exp Med 150:919, 1979.
8. Lichtman, MA, Chamberlain, JK, Simon, W, et al: Parasinusoidal location of megakaryocytes in marrow. A determinant of platelet release. Am J Hematol 4:303, 1978.
9. Claman, HN, Chaperon, EA, and Triplett, RF: Immunocompetence of transferred thymus–marrow cell combinations. J Immunol 97:828, 1966.
10. Hassett, JM: Humoral immunodeficiency: A review. Pediatr Ann 16:404, 1987.
11. Gordon, MY: Annotation. Extracellular matrix of the marrow microenvironment. Br J Haematol 70:1, 1988.
12. Clark, SC and Kamen, R: The human hematopoietic colony-stimulating factors. Science 236:1229, 1987.
13. Neinhuis, AW: Hematopoietic growth factors. Biologic complexity and clinical practice. N Engl J Med 318:916, 1988.
14. Iscove, NN: Erythropoietin-independent stimulation of early erythropoiesis in adult marrow cultures by conditioned media from lactin-stimulated mouse spleen cells in hematopoietic cell differentiation. In Golde, DW, Cline, MJ, Metcalf, D, and Fox, CJ (eds): ICN-UCLA Symposium on Hematopoietic Cell Differentiation: Academia, NY, 1978, p 25.
15. Erslev, AJ: Humoral regulation of red cell production. Blood 8:349, 1953.
16. Erslev, AJ: Erythropoietin coming of age. N Engl J Med 316:101, 1987.
17. Camille, AN and Marshall, AL: Structure of marrow. In Beutler, E, Lichtman, ME, Coller, BS, and Kipps, TJ (eds): Williams Hematology, ed 5. McGraw-Hill, New York, 1995, p 31.
18. Becker, RP, and de Bruyn, PPH: The transmural passage of blood cells into myeloid sinusoids and the entry of platelets into the sinusoidal circulation. A scanning electron microscopic investigation. Am J Anat 145:183, 1976.
19. de Bruyn, P, et al: The migration of blood cells of the bone marrow through the sinusoidal wall. J Morphol 133:417, 1971.
20. Arinkin, MJ: Intravitale Untersuchungsmethodik der Knochenmarks. Folia Haematol (Leipz) 38:233, 1929.
21. Nelson, DA: Hematopoiesis. In Henry, JB (ed): Clinical Diagnosis and Management by Laboratory Methods, ed 16. WB Saunders, Philadelphia, 1979, p 956.
22. Rywlin, AM, Marvan, P, and Robinson, MJ: A simple technique for the preparation of bone marrow smears and sections. Am J Clin Pathol 53:389, 1970.
23. Brynes, RK, McKenna, RW, and Sundberg, RD: Bone marrow aspiration and trephine biopsy, an approach to a thorough study. Am J Clin Pathol 70:753, 1978.
24. Sheeham, DC and Hrapchak, BB: Theory and Practice of Histotechnology. CV Mosby, St Louis, 1980, pp 46, 94.
25. Carson, FL: Histotechnology—A Self-Instructional Text. ASCP Press, Chicago, 1990, pp 10, 38.
26. Wilkins, BS, and O'Brien, CJ: Techniques for obtaining differential cell counts from bone marrow trephine biopsy specimens. J Clin Pathol 41:558, 1988.
27. Williams, WJ and Douglas, NA: Examination of the marrow. In Beutler, E, Lichtman, ME, Coller, BS, and Kipps, TJ (eds): Williams Hematology, ed 5. McGraw-Hill, New York, 1995, p 18.
28. Rosse, C, Kraemer, MJ, Dillon, TL, et al: Bone marrow cell population of normal infants: The predominance of lymphocytes. J Lab Clin Med 89:1225, 1977.
29. Oski, FA and Naiman, LJ: Hematologic Problems of the Newborn. WB Saunders, Philadelphia, 1982, p 21.
30. Longacre, TA, Foucar, K, Crago, S, et al: Hematogones: A multiparameter analysis of bone marrow precursor cells. Blood 73:543, 1989.
31. Rubinstein, MA: Aspiration of bone marrow from iliac crest comparison of iliac crest and sternal bone marrow studies. JAMA 137:1821, 1948.
32. Hartsock, RJ, Smith, EB, and Petty, SC: Normal variations with aging of the amount of hematopoietic tissue in bone marrow from anterior iliac crest. Am J Clin Pathol 43:326, 1965.
33. Lee, R: Microcystosis and the anemias associated with impaired hemoglobin synthesis. In Wintrobe's Clinical Hematology, ed 9, vol I. Lea & Febiger, Philadelphia, 1993, pp 799, 800.

ADDITIONAL RECOMMENDED READINGS

1. Hanson, CA: Bone marrow examination in clinical laboratory medicine. In McClatchey, KD (ed): Clinical Laboratory Medicine. William & Wilkins, Baltimore, 1994, pp 848–851.
2. Weitberg, AB: Study of bone marrow. In Handin, RI, Lux, SE, and Stossel, TP (eds): Blood, Principles and Practice of Hematology. JB Lippincott, Philadelphia, 1995, pp 61–79.

QUESTIONS

1. Which of the following is most variable in normal marrow?
   a. Differential count of 500 cells
   b. M:E ratio
   c. Cellularity
   d. Iron storage

2. Bone marrow aspirate smears are preferred to bone biopsy in diagnosis and classification of:
   a. Granulomatous diseases
   b. Acute leukemias
   c. Metastatic carcinomas
   d. Gaucher's disease

3. When quantitative measurement of bone marrow is performed, the layer most suitable for iron study is:
   a. Fat and perivascular cells
   b. Plasma
   c. Buffy coat of nucleated myeloid and erythroid cells
   d. Erythrocytes

4. Occasionally, nonhemopoietic cells are seen in marrow aspirates. Which of the following is most likely to be misidentified as megakaryocyte?
   a. Reticular cell
   b. Storage histiocyte
   c. Osteoclast
   d. Endothelial cell

5. Trephine marrow biopsy is most useful in the initial diagnosis of all of the following diseases except:
   a. Refractory anemia
   b. Disseminated tuberculosis
   c. Staging renal cell carcinoma
   d. Staging lymphoma

6. In early infancy the most numerous cells of the bone marrow are:
   a. Erythroblasts
   b. Granulocytic precursors
   c. Lymphocytes
   d. Histiocytes-monocytes

ANSWERS

1. **c** (p. 50)
2. **b** (p. 46)
3. **a** (p. 46)
4. **c** (p. 43)
5. **a** (p. 47)
6. **c** (p. 49)

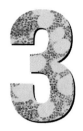

The Red Blood Cell: Structure and Function

Denise M. Harmening, PhD, MT(ASCP), CLS(NCA)

Objectives

At the end of this chapter, the learner should be able to:

1 List the areas of red cell metabolism that are crucial to normal red cell survival and function.
2 List the two most important red blood cell (RBC) membrane proteins and describe their function and the characteristics of deformability and permeability.
3 List the abnormalities that may lead to a change in RBC structure and name the associated RBC morphology.
4 List the criteria for normal hemoglobin synthesis and describe hemoglobin formation.
5 List the structural components of normal hemoglobin.
6 List the globin chains found in HbA, HbA_2, and HbF and their respective concentrations (%) found in vivo.
7 Define "shift to the left" and "shift to the right" in relation to the hemoglobin-oxygen dissociation curve.
8 Define P_{50} and state normal in vivo levels.
9 Define the toxic levels for abnormal hemoglobins of clinical importance.
10 List the various metabolic pathways involved in red cell metabolism, stating the specific function of each one.
11 List and compare the steps in the extravascular and intravascular breakdown of senescent RBCs.

Three areas of red blood cell (RBC) metabolism are crucial for normal erythrocyte survival and function: the RBC membrane, hemoglobin structure and function, and cellular energetics (Table 3–1). Defects or problems associated with any of these areas will result in impaired RBC survival. A thorough working knowledge of these areas of RBC physiology will ensure basic understanding of the various complex erythrocyte functions.

RED BLOOD CELL MEMBRANE

The actual biochemical structure and organization of the RBC membrane still remains to be elucidated;

however, our general knowledge of all plasma membranes has been expanded. The RBC membrane viewed by transmission electron microscopy (TEM) appears as a trilaminar structure consisting of a dark-light-dark band arrangement of layers (Fig. 3–1). These layers represent: (1) an outer hydrophilic portion chemically composed of glycolipid, glycoprotein, and protein; (2) a central hydrophobic layer containing protein, cholesterol, and phospholipid; and (3) an inner hydrophilic layer containing protein. The RBC membrane is highly elastic, responds rapidly to applied stresses of fluid forces, and is capable of undergoing large membrane extensions without fragmentation.[1]

The RBC membrane represents a semipermeable

TABLE 3–1 **Areas of Red Cell Metabolism Important in Normal RBC Survival and Function**

- RBC membrane
- Hemoglobin structure and function
- RBC metabolic pathways

lipid bilayer supported by a meshlike cytoskeleton structure (Fig. 3–2). The RBC membrane cytoskeleton is a network of proteins on the inner surface of the plasma membrane that is responsible for maintaining the shape, stability, and deformability of the RBC.[1] This fluid lipid matrix contains equal amounts of cholesterol and phospholipids with a mosaic of proteins interspersed throughout at various intervals. Those proteins that extend from the outer surface and traverse the entire membrane to the inner cytoplasmic side of the RBC are termed *integral* membrane proteins. The other class of RBC membrane proteins, called *peripheral* proteins, is limited to the cytoplasmic surface of the membrane, which is beneath the lipid bilayer and forms the RBC cytoskeleton. Both the protein and the lipids are organized asymmetrically within the RBC membrane. The chemical composition of the membrane mass is approximately 40% lipids, 52% proteins, and 8% carbohydrates.[2]

Red Blood Cell Membrane Proteins

It is estimated that 10 major and 200 minor proteins are asymmetrically organized within the RBC membrane.[3] After solubilization of the RBC membrane with

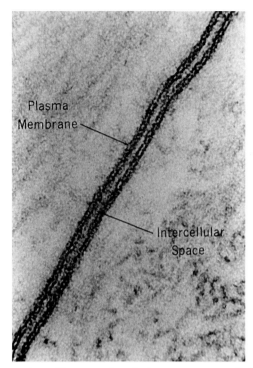

FIGURE 3–1 Transmission electron microscopy of plasma membrane.

the detergent sodium dodecyl sulfite (SDS), membrane proteins can be separated by polyacrylamide gel electrophoresis and stained.[4] The separated RBC membrane proteins are numbered 1 through 8 when stained with Coomassie blue and 1 through 4 when

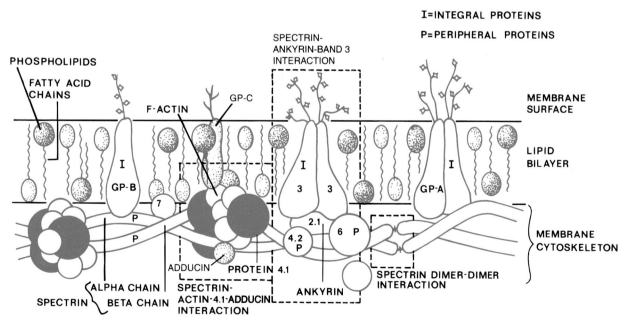

FIGURE 3–2 Schematic illustration of red blood cell membrane depicting the composition and arrangement of red cell membrane proteins. GP-A = glycophorin A; GP-B = glycophorin B; GP-C = glycophorin C; G = globin. Numbers refer to pattern of migration of SDS (sodium, dodecyl, sulfite) polyacrylamide gel pattern stained with Coomassie brilliant blue. Relations of protein to each other and to lipids are purely hypothetical; however, the positions of the proteins relative to the inside or outside of the lipid bilayer are accurate. (Note: proteins are not drawn to scale and many minor proteins are omitted.)

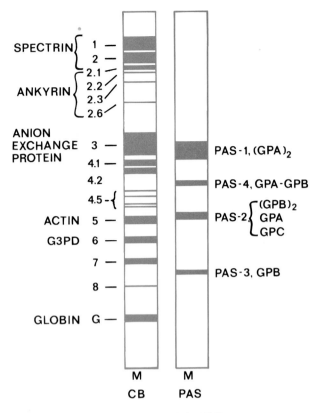

FAIRBANKS-STECK

FIGURE 3–3 Schematic illustration of SDS (sodium, dodecyl, sulfite) polyacrylamide gel electrophoresis patterns of red cell membrane proteins stained with Coomassie brilliant blue (CB) and sialoglycoproteins stained with periodic acid-Schiff (PAS) stain. GPA, GPB, and GPC refer to glycophorins A, B, and C, respectively. (GPA)$_2$ and (GPB)$_2$ are the dimers, and GPA-GPB is the heterodimer of GPA and GPB.

TABLE 3–2 **Red Cell Membrane Integral and Peripheral Proteins**	
Integral Proteins	**Peripheral Proteins**
Glycophorin A	Spectrin
Glycophorin B	Actin (band 5)
Glycophorin C	Ankyrin (band 2.1)
Anion-exchange-channel protein (band 3)	Band 4.1 and 4.2
	Band 6
	Adducin

outer RBC membrane surface and migrate primarily in band 3 of the SDS gel electrophoretic pattern stained with Coomassie blue (see Fig. 3–3). Most of these proteins, as mentioned previously, carry RBC antigens and are receptors (such as the glycophorins) or transport proteins (such as band 3, the anion exchange-channel glycoprotein). The plasma membrane envelope is anchored to the RBC cytoskeleton network of proteins through tethering sites of integral (transmembrane) proteins located in the lipid bilayer.[1] The condensed-fluid lipid bilayer plus integral (transmembrane) proteins chemically isolates and regulates the cell interior. The RBC cytoskeleton network of proteins provides rigid support and stability to the lipid bilayer and is responsible for the deformability properties of the RBC membrane, leading to shape change. It is speculated that band 3 and the glycophorins play a major role in anchoring the RBC membrane cytoskeleton to the lipid bilayer. As a result, lateral mobility of these integral proteins within the lipid bilayer is relatively restricted. Transmembrane (integral) proteins can also greatly influence mechanical stability and membrane rigidity.[5,6]

Peripheral Proteins

The major components of the red cell cytoskeleton include spectrin, ankyrin, protein 4.1, actin, and adducin.[7] Spectrin is clearly the most abundant peripheral protein of the RBC membrane cytoskeleton, comprising approximately 25% to 30% of the total membrane protein and 75% of the peripheral protein.[8]

Spectrin, a flexible rodlike molecule, is composed of a helix of two polypeptide chains, an alpha chain (band 1, molecular weight 240,000 d) and a beta chain (band 2, molecular weight 225,000 d).[3] These chains intertwined side-to-side form heterodimers, which link together with other alpha-beta chains to form $(\alpha\beta)_2$ tetramers. Spectrin is an important factor in RBC membrane integrity because it binds with other peripheral proteins such as actin (band 5), ankyrin (band 2.1), band 4.1, and adducin to form a skeletal network of microfilaments on the inner surface of the RBC membrane (see Fig. 3–2). These microfilaments strengthen the membrane, protecting the cell from being broken by circulatory shear forces, and also control the biconcave shape and deformability of the cell. In addition, the cytoskeletal network provides stability to the lipid bilayer interface.[1] Two sets of spectrin complexes tie the RBC cytoskeleton network together and stabilize the spectrin-actin junction. A spectrin–actin–

stained with periodic acid-Schiff (PAS) stain, which is the basis of their nomenclature (Fig. 3–3).[4] The proteins range in molecular weight from 16,000 to 244,000 daltons (d).

Two of the most important protein constituents include glycophorin, an integral membrane protein, and spectrin, a peripheral membrane protein. Table 3–2 lists the integral and peripheral membrane proteins.

Integral Membrane Proteins

Glycophorin, a major integral membrane protein, is the principal RBC glycoprotein, representing approximately 20% of the total membrane protein.[2] The molecule contains approximately 60% carbohydrate and accounts for most of the membrane sialic acid, which gives the erythrocyte its negative charge. Glycophorin, similar to other integral membrane proteins, spans the entire thickness of the lipid bilayer and appears on the external surface of the RBC membrane, accounting for the location of many RBC antigens. Three types of glycophorins have been described—glycophorin A, B, and C (see PAS bands 1, 2, and 3). A glycophorin D has also been described.[2] All glycoproteins are exposed on the

TABLE 3–3   **Characteristics of the Major Components of the Red Cell Membrane**

Protein	Size	Function
*Spectrin	0.1-μm heterodimeric filamentous protein consisting of a 240-kd α chain and a 220-kd β chain constitutes 20–25% of the mass of membrane proteins	Principal structural element of RBC membrane that plays a major role in the RBC cytoskeleton membrane organization
*Ankyrin	210-kd globular protein composed of 1879 amino acids	Primary determinant of mechanical coupling of the lipid bilayer to the membrane skeleton
*Adducin	Protein doublet of approximately 97 and 103 kd	Promotes the association of spectrin with F-actin in a manner similar to band 4.1
*Band 4.1	Composed of 622 amino acids, constitutes 5% of the mass of membrane proteins	Dual functions: promotes high-affinity association between spectrin and F-actin and may link the skeleton to the membrane by virtue of its associations with glycophorin and band 3
Band 3	Major RBC transmembrane protein and major integral protein that has two distinct domains: the transmembrane and cytoplasmic; 911 amino acid protein, comprising 15–20% of the total membrane protein	Two separate functions: catalyzes chloride-bicarbonate exchange and contains binding sites for ankyrin, band 4.1, band 4.2, and several glycolytic enzymes
Band 4.2	Known to associate with the cytoplasmic domain of band 3	Actual function unknown; however, a deficiency of the protein is associated with several types of inherited hemolytic anemias

*Denotes major components of the red cell cytoskeleton
Source: Data from Mohandas and Chasis,[1] and Cohen and Gascard.[8]

band 4.1–adducin complex and a spectrin-ankyrin complex bind to the integral protein, band 3, to anchor the skeleton to the overlaying lipid bilayer (see Fig. 3–2).[1] In addition, spectrin is also linked to the RBC lipid bilayer through the bonding between band 4.1 and the integral protein, glycophorin C. The preservation of the spectrin–actin–band 4.1–adducin and spectrin-ankyrin network, and thus the integrity of the RBC membrane, requires phosphorylation of spectrin by a protein kinase present in the membrane, which is energy-dependent, being catalyzed by adenosine triphosphate (ATP). Other peripheral membrane proteins that lack carbohydrates and are confined to the cytoplasmic membrane surface include certain enzymes such as glyceraldehyde-3-phosphate dehydrogenase (band 6) and structural proteins such as hemoglobin.

As mentioned earlier, the normal chemical composition, structural arrangement, and molecular interactions of the erythrocyte membrane are crucial to the normal RBC survival in circulation of 120 days. In addition, they play a critical role in two important RBC characteristics: deformability and permeability. Table 3–3 lists characteristics of the major components of the red cell membrane.

Deformability

RBC's membrane deformability or pliability is critical not only to RBC survival as it travels through the microvasculature, but also for its function of oxygen delivery.[1] Decreased cellular deformability and red cell shape changes have been recognized as distinguishing features of a number of congenital or hereditary hemolytic anemias leading to decreased RBC survival in these disorders. (See Chaps. 9 and 10.)

It has already been mentioned that a loss of ATP (energy) levels leads to a decrease in the phosphorylation

of spectrin and, in turn, a loss of membrane deformability. An accumulation or increase in deposition of membrane calcium also results, causing an increase in membrane rigidity and loss of pliability. These cells are at a marked disadvantage when they pass through the small (3- to 5-μm-diameter) sinusoidal orifices of the spleen, one of whose functions is extravascular sequestration and removal of aged, damaged, or less deformable RBC or fragments of their membrane (Fig. 3–4). The loss of RBC membrane is exemplified by the formation of spherocytes (Fig. 3–5), cells with a reduced surface-to-volume ratio, and "bite cells" (Fig. 3–6), in which the removal of a portion of membrane has left a permanent indentation in the remaining cell

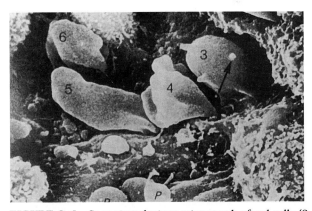

FIGURE 3–4   Scanning electron micrograph of red cells (3 to 6) squeezing through fenestrated wall in transit from splenic cords to sinus. Epithelial linings of sinus wall, to which platelets (P) adhere, along with "hairy" white cells, probably macrophages, are shown. (From Weiss, L: A scanning electron microscopic study of the spleen. Blood, 43:665, 1974, with permission.)

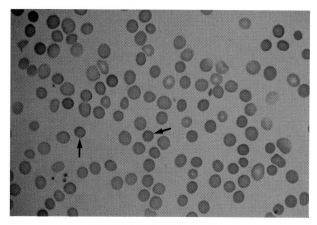

FIGURE 3–5   Spherocytes.

TABLE 3–4   **Biochemical Changes That Can Transform RBC Discs into Crenated Forms**
• Low concentration of fatty acids and phospholipids
• A variety of amphoteric agents
• Elevated intracellular calcium concentration
• Decreased adenosine triphosphate (ATP) levels

membrane. The survival time of these forms is also shortened. Shape change from the normal symmetric and resilient discoid shape of the RBC can be stimulated by a variety of factors, which include both mechanically induced and chemically induced forces.[3] Spectrin molecules exist in a folded conformation in the membrane of the nondeformed red cell. During reversible membrane deformability, certain spectrin molecules become uncoiled and extended, whereas others become more compressed and folded, resulting in a rearrangement of the cytoskeletal network.[1] This reversible RBC membrane deformability results in a shape change while maintaining a constant surface area. The limit to reversible RBC membrane deformability occurs when applied forces break the protein-to-protein associations necessitating an increase in surface area.[9] The RBC membrane fails, resulting in irreversible deformability, when red cells are exposed to forces great enough to require an increase in surface area, leading to membrane fragmentation.[1] Table 3–4 lists a wide variety of chemical changes that can induce shape changes in the red cell.

Permeability

The RBC membrane is freely permeable to water and anions; chloride (Cl^-) and bicarbonate (HCO_3^-) tra-

verse the membrane in less than a second. It is speculated that this massive exchange of HCO_3^- and Cl^- ions occurs through a large number of exchange channels formed by the integral membrane protein, band 3, a glycoprotein previously described (see section on RBC integral membrane proteins). In contrast, the RBC membrane is relatively impermeable to cations, with a half-time exchange of sodium (Na^+) and potassium (K^+) of more than 30 hours. It is primarily through the control of the sodium and potassium intracellular concentrations that the RBC maintains its volume and water homeostasis. The erythrocyte intracellular-to-extracellular ratios for sodium and potassium are 1:12 and 25:1, respectively. The passive influx of sodium and potassium is controlled by as many as 300 cationic pumps that actively transport sodium out of the cell and potassium into the cell. Like other cationic pumps, these sodium-potassium pumps are energy-dependent, requiring ATP. The functional active transport of these particular cations by these cationic pumps also requires the membrane enzyme sodium-potassium ATPase. It is interesting to note that full activation of the sodium-potassium-ATPase pumps requires the presence of the RBC membrane amino phospholipid phosphatidyl serine. Similarly, calcium (Ca^{2+}) is also actively pumped from the interior of the RBC through the energy-depenent calcium-ATPase cationic pump. Calmodulin, a cytoplasmic calcium-binding protein, is speculated to control these calcium-ATPase pumps, preventing excessive intracellular calcium buildup, which is deleterious to the RBC, resulting in shape changes and loss of deformability.[8] The permeability properties of the RBC membrane, as well as active cation transport, are crucial to the prevention of colloid osmotic hemolysis and controlling the volume of the RBC. In addition, ATP-depleted cells allow the accumulation of excess intracellular calcium and sodium followed by potassium and water loss, resulting in a dehydrated, rigid cell subsequently sequestered by the spleen. The energy required for active transport and maintenance of membrane electrochemical gradients is provided by ATP. Any abnormality that increases membrane permeability or alters cationic transport may lead to a decrease in RBC survival.

Red Blood Cell Membrane Lipids

Phospholipids

The erythrocyte membrane lipid consists of a bilayer of phospholipids interspersed with molecules of unesterified cholesterol and glycolipids that are present in nearly equimolar quantities.[2] Free fatty acid and glycolipids are present in small quantities.[2] Two groups

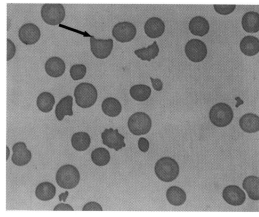

FIGURE 3–6   Bite cells.

of phospholipids, choline phospholipids and amino phospholipids, are known to possess a distinct asymmetry within the bilayer matrix of the RBC.

Choline phospholipids, consisting of phosphatidyl choline and sphingomyelin, are primarily located on the outside half of the lipid bilayer, readily accessible to the external environment.[3] Because of their outward orientation in the lipid bilayer, the choline phospholipids may represent controlling points in the major pathways of lipid renewal, since there is an exchange between plasma fatty acids and the RBC membrane. Fatty acids are incorporated through an energy-dependent process into membrane phospholipids. Therefore, changes in body lipid transport and metabolism may cause abnormalities in the plasma phospholipid concentration that may alter the RBC membrane composition, resulting in a decreased RBC survival in circulation. In addition, research suggests that the interaction of these phospholipids with cholesterol may play a role in cholesterol homeostasis in the RBC membrane.

In contrast, amino phospholipids, consisting of phosphatidylethanolamine and phosphatidylserine, are located almost exclusively on the inside half or cytoplasmic side of the RBC membrane along with phosphatidylinositol. This specific orientation of these phospholipids maintains a precise lipid pattern that is critical to normal RBC survival in circulation. Alteration of this arrangement, leading to the abnormal appearance of these amino phospholipids on the outer surface of the lipid bilayer, promotes activation of the clotting cascade and may result in extravascular hemolysis. Stabilization of this phospholipid asymmetry in the erythrocyte membrane is maintained through the interaction with specific peripheral proteins (see "RBC Membrane Proteins").

Glycolipids and Cholesterol

Most of the glycolipids are located in the outer half of the lipid bilayer and interact with glycoproteins to form many of the RBC antigens. Cholesterol is approximately equally distributed, being located on both sides of the lipid bilayer inserted between the choline and amino phospholipids. Cholesterol composes 25%

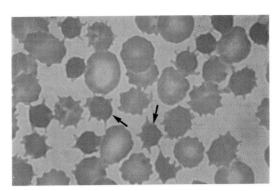

FIGURE 3–8   Acanthocytes.

of the RBC membrane lipid and is present in a 1:1 molar ratio with phospholipids. RBC membrane cholesterol is in continual exchange with plasma cholesterol and is therefore affected by changes in body lipid transport.

Accumulation of cholesterol results in morphological changes in the RBCs, such as target cells (Fig. 3–7), and may cause RBC membrane damage. Acanthocytes, RBCs with irregular, spiny projections called *spicules* (Fig. 3–8), have also been associated with an excess accumulation of membrane cholesterol in association with liver disease and particular lipid disorders such as abetalipoproteinemia. All of these RBCs have a decreased survival rate because the excess lipid makes the cell membrane less deformable.

Another example, the congenital deficiency of the plasma enzyme LCAT (lecithin-to-cholesterol acyltransferase), leads to an excess of free cholesterol in both the plasma and the RBC membrane, resulting in, among other problems, a chronic hemolytic anemia. In general, all of these lipids are mobile within the plane of the erythrocyte membrane, and, as a result of this phenomenon, the RBC membrane is characteristically a viscous, two-dimensional fluid. This lipid bilayer also acts as an impenetrable barrier. Consequently, most transport across the RBC membrane occurs through transport protein globules. Table 3–5 summarizes the

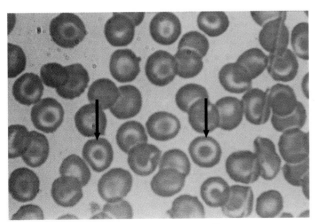

FIGURE 3–7   Target cells.

TABLE 3–5 **Abnormalities That Can Lead to a Change in RBC Morphology**	
Abnormality	**RBC Morphology**
Cholesterol accumulation in the RBC membrane (i.e., liver disease)	Target cells
Abetalipoproteinemia with cholesterol accumulation	Acanthocytes
LCAT deficiency with cholesterol accumulation	Hemolysis with red cell fragmentation
Decreased phosphorylated spectrin or altered spectrin	Bite cells and spherocytes

abnormalities that can lead to a change in RBC morphology.

HEMOGLOBIN STRUCTURE AND FUNCTION

Hemoglobin, a conjugated globular protein with a molecular weight of approximately 64.4 kilodaltons (kd), constitutes 95% of the RBC's dry weight, or 33% of the RBC's weight by volume.[10] Approximately 65% of the hemoglobin synthesis occurs during the nucleated stages of RBC maturation, and 35% occurs during the reticulocyte stage. Normal hemoglobin consists of globin (a tetramer of two pairs of unlike globin polypeptide chains) and four heme groups, each of which contains a protoporphyrin ring plus iron (Fe^{2+}).

Hemoglobin Synthesis

Normal hemoglobin production is dependent on three processes (Fig. 3–9):
1. Adequate iron delivery and supply
2. Adequate synthesis of protoporphyrins (the precursor of heme)
3. Adequate globin synthesis

Iron Delivery and Supply

Iron is delivered to the membrane of the RBC precursor by the protein carrier transferrin. Most of the iron that crosses the membrane and enters the cytoplasm of the cell is committed to hemoglobin synthesis and thereby proceeds to the mitochondria for insertion into the protoporphyrin ring to form heme. Excess iron in the cytoplasm aggregates as ferritin, the amount of which depends on the ratio between the level of plasma iron and the amount of iron required by the erythrocyte for hemoglobin synthesis.[11] Two thirds of the total body iron supply is bound to heme in the hemoglobin molecule (see Chap. 6 for a discussion of iron kinetics).

Synthesis of Protoporphyrins

Protoporphyrin synthesis begins in the mitochondria with the formation of delta-aminolevulinic acid (δALA) from glycine and succinyl coenzyme A (CoA), which is the major rate-limiting step in heme biosynthesis (Fig. 3–10).[12] The mitochondrial enzyme, δALA synthetase, which mediates this reaction, is influenced by erythropoietin and requires the presence of the cofactor pyridoxal phosphate (vitamin B_6).[13]

Porphyrinogens, not porphyrins, are the intermediates of heme synthesis. Porphyrinogens are unstable tetrapyrroles that are readily and irreversibly oxidized to form porphyrins. In contrast, porphyrins are highly stable resonating molecules that are normally found in small quantities in the urine as a result of normal RBC catabolism.[14,15]

Excessive formation of porphyrins can occur if any one of the normal enzymatic steps in heme synthesis is blocked and can result in one of a number of metabolic disorders collectively called the porphyrias.[16]

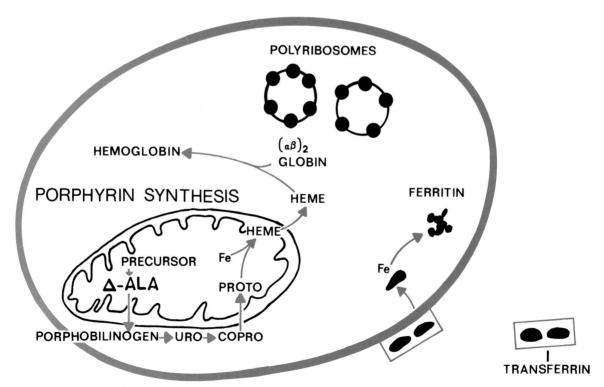

FIGURE 3–9 Hemoglobin synthesis in the reticulocyte.

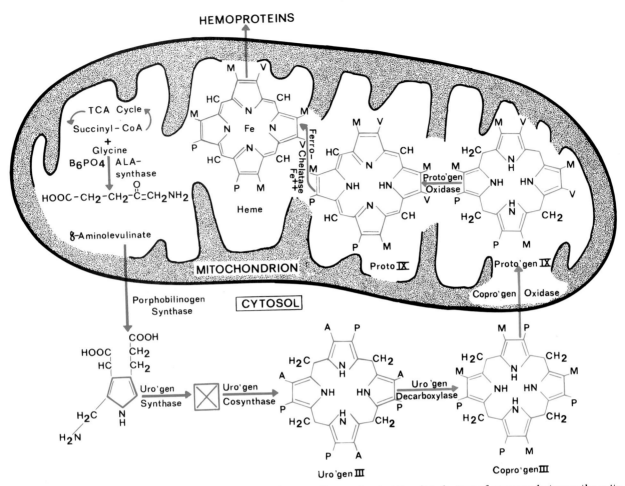

FIGURE 3–10 Synthesis of heme. The heme biosynthetic pathway showing the distribution of enzymes between the mitochondria and the cytoplasm. Intermediates between uroporphyrinogen and coproporphyrinogen, designated by X, remain unidentified. B_6PO_4 = pyridoxal phosphate. (From Tietz, MW: Textbook of Clinical Chemistry. WB Saunders, Philadelphia 1986, with permission.)

Globin Synthesis

Globin chain synthesis occurs on RBC-specific cytoplasmic ribosomes, which are initiated from the inheritance of various structural genes. Each gene results in the formation of a specific polypeptide chain. Each somatic diploid cell, including the RBC, contains four alpha (α), two zeta (ζ), two beta (β), two delta (δ), two epsilon (ϵ), and four gamma (γ) genes.[17] The alpha and zeta genes are located on chromosome 16, and the beta, delta, epsilon, and gamma genes on chromosome 11 (Fig. 3–11). The resulting gene products formed have been called alpha, zeta, beta, delta, epsilon, and gamma globin chains. Throughout embryonic and fetal development, activation of the globin genes progresses from the zeta to the alpha gene and from the epsilon to the gamma, delta, and beta genes.[17]

The epsilon and zeta chains normally appear only during embryonic development (Table 3–6). These two chains, plus the alpha and gamma chains, are con-

stituents of embryonic hemoglobins: Hb Gower 1 ($\zeta_2\epsilon_2$), Hb Gower 2 ($\alpha_2\epsilon_2$), and Hb Portland ($\zeta_2\gamma_2$). The epsilon and zeta chains are produced up to approximately 3 months following conception. The alpha chain is always present. Gamma chain production is active from the third fetal month until 1 year postnatally. In the fetus, the major hemoglobin is $\alpha_2\gamma_2$ (hemoglobin F). The gamma chains occur as a mixture of two types of chains, differing only by one amino acid at position 136. G-gamma ($^G\gamma$) contains glycine, whereas A-gamma ($^A\gamma$) has alanine at that position.[17] The ratio of G-gamma to A-gamma is approximately 3:1 at birth and 2:3 by 1 year of age.[17] By the age of 2 years, hemoglobin F comprises less than 2% of the total hemoglobin. Beta-chain production rises gradually prenatally and reaches adult percentages between 3 and 6 months postnatally.[17] Figure 3–12 depicts the time sequence of globin chain synthesis during fetal development, birth, and infancy.

All normal adult hemoglobins are formed as tetrameres consisting of two alpha chains plus two (non-

GENE PRODUCTS (GLOBIN CHAINS)
HEMOGLOBINS (Hb)

Genes   Genes

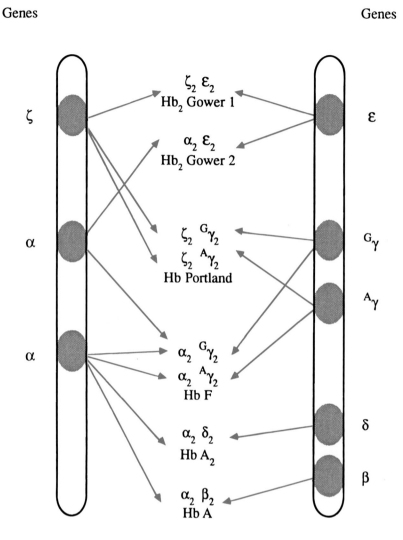

Chromosome 16   Chromosome 11

FIGURE 3–11 Genetic control and formation of human hemoglobins.

alpha) globin chains. Normal adult RBCs contain the following types of hemoglobin:

95% to 97% of the hemoglobin is HbA, which consists of $\alpha_2\beta_2$ chains.

2% to 3% of the hemoglobin is HbA$_2$, which consists of $\alpha_2\delta_2$ chains.

1% to 2% of the hemoglobin is HbF (fetal hemoglobin), which consists of $\alpha_2\gamma_2$ chains.

Each synthesized globin chain links with heme (ferroprotoporphyrin IX) to form hemoglobin, which primarily consists of two alpha chains, two beta chains, and four heme groups. Normal alpha chains consist of 141 amino acid residues linked together in a linear fashion, whereas normal beta chains (as well as δ, γ, and ϵ) consist of 146 amino acid residues. Table 3–6 shows the composition of hemoglobin found during

normal human development. The precise order of amino acids is critical to the hemoglobin molecule's structure and function.

The rate of globin synthesis is directly related to the rate of porphyrin synthesis, and vice versa: protoporphyrin synthesis is reduced when globin synthesis is impaired. There is, however, no such relationship with iron uptake when either globin or protoporphyrin synthesis is impaired; iron accumulates in the RBC cytoplasm as ferritin aggregates. The iron-laden, nucleated RBC is termed a *sideroblast*, and the anucleated form a *siderocyte*, when stained with Prussian blue for visualization of iron (see Chap. 6, Fig. 6–5). When protoporphyrin synthesis is impaired, the mitochondria become encrusted with iron, which is visible around the nucleus of the RBC precursor when stained with

TABLE 3-6   Composition of Hemoglobin Found in Normal Human Development

Globin Chains	Hemoglobin	Stage of Development
$\alpha_2\epsilon_2$	Gower 2	
$\zeta_2\epsilon_2$	Gower 1	Embryo
$\zeta_2\gamma_2$	Portland	
$\alpha_2^{\ A}\gamma_2$	F	Fetus
$\alpha_2^{\ G}\gamma_2$	F	
$\alpha_2\beta_2$	A	Adult
$\alpha_2\delta_2$	A_2	

Prussian blue. Such an RBC is termed a *ringed sideroblast* and is diagnostic for a pathogenesis linked to deficient protoporphyrin synthesis (see Fig. 6–5).

Hemoglobin Function

Hemoglobin's primary function is delivery and release of oxygen to the tissues and facilitation of carbon dioxide excretion. Because of hemoglobin's multichain structure, the molecule is capable of a considerable amount of allosteric movement as it loads and unloads oxygen. One of the most important controls of hemoglobin affinity for oxygen is the RBC organic phosphate 2,3-diphosphoglycerate (2,3-DPG). The unloading of oxygen by hemoglobin is accompanied by the widening of the space between beta chains and the binding of 2,3-DPG, on a mole-for-mole basis, with the formation of anionic salt bridges between the beta chains.[18] The resulting conformation of the deoxyhemoglobin molecule is known as the tense (T) form, which has a lower affinity for oxygen. When hemoglobin loads oxygen and

becomes oxyhemoglobin, the established salt bridges are broken and beta chains are pulled together, expelling 2,3-DPG. This relaxed (R) form of the hemoglobin molecule has a higher affinity for oxygen.

These allosteric changes that occur as the hemoglobin loads and unloads oxygen are referred to as the *respiratory movement.*[18] The dissociation and binding of oxygen by hemoglobin are not directly proportional to the P_{O_2} of its environment, but instead exhibit a sigmoid-curve relationship—the hemoglobin-oxygen dissociation curve depicted in Fig. 3–13. The shape of this curve is very important physiologically because it permits a considerable amount of oxygen to be delivered to the tissues with a small drop in oxygen tension. For example, in the environment of the lungs, where the P_{O_2} (oxygen tension), measured in millimeters of mercury (mmHg), is nearly 100 mmHg, the hemoglobin molecule is almost 100% saturated with oxygen (Fig. 3–13, point A). As the RBCs travel to the tissues where the P_{O_2} drops to an average 40 mmHg (mean venous oxygen tension), the hemoglobin saturation drops to approximately 75% saturation, releasing approximately 25% of the oxygen to the tissues (point B).

This is the normal situation of oxygen delivery at basal metabolic rate. In conditions such as hypoxia, a compensatory "shift to the right" of the hemoglobin-oxygen dissociation curve (Fig. 3–14) occurs to alleviate a tissue oxygen deficit. This rightward shift of the curve, mediated by increased levels of 2,3-DPG, results in a decrease in hemoglobin's affinity for the oxygen molecule and an increase in oxygen delivery to the tissues. Note that the oxygen saturation of hemoglobin in the environment of the tissues [40 mmHg P_{O_2} (Fig. 3–13, point B)] is now only 50%; the other 50% of the oxygen is being released to the tissues. The RBCs thus have become more efficient in terms of oxygen delivery.

Therefore, a patient who is suffering from an anemia caused by a loss of RBCs may be able to compensate by shifting the oxygen dissociation curve to the right, making the RBCs, though fewer in number, more efficient. Some patients may be able to tolerate anemia better than others because of this compensatory mechanism. A shift to the right also may occur in response to acidosis or a rise in body temperature.[18] The shift to the right of the hemoglobin-oxygen dissociation curve is only one way in which patients may compensate for various types of hypoxia; other ways include increases in total cardiac output and in erythropoiesis.

A "shift to the left" of the hemoglobin-oxygen dissociation curve conversely results in an increase in hemoglobin-oxygen affinity and a decrease in oxygen delivery to the tissues (Fig. 3–15). With such a dissociation curve, RBCs are much less efficient because only 12% of the oxygen can be released to the tissues (point B). Among the conditions that can shift the oxygen dissociation curve to the left are alkalosis; increased quantities of abnormal hemoglobins, such as methemoglobin and carboxyhemoglobin; increased quantities of hemoglobin F; or multiple transfusions of 2,3-DPG–depleted stored blood (attesting to the importance of 2,3-DPG in oxygen release).[18]

Hemoglobin-oxygen affinity also can be expressed by P_{50} values, which designate the P_{O_2} at which hemoglo-

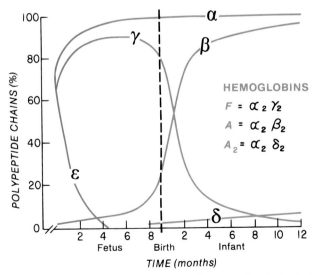

FIGURE 3–12 Changes in globin chain synthesis during fetal development, birth, and infancy. (From Hillman, RF and Finch, CA: Red Cell Manual, ed 5. FA Davis, Philadelphia, 1985, with permission.)

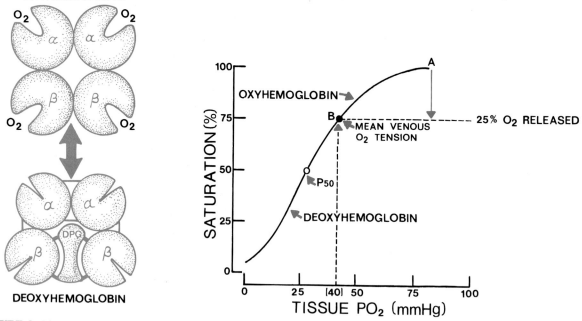

FIGURE 3-13   Normal hemoglobin-oxygen dissociation curve. (From Hillman, RF and Finch, CA: Red Cell Manual, ed 5. FA Davis, Philadelphia, 1985, with permission.)

bin is 50% saturated with oxygen under standard in vitro conditions of temperature and pH.[12] The P_{50} of normal blood is 26 to 30 mmHg.[10] An increase in P_{50} represents a decrease in hemoglobin-oxygen affinity or a shift to the right of the oxygen dissociation curve. A decrease in P_{50} represents an increase in hemoglobin-oxygen affinity or a shift to the left of the oxygen dissociation curve. In addition to the reasons listed previously for shifts in the curve, inherited abnormalities of the hemoglobin molecule can result in either situation. These abnormalities are described by the P_{50} measurements. Abnormalities in hemoglobin structure or function can therefore have profound effects on the RBC's ability to provide oxygen to the tissues.

Abnormal Hemoglobins of Clinical Importance

The hemoglobins previously described—oxyhemoglobin and reduced hemoglobin—are physiologic hemoglobins because they function in the transport and delivery of oxygen within the circulation. Abnormal hemoglobins of clinical significance that are unable to transport or deliver oxygen include the following:

1. Carboxyhemoglobin
2. Methemoglobin
3. Sulfhemoglobin

In carboxyhemoglobin, the oxygen molecules bound to heme have been replaced with carbon monoxide

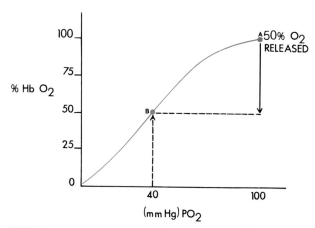

FIGURE 3-14   Right-shifted hemoglobin-oxygen dissociation curve.

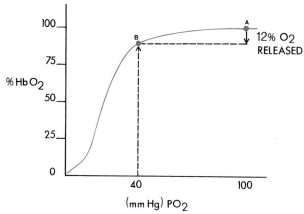

FIGURE 3-15   Left-shifted hemoglobin-oxygen dissociation curve.

TABLE 3–7 **Toxic Levels for Abnormal Hemoglobins of Clinical Importance**	
Abnormal Hemoglobin	**Toxic Level (g%)**
Carboxyhemoglobin	5.0
Methemoglobin	1.5
Sulfhemoglobin	0.5

(CO). This replacement process is relatively slow and dependent upon the concentration of carbon monoxide in the blood. Once attached, however, the binding of carbon monoxide to the heme of the hemoglobin molecule is 200 times tighter than the binding of oxygen to heme.[12] The concentration of carbon monoxide can be increased in a number of conditions, including that of chronic heavy smokers.

Methemoglobin is formed when the iron of the hemoglobin molecule is oxidized to the ferric (Fe^3) state.[12] Normally, less than 1% of the total circulating hemoglobin is in the methemoglobin form. Increased formation of methemoglobin can occur as a result of an overload of oxidant stress, owing to the ingestion of strong oxidant drugs or to an enzyme deficiency (see the following section on RBC metabolic pathways).[17]

Sulfhemoglobin is formed when a certain situation or condition, such as ingestion of a sulfur-containing drug or chronic constipation, builds up the sulfur content of the blood.[12] Sulfhemoglobin is incapable of carrying oxygen and represents an irreversible change of the hemoglobin molecule that persists until the RBCs are removed from the circulation. Both carboxyhemoglobin and methemoglobin, however, can be reverted to oxyhemoglobin through the use of oxygen inhalation and the administration of strong reducing substances, respectively. Table 3–7 lists the toxic levels for each abnormal hemoglobin at which cyanosis, anemia, and death may result from a tissue oxygen deficit and increased concentration of circulating abnormal hemoglobin.

MAINTENANCE OF HEMOGLOBIN FUNCTION: ACTIVE RED BLOOD CELL METABOLIC PATHWAYS

Active erythrocyte metabolic pathways are necessary for the production of adequate ATP levels. Such generated energy is crucial to RBC survival and function in that it is necessary for maintaining: (1) hemoglobin function, (2) membrane integrity and deformability, (3) RBC volume, and (4) adequate amounts of reduced pyridine nucleotides.

RBCs generate energy almost exclusively through the anaerobic breakdown of glucose because the metabolism of the anucleated erythrocyte is more limited than that of other body cells. The adult RBC possesses little ability to metabolize fatty acids and amino acids. Additionally, mature RBCs contain no mitochondrial apparatus for oxidative metabolism (Table 3–8 compares RBC metabolism during various stages of maturation). The RBC's metabolic pathways are mainly anaerobic, fortunately, because the function of the RBC is to deliver oxygen and not to consume it. Four pathways of RBC metabolism will be considered: the anaerobic glycolytic pathway and three ancillary pathways that serve to maintain the function of hemoglobin (Fig. 3–16). All of these processes are essential if the RBC is to transport oxygen and maintain the physical characteristics required for its survival in circulation.

Of the ATP needed by RBCs, 90% is generated by the Embden-Meyerhof glycolytic pathway.[12] Here, the metabolism of glucose results in the net generation of two molecules of ATP. Although this ATP synthesis is inefficient when compared with cells that use the Krebs cycle (aerobic metabolism), it provides sufficient ATP for the RBC's requirements. Glycolysis also generates NADH from NAD^+, which is important in some of the RBCs' other metabolic pathways.

Another 5% to 10% of glucose is metabolized by the hexose monophosphate shunt (also called the *phosphogluconate pathway*).[12] This pathway produces the pyridine nucleotide NADPH from $NADP^+$. NADPH, together with reduced glutathione, provides the main line of defense for the RBC against oxidative injury.[17]

TABLE 3–8 **Comparison of Red Blood Cell Metabolic Activities During Various Stages of Maturation**			
	Nucleated RBC	**Reticulocyte**	**Adult RBC**
Replication	+	0	0
DNA synthesis	+	0	0
RNA synthesis	+	0	0
Lipid synthesis	+	+	0
RNA present	+	+	0
Heme synthesis	+	+	0
Protein synthesis	+	+	0
Mitochondria	+	+	0
Krebs' tricarboxylic acid cycle	+	+	0
Embden-Meyerhof pathway	+	+	+
Pentose phosphate pathway	+	+	+
Maturation and/or senescence	+	+	+

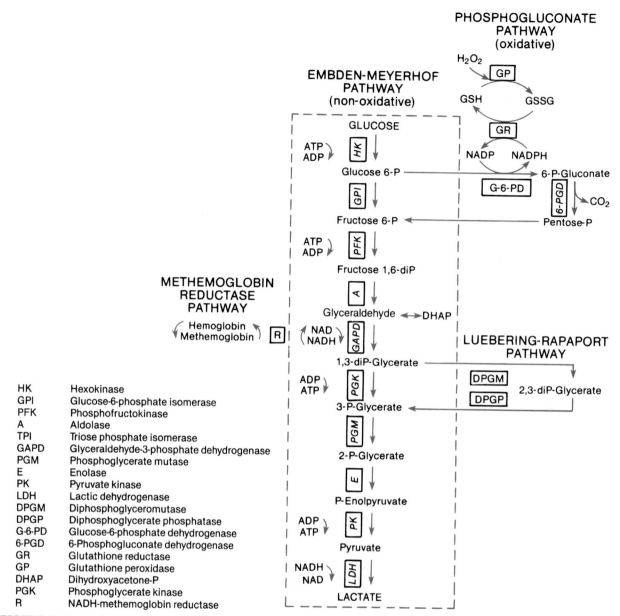

FIGURE 3–16 Red cell metabolism. (From Hillman, RF and Finch, CA: Red Cell Manual, ed 7. FA Davis, Philadelphia, 1996, with permission.)

Oxidant drugs, as well as infections, can cause the accumulation of hydrogen peroxide and other oxidants, which can be toxic to cell proteins. The sequence of biochemical reactions shown in Figure 3–17 occurs within the normal RBC with adequate levels of appropriate enzymes and substrate to prevent the accumulation of these agents.

When the hexose monophosphate pathway is functionally deficient, the amount of reduced glutathione becomes insufficient to neutralize intracellular oxidants. This results in globin denaturation and precipitation as aggregates (Heinz bodies) within the cell. If this process sufficiently damages the membrane, cell destruction occurs. Inherited defects in the pentose phosphate glutathione pathway, the most common of

which is glucose-6-phosphate dehydrogenase (G6PD) deficiency, result in the formation of Heinz bodies with subsequent extravascular hemolysis.[12] (Glutathione is not only crucial to keeping hemoglobin in a functional state but it is also important in maintaining RBC integrity by reducing sulfhydryl groups of hemoglobin, membrane protein, and enzymes subsequent to oxidation.)

The methemoglobin reductase pathway is another important component of RBC metabolism. Two methemoglobin reductase systems are important in maintaining heme iron in the reduced (Fe^{2+}, ferrous) functional state.[12] Both pathways depend on the regeneration of reduced pyridine nucleotide and are referred to as the NADH and NADPH methemoglobin

Reaction A. RBC + infection or oxidant $\longrightarrow H_2O_2$

Reaction B. H_2O_2 + 2GSH (reduced glutathione) $\xrightarrow[\text{peroxidase}]{\text{Glutathione}}$ GSSG (oxidized glutathione)+$2H_2O$

Reaction C. GSSG + NADPH (reduced form) + H^+ $\xrightarrow[\text{reductase}]{\text{Glutathione}}$ 2GSH+ $NADP^+$ (oxidized form)

Reaction D. G-6-P (glucose-6-phosphate) + $NADP^+$ $\xrightarrow[\substack{\text{Phosphate}\\\text{dehydrogenase}}]{\text{Glucose-6-}}$ 6-PG (6-phosphogluconate) + NADPH + H^+

FIGURE 3–17   Reactions within erythrocytes to prevent accumulation of oxidants.

reductase pathways. In the absence of the enzyme methemoglobin reductase and the reducing action of the pyridine nucleotide NADH, there is an accumulation of methemoglobin, resulting from the conversion of the ferrous iron of heme to the ferric form (Fe^{3+}). Methemoglobin is a nonfunctional form of hemoglobin, having lost oxygen transport capabilities, as the metheme portion cannot combine with oxygen. Normal efficiency of the methemoglobin reductase pathway is exemplified by the fact that usually no more than 1% of RBC hemoglobin exists as methemoglobin in the RBCs of healthy individuals.[17]

Another important pathway that is crucial to RBC function is the Leubering-Rapoport shunt. This pathway causes an extraordinary accumulation of the RBC organic phosphate 2,3-DPG, which is important because of its profound effect on hemoglobin's affinity for oxygen. Stores of this organic phosphate can serve as a reserve for additional ATP generation.

ERYTHROCYTE SENESCENCE

The RBC, a 6 to 8 μm biconcave disc, travels 200 to 300 miles during its 120-day life span. During this time, circulating RBCs undergo the *process* of senescence or aging. Various metabolic and physical changes associated with the aging of RBCs are listed in Table 3–9. Each day 1% of the old RBC's in circulation are taken out by a system of fixed macrophages in the body known as the *reticuloendothelial system*

(RES). These RBCs are replaced by the daily release of 1% of the younger RBC's reticulocytes, from the bone marrow storage pool. As erythrocytes become old, certain glycolytic enzymes decrease in activity, resulting in a decrease in the production of energy and loss of deformability. At a certain critical point, the RBCs are no longer able to traverse the microvasculature and are phagocytized by the RES cells. Although RES cells are located in various organs and throughout the body, those of the spleen, called *littoral cells*, are the most sensitive detectors of RBC abnormalities.[19]

Extravascular Hemolysis

Ninety percent of the destruction of senescent RBCs occurs by the process of extravascular hemolysis (Fig. 3–18). During this process, old or damaged RBCs are phagocytized by the RES cells and digested by their lysosomes. The hemoglobin molecules are disassembled and broken down into their various components. The iron recovered is salvaged and returned by the plasma protein carrier, transferrin, to the erythroid precursors in the marrow for synthesis of the new hemoglobin. Globin is broken down into amino acids and redirected to the amino acid pool of the body. Finally, the protoporphyrin ring of heme is disassembled, its alpha carbon exhaled in the form of carbon monoxide. The opened tetrapyrrole, biliverdin, is converted to bilirubin and carried by the plasma protein albumin to the liver.[12] In the liver, bilirubin is conjugated to bilirubin glucuronide and excreted along with bile into the intestines. Here it is further converted through bacterial action into urobilinogen (stercobilinogen) and excreted in the stool. A small amount of urobilinogen is reabsorbed through enterohepatic circulation, filtered by the kidneys, and excreted in small amounts in the urine. Both unconjugated (prehepatic) and conjugated (posthepatic) bilirubin can be measured in the plasma as indirect and direct bilirubin, respectively, and used to monitor the amount of hemolysis.[12]

TABLE 3–9 **Changes Occurring During Aging of RBCs**	
Increases	**Decreases**
Membrane-bound IgG	Several enzyme activities
Density	Sialic acid
Spheroidal shape	Deformability
MCHC	MCV
Internal viscosity	Phospholipid
Agglutinability	Cholesterol
Na^+	K^+
Methemoglobin	Protoporphyrin
Oxygen affinity	

MCHC = mean cell hemoglobin concentration.
MCV = mean cell volume.
Source: Garratty, G: Basic mechanisms of in vivo cell destruction. In Bell, C (ed): A Seminar in Immune-Mediated Cell Destruction. American Association of Blood Banks, 1981, with permission.

Intravascular Hemolysis

Only 5% to 10% of normal RBC destruction occurs through intravascular hemolysis (Fig. 3–19).[12] During this process, RBC breakdown occurs within the lumen of the blood vessels. The RBC ruptures, releasing hemoglobin directly into the bloodstream. The hemoglobin molecule dissociates into alpha-beta dimers and is picked up by the protein carrier, haptoglobin.[12] The haptoglobin-hemoglobin complex prevents renal excretion of hemoglobin and carries the dimers to the

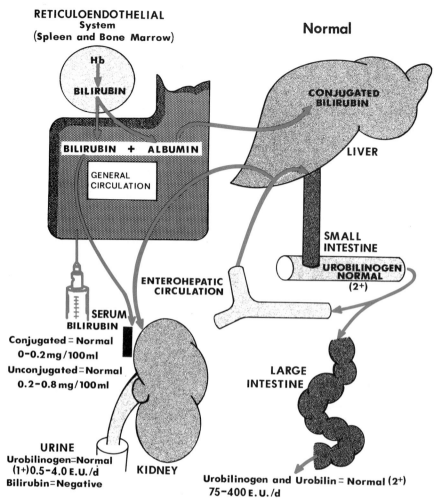

FIGURE 3–18   Normal extravascular hemolysis. (From Tietz, MW: Textbook of Clinical Chemistry. WB Saunders, Philadelphia, 1986, with permission.)

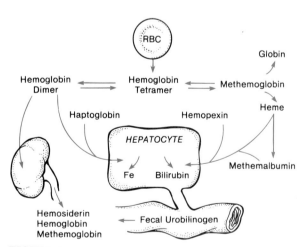

FIGURE 3–19   Intravascular hemolysis. (From Hillman, RF and Finch, CA: Red Cell Manual, ed 5. FA Davis, Philadelphia, 1985, with permission.)

liver cell for further catabolism. The hepatocyte uptake and processing are identical at this point to the process previously described for extravascular hemolysis (see Fig. 3–18). Haptoglobin levels, therefore, fall in plasma as haptoglobin is removed as the hemoglobin-haptoglobin complex. It is estimated that as little as 1 to 2 mL of RBC intravascular hemolysis can totally deplete the amount of plasma haptoglobin.[12] Normally, 50 to 200 mg/dL of plasma haptoglobin is available and represents the hemoglobin-dimer binding capacity.[12] As haptoglobin is depleted, unbound hemoglobin dimers appear in the plasma (hemoglobinemia) and are filtered through the kidneys and reabsorbed by the renal tubular cells. The renal tubular uptake capacity is approximately 5 g per day of filtered hemoglobin.[12] Beyond this level, free hemoglobin appears in the urine (hemoglobinuria).

Hemoglobinuria is always associated with hemoglobinemia. A normal plasma hemoglobin level is approximately 2 to 5 mg/dL, which is released as a result of excessive intravascular hemolysis.[12] Depending on the amount of hemolysis and type of hemoglobin, the plasma may be pink, red, or brown. Likewise, in he-

TABLE 3–10	**Protein Carriers**
Protein	**Substance Carried**
Transferrin	Iron
Haptoglobin	Hemoglobin dimers
Hemopexin	Metheme
Albumin	Billirubin

moglobinuria the urine also may be pink, red, brown, or black. Two hemoglobin pigments, oxyhemoglobin and methemoglobin, are produced by auto-oxidation of the hemoglobin in the urinary tract when the urine is acidic.[12] Oxyhemoglobin is bright red and methemoglobin is dark brown. The color of the urine, therefore, depends on the amount of hemolysis and concentration and relative proportions of these two pigments. Oxyhemoglobin predominates in alkaline urine, and methemoglobin predominates in acidic urine.

Hemoglobin that is neither processed by the kidneys nor bound to haptoglobin is oxidized to methemoglobin, which is further disassembled as metheme groups are released and globin degraded. Free metheme is quickly bound by another transport protein, hemopexin, and is carried to the liver cell to be catabolized, as previously described. The heme-binding capacity of hemopexin is approximately 50 to 100 mg/dL; when this is exceeded, the metheme groups combine with albumin to form methemalbumin.[12] Albumin cannot transfer the metheme across the membrane of the hepatocyte for subsequent degradation. As a result, the methemalbumin circulates until additional hemopexin is produced by the liver to serve as the protein carrier. It is this circulating methemalbumin that imparts a brown tinge to the plasma or blood. (Table 3–10 provides a review of the various protein carriers discussed regarding hemolysis.) Intravascular hemolysis that occurs as a result of RBC senescence is so minimal that it is limited to the involvement of only haptoglobin, which is rarely depleted. Hemoglobinemia and hemoglobinuria, as well as the other processes discussed, come into play only with excessive intravascular hemolysis, which can occur in patients having various hemolytic anemias (see Chaps. 9 through 14).

CONCLUSION

This chapter has outlined and described three important areas of RBC structure and metabolism: the red cell membrane, hemoglobin structure and function, and red cell metabolic pathways. An understanding of these aspects of the RBC is important to appreciating the development and pathogenesis of the many forms of inherited and acquired RBC defects that result in hemolytic anemias.

REFERENCES

1. Mohandas, N and Chasis, JA: Red blood cell deformability, membrane material properties and shape: Regulation by transmembrane, skeletal and cytosolic proteins and lipids. Semin Hematol 30:171–192, 1993.
2. Mohandas, N and Evans, E: Mechanical properties of the red cell membrane in relation to molecular structure and genetic defects. Ann Rev Biophys Biomol Struct 23:787–818, 1994.
3. Lui, SC and Derick, LH: Molecular anatomy of the red blood cell membrane skeleton: Structure-function relationships. Semin Hematol 29:231–243, 1992.
4. Gallagher, PG and Forget, BG: Spectrin genes in health and disease. Semin Hematol 30:4–21, 1993.
5. Mohandas, N, Winardi, R, Knowles, D, et al: Molecular basis for membrane rigidity of hereditary ovalocytosis: A novel mechanism involving the cytoplasmic domain of band 3. J Clin Invest 89:686–692, 1992.
6. Schofield, AE, Tanner, MJA, Pinder, JC, et al: Basis of unique red cell membrane properties in hereditary ovalocytosis. J Mol Biol 223:949–958, 1992.
7. Derick, LH, Liu, SC, Chishti, AH, et al: Protein immunolocalization in the spread erythrocyte membrane skeleton. Eur J Cell Biol 57:317–320, 1992.
8. Cohen, CM and Gascard, P: Regulation and post-translated modification of erythrocyte membrane and membrane-skeletal proteins. Semin Hematol 29:244–292, 1992.
9. Maeda, N, Nakajima T, Izumida, Y, et al: Decreased deformability of red cells in refractory anemia and the abnormality of the membrane skeleton. Biorheology 31:395–405, 1994.
10. Bunn, HF: Hemoglobin structure, function and assembly. In Embury, SH, Hebbel, RP, Mohandas, N, and Steinberg, MH (eds): Sickle Cell Disease: Basic Principles and Clinical Practice. Raven Press, New York, 1994.
11. Hillman, RS and Finch, CA: Red Cell Manual, ed 6. FA Davis, Philadelphia, 1994.
12. Burtis, CA and Ashwood, ER: Tietz Textbook of Clinical Chemistry, ed 2. WB Saunders, Philadelphia, 1994.
13. Adas, IZ: Heme production in animal tissues: The regulation of biogenesis of δ-aminolevulinate synthase. Int J Biochem 22:565, 1990.
14. Warren, MJ and Scott, AI: Tetrapyrrole assembly and modification into the ligands of biologically functional cofactors. Trends Biochem Sci 15:486, 1990.
15. van Pelt, J, Verheesen, PE, and van Oosterhout, AGM: Interference of dipyridamole in the analysis of porphyrins by HPLC. Ann Clin Biochem 29:347–348, 1992.
16. Straka, JG, Hill, HD, Krikava, JM, et al: Immunochemical studies of ferrochelatase protein: Characterization of the normal and mutant protein in bovine and human protoporphyria. Am J Hum Genet 48:72–78, 1991.
17. Williams, WJ, Beutler, E, Erslev, AJ, et al: Hematology, ed 5. McGraw-Hill, New York, 1995.
18. Green, R and DeLoach, JR: Resealed erythrocytes as carriers and bioreactors. Proceedings of the Third International Meeting held at the Gwinn Estate, Cleveland, OH, Pergamon Press, New York, 1991.
19. Cotran, RS, Kumar, V, Robbins, SL, et al: Robbins' Pathologic Basis of Disease, ed 5. WB Saunders, Philadelphia, 1994.

QUESTIONS

1. Which of the following is not a crucial area of RBC survival and function?
   a. Integrity of RBC cellular membrane
   b. Cell metabolism
   c. Intravascular hemolysis
   d. Hemoglobin structure

2. Which abnormal RBC is not caused by a structural membrane defect?
   a. Spherocytes
   b. Target cells
   c. Siderocytes
   d. Acanthocytes

3. Which list represents the complete set of processes necessary for normal hemoglobin production?
   a. Iron delivery and supply, synthesis of protoporphyrins, globin synthesis
   b. Iron salvage, synthesis of conjugated bilirubin, haptoglobin synthesis
   c. Iron accumulation, synthesis of hemoplexin, globin catabolism
   d. Iron catabolism, synthesis of uroporphyrinogen, ferritin synthesis

4. What is the correct list for the number and type of globin chains in normal adult hemoglobin?
   a. 4 alpha, 2 beta, 2 delta chains
   b. 2 alpha, 2 nonalpha chains
   c. 2 alpha, 4 beta, 1 delta, and 1 epsilon chain
   d. 4 alpha, 2 beta, 2 delta, and 1 epsilon chain

5. What is the composition of normal adult hemoglobin?
   a. 92–95% HbA; 5–8% HbA$_2$; 1–2% HbF
   b. 90–92% HbA; 2–3% HbA$_2$; 2–5% HbF
   c. 80–85% HbA; 2–3% HbA$_2$; 1–2% HbF
   d. 95–97% HbA; 2–3% HbA$_2$; 1–2% HbF

6. Which of the following cells is caused by iron accumulation?
   a. Acanthocyte
   b. Ringed sideroblast
   c. Burr cell
   d. Bite cell

7. Which of the following is a complete list of abnormal hemoglobins that are unable to transport or deliver oxygen?
   a. Carboxyhemoglobin and methemoglobin
   b. Methemoglobin and fetal hemoglobin
   c. Carboxyhemoglobin, sulfhemoglobin, and fetal hemoglobin
   d. Carboxyhemoglobin, methemoglobin, and sulfhemoglobin

8. Which metabolic pathway generates 90% of the ATP needed by RBCs?
   a. Methemoglobin reductase pathway
   b. Hexose monophosphate shunt
   c. Embden-Meyerhoff pathway
   d. Leubering-Rapoport shunt

9. What steps occur in the extravascular breakdown of senescent RBCs?
   a. RES cells phagocytize red cells; iron is coupled to transferrin and returned to marrow; globin is returned to amino acid pool; biliverdin is converted to bilirubin; bilirubin is coupled to albumin and transported to liver; bilirubin glucuronide is converted to urobilinogen and excreted.
   b. RBCs break down in lumen of vessel; haptoglobin-hemoglobin complex goes to liver; unbound hemoglobin dimers are excreted through kidney as hemosiderin, hemoglobin, or methemoglobin; haptoglobin is broken down to be excreted as urobilinogen.
   c. RES cells phagocytize red cells; iron is coupled to transferrin and returned to marrow; globin is returned to amino acid pool; haptoglobin-hemoglobin complex goes to liver; unbound hemoglobin dimers are excreted through kidney as hemosiderin, hemoglobin, or methemoglobin; haptoglobin is broken down to be excreted as urobilinogen.
   d. RBCs break down in lumen of vessel; haptoglobin picks up dissociated hemoglobin; haptoglobin-hemoglobin complex goes to liver; biliverdin is converted to bilirubin; bilirubin is coupled to albumin and transported to liver; bilirubin glucuronide is converted to urobilinogen and excreted.

10. What steps occur in the intravascular breakdown of senescent RBCs? (Use answer choices for question 9).

ANSWERS

1. **c** (p. 54)
2. **c** (pp. 57, 58)
3. **a** (p. 60)
4. **b** (pp. 61, 62)
5. **d** (p. 62)
6. **b** (pp. 62, 63)
7. **d** (p. 64)
8. **c** (p. 65)
9. **a** (p. 67)
10. **b** (pp. 67, 68)

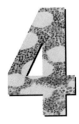

4 Anemia: Diagnosis and Clinical Considerations

Armand B. Glassman, MD

Definition of Anemia

Considerations by Age, Sex, and Other Factors

Causes of Anemia

Significance of Anemia and Compensatory Mechanisms

Clinical Diagnosis of Anemia

Classification of Anemia

Differential Diagnosis of Anemia

Overview of the Treatment of Anemias

Tests in the Diagnosis of Anemia

Summary

Patient Studies of Anemia

Objectives

At the end of this chapter, the learner should be able to:
1 Use laboratory criteria for the diagnosis of anemia.
2 List causes of anemia.
3 Describe clinical signs of anemia.
4 Explain the most common method for measuring hemoglobin.
5 Explain how the hematocrit is calculated on automated hematology instruments.
6 Calculate and state the significance of red blood cell indices as related to the diagnosis of anemia.
7 Describe the appearance of the peripheral blood smear in anemia.
8 Explain the diagnostic value of the reticuloycte count.
9 List factors to be evaluated in the interpretation of a bone marrow aspirate smear.

DEFINITION OF ANEMIA

Anemia in its broadest sense is the inability of the blood to supply the tissue with adequate oxygen for proper metabolic function.[1] Clinically, the diagnosis of anemia is made by patient history, physical examination, signs and symptoms, and hematologic laboratory findings. Determining the specific cause of an anemia is important to the physician in applying to the specific patient the appropriate therapy and prognosis related to the natural history of the disease. Anemia is usually associated with decreased levels of hemoglobin or a decreased packed red blood cell (RBC) volume, also known as the *hematocrit*. Under rare circumstances, certain abnormal hemoglobins have very strong oxygen-binding capacities, or oxygen is not released nor-

mally to tissue, resulting in all the clinical signs and symptoms of anemia even though the hemoglobin or hematocrit value is normal or even raised. From a practical laboratory standpoint, however, the usual diagnostic criteria for anemia are decreased hemoglobin (Hgb), hematocrit (Hct), or RBC count.[2]

Because most patients with anemia have lowered hemoglobin levels, the anemia may be classified arbitrarily as either moderate (7 to 10 g of hemoglobin per deciliter) or severe (less than 7 g of hemoglobin per deciliter). Moderate anemias do not usually produce clinically evident signs or symptoms, especially if the onset is slow. However, depending on the patient's age or cardiovascular condition, even moderate amounts of anemia may be associated with exertional dyspnea (difficulty breathing), lightheadedness, vertigo, muscle weakness, headache, or general lethargy. Anemia of rapid onset, such as that resulting from gastrointestinal hemorrhage, may be associated with significant clinical symptoms such as hypotension, tachycardia, and dyspnea. These symptoms are usually associated with the precipitous loss of intravascular volume as well as the oxygen-carrying capacity of the RBCs.

CONSIDERATIONS BY AGE, SEX, AND OTHER FACTORS

Newborn infants (less than 1 week old) have a hemoglobin of 18 ± 4 g/dL as a reference range. At approximately 6 months of age, the reference range is 12.5 ± 1.5 g/dL. Childhood levels from the ages of 1 to 15 years have a reference range of approximately 13.0 ± 2 g/dL. Adult hemoglobin reference ranges are approximately 15.0 ± 2 g/dL for men and 14.0 ± 2 g/dL for women (Table 4–1). In the geriatric age group, the difference between the hemoglobin levels of men and women narrows. Hemoglobin levels of geriatric men usually decrease slightly and those of postmenopausal women approach those of men. The reference ranges of each laboratory should be obtained because they best reflect the patient population served.

Many other factors, including geographic elevation, influence individual "normal" hemoglobin levels. Persons living at elevations above 8000 feet may have persistently increased hemoglobin values secondary to decreased oxygen saturation in the ambient atmosphere. Lung diseases may alter oxygen diffusion at the lung alveolar membranes. A compensatory sequence to chronic lung disease may result in increased hemoglobin levels (secondary polycythemia).

Various other diseases and disorders are associated with lower-than-usual hemoglobin levels; these include nutritional deficiencies; external or internal blood loss; accelerated destruction of RBCs; ineffective or decreased production of RBCs; abnormal hemoglobin synthesis; bone marrow replacement by infection or tumor; and bone marrow suppression by toxins, chemicals, or radiation.[3]

CAUSES OF ANEMIA

Anemia has many causes (Table 4–2). These can be broadly classified as nutritional deficiency (e.g., folate

TABLE 4–2 **Categories of Anemia by Cause**
Blood loss (hemorrhage)
Accelerated destruction of RBCs (immune and nonimmune hemolytic)
Nutritional deficiency (folate or B_{12})
Bone marrow replacement (e.g., by cancer)
Infection
Toxicity
Hematopoietic stem cell arrest or damage
Hereditary or acquired defect
Unknown

or B_{12} deficiencies), blood loss (hemorrhage), accelerated destruction of RBCs (immune and nonimmune hemolysis), bone marrow replacement (e.g., by cancer), infection, toxicity, hematopoietic stem cell arrest or damage, and hereditary or acquired defect. Categories may be simplified to embrace conditions of increased RBC destruction, abnormal or decreased production, or some combination thereof.[2,4]

SIGNIFICANCE OF ANEMIA AND COMPENSATORY MECHANISMS

RBC and Hemoglobin Production

In a healthy ambulatory person, approximately 1% of the senescent circulating RBCs are lost daily. Normally, the bone marrow continues to produce RBCs. A laboratory measure of this replacement is the reticulocyte count. In healthy people, reticulocytes, early circulating RBCs containing residual ribonucleic acid (RNA), account for 0.5% to 1.5% of the circulating RBCs. Replacement of RBCs requires a bone marrow with adequate functioning stem cells, normal RBC maturation processes, and the ability to release mature RBCs from the bone marrow. Proper hemoglobin and RBC production requires a variety of nutritional factors, including iron, vitamin B_{12}, and folic acid, and normal hemoglobin synthesis pathways. The role of hemoglobin synthesis in anemias is covered in greater detail in the chapter on hemoglobinopathies (see Chap. 11).

In severe anemias (less than 7 g hemoglobin per deciliter), symptoms of functional impairment of a number of organ systems may be evident. With minimal exercise, the patient's cardiac and respiratory rates may increase dramatically. If the anemia is secondary to blood loss and decreased intravascular volume, the patient's blood pressure may drop significantly when he or she is raised from reclining to a sitting or standing position. The heart rate will increase to elevate the cardiac output to keep pace with peripheral tissue oxygen demands in the face of a decreased oxygen-carrying capacity of the lowered hemoglobin level. Respiratory symptoms, including dyspnea on exertion, may also occur with anemia.

An interesting compensatory mechanism to anemia that occurs is an increase in the 2,3-diphosphoglycerate (2,3-DPG) levels. This compound is a remark-

TABLE 4–1 **Reference Range Values for Hemoglobin**	
Age Group	**Hemoglobin (g/dL)**
Infants	
Newborns (<1 week old)	14.0–22.0
6 months old	11.0–14.0
Children (1–15 years old)	11.0–15.0
Adults	
Men	13.0–17.0
Women	12.0–16.0

able physiologic regulator of normal hemoglobin's oxygen-carrying capacity and tissue oxygen delivery. In the presence of 2,3-DPG, hemoglobin can more readily release the oxygen it is carrying to peripheral tissues. This enhanced release occurs regardless of pH or blood arterial oxygen level.

A normal individual responds to anemia with elevated levels of erythropoietin (Epo) (see Chap. 1). The Epo level is sometimes used as an ancillary diagnostic aid in the differential diagnosis of anemia. Epo is a hormone of approximately 31,000 daltons (d). It has a plasma half-life of between 6 and 9 hours and is produced by the peritubular complex of the kidney. In patients with anemia, Epo levels vary as a result of altered oxygen tension in the tissues of the kidney. Increased Epo production occurs when there is a decreased hemoglobin level, a hemoglobin structural problem in which oxygen is not released, or low ambient oxygen tension at high altitude. On the other hand, high oxygen levels in the kidney result in a decrease in Epo production. Recombinant Epo is now available for treatment of certain types of anemias, particularly end-stage renal disease, anemia associated with human immunodeficiency virus, and certain other chronic disorders.[5] The bone marrow's production of new RBCs when receiving proper nutrients, vitamins, and other factors may be evaluated by the reticulocyte count.

CLINICAL DIAGNOSIS OF ANEMIA

The clinical diagnosis of anemia is made by a combination of factors including patient history, physical signs, and changes in the hematologic profile. The signs and symptoms of anemia are generally nonspecific, such as fatigue and weakness, and may include gastrointestinal symptoms such as nausea, constipation, or diarrhea. The patient may complain of dypsnea after a level of exertion that previously had not caused any problems.[6–9]

A patient example may be useful here. A man who had been able to climb two flights of stairs with neither difficulty nor significant shortness of breath might report that now he must stop after climbing one flight of stairs and is then very short of breath. Subsequent information indicates that the patient has passed very dark stools (melena) over the past week. Measurement of his hemoglobin reveals a level of 8 g/dL. The diagnostic impression from the clinical information is that the patient's anemia is secondary to gastrointestinal bleeding.

Physical signs of anemia are usually not specific for the underlying disease. Occasionally, however, the underlying diagnosis may be suspected from certain physical findings. One example would be signs of malnutrition and neurologic changes with loss of proprioception (position sense) and vibration awareness in a patient with vitamin B_{12} deficiency. Another example would be severe pallor, smooth tongue, and an esophageal web seen in a patient with severe iron-deficiency anemia. Light-skinned patients who are anemic may appear to have pale coloration of mucosal membranes,

nailbeds, and skin. Occasionally, the temperature may be slightly elevated, particularly in patients having certain types of hemolytic anemia. In the presence of anemia, heart murmurs may be heard; these are sometimes secondary to the cause of the anemia and sometimes related to the increased cardiac workload required to bring oxygen to the tissues. Patients with bacterial endocarditis have fever, heart murmurs, and anemia. Bacterial endocarditis is a clinical example in which the damaged myocardial valve and heart murmur are related etiologically to the anemia. Prosthetic heart valves, arterial grafts, or disseminated intravascular coagulation (DIC) can cause a form of mechanical hemolytic anemia also known as *microangiopathic hemolytic anemia.*

CLASSIFICATION OF ANEMIA

The individual types of anemias can be classified according to several different criteria. A functional classification would be hypoproliferative or accelerated destruction (hemolytic), or a combination of the two (sometimes called *ineffective hematopoiesis*). Anemias are often classified clinically according to their associated causes such as blood loss, iron deficiency, hemolysis, infection, metastatic bone marrow replacement, or nutritional deficiency. Anemias can also be categorized quantitatively by their hematocrit, hemoglobin level, blood cell indices, and/or reticulocyte count.[7–9] The clinical laboratory scientist is frequently involved in these quantitative measurements and in subsequent evaluations.

Hemoglobin and Hematocrit

Measurement of the hemoglobin level or packed cell volume is the usual method of determining whether a patient has anemia. As discussed earlier, reference ranges may vary by age, sex, state of hydration, patient positioning, and local laboratory patient population determinations (see Table 4–1). Hemoglobin assays are based on the spectrophotometric absorbance readings of cyanmethemoglobin compared with known amounts (a standard curve). Several companies manufacture automated instruments that include these determinations as part of a hematologic profile. The hematocrit, or packed red blood cell volume (PCV), is determined by centrifugation of blood of either capillary or venous origin or can be calculated on some automated instruments. The reference PCV for adult men varies by institution (i.e., 43% ± 3%). For adult women during the reproductive years, the PCV reference range is 42% ± 4%. On the basis of hemoglobin or PCV values and the duration of onset, anemias may be classified as mild, moderate, or severe and as either acute or chronic. The approximate relationship of the hemoglobin level to hematocrit is 1:3, a ratio that may vary with the cause of the anemia and the effect of that cause on the RBC indices, particularly the mean corpuscular volume (MCV).

Microscopic examination of a properly prepared peripheral blood smear is a requirement for the clinical and laboratory evaluation of anemia. This technique is discussed later under the tests in the diagnosis of anemia. Histologic examinations of the bone marrow smear and aspirate are adjuncts to further elucidate the cause of the anemia.

RBC Indices

The RBC indices are the mean corpuscular volume (MCV), mean cell hemoglobin (MCH), and mean cell hemoglobin concentration (MCHC).[10] The MCV is used as an estimation of the average size of the RBC, and may be calculated by dividing the hematocrit by the number of RBCs or measured directly using automated cell counters. If the MCV is within the reference range, the RBCs are considered normocytic; if less than normal, microcytic; and if greater than normal, macrocytic. Both MCH and MCHC values are used to determine the content of hemoglobin in RBCs. Most automated hematology instruments also provide an RBC distribution width (RDW) value. The RDW is an index of size variation and has been used to quantitate the amount of anisocytosis seen on a peripheral blood smear. The reference range for RDW is 11.5% to 14.5% for both men and women. The MCV is not dependable when RBCs vary markedly in size. If MCHC is normal, the RBCs are referred to as *normochromic*; hypochromic RBCs have a less than normal MCHC, and there are no truly hyperchromic RBCS.

RBC Indices and Other Tests

The RBC indices are accurately calculated by the automated blood-profiling machines. These instruments provide precise numeric values for hemoglobin levels, the numbers of RBCs, and the MCV. Although less precise, careful microscopic examination of a peripheral blood smear can tell the examiner whether the RBCs are normocytic, microcytic, macrocytic, normochromic, or hypochromic. A proper specimen is required to obtain accurate answers.[11] RBC index calculations and reference ranges are

1. MCV equals the Hct (%) $\times$ 10, divided by RBC count (millions/μL); reference range: 90 $\pm$ 10 fL.

$$MCV = \frac{Hct \times 10}{RBC \text{ count (millions per } \mu L)}$$

2. MCH equals the Hgb (g/dL) $\times$ 10 divided by RBC count (millions per μL); reference range: 29 $\pm$ 2 pg

$$MCH = \frac{Hgb \text{ (g/L)} \times 10}{RBC \text{ count (millions per } \mu L)}$$

3. MCHC equals the Hgb (g/dL) $\times$ 100, divided by Hct (%); reference range: 34 $\pm$ 2%

$$MCHC = \frac{Hgb \text{ (g/dL)} \times 100}{Hct \text{ (%)}}$$

Use of the RBC indices in the differential diagnosis of anemia can provide a general idea as to what is occurring clinically (Table 4–3). A normocytic-normochromic anemia may be the result of bone marrow failure, hemolytic anemia, or some subset of either of these conditions.

Making the differential diagnosis of bone marrow failure requires information about RBC production. This information can be gotten from the reticulocyte count, which indicates whether there is bone marrow capacity for increased RBC production. Since RBC destruction may exceed production, the reticulocyte count measures effective RBC production. Hemolytic anemia occurs when there is decreased RBC survival, which in turn may be the result of extravascular elimination, intravascular elimination, or a combination of the two.

Macrocytic-normochromic anemias usually occur in association with folate or vitamin B_{12} deficiency. The most commonly encountered anemias are the microcytic-hypochromic anemias, usually related to iron-deficiency anemia. Beta thalassemia, an inherited defect of hemoglobin synthesis, is another cause of microcytosis. Less frequently seen are the sideroblastic anemias, which are also associated with decreased MCV.

DIFFERENTIAL DIAGNOSIS OF ANEMIA

The differential diagnosis of anemia is based on a combination of the clinical and laboratory findings (Table 4–3). An abbreviated flowchart for the diagnosis of anemia using the RBC indices is provided in Figure 4–1.

OVERVIEW OF THE TREATMENT OF ANEMIAS

Anemia is treated according to its causes. The cause should be considered before beginning either supportive therapy (such as a transfusion) or replacement therapy. Table 4–3 and Figure 4–1 represent only some of the possible causes of anemia. Indeed, more than one cause of anemia can exist in a patient. Obtaining the proper diagnostic studies in the shortest and most cost-effective manner is the responsibility of the attending physician and the laboratory professionals. More details concerning the appropriate treatment of anemias are provided in Chapters 6 to 15.

The natural history of anemia depends on its cause. For example, a patient with an iron-deficiency anemia associated with carcinoma of the colon may present with signs of an iron-deficiency anemia associated with blood loss from the tumor. Later, with more extensive tumor involvement, the anemia may have a bone marrow failure component because of bone marrow replacement by the tumor (a myelophthisic anemia). Patients with pernicious anemia require lifelong parenteral vitamin B_{12} supplementation. Patients with other forms of megaloblastic anemia may need only a balanced diet and replacement of folic acid.[9]

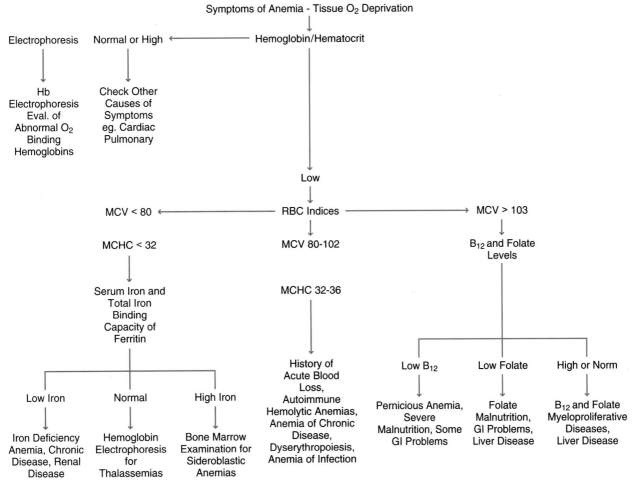

FIGURE 4–1 Anemia: abbreviated diagnostic tests and clinical possibilities.

Transfusions can obscure and confuse the findings of diagnostic tests in patients with anemia. Transfusions can suppress erythropoiesis; alter vitamin B_{12}, folate, and iron levels; and thwart the interpretation of diagnostic tests seeking the specific cause of the anemia. It is important that a diagnosis be made, if at all possible, before transfusions are given.

TESTS IN THE DIAGNOSIS OF ANEMIA

Hemoglobin

Hemoglobin is the main component of the RBC. It is the physiologic carrier of oxygen to tissues and acts as a buffer to handle carbon dioxide formed in metabolic

TABLE 4–3	**Classification of Anemia by RBC Indices**	
Size (MCV) **(μM^3 or fL)**	Hgb Content (MCHC) (g/dL)	Possible Causes
Normocytic (80–100)	Normochromic (32–36)	Bone marrow failure, hemolytic anemia, chronic renal disease, leukemia, metastatic malignancy
Macrocytic (>100)	Normochromic (32–36)	Megaloblastic and nonmegaloblastic macrocytic anemias (e.g., liver disease, myelodysplasias)
Microcytic (<80)	Hypochromic (<32)	Iron deficiency, sideroblastic anemia, thalassemia, lead poisoning, chronic diseases, chronic infection or inflammation, unstable hemoglobins

μm^3 = cubic microns

activities.[12] The three methods of measuring hemoglobin are the cyanmethemoglobin method, the oxyhemoglobin method, and the method in which iron content is measured. The cyanmethemoglobin method as modified in 1978 is recommended by the International Committee for Standardization in Hematology and will be the only one discussed. In this technique, blood is diluted in a solution of potassium ferricyanide and potassium cyanide, which oxidizes the hemoglobin to form methemoglobin. Subsequently, methemoglobin forms cyanmethemoglobin in the presence of the potassium cyanide. Because the absorption maximum occurs at wavelength 540 nm, the absorbance of the solution is read in a spectrophotometer at 540 nm and compared with a standard cyanmethemoglobin solution. The advantages of this method are that most forms of hemoglobin are measured, the sample can be directly compared with a standard, the solutions are stable, and the coefficient of variation for the method is less than 2% at physiologic ranges.

Errors in the measurement of hemoglobin can be produced by improperly drawing or handling the specimen, by poorly prepared or stored reagents, faulty equipment, or operator error.

Hematocrit

The hematocrit, or packed RBC volume, is the ratio of the volume of RBCs to the volume of whole blood. Hematocrit is usually expressed as a percentage (e.g., 42%) but is expressed in the Système International d'Unités (SI) as a decimal fraction (e.g., 0.42). The venous hematocrit agrees closely with the central blood hematocrit but is greater than the total body hematocrit. Anticoagulants—usually ethylenediaminetetraacetic acid (EDTA), oxalate, or heparin—are used to prevent the blood from clotting.

Measurement of the hematocrit may be done by centrifugation or through calculations performed on many automated hematology instruments. The calculated hematocrit is the product of the mean corpuscular volume (MCV) and the RBC count.

The adult reference range for hematocrit is 40% to 46% in men and 38% to 44% in women. Different reference ranges are required for neonates, very young children, and male and female patients, and may vary among institutions.

Problems in the measurement of the hematocrit include incorrect centrifuge calibration, choice of sample site, incorrect ratio of improper anticoagulant to blood owing to improper amount of blood drawn, and reading error—particularly for hematocrits determined after centrifugation. In our laboratory, the coefficient of variation for hematocrit, within the reference range, is approximately 2%. With centrifuge hematocrit techniques, the lower hematocrit values are associated with the higher coefficients of variation.

Red Blood Cell Indices

RBC indices were introduced previously. The MCV is the average volume, expressed in femtoliters, of RBCs, and is measured directly or calculated from the hematocrit and RBC count. The MCH is the content of hemoglobin in the average RBC. MCH is calculated from the hemoglobin concentration and the RBC count. MCHC, the average concentration of hemoglobin in a volume of packed RBCs, is calculated from the hemoglobin concentration and the hematocrit.[10]

RBC indices are readily available from the automated hematology counting devices. In devices in which the MCV is derived from the voltage changes formed during the RBC count and the hemoglobin is measured by spectrophotometric determination of the cyanmethemoglobin, the values are calculated as follows: the hemotocrit equals the MCV times the RBC count, the MCH equals the hemoglobin divided by the RBC count, and the MCHC equals the hemoglobin divided by the hematocrit. The reference range for MCV is 80 to 100 fL; for MCH it is 27 to 31 pg; and for MCHC it is 32% to 36%.

In various anemic states, the indices may be altered as follows: Microcytic anemia, from an MCV of less than 80 fL down to a low of approximately 50 fL; from an MCH of less than 25 pg to approximately 15 pg; and from an MCHC of less than 30% to 22%. In the macrocytic anemias, MCV values are usually greater than 100 fL and may be as high as, and sometimes even higher than, 120 fL; the MCHC may be normal or decreased. The MCHC may be increased only in the presence of spherocytosis, if at all.

Peripheral Blood Smear

Much information concerning the cause of an anemia can be determined from a peripheral blood smear. Coexistent neutropenia, thrombocytopenia, and anemia may indicate bone marrow failure or a lack of a nutritional substance to provide adequate bone marrow production. The size and shape of the RBCs can be noted. Alteration in size of the RBCs results in anisocytosis; alterations in their shape result in poikilocytosis. The hemoglobin (chromatic) content of the RBCs can be inspected visually on the peripheral smear. In addition, cytologic details on the peripheral smear may provide clues to the cause of the anemia, the bone marrow response, or both. The white cells may be evaluated. For example, excess lobulations of the polymorphonuclear leukocytes are seen in the hypersegmented granulocytes of macrocytic anemias (see Chap. 7).

Basophilic stippling in the RBCs may suggest the presence of increased bone marrow production and reticulocytosis (see Fig. 1–16). It may also indicate that there are remnants of ribonucleic acid (RNA), which may be associated with lead poisoning and some malignancies. Howell-Jolly bodies (see Chap. 12), which are small, round, blue inclusions seen in RBCs, are the result of leftover fragments of deoxyribonucleic acid (DNA). Howell-Jolly bodies are often seen in hyposplenism or asplenism, pernicious anemia, and some hemoglobinopathies, particularly thalassemia.[13–16] Pappenheimer bodies, which are iron-containing or siderotic granules, appear as purplish-blue granules with Wright's stain and as coarse blue granules with Prussian blue iron stain. The clinical disorders associated with Pappenheimer bodies include sideroblastic anemia, alcoholism, thalassemia, and some myelodysplastic syndromes. Nucleated RBCs with iron

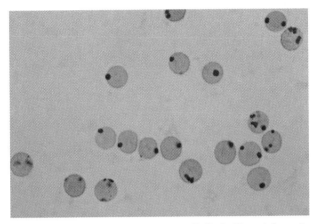

FIGURE 4-2 Heinz bodies. From Bell, A: Hematology. In Listen, Look and Learn. Health and Education Resources, Inc., Bethesda, Md., with permission.

granules are known as *sideroblasts*, and RBCs containing iron granules but without a nucleus are referred to as *siderocytes*. Ringed sideroblasts are those in which more than five granules are arranged in a ring around the nucleus of an orthochromatic normoblast (see Chap. 6, Fig. 6–8). Ringed sideroblasts are indicative of ineffective erythropoiesis.

A threadlike blue ring contained entirely within an abnormal RBC, which may or may not have a "figure-8" and a round or oval configuration, is known as a Cabot ring (see Chap. 7, Fig. 7–6). This is a remnant of the nuclear membrane. This infrequent finding may be seen in several clinical disorders, including pernicious anemia, lead poisoning, and other severe anemias. Heinz bodies (Fig. 4–2) are small, rounded, angular inclusions about 1 μm in diameter that are aggregates of denatured hemoglobin and are negative when stained with Prussian blue or other iron stains. Heinz bodies can be demonstrated only by using supravital stains (e.g., methylene blue) and are not visible with the usual Wright's stain. The clinical disorders that have been associated with Heinz bodies include glucose-6-phosphate dehydrogenase (G6PD) deficiency after exposure to oxidizing drugs, a variety of unstable hemoglobinopathies, and α thalassemia; they can also be seen after splenectomy.

Reticulocyte Count

The reticulocyte count is useful in determining the response and potential of the bone marrow. Reticulocytes are nonnucleated RBCs that still contain RNA. Reticulocytes can be visualized after incubation with a variety of so-called supravital dyes, including new methylene blue or brilliant cresyl blue (see Chap. 31). RNA is precipitated as a dye-protein complex. Reticulocytes under normal circumstances lose their RNA a day or so after reaching the bloodstream from the marrow. Reticulocyte activity can be expressed as an absolute count, a production index, or a percentage. The reference values for reticulocytes range from 0.5% to 1.5% as a percentage of all RBCs. Because anemia should be accompanied by increased bone marrow ac-

tivity, the reticulocytes should be expected to increase. One may correct the reticulocyte count for the following formula:

$$\text{Corrected reticulocyte \%} = \frac{\text{Patient PCV}}{\text{Reference PCV mean}} \times \text{Reticulocyte \%}$$

Manual reticulocyte counting is associated with poor reproducibility. In the reference range the coefficient of variation is said to be as great as 50%. Automated reticulocyte counting using fluorescent compounds and automated instruments results in better reproducibility.[2,10]

Interpretation of the reticulocyte count must take into account the age and nutritional status of the patient. Normal adults have a reticulocyte count between 0.5% and 1.5%, or from 24 to 84 $\times$ 10^9 reticulocytes per liter. The newborn infant has a higher reticulocyte count, which falls to the adult range usually by the second or third week of life. Sources of error in the reticulocyte count include sampling error resulting from counting relatively few reticulocytes in a large number of erythrocytes. The 95% confidence level when counting 100 RBCs, where the true reticulocyte count is 1%, ranges from 0.4% to 1.6%; obviously, there is a very high coefficient of variation unless large numbers of RBCs are counted. Usually 1000 cells are counted for a reticulocyte count.

Bone Marrow Smear and Biopsy

Bone marrow aspiration and biopsy are important diagnostic tools in the determination of anemia. Bone marrow interpretation and evaluation is covered in Chapter 2. Factors to be evaluated in interpretation of a bone marrow aspirate smear and biopsy include maturation of the red and white cell series, presence of megakaryocytes, ratio of myeloid to erythroid series, abundance of iron stores, presence or absence of granulomas, tumor cells, and overall estimate of bone marrow activity.

Interpretation requires a differential count of the myeloid, lymphoid, and erythroid series; an iron stain; and other appropriate techniques such as immunohistochemical stains if a differential diagnosis of lymphoproliferative or myeloproliferative disorders is being considered. Other specific stains may be indicated if metastatic tumor or infection is suspected or being evaluated.[17-19] Table 4–4 lists the other tests that may be performed in the diagnosis of anemias and the chapters in which these tests are discussed.

SUMMARY

Anemia has physiologic, functional, and quantitative parameters that may be related to hemoglobin or hematocrit levels. The differential diagnosis of anemia requires careful consideration of a wide variety of marrow, extramedullary, and interrelating disease states. A large armamentarium of tests is available to aid in the differential diagnosis of the spectrum of anemias. Successful studies of anemia require broad knowledge

TABLE 4–4   Other Tests That May Be Performed in the Diagnosis of Anemias

Test	Diagnostic Use	Chapter
Hemoglobin electrophoresis	Hemoglobinopathies Thalassemia syndromes	11, 31
Antiglobulin testing	Hemolytic anemias	14
Osmotic fragility test	Hereditary spherocytosis* Severe iron deficiency Sickle-cell disease β-thalassemia	9, 31
Sucrose hemolysis test (sugar-water test)	Paroxysmal nocturnal hemoglobinuria* Hypoplastic anemias Myelodysplastic syndromes	13, 31
Acidified serum test (Ham's test)	Paroxysmal noctural hemoglobinuria Dyserythropoietic anemia, type II	13, 31
Tests for red blood cell enzymes	Hemolytic anemias G-6-PD deficiency PK deficiency	10
Serum iron and iron-binding capacity	Iron-deficiency anemia	6
Folate and B_{12} measurements	Megaloblastic anemias	7

*Primary use
G-6-PD = glucose 6 phosphate dehydrogenose, PK = pyruvate kinase

of clinical laboratory techniques and the practice of medicine.

PATIENT STUDIES OF ANEMIA

Individual patient studies of anemia are addressed in Chapters 6 to 15.

REFERENCES

1. Beck, WS: Hematology, ed 3. MIT Press, Cambridge, MA, 1981, p 16.
2. Reiss, RF: Laboratory Diagnosis of erythroid disorders. In Tilton, RC, Balows, A, Hohnadel, DC, and Reiss, RF (eds): Clinical Laboratory Medicine. Mosby–Year Book, St Louis, 1992, pp 898–937.
3. Hoffbrand, AV, et al: Erythropoiesis and general aspects of anaemia. In Hoffbrand, AV and Pettit, JE (eds): Essential Haematology, ed 3. Blackwell Scientific, Oxford, 1993, pp 12–35.
4. Woodson, RD, et al: Introduction to hemopoiesis. In MacKinney, AA, Jr (ed): Pathophysiology of Blood. John Wiley, New York, 1984, pp 12–15.
5. Nathan, DG: Hematologic diseases. In Wyngaarden, JB, Smith, LH, and Bennett, JC (eds): Cecil Textbook of Medicine, vol 1, ed 19. WB Saunders, Philadelphia, 1992, pp 817–822.
6. Lindenbaum, J: An approach to the anemias. In Wyngaarden, JB, Smith, LH, and Bennett, JC (eds): Cecil Textbook of Medicine, vol 1, ed 19. WB Saunders, Philadelphia, 1992, pp 822–831.
7. Kushner, JP: Normochromic, normocytic anemias. In Wyngaarden, JB, Smith, LH, and Bennett, JC (eds): Cecil Textbook of Medicine, vol 1, ed 19. WB Saunders, Philadelphia, 1992, pp 837–839.
8. Kushner, JP: Hypochromic anemias. In Wyngaarden, JB, Smith, LH, and Bennett, JC (eds): Cecil Textbook of Medicine, vol 1, ed 19. WB Saunders, Philadelphia, 1992, pp 839–846.
9. Allen, RH: Megaloblastic anemias. In Wyngaarden, JB, Smith, LH, and Bennett, JC (eds): Cecil Textbook of Medicine, vol 1, ed 19. WB Saunders, Philadelphia, 1992, pp 846–856.
10. Savage, RA, et al: The red cell indices: Yesterday, today and tomorrow. Clin Lab Med, Routine Hematologic Testing 13:773–785, 1993.
11. Jones, BA, et al: Complete blood count specimen acceptability. A College of American Pathologists Q-probes study of 703 laboratories. Arch Pathol Lab Med 119:203–208, 1995.
12. Benz, EJ: Structure, function, and synthesis of the human hemoglobins. In Wyngaarden, JB, Smith, LH, and Bennett, JC (eds): Cecil Textbook of Medicine, vol 1, ed 19. WB Saunders, Philadelphia, 1992, pp 872–877.
13. Benz, EJ: Classification and basic pathophysiology of the hemoglobinopathies. In Wyngaarden, JB, Smith, LH, and Bennett, JC (eds): Cecil Textbook of Medicine, vol 1, ed 19. WB Saunders, Philadelphia, 1992, pp 877–879.
14. Benz, EJ: Hemoglobinopathies with altered solubility or oxygen affinity. In Wyngaarden, JB, Smith, LH, and Bennett, JC (eds): Cecil Textbook of Medicine, vol 1, ed 19. WB Saunders, Philadelphia, 1992, pp 879–883.
15. Nienhuis, AW: The thalassemias. In Wyngaarden, JB, Smith, LH, and Bennett, JC (eds): Cecil Textbook of Medicine, vol 1, ed 19. WB Saunders, Philadelphia, 1992, pp 883–888.
16. Forget, BG: Sickle cell anemia and associated hemoglobinopathies. In Wyngaarden, JB, Smith, LH, and Bennett, JC (eds): Cecil Textbook of Medicine, vol 1, ed 19. WB Saunders, Philadelphia, 1992, pp 888–893.
17. Brunning, RD and McKenna, RW: Atlas of Tumor Pathology. Tumors of the Bone Marrow. Armed Forces Institute of Pathology, Washington DC, 1994, p 496.
18. Young, NS: Aplastic anemia and related bone marrow failure syndromes. In Wyngaarden, JB, Smith, LH, and Bennett, JC (eds): Cecil Textbook of Medicine, vol 1, ed 19. WB Saunders, Philadelphia, 1992, pp 831–837.
19. Ross, DW: Laboratory evaluation of the patient with hematologic disease. In Bick, RL, et al (eds): Hematology. Clinical and Laboratory Practice, vol I. Mosby–Year Book, St Louis, 1993, pp 7–16.

QUESTIONS

1. Which of the following laboratory results would not be a usual diagnostic criterion for a patient with anemia?
   a. Decreased hemoglobin level
   b. Decreased hematocrit level
   c. Decreased platelet count
   d. Decreased RBC count

2. What condition is not a cause of anemia?
   a. Dietary deficiency
   b. Moderate exercise
   c. Decreased RBC production
   d. Increased RBC destruction or loss

3. Which response represents the most complete and correct listing of the most common clinical signs of anemia?
   a. Fatigue, weakness, gastrointestinal symptoms, dypsnea, pallor
   b. Urticaria, hypertension, inflammation, nausea
   c. Nausea, hypertension, temperature elevation, melena
   d. Rapid pulse, inflammation, temperature elevation, dehydration

4. What is the most commonly accepted method of measuring hemoglobin?
   a. Conversion of hemoglobin to oxyhemoglobin, followed by spectrophotometric measurement
   b. Iron content measured by RIA technique
   c. Copper sulfate measured by specific gravity
   d. Conversion of hemoglobin to cyanmethemoglobin followed by spectrophotometric measurement.

5. How is hematocrit determined on automated hematology instruments?
   a. Centrifugation
   b. Photometrically
   c. Calculation (MCV × RBC count)
   d. Calculation (MCH × Hgb)

6. A patient has the following results: Hct 26%; Hgb 8 g/dL; and RBC count $3.5 \times 10^6/\mu L$. Calculate the RBC indices—MCV, MCH, and MCHC—and determine the classification of the anemia.
   a. MCV 88 m³; MCH 30 pg; MCHC 33 g/dL; normocytic, normochromic
   b. MCV 101 m³; MCH 33 pg; MCHC 35 g/dL; macrocytic, normochromic
   c. MCV 74 m³; MCH 22 pg; MCHC 31 g/dL; microcytic, hypochromic

7. Which of the following would not be characteristically found on a peripheral blood smear in a case of anemia?
   a. Anisocytosis and/or poikilocytosis
   b. Basophilic stippling, Howell-Jolly bodies, and Pappenheimer bodies
   c. Cabot rings and Heinz bodies
   d. Rouleaux and Döhle bodies

8. What is the diagnostic value of the reticulocyte count in the evaluation of anemia?
   a. Determines response and potential of the bone marrow
   b. Determines compensation mechanisms for anemia
   c. Determines the corrected RBC count after calculation
   d. Determines the potential sampling error for RBC count

9. Which of the following is not a factor to be evaluated in the interpretation of a bone marrow aspirate smear?
   a. Maturation of red and white blood cell series
   b. M:E ratio
   c. Type and amount of hemoglobin
   d. Estimate of bone marrow activity

ANSWERS

1. **c** (p. 71)
2. **b** (p. 72)
3. **a** (p. 73)
4. **d** (p. 73)
5. **c** (p. 74)
6. **c** (p. 74)
7. **d** (pp. 76, 77)
8. **a** (p. 77)
9. **c** (p. 78)

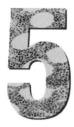

Morphological Changes Associated with Disease

Betty E. Ciesla, MS, MT(ASCP)SH

Objectives

At the end of this chapter, the learner should be able to:

1 Define *anisocytosis* and *poikilocytosis*.
2 List the clinical conditions in which a variable red cell size is observed.
3 Define the terms *normochromic* and *hypochromic* according to red cell indices.
4 Name and describe the clinical disorders that result in hypochromia.
5 Describe the clinical conditions that may produce polychromatophilic cells.
6 Indicate which clinical conditions may show target cells, spherocytes, ovalocytes, elliptocytes, and stomatocytes.
7 List diseases that may show fragmented red cells and describe their pathophysiology.
8 Discuss agglutination and rouleaux and specify the particular clinical conditions associated with these abnormalities.
9 Describe the most common red blood inclusions and relate each inclusion to a clinical condition.
10 Describe normal platelet morphology and specify some platelet abnormalities seen in pathologic conditions.

Automation has distinctly modified the responsibilities of staff technologists in hematology laboratories. Ten years ago there were *no* automated leukocyte differential instruments. Presently, more than 20 manufacturers offer this type of technology. More than any other hematologic innovation, this technology has shifted work patterns. Less and less time is spent reviewing blood smears, since according to the flagging codes of most automated instruments, only those samples with quantitative abnormalities and some qualitative abnormalities are "flagged" (held out for a manual review). This practice has significant implications for educators and practitioners of hematology.

From the educational perspective, it is essential that

we train our students to recognize cellular abnormalities, because most of the blood smears that they review will be abnormal. From the practitioner's perspective, students graduating from most programs will be unfamiliar with operator responsibilities and flagging codes delineated by automated differential instruments, since these criteria vary from manufacturer to manufacturer. Because of the high cost of purchasing automated differential instruments, few hematology programs will have the luxury of owning automated cell equipment and subsequently training their students on it. The easy and natural progression from student lab to training or clinical affiliate lab will be lost. Training at the laboratory site will need to include com-

TABLE 5–1	Grading Scale for Anisocytosis and Poikilocytosis

Normal = 5% of cells differ in size or shape from normal red cell
Slight = 5%–10% of cells differ in size or shape from normal red cell
1+ = 10%–25% of cells differ in size or shape from normal red cell
2+ = 25%–50% of cells differ in size or shape from normal red cell
3+ = 50%–75% of cells differ in size or shape from normal red cell
4+ = >75% of cells differ in size or shape from normal red cell
At the level of 4+ the suffix "-cytosis," rather than numerical grading, is acceptable.

Sample Situations

2+ microcytes	Few schistocytes
1+ macrocytes	Few burr cells
3+ anisocytosis	1+ target cells
	2+ poikilocytosis

prehensive and detailed training on automated instruments.

This chapter will guide the student in interpretation of red cell, white cell, and platelet morphology. Basic mechanics in assessing morphology will be reviewed (Table 5–1); however, the emphasis will be on recognizing a distinct morphology and relating it to the clinical condition. *Physiologic mechanisms* will be explained for each morphology to give the reader a better understanding of a particular cellular structure. This description of blood cell morphology will maximize the ability of each slide reviewer to recognize and correlate the blood morphology to the clinical pathology.

THE NORMAL RED BLOOD CELL

The mature erythrocyte (red blood cell, normocyte) is a remarkable structure. Its simplistic appearance is deceiving. It is one of the few cells that pass from a nucleated to a nonnucleated status upon maturity, with decreasing size and a dramatic change in cytoplasmic color. On a Wright-stained blood smear, this mature red cell has a reddish-orange appearance.

The average diameter of the red cell is from 6.0 to 8.0 μm, and the average volume is 90 fL. The area of central pallor is approximately 2 to 3 μm in diameter (Fig.

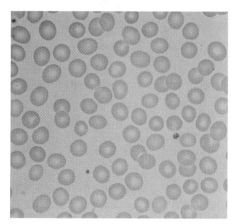

FIGURE 5–1 Normal red blood cell morphology.

5–1). In the average patient, red cells vary in size over a range of about 5%. As a rule of thumb, the normal red blood cell (RBC) is about the same size as a small lymphocyte (e.g., see Fig. 1–39).

The fundamental purpose of the RBC is the formation of hemoglobin, which functions primarily as the oxygen-carrying component of the cell. Additionally, a minimum amount of hemoglobin is required for maintenance of structural integrity. The red cell membrane is a lipid bilayer whose skeleton is composed of glycophorin and spectrin. Glycophorin, an integral red cell membrane protein, spans the entire diameter of the red cell membrane and contains most of the membrane sialic acid, upon which many red cell antigens are located. Spectrin, the dominant peripheral membrane protein, consists of two high-molecular-weight polypeptides and functions prominently in the maintenance of cell shape and deformability.

ASSESSMENT OF RED CELL ABNORMALITY

A well-stained and well-distributed blood smear is essential for any peripheral blood smear review. When inspecting a blood smear for abnormal morphology, two criteria must be met:

1. Is the abnormal morphology seen in every field to be examined?
2. Is the morphology pathologic and not artificially induced?

If these criteria are met, then the reviewer must make an assessment of anisocytosis and poikilocytosis. By definition, anisocytosis implies a variation in size of erythrocytes *(from the normal red cell size)*. Most assessments of anisocytosis are done in concert with the red cell indices and the red cell distribution width (RDW) rating. The RDW is a measure of the variation in the red cell volume distribution. The normal value for RDW is 11.5% to 14.5%, and this value is calculated by dividing the standard deviation of the red cell population by its mean. An increased value in this parameter may indicate anisocytosis resulting from a heterogeneous population of cells and also may indicate that poikilocytosis is present.

In scanning a peripheral smear, a reviewer takes into account the percentage of cells that vary in size in at

RED BLOOD CELL MORPHOLOGY

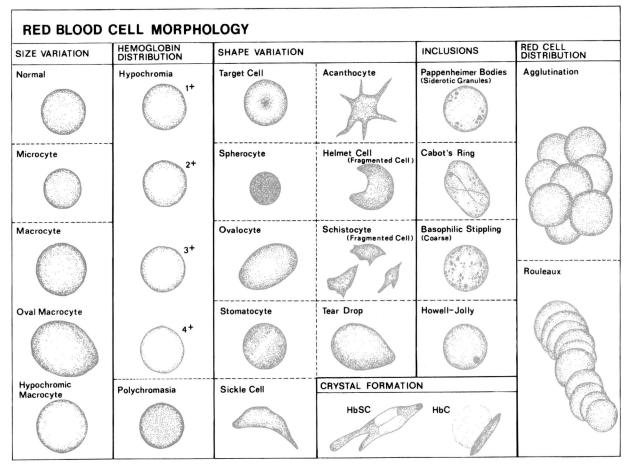

FIGURE 5-2 Normal and abnormal red blood cell morphology.

least ten oil immersion fields. For example, if the MCV is 65 fL, the reviewer would expect to see a majority of small cells. If, however, the MCV is 80 with a high RDW rating (normal RDW 11.5% to 14.5%), the reviewer would expect to see a mixture of large and small cells.

Poikilocytosis, on the other hand, implies a variation from the normal red cell shape. Most institutions use either qualitative remarks (few or marked) or a numerical grading (1+ to 4+) based upon percentage of variation to describe anisocytosis and poikilocytosis. Once an anisocytosis or poikilocytosis rating has been assigned, that rating is validated by observing and recording the *type of cell or cells* that have caused the variation from the normal. Using this method, a reviewer can present to the clinician a series of objective ratings that can translate to a visual impression of a patient's peripheral smear. See Table 5–1 for guidelines in grading anisocytosis and poikilocytosis. Figure 5–2 is a composite chart of abnormal red cell morphology.

Included in this chapter are flowcharts correlating the abnormal morphology with a possible pathology. This scheme should enable the learner to more easily associate an abnormal morphology to the clinical condition.

SIZE VARIATIONS

Macrocyte

Macrocytes may be defined as cells approximately 9 μm or larger in diameter, having an MCV of greater than 100 fL. They may arrive in the peripheral circulation by several mechanisms. Three of the most distinct are:

1. Impaired DNA synthesis leading to a decreased number of cellular divisions, consequently a larger cell (megaloblastic erythropoiesis).
2. Accelerated erythropoiesis yielding a premature release of reticulocytes. In the Wright-stained smear this is manifested as polychromatophilic macrocytes.
3. In conditions where membrane cholesterol and lecithin levels are increased; however, this mechanism may not be reflective of a "true" macrocytosis (obstructive liver disease).

Macrocytes should be evaluated for shape (oval vs. round, Fig. 5–3), color (red vs. blue), pallor (if present), and the presence or absence of inclusions.

Figure 5–4 lists the more common conditions in which macrocytes may be seen: the megaloblastic pro-

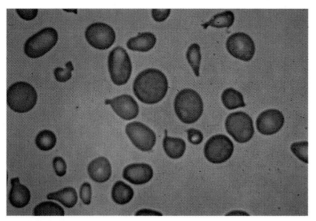

FIGURE 5-3 Extreme degree of anisocytosis (+ 4) and poikilocytosis (+ 3) with oval macrocytosis in a case of severe pernicious anemia.

cesses, liver disease, and regenerative bone marrow. Additionally, macrocytic cells may be seen in metastatic marrow infiltration, neonatal blood, and hypothyroidism.

Microcyte

A microcyte is defined as a small cell having a diameter of less than 7 μm and an MCV of less than 80F fL. See Figure 20–7F for an example of microcytic RBCs in relation to a normal lymphocyte. Any defect that results in impaired hemoglobin synthesis will result in a microcytic, hypochromic blood picture. When developing erythroid cells are deprived of any of the "essentials" in hemoglobin synthesis (see Chap. 6), the result is increased cellular divisions, consequently a smaller cell in the peripheral blood. Hemoglobin synthesis involves multiple steps and microcytosis develops from: (1) ineffective iron utilization, absorption, or release; and (2) decreased or defective globin synthesis. Effective porphyrin synthesis is, of course, vital for hemoglobinization; however, the porphyrias generally do not cause a microcytic erythrocyte. Figure 5–5 shows the clinical conditions in which microcytes may be seen as the predominant cell morphology.

STAIN VARIATIONS

Hypochromia

Any RBC having a central area of pallor of greater than 3 μm is said to be hypochromic. There is a direct relationship between the amount of hemoglobin deposited in the red cell and the appearance of the red cell when properly stained. For this reason, any irregularity in hemoglobin synthesis will lead to some degree of hypochromia. Most clinicians choose to assess hypochromia based on the MCHC (mean corpuscular hemoglobin content), which by definition measures hemoglobin content in a given volume of red cells (100 mL). In general, this is very reliable; however, it does not take into account the situation when a true hypochromia is observed in the presence of a normal MCHC. It is sufficient to say that not all hypochromic cells are microcytic. Target cells possess some degree

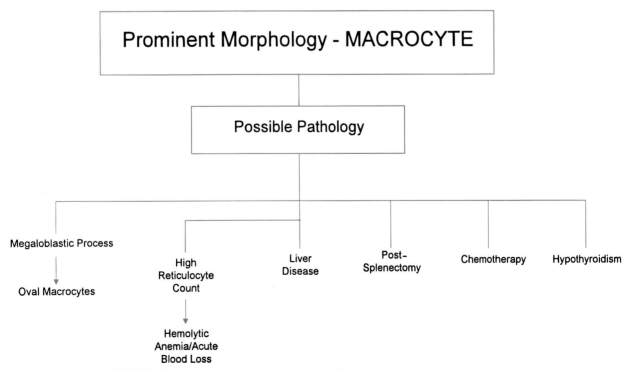

FIGURE 5-4 Correlation of the presence of macrocytes to pathologic processes.

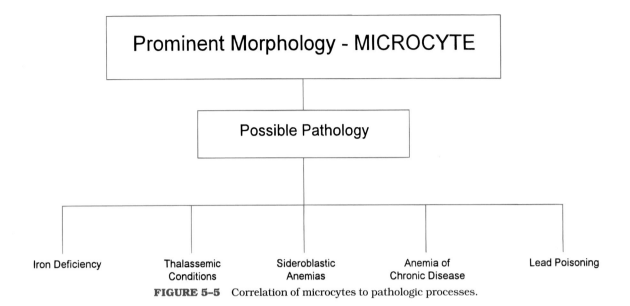

FIGURE 5–5   Correlation of microcytes to pathologic processes.

of hypochromia, and some macrocytes and normocytes can be distinctly hypochromic.

Peripheral Blood Observations

The most common and severe changes manifesting hypochromia are seen in patients with iron-deficiency anemia. In severe cases of iron-deficiency anemia, red cells exhibit an inordinately thin band of hemoglobin. Patients with iron deficiency have many hypochromic cells, depending on the magnitude of the deficiency. Hypochromia in thalassemia syndromes is much less pronounced. In the alpha thalassemias and beta-thalassemia trait, the MCHC is normal. The sideroblastic anemias show a prominent dimorphic blood picture—macrocytic, normocytic, and microcytic cells together, only some of which show genuine hypochromia. Some hypochromic cells can be seen in victims of lead poisoning; however, the association of microcytosis with lead poisoning irrespective of any other underlying process is being questioned. The morphologist should not be unduly influenced by the RBC indices in the evaluation of hypochromia. In many cases, the MCHC will not be concordant with what is observed on the peripheral smear. True hypochromia will appear as a delicate shaded area of pallor as opposed to pseudo-hypochromia (the water artifact), in which the area of pallor will be distinctly outlined (see Fig. 6–9). Table 5–2 lists the guidelines for grading hypochromia.

Polychromasia

When RBCs are delivered to the peripheral circulation prematurely, their appearance in the Wright-stained smear is distinctive. Red cells showing polychromatophilia are gray-blue in color and are usually larger than normal red cells. The basophilia of the red cell is the result of the residual RNA involved in hemoglobin synthesis. Polychromatophilic macrocytes are actually reticulocytes; however, the reticulum cannot be visualized without supravital staining (see Fig. 1–16).

Peripheral Blood Observations

It is not uncommon to find a few polychromatophilic cells in a normal peripheral blood smear, since regeneration of red cells is a dynamic process. The reticulocyte count should reflect the degree of polychromasia (normal adult value, 0.5 to 2.5%). In the blood smear, polychromatophilic red cells come in varying shades of blue. Any clinical condition in which the marrow is stimulated, particularly RBC regeneration, will produce a polychromatophilic blood picture, and the reticulocyte count should be increased proportionately. This represents effective erythropoiesis. Examples of several conditions in which polychromasia is noted include acute and chronic hemorrhage, hemolysis, and any regenerative red cell process. The degree of polychromasia is an excellent indicator of therapeutic ef-

TABLE 5–2   **Hypochromia Grading**
1+ = area of central pallor is ½ of cell diameter
2+ = area of central pallor is ⅔ of cell diameter
3+ = area of central pallor is ¾ of cell diameter
4+ = thin rim of hemoglobin

TABLE 5–3   **Polychromatophilia Grading**
Slight = 1% of red cells are polychromatophilic
1+ = 3% of red cells are polychromatophilic
2+ = 5% of red cells are polychromatophilic
3+ = 10% of red cells are polychromatophilic
4+ = >11% of red cells are polychromatophilic

fectiveness when a patient is given iron or vitamin therapy as a treatment for his or her anemia. Table 5–3 lists guidelines for polychromasia grading.

SHAPE VARIATIONS

Target Cells (Codocytes)

Target cells appear in the peripheral blood as a result of increase in red cell surface membrane or decreased intracellular hemoglobin. Their true circulating form is a bell-shaped cell. In air-dried smears, however, they appear as "targets" with a large portion of hemoglobin displayed at the rim of the cell and a portion of hemoglobin either central, eccentric, or banded (Fig. 5–6). Target cells are always hypochromic.

The mechanism of targeting is related to excess membrane cholesterol and phospholipid and decreased cellular hemoglobin. This is well documented in patients with liver disease in which the cholesterol-phospholipid ratio is altered. Mature red cells are unable to synthesize cholesterol and phospholipid independently. As cholesterol accumulates in the plasma, as is the case with liver dysfunction, the red cell is expanded by increased membrane lipid, resulting in increased surface area. Consequently, the osmotic fragility is also decreased. Figure 5–7 shows the more common conditions in which target cells are observed.

Spherocytes

Spherocytes (see Chap. 9) have several distinctive properties and, in contrast to the target cell, the lowest surface area–volume ratio. They appear smaller than the normal red cell and their hemoglobin content

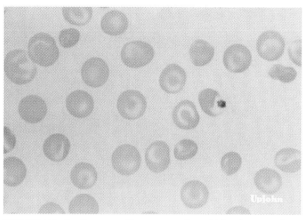

FIGURE 5–6 Target cells in a peripheral blood smear from a patient with liver disease.

seems to be relatively concentrated. Because there is no visible central pallor, they are easily distinguished in a peripheral smear. Their shape change is irreversible. There are several mechanisms for the production of spherocytes, each sharing the mutual defect of loss of membrane. In the normal aging process of red cells, spherocytes are produced as a final stage before senescent red cells are detained in the spleen and trapped by the reticuloendothelial system. Red cells coated with antibodies become spherocytes as the red cell membrane loses cholesterol and surface area as a result of splenic sequestration.

Perhaps the most detailed mechanism for sphering is the congenital condition known as *hereditary spherocytosis*. This condition is inherited as an autosomal dominant trait and it is an intrinsic defect in the red

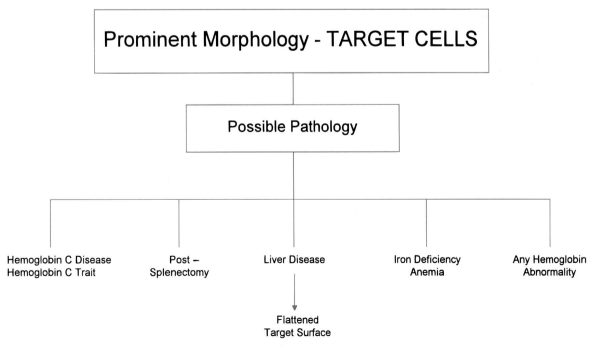

FIGURE 5–7 Correlation of target cells to pathologic processes.

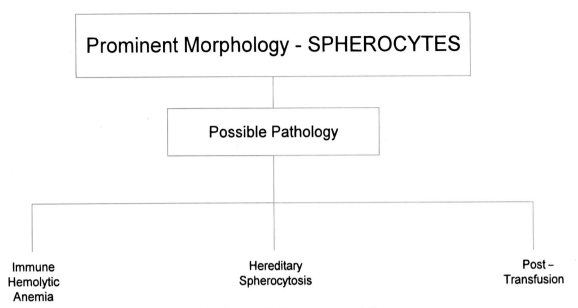

FIGURE 5-8 Correlation of spherocytes to pathologic processes.

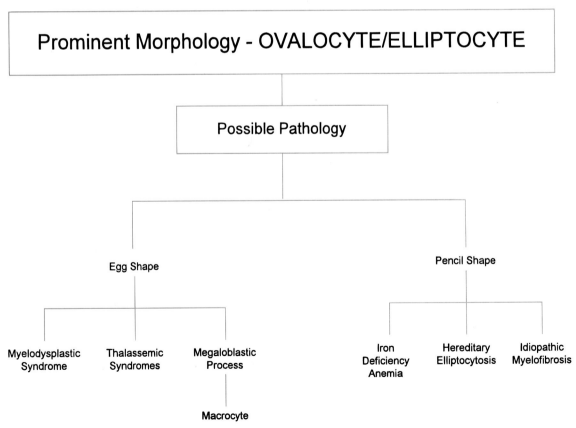

FIGURE 5-9 Correlation of ovalocytes/elliptocytes to pathologic processes.

cell membrane that causes the spheroidal red cell to be prematurely trapped and destroyed in the spleen. Erythrocytes from patients with hereditary spherocytosis have a mean influx of sodium twice that of normal cells. It is thought that this increased permeability to sodium results from some sort of membrane "lesion." As these cells travel through plasma, they are able to handle their increased sodium content because it has been documented that spherocytes have 35 times the ability to metabolize glucose, producing enough energy to pump sodium out of the cell. However, once these cells reach the microenvironment of the spleen, where glucose is deficient, the active-passive transport system is invariably "hurt" and the cells swell and hemolyze. The MCV of patients with hereditary spherocytosis is normal to low normal, but the MCHC is over 36% (see Chap. 9). Figure 5–8 lists the more common pathologic conditions in which spherocytes are seen. (See Fig. 9–4, which is a smear from a patient with hereditary spherocytosis.)

Ovalocytes and Elliptocytes

The ovalocyte is a cell of many capabilities (see Fig. 9–7). It can appear normochromic or hypochromic, normocytic or macrocytic. The exact physiologic mechanism is not well defined. When these erythrocytes are incubated in vitro, they reduce adenosine triphosphate (ATP) and 2,3-diphosphoglycerate (2,3-DPG) more rapidly than do normal cells. Hemoglobin seems to have a bipolar arrangement in these cells and there seems to be a reduction in membrane cholesterol.

Many investigators consider ovalocytes and elliptocytes as interchangeable terms; however, these two items will be dealt with distinctly and separately. Ovalocytes are more egg-shaped and have a greater tendency to vary in their hemoglobin content. Elliptocytes, on the other hand, are pencil-shaped and invariably not hypochromic. Figure 5–9 lists the pathologic processes associated with these morphologies.

Stomatocytes

The stomatocyte is defined as a red cell of normal size that appears bowl-shaped in wet preparation (Fig. 5–10). This peculiar shape is manifested in air-dried smears as a "slitlike" area of central pallor. The exact physiologic mechanism of stomatocytosis has yet to be clarified. Many chemical agents (e.g., phenothiazine and chlorpromazine) may induce stomatocytosis in vitro; however, these changes are reversible. Stomatocytes are known to have an increased permeability to sodium; consequently, their osmotic fragility is increased.

Stomatocytes are more often artifactual than a true manifestation of a particular pathophysiologic process. The artifactual stomatocyte has a distinct slit-like area of cenral pallor, whereas the area of pallor in the genuine stomatocyte appears shaded. Several of the associated disease states in which stomatocytes may be found are hereditary spherocytosis (the stomatospherocyte viewed best in wet preparations), he-

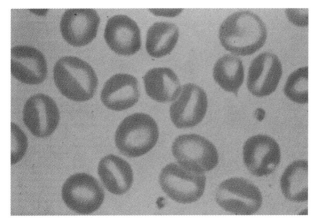

FIGURE 5–10   Stomatocytes (peripheral blood).

reditary stomatocytosis, which is usually a benign condition, occasionally hemolytic; acute alcoholism; and the Rh null phenotype.

Sickle Cells (Drepanocytes)

Sickle cells, or drepanocytes, are red cells that have been transformed by hemoglobin polymerization into rigid, inflexible cells with at least one pointed projection (see Figs. 5–2 and 11–5). Patients may be homozygous or heterozygous for the presence of the abnormal hemoglobin, hemoglobin S. Conditions of low oxygen tension (in vivo or in vitro) cause the abnormal hemoglobin to polymerize, forming tubules that line up in bundles to deform the cell. The surface area of the transformed cell is much greater, and the normal elasticity of the cell is severely restricted. Most sickled cells possess the ability to revert to the discocyte shape when oxygenated, and these are seen in peripheral smears as oat-shaped cells. However, approximately 10% of these cells are incapable of reverting to their normal shape. These irreversibly sickled cells (ISCs) are the result of repeated sickling episodes. In the peripheral smear they appear as crescent-shaped cells with long projections. When reoxygenated, these ISCs may undergo fragmentation.

Classically, sickled cells are best seen in wet preparations. Many of the cells observed in the Wright-Giemsa stain are the oat cell or the boat-shaped form of the sickled cell. In this form, the projections are much less pronounced and the central area of the cell is fairly broad. This shape is reversible. During a symptomatic period, the percentages of irreversibly sickled cells vary tremendously, and consequently do not correlate with symptomatology.

Figure 5–11 lists some of the more prominent pathologic conditions in which sickle cells may be observed. In this figure, a morphological distinction is made between ISCs and reversibly sickled cells.

Acanthocytes

An acanthocyte is defined as a cell of normal or slightly reduced size possessing three to eight spicules

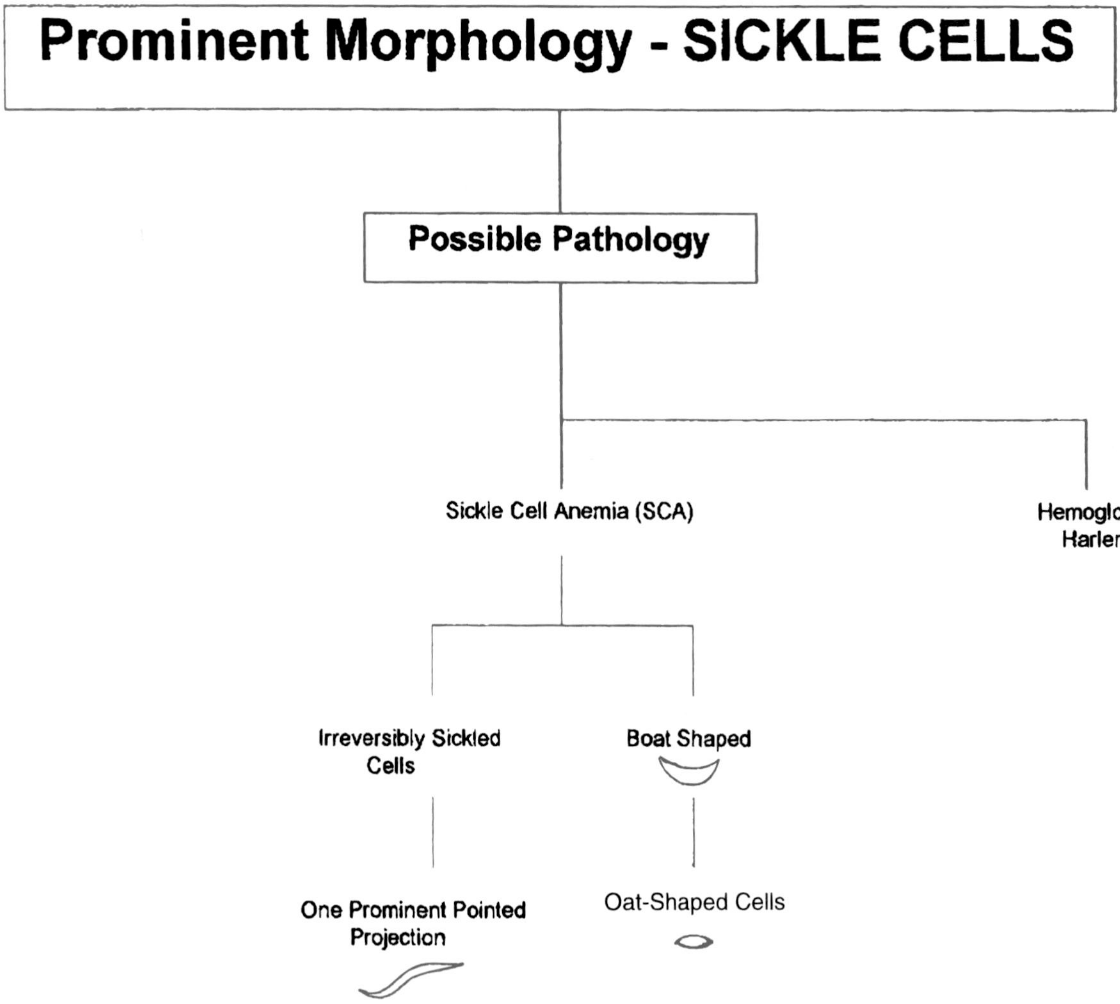

Prominent Morphology - SICKLE CELLS

Possible Pathology

Sickle Cell Anemia (SCA)

Hemoglobin C Harlem

Irreversibly Sickled Cells

Boat Shaped

One Prominent Pointed Projection

Oat-Shaped Cells

FIGURE 5-11   Correlation of sickle cells to pathologic processes.

of uneven length distributed along the periphery of the cell membrane (see Fig. 5–2). The uneven projections of the acanthocyte are rather pointed, and the acanthocyte can easily be distinguished from the peripheral smear background because it appears to be saturated with hemoglobin. The MCHC is, however, always within the normal range.

A specific mechanism related to the formation of acanthocytes is unknown. However, some details about these peculiar cells are of interest. Acanthocytes contain excess cholesterol and have an increased cholesterol:phospholipid ratio. Their surface area is increased. The lecithin content of acanthocytes is decreased. The only inherited condition in which acanthocytes are seen in numerous numbers is congenital abetalipoproteinemia. Most cases of acanthocytosis are acquired, such as the deficiency of LCAT (lecithin-cholesterol acyltransferase), which has been well documented in patients with severe hepatic disease. This enzyme is synthesized by the liver and is directly responsible for esterifying free cholesterol;

when this enzyme is deficient, cholesterol builds in the plasma.

The red cell responds to this excess cholesterol in one of two ways, depending on the balance of other lipids in the membrane. It becomes a target cell or an acanthocyte. Once an acanthocyte is formed, it is very liable to undergo splenic sequestration and fragmentation, and the fluidity of the membrane is directly affected. Figure 5–12 lists the most prominent pathologies in which acanthocytes are observed.

Fragmented Cells (Schistocytes, Burr Cells, Helmet Cells)

It may seem unusual to have these three red cell forms under the same heading; however, the choice for such a grouping becomes reasonable with an expanded definition of fragmentation. Fragmentation may be defined as "loss from the cell of a piece of membrane that may or may not contain hemoglobin." These events may occur repeatedly without the loss of he-

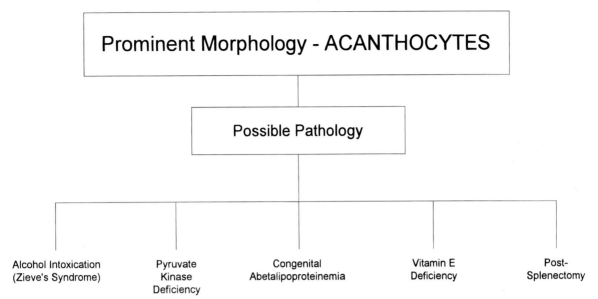

FIGURE 5-12   Correlation of acanthocytes to pathologic processes.

moglobin. However, each successive loss of membrane (each fragmentation that occurs) leaves the red cell more rigid and more likely to become entrapped in the splenic sinuses. It is recognized that not all membrane alterations occur pathologically. Indeed, the echinocytic transformation of normal red cells in stored plasma is known to be reversible. Likewise, discocyte-to-echinocyte transformation is part of normal red cell senescence. However, there are certain triggering events in disease that invariably lead to fragmentation. Two pathways are recognized. First, alteration of normal fluid circulation occurs, which may predispose to fragmentation. Examples of this include vasculitis, malignant hypertension, thrombotic thrombocytopenic purpura, and heart valve replacement.

Second, intrinsic defects of the red cell make it less deformable and therefore more likely to be fragmented as it traverses the microvasculature of the spleen. Spherocytes, antibody-altered red cells, and red cells containing inclusions have significant alterations that decrease their red cell survival, and these serve as examples of the second pathway.

Burr or crenated cells (echinocytes) are red cells with approximately 10 to 30 rounded spicules evenly placed over the surface of the red cells (Fig. 5–13). They are normochromic and normocytic for the most part. They may be observed as an artifact, usually as a result of specimen contamination, in which case they will appear in large numbers and will present with spiky projections. "True" burr cells occur in small numbers in uremia, heart disease, cancer of the stomach, bleeding peptic ulcer, immediately following an injection of heparin, and in a number of patients with untreated hypothyroidism. In general, they may occur in situations that cause a change in tonicity of the intravascular fluid (e.g., dehydration and azotemia).

Helmet or bite cells are recognized by their distinctive projections, usually two, surrounding an empty area of the red cell membrane that looks as if it has been bitten off (see Fig. 5–13). In hematologic conditions in which large inclusion bodies are formed (Heinz bodies), helmet cells are visible in the peripheral smear. Fragmentation occurs by the pitting mechanism of the spleen. Helmet cells may also be seen in pulmonary emboli, myeloid metaplasia, and DIC (disseminated intravascular coagulation).

Schistocytes are the *extreme* form of red cell fragmentation (see Fig. 5–13). Whole pieces of red cell membrane appear to be missing and very bizarre red cells are apparent. Schistocytes may be seen in microangiopathic hemolytic anemia, DIC, heart valve surgery, hemolytic uremic syndrome, and thrombotic thrombocytopenic purpura, as well as severe burn cases. Figure 5–14 correlates the fragmented cells to the pathologic processes in which they may be observed.

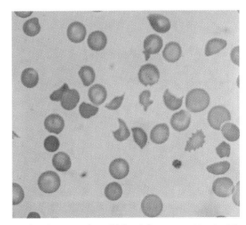

FIGURE 5-13   Peripheral blood from a patient with malignant hypertension. Note presence of schistocytes, helmet cells, and a burr cell. (From Bell, A: Hematology. In Listen, Look, and Learn. Health and Education Resources, Inc., Bethesda, Md., with permission.)

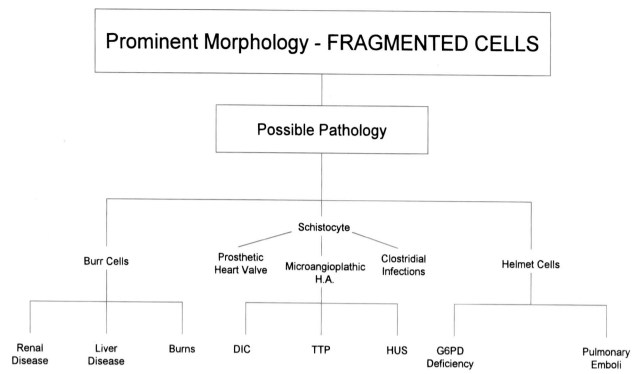

FIGURE 5-14   Correlation of fragmented cells to pathologic processes.

Teardrop Cells

Teardrop cells appear in the peripheral circulation as pear-shaped red cells. The extent to which a portion of the red cells form tails is variable, and these cells may be normal, reduced, or increased in size (Fig. 5–15). The exact physiologic mechanism is unknown, yet teardrop formation from inclusion-containing red cells is well documented. As cells containing large inclusions attempt to pass through the microcirculation, the portion of the cells containing the inclusion gets pinched, leaving a tailed end as it continues its journay. For some reason, the red cell is unable to maintain the discocyte shape once this has occurred.

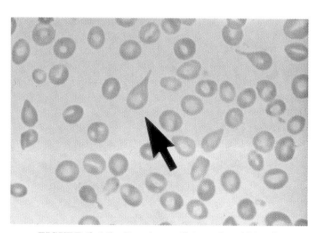

FIGURE 5-15   Teardrop cell (peripheral blood).

Teardrop cells are seen most prominently in idiopathic myelofibrosis with myeloid metaplasia (see Chap. 21). This type of morphological finding can also be seen in the thalassemia syndromes, in iron deficiency, and in conditions in which inclusion bodies are formed. Refer to Figure 5–2 for a composite of abnormal red cell morphology.

VARIATIONS IN RED CELL DISTRIBUTION

Agglutination

If an erythrocyte antibody is present in a patient's plasma and a corresponding erythrocyte antigen is represented, agglutination will take place. This is the case with cold antibody syndromes such as cold hemagglutination disease and paroxysmal cold hemoglobinuria. The agglutination occurs at room temperature in sample preparation and will appear as interspersed areas of clumping throughout the peripheral smear (see Fig. 14–3). The use of saline does not disperse these agglutinated areas; however, warming the sample helps to break up the agglutinins.

Rouleaux

Rouleaux formation is the result of elevated globulins or fibrinogen in the plasma. Red cells that are constantly bathed in this abnormal plasma appear as stacks of coins in the peripheral smear (see Fig. 22–11). These stacks are rather evenly dispersed throughout the smear. The use of a saline dilution of the plasma disperses rouleaux. Rouleaux formation correlates well with a high erythrocyte sedimentation rate and occurs as a direct result of protein deposition or adsorption on the erythrocyte membrane. This lowers the zeta potential, the difference in charge of red cells in an electrolyte solution, thus facilitating the stacking effect.

Patients with multiple myeloma, Waldenstrom's macroglobulinemia, chronic inflammatory disorders, and some lymphomas demonstrate rouleaux.

RED CELL INCLUSIONS

Howell-Jolly Bodies

Howell-Jolly bodies (Fig. 5–16B) are nuclear remnants containing DNA. They are 1 to 2 μm in size and may appear singly or doubly in an eccentric position on the periphery of the cell membrane. They are thought to develop in periods of accelerated or abnormal erythropoiesis. A fragment of the chromosome becomes detached and is left floating in the cytoplasm after the nucleus has been extruded. Under ordinary circumstances, the spleen effectively pits these nondeformable bodies from the cell. However, during periods of erythroid stress, the pitting mechanism cannot keep pace with inclusion formation. Howell-Jolly bodies may be seen following splenectomy and in thalassemic syndromes, hemolytic anemias, megaloblastic anemias, and functional hyposplenia.

Basophilic Stippling

Red cells that contain ribosomes can potentially form stippled cells (see Fig. 6–16). However, it is thought that the actual stippling is the result of the drying of cells in preparation for microscopic examination. Coarse, diffuse, or punctate basophilic stippling may occur and consist of ribonucleoprotein and

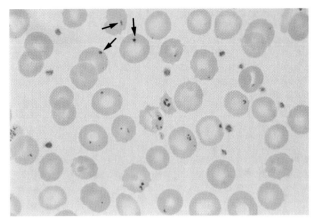

FIGURE 5-17 Pappenheimer bodies (peripheral blood, Wright's stain).

mitochondrial remnants. Diffuse basophilic stippling appears as a fine blue dusting, whereas coarse stippling is much more outlined and easily distinguished. Punctate basophilic stippling is a coalescing of smaller forms and is very prominent and easily identifiable. Stippling may be found in any condition showing defective or accelerated heme synthesis, lead intoxication, and thalassemia syndromes.

Siderotic Granules and Pappenheimer Bodies

Siderotic granules are small, irregular magenta inclusions seen along the periphery of red cells (Fig. 5–17). They usually appear in clusters, as if they had been gently placed on the red cell membrane. Their presence is presumptive evidence for the presence of iron. However, the Prussian blue stain is the confirmatory test for determining the presence of these inclusions. These granules in red blood cells are non-heme iron resulting from an excess of available iron throughout the body. They are designated *Pappenheimer bodies* when seen in a Wright-stained smear and *siderotic granules* when seen in Prussian blue stain. RBCs containing Pappenheimer bodies are referred to as *siderocytes*.

Siderotic granules are found in sideroblastic anemias and in any condition leading to hemochromatosis or hemosiderosis. They may also be seen in the hemoglobinopathies (e.g., sickle cell anemia and thalassemia) and in splenectomized patients.

Heinz Bodies

Heinz bodies are formed as a result of denatured or precipitated hemoglobin. They can be formed experimentally by incubation with phenylhydrazine. They are large (0.3 to 2 μm) inclusions that are rigid and severely distort the cell membrane. On initial exposure to phenylhydrazine, small crystalline bodies appear, coalesce, and migrate to an area beneath the cell membrane. They may not be visualized in Wright's stain but

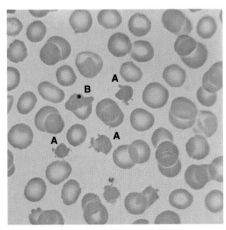

FIGURE 5-16 Peripheral blood of a patient after kidney transplantation and splenectomy. Note *(A)* small, condensed, irregularly shaped cells and *(B)* presence of a Howell-Jolly body.

may be seen with crystal violet and brilliant cresyl blue (see Fig. 4–2).

Heinz bodies may be seen in the alpha-thalassemic syndromes, G6PD deficiency under oxidant stress, and in any of the unstable hemoglobin syndromes (hemoglobin Koln, hemoglobin Zurich). They may also be seen in red cell inury resulting from chemical insult.

Cabot Rings

The exact physiologic mechanism in Cabot ring formation has yet to be elucidated. Cabot rings are found in heavily stippled cells and appear in a figure-eight conformation like the beads of a necklace (see Fig. 7–6). They are not composed of DNA, but they do contain arginine-rich histone and nonhemoglobin iron.

Cabot rings may be found in megaloblastic anemias and homozygous thalassemia syndromes, as well as after splenectomy.

EXAMINATION OF PLATELET MORPHOLOGY

The normal platelet has several distinctive morphological characteristics. This structure measures approximately 1 to 4 μm, with a discoid shape and even blue granules dispersed throughout a light-blue cytoplasm. In pathological states, platelets may appear as blue or gray agranular discs; they may be extremely large (see Fig. 1–51) and may show tailing or streaming of the cytoplasm. In rare instances, one may see megakaryocytic fragments in the peripheral circulation (see Fig. 1–51).

A close and thorough examination of platelet morphology will provide important information as to the patient's hemostatic capability. Gross variation in platelet morphology may be seen in infiltrative disease of the bone marrow (e.g., idiopathic myelofibrosis or metastatic infiltrates). Large platelets may be seen in any disorder associated with increased platelet turnover as may occur with idiopathic thrombocytopenic purpura or bleeding disorders. In addition to the elevated platelet count, morphological changes may also occur after splenectomy.

SUMMARY

The study of red cell morphology is an interpretive science and gives the evaluator many opportunities to negotiate through to diagnostic impressions. Although automated instruments, three- and five-part differentials, and flagging codes may improve productivity, there is no substitute for a peripheral smear evaluator with finely tuned morphological skills. Hopefully, this chapter will provide a solid foundation from which to develop and expand on this knowledge base.

CASE STUDY

A 28-year-old man presented to the emergency room with a complaint of abdominal pain. He appeared quite ill, with nausea, cold sweats, and tachycardia. The patient appeared slightly jaun-

diced, and on further questioning admitted that his urine had been dark and discolored that day. He had been treated with a sulfanomide drug for an undisclosed illness. The preliminary impression was of acute appendicitis. The laboratory results are as follows:

Test Ordered	Value	Normal Value
Amylase	<31	30–110 U/L
WBC	6.3	4.5–10.5×10^9/L
RBC	1.00	4.20–5.80×10^{12}/L
HGB	4.4	13.5–16.5 g/dL
HCT	12.6	40%–49%
MCV	126	80–100 fL
MCH	43.9	27.0–34.0 pg
MCHC	34.8	32.0–36.5%
Platelets	209	150–450×10^9/L
RDW	23.5	0%–16.5%
Direct bilirubin	0.7	0.0–0.4 mg/dL
Total bilirubin	7.9	0.1–1.4 mg/dL
SGOT	567	0–100 IU/L
LDH	2844	0–100 IU/L
Haptoglobin	0.1 g/L	0.4–3.6 g/L
Manual Differential		
Segments	60	35%–70%
Bands	5	2%–7%
Lymphocytes	32	15%–55%
Monocytes	1	0%–10%
Eosinophil	1	0%–15%
Basophil	1	0%–3%
Platelet estimate	Increased	
NRBC	8	
RBC morphology	Mkd. aniso, mod poikilo, occ. basophilic stippling, S1-mod polychromasia, mod. teardrop cells, occ. schistocytes, bites, occ. ovalocytes	

Questions

1. Based on the serum chemistries, is the patient experiencing a hemolytic episode?
2. Are there any pertinent morphologies in the peripheral smear?
3. Why is the MCV macrocytic?

This case is an example of a patient with G6PD deficiency. He has suffered a violent episode as a result of exposure to drugs. The inheritance of G6PD is X-linked, with mother-to-son transmission. The red cell indices show a normocytic, normochromic picture with striking poikilocytosis, including irregular contracted cells, *bite cells*, teardrops, and moderate polychromasia. The patient may need to have transfusion support; however, the hemolytic state is self-limiting. The hemolysis is primarily intravascular, as noted by the decreased haptoglobin, hemoglobinurea, and hemoglobinemia. Our patient shows a classic drug-induced G6PD episode. His hemoglobin and hematocrit are precipitously low and his smear shows evidence of marrow response with NRBCs, moderate polychromasia, and marked anisopoikilocytosis. The high MCV can be expected in view of the high level of polychromasia, indicating a high level of polychromatophilic macrocytes (reticulocytes). A Heinz body preparation was performed by allowing equal volumes of EDTA blood to mix with crystal violet stain for 20 minutes. One drop of well-mixed blood was cover-slipped and observed under oil immersion, and occasional Heinz bodies were seen. Bite cells are formed as Heinz bodies are pitted from the red cell by the spleen, but in G6PD this may be a highly transient finding. This patient's laboratory results returned to normal in 48 hours once the drug had cleared from his system. Other clinical conditions associated with G6PD deficiency are favism, neonatal jaundice, and congenital nonspherocytic anemia.

BIBLIOGRAPHY

Agre, P: Hereditary spherocytosis. JAMA 262:2887, 1989.

Babior, B and Stossel, T: Hematology—A Pathophysiological Approach. Churchill-Livingstone, New York, 1994.

Backman, L: Shape control in the human red cell. J Cell Sci 80:281, 1986.

Ballis, SK: Sickle cell anemia with few painful crises is characterized by decreased red cell deformability and increased number of dense cells. Am J Hematol 36:122, 1991.

Bartels, PC and Roijers, AF: Effects of ageing on preserved red blood cell populations as measured by light scattering. J Clin Chem Clin Biochem 26:29, 1988.

Bator, JM, Groves, MR, Price, BJ, et al: Erythrocyte deformability and size measured in a multiparameter system that includes impedance sizing. Cytometry 5:34, 1984.

Bessis, M, Weed, RI, and Leblond, PF: Red Cell Shape Physiology Pathology, Ultrastructure. Springer-Verlag, New York, 1973.

Bick, R (ed): Hematology, Clinical and Laboratory Practice. Mosby-Year Book, St Louis, 1993.

Branton, D: Erythrocyte membrane protein associations and erythrocyte shape. Harvey Lect 77:23, 1981–1982.

Chasis, JA and Schrier, SL: Membrane deformability and the capacity for shape change in the erythrocyte. Blood 74:2562, 1989.

Cohen, AR, Trotzky, MS, and Pincus, D: Reassessment of the microcytic anemia of lead poisoning. Pediatrics 67:904, 1981.

Crouch, JY and Kaplow, LS: Relationship of reticulocyte age to polychromasia, shift cells, and shift reticulocytes. Arch Pathol Lab Med 109:325, 1985.

deHaan, LD, Werre, JM, Ruben, AM, et al: Alteration in size, shape and osmotic behavior of red cells after splenectomy: A study of their age dependence. Br J Hematol 69:71, 1988.

Fairbanks, VF: Hemoglobinopathies and Thalassemias, Laboratory Methods and Clinical Cases. Thieme-Stratton, New York, 1992.

Fukushima, Y and Kon, H: On the mechanism of loss of deformability in human erythrocytes due to Heinz body formation: A flow EPR study. Toxicol Appl Pharmacol 102:205, 1990.

Hecner, F, Lehmann, HP, and Kao, YS: Practical Microscopic Hematology, ed 4. Williams & Wilkins, Philadelphia, 1994.

Hillman, RS and Finch, CA: Red Cell Manual, ed 6. FA Davis, Philadelphia, 1992.

Hoffbrand, AV and Pettit, JE: Essential Hematology, ed 3. Blackwell Scientific. St Louis, 1993.

Johnson, CS, Tegos, C, and Beutler, E: Thalassemia minor: Routine erythrocyte measurements and differentiation from iron deficiency. Am J Clin Pathol 80:31, 1983.

Kapff, CT: Blood Atlas and Sourcebook of Hematology. Little, Brown, Boston, 1981.

Krogstad, DJ, Sutera, SP, Boylan, CW, et al: Intraerythrocytic parasites and red cell deformability: *Plasmodium berghei* and *Babeisa microti*. Blood Cells 17:209, 1991.

Lange, Y and Stech, TL: Mechanism of red blood cell acan-thocytosis and echinocytosis in vivo. J Membr Biol 77:153, 1984.

Leiter, SS: The human blood platelet: Its derivation from the red cell. Folia Hematol 111:60, 1984.

Linde, T, Sandhagen, B, Danielson, BG, et al: Impaired erythrocyte fluidity during treatment of renal anaemia with erythropoietin. J Intern Med 231:601, 1992.

O'Conner, BH: A Color Atlas and Instruction Manual of Peripheral Blood Cell Morphology. Williams & Wilkins, Baltimore, 1984.

Mohandas, N and Chasis, JA: Red cell deformability, membrane material properties and shape: Regulation by transmembrane, skeletal, and cytosolic proteins and lipids. Semin Hematol 30:171, 1993.

Nathan, DG and Oski, FA (eds): Hematology of Infancy and Childhood. WB Saunders, Philadelphia, 1993.

Norton, JM: The effect of macrocytosis on rate erythrocyte deformability during recovery from phenylhydrazine-induced anemia. Biorheology 27:21, 1990.

Powell, RJ, Macheido, GW, and Rush, BF, Jr: Decreased red blood cell deformability and impaired oxyten utilization during human sepsis. Am Surg 59:65, 1993.

Rao, KR and Patel, AR: Erythrocytic ecdysis in shears of EDTA venous blood in eight patients with sickle cell anemia. Blood cells 12:543, 1987.

Reich, PR and Robinson, SH: Hematology: Physiopathologic Basis for Clinical Practice, ed 3. Little, Brown, Boston, 1993.

Reinhart, WH and Singh, A: Erythrocyte aggregation: the roles of cell deformability and geometry. Eur J Clin Invest 20:458, 1990.

Reinhart, WH: The influence of iron deficiency on erythrocyte deformability. Br J Haematol 80:550, 1992.

Salt, HB and Wolf, OH: On having no beta lipoprotein: A syndrome comprising a beta-lipoproteinemia acanthocytosis and steatorrhea. Lancet 2:323, 1968.

Schilling, RF: Anemia of Chronic Disease: A Misnomer. Ann Intern Med 115:572, 1991.

Scott, MD, Rouyer-Fessard, P, Ba, MS, et al: Alpha and beta hemoglobin chain induced changes in normal erythrocyte deformability: Comparison to beta thalassemia intermedia and Hgb H disease. Br J Haematol 80:519, 1992.

Silinsky, JJ: Understanding red cell morphology. RN 47:99, 1984.

Spivak, JL: Fundamentals of Clinical Hematology, ed 3. Johns Hopkins University Press. Baltimore, 1993.

Stewart, GW, O'Brien, H, Morris, SA, et al: Stomatocytosis, abnormal platelets and pseudohomozygous hypercholesterolemia. Eur J Hematol 38:376, 1987.

Stuart, J and Nash, GB: Red cell deformability and haematological disorders. Blood Rev 4:141, 1990.

Todd, JC, 3d, Poulos, ND, Davidson, LW, et al: Role of the leukocyte in endotoxin induced alterations of the red cell membrane. Am Surg 59:9, 1993.

Westerman, MP and Bacus, JW: Red blood cell morphology in sickle cell anemia as determined by image processing analysis: The relationship to painful crisis. Am J Clin Pathol 79:667, 1983.

Williams, WJ, Beutler, E, et al: Hematology. McGraw-Hill, New York, 1990.

Wolf, BC and Neiman, RS: Disorders of the Spleen. WB Saunders, Philadelphia, 1989.

QUESTIONS

1. The elliptocyte is a prominent morphology in:
   a. Myeloid metaplasia
   b. Hemolytic anemia
   c. Iron-deficiency anemia
   d. Sickle cell anemia

2. The blood smear of a patient with a prosthetic heart valve may show:
   a. Target cells
   b. Burr cells
   c. Schistocytes
   d. Elliptocytes

3. How would a cell that has a diameter of 9 μm and an MCV of 104 be classified?
   a. Macrocyte
   b. Microcyte
   c. Normal
   d. Either normal or slightly microcytic

4. Which type of red cell inclusion is a DNA remnant?
   a. Heinz bodies
   b. Howell-Jolly bodies
   c. Pappenheimer bodies
   d. Cabot rings

5. In a patient with an MCHC >36%, one would expect to observe:
   a. Target cells
   b. Spherocytes
   c. Helmet cells
   d. Elliptocytes

6. A microcytic cell can be described as possessing:
   a. A thin rim of hemoglobin
   b. A blue-gray color
   c. A size of less than 7 μm
   d. An oval shape

7. Basophilic stippling is composed of:
   a. DNA
   b. Precipitated stain
   c. Denatured hemoglobin
   d. RNA

8. Which inclusion cannot be visualized on Wright's stain?
   a. Basophilic stippling
   b. Pappeheimer bodies
   c. Howell-Jolly bodies
   d. Heinz bodies

9. Which morphologies would be prominent on a smear of a patient with severe liver disease?
   a. Target cells, macrocytes
   b. Microcytes, elliptocytes
   c. Schistocytes, bite cells
   d. Sickle cells, crystals

ANSWERS

1. **c** (p. 86, Fig. 5–9)
2. **c** (p. 89)
3. **a** (p. 82)
4. **b** (p. 91)
5. **b** (p. 87)
6. **c** (p. 83)
7. **d** (p. 91)
8. **d** (pp. 91, 92)
9. **a** (pp. 83, 85, Figs. 5–4, 5–7)

Part II

ANEMIAS

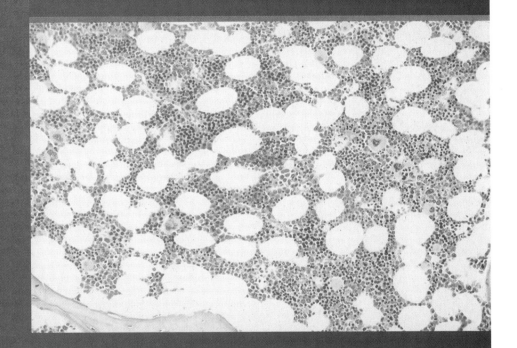

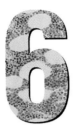

6

Iron Metabolism and Hypochromic Anemias

Susan J. Leclair, MS, CLS(NCA)

Objectives

At the end of this chapter, the learner should be able to:

1 State the primary function of iron in the body.
2 List factors that influence iron absorption.
3 Trace iron transport from ingestion to tissue and hemoglobin incorporation.
4 Name three stages of iron deficiency and describe findings associated with each stage.
5 List two major categories of iron deficiency.
6 Name the most diagnostic laboratory finding for iron-deficiency anemia.
7 List laboratory test results that help to distinguish iron-deficiency anemia from anemia of chronic disease.
8 Define *hemosiderosis*.
9 Describe typical laboratory findings for patients with sideroblastic conditions.
10 Specify characteristic findings in lead poisoning.

Evaluation of the hemoglobin molecule includes looking at the molecule as a set of three separate but interdependent components: iron, protoporphyrin IX, and globin chains. Deficiency in any hemoglobin component results in the development of a hemoglobin-deficient state and microcytic erythrocytes demonstrating hypochromia. Because globin chain abnormalities are presented in Chapter 12, only iron and protoporphyrin are discussed here. The first part of the chapter is a consideration of normal iron metabolism. In the second part, iron-deficiency anemia and iron utilization dysfunction are covered. The third part of the chapter presents a discussion of the hereditary porphyrias and the most common acquired heme disorder, lead poisoning or intoxication. The chapter ends with case histories that illustrate some of these conditions.

NORMAL IRON METABOLISM

In humans, the primary function of iron is oxygen transport; a lesser function is participation in catalytic energy transfer and reactions. The average adult has a total body iron content between 3500 and 4000 mg. Found in a variety of sites in the human body, approximately two thirds (2500 mg) of this iron is found in hemoglobin, with the remainder found in storage pools of the marrow, spleen, and liver and in such compounds as myoglobin, myeloperoxidase, and certain

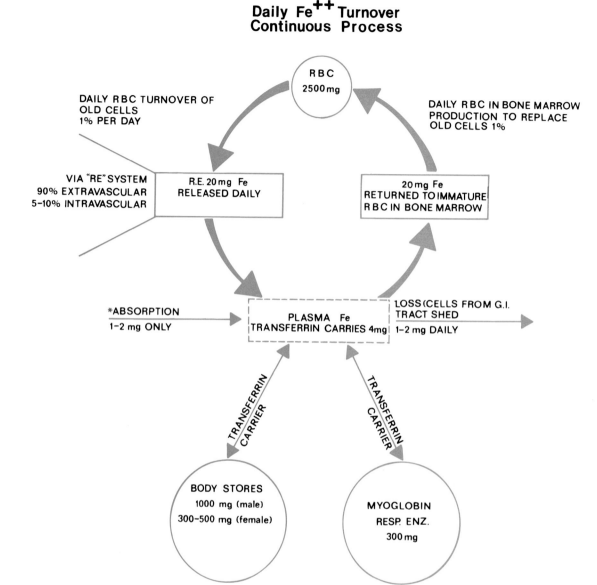

Daily Fe^{++} Turnover
Continuous Process

RBC
2500 mg

DAILY RBC TURNOVER OF
OLD CELLS
1% PER DAY

DAILY RBC IN BONE MARROW
PRODUCTION TO REPLACE
OLD CELLS 1%

VIA "RE" SYSTEM
90% EXTRAVASCULAR
5-10% INTRAVASCULAR

R.E. 20 mg Fe
RELEASED DAILY

20 mg Fe
RETURNED TO IMMATURE
RBC IN BONE MARROW

*ABSORPTION
1-2 mg ONLY

PLASMA Fe
TRANSFERRIN CARRIES 4 mg

LOSS (CELLS FROM G.I.
TRACT SHED
1-2 mg DAILY

TRANSFERRIN
CARRIER

TRANSFERRIN
CARRIER

BODY STORES
1000 mg (male)
300-500 mg (female)

MYOGLOBIN
RESP. ENZ.
300 mg

FIGURE 6-1 Daily turnover and pathways of internal iron exchanges.

electron transfer proteins. Figure 6–1 illustrates the continuous process of daily iron turnover. Iron's importance in humans cannot be overstated. Studies have indicated that damage caused during gestation by iron deficiency may be life long. Iron deficiency in adults is a major cause of morbidity and mortality—a significant statement because 10% to 30% of the world's population is believed to be iron-deficient.[1]

Iron is more stable in the ferric (Fe^{3+}) state than in the ferrous (Fe^{2+}) state. Most of the iron in organic compounds, such as protein, is in the ferric state. Reduction of iron from the ferric to the ferrous state is accomplished by the RBCs methemoglobin reductase metabolic pathway[3] (see Chap. 3).

Iron-Containing Compounds

Iron is found in a wide variety of animal and plant tissues. Significant iron concentration exists in both vegetables and meats. Plant tissue is a less accessible source of iron because vegetables contain less iron on a weight basis. In addition, spinach and other green leafy vegetables contain insoluble substances such as phytates and phosphates that greatly interfere with iron absorption. Iron is in a more accessible form in meats because this source contains few insoluble complexes. Foods high in available iron include organ meats, wheat germ, brewer's yeast, and certain legumes. Foods with a moderate amount of iron include muscle meats such as beef, fish, and fowl; prunes; some green vegetables; and most cereals. Milk and nongreen vegetables contain little available iron. Preparation of foods may also affect iron content. For example, pasta contains more iron when cooked in an iron container than when cooked in glass. Low-molecular-weight compounds such as fructose, amino acids, and organic acids such as ascorbic acid (vitamin C) facilitate iron absorption.[4] However, despite the abundance of dietary iron, iron deficiency is the world's most common cause of anemia.

Iron-containing compounds are typically divided into two categories: heme and nonheme. The term *heme compound* refers to those proteins in which iron is complexed to a porphyrin. The most important of these are the oxygen carriers, hemoglobin and myoglobin. Figure 6–2 illustrates the iron-porphyrin bond (A) and compares it to a compound in which iron is not bound to a porphyrin (B). Nonheme-iron-containing compounds include a large number of transfer and storage compounds such as transferrin, lactoferrin,

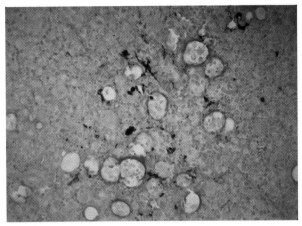

FIGURE 6–3 Bone marrow aspirate stained positively with Prussian blue. (From the American Society of Hematology Slide Bank, ed 2, #IOA-02-04-01, with permission.)

and ferritin. Nonheme iron is sometimes visible in developing erythroid cells as inclusions sometimes called *Pappenheimer bodies*. Only when these inclusions have been stained positively with an iron-specific stain such as Perl's Prussian blue should they be called *siderotic granules*. (Figs. 6–3 and 6–4 demonstrate bone marrow samples stained positively and negatively with Prussian blue.) At a higher magnification, nonheme iron can be seen in close to the nucleus (inside nonstained mitochrondria) of the developing red cells. These nucleated red cells containing stainable nonheme iron are called *sideroblasts*; nonnucleated red cells containing stainable iron are called *siderocytes* (Fig. 6–5).

Iron Requirements

A minor but sometimes confusing point is that of nomenclature. Iron is expressed in milligrams when the element is being described, whereas erythroid cells (which contain iron) are usually quantified in millili-

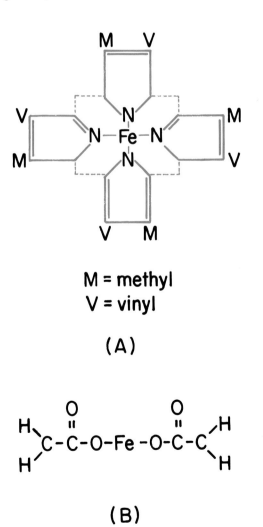

M = methyl
V = vinyl

(A)

(B)

FIGURE 6–2 A heme iron is an iron bound within a porphyrin. *A.* Heme iron compound. *B.* Nonheme iron compound.

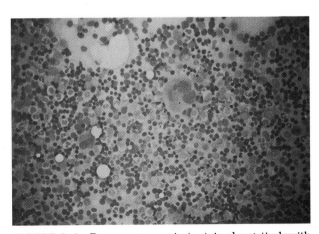

FIGURE 6–4 Bone marrow aspirate stained negatively with Prussian blue. (From the American Society of Hematology Slide Bank, ed 2, #I1A-01-04-01, with permission.)

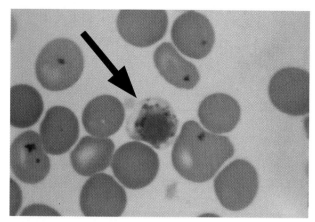

FIGURE 6–5 Ringed sideroblast (center) and siderocytes (surrounding cells). (From Bell, A: Hematology. In Listen, Look and Learn. Health and Education Resources, Inc., Bethesda, MD, with permission.)

TABLE 6–2 **Minimum Daily Requirements (MDR) for Iron (assuming a 10% absorption)**		
	MDR (mg)	Iron Content of Food (mg)
Infant	1.0	10
Child	0.5	5
Premenopausal woman	2.0	20
Pregnant or lactating woman	3.0	30
Adult man or postmenopausal woman	1.0	10

ters. Because 1 mg of iron is needed to produce 1 mL of erythrocytes, it is easy to become confused about whether one is speaking of iron or hemoglobin. Healthy individuals average 1% (approximately 20 to 25 mL) red cell loss each day. This translates into 20 to 25 mg of iron needed to maintain consistent total body iron concentration. However, humans typically absorb only 1 mg of dietary iron, or 5% of the required amount, each day. Therefore, homeostasis requires that the 95% of the total iron used for new red cell development each day must be recycled from normal RBC senescence (Table 6–1). Iron recycling in the normal individual is extraordinarily efficient and recovers all iron except that lost through sweating, desquamated skin or fecal and urinary excretion, and, in women of reproductive age, menstruation.

Iron Absorption and Storage

Iron absorption responds to daily need and is influenced by: (1) the amount and type of iron accessible from food, (2) the functional state of the gastrointestinal mucosa and pancreas, (3) current iron stores, and (4) erythropoietic needs. As mentioned previously, iron exists in a wide variety of foods, although it may be more or less accessible for human absorption. Absorption is increased by ingestion of acidic foods such as citrus fruit juices along with the iron-containing foods.[5] Conversely, absorption is decreased by eating foods containing phosphates, phytates, or other compounds that form insoluble iron complexes.[6] Large amounts of dairy products also interfere with the conversion of ferric iron to ferrous iron. Although both the ferric (Fe^{3+}) and ferrous (Fe^{2+}) states of iron are biologically active, the small intestine preferentially absorbs ferrous iron. The entire gastrointestinal (GI) tract has the capacity to absorb iron, but optimal absorption occurs in the duodenum and jejunum. The strongly acidic pH of the stomach in conjunction with pancreatic enzymes contributes to a favorable microenvironment for increased iron absorption. Thus iron absorption can be increased by maintaining a healthy gastric pH or decreased by an injudicious use of antacids.

In most developed countries, a typical diet contains less than 20 mg of elemental iron. Because only 10% of ingested iron is typically absorbed, the average daily absorption does not reach more than 2 mg of iron.

TABLE 6–1 **Daily Iron Turnover**			
Turnover Rate	**Cells**	**Replacement Source**	
1%	Loss from RBC death, blood loss, desquamation, fecal and/or urinary excretion, menstruation	Dietary sources Recycling in spleen or liver	5% 95%
If a person maintains a 15% g/dL hemoglobin, this translates to			
Turnover	**Cell Loss**	**Replacement Quantity and Sources**	
1% or 25 mg of iron or 0.15 g/dL of HB	0.45×10^{12}/L	1 mg, dietary sources 24 mg, recycled RBC iron	

Source	Iron State	Site	Action Required for Iron to Be Utilized and Available for Next Step or Process
Foodstuffs	Ferrous or ferric	Upper GI tract	
	Ferrous	Stomach	Reduction by HCl
	Ferrous	Duodenum and jejunum	Absorption by mucosal cells
Transferrin	Ferric	Liver	Protein carrier for iron
Ferritin	Ferric	Storage sites	Action by ferrochelatases
Hemoglobin	Ferrous	RBC	Required for O_2 uptake
Hemosiderin	Ferric	RBC	Occurs at release of O_2 at cell level—action of methemoglobin reductase to allow for return to ferrous state

TABLE 6–3 **Iron States**

Most well-nourished adult men absorb at least 1 mg of iron per day. Premenopausal women absorb approximately the same amount of iron but do so as a result of different conditions. They tend to eat less than men, but because the typical premenopausal women's iron stores are lower than normal, the GI tract responds to the stress and increases iron absorption (Table 6–2). Circumstances such as pregnancy or recovery from anemia can cause the GI tract to absorb as much as 20% of ingested elemental iron. Routinely supplementing foods such as bread flour with iron helps to prevent dietary iron deficiency on a national scale but may cause iron overload in susceptible people.

Although the most common dietary form of iron is in the ferric state, it is converted to the ferrous state when the gastric acid pH is less than 4.0 and in the presence of reducing substances such as ascorbic acid or glutathione. This ferrous form is absorbed through the mucosal cells of the duodenum and jejunum. Once in the bloodstream, ferrous iron is reconverted to the ferric state by serum ferroxidases. This reconversion allows iron to be carried by a transport protein specific for iron called *transferrin*. Transferrin is a beta globulin synthesized in the liver and weighs approximately 80,000 daltons (d). Two atoms of ferric iron can bind to each transferrin molecule, giving the protein a total binding capacity of 240 to 280 mg/dL. Because transferrin has a short half-life (8 to 10 days), any hepatic dysfunction that interferes with the liver's synthetic pathways will result in a relatively quick decrease in serum transferrin. Usually saturation of transferrin is approximately 30%; saturation of the two available binding sites, however, occurs in only 10% of transferrin. Table 6–3 lists the electron changes that iron experiences from dietary source to hemoglobin molecule. Figure 6–6 illustrates the relationship of iron and transferrin in a variety of conditions. Following absorption and transferrin binding, iron is delivered to body tissues because transferrin is freely distributed in extravascular fluids.[7] Transferrin can also directly release its iron content to developing red cells.

Once all immediate iron needs are satisfied, transferrin releases iron in the liver, where it is bound to ferritin, the major storage compound. An equilibrium between intracellular ferritin and serum ferritin exists.

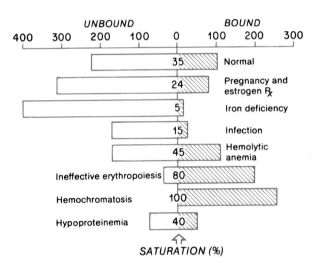

FIGURE 6–6 Transferrin and its iron. The reference range for serum iron is from 50 to 150 μg/dL of plasma, with 10μg/dL an average normal value. This represents only about one-third of the binding capacity of transferrin, so the saturation is about 30 percent. Both the serum iron and the total iron-binding capacity are altered by disease states. Pregnancy is associated with a modest reduction in the serum iron and an increase in the total iron-binding capacity. Iron deficiency shows an even more striking change with a major reduction in the serum iron and a dramatic increase in the total iron-binding capacity, giving a percent saturation below 10 percent. In contrast, infection reduces both the serum iron and the total iron-binding capacity. The pattern observed with most hemolytic anemias is quite different from that observed with marked ineffective erythropoiesis. In hemolytic anemias, the plasma iron is relatively normal, whereas with ineffective erythropoiesis there may be an increase in the serum iron with near total saturation of the iron-binding capacity. A similar pattern is seen with hemochromatosis. Severe starvation, nephrotic syndrome, and chronic inflammatory disease can result in marked hypoproteinemia with pronounced reductions in transferrin. (From Hillman, RS and Finch, CA: Red Cell Manual, ed 5. FA Davis, Philadelphia, 1985, p 53, with permission.)

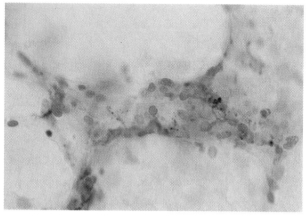

FIGURE 6–7 Iron stain of bone marrow smear shows the processes of the nutrient histiocytes surrounding the erythrocyte precursors.

Thus, serum ferritin reflects the dynamic equilibrium of total iron stores and cellular requirements.[8] Quantitative serum ferritin assays were once thought to be a sensitive measure of iron metabolism. However, experience suggests that this test is an unreliable indicator if the patient is experiencing an acute inflammatory condition or hepatic injury. In either situation, ferritin levels are unusually elevated and values may be misleading.[9]

Another compound involved in iron storage is hemosiderin. Hemosiderin is a water-insoluble ferric hydroxide and partial apoferritin complex in a pseudocrystalline form found in lysosomal membranes of macrophages. Temporary hemosiderin storage occurs commonly during hemoglobin degradation after senescent red cells have been phagocytized by macrophages. Less commonly, a more prolonged storage occurs after ferritin capacity has been reached. Hemosiderin can be visualized in bone marrow aspirates by staining with Prussian blue (Fig. 6–7).

Since only 1 mg of elemental iron is absorbed from dietary sources each day and approximately 20 mg of iron is needed to synthesize hemoglobin in replacement red cells, it is clear that the major source of the daily iron requirement is recycled iron liberated from senescent red cells. Dying red cells are phagocytized by cells of the mononuclear phagocytic system (MPS) and hemoglobin's degradation into bilirubin is begun.

Microsomal enzymes within the macrophage allow the now nonheme iron to bind to transferrin, which in turn transfers it back to developing erythroid cells. This efficient system allows for the recycling of approximately 80% of iron released from hemoglobin. Ferrous iron released from hemoglobin through hemolysis rather than phagocytosis is converted to ferric iron by serum ferroxidases. This ferric iron is then bound to transferrin, and the cycle continues.

CLINICAL SYNDROMES OF IRON METABOLISM

Causes of Iron Deficiency

Iron deficiency may be grouped into two major categories: low availability of iron and increased loss of iron-containing compounds or cells. Since iron requirements vary throughout life, these categories are further subdivided by age and sex (Table 6–4).

Assuming adequate prenatal care and maternal stores, the typical neonate has approximately 300 mg in total body iron, all of which was transferred to the developing fetus from maternal stores during pregnancy. Inadequate maternal stores prevent a fetus from acquiring adequate iron, which will compound the increased need for iron during the growth spurt of the first 2 years of life. Low iron availability in children would include dietary inadequacy during times of growth and/or stress occurring in premature births, immediately postpartum, and during growth spurts in infancy.[10] Low availability also includes those conditions that interfere with the absorption of iron from the GI tract, such as celiac disease, defective gastric function, or achlorhydria, or following gastrectomy. Less common causes include copper deficiency, inherited or acquired inadequate production of transferrin, and steatorrhea. Both children and adults commonly fail to achieve adequate dietary iron intake during weight-reduction diets, particularly fad-type diets. Recent findings suggest that iron deficiency is causally related to a decline in early psychomotor skill development.[11]

The need for iron in premenopausal adult women is variable because it is affected by both menstrual blood loss and pregnancy. In menstruating women, approximately 60 to 80 mL of blood is lost per month; therefore, an additional 1 to 1.5 mg of iron is needed daily

TABLE 6–4	**Common Causes of Iron Deficiency**			
Neonates	**Infants, Children and Adolescents**	**Premenopausal Women**	**Adult Males and Postmenopausal Women**	**Not Specifically Age- or Sex-Related Causes**
Maternal iron deficiency	Growth spurts	Menstrual blood loss, inadequate diet, pregnancy, fetomaternal hemorrhage, multiple births, malabsorption	Inadequate diet, blood loss, typically chronic malabsorption	Inadequate diet, repetitive phlebotomies, inherited or acquired bleeding disorder, repetitive blood donations, various forms of GI disease, atransferrinemia

to maintain iron balance. Approximately 2 mg of iron is lost daily during an uncomplicated pregnancy.[12] Compared with adult men and postmenopausal women, premenopausal women typically have both decreased iron ingestion and increased loss and, as a result, have lower storage iron concentrations, ranging from 100 to 400 mg. Pregnant women are especially vulnerable to iron deficiency because they lose some maternal iron stores to the developing fetus. Repeated pregnancies and lactation cause a further drain on maternal supplies.

Boys are at risk for iron deficiency during peak adolescent growth years. In men, this need for daily replacement levels off after adolescence and remains a constant requirement of 1 mg per day. The total body iron content for a man remains at approximately 2.5 to 4.0 g throughout adult life.

Because postmenopausal women do not have these increased losses, they have the same iron requirements as adult men, although they often have lower iron stores than men of the same age.[13] Finally, many older people, especially those living alone, find it difficult to cook adequate meals and fall into the habit of a diet of tea and toast or milk and crackers.

The two most common conditions that result in iron deficiency because of increased iron loss are menstrual bleeding and chronic bleeding, most often in, but not limited to, the GI tract. Menstrual bleeding is the most common cause of iron deficiency in premenopausal American women. One common problem in confirming the etiology of iron-deficiency anemia from menstrual blood loss is the inability of women to estimate normality of menstrual flow. Although the "normal" menstrual flow range is as large as 35 to 80 mL of blood per day, approximately 60 to 80 mL is considered average. In adult men and postmenopausal women, the most common cause of increased iron loss is GI bleeding.[14] Indeed, a commonly held assumption is that any man with hematologic values suggesting an iron-deficient state must have GI bleeding. GI bleeding occurs commonly in all of the following intestinal diseases and disorders: malignancy, ulceration, inflammation, diverticulosis, infestation of certain parasites, and hemorrhoids. Causes of blood loss unrelated to the GI tract include parasite infestation or infection from *Plasmodium* spp., *Babesia* spp., or *Bartonella bacilliformis* (these organisms produce hemolysis). Other conditions that lead to increased blood loss include inherited or acquired bleeding disorders, hemoptysis (expectoration of blood), nosebleeds, and hematuria. Other activities that can result in increased loss include hemodialysis and repeated blood donations.

Iron Deficiency and Iron-Deficiency Anemia

Iron deficiency is a state in which iron stores in the body are inadequate to preserve homeostasis. Because this condition is acquired and progressive, the signs and symptoms range from asymptomatic to severe. Three stages can be defined in the development of iron-deficiency anemia (IDA) (Table 6–5).

At the mildest extreme (stage I), in the face of a negative iron balance, iron stores are mobilized first and then body iron is depleted. In stage I, iron depletion, the hemosiderin content of the cells of the MPS in the marrow aspirate is decreased or absent. Serum ferritin levels (the storage form of iron) are decreased during this stage. An individual may not have any iron reserves yet be able to maintain a minimum equilibrium by increasing mucosal absorption of iron. This person

TABLE 6–5	Three Stages in the Development of Iron-Deficiency Anemia			
Tests	Normal	Stage I: Iron Depletion	Stage II: Iron-Deficient Erythropoiesis	Stage III: Iron-Deficiency Anemia
Peripheral Blood				
HB	N	N	>10 g/dL	<10 g/dL
HCT	N	N	N	DEC
RBC count	N	N	N	DEC
RBC morphology	N/N	N/N	N/N to M/N	M/N TO M/H
Reticulocyte count (%)	N	N	SLT>	INC 2–5%
Bone Marrow				
Stainable iron stores	N	N to DEC	0	0
Erythrocyte cellularity	N	N	HYPER	HYPER/INEFF
Sideroblasts (%)	40–60	N	DEC	DEC
Fe Studies				
Serum iron	N	N	DEC	DEC
Total iron-binding capacity	N	N	N/INC	N/INC
Saturation (%)	N	N	DEC	DEC
Ferritin	N	DEC	DEC	DEC
Hemosiderin	N	DEC	DEC	DEC
FEP	N	N	INC	INC
Iron absorption (%)	5–10	INC	INC	INC
Ferrokinetics*	N	N	Shortened	Shortened

*Half life plus clearance from plasma.
Abbreviations: N = within expected limits; SLT = slight; M = microcytic; H = hypochromic; DEC = decreased; INC = increased; HYPER = hyperplastic; INEFF = ineffective.

is capable of maintaining homeostasis by mobilizing all available iron but is incapable of responding to any alteration in demand. As soon as this person fails to respond adequately to a challenge that increases iron utilization, a series of physiologic corrections is initiated.

Stage II is known as iron-deficient erythropoiesis. During this stage, transferrin levels, reflected in total serum iron-binding capacities (TIBC), are increased in order to increase the absorption of dietary iron. In addition there is a fall in plasma iron, and transferrin saturation drops to less than 15% with an accompanying increase in red cell protoporphyrin concentration that increases because there is insufficient iron to convert protoporphyrin to heme. The decreased available iron limits hemoglobin synthesis even though there is no recognizable abnormality present on the peripheral blood smear; the red cells still appear normocytic and normochromic (Table 6–5).

Stage III, iron-deficiency anemia, represents the very last stage and is characterized by a decrease in hemoglobin, hematocrit, and mean corpuscular volume (MCV). As a result, the process of red cell development becomes less efficient and is termed *ineffective erythropoiesis* (Fig. 6–8). Hemoglobin formation is delayed, additional red cell division occurs during development, and microcytes result. The anemia of iron deficiency is morphologically classified as microcytic hypochromic anemia with a decrease in red cell indices (Fig. 6–9). Iron-deficiency anemia is also characterized by an increased red cell distribution width (RDW).[15] The diminished number of RBCs will stimulate an increase in erythropoietin activity and a slight to moderate reticulocytosis will occur. Figure 6–10 illustrates the relationship of iron, anemia, and bone marrow response capability. If the primary cause of the IDA is bleeding, leukocytosis and thrombocytosis are possible. If the anemia continues to progress beyond this point, abnormal shapes of RBC (poikilocytosis) will appear in the circulation. In the bone marrow, normoblasts will show decreased hemoglobinization and ragged cytoplasm (see Fig. 6–8).

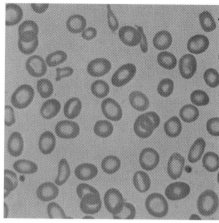

FIGURE 6–9 Peripheral blood smear in iron-deficiency anemia showing microcytosis and hypochromia and poikilocytosis. Note the occasional thin ovalocyte or pencil cell. (From Bell, A: Hematology. In Listen, Look and Learn. Health and Education Resources, Inc., Bethesda, MD, with permission.)

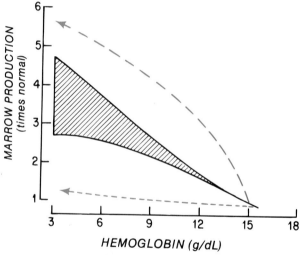

FIGURE 6–10 The role of iron supply and the degree of anemia in determining the erythroid marrow response. Moderate reductions in the hemoglobin level are largely compensated for by a shift in hemoglobin-oxygen affinity and do not elicit a maximal marrow response. With more severe anemia, the most important factor in determining the marrow production is the level of iron supply. When iron stores are exhausted (lower dashed curve), the erythroid marrow will not proliferate despite increased erythropoietin stimulation. In the presence of moderate to abundant iron stores, marrow production can increase from as little as two to as much as four times basal (shaded area). In contrast, patients with acute hemolytic anemia who have an ample iron supply from catabolized red cells will show production levels in excess of five times basal. With chronic hemolysis, sustained higher production levels with only moderate anemia are seen (upper curve). (From Hillman, RS and Finch, CA: Red Cell Manual, ed 5. FA Davis, Philadelphia, 1985, p 31, with permission.)

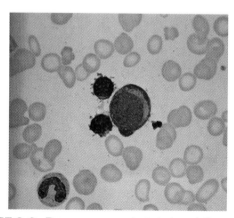

FIGURE 6–8 Bone marrow aspirate in iron-deficiency anemia showing ineffective erythropoiesis, "ragged" erythroid precursors. (From Bell, A: Hematology. In Listen, Look and Learn. Health and Education Resources, Inc., Bethesda, MD, with permission.)

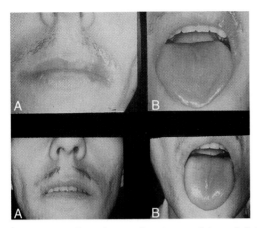

FIGURE 6–11   Clinical manifestations of iron-deficiency anemia. *A.* cheilitis and *B.* glossitis, before and after therapy.

Clinical Signs and Symptoms

The clinical disease state begins when a patient begins to experience the classic signs and symptoms of anemia. Clinical symptoms of fatigue, lethargy, and dizziness are common. Elderly patients complain of palpitations, shortness of breath, and possibly chest pain. Clinical signs might include pallor of mucous membranes, cheilitis (Fig. 6–11), koilonychia (spooning of the nails, Fig. 6–12), and/or an apical systolic, or "hemic," heart murmur. Occasionally neurologic signs and symptoms are seen. Peculiar cravings for unusual "foods" such as ice (pagophagia), clay (pica), dirt (geophagia), starch, or pickles is common in patients with iron-deficiency anemia. This manifestation is also seen in certain cultural subpopulations, however, and therefore cannot be used as primary evidence of an iron-deficient state.[16]

Although the initial red cell values are within normal limits, they eventually become the classic hematologic values of moderate to severe anemia (Hb less than 10 g/dL) and microcytic (MCV less than 80 fL), hypochromic (MCHC less than 30%) red cell morphology.

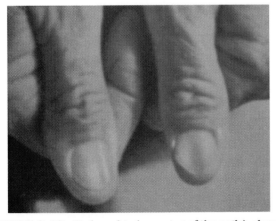

FIGURE 6–12   Koilonychia (spooning of the nails), characteristic of iron-deficiency anemia.

Laboratory Values

Clinically, iron deficiency can be characterized by three levels of severity. In the first, iron stores may be unacceptably low or even absent, while no clinical state of anemia exists. Unless the patient is investigated for some other complaint, the condition is typically not recognized by the physician or identified by the laboratory. There is adequate iron to maintain almost-normal red cell production. This subtle condition often goes undetected, for it would be difficult to know a priori that a person's hemoglobin value of 13.5 g/dL really should be 15.0 g/dL. The traditional laboratory-based definition of iron deficiency includes the absence of stainable iron in the bone marrow as the *sine qua non* of the condition; yet many premenopausal women who have no stainable iron do not have iron-deficiency anemia. Physicians treating patients who are at risk for iron deficiency without anemia are left with two unacceptable alternatives: prophylactic intervention with supplemental iron on the assumption of iron deficiency or no intervention until the condition becomes severe enough to demonstrate RBC numeric abnormalities.

Unless there is some intervention, the patient will eventually proceed from iron deficiency without anemia to the more serious state of IDA.[17] Although anemia is a major consequence of the iron-deficient state, many other deficits occur as a result of decreased iron. Patients with IDA may show decreased or inefficient activity of other compounds that require iron for biologic activity. For example, decreased myeloperoxidase activity or a diminished T-cell function may be seen in conjunction with IDA. These deficits are usually not seen as critical in making the diagnosis or determining treatment. Moreover, many of the nonerythroid iron compounds are difficult to sample or measure. From the laboratory's standpoint, it becomes useful then to evaluate a patient's overall condition by the use of a few narrowly defined aspects (such as hemoglobin value, erythrocyte morphology, iron stores in the marrow) of iron deficiency.

Using these quantitative aspects as a guide, parameters available in modern hematology instruments can identify iron-deficient states at a much earlier stage of progression (Table 6–6). An elevated RDW in the absence of any other RBC numeric abnormalities is seen as a major diagnostic tool in the evaluation of iron-deficient states. Classic laboratory values for IDA include a hemoglobin value of less than 10 g/dL and an RBC morphology consistent with an elevated RDW and low MCV, MCH, and MCHC values. Peripheral blood morphology should demonstrate microcytic hypochromic cells and a mild to moderate poikilocytosis (ovalocytes, elliptocytes, folded forms, and so on). The reticulocyte count will be within normal range to slightly elevated, providing the end test result of the ineffective erythropoiesis of the bone marrow. Evaluation of the bone marrow is not necessary for the diagnosis of iron deficiency.

When performed, however, the bone marrow aspirate illustrates morphologic changes associated with faulty hemoglobin synthesis and increased cell death resulting in ineffective erythropoiesis. The aspirate

TABLE 6–6 **Typical Peripheral Blood Values in Patients with Mild, Moderate, and Severe Iron Deficiency**			
Test	Mild IDA	Moderate IDA	Severe IDA
Hemoglobin	>11 g/dL; may be within reference ranges	<10 g/dL	<10 g/dL
Hematocrit	>36 g/dL; may be within reference ranges	<30 g/dL	<30%
Red blood cell count	May be within reference ranges	May be within reference ranges	Decreased
MCV	May be within reference ranges	Microcytic; <80 fL	Microcytic; <80 fL
MCH	May be within reference ranges	<27 pg	<27 pg
MCHC	May be within reference ranges	Normochromic to hypochromic	Hypochromic
RDW	Slightly elevated	Frankly elevated	Frankly elevated
Reticulocyte count	Elevated	Elevated	Elevated

shows a moderate increase in cellularity with erythroid hyperplasia that decreases the myeloid-to-erythroid (M:E) ratio in favor of the erythroid component. Normoblasts are smaller than normal. The cytoplasm is typically described as scanty. The usual comparison of hemoglobin content to nuclear maturity reveals an increase in the number and variety of cellular abnormalities as well, including karyorrhexis and nuclear fragmentation. As stated before, in iron deficiency, sideroblasts are reduced or absent and the corresponding special stain for iron (Prussian blue) will be negative. Serum iron concentration is usually below 50 mg/dL. TIBC may be normal to elevated, with the percent saturated usually decreased below 15% (Table 6–7).

Treatment

Therapy of IDA demands the correction of the underlying cause. Dietary deficiencies can be corrected through nutrition counseling or oral medication. Malabsorption syndromes may or may not be corrected by diet alone. Correction of the primary disease state is the first choice, but if uncorrectable (e.g., because of surgical loss of duodenal or jejunal tissue from some other disease), then supplementary iron in oral or intramuscular from is required. Recovery from anemia is first seen on the peripheral blood smear by the presence of a dual population of red cells: older cells that are microcytic and hypochromic as a result of iron deficiency and a younger, normochromic-normocytic cell group able to make use of supplemental iron (Fig. 6–13). The second stage of recovery is equated with the re-establishment of normal hemoglobin concentration and marrow iron stores. Whenever iron supplements are given, they should be considered as part of the therapeutic regimen. Any underlying disorders must be corrected if iron supplementation is to be effective. Typically, appropriate therapy consists of ferrous sul-

TABLE 6–7 **Summary of Other Laboratory Values Found Commonly in Iron Deficiency States**		
Tests	Values	Comments
Peripheral Blood		
WBC and PLT counts	Increased	May be increased if associated with bleeding (mature neutrophilia predominates)
Bone Marrow		
Cellularity	Normal to hypercellular	
Morphology	RBC precursors are increased in number but have skimpy cytoplasm	
Iron stain	Negative	
Chemical Testing on Serum		
Serum iron	Decreased	
Transferrin/TIBC	Normal to increased	
% saturation	Decreased	
Serum ferritin	Decreased	

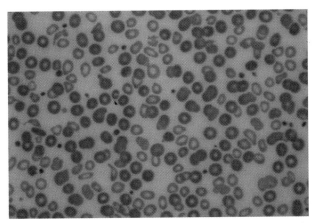

FIGURE 6-13 Peripheral blood of patient with iron-deficiency anemia following therapy. Note the two populations of red cells.

fate tablets or elixir. Parenteral therapy is available but not frequently used. Because iron absorption in the iron-deficiency patient is increased, as much as 20% absorption should occur, provided absorption is not impaired. Iron supplements can cause side effects (e.g., nausea, diarrhea, constipation), and many patients prefer to take the medication with meals rather than before eating.[18] Assuming that absorption is adequate, quantifiable changes will be seen quickly, regardless of the route of administration.[19]

Dysfunction of Iron Utilization

Usually secondary to another disease, iron deficiency may be caused by an inability of erythroid cells to access iron stored within macrophages. One common cause involves a blockage within mitochondria that prevents nonheme iron from being used by the developing red cell; another involves dysfunctional serum transferrin receptors on the developing cells.[20]

Known as the anemia of chronic disease, this condition is thought to be influenced by the strong inflammatory component and suppressive effect found in diseases such as rheumatoid arthritis, Crohn's disease, or increased immune hemolysis through agglutinins such as those found in infectious mononucleosis (anti-i) and infections by *Mycoplasma pneumoniae* (anti-I).[21] Much less frequently, iron deficiency–like states can be caused by direct infection of red cell precursors by hepatitis B virus or parvovirus B19.[22] A primary chronic inflammatory disease with secondary microcytic hypochromic anemia is important to distinguish from a microcytic hypochromic anemia caused by iron deficiency from nutritional deficit or blood loss. A more thorough discussion of anemia of chronic disease is found in Chapter 15.

Laboratory values for an iron deficiency–like anemia are less dramatic than those of iron deficiency. Typically, the whole blood hemoglobin is between 9 and 12 g/dL. The red cells are normocytic, normochromic, with some anisocytosis. The RDW is usually within reference limits. Important biochemistry test results include a decreased serum iron and a decreased TIBC. The decreased TIBC is important inasmuch as it helps distinguish this condition from IDA, which typically has a high-normal to elevated TIBC (Table 6–8).

Iron Excess and Sideroblastic States

Although the absorption of iron is carefully regulated to prevent overload, the sideroblastic state still occurs. Increased iron absorption and storage are seen in patients with inherited disorders and malignancies, and in those following fad diets (Table 6–9). Regardless of cause, similarities in morphology and hemogram (complete blood count, CBC) values exist.

Hemosiderosis

Hemosiderosis is the accumulation of excess iron in macrophages in varying tissues. Most often, hemosiderosis has no significant signs or symptoms of its own

TABLE 6–8 **Differential Diagnosis of Iron Deficiency and Anemia Because of Chronic Disease**		
	Iron Deficiency	Anemia Because of Chronic Inflammation
Peripheral Blood		
Anisopoikilocytosis	Variable	Usually absent
Target cells	Few	Absent
Basophilic stippling	Absent	Usually absent
Bone Marrow		
Marrow iron	Decreased	Normal to increased
Marrow sideroblasts	Decreased	Decreased
Serum Levels		
Serum ferritin	Decreased	Increased/normal
Serum iron	Decreased	Decreased
Total iron-binding capacity (TIBC)	Increased	Decreased
% iron saturation of transferrin	Decreased	Decreased
Free erythrocyte protoporphyrin (FEP)	Increased	Increased

TABLE 6–9 Categories of Sideroblastic Anemias

Primary
Sideroblastic anemia—autosomal recessive
Congenital sideroblastic anemia—sex-linked
Idiopathic sideroblastic anemia (RARS)

Secondary
To Other Disease States:
    Infections
    Neoplasms
    Acute or chronic inflammation
To Toxic Exposure:
    Chronic alcohol abuse
    Unusual dietary habits or culture
    Lead poisoning
Iatrogenic:
    Chronic transfusion support
    Antitubercular medications (e.g., isoniazid)
    Antibiotics (e.g., choramphenicol)

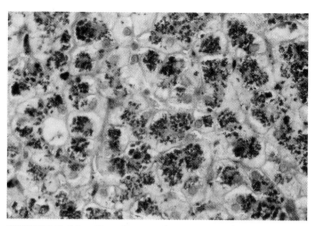

FIGURE 6–14. Liver biopsy of a patient with idiopathic hemochromatosis and cirrhosis. Note the excess deposits of iron (ferric ferricyanide stain).

but can occur secondary to bleeding into an organ such as the lungs or kidneys. For example, pulmonary hemosiderosis results from an accumulation of iron in the pulmonary macrophages after episodes of bleeding into the lungs and is found as a complication of the primary condition. This iron is bound to hemosiderin but is unavailable to the recycling process. The hemosiderin found in patients with primary or secondary hemochromatosis has an altered molecular structure compared with the hemosiderin found in healthy persons.[23]

Hemochromatosis

Hereditary hemochromatosis, on the other hand, is a significant and common disease in its own right.[24] This autosomal-recessive disease is characterized by an iron absorption rate of up to 4 g daily.[25] Although this disease may actually begin early in childhood, the accumulation of iron occurs slowly and the complications of that accumulation often take time to become apparent. As a consequence, most patients with hemochromatosis are adults in their 50s or 60s. Men are more often afflicted than women. It is unknown whether this is due to some genetic predisposition or to the fact that women typically ingest less iron and eliminate more iron through menstrual bleeding, pregnancy, or both. The major concern is the location of the iron deposits. Hemosiderosis occurs in the reticuloendothelial system (RES); hemochromatosis occurs in the parenchymal tissues of organs such as the pancreas, liver, and spleen, where it initiates a fibrotic process. This disease is often referred to as *bronze diabetes*, because a major presenting syndrome consists of a type of adult-onset diabetes caused by fibrosis in the pancreas and a peculiar skin discoloration. The signs of bronze diabetes include weakness and weight loss (probably because of the diabetes) and excessive melanin deposits in the skin most frequently exposed to sunlight. These patients can also develop cirrhosis of the liver (Fig. 6–14) and heart failure. Therapeutic removal of iron, by either phlebotomy or chelating

agents, may lessen the degree of diabetes or heart failure. Repeated phlebotomies are the treatment of choice in patients with a hemoglobin value greater than 10 g/dL. Fewer donations are needed once an acceptable serum iron level is reached. The frequency is regulated by the need to keep the serum iron within acceptable limits. For patients who have a hemoglobin level of less than 10 g/dL or who show a decreased marrow response, the chelating agent desferoxamine is the treatment of choice.[26]

Sideroblastic States

Primary sideroblastic anemia (Fig. 6–15) may be either inherited or acquired (see Table 6–9). Hereditary sideroblastic anemia is a sex-linked disorder usually affecting men, although women also may develop some abnormalities. Some patients demonstrate hepatosplenomegaly. Approximately 50% of these patients respond to vitamin B_6 (pyridoxine) therapy. Idiopathic or acquired sideroblastic anemia, a type of myelodysplastic disorder, is discussed in Chapter 19.

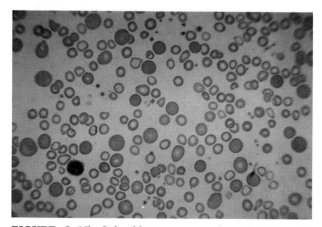

FIGURE 6–15 Sideroblastic anemia (peripheral blood). Note the characteristic dimorphic blood picture. (Magnification × 500)

Secondary sideroblastic anemia actually comprises a group of diseases with several different acquired mechanisms of iron overload. Some are acute, others chronic. Acute iron intoxication may be found in cases involving suicide attempts or accidental poisoning in children and will not be discussed here.

Clinical Signs and Symptoms An iatrogenic secondary sideroblastic state is seen in patients taking antitubercular, antimicrobial, or antiparkinsonian drugs (inhibitors of pyridoxine metabolism). Chloramphenicol treatment also causes iron overload. Iatrogenic sideroblastosis occurs also in patients who need chronic transfusions, such as those with aplastic anemia, thalassemia, and leukemia. Because these patients usually have a normal dietary intake of iron, the combination of normal intake and increased iron from transfusions results in increased absorption and storage.

Chronic iron overload is achieved by an increased iron uptake accompanied by increased iron absorption. Alcoholics may have an increased iron absorption (alcoholic beverages have an iron content that ranges from 5 to 20 mg/L), although their condition may be complicated by folate deficiency, cirrhosis, or lead poisoning. This condition is much more commonly seen in the developed countries in persons who are food faddists and take megavitamins or mineral supplements, but it is also seen among such cultural groups as the Bantu tribe of South Africa (because of use of iron utensils) and certain tribes of Manchurian hunters (because of Kashin-Beck disease, iron utensils, and heavy concentration of iron in well water).

Laboratory Values A patient with any of these sideroblastic conditions typically presents with mild to moderate anemia, variable red cell indices, and an elevated RDW with a significant widening of the RBC histogram. This suggestion of a dimorphic red cell population is seen in the evaluation of the peripheral blood smear (see Fig. 6–15). In addition, anisopoikilocytosis and Pappenheimer bodies are usually observed. Care must be used to differentiate Pappenheimer bodies from basophilic stippling, which also occurs in these patients. Reticulocyte counts are decreased. Microscopic examination of the bone marrow aspirate shows erythroid hyperplasia resulting from ineffective erythropoiesis. Since mitochondria are usually located around the nucleus of developing normoblasts and the iron is entrapped within them, Prussian blue staining sometimes creates a halolike effect around the negatively stained nucleus. Ringed sideroblasts are found in normal bone marrow aspirates, but patients with any of the sideroblastic anemias commonly have a significant increase in the number of ringed sideroblasts (see Fig. 6–5). Furthermore, these patients have a significant number of siderotic granules in peripheral blood erythrocytes. Greater than 10% positive-staining cells is common. In addition to the increased iron absorption seen in many of these patients, there is also an ineffective erythropoiesis because of the failure to utilize iron trapped in the mitochondria. As a consequence of the engorgement of the normal iron deposits, the serum iron and marrow iron stores are elevated and additional deposit sites in the liver and spleen occur. Tables 6–10 and 6–11 compare the most common presentations of microcytic hypochromic states.

Treatment Treatment of these secondary disease states must be directed at the primary cause. Simple steps include diet modification or changes in therapeutic regimens requiring antimicrobial agents or transfusions. Aggressive therapies include repeat phlebotomies or chelation agents, or both.

Lead Poisoning (Acquired Sideroblastic Anemia or Acquired Porphyria)

Similar to both porphyria and sideroblastic anemia, lead intoxication produces a microcytic hypochromic anemia, skin lesions, and neurologic dysfunctions.[27] Lead consumption produces two coincidental and synergistic effects. First, it interferes with iron storage in the mitochondria, thus producing a classic sideroblastic anemia. When severe enough, the mitochondrial buildup of iron can be shown by Prussian blue staining.[28] Second, lead has a damaging effect on the ac-

TABLE 6–10 **Differential Diagnosis of Iron Deficiency and Sideroblastic Anemia**		
	Iron Deficiency	Sideroblastic Anemia
Peripheral Blood		
Anisopoikilocytosis	Variable	Variable
Target cells	Few	Absent
Basophilic stippling	Absent	Mild to moderate
Bone Marrow		
Marrow iron	Decreased	Increased
Marrow sideroblasts	Decreased	Increased (ringed sideroblasts)
Serum Levels		
Serum ferritin	Decreased	Increased
Serum iron	Decreased	Increased
Total iron-binding capacity (TIBC)	Increased	Normal
% iron saturation of transferrin	Decreased	Increased
Free erythrocyte protoporphyrin (FEP)	Increased	Increased

TABLE 6–11   **Differential Diagnosis of Iron Deficiency and Anemia from Chronic Disease and Sideroblastic Anemia**

	Iron Deficiency	Anemia from Chronic Inflammation	Sideroblastic Anemia
Peripheral Blood			
Anisopoikilocytosis	Variable	Usually absent	Variable
Target cells	Few	Absent	Absent
Basophilic stippling	Absent	Usually absent	Mild to moderate
Bone Marrow			
Marrow iron	Decreased	Increased/normal	Increased
Marrow sideroblasts	Decreased	Decreased	Increased (ringed sideroblasts)
Serum Levels			
Serum ferritin	Decreased	Increased/normal	Increased
Serum iron	Decreased	Decreased	Normal or increased
Total iron-binding capacity (TIBC)	Increased	Decreased	Normal or increased
% Iron saturation of transferrin	Decreased	Decreased	Normal or increased
Free erythrocyte protoporphyrin (FEP)	Increased	Increased	Increased

tivity of at least six of the enzymes used in heme synthesis: δ-aminolevulinic acid (δ-ALA) dehydrogenase synthetase, ALA dehydrase, porphyrinogen oxidase, uroporphyrinogen decarboxylase, coproporphyrinogen oxidase, and heme synthetase. δ-Aminolevulinic dehydrase (δ-ALA) is most sensitive to the presence of lead, and the resultant elevations in ALA are an early sign of lead intoxication.[29] Although other precursors may also be elevated, measurement of increased quantities of zinc-bound protoporphyrin (also known as free erythrocyte protoporphyrin, or FEP) caused by dysfunctional heme synthetase within the red cell is widely used as a diagnostic tool.

It was hoped that lead poisoning as a major disease could be diminished through the enactment of laws regulating the manufacture of lead-based paint and other lead-based substances. Lead intoxication occurs in both children and adults, although the mechanism of exposure and clinical sequelae of that exposure are quite different.[30] Children may be exposed to lead by eating sweet-tasting lead-based paint that is flaking or by inhaling the powdery residue from lead-based paint.[31] This paint, sometimes hidden under several layers of newer paints, can often be found in older homes. Infants and toddlers are particularly sensitive to the effects of lead exposure, and moderate to severe mental retardation can result. There may also be abdominal pains and cramping (abdominal colic) following lead exposure of this type.[32] Adults may be exposed to lead in the workplace (e.g., in the manufacture of batteries or decoration of pottery in which lead is used in the underglazing processes). Adults also tend to complain of peripheral neuropathy and skin lesions as well as abdominal pains, but mental retardation is not an issue in adult-onset lead poisoning.[33]

Another difference between adult and pediatric patients with lead intoxication is the complicating state

of iron deficiency. Many infants and toddlers also have iron deficiency because of poor nutrition during gestation and during the formative growth spurt of the first 2 years.[34]

The interference of lead with heme synthesis results in an ineffective erythropoietic state in which shortened red cell survival and difficulty in heme synthesis produce a mild microcytic hypochromic anemia. Basophilic stippling is found in many circulating RBCs and may occur as a result of other lead-induced enzyme dysfunctions (Fig. 6–16). As a result of RBC inclusions, damaged enzymes, and inadequate hemoglobinization, erythrocyte osmotic fragility may be decreased. Leukocytosis may be present, showing increased numbers of eosinophils and reactive lymphocytes. Reticulocytosis may or may not be present. He-

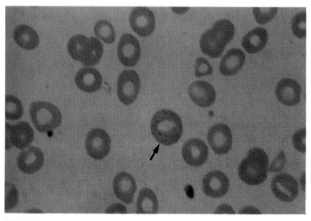

FIGURE 6–16   Basophilic stippling in lead poisoning (arrow).

moglobin A_2 or F may be elevated and ineffective erythroid hyperplasia is seen in the marrow.

Both children and adult victims of lead poisoning are usually treated with chelation therapy. Ethylenediaminetetraacetic acid (EDTA) binds irreversibly to lead to produce a lead chelate that is neurologically toxic but rapidly excreted in the urine. Therapy will eliminate the lead; however, those cells that have been damaged will remain in that state until senescence. Some studies now indicate that damage sustained during the acute phase of lead inotoxication is never completely repaired, regardless of therapy.[35,36]

HEME SYNTHESIS AND RELATED DISORDERS

Normal Heme Synthesis

The term *heme synthesis* is reserved for those steps involving the synthesis of protoporphyrin IX (heme without the iron). Heme synthesis is a series of eight enzymatic reactions that involve time- and concentration-dependent equilibrium among substrates, enzymes, and cofactors, with each product acting as the substrate for the next step. A defect causing a slower reaction rate or a lessened amount of product results in the accumulation of substrate. Some accumulated substrates are inherently unstable and metabolize into porphyrins, a class of stable but highly resonating compounds. Defects occurring in either of the first two steps result in the formation of compounds loosely called *porphyrin precursors*.

The intermediate substrates occurring after the second step in the pathway are forms of porphyrinogen, which, if unused in normal heme synthesis, degrade into small amounts of porphyrins easily excreted in the urine.[37] Excessive formation of porphyrins occurs if any one of the normal enzymatic steps in heme synthesis is blocked and results in one of a number of metabolic disorders collectively called the porphyrias. (For a more detailed explanation of heme synthesis, see Chap. 2.)

Abnormal Heme Synthesis

Disorders of heme synthesis (porphyrias) can be either inherited or acquired. In either case, abnormal accumulation of porphyrin precursors or porphyrins occurs in the two major sites of heme synthesis—the bone marrow and the liver. The inherited porphyrias are uncommon and are classically categorized by the mode of transmission, the defective enzyme, and the porphyrin allowed to accumulate. Clinically, these disorders are categorized by site of accumulation and major signs and symptoms.[38] Using this method, porphyrias are divided into three major classes: (1) erythropoietic porphyrias—accumulation of porphyrins in the bone marrow associated with high incidence of photosensitivity and dermatitis; (2) hepatic porphyrias—accumulation of porphyrin precursors in the liver associated with neurologic deficit; and (3) mixed porphyrias—accumulation in both bone marrow and liver resulting in both neurologic and dermatologic involvement (Table 6–12).

TABLE 6–12 **Inherited Heme Synthesis Disorders**

Erythropoietic Porphyrias (hematology and/or skin manifestations)
     Congenital erythropoietic porphyria (congenital photosensitive porphyria)
     Porphyria cutanea tarda

Hepatic Porphyrias (neurologic and/or hepatic manifestations)
     Acute intermittent hepatic porphyria (acute or Swedish-type porphyria)
     Hereditary coproporphyria (benign coproporphyria)
     Erythropoietic protoporphyria (congenital erythropoietic protoporphyria)

Mixed Porphyrias (variable manifestations)   Variegated porphyria (mixed hepatic porphyria)

Erythropoietic Porphyrias

Congenital erythropoietic porphyria (Fig. 6–17) is the least common of these rare disorders and occurs when the defective enzyme is uroporphyrinogen III cosynthetase, with a resultant buildup of uroporphyrin II and III and coproporphyrin in the bone marrow, with onset in early childhood or infancy.[39] Because this disease involves an accumulation of porphyrins in developing RBCs, RBC survival time is shortened. The hemolytic process develops into a hemolytic anemia with splenomegaly and ineffective erythropoiesis. Dermal photosensitivity occurs as a result of the accumulation of fluorescing compounds such as coproporphyrin.

In erythropoietic protoporphyria, dermal photosensitivity and solar erythema, urticaria, and eczema with onset in childhood characterize the loss of heme synthetase and the buildup of protoporphyrin. Possibly inherited as an autosomal-dominant disorder, it is seen throughout the world. Protoporphyria is usually

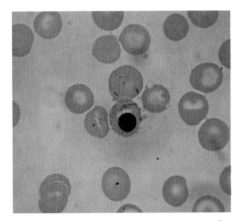

FIGURE 6–17 Erythropoietic porphyria. Note the precipitated porphyrins in the cytoplasm. (From Bell, A: Hematology. In Listen, Look and Learn. Health and Education Resources, Inc., Bethesda, MD, with permission.)

considered a relatively benign disorder, concentrated in skin lesions, although many patients also have liver and biliary tract dysfunctions.

CASE STUDY 1

An 18-year-old woman came to her physician for a routine physical examination before entering college. Her family history was unremarkable. Her personal history revealed that she had begun menstruation at the age of 13 and had experienced no complaints other than cramping. Other than an occasional cold, she stated that she was perfectly healthy.

On physical examination, she appeared to be well nourished and looked her stated age. Mucous membranes were pale. Her overall muscle tone was poor, but she explained that "she just wasn't very athletic." Her pulse was 80 beats per minute and her blood pressure within normal limits. A grade I apical murmur was noted.

Results of laboratory tests included: WBC, 11.4×10^9/L; Hb, 10.0 g/dL; MCV, 79 fL; RDW, 14.8%; PLT, 400×10^9/L. Microcytes, some hypochromic cells, and polychromatophilic RBCs were seen on the peripheral blood smear. The reticulocyte count was 2.5%.

Questions

1. What is the most likely explanation of this presentation?
   a. Iron-deficiency anemia
   b. Lead poisoning
   c. Hemochromatosis
   d. Acute intermittent porphyria
2. What are the next laboratory tests that need to be performed?
   a. Bone marrow aspiration
   b. Hemoglobin electrophoresis
   c. Serum iron and TIBC
   d. Serum lead and FEP
3. If the serum iron was abnormally low and the TIBC slightly elevated, what would you conclude about the state of iron storage in the bone marrow?
   a. Iron stores are adequate.
   b. Iron stores are absent.
   c. Bone marrow hemosiderin is adequate.
   d. Insufficient information is given to answer the question.
4. What questions need to be asked before initiation of any therapy?
   a. Questions concerning her dietary habits.
   b. Questions concerning exposure to any chemicals, lead, and so forth.
   c. Questions that would elicit more detailed information concerning the frequency, duration, and severity of menstrual blood loss.
   d. Questions regarding possible allergy or extreme sensitivity to ferrous sulfate medication.
5. Assuming that the correct medications have been given and it is 1 month later, what statement could be made about this young woman's condition?

   a. Her hemoglobin concentration is now above 12.0 g/dL.
   b. Iron stores have been replenished in the bone marrow.
   c. Serum ferritin is increased but plasma iron is not.
   d. The TIBC is completely saturated.

Answers

1. a (p 105)
2. c (p 106)
3. b (p 105)
4. c (p 103)
5. b (p 106)

CASE STUDY 2

A 36-month-old boy of Sicilian ancestry was seen by his pediatrician to investigate a complaint of irritability and "coliclike pain." The child's birth weight was 7 pounds, 9 ounces. The mother's pregnancy and delivery had been without complication. Early developmental milestones were achieved without incident. Approximately 1 month earlier, the child had become unusually irritable in response to otherwise normal activity. This had been accompanied by signs of abdominal discomfort and diarrhea.

Physical findings included pale mucous membranes and a thin, dark line around the gums. Neurologic examination showed increased irritability and decreased ability to maintain normal concentration. The rest of the examination was unremarkable.

Hematologic test results included: WBC, 14.5×10^9/L; Hb, 9.7 g/dL; MCV, 77 fL; and RDW, 15.5%. Peripheral blood morphology demonstrated the presence of microcytic, hypochromic cells; normocytic, normochromic cells; basophilic stippling; and nonspecific poikilocytosis. Rare nucleated RBCs were seen on microscopic scan of Wright-stained peripheral blood smear.

Questions

1. What is the best explanation of this child's condition?
   a. Iron-deficiency anemia
   b. Lead poisoning
   c. Hemochromatosis
   d. Acute intermittent porphyria
2. What are the next laboratory tests that need to be performed?
   a. Bone marrow aspiration
   b. Hemoglobin electrophoresis
   c. Serum iron and TIBC
   d. Serum lead and FEP
3. If the serum lead and FEP were elevated, what would you conclude about the state of iron storage in the bone marrow?
   a. Iron stores are adequate.
   b. Iron stores are absent.
   c. Bone marrow hemosiderin is adequate.
   d. Insufficient information is given to answer the question.
   e. All of the above.

4. Which of the following enzymes needed for heme synthesis is altered in lead poisoning?
   a. δ-Aminolevulinic acid synthetase
   b. Uroporphyrinogen decarboxylase
   c. Coproporphyrinogen oxidase
   d. Heme synthetase
   e. All of the above
5. Why does treatment of lead poisoning involve chelation therapy and iron supplements?
   a. Chelation drugs always interfere with iron metabolism.
   b. Many children who have lead poisoning also have a dietary iron deficiency.
   c. Iron supplements help to re-establish the normal iron concentrations.
   d. Iron supplements bind to excess chelation agents.

Answers

1. b (p 109–110)
2. d (p 110)
3. d (p 110)
4. e (p 110)
5. b (p 110)

CASE STUDY 3

A 72-year-old woman was admitted to the hospital with a complaint of rectal bleeding. She had a 40-year history of progressive rheumatoid arthritis that resulted in artificial knee, elbow, and shoulder replacement surgery. Past drug history includes aspirin, naproxen sodium, and ibuprofen. Currently she takes a high anti-inflammatory dose of ibuprofen. Her admission CBC demonstrates:

RBC: 4.98×10^{12}/L   MCV: 64 fL
Hb: 9.7 g/dL   MCH: 19.4 pg
Hct: 32%   MCHC: 30.3%
RDW: 16%   PLT: 490×10^9/L
WBC: 13.0×10^9/L

Differential blood examination shows a mild neutrophilia, slight thrombocytosis, and microcytic hypochromic red blood cells; 4+ poikilocytosis and 3+ microcytosis are seen, along with occasional basophilic stippling and rare Pappenheimer bodies.

Questions

1. What is the best explanation for this presentation?
   a. Iron deficiency
   b. Beta thalassemia minor
   c. Anemia because of inflammatory disease
   d. Sideroblastic anemia
2. Her serum iron level is at the low end of the reference range, although the TIBC is slightly increased. Serum ferritin levels are increased. One explanation for this is:
   a. The inflammatory block prevents iron absorption from the GI tract.
   b. She is also experiencing chronic blood loss, which adds an absolute iron deficiency on top of the inflammatory block's inability to use iron.
   c. Available iron stores are being mobilized in the ferritin, thus providing false results.

   d. High-dose ibuprofen ingestion interferes with serum iron results.
3. Treatment for this woman should include:
   a. Daily iron injections to eliminate the inflammatory block
   b. High-dose iron supplements taken with antacids to prevent stomach upset
   c. Correction of the GI bleeding
   d. Eliminating the ibuprofen in favor of aspirin to control the inflammation
4. If a bone marrow aspirate were performed, the Prussian blue stain would show:
   a. Stainable iron in both red cell precursors and macrophages
   b. No stainable nonheme iron
   c. Stainable iron in red cell precursors
   d. Stainable iron in macrophages only
5. Correction of the microcytic anemia will occur with:
   a. Absorption of adequate iron
   b. Correction of the rectal bleeding
   c. Increased iron supplementation
   d. Suppression of the inflammation

Answers

1. c (p 107)
2. b (p 107 [Table 6–8])
3. c (p 103)
4. d (p 106)
5. d (p 106)

REFERENCES

1. Dallman, PR: Iron deficiency: Does it matter. J Intern Med 226:367, 1989.
2. Weinberg, ED: Cellular regulation of iron assimilation. Q Rev Biol 64:261, 1989.
3. Bhagavan, NV: Biochemistry, ed 2. JB Lippincott, Philadelphia, 1978, p 676.
4. Bothwell, TH, et al: Nutritional iron requirements and food iron absorption. J Int Med Res (Engl) 226:357, 1989.
5. Hallberg, L, Brune, M, and Rossander, L: The role of vitamin C in iron absorption. Int J Vitam Nutr Res (suppl) 30:103, 1989.
6. Conrad, ME and Barton, JC: Factors affecting iron balance. Am J Hematol 10:199, 1981.
7. Nimeh, N and Bishop, RC: Disorders of iron metabolism. Med Clin North Am 64:631, 1980.
8. Finch, CA and Huebers, H: Perspectives in iron metabolism. N Engl J Med 306:1520, 1981.
9. Ahmadzadeh, N, Shingu, M, and Nobunaga, M: Iron binding proteins and free iron in synovial fluids of rheumatoid arthritis patients. Clin Rheumatol (Belg) 8:345, 1989.
10. Dallman, PR, Simes, MA, and Stekjel, A: Iron deficiency in infancy and childhood. Am J Clin Nutr 33:86, 1980.
11. Major, P: Iron deficiency anemia and psychomotor development in infants. Tidsskr Nor Laegeforen (Norway) 114(7): 1995, 1994.
12. Beck, WS (ed): Hematology. MIT Press, Cambridge, MA, 1985.
13. Johnson, MA, Fischer, JG, Bowman, BA, and Gunter, EW: Iron nutrition in elderly individuals. FASEB-J 8:609, 1994.
14. Fairbanks, VF and Beutler, E: Iron deficiency. In Williams WWJ, et al (eds): Hematology, ed 3. McGraw-Hill, New York, 1983, p 300.
15. Qurtom, HA, et al: The value of red cell distribution width in the diagnosis of anaemia in children. Eur J Pediatr 148:745, 1989.

16. Moore, DF, Jr and Sears, DA: Pica, iron deficiency, and the medical history. Am J Med 97:390, 1994.

17. Brekelmans, P, van Soest, P, Leenen, PJ, and van Ewijk, W: Inhibition of proliferation and differentiation during early T cell development by anti-transferrin receptor antibody. Eur J Immunol 24:2896, 1994.

18. Galloway, R and McGuire, J: Determinants of compliance with iron supplementation: Supplies, side effects, or psychology? Soc Sci Med 39:381, 1994.

19. McCurdy, PR: Oral and parenteral iron therapy: A comparison. JAMA 191:859, 1965.

20. Zoli, A, et al: Serum transferrin receptors in rheumatoid arthritis. Ann Rheum Dis 53:699, 1994.

21. Gasche, C, et al: Anemia in Crohn's disease: Importance of inadequate erythropoietin production and iron deficiency. Dig Dis Sci 39:1930, 1994.

22. Tchernia, G, Dussaix, E, and Laurian, Y: Parovirus B 19 and pediatric pathology. Arch Pediatr 1:508, 1994.

23. Ward, RJ, et al: Biochemical studies of the iron cores and polypeptide shells or haemosiderin isolated from patients with primary or secondary haemochromatosis. Biochem Biophys Acta 993:131, 1989.

24. Haddy, TB, Castro, OL, and Rana, SR: Hereditary hemochromatosis in children, adolescents, and young adults. Am J Pediatr Hematol Oncol 10:23, 1988.

25. Lynch, SR, Skikne, BS, and Cook, JD: Food iron absorption in idiopathic hemochromatosis. Blood 74:2187, 1989.

26. Pippard, MJ: Desferrioxamine-induced excretion in humans. Baillieres Clin Haematol 2:232, 1989.

27. Dagg, JG, et al: The relationship of lead poisoning to acute intermittent porphyria. Q J Med 34:163, 1965.

28. Albahary, C: Lead and hemopoiesis. Am J Med 52:369, 1972.

29. Lichtman, HC and Feldman, F: In vitro pyrrole and porphyrin synthesis in lead poisoning. Pediatrics 31:996, 1963.

30. Philip, AT and Gerson, B: Lead poisoning—Part I, incidence, etiology and toxicokinetics. Clin Lab Med 14:423, 1994.

31. Casey, R, Wiley, C, Rutstein, P, and Pinto-Martin, J: Prevalence of lead poisoning in an urban cohort of infants with high socioeconomic status. Clin Pediatr 33:480, 1994.

32. Wasserman, GA, et al: Consequences of lead exposure and iron supplementation on childhood development at age 4 years. Neurotoxicol Teratol 16:233, 1994.

33. Chao, KY and Wang, JD: Increased lead absorption caused by working next to a lead recycling factory. Am J Ind Med. 26:229, 1994.

34. Committee on Nutrition (American Academy of Pediatrics): Iron Supplmentation for Infants. Pediatrics 58:765, 1976.

35. Needleman, HL, et al: The long term effects of exposure to low doses of lead in childhood. N Engl J Med 322:83, 1990.

36. Minder, B, Das-Smaal, EA, Brand, EF, and Orlebeke, JF: Exposure to lead and specific attention deficit problems in school children. J Learn Disabil 27:393, 1994.

37. Robinson, SH and Glass, J: Disorders of heme metabolism: Sideroblastic anemia and the porphyrias. In Nathan DG, and Oski, FA (eds): Hematology of Infancy and Childhood, ed 2. WB Saunders, Philadelphia, 1981, p 336.

38. Thompson, RB and Procter, SJ: A Concise Textbook of Hematology, ed 6. Urban and Schwarzenberg, Baltimore, 1984, p 48.

39. Meyers, US and Schmid, R: The porphyrias. In Stanbury, JB, Wyngaarden, JB, and Fredrickson, DS (eds): The Metabolic Basis of Inherited Disease, ed 4. McGraw-Hill, New York, 1978, p 1166.

40. Dean, G and Barnes, HB: The Porphyrias: A Story of Inheritance and Environment. Pitman, London, 1963.

QUESTIONS

1. What is the primary function of iron?
   a. Molecular stability
   b. Oxygen transport
   c. Cellular metabolism
   d. Cofactor

2. Which of the following influence(s) iron absorption?
   a. Amount and type of iron in food
   b. Function of GI mucosa and pancreas
   c. Erythropoietic needs and iron stores
   d. All of the above

3. What is the correct sequence for iron transport?
   a. Ingestion, conversion to ferrous state in stomach, reconversion to ferric state in bloodstream, transport by transferrin, incorporation into cells and tissues
   b. Ingestion, transport by transferrin to liver, conversion in liver to ferric state, transport in ferrous state to cells and tissues for incorporation
   c. Ingestion, conversion to ferrous state in stomach, transport in bloodstream to cells and tissues, conversion to ferric state prior to incorporation into cells and tissues
   d. Ingestion, transport by transferrin to cells and tissues, conversion to ferrous state prior to incorporation into cells and tissues

4. Which of the following is *not* consistent with the finding for a stage of iron deficiency?
   a. State I: Iron depletion; decreased serum ferritin levels; depletion of stored iron; equilibrium maintained through compensation mechanisms
   b. Stage II: Iron-deficient erythropoiesis; increased TIBC; decreased plasma iron and transferrin saturation; normocytic, normochronic RBCs
   c. Stage III: Iron-deficiency anemia; decreased hemoglobin, hematocrit, and MCV; microcytic, hypochromic anemia; increased RDW
   d. Stage IV: Chronic iron-deficiency anemia; decreased hemoglobin, hematocrit; increased MCV; macrocytic, hypochromic anemia; decreased RDW

5. What are the two major categories of iron deficiency?
   a. Defects in globin synthesis and iron incorporation
   b. Low availability and increased loss of iron
   c. Defective RBC catabolism and recovery of iron
   d. Problems with transport and storage of iron

6. Which are characteristic laboratory finding(s) for IDA?
   a. Increased RDW
   b. Decreased MCV, MCH, MCHC
   c. Ovalocytes, elliptocytes, microcytes
   d. All of the above

7. Which laboratory test results would be most helpful in distinguishing IDA from anemia of chronic disease?
   a. Decreased MCV, MCH; marked poikilocytosis
   b. Increased MCV, MCH, MCHC; decreased RDW
   c. Increased RDW and TIBC
   d. Decreased RDW and TIBC

8. What term refers to the accumulation of excess iron in macrophages?
   a. Sideroblastic anemia
   b. Hemosiderosis

c. Porphyria
d. Thalassemia

9. Which of the following findings would *not* be seen in sideroblastic conditions?
a. Increased RDW
b. Pappenheimer bodies
c. Ringed sideroblasts
d. Decreased serum iron

10. What is a characteristic finding in lead poisoning?
a. Basophilic stippling
b. Target cells
c. Sideroblasts
d. Spherocytes

ANSWERS

1. **b** (p 97)
2. **d** (p 100)
3. **a** (p 101)
4. **d** (p 103 [Table 6–5])
5. **b** (p 102)
6. **a** (p 105)
7. **c** (p 107 [Table 6–8])
8. **b** (p 107)
9. **d** (p 109)
10. **a** (p 110)

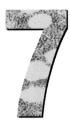

7

Megaloblastic Anemias

Mitra Taghizadeh, MS, MT(ASCP), CLS(NCA)

Objectives

At the end of this chapter, the learner should be able to:

1. Define *megaloblastic anemia*.
2. Compare and contrast the morphologic characteristic of megaloblasts and normoblasts.
3. Characterize the peripheral blood morphology of megaloblastic anemia.
4. Identify the bone marrow morphology of megaloblastic anemia.
5. Describe pernicious anemia, including the pathophysiology and clinical and laboratory findings.
6. Describe the Schilling test as a diagnostic tool for pernicious anemia.
7. List the causes of vitamin B_{12} and folate deficiencies.
8. Evaluate laboratory tests used for differential diagnosis of megaloblastic anemia.
9. Compare and contrast the treatment for vitamin B_{12} and folate deficiencies.
10. Using the peripheral blood findings, differentiate the anemia of liver disease from a megaloblastic anemia caused by vitamin B_{12} or folate deficiency.

Megaloblastic anemias are a group of disorders characterized by defective nuclear maturation caused by impaired deoxyribonucleic acid (DNA) synthesis. This defect is manifested by the presence of megaloblasts (large and abnormal red cell precursors) in the bone marrow and macro-ovalocytes in the peripheral blood. The granulocyte precursors tend to be larger than normal, with giant metamyelocytes being a striking feature. An abnormal nuclear pattern in megakaryocytes may also be seen in severe anemia. The megaloblastic changes are not limited to the hematopoietic cells; changes are also present in other nucleated actively proliferating cells, such as skin, vaginal, uterine, cervical, and buccal cells.

BIOCHEMICAL ASPECT

The defective nuclear maturation and the megaloblastic morphology are caused by a decrease in thymidine triphosphate (TTP) synthesis from uridine monophosphate (UMP). This deficiency interferes with nuclear maturation, DNA replication, and cell division. When thymidine triphosphate is not present in adequate amounts, deoxyuridine triphosphate incorporates into the DNA instead[1,2] (Fig. 7–1). This misincorporation causes fragmentation of the nucleus and ultimately immature cell destruction.

The primary causes for lack of thymidine and consequently defective DNA synthesis are vitamin B_{12} and folic acid deficiencies. These vitamins, in the form of cofactors, play important roles in some key reactions involved in DNA synthesis. In addition, drugs that interfere with the metabolism of these vitamins also cause DNA impairment.

CLINICAL MANIFESTATIONS OF MEGALOBLASTIC ANEMIA

Certain clinical manifestations are common to all patients with megaloblastic anemias regardless of the cause. The degree of anemia may be mild to severe with the symptoms of weakness, fatigue, shortness of breath, and lightheadedness. Congestive heart failure may or may not be present, depending upon the degree of anemia. In severe anemia, the patient may have a lemon-yellow skin tint because of mild jaundice and pallor. Increased bilirubin is reported in about 30% of patients as a result of intramedullary hemolysis caused by ineffective erythropoiesis.[3]

HEMATOLOGIC FEATURES

Ineffective Hematopoiesis

Megaloblastic anemia is associated with ineffective erythropoiesis and hemolysis. The mean corpuscular volume (MCV) is greater than 100 femtoliters (fL). Patients with megaloblastic anemia may have MCV values as high as 160 fL. This elevated MCV reflects the megaloblastic picture of the bone marrow. Increased erythrocyte precursors in the bone marrow and their decreased release into the peripheral blood indicate ineffective erythropoiesis, which is supported by decreased reticulocytes.

The megaloblastic erythrocytes have much shorter life spans than do normal erythrocytes. They are more fragile and, therefore, die prematurely in the marrow. Evidence of intramedullary hemolysis includes increased values for serum bilirubin, serum lactate dehydrogenase (LDH) (in particular LDH-1 and LDH-2 isomers), and serum iron.[1]

Ineffective granulopoiesis is defined by increased bone marrow white cell precursors and failure in release of mature forms into the peripheral blood. The giant metamyelocytes do not mature to circulating neutrophils but, rather, die prematurely in the bone marrow. The elevated serum muramidase is a result of this increased turnover of white cells.

Ineffective thrombopoiesis is manifested by the presence of increased abnormal megakaryocytes in the bone marrow and thrombocytopenia in the peripheral blood.

Bone Marrow Morphology

Patients with megaloblastic anemia have a hypercellular bone marrow. The myeloid-to-erythroid (M:E) ratio is decreased (Fig. 7–2) and may be as low as 1:1 to 1:3. The degree of increased cellularity (megaloblas-

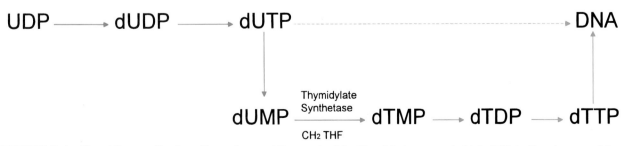

FIGURE 7–1 Thymidine synthesis pathway from uridine nucleotide. Uracil is incorporated into DNA in the absence of thymine. UDP = uridine diphosphate; dUDP = deoxyuridine diphosphate; dUTP = deoxyuridine triphosphate; dUMP = deoxyuridine monophosphate; dTMP = deoxythymidine monophosphate; dTDP = deoxythymidine diphosphate; dTTP = deoxythymidine triphosphate; CH_2THF = methylene tetrahydrofolate.

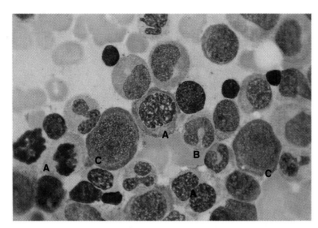

FIGURE 7–2 *A.* Mitotic figures in megaloblastic marrow. *B.* Large megaloblastic band neutrophil. *C.* Megaloblastic pronormoblast with open, sievelike chromatin.

tic picture) is dependent upon the severity of the anemia. Megaloblasts are large cells with increased ribonucleic acid (RNA) per DNA unit. Their nuclear chromatin appears loose and less mature than nuclear chromatin of the normal red cells at the same stage of maturation (Fig. 7–3; see also Fig. 1–3). The cytoplasm maturation is, however, normal. This phenomenon is referred to as nuclear to cytoplasm asynchrony. The mature megaloblastic red cells entering the circulation usually have a shorter life span than normal, mature red cells.

Megaloblastic changes are manifested in white cell precursors by the presence of giant bands and giant metamyelocytes in the bone marrow (see Fig. 7–2). The nucleus of the giant bands may show abnormal staining characteristics. These white cell abnormalities are not seen in the megaloblastic bone marrow present in patients with myelodysplastic syndrome or erythroleukemia.[4]

Megakaryocytes are also affected in severe megaloblastic anemia. They may have abnormal nuclear and/

or cytoplasm morphology, such as increased nuclear lobulation and hypogranulation.[5]

Peripheral Blood Morphology

Megaloblastic anemia is a macrocytic, normochromic anemia. Depending on the degree of anemia, the MCV may range from 100 to 160 fL. The mean corpuscular hemoglobin (MCH) is elevated but the mean corpuscular hemoglobin concentration (MCHC) is normal. Not all patients with macrocytosis have megaloblastic anemia (i.e., alcoholism and liver disease) and not all megaloblastic anemias are macrocytic. A normal MCV may be present in patients with megaloblastic anemia and coexisting iron deficiency or thalassemia.

The hemoglobin value may be normal to low. The erythrocyte count is generally decreased. The leukocyte count may be normal at the early stage of anemia but may decrease to as low as 2 to 4 × 10⁹/L. Although platelets are the least affected cell line, platelet counts below 100 × 10⁹/L have been reported in patients with severe anemia.[6]

The peripheral smear is hypocellular with the presence of macrocytes and macro-ovalocytes (Fig. 7–4). The degree of anisocytosis and poikilocytosis varies with the severity of anemia. Other poikilocytes such as schistocytes, tear-drop-shaped cells, spherocytes, and target cells may also be seen on the peripheral blood smear.[5] Increased anisocytosis causes an elevated red cell distribution width (RDW) as determined by an automated cell counter. Dimorphic red cell morphology may be present in patients who have iron-deficiency anemia, thalassemia, anemia of chronic diseases, or hyperthyroidism in addition to the megaloblastic anemia. Trimorphic blood smear may be seen in transfused patients. Red cell inclusions such as Howell-Jolly bodies and basophilic stippling are frequently present (Fig. 7–5 and see Fig. 6–16). Cabot rings and megaloblastic nucleated red cells may be seen on the peripheral blood smear (Fig. 7–6). The absolute reticulocyte count is decreased with a reticulocyte produc-

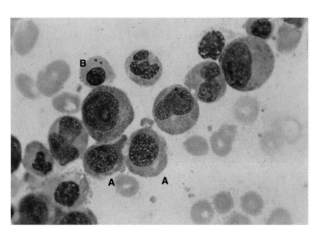

FIGURE 7–3 Bone marrow. *A.* Polychromatophilic megaloblasts. *B.* Orthochromic megaloblast with multiple Howell-Jolly bodies.

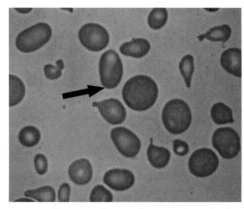

FIGURE 7–4 Extreme degree of anisocytosis (+4) and poikilocytosis (+4) with oval macrocytosis (*arrow*) in a severe pernicious anemia case. (From Bell, A: Hematology. In Listen, Look and Learn. Health and Education Resources, Inc., Bethesda, MD, with permission.)

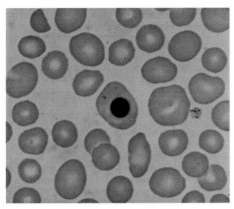

FIGURE 7–5 Howell-Jolly body in an orthochromic megaloblast in pernicious anemia (center). (From Bell, A: Hematology. In Listen, Look and Learn. Health and Education Resources, Inc., Bethesda, MD, with permission.)

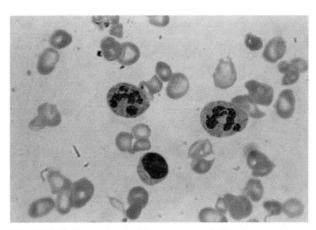

FIGURE 7–7 Neutrophil hypersegmentation in pernicious anemia.

tion index (RPI) of less than 2, indicating ineffective erythropoiesis. With treatment, the number of reticulocytes increases along with increased numbers of nucleated red cells.

In patients with untreated megaloblastic anemia, the macrocytes have a shortened survival time (28 to 75 days) compared to the survival time of normal red cells (110 to 120 days). The survival of normal red cells is shortened when transfused to a patient with severe and untreated megaloblastic anemia. Although the exact cause is unknown, it is an indication of extracorpuscular hemolysis.[6]

Multilobed neutrophils, termed *hypersegmented neutrophils*, are seen in the peripheral smear in 98% of cases (Fig. 7–7).[7] Hypersegmented neutrophils refer to neutrophils with more than five lobes. They are larger than normal mature neutrophils. The number of the hypersegmented neutrophils counted per 100 white cells as determined by the differential should be reported. Although hypersegmented neutrophils appear early in the peripheral blood, they are the last morphologic feature to disappear. Their absence does not rule out the diagnosis of megaloblastic anemia.

The diagnosis of megaloblastic anemia is usually based on the morphologic characteristics of the peripheral blood, and the results of other biochemical tests. The bone marrow examination is generally not required. Bone marrow aspirates are performed for diagnosis of other disorders with a megaloblastic picture such as myelodysplastic syndrome or erythroleukemia. The clinical features of megaloblastic anemia are summarized in Table 7–1.

ETIOLOGY

The major causes of the megaloblastic anemias are vitamin B_{12} deficiency, folic acid deficiency, or a combination of both. Megaloblastic anemia can also be present in non–vitamin-deficient diseases, such as myelodysplastic syndromes and acute leukemias. Drug-induced megaloblastic anemia is caused by those drugs that interfere with the metabolism of either vitamin B_{12} or folic acid. Examples of these drugs include chemotherapeutic agents and anticonvulsants.

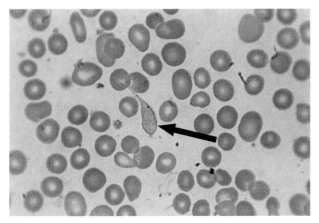

FIGURE 7–6 Cabot ring in pernicious anemia (*center*).

TABLE 7–1 **Clinical Features of Megaloblastic Anemia**
Bone Marrow
Hypercellular
Low M:E ratio
Megaloblasts
Giant bands and metamyelocytes
Peripheral Blood
Pancytopenia
Macro-ovalocytes
Hypersegmented neutrophils
Biochemical Changes
Elevated LDH
Elevated indirect bilirubin
Increased serum iron and ferritin

VITAMIN B$_{12}$ DEFICIENCY

Sources and Requirements

Vitamin B$_{12}$ is produced by micro-organisms and fungi.[4] It is present in foods of animal origin such as liver, fish, poultry, meat, eggs, and dairy products. Liver is a major source of vitamin B$_{12}$. Vegetables do not contribute B$_{12}$ to the diet. Vitamin B$_{12}$ is commercially available for treatment of deficiencies.

In the United States, the daily diet has an average of 5 to 20 μg of vitamin B$_{12}$,[3] of which 70% is absorbed. The recommended dietary intake of vitamin B$_{12}$ for adults is 2 μg/day.[3] This requirement increases in pregnancy, infancy, during growth, and during increased metabolic stages. Vitamin B$_{12}$ is lost through the urine and feces. The rate of loss is about 0.1% per day. Body storage of vitamin B$_{12}$ is about 2 to 5 mg, of which approximately 1 to 2 mg is stored in the liver.[3]

Since the daily requirement of vitamin B$_{12}$ is low and the storage rate is high, it takes about 2 to 7 years for one to develop vitamin B$_{12}$ deficiency in the case of malabsorption.[8]

Structure

Vitamin B$_{12}$ (cobalamin) is a large water-soluble molecule with a molecular weight of 1335 daltons (d).[6] It is made of a corrin nucleus composed of four pyrrol rings (A to D) and a cobalt atom at the center (Fig. 7–8), similar to porphyrin nucleus (refer to Chap. 6).

The corrin ring is attached to the nucleotide 5,6-dimethylbenzimidazole. The cobalt atom can be attached to several different molecules such as adenosyl (5-deoxyadenoside), methyl, cyanide, and hydroxy to form the biologically active forms of cobalamins (see Fig. 7–8).

Transport and Metabolism

There are two important proteins involved in the transport of vitamin B$_{12}$ from diet to ileum and from ileum to tissues. These proteins are the intrinsic factor and transcobalamin II.[4,7]

The dietary cobalamin is released from the food by gastric acids and intestinal enzymes. On release, it binds to a binding protein called *intrinsic factor* (IF). IF is a glycoprotein with molecular weight of 45,000 d.[6] It is secreted by parietal cells of the stomach. The parietal cells also secrete hydrochloric acid and other gastric juices. IF binds to vitamin B$_{12}$ and forms B$_{12}$-IF complex. This complex allows vitamin B$_{12}$ to be absorbed through the receptors present on the brush borders of the ileum (the distal half of the small intestine) (Fig. 7–9). The intrinsic factor is not absorbed by the ileum and therefore cannot be reutilized. It is degraded on release from vitamin B$_{12}$.[1,9] The released vitamin B$_{12}$ then enters the portal vein.

When vitamin B$_{12}$ leaves the ileum and enters the portal vein, it attaches to three proteins, transcobalamin I (TC I), transcobalamin II (TC II), and transcobalamin III (TC III). Transcobalamin II is the main

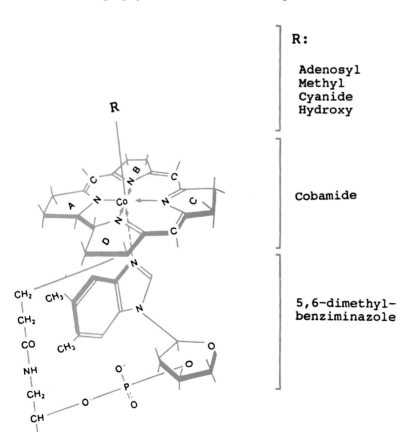

R:

Adenosyl
Methyl
Cyanide
Hydroxy

Cobamide

5,6-dimethyl-benziminazole

FIGURE 7–8 Structure of vitamin B$_{12}$ (cobalamin). When R is adenosyl, the compound is adenosylcobalamin (AdoCb); when R is methyl, it is methylcobalamin (MeCB); when R is cyanide, it is cyanocobalamin (CNCb); and when R is hydroxy, it is hydroxocobalamin (OHCb).

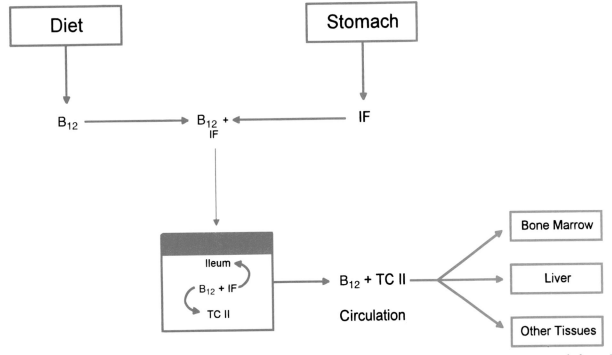

FIGURE 7-9   Transportation path of vitamin B_{12} from the diet to the tissues. IF = intrinsic factor; TC II = transcobalamin II.

transport protein of cobalamin. It is a polypeptide with a molecular weight of 38,000 d.[6] TC II is synthesized by ileal cells, endothelial cells, liver, and macrophages and secreted into the plasma.[4,6,7] Transcobalamin II transports vitamin B_{12} to the liver for storage and to the bone marrow and other tissues for DNA synthesis (see Fig. 7–9). The deficiency of TC II causes megaloblastic anemia, but the functions of TC I and TC III are not exactly known.[10]

Vitamin B_{12} plays an important role in two key reactions in the body. First, it is necessary in the synthesis of methionine from homocysteine. In this biochemical reaction, both vitamin B_{12} and folic acid are involved. Vitamin B_{12} acts as a coenzyme, methylcobalamin (MeCb) for the enzyme methyltransferase (Fig. 7–10). Secondly, vitamin B_{12} is important in conversion of methylmalonyl CoA, a Krebs cycle intermediate, to succinyl CoA. In this reaction vitamin B_{12} also acts as a coenzyme, adenosylcobalamin (AdoCb) for the enzyme methylmalonyl CoA mutase. Adenosylcobalamin acts as a hydrogen (H) carrier, taking the H from methylmalonyl CoA to make succinyl CoA (Fig. 7–11).

Causes of Vitamin B_{12} Deficiency

Vitamin B_{12} deficiency progresses through four stages. Stage I, negative vitamin B_{12} balance; stage II, vitamin B_{12} depletion; stage III, vitamin B_{12}–deficient erythropoiesis; stage IV, vitamin B_{12}–deficient anemia. Stages I and II are referred to as the depletion stages. Stages III and IV are referred to as the deficient stages.[11]

Nutritional vitamin B_{12} deficiency is uncommon in western countries and is limited to strict vegetarians. In this group, the decrease in vitamin B_{12} is accompanied by an increased plasma folate level.[11]

It is worth noting that the children born to a "vegan" mother (no animal food) or to a mother who has an untreated vitamin B_{12} deficiency are B_{12} deficient, especially if they are breast-fed.[4] Untreated infants are severely megaloblastic, with retarded growth and psychomotor development. Neurologic complications such as irritability, anorexia, and failure to thrive have been reported in severe vitamin B_{12}–deficient infants.[4,12]

The major cause of vitamin B_{12} deficiency is malabsorption. The most common form of intestinal malabsorption is pernicious anemia. Other causes of vitamin B_{12} deficiency are summarized in Table 7–2 and will be discussed later.

Pernicious Anemia

Definition   Pernicious anemia is a disease characterized by gastric parietal cell atrophy. This defect causes decreased secretion of IF and other gastric juices. Lack of IF leads to defective vitamin B_{12} absorption and consequently megaloblastic anemia.

Pernicious anemia is more common in people of Scandinavian, English, and Irish descent, with 0.13 to 0.20% of the population having been diagnosed with the disease.[3]

Pernicious anemia is more common after age 50. In blacks, the disease may start earlier, with a mean of 53 years.[13,14] Pernicious anemia is rare in children, and, if it occurs, it may be in the congenital form. Congenital pernicious anemia is characterized by the total

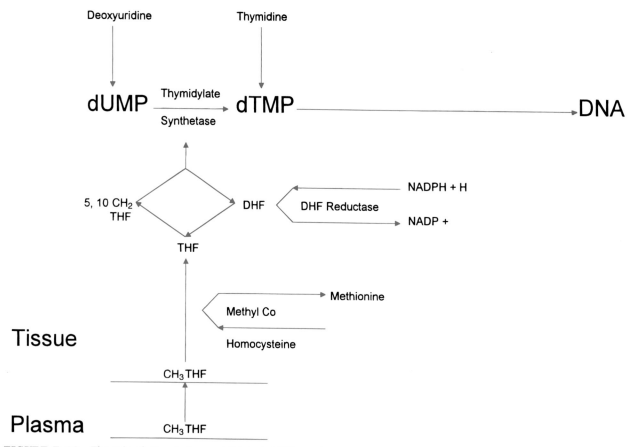

FIGURE 7-10   The role of vitamin B_{12} and folate in DNA synthesis. CH_2THF = methylene tetrahydrofolate; THF = tetrahydrofolate; DHF = dihydrofolate; CH_3THF = methyl tetrahydrofolate; dUMP = deoxyuridine monophosphate; dTMP = deoxythymidine monophosphate.

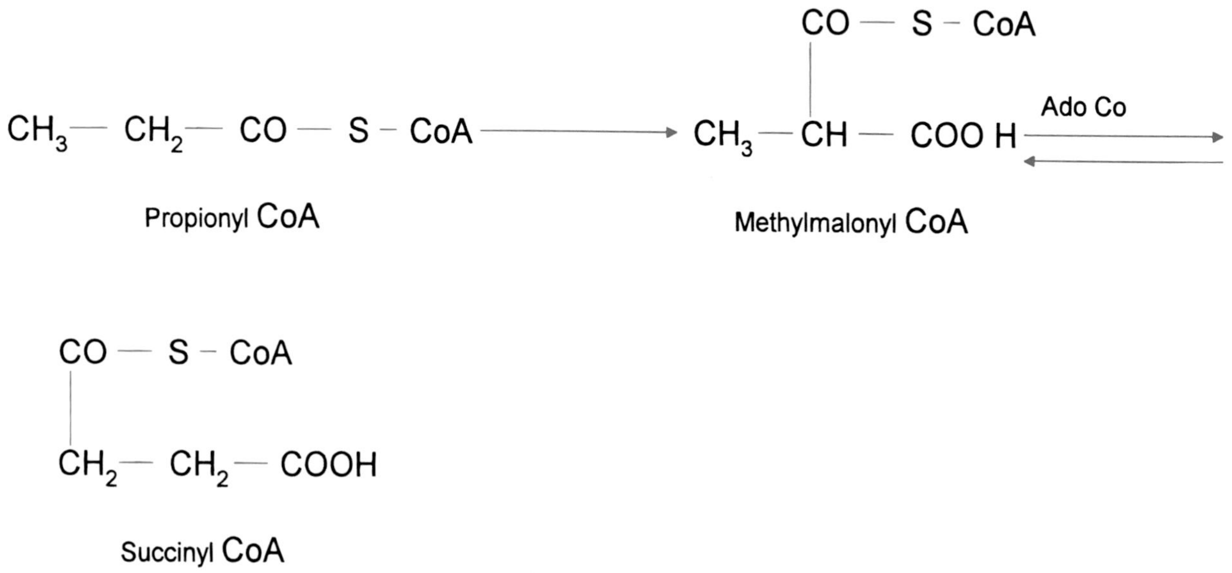

FIGURE 7-11   Conversion of methylmalonyl CoA to succinyl CoA. AdoCo = adenosylcobalamin.

TABLE 7–2 Causes of Vitamin B$_{12}$ Deficiency

Dietary Deficiency
Strict vegans

Malabsorption
Pernicious anemia
Gastrectomy (total or partial)
Blind loop syndrome
Fish tapeworm (*Diphyllobothrium latum*)
Diseases of ileum
Chronic pancreatic disease

Drugs
Alcohol
Nitrous oxide (N$_2$O)
Para-aminosalycylic acid (PAS)

absence of IF and normal secretion of other gastric juices. There are no antibodies present against IF or the parietal cells. Juvenile pernicious anemia is similar to adult pernicious anemia, with the age of onset in the second decade.[3]

Pathophysiology The main cause of pernicious anemia is atrophic gastritis characterized by atrophy of the gastric mucosa with decrease of gastric secretions and IF. The cause of gastric atrophy, however, is not clearly known.[3] It is postulated that genetic, immunologic, and environmental factors all play a role. IF is essential for absorption of vitamin B$_{12}$. In absence of IF, only a small amount of vitamin B$_{12}$ is absorbed.

The congenital form of pernicious anemia is inherited as an autosomal-recessive trait.[3] The genetic contribution to the adult form of pernicious anemia is supported by: (1) the concordant presence of pernicious anemia in identical twins, (2) the increased risk in relatives of patients with pernicious anemia, (3) the presence of achlorhydria with or without malabsorption in relatives of patients with pernicious anemia, and (4) the relatives of patients with pernicious anemia may produce antibody to gastric parietal cells.[1,3,10]

The cause for the genetic predisposition of pernicious anemia is not yet clear. The association of pernicious anemia and the human leukocyte antigen (HLA) is not conclusive. Association of HLA-B7 and pernicious anemia has been reported in whites. The association of HLA-D antigens, Dw2, Dw5, and DR2 with pernicious anemia is more significant than other HLA antigens.[3,10]

The serum of patients with pernicious anemia contains autoantibodies to parietal cells, to IF, and to thyroid tissue. The parietal cell antibody is found in the serum of approximately 84% of all patients with pernicious anemia and in 50% of patients with atrophic gastritis. The antibody is also present in the gastric juices of 75% of patients with pernicious anemia. This antibody is specific for the parietal cells only and does not show any cross-reactivity.

Antibodies to IF are demonstrated in the serum of approximately 56% of patients with pernicious anemia. These antibodies are more specific for diagnosis of anemia than antiparietal antibodies. Two types of IF antibodies have been reported. Type I, or blocking antibodies, prevent IF-B$_{12}$ complex formation. Type II, or

binding antibodies, are usually present with blocking antibodies. Binding antibodies are of two varieties. One type binds to free IF and IF-B$_{12}$ complex, and the other binds to the complex only.[3,10]

Thyroid antibody has often been found in the serum of patients with pernicious anemia or their relatives.[3]

Lymphocytotoxic antibodies have also been detected in one third of patients with pernicious anemia. A decrease in suppressor T cells and increase in CD4:CD8 ratio supports the presence of cell-mediated immunity in patients with pernicious anemia.[3]

An association between pernicious anemia and other autoimmune diseases such as thyroid disease, diabetes mellitus, and rheumatoid arthritis has also been noted.[3] The positive response to steroids in some patients with pernicious anemia supports the autoimmune mechanism.[3,8]

Clinical Manifestations of Vitamin B$_{12}$ Deficiency

The onset of pernicious anemia is generally insidious. Patients with pernicious anemia and other vitamin B$_{12}$ deficiencies have all the signs and symptoms of megaloblastic anemia mentioned earlier. Fever is usually present in severe anemia. Loss of appetite is a common complaint. Glossitis (sore tongue) is reported in 50% of patients.[3]

The bone marrow morphology of patients with vitamin B$_{12}$ deficiency is megaloblastic, and the peripheral smear has macro-ovalocytes.

Neurologic problems are more common in pernicious anemia than in other types of vitamin B$_{12}$ deficiencies. The degree of neurologic involvement is not directly related to the degree of anemia. Neurologic manifestations in the absence of hematologic abnormalities have been reported in many cases.[15]

The neurologic abnormalities may be mild, moderate, or severe and may involve degeneration of peripheral nerves, posterior columns of the spinal cord, and posterior and lateral columns of the spinal cord (Table 7–3). Because multiple neuropathies are involved, the terms *subacute combined degeneration* and *combined system disease* may be used.[3]

In the earlier stage of pernicious anemia, the patient often experiences symmetric tingling or "pins-and-needle sensations" in the toes and later in all four limbs. Less often, the patient may complain of numbness. At the later stage, the postal spinal columns may be involved. At this stage, the patient may complain of clumsiness and have an incoordinate gait. The lateral spinal columns become involved in the most severe stage of illness, with manifestations of severe weakness and stiffness of limbs, impairment of memory,

TABLE 7–3 Neurologic Manifestations in Pernicious Anemia

- Peripheral nerves
- Degeneration of posterior columns
- Degeneration of posterior and lateral columns

and depression. Severe psychiatric symptoms are less common and include stupor, hallucinations, paranoia, and severe depression, referred to as "megaloblastic madness." Less frequent neurologic problems include ophthalmoplegia. Bilateral retinal bleeding in severe anemia with thrombocytopenia has been reported in some patients.[3,8,16,17] The basic underlying cause for the neuropathy associated with vitamin B_{12} deficiency is not exactly known. For many years, it was postulated that the deficiency of adenosylcobalamin in the methyl-malonyl CoA reaction was responsible for the neurologic defects. Recently, however, more attention has been given to impairment of methionine synthetase reaction as a possible cause for the neuropathy. The rationale for this hypothesis is that the deficiency of methionine leads to decreased production of S-adenosyl methionine (SAM), a key intermediate in methylation reactions of myelin. The impairment of methylation in myelin could result in demyelination and consequently clinical neuropathy.[3,18,19]

Since the methionine synthesis reaction is both vitamin B_{12}– and folate-dependent and the rate of neuropathy is low in folate-deficient patients, more research is needed to support the validity of this hypothesis.

Other Causes of Vitamin B_{12} Deficiency

There are many other causes of malabsorption that lead to vitamin B_{12} deficiency (see Table 7–2). In a gastrectomy procedure, the IF-producing cells are removed. Vitamin B_{12} deficiency develops in these patients within several years in the absence of vitamin B_{12} therapy. Vitamin B_{12} deficiency has been reported in 30% to 40% of patients with partial gastrectomy.[3]

In blind loop syndrome, an anatomic abnormality of the small intestine, there is an overgrowth of bacteria in the small bowel. These micro-organisms take up the vitamin B_{12} and make it unavailable for absorption by the ileum. Tetracycline therapy for 10 days will normalize the vitamin B_{12} level.[3,10]

Fish tapeworm (*Diphyllobothrium latum*) is a parasite that competes for vitamin B_{12} by splitting vitamin B_{12} from IF. This type of vitamin B_{12} deficiency is common in Scandinavian countries and is reported in 1.9% to 3.0% of carriers of the fish tapeworm.[3,10] The malabsorption type of vitamin B_{12} deficiency is normally corrected when vitamin B_{12} or vitamin B_{12} and IF are given to the patients.

Vitamin B_{12} deficiency can also be seen in diseases of the ileum such as ileal resection or bypass, and in regional enteritis.[3]

In pancreatic disease, vitamin B_{12} deficiency develops as a result of a decrease in the proteases necessary for release of vitamin B_{12} from salivary and gastric R proteins for absorption. A low level of free calcium, which is necessary for calcium-dependent ileal absorption, can cause B_{12} deficiency in patients with chronic pancreatic disease.[3,11]

Other causes of vitamin B_{12} deficiency are drugs such as alcohol, anesthetics, nitrous oxide (N_2O), and the antituberculosis drug para-aminosalicyclic acid (PAS).[4,11,19] Vitamin B_{12} deficiency has also been reported in patients who are on hemodialysis.[3]

FOLIC ACID DEFICIENCY

Sources and Requirements

Folic acid, also known as folate or pteroylglutamic acid, is a water-soluble vitamin present in a variety of foods. The highest concentration is present in green leafy vegetables, fruits, dairy products, cereals, and also in animal foods such as liver and kidney. It is a heat-labile vitamin and, therefore, is easily destroyed (50% to 90%) in overcooked vegetables. The recommended dietary intake of folic acid for adults is approximately 3 µg/kg per day.[3] This requirement increases many times during infancy, pregnancy, and lactation. Folate deficiency during early pregnancy can have adverse effects on the fetus.[20–22] The body storage is about 5 to 10 mg,[3] of which almost 80% is stored in the liver. The amount of folic acid absorbed is about 80% of intake. It is absorbed through the duodenum and jejunum. Folate is lost via body secretions such as bile, urine, sweat, and saliva.[8] Folic acid has a higher turnover time and a higher rate of loss compared to vitamin B_{12} and, therefore, it takes only a few months to develop folate deficiency.

Structure

Folic acid is made of three components: pteridine, aminobenzoic acid, and glutamic acid (Fig. 7–12). Folic acid derived from the diet is not biologically active. Once absorbed through the intestinal lumen, it is hydrolyzed, reduced, and methylated to form methyltetrahydrofolate (CH_3THF). Other biologically active forms of folic acid are tetrahydrofolate (THF) and its coenzyme, N^5N^{10}-methylenetetrahydrofolate (N^5N^{10}-CH_2THF).

Serum folate is in the form of CH_3THF and enters all tissue cells in this form.

Absorption and Metabolism

Dietary folic acid is in the form of polyglutamic acid (many glutamic acid residues). Once in the intestinal lumen, it is acted upon by the enzyme folate deconjugase, which is present in the epithelial cells of intestine, to form monoglutamic acid (single glutamic acid residue). Monoglutamic acid is then reduced and methylated to CH_3THF (Fig. 7–13). This compound is then released into the circulation (Fig. 7–14). Most of the circulatory folic acid is in the form of CH_3THF.[9] When CH_3THF is absorbed from the circulation into the tissue cells, it transfers its methyl group to homocysteine to form methionine and THF. The THF formed reconjugates with additional glutamic acid residues to form the cellular THF (see Figs. 7–12 and 7–13). The THF is then methylated to form coenzyme methylene-THF, N^5N^{10}-CH_2THF, necessary for the formation of thymidine monophosphate from uridine monophosphate. This is the key reaction for DNA synthesis (see Fig. 7–10).

Causes of Folic Acid Deficiency

The main cause of folic acid deficiency is decreased dietary intake. Other causes are malabsorption, in-

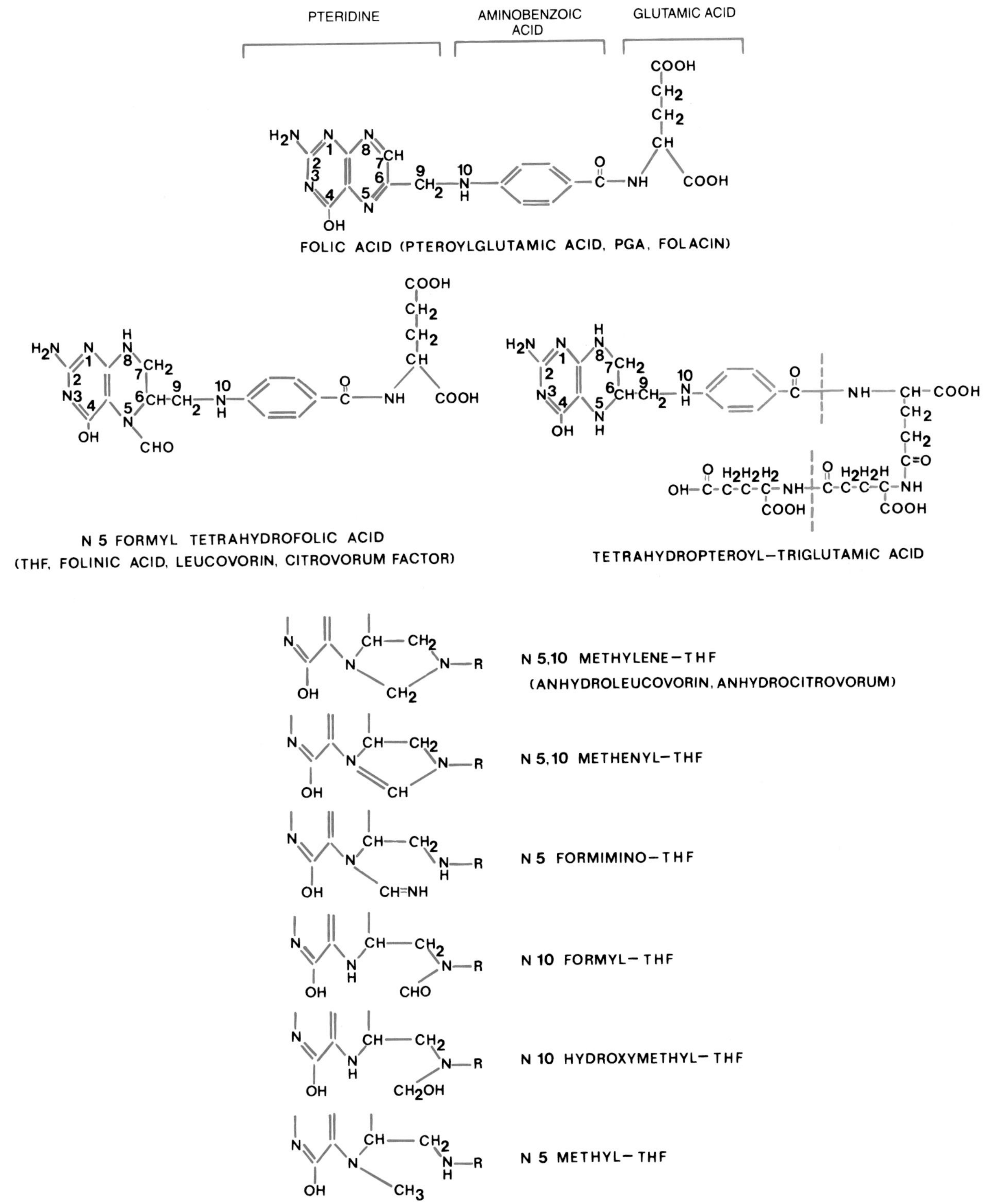

FIGURE 7-12 Structure of folic acid and its derivatives. THF = tetrahydrofolate. (From Harris, JW and Kellerman, RW: The Red Cell. Harvard University Press, Cambridge, MA, 1970, p 395, with permission.)

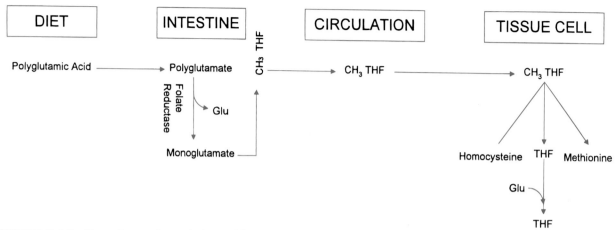

FIGURE 7-13 Absorption and metabolism of folic acid. Glu = glutamic acid; CH₃THF = methyl tetrahydrofolate; THF = tetrahydrofolate.

creased requirement, and drug-induced folate deficiencies (Table 7–4).

Nutritional folate deficiency is usually a consequence of poverty, old age, alcoholism, and chronic diseases.

The most common causes of folate malabsorption are tropical sprue and gluten-sensitive enteropathy. Tropical sprue is an infection that causes intestinal atrophy with clinical manifestations of weakness, weight loss, and steatorrhea. Tropical sprue affects the entire intestine and, therefore, causes a wide variety of nutritional deficiencies, including vitamin B_{12} deficiency.[3,23] Affected individuals respond well to antibiotics.

Gluten-sensitive enteropathy has the same clinical manifestations as those mentioned in tropical sprue. It includes both nontropical sprue and childhood celiac disease. Affected individuals cannot digest gluten, a protein found in wheat and other grains. Lesions are most severe in the proximal intestine. Childhood celiac disease is a malabsorption syndrome resulting in anemia caused by iron deficiency and to a lesser degree by vitamin B_{12} and folate deficiencies.

The requirement for folic acid increases during rapid cellular proliferation in hematologic diseases such as sickle cell anemia, thalassemia, hereditary spherocytosis, and autoimmune hemolytic anemia.[10]

Drug-induced folate-deficient megaloblastic anemia has been reported with a variety of drugs such as methotrexate, pyrimethamine, phenytoin, alcohol, isoniazid, and oral contraceptives.[3,10]

Clinical Manifestations of Folic Acid Deficiency

Clinical manifestations of folate deficiency are the same as those in vitamin B_{12} deficiency mentioned earlier. The onset of anemia is insidious, with the distinct

ERYTHROCYTES

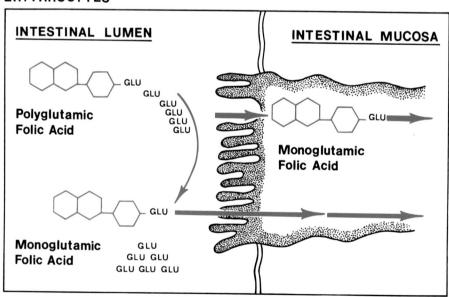

FIGURE 7-14 Intestinal absorption of the folate derivatives of food. (From Streiff, RR: Intestinal absorption of the folate derivatives of food. JAMA 214:105, 1970, with permission.)

TABLE 7-4   Causes of Folic Acid Deficiency

Dietary Deficiency
Poverty
Old age
Alcoholism
Chronic diseases

Malabsorption
Tropical sprue
Gluten-sensitive enteropathy
Childhood celiac

Increased Requirement
Pregnancy
Infancy
Malignancy

Drugs
Methotrexate
Pyrimethamine
Phenytoin
Alcohol
Isoniazid
Oral contraceptives

morphology characteristic of megaloblastic anemia in the bone marrow and in the peripheral blood. Although neuropathy is mainly characteristic of vitamin B_{12} deficiency, several cases of neurologic abnormalities, depression, and dementia associated with folic acid deficiency have been reported. Some of these neuropathies responded favorably to treatment with folate.[24,25] The association of folate deficiency and neurologic abnormalities needs further investigation. Some investigators believe that in addition to folate deficiency, vitamin B_{12} deficiency or other factors may play a role in this type of neuropathy.[10]

LABORATORY DIAGNOSIS OF MEGALOBLASTIC ANEMIA

Several important factors in differential diagnosis of megaloblastic anemias are the patient's physical examination, medical history, drug history, family history, and laboratory tests.[19,24]

The most common laboratory screening tests and results that are used in the diagnosis of megaloblastic anemias are low hemoglobin level, elevated MCV, and peripheral smear morphology such as macro-ovalocytes and hypersegmented neutrophils.[15] Once the diagnosis of megaloblastic anemia is established, the exact cause of the anemia should be determined for appropriate and effective treatment. Figure 7-15 demonstrates the proper selection and interpretation of laboratory tests in the differential diagnosis of megaloblastic anemia.

Diagnostic tests used for vitamin B_{12} and folate deficiencies are serum B_{12} and serum and red cell folate levels. Red cell folate is a better indicator of tissue folate levels (Table 7-5).

The methods available for quantitation of these vitamins are microbiologic assay and immunoassays (radioimmunoassay and chemiluminescence). Vitamin B_{12} and folic acid can be measured simultaneously by both immunoassay methods.

Low levels of serum B_{12} in the absence of vitamin B_{12} deficiency have been reported in patients with folate deficiency, pregnancy, oral contraceptive use, and decreased TC I level. Normal or elevated serum B_{12} is associated with myeloproliferative disorders, chronic myelocytic leukemia, and liver disease.[7,10,11]

In patients with folate deficiency, both serum folate and red cell folate are decreased. However, in patients with B_{12} deficiency, the serum folate is increased while the red cell folate is decreased. The increased serum folate level is the result of increased CH_3THF in the serum (methyl trap hypothesis) resulting from the lack of vitamin B_{12} necessary for conversion of homocysteine to methionine and methyl-THF to THF (see Fig. 7-10). Serum folate may also increase following ingestion of foods high in folate. Occasionally, serum folate may be decreased in vitamin B_{12}-deficient patients. The cause is not known.[3] False low serum folate levels have also been reported in patients on antibiotics or certain cytotoxic drugs.[17]

Other laboratory tests that may support a diagnosis of vitamin B_{12} or folate deficiency are gastric achlorhydria, antibodies to IF, vitamin B_{12} absorption (Schilling) test, methylmalonic acid (MMA) assay, homocysteine assay, and the deoxyuridine (du) suppression test. These tests are useful when the other laboratory tests are inconclusive.

Gastric achlorhydria (low gastric acidity) is present in almost all patients with pernicious anemia. Achlorhydria following histamine stimulation supports the diagnosis of pernicious anemia. However, this test is not specific, since achlorhydria has also been reported in patients without pernicious anemia.

Antibodies to IF are present in the serum of about 56% of patients with pernicious anemia. Although testing for the presence of antibodies is not sensitive, it is specific for the diagnosis of pernicious anemia. Decreased serum B_{12} and the presence of the antibody to IF is indicative of pernicious anemia.

The Schilling test evaluates absorption of vitamin B_{12} from the intestinal tract. The test is specific for vitamin B_{12} and is done to pinpoint the cause of vitamin B_{12} malabsorption.

The Schilling test is done in two parts (Fig. 7-16). In part I, the patient is given 0.5 to 2.0 μg of labeled (^{57}Co or ^{58}Co) vitamin B_{12} orally. Two hours later, a flushing dose (1000 μg) of unlabeled vitamin B_{12} is injected intramuscularly to saturate all of the circulating cobalamin binders. The amount of the labeled vitamin B_{12} is then measured in a 24-hour urine collection. If the IF is present and the normal absorption takes place, the labeled vitamin B_{12} absorbed through the intestine is rapidly excreted into the urine. The urinary excretion varies depending on the dosage given. In normal absorption, about 5% to 35% of labeled B_{12} is excreted in the urine.[4]

An abnormal result in part I indicates that B_{12} was not absorbed through the intestine. In this case, testing will proceed to part II to find the cause of malabsorption (see Fig. 7-16).

In part II, the test is repeated with the addition of IF to the oral dose to determine if malabsorption is

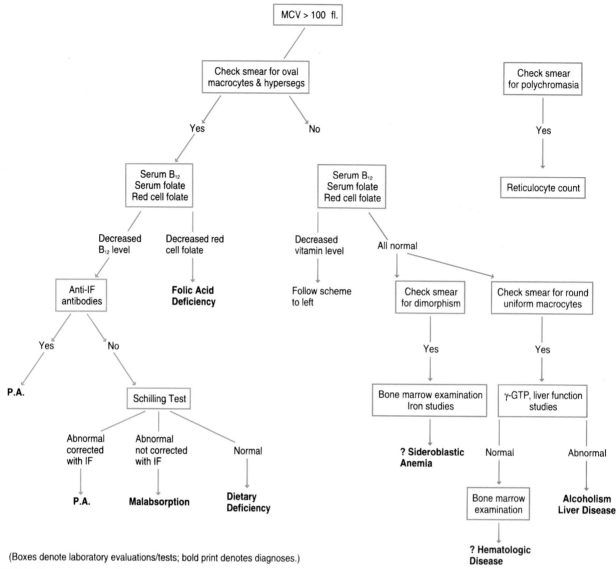

FIGURE 7–15 Logical scheme of laboratory testing in cases of macrocytosis. Boxes denote laboratory evaluations and/or tests; bold type denotes diagnoses.

caused by the lack of IF. If the Schilling test is corrected in part II, a deficiency of IF is confirmed. If the Schilling test is still abnormal, other causes of malabsorption should be investigated (see Fig. 7–16). Parts I and II can be done simultaneously if B_{12} and B_{12} + IF are labeled with different isotopes. Reliability of the Schilling test depends on normal renal function and proper urine collection.

Serum and urine methylmalonic acid (MMA) levels are both elevated in patients with vitamin B_{12} deficiency. As discussed earlier, vitamin B_{12} in the form of adenosylcobalamin is necessary for conversion of methylmalonyl CoA to succinyl CoA (see Fig. 7–11). In the absence of vitamin B_{12}, the level of methylmalonyl CoA will be increased in the serum and consequently in the urine. Falsely elevated results have been reported in non–vitamin-deficient patients with renal disease and with inborn errors of metabolism.

TABLE 7–5	**Diagnosis of Vitamin Deficiencies**		
	Serum B_{12}	**Serum Folate**	**Red Cell Folate**
B_{12} deficiency	Decreased	Increased, normal	Decreased, normal
Folate deficiency	Normal	Decreased	Decreased
B_{12} and folate deficiencies	Decreased	Decreased	Decreased

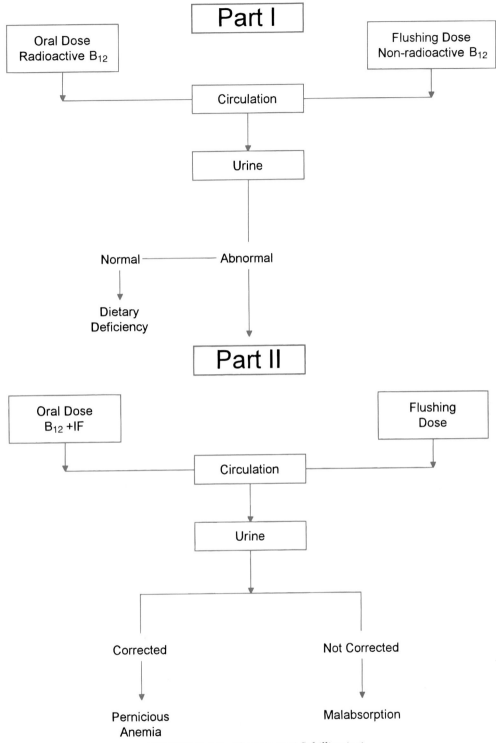

Part I

Oral Dose Radioactive B_{12}

Flushing Dose Non-radioactive B_{12}

Circulation

Urine

Normal ——————— Abnormal

Dietary Deficiency

Part II

Oral Dose B_{12} +IF

Flushing Dose

Circulation

Urine

Corrected

Not Corrected

Pernicious Anemia

Malabsorption

FIGURE 7–16   The two-part Schilling test.

Measurement of urinary MMA by a gas chromatograph–mass spectrophotometer (GC–MS) is a highly specific and sensitive test. This test can be used for evaluation of tissue vitamin B_{12} deficiency in the absence of decreased serum B_{12} and lack of clinical manifestations of megaloblastic anemia.[26]

Normal individuals excrete approximately 9 mg MMA in the urine in 24 hours. Patients with B_{12} deficiency may excrete as much as 300 mg/day.[3]

Serum and urine homocysteine levels are elevated in patients with both vitamin B_{12} and folate deficiencies, since both vitamins are necessary in the conversion of homocysteine to methionine. Serum homocysteine is also increased in short-term folate restriction diet and in patients with congenital homocysteinuria.[2,27-29]

The du suppression test measures the level of 5,10-CH_2THF. It is an indirect measurement of thymidylate synthesis in vitro and is abnormal in both vitamin B_{12} and folate deficiencies (see Fig. 7–10). The principle of this test is based on the fact that B_{12} or folate-deficient cells cannot convert deoxyuridine to deoxythymidine and, therefore, the radioactive-labeled thymidine will be incorporated into DNA. In patients with normal levels of B_{12} or folate, deoxyuridine is converted to thymidine. This conversion suppresses the labeled thymidine incorporation into the DNA.[7,19] Specificity of the deficient vitamin can be determined by addition of vitamin B_{12} or folate to the test system and a correction of the original abnormal result. This test is relatively time-consuming and therefore, despite its sensitivity, is not used as a diagnostic test.

Many studies have shown that some patients with vitamin B_{12} deficiency may seek medical help because of complications other than the classical features of megaloblastic anemia. Examples of these complications are retinopathy, neuropathy, vascular disorders, infertility, and physical and mental growth retardations in infancy.[12,16,27,30,31] However, these conditions have been reversed upon early treatment with vitamin B_{12}. To prevent these complications, numerous attempts have been made for early diagnosis of vitamin B_{12} and folate deficiencies.

The laboratory tests that are helpful for early detection of vitamin B_{12} and folate deficiencies are urinary methylmalonyl assay and serum homocysteine assay, respectively.[26,29]

TREATMENT

Vitamin B_{12} Deficiency

Most people with vitamin B_{12} deficiency require lifelong vitamin therapy. Cyanocobalamin and hydroxocobalamin are the two therapeutic forms of vitamin B_{12}. Hydroxocobalamin is preferred by some physicians because it has a longer half-life. Cyanocobalamin is less expensive and will convert to the physio-

logic form. Vitamin B_{12} is injected intramuscularly or subcutaneously. The initial dose administered is higher in order to saturate the body storage. Vitamin B_{12} is given in 6 injections of 1000 μg per dose over a 2- to 3-week period. The maintenance dose is injected in 100 to 1000 μg doses every 1 to 3 months[4,19] (Table 7–6).

Folic Acid Deficiency

The recommended therapeutic dose for folate deficiency is 5 mg/day over 3 to 4 months.[19] Folic acid vitamin is water-soluble and is given orally. Lifelong therapy is not required since it is usually possible to treat folate deficiency in a short period of time.[19] Folic acid may be given along with vitamin B_{12} when both vitamins are deficient or when the exact cause of megaloblastic anemia is not known. Folic acid given as prophylaxis is recommended during pregnancy and dialysis and may be required in patients with sickle cell anemia and thalassemia.[10]

RESPONSE TO THERAPY

The initial sign of a positive response to therapy is an increase in the reticulocyte count. The number of circulatory reticulocytes increase 2 to 3 days after therapy with a peak at about 7 days. The reticulocyte count may increase to 50% to 70% initially.[7] The megaloblastic morphology of the bone marrow disappears within the first 24 to 48 hours after therapy. The hematocrit rises in about 5 to 7 days after therapy, reaching normal levels in 4 to 8 weeks. Giant metamyelocytes and hypersegmented neutrophils disappear within 2 weeks. The entire therapeutic response process may take only 3 to 6 weeks, depending on the severity of the disease.[7,9]

VITAMIN-INDEPENDENT MEGALOBLASTIC CHANGES

This group of disorders is characterized by the presence of megaloblastic changes in the bone marrow and

TABLE 7–6	Treatment of Megaloblastic Anemia	
	Vitamin B_{12} Deficiency	**Folic Acid Deficiency**
Source	Hydroxocobalamin Cyanocobalamin	Folic acid
Route	Intramuscularly Subcutaneously	Oral
Initial dose	6 × 1000 μg over 2–3 weeks	5 mg/day for 4 months
Maintenance dose	100–1000 μg every 1–3 months	<5 mg
Prophylactic treatment	Total gastrectomy Partial gastrectomy Ileal resection	Pregnancy Sickle cell anemia Thalassemia Hemodialysis

TABLE 7–7 Vitamin-Independent Megaloblastic Anemias

Inherited
Orotic aciduria
Lesch-Nyhan syndrome
Dihydrofolate reductase deficiency
Transcobalamin deficiency
Abnormal cobalamin molecule
Congenital dyserythropoiesis

Acquired
Myelodysplastic syndrome
Erythroleukemia

Drugs
Folate antagonist (Methotrexate)
Purine or pyrimidine antagonists (6-mercaptopurine, cytosine arabinoside, and hydroxyurea)
Nitrous oxide

Toxic Materials
Arsenic
Chlordane

TABLE 7–8 Causes of Macrocytic Nonmegaloblastic Anemias

Chronic liver disease
Alcoholism
Acute hemorrhage
Hypothyroidism
Hematologic disorders
    Hemolytic anemia
    Aplastic anemia
    Chronic myeloproliferative disorders
Immunosuppressive drugs
Arsenic and chlordane intoxications

in the peripheral blood that are refractory to vitamin B_{12} and folic acid treatments. The megaloblastic changes in this group of patients may occur because of an inherited or acquired predisposition, or may be drug-induced (Table 7–7).

Orotic aciduria is a rare inherited disorder of pyrimidine metabolism characterized by increased excretion of orotic acid in the urine. Lesch-Nyhan syndrome is an X-linked disorder of purine metabolism. Megaloblastic changes are also noted in inherited dihydrofolate reductase deficiency, a disorder of folate metabolism. Inherited disorders of transcobalamin II deficiency or abnormal transcobalamin II molecule are associated with megaloblastic anemia. In congenital dyserythropoiesis, the megaloblastic changes are limited only to erythrocyte precursors of the bone marrow and red cells in the peripheral smear. White blood cells and platelets are normal.[7]

Megaloblastic changes may also be present in association with hematologic disorders such as myelodysplastic syndromes and erythroleukemia. The exact mechanism responsible for the defects in these disorders is not known.[19]

A wide variety of drugs with differing modes of action are associated with megaloblastic anemia. Methotrexate is an example of a folate antagonist drug. Drugs such as 6-mercaptopurine, cytosine arabinose, and hydroxyurea interfere with purine or pyrimidine metabolism. Nitrous oxide (N_2O), an anesthetic gas, inactivates vitamin B_{12}.[7,19]

Exposure to toxic materials such as arsenic and chlordane can also cause megaloblastic anemia.[7]

MACROCYTIC NONMEGALOBLASTIC ANEMIAS

Macrocytic anemias may be megaloblastic or nonmegaloblastic. Differentiation between the two is important. In macrocytic normoblastic anemias, the MCV is above 100 fL, but not as high as the MCV in megaloblastic anemias (MCV above 110 fL). The red cells on the peripheral blood smear appear large and round, but not oval. The neutrophils are not hypersegmented. The red cell precursors in the marrow are normoblastic and not megaloblastic. The mechanism responsible for the macrocytic morphology is not exactly known. Increased lipid deposition onto the red cell membrane or altered maturation time of the red cell precursors are among the possible causes.[19]

The most common causes of macrocytic anemia are chronic liver disease and alcoholism. In 40% to 96% of alcoholics, macrocytosis is present in the absence of anemia. In this case, alcohol has a direct toxic effect on the red cells rather than causing folate deficiency. The finding of macrocytosis is a valuable screening test for early detection of alcoholism.[3,10] Liver function tests such as serum LDH and bilirubin are helpful in the diagnosis.

Macrocytic anemia with an elevated reticulocyte count is associated with hemolytic anemia or acute blood loss. Macrocytic anemia may also be associated with aplastic anemia, chronic myeloproliferative disorders, and sideroblastic anemia. In sideroblastic anemia, a dimorphic red cell population may be observed (see Fig. 7–15). Bone marrow examination is often required for differential diagnosis.

Macrocytosis has also been reported in patients taking immunosuppressive drugs as well as arsenic and chlordane intoxification. Causes of macrocytic nonmegaloblastic anemia are summarized in Table 7–8.

CASE STUDY

A 50-year-old woman visited her doctor because she had experienced weakness, fatigue, and shortness of breath for the past few months.

Physical examination revealed a tall, slender woman with "lemon-yellow skin" and a smooth, red tongue. No hepatosplenomegaly was noted. She had experienced a loss of vibratory sense and had some problem with gait coordination.

Her family history and her past medical history were unremarkable. The patient was not on any medications.

A complete blood count with WBC differential was ordered and the results were as follows:

$$WBC = 7.4 \times 10^9/L \ (4.4-11)$$
$$RBC = 2.2 \times 10^{12}/L \ (4.1-5.1)$$
$$Hgb = 8.5 \ g/dL \ (12.3-15.3)$$
$$Hct = 25\% \ (36-45)$$
$$MCV = 114 \ fL \ (87-98)$$
$$MCHC = 34\% \ (32-36)$$
$$RDW = 15.2\% \ (11.5-14.5)$$
$$Platelet = 170 \times 10^9/L \ (150-400)$$

Differential
- = 67% segmented neutrophils (5% hypersegmented)
- = 25% lymphocytes
- = 5% monocytes
- = 3% eosinophils

RBC morphology = macrocytic with few macro-ovalocytes and few schistocytes.

RBC inclusions = few Howell-Jolly bodies

Reticulocytes = 0.2% (0.5–1.5)

Chemistry test results were as follows:

$$Total \ bilirubin = 4.0 \ mg/dL \ (0.2-1.0)$$
$$Indirect \ bilirubin = 2.9 \ mg/dL \ (0.2-0.8)$$
$$Serum \ LDH = 720 \ U/L \ (100-190)$$
$$Serum \ iron = 220 \ \mu g/dL \ (50-170)$$
$$TIBC = 215 \ \mu g/dL \ (250-450)$$
$$Serum \ B_{12} = 50 \ pg/dL \ (100-700)$$
$$Red \ cell \ folate = 200 \ ng/mL \ (130-628)$$

Questions

1. These laboratory findings are representative of what type of anemia?
2. How would you classify this anemia based upon the RBC indices?
3. What does the decreased reticulocyte count represent?
4. What is the cause of this anemia?
5. What test is used to evaluate B_{12} malabsorption?

Comments

The diagnosis of megaloblastic anemia was made based on the patient's physical examination and the highlights of the laboratory results. Physical findings reveal that the patient had the signs and symptoms of anemia, with the "lemon-yellow skin" caused by anemia and jaundice. The low hemoglobin and hematocrit levels in combination with an elevated MCV and normal MCHC are suggestive of macrocytic, normochromic anemia, a characteristic of megaloblastic anemia. The macro-ovalocytes and hypersegmented neutrophils present on the peripheral smear are striking features of megaloblastic anemia. Howell-Jolly bodies are the red cell inclusions commonly seen in this type of anemia. The low reticulocyte value is indicative of ineffective erythropoiesis. The WBC and platelet counts are normal in this patient, as is expected in early stages of megaloblastic anemia.

The elevated bilirubin, serum LDH, and serum iron levels can all be attributed to red cell hemolysis. In megaloblastic anemia, the red cells are fragile and have a shortened life span, and are thus prematurely destroyed in the bone marrow and in the peripheral blood.

The most common causes for megaloblastic anemia are vitamin B_{12} and folate deficiencies. In this patient,

the serum B_{12} level was decreased, whereas the red cell folate level was normal. These findings indicate that B_{12} deficiency was the probable cause for the megaloblastic anemia. The patient was on a good balanced diet and had no past medical history. Vitamin B_{12} deficiency because of malabsorption was suspected, and a two-part Schilling test was ordered to evaluate the cause of B_{12} malabsorption. In part I, the patient excreted 2% labeled B_{12} in her 24-hour urine, and in part II, she excreted 8%. This result supported the diagnosis of pernicious anemia.

The initial doses of hydroxocobalamin were administered intramuscularly for several weeks, followed by maintenance doses. After 2 months of therapy, the patient had completely recovered. Her hemoglobin and hematocrit had returned to normal and her abnormal blood cell morphologies had disappeared. The patient was advised to continue the vitamin B_{12} therapy to prevent relapse of the symptoms, since lack of IF in patients with pernicious anemia prevents absorption of dietary B_{12}.

REFERENCES

1. Williams, WJ, et al: Hematology, ed 4. McGraw-Hill, New York, 1990, pp 345, 453–460.
2. Wickramasinghe, SN and Fida, S: Bone marrow cells from vitamin B_{12} and folate deficient patients misincorporate uracil into DNA. Blood 83:1656, 1994.
3. Lee, GR, et al: Wintrobe's Clinical Hematology, ed 9, vol 1. Lea & Febiger, Philadelphia, 1993, pp 161–165, 749–776.
4. Nathan, DG and Oski, AF: Hematology of Infancy and Childhood, ed 4, vol 1. WB Saunders, Philadelphia, 1993, p 356.
5. Heckner, F, Lehmann, HP, and Kao, YS: Practical Microscopic Hematology, ed 4. Lea & Febiger, Philadelphia, 1994, pp 47, 50–53.
6. Chanarin, I: The Megaloblastic Anemia, ed 3. Blackwell, 1990, pp 10–11, 21–28.
7. Bick, RL: Hematology, Clinical and Laboratory Practice, vol 1. CV Mosby, St Louis, 1993, p 460.
8. Hughes-Jones, NC and Wickramasinghe, SN: Lecture Notes on Haematology, ed 5. Blackwell Scientific, Oxford, 1991, p 88.
9. Babior, BM and Stossel, TP: Hematology, A Pathophysiological Approach, ed 3. Churchill Livingstone, New York, 1994, p 87.
10. Spivak, JL and Eichner, ER: The Fundamentals of Clinical Hematology, ed 3. Johns Hopkins University Press, Baltimore, 1993, p 31.
11. Herbert, V: Staging vitamin B_{12} (cobalamin) status in vegetarians. Am J Nutr 59:1214S, 1994.
12. Graham, SM, Arvela, OM, and Wise, GA: Long-term neurologic consequences of nutritional vitamin B_{12} deficiency in infants. J Pediatr 121:710, 1992.
13. Pippard, MJ: Megaloblastic anemia: geography and diagnosis. Lancet 344:7, 1994.
14. Akinyanju, OO and Okany CC: Pernicious anemia in Africa. Clin Lab Haematol 14:33, 1992.
15. Van Den Berg, H: Vitamin B_{12}. Int J Vitamin Nutr Res 63:283, 1993.
16. Lam, S and Lam, BL: Bilateral retinal hemorrhages from megaloblastic anemia. Ann Ophthalmol 24:86, 1992.
17. Hoggarth, K: Macrocytic anemia. Practitioner 237:331, 1993.
18. Metz, J: Pathogenesis of cobalamin neuropathy: Deficiency of nervous system s-adenosylmethionin. Nutr Rev 51:12, 1993.

19. Hoffbrand, AV and Pettit, JE: Essential Haematology, ed 3. Blackwell Scientific, Oxford, 1993, p 64.
20. Hibbard, BM: Folate and fetal development. Br J Obstet Gynaecol 100:307, 1993.
21. Wald, NJ and Bower, C: Folic acid, pernicious anaemia, and prevention of neural tube defects. Lancet 343:307, 1994.
22. Lockith, G: Handbook of Diagnostic Biochemistry and Hematology in Normal Pregnancy. CRC Press, Ann Arbor, 1993, p 125.
23. Lotspeich-Steininger, CA, Steine-Martin, EA, and Koepke, JA: Clinical Hematology. Principles, Procedures, Correlations. JB Lippincott, Philadelphia, 1992, p 165.
24. Wevers, RA, et al: Folate deficiency in cerebrospinal fluid associated with a defect in folate binding protein in the central nervous system. J Neurol Neurosurg Psychiatry 57:223, 1994.
25. Crellin, R, Bottiglieri, T, and Reynolds, EH: Folate and psychiatric disorders, clinical potential. Drugs 45:624, 1993.
26. Norman, EJ: Detection of cobalamin deficiency using the urinary methylmalonic acid test by gas chromatography mass spectrometry. J Clin Pathol 45:382, 1992.
27. Ubbnik, JB, et al: Vitamin B_{12}, vitamin B_6, and folate nutritional status in men with hyperhomocysteinemia. Am J Clin Nutr 57:47, 1993.
28. Savage, DG, et al: Sensitivity of serum methylmalonic acid and total homocysteine determinations for diagnosing cobalamin and folate deficiencies. Am J Med 96:239, 1994.
29. Joostan, E, et al: Metabolic evidence that deficiencies of vitamin B_{12} (cobalamin), folate, and vitamin B_6 occur commonly in elderly people. Am J Clin Nutr 58:468, 1993.
30. Rees, MM, and Rodgers, GM: Homocysteinemia: Association of a metabolic disorder with vascular disease and thrombosis. Throm Res 71:337, 1993.
31. Menachem, Y, Cohen, AM, and Mittelman, M: Cobalamin deficiency and infertility. Am J Hematol 469:152, 1994.

BIBLIOGRAPHY

Allen, RH, et al: Metabolic abnormalities in cobalamin (vitamin B_{12}) and folate deficiency. FASEB J 7:1344, 1993.
Affronti, J and Baillie, J: Gastroscopic follow-up of pernicious anemia patients. Gastrointestinal Endoscopy 40:129, 1994.
Beck, WS: Hematology, ed 5. MIT Press, Cambridge, 1991, pp 84–110, 113–131.
Chanarin, I, et al: Cobalamin and folate: Recent developments. J Clin Pathol 45:277, 1992.
Curtis, D, et al: Elevated of serum homocysteine as a predictor for vitamin B_{12} or folate deficiency. Eur J Haematol 52:227, 1994.
Eastham, RD and Slade, RR: Clinical Hematology, ed 7. Butterworth-Heinemann, Oxford, 1992, p 26.
Flippo, TS and Holder, WD: Neurologic degeneration associated with vitamin B_{12} deficiency. Arch Surg 128:1391, 1993.
Goodman, KI and Salt, WB: Vitamin B_{12} deficiency. Important new concepts in recognition. Postgrad Med 88:147, 1990.
Healton, EB, et al: Neurologic aspects of cobalamin deficiency. Medicine 70:229, 1991.
Hoffbrand, AV and Jackson, BF: Correction of the DNA synthesis defect in vitamin B_{12} deficiency by tetrahydrofolate: Evidence in favor of the methyl-folate trap hypothesis as the cause of megaloblastic anemia in vitamin B_{12} deficiency. Br J Haematol 83:643, 1993.
Hsing, AW, et al: Pernicious anemia and subsequent cancer. A population-based cohort study. Cancer 71:745, 1993.
Jacob, RA, et al: Homocysteine increases as folate decreases in plasma of healthy men during short-term dietary folate

and methyl group restriction. J Nutr 124:1072, 1994.
Mukiibi, JM, Makumbi, FA, and Gwanzura, C: Megaloblastic anemia in Zimbabwe: spectrum of clinical and haematological manifestations. East Afr Med J 69:83, 1992.
Norman, EJ and Morrison, JA: Screening elderly populations for cobalamin (vitamin B_{12}) deficiency using the urinary methylmalonic acid assay by gas chromatography mass spectrometry. Am J Med 94:589, 1993.
Otega, RM, et al: Nutritional assessment of folate and cyanocobalamin status in a spanish elderly group. Int J Vitam Nutr Res 63:17, 1993.
Robinson, SH, Reich, PR: Hematology, Pathophysiologic Basis for Clinical Practice, ed 3. Little, Brown, Boston, 1993, pp 75–103.
Shevell, MI and Rosenblatt, DS: The neurology of cobalamin. Can J Neurol Sci 19:472, 1992.
Span, J, Koopmans, P, and Jansen, J: A reversible case of pernicious anemia. Am J Gastroenterol 88:1277, 1993.
Tungtrongchitr, R, et al: Vitamin B_{12}, folic acid and haematological status of 132 Thai vegetarians. Int J Vitam Nutr Res 63:202, 1993.
Wild, J, et al: Investigation of folate intake and metabolism in women who have had two pregnancies complicated by neural tube defects. Br J Obstet Gynaecol 101:197, 1994.
Wickramasinghe, SN and Fida, S: Correlations between holo-transcobalamin II, holo-haptocorrin, and total B_{12} in serum samples from healthy subjects and patients. J Clin Pathol 46:537, 1993.
Waters, HM, et al: High incidence of type II autoantibodies in pernicious anemia. J Clin Pathol 46:45, 1993.
Wood, ME, and Bunn, PA: Hematology/Oncology Secrets. Hanley and Belfus, Philadelphia, 1994, pp 34–38.
Young, SN: The use of diet and dietary components in the study of factors controlling affect in humans: a review. J Psychiatry Neurosci 18:235, 1993.

QUESTIONS

1. The pathophysiology of megaloblastic anemia is:
   a. Defective RNA synthesis and abnormal cytoplasm maturation
   b. Defective DNA synthesis and abnormal nuclear maturation
   c. Defective RNA synthesis and abnormal nuclear maturation
   d. Defective DNA synthesis and abnormal cytoplasm maturation

2. All of the following laboratory findings coincide with megaloblastic anemia except:
   a. Increased serum bilirubin
   b. Increased serum iron
   c. Decreased muramidase
   d. Increased LDH-1

3. Megaloblastic anemia is associated with:
   a. Ineffective erythropoiesis and increased reticulocytes
   b. Ineffective erythropoiesis and decreased reticulocytes
   c. Ineffective erythropoiesis and decreased LDH
   d. Ineffective erythropoiesis and decreased erythropoietin

4. According to the morphological classification of anemias, megaloblastic anemia is a:
   a. Macrocytic, hypochromic anemia
   b. Macrocytic, hyperchromic anemia
   c. Macrocytic, normochromic anemia
   d. Normocytic, normochronic anemia

5. Which of the following is not seen on the peripheral smear of a patient with megaloblastic anemia?
   a. Macro-ovalocytes

b. Hypersegmented neutrophils
c. Hyposegmented neutrophils
d. Howell-Jolly bodies

6. Which of the following are the characteristic findings of the bone marrow in a patient with megaloblastic anemia?
a. Hypercellular with low M:E ratio
b. Hypercellular with high M:E ratio
c. Hypocellular with high M:E ratio
d. Hypercellular with low M:E ratio

7. The glycoprotein necessary for absorption of vitamin B_{12} is:
a. Albumin
b. Transcobalamin II
c. Haptocorrin
d. Intrinsic factor

8. All of the following are clinical manifestations of both B_{12} deficiency and folate deficiency *except*:
a. Anemia and jaundice
b. Weakness and shortness of breath
c. Thrombocytopenia and bleeding
d. Hemoglobinuria

9. Which of the following Schilling test results corresponds to a diagnosis of pernicious anemia?
a. Part I abnormal, part II not corrected
b. Part I abnormal, part II corrected
c. Part I and part II are abnormal
d. Part I normal, part II corrected

10. Which of the following *is not* a cause of vitamin B_{12} deficiency?
a. Atrophic gastritis
b. Total gastrectomy
c. Blind loop syndrome
d. Chronic glossitis

ANSWERS

1. **b** (p 117)
2. **c** (p 117)
3. **b** (p 117)
4. **c** (p 118)
5. **c** (pp 118–119)
6. **a** (p 119 (Table 7–1))
7. **d** (p 120)
8. **d** (pp 117, 123, 126)
9. **b** (pp 127–128)
10. **d** (pp 121, 123–124)

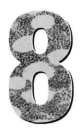

8 Aplastic Anemia (Including Pure Red Cell Aplasia and Congenital Dyserythropoietic Anemia)

Sherrie L. Perkins, MD, PhD

Objectives

At the end of this chapter, the learner should be able to:
1. Define aplastic anemia
2. List the etiologic classifications for aplastic anemia.
3. List four causes of acquired aplastic anemia.
4. Identify the most common cause of aplastic anemia.
5. Name the most common congenital disorder associated with development of aplastic anemia.
6. Describe the clinical and laboratory features associated with aplastic anemia.
7. Describe the bone marrow findings in aplastic anemia.
8. List the treatment modalities used in aplastic anemia and identify the best therapy for younger patients.
9. Define pure red cell aplasia and list clinical and laboratory features associated with this disorder.
10. Describe the common characteristics seen in all types of congenital dyserythropoietic anemias (CDAs).

DEFINITION

Aplastic anemia is a disorder (or group of disorders) characterized by cellular depletion and fatty replacement of the bone marrow and concomitant decreases in production of erythrocytes, leukocytes, and platelets leading to pancytopenia. The loss of functional bone marrow may be caused by a variety of pathogenetic mechanisms, including drugs, chemicals, irradiation, infections, and immune dysfunction. These processes all lead to loss of bone marrow precursor cells or damage of the bone marrow microenvironment, which is required to sustain bone marrow cell growth and differentiation. Thus, the progenitor cells that give rise to the various peripheral blood elements lose their ability to renew themselves and produce progeny, leading to a loss of bone marrow cellular mass.

PATHOGENESIS

The basic defect in aplastic anemia is a failure of blood cell production by the bone marrow involving erythrocytes, leukocytes, and platelets. Blood cell production within the bone marrow is dependent on the growth, differentiation, and self-renewal of a common, pluripotential stem cell or CFU–S.[1,2] In order to proliferate and differentiate into mature blood elements, the CFU–S responds to cytokines and other factors produced by cells in the bone marrow microenvironment.[3] Thus, bone marrow failure may develop as a consequence of a failure of blood cell formation at the level of the stem cell or a disturbance of the bone marrow microenvironment (Fig. 8–1).[4-6] Because the bone marrow is unable to respond to the developing peripheral blood cytopenias, it has been classified as a refractory or aregenerative anemia.

ETIOLOGY

Aplastic anemia may be acquired or congenital (hereditary) (Table 8–1). The vast majority of the cases are acquired, and of these cases most (40% to 70%) are primary or idiopathic in nature. The remaining cases of acquired aplastic anemia are considered secondary, resulting from exposure to chemicals or drugs, irradiation, or infection. In addition, aplastic anemia has been described as a result of immune dysfunction leading to immunologic "rejection" of the bone marrow.[7] Hereditary cases of aplastic anemia are extremely rare, and are grouped under the designation of Fanconi's anemia. These are usually associated with other genetic anomalies.

TABLE 8–1   Factors Associated with Development of Aplastic Anemia
Acquired
Idiopathic or primary
Secondary
Chemical agents
Drugs
Ionizing radiation
Infections
Miscellaneous causes
Congenital (Hereditary)
Fanconi's anemia

ACQUIRED APLASTIC ANEMIA

Idiopathic or Primary

Aplastic anemia is most often thought to be idiopathic in nature, because no clear-cut cause of the bone marrow failure is suspected or can be identified despite a careful search. Idiopathic aplastic anemia makes up about 50% of the cases of acquired aplastic anemia seen in western populations.

Secondary Causes

A wide variety of agents have been associated with the development of aplastic anemia (Table 8–2). Usually these agents can be divided into one of two categories: those that regularly produce bone marrow aplasia on sufficient exposure (e.g., benzene, irradiation) and those in which development of aplasia is considered a rare or idiosyncratic event (e.g., chloramphenicol, phenylbutazone).

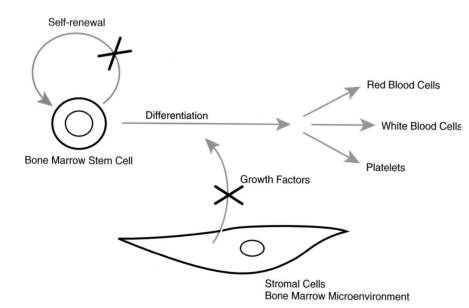

FIGURE 8–1 Schematic representation of possible defects in hematopoiesis that may give rise to aplastic anemia. It is postulated that inhibition of bone marrow stem cell self-renewal and/or changes in the bone marrow microenvironment that alter cytokine levels may cuase aplasia to develop.

TABLE 8–2 Causes of Secondary Acquired Aplastic Anemia

- Chemical agents: Benzene, insecticides, weed killers
- Drugs: Chloramphenicol, phenylbutazone, anticonvulsants, sulfonamides, gold
- Ionizing radiation
- Infections: Hepatitis, Epstein-Barr virus, cytomegalovirus, human immunodeficiency virus
- Miscellaneous causes: Pregnancy, malnutrition, immunologic dysfunction

Chemical Agents

Several chemical agents have been associated with the development of aplastic anemia, including benzene, trinitrotoluene, arsenic, insecticides, and weed killers (Table 8–2). Many of these compounds have a benzene ring as a part of their chemical structure. Modification of this benzene ring moiety with a nitroso or nitro group is highly associated with the development of aplastic anemia.[8,9]

Benzene has been known to cause varying degrees of bone marrow failure for nearly 100 years, since the original description by Santesson of four cases of fatal aplastic anemia occurring in workers in a bicycle tire factory. Benzene is used in a variety of industrial applications including as a solvent for rubber, fats, and alkaloids, as well as in the manufacture of drugs, dyes, and explosives. Because most benzene compounds are volatile, they are easily absorbed by inhalation.

It should be noted that benzene may cause a wide spectrum of bone marrow suppression, ranging from anemia or thrombocytopenia to severe aplastic anemia and fatal pancytopenia. There appears to be a wide variation in individual susceptibility to benzene, with bone marrow suppression occurring shortly after exposure in some people, or up to as long as 10 years after exposure in others.[10] Often the bone marrow suppression is reversible following discontinuation of benzene exposure. It is thought that benzene acts to inhibit DNA and RNA synthesis by the bone marrow cells, inhibiting cellular proliferation and differentiation.[11,12] In addition to the development of bone marrow aplasia by benzene, it has been associated with accumulation of chromosomal abnormalities and the ultimate development of an acute leukemia in some patients.[13]

Drugs

A wide number of drugs have been associated with development of aplastic anemia,[14] often as the result of an idiosyncratic reaction (Table 8–3). Of these drugs, the antibiotic choramphenicol and the anti-inflammatory drug phenylbutazone are probably the best known. Usually the toxicity associated with these drugs is *not* related to the dosage of the drug received, and it is often difficult to establish a relationship between the development of aplastic anemia and drug ingestion. Often such an association is dependent on epidemiologic data and a temporal relationship to ingestion of the drug. The mechanism by which these drugs cause the bone marrow suppression is often unknown, and it is impossible to identify which patients will react adversely to the drug. Such idiosyncratic reactions to drugs are relatively rare. It is estimated that 1 person in 20,000 to 30,000 may have an idiosyncratic reaction to chloramphenicol, which is about 10 times the incidence of developing aplastic anemia for the general population not taking chloramphenicol.[15]

Idiosyncratic or nonpredictable reactions to choramphenicol have been shown to be of two types.[16] One is a reversible bone marrow suppression that occurs while the patient is receiving the drug. This reaction is observed in many patients and is associated with vacuolization of bone marrow precursor cells (Fig. 8–2) and increased serum iron concentrations. The second type of reaction to chloramphenicol is development of an irreversible aplastic anemia weeks to months after drug exposure. This type of idiosyncratic reaction cannot be predicted by the dose, duration of drug use, or route of administration. Because of chloramphenicol's strong association with aplastic anemia, its use has decreased, and it is used only for specific indications where no other reasonable alternative drug exists.

A wide variety of other drugs have been implicated as suppressors of hematopoiesis (see Table 8–3). Knowledge of this potential side effect must be kept in mind when using these drugs, and appropriate monitoring of peripheral blood indices performed. Other drugs, such as chemotherapeutic agents, are well known to cause bone marrow hypoplasia when used in sufficient dosages. Usually this type of drug-induced bone marrow hypoplasia is fully reversible.

Ionizing Radiation

It is well known that ionizing radiation has an acute destructive effect on the rapidly dividing cells of the bone marrow, an effect which is fairly predictable based on the radiation dosage.[17] High doses of radiation, in the range of 300 to 500 rads (3 to 5 Gy), lead to a complete loss of hematopoietic cells that is irreversible and lethal. Lesser doses may lead to a reversible anemia, leukopenia, and thrombocytopenia with recovery of counts in 4 to 6 weeks. Hematopoietic cells are most susceptible to penetrating forms of radiation, such as those found in gamma rays and x-rays. However, chronic ingestion of lower-energy radiation sources (such as that seen many years ago in the painters of watch dials who ingested radium by wetting their brushes in their mouths and inhaling radium dust) may also cause toxic effects in bone marrow.[18]

Ionizing radiation affects the bone marrow and other rapidly proliferating cells within the body by disrupting chemical bonds and leading to the formation of free radicals and other ions. These interact with DNA that is being replicated within the cell, causing breaks or crosslinking of the DNA strands and leading to cellular death or genetic abnormalities.[19]

In addition to the immediate effects of irradiation on hematopoietic cells, there may also be delayed or long-term effects that are less predictable. Aplastic anemia

TABLE 8–3	Agents Associated with Aplastic Anemia

Agents That Regularly Produce Bone Marrow Hypoplasia with Sufficient Doses
Ionizing radiation
Benzene and benzene derivatives
Cytostatic agents (e.g., busulfan, vincristine)

Agents That Produce Bone Marrow Hypoplasia in an Idiosyncratic Manner		
Type of Drug	Relatively Frequent	Rare
Antimicrobials	Chloramphenicol, penicillin, tetracycline	Streptomycin, amphotericin B, sulfonamides
Anticonvulsants (Dilantin)	Methylphenylethylhydantoin, trimethadione	Methylphenylhydantoin, diphenylhydantoin, primidone
Analgesics	Phenylbutazone	Aspirin, tapazole
Hypoglycemic		Tolbutamide, chlorpropamide
Antianxiety		Chlorpromazine, chlordiazepoxide
Insecticide		Chlorophenothane (DDT), parathion
Miscellaneous		Colchicine, acetazolamide, hair dyes

may occur months to years after the radiation exposure, although development of bone marrow hyperplasia and acute leukemias is more common. Usually the bone marrow will develop abnormalities in maturation or dysplastic changes, which become more severe with time, culminating in bone marrow aplasia.[20]

Infections

Many infections have myelosuppressive effects on the bone marrow. Acute, self-limited infections may suppress bone marrow activity for 10 to 14 days with minor effects on the peripheral blood counts. Chronic infections may have more severe effects on hematopoiesis. Several viral infections, including hepatitis,[21,22] Epstein-Barr virus,[23] cytomeglovirus,[22] and HIV infection,[24] have been associated with the development of aplastic anemia. Of these, hepatitis C has the strongest association with development of a refractory aplastic anemia.[25,26] Although the mechanism whereby viruses cause aplastic anemia is unknown, it

has been suggested that the virus may directly infect the hematopoietic stem cell or induce an autoimmune reaction when the virus interacts with bone marrow cells, thereby causing the patient's immune system to damage the infected cell.[22] Other infections, such as miliary tuberculosis[27] and dengue fever, have also been associated with the development of aplastic anemia or bone marrow dysfunction.

Miscellaneous Causes

Aplastic anemia has been associated with a number of conditions of altered immunity, including eosinophilic fasciitis,[28] pregnancy,[29] and graft-versus-host disease.[30] This suggests that autoimmune targeting of the hematopoietic stem cell may provide a cause for development of the disease. Other cases of aplastic anemia have been associated with malnutrition, such as that seen in cases of anorexia nervosa[31,32] or pancreatic insufficiency.[33] These are associated with stem cell necrosis and degenerative changes within the bone marrow stromal cells that are termed *gelatinous transformation*.

CONGENITAL APLASTIC ANEMIA

Fanconi's Anemia

Congenital aplastic anemia is characterized by hematologic abnormalities that have been present since birth, a familial occurrence, and the presence of associated congenital defects. Several identifiable clinical entities are known, of which the best described is Fanconi's anemia.[34] Over 400 cases have been reported in the literature and show a variable clinical picture and autosomal recessive inheritance. Usually these patients have a variety of physical abnormalities that may include one or more of the following: skeletal defects (usually aplasia or hypoplasia of the thumb), cutaneous hyperpigmentation, renal abnormalities, microcephaly, mental retardation, and poor growth.

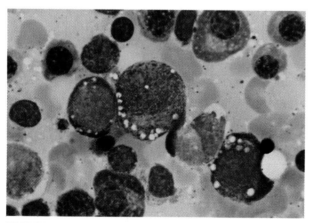

FIGURE 8–2 Vacuolation of bone marrow hematopoietic precursor cells indicating toxicity in a patient being treated with chloramphenicol. (Wright's stain, magnification ×250)

The patients have pancytopenia, which becomes progressively worse with age. Patients are usually symptomatic from the pancytopenia by 5 to 10 years of age. The bone marrow may be originally normocellular or hypercellular, but over time hypoplasia develops. Fanconi's anemia is characterized by a number of chromosomal abnormalities as determined by cytogenetic analysis, and special studies show a high number of chromosomal breakages and defective DNA repair.[35] It is therefore not surprising that these patients also have an increased incidence of acute myelogenous leukemia.

Untreated patients with Fanconi's anemia usually die of infections or hemorrhage. Some respond to androgen and corticosteroid therapy, but this therapy has been associated with development of hepatocellular carcinomas. Currently, most patients are treated with allogeneic bone marrow transplantation.[35,36]

Other congenital causes of aplastic anemia are much more rarely seen than Fanconi's anemia. Dyskeratosis congenita is an X-linked disorder where approximately half of the affected patients will develop aplastic anemia. It is not associated with chromosomal instability or development of acute leukemia.[37]

CLINICAL MANIFESTATIONS

Aplastic anemia often presents as an insidious process because of the gradual decrease in bone marrow production of red blood cells, leukocytes, and platelets. It may occur in all age groups. Most patients present with symptoms of progressive fatigue, dyspnea, and palpitations. However, bleeding or infection may occasionally be seen. Physical examination may reveal pallor secondary to the anemia or evidence of thrombocytopenia including petechiae, purpura, ecchymoses, and mucosal bleeding. Signs of infection because of the decrease in leukocytes are usually late manifestations of the disease. Other physical findings are minimal. Mild lymphadenopathy may be seen, but splenomegaly is very unusual.

LABORATORY EXAMINATION

The complete blood count (CBC) shows pancytopenia of varying degrees, often with anemia being the most notable (Table 8–4). The hemoglobin concentration is usually 70 g/L or lower, and the anemia is usu-

TABLE 8–5 Differential Diagnosis for Pancytopenia

- Infiltration of the Bone Marrow
  - Tumors—leukemias, lymphomas, metastatic disease
  - Fibrosis—myelofibrosis
  - Infections—mycobacteria
  - Other processes—granulomas of sarcoid, storage disorders such as Gaucher's disease
- Inhibition of Hematopoiesis or Ineffective Hematopoiesis
  - Myelodysplasia or paroxysmal nocturnal hemoglobinuria
  - Vitamin B_{12} or folate deficiency
  - Myelosuppressive drugs
- Increased Splenic Activity (hypersplenism)
  - Congestion
  - Tumors—leukemias, lymphomas
  - Infiltrative disorders—Gaucher's disease, Niemann-Pick disease
  - Infections
  - Primary hypersplenism
- Aplastic Anemia

ally characterized as normochromic and normocytic, although the cells may occasionally be macrocytic with moderate anisocytosis and poikilocytosis. The corrected reticulocyte count is characteristically normal or low (<1%, or <25 × 10^9/L), reflecting the lack of bone marrow regenerative activity. The white cells, in particular the myeloid and monocytic cells, as well as platelets are decreased.

There is no specific morphological abnormality of the peripheral blood smear that is associated with aplastic anemia. Examination of the peripheral blood smear will confirm a normochromic, normocytic anemia with little or no evidence of regeneration such as polychromatophilic cells, basophilic stippling, or nucleated red cells seen. The white cells usually show a relative lymphocytosis of up to 70% to 90%, and decreased numbers of myeloid and monocytic cells. If the white cell count falls below 1.5 × 10^9/L, an absolute lymphopenia may also be present. Rarely, immature myeloid cells such as myelocytes and metamyelocytes are seen, but large numbers of these cells would call into doubt

TABLE 8–4 Characteristic Abnormal CBC Values Seen in Severe Aplastic Anemia

Red Blood Cells
Hematocrit ≤ 0.20–0.25 (L/L) or 20%–25%
Hemoglobin concentration ≤ 70 g/L
Absolute reticulocyte count ≤ 25 × 10^9/L
Corrected reticulocyte count <1%

White Blood Cells
Total leukocyte count ≤ 1.5 × 10^9/L
Absolute neutrophil count ≤ 0.5 × 10^9/L

Platelets
Platelet Count ≤ 20–60 × 10^9/L

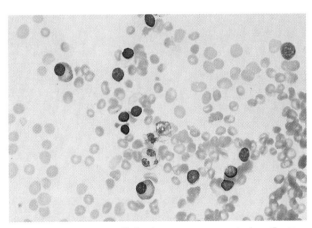

FIGURE 8–3 Hypocellular bone marrow aspirate reflecting bone marrow aplasia. (Wright's stain, magnification ×125)

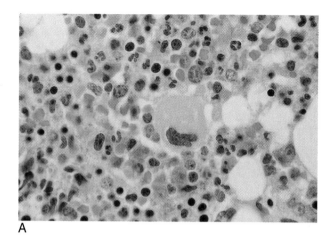
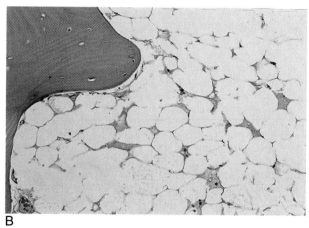

A   B

FIGURE 8–4 **Panel A**: Normocellular bone marrow. **Panel B**: Markedly hypocellular bone marrow biopsy associated with aplastic anemia. (Hematoxylin and eosin stain, magnification ×50)

the diagnosis of aplastic anemia. Platelets are often decreased, and it is unusual to find large or abnormal forms. Platelet function tests, such as bleeding time and clot retraction, are normal.

Because of the lack of specific features in the CBC data and peripheral smear, a wide differential diagnosis for causes of pancytopenia must usually be considered (Table 8–5) and a bone marrow examination must be performed. The bone marrow aspiration is often markedly hypocellular or a dry tap (Fig. 8–3). Small numbers of lymphocytes and rare hematopoietic precursor cells are seen. The bone marrow biopsy will most commonly show a very hypocellular bone marrow with reductions in the myeloid, erythroid, and megakaryocytic lineages. Often one sees only residual stroma and fat (Fig. 8–4). Scattered lymphocytes and plasma cells (Fig. 8–5) or occasional lymphoid aggregates may be seen (Fig. 8–6). It should be noted that patients with aplastic anemia often have residual islands of normal marrow or focal areas of bone marrow hyperplasia, which may mimic the findings of myelodysplasia or other processes (Fig. 8–7). It is crucial to

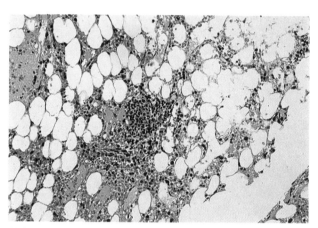

FIGURE 8–6 Lymphoid aggregate seen in a bone marrow biopsy for aplastic anemia. (Hematoxylin and eosin stain, magnification ×50)

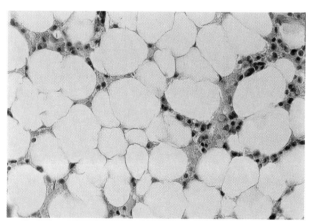

FIGURE 8–5 Residual lymphocytes, plasma cells, and bone marrow stroma in bone marrow biopsy for aplastic anemia. (Hematoxylin and eosin stain, magnification ×100)

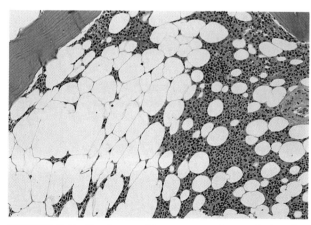

FIGURE 8–7 Focal area of bone marrow hyperplasia adjacent to a hypoplastic area in early aplastic anemia. (Hematoxylin and eosin stain, magnification ×50)

remember that there may be variations within each bone marrow biopsy specimen and between different biopsy sites in aplastic anemia, perhaps necessitating multiple or sequential biopsies to establish the diagnosis.

TREATMENT, CLINICAL COURSE, AND PROGNOSIS

Untreated aplastic anemia has an extremely poor prognosis, as the patients undergo progressive decrease in counts and subsequent lethal infection or bleeding.[38] However, some patients recover spontaneously. Until the early 1970s, patients with severe aplastic anemia were treated by supportive transfusions, possible treatment with androgens and anabolic steroids to stimulate hematopoiesis, and an extensive search for the possible causative agent in order to prevent further exposure.[39] Even so, the course was usually progressive with a 5-year mortality of about 70% and only 10% of patients fully recovering.

Currently, the treatment of choice for aplastic anemia in patients under age 50 years is bone marrow transplantation. This therapy is optimal if bone marrow from an HLA-matched sibling is used, although unrelated donors are becoming more readily available. Long-term survival rates of 60% to 80% have been reported following bone marrow transplantation, usually with full bone marrow recovery.[40,41] It should be noted that the chances of a successful transplant diminish in patients that have received multiple transfusions (>20), probably because of autoimmunization that leads to graft rejection; hence there is a tendency to minimize the number of supportive transfusions as much as is possible.[40]

In patients who are unable to receive a bone marrow transplant because of age or lack of a suitable donor, immunomodulatory therapy has been utilized. This type of therapy uses antithymocyte or antilymphocyte globulin, cyclosporine, or cyclophosphamide in an attempt to inhibit a presumed immune attack on the bone marrow stem cell. Up to a 60% 5-year survival rate has been seen, although a large number of these patients (up to 40%) will eventually develop a clonal disorder, such as myelodysplasia or paroxysmal nocturnal hemoglobinuria, which may eventually terminate in an acute leukemia.[42]

The prognosis of aplastic anemia has markedly improved with the advent of such therapeutic options as bone marrow transplant. The outcome is still variable and depends primarily on the severity of the anemia at the time of presentation, supportive care such as blood product transfusions, and the treatment modality employed.

RELATED DISORDERS

Pure Red Cell Aplasia

Pure red cell aplasia is an uncommon disorder in which the erythroid cells in the bone marrow are selectively decreased, giving rise to an anemia without other associated cytopenias. Over 600 cases have been

TABLE 8–6   **Causes of Pure Red Cell Aplasia**
Congenital
Diamond-Blackfan anemia
Acquired
Aplastic crisis in hemolytic disorders
Infection—parvovirus B19
Malnutrition
Drugs
Thymoma or other neoplasms
Idiopathic

reported in the world's literature.[43] This may be an acquired or congenital process (Table 8–6). The disease is characterized by a severe, chronic normocytic to slightly macrocytic anemia. Reticulocyte numbers are decreased, and may even be absent. There is no evidence of hemolysis or hemorrhage. White cells and platelets are normal. A bone marrow biopsy usually demonstrates normal cellularity with an absence of erythroid precursor cells. Erythropoietin levels are often markedly increased as the body attempts to compensate for the profound anemia.

Acquired causes of pure red cell aplasia are the most commonly seen, and may be either acute or chronic in onset and duration. Viral-type illnesses have been associated with development of a transient cessation of red cell production and disappearance of erythroblasts from the bone marrow in patients with longstanding hemolytic disease (e.g., sickle cell disease, hereditary spherocytosis). This loss of red cell production, termed an *aplastic crisis*, has in some cases been associated with infection by parvovirus B19 (the causative agent of erythema infectiosum or fifth disease, observed in children).[22] Parvovirus B19 selectively infects red blood cell precursors, leading to an absence of late erythroblasts and subsequent stages of erythoid differentiation.[44] Some erythroblasts may contain viral inclusions (Fig. 8–8). Parvovirus B19 infection may also cause a transient anemia in immunocompromised patients or patients with severe malnutrition. Usually the patient recovers erythropoietic capacity,

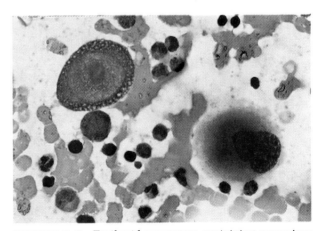

FIGURE 8–8 Erythroid precursors containing parvovirus B19 viral inclusions. (Wright's stain, magnification ×250)

as evidenced by the appearance of reticulocytes, within 7 to 10 days, although a chronic anemia may persist.[45]

Another frequent cause of pure red cell aplasia is an idiosyncratic reaction to drug therapy. Several drugs have been implicated, and these are usually the same drugs that may give rise to aplastic anemia, including sulfamides, anticonvulsants, isoniazid, phenylbutazone, and quinicrine. Usually the red cell aplasia resolves on discontinuation of the drug.[43] Other causes associated with development of pure red cell aplasia include malnutrition, chronic infection, and vitamin deficiency in children and the presence of a thymoma in adults.[43] In adult patients with a chronic red cell aplasia, more than 50% will also have a thymoma, although it may not be detected until several years after the development of the anemia. Removal of the thymic tumor will cause resolution of the anemia in about one third of the patients.[46] Occasionally, pure red cell aplasia has been associated with T-cell chronic lymphocytic leukemias. This association with T-cell disorders suggests that these cases of red cell aplasia may have an immune etiology, and some response to immunosuppressive therapies has been noted in these patients.

A congenital form of pure red cell aplasia was described in 1938 by Diamond and Blackfan and bears the name Diamond-Blackfan anemia. It is characterized by a moderate to severe chronic anemia that appears early in infancy and is associated with normal white cells and platelets. Minor congenital abnormalities may be present, as in Fanconi's anemia. The mode of inheritance is uncertain, and there are wide variations in the age of onset, severity of the disease, and the natural course of the disease. Spontaneous remissions have been noted in up to 25% of patients, often following many years of anemia. Most patients are treated with steroids and are able to maintain adequate hemoglobin levels, but some patients may become transfusion-dependent. A few patients develop acute leukemia late in the course of their disease.[47]

Congenital Dyserythropoietic Anemias

Congenital dyserythropoietic anemias (CDAs) make up a rare group of familial disorders in which anemia and ineffective erythropoiesis are associated with bizarre binuclear and multinuclear erythroblasts[48] (Fig. 8–9). Three types of CDAs have been well described

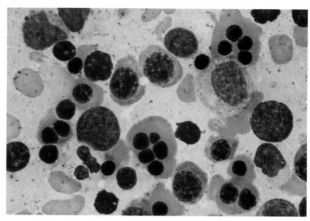

FIGURE 8–9 Multinucleated erythroid precursors in congenital dyserythropoietic anemia, type 2. (Wright's stain, magnification ×250)

(Table 8–7), although other forms have also be proposed. All of the CDAs are characterized by anemia, erythroid hyperplasia, and indirect hyperbilirubinemia or mild jaundice.

CDA type 1 is characterized by a mild to moderate macrocytic anemia with prominent anisocytosis and poikilocytosis. The bone marrow erythroblasts show megaloblastic maturation and the presence of a small number (1 to 3%) of marrow erythroblasts that are binucleated or contain chromatin bridges (thin, fiberlike connections between the nuclei). It is inherited as an autosomal recessive trait. Type 2 CDA gives rise to a mild to severe normocytic anemia with 10% to 50% of the erythroblasts in the marrow being binucleated or multinucleated. This form is also characterized by an autosomal recessive mode of inheritance and is the most commonly seen form of CDA. Type 2 CDA red cells will lyse in acidified serum, giving rise to an alternative name for this disease of HEMPAS (hereditary erythroblast multinuclearity with a positive acid serum test). Because of the cellular lysis in acidified serum, a diagnosis of paroxysmal nocturnal hemoglobinuria (PNH) may be entertained. However, unlike the cells of PNH, the cells in CDA type 2 will not lyse in the sugar water test. In addition, the type 2 CDA cells have been found to be strongly agglutinated by anti-i, and the i antigen is expressed on all of the erythrocytes in

TABLE 8–7	**Congenital Dyserythropoietic Anemias**		
	Type 1	**Type 2 (HEMPAS)**	**Type 3**
Degree of anemia	Mild to moderate	Mild to severe	Mild
Red blood cell size	Macrocytic	Normocytic	Macrocytic
Bone marrow features	Megaloblastic maturation 1%–3% binucleated erythroid or precursors cells with chromatin bridges	10%–50% binucleated or multinucleated erythroid precursors	Extreme multinucleation of erythroid precursors "gigantoblasts"
Genetic inheritance pattern	Autosomal recessive	Autosomal recessive	Autosomal dominant
Acid serum test	Negative	Positive	Negative
Sugar water test	Negative	Negative	Negative

Abbreviation: HEMPAS = hereditary erythroblast multinuclearity with a positive acid serum test

HEMPAS. Most patients with type 2 CDA have a relatively benign course, although some may require transfusions or splenectomy if splenomegaly develops. Type 3 CDA presents as a mild to moderate macrocytic anemia. It is differentiated from type 1 CDA by the presence of as many as 30% of the erythroid cells being multinucleated, some containing as many as 12 nuclei (gigantoblasts). This disorder appears to be inherited in an autosomal dominant fashion.

CASE STUDY

A 20-year-old woman was seen by her physician for fatigue, pallor, and easy bruising. Physical examination was unremarkable except for pallor, widespread petechiae and ecchymoses, and bleeding gums. The spleen was not enlarged. There was no history of recent exposures to drugs, toxins, or radiation. There was no history of any other illnesses, and she had been in good health until the past 2 weeks.

Laboratory data revealed a normochromic, normocytic anemia with a hematocrit of 20%, WBC of $2.0 \times 10^9/L$, and platelets of $20 \times 10^9/L$. The peripheral blood differential showed 9% neutrophils, 90% lymphocytes, and 1% monocytes. The corrected reticulocyte count was 1.1%. The bone marrow biopsy was hypocellular with less than 5% cellularity. Increased numbers of lymphocytes were noted in the aspirate admixed with a rare myeloid or erythroid precursor. No megakaryocytes were noted. No dysplastic changes were noted in the few hematopoietic cells seen, and there was no increase in the numbers of blasts. Further studies and historical information pertaining to infections, drug ingestion, and toxic exposures failed to identify an underlying cause for the patient's aplastic anemia. The patient was followed for the next 3 months with no resolution of her symptoms and no improvement in her blood counts. She received two transfusions of red blood cells for worsening anemia.

The patient's family was tested and a sister who was HLA-compatible was found. The sister had her bone marrow harvested, and it was infused into the patient following conditioning with cyclophosphamide to deplete the patient's immune cells. Approximately 35 days after her transplant, the patient had one bout of acute graft-versus-host disease, which was successfully treated with cyclosporin therapy. Her counts 1 year after transplant showed a hematocrit of 42%, WBC of $6.0 \times 10^9/L$, and platelets of $210 \times 10^9/L$. The WBC differential showed 71% neutrophils, 21% lymphocytes, 6% monocytes, and 2% eosinophils. A bone marrow biopsy showed a bone marrow cellularity of 50%, with all cell lineages present and maturing normally. The patient has had no further episodes of graft-versus-host disease, bleeding, or infection.

This is a fairly typical history for development of an idiopathic aplastic anemia. Currently, if an HLA-related bone marrow donor can be found, most of these patients proceed to bone marrow transplantation. Physicians usually prefer this procedure to be done relatively early in the course of the disease to minimize the numbers of transfusions, because

these have been found to have a negative effect on the survival of the bone marrow graft. If the transplant is successful, these patients often lead normal lives with no need for chronic immunosuppression or development of other hematologic problems.

Questions

1. What word can be used to classify the blood cell counts in this patient?
2. Does this anemia appear to be acquired or congenital?
3. What other treatment modality would be advised if an HLA-compatible bone marrow were not available?
4. What type of lymphocytosis is present here?
5. What is the basis for performing a corrected reticulocyte count?

REFERENCES

1. Spangrude, GJ, et al: Mouse hematopoietic stem cells. Blood 78:1395, 1991.
2. Iscove, N: Hematopoiesis. Searching for stem cells. Nature 347:126, 1990.
3. Holbrook, ST and Christensen, RD: Hematopoietic growth factors. Adv Pediatr 38:23, 1991.
4. Holmberg, LA, et al: Aplastic anemia: Analysis of stromal cell function in long-term marrow cultures. Blood 84:3585, 1994.
5. Boggs, DR and Boggs, SS: The pathogenesis of aplastic anemia. Blood 48:71, 1976.
6. Nissen, C: The pathophysiology of aplastic anemia. Semin Hematol 28:313 1991.
7. Parkinson, R: The immunopathology of bone marrow failure. Clin Hematol 7:475, 1978.
8. Kalf, GF: Recent advances in the metabolism and toxicity of benzene. CRC Crit Rev Toxicol 18:141, 1987.
9. Moeschlin, S and Speck, B: Experimental studies on the mechanism of action of benzene on the bone marrow (radioautographic studies using ^{3}H-thymidine). Acta Haematol 38:104, 1967.
10. Goldstein, BD: Benzene toxicity. Occup Med 3:541, 1988.
11. Kalf, GF, Rushmore T, and Snyder R: Benzene inhibits RNA synthesis in mitochondria from liver and bone marrow. Chem Biol Interact 42:353, 1982.
12. Thnek, A, Hogstedt, B, and Orofosson, T: Mechanisms of benzene toxicity: Effects of benzene and benzene metabolites on bone marrow cellularity, number of granulopoietic stem cells and frequency of micronuclei in mice. Chem Biol Interact 39:129, 1982.
13. Vigliani, ED: Leukemia associated with benzene exposure. Ann NY Acad Sci 271:143, 1976.
14. Appelbaum, FR and Fefer, A: The pathogenesis of aplastic anemia. Semin Hematol 4:241, 1981.
15. Weisenberger, AS: Mechanism of action of chloramphenicol. JAMA 209:97, 1969.
16. Yunis, AA and Bloomberg, GR: Chloramphenicol toxicity: Clinical features and pathogenesis. Prog Hematol 4:138, 1964.
17. Dunlap, CE: Effects of radiation on the blood and the hematopoietic tissues, including the spleen, the thymus and the lymph nodes. Arch Pathol Lab Med 34:562, 1942.
18. Martland, HS: Occupational poisoning in manufacture of luminous watch dials. JAMA 92:466, 1929.
19. Puck, TT: The action of radiation on mammalian cells. Am Naturalist 95:94, 1960.
20. Cronkite, EP: Radiation-induced aplastic anemia. Semin Hematol 4:273, 1967.

21. Hagler, L, Pastore, RA, and Bergin, JJ: Aplastic anemia following viral hepatitis: Report of two fatal cases and literature review. Medicine 54:139, 1975.
22. Young, N and Mortimer, P: Viruses and bone marrow failure. Blood 63:729, 1984.
23. Grishaber, JE, et al: Successful outcome of severe aplastic anemia following Epstein-Barr virus infection. Am J Hematol 28:273, 1988.
24. Spivak, JL, et al: Hematologic abnormalities in the acquired immune deficiency syndrome. Am J Med 77:224, 1984.
25. Zeldis, JB, et al: Aplastic anemia and non-A, non-B hepatitis. Am J Med 74:64, 1983.
26. Campell, AN and Freedman, MF: Fatal aplasia associated with non-A non-B hepatitis. Br Med J 286:1820, 1983.
27. Knobel, B, et al: Pancytopenia: A rare complication of miliary tuberculosis. Isr J Med Sci 19:555, 1983.
28. Debusscher, L, et al: Eosinophilic fasciitis and severe aplastic anemia: Favorable response to either antithymocyte globulin or cyclosporine A in blood and skin disorders. Transplant Proc 20:310, 1988.
29. Suda, T, et al: Prognostic aspects of aplastic anemia in pregnancy. Experience on six cases and review of the literature. Blut 36:285, 1978.
30. Hathaway, WE, et al: Graft vs. host reaction (human runt disease) following a single blood transfusion. JAMA 201:1015, 1967.
31. Pearson, HA: Marrow hypoplasia in anorexia nervosa. J Pediatr 71:211, 1967.
32. Smith, RRL and Spivak, JL: Marrow cell necrosis in anorexia nervosa and involuntary starvation. Br J Haematol 60:525, 1985.
33. Shwachman, H, et al: The syndrome of pancreatic insufficiency and bone marrow dysfunction. J Pediatr 65:645, 1964.
34. Nilsson, LR: Chronic pancytopenia with multiple congenital abnormalities (Fanconi's anemia). Acta Pediatr. 49:518, 1960.
35. Lui, JM, et al: Fanconi's anemia and novel strategies for therapy. Blood 84:3995, 1994.
36. Deeg, HJ, et al: Fanconi's anemia treated by allogeneic bone marrow transplantation. Blood 61:954, 1983.
37. Trowbridge, AA, et al: Dyskeratosis congenita: hematologic evaluation of a siblingship and review of the literature. Am J Hematol 3:143, 1977.
38. Najean, Y and Pecking, A: Prognostic factors in aplastic anemia. Am Med J 67:564, 1979.
39. Shahidi, NT and Diamond, LK: Testosterone-induced remission in aplastic anemia of both acquired and congenital types. N Engl J Med 264:953, 1961.
40. Speck, B: Allogeneic bone marrow transplantation for severe aplastic anemia. Semin Hematol 28:319, 1991.
41. Gluckman, E: Current status of bone marrow transplantation for severe aplastic anemia. A preliminary report from the International Bone Marrow Transplant Registry. Transplant Proc 19:2597, 1987.
42. Tichelli, A, et al: Morphology in patients with severe aplastic anemia treated with antilymphocyte globulin. Blood 80:337, 1992.
43. Dessypris, EN: The biology of pure red cell aplasia. Semin Hematol 28:275, 1991.
44. Young, N: Hematologic and hematopoietic consequences of B19 parvovirus infection. Semin Hematol 25:159, 1988.
45. Kurtzman, GJ, et al: Chronic bone marrow failure due to persistent B19 parvovirus infection. N Engl J Med 317:287, 1987.
46. Dameshek, W, Brown SM, and Rubin, AD: Pure red cell aplasia (erythroblastic hypoplasia) and thymoma. Semin Hematol 4:222, 1967.
47. Alter, BP: Childhood red cell aplasia. Am J Pediatr Hematol Oncol 2:121, 1980.
48. Heimpel, H and Wendt, F: Congenital dyserythropoietic anemia with karyorrhexis and multinuclearity of erythroblasts. Helv Med Acta 34:103, 1968.

BIBLIOGRAPHY

Adamson, JW and Erslev, AJ: Aplastic anemia. In Williams, WJ, Beutler, E, Erslev, AJ, and Lichtman, MA (eds): Hematology. McGraw-Hill, New York, 1990, p 158.
Jandl, JH: Aplastic anemias. In Blood. Little, Brown, Boston, 1987, p 115.
Jandl, JH: Aplastic and dysplastic anemias. In Blood: Pathophysiology. Blackwell Scientific, Boston, 1991, p 91.
Williams, DM: Pancytopenia, aplastic anemia, and pure red cell aplasia. In Lee, GR, Bithell, TC, Foerster, J, et al (eds): Wintrobe's Clinical Hematology. Lea & Febiger, Philadelphia, 1993, p 911.

QUESTIONS

1. How is aplastic anemia best defined?
   a. A condition in which bone marrow production of red blood cells, white blood cells, and platelets has failed.
   b. A condition in which a severe anemia is seen.
   c. A condition where platelet numbers are decreased.
   d. A condition where there are reversible increases in bone marrow elements.

2. Which is the most common cause of aplastic anemia?
   a. Drug ingestion
   b. Toxin exposure
   c. Idiopathic
   d. Ionizing radiation

3. Which of the following represents the most complete list of causes of aplastic anemia?
   a. Secondary and congenital
   b. Idiopathic and congenital
   c. Secondary and idiopathic
   d. Secondary, idiopathic, and congenital

4. Which of the following has *not* been associated with an acquired type of aplastic anemia?
   a. Ionizing radiation
   b. Increased chromosomal breakage
   c. Chemical agents
   d. Drugs

5. The aplastic anemia associated with benzene exposure is characterized by which of the following statements?
   a. Always occurs while the exposure to benzene is occurring
   b. Is always irreversible
   c. Always causes fatal, severe aplastic anemia
   d. May cause a spectrum of disease that may not manifest until several years following the benzene exposure

6. Chloramphenicol-induced aplastic anemia is associated with which of the following statements?
   a. The onset of the bone marrow aplasia is not predictable by the dose or the duration of drug exposure.
   b. Low doses of chloramphenicol never lead to aplastic anemia.
   c. People who receive chloramphenicol are 50 times more likely to develop aplastic anemia than the general population.
   d. The longer a patient receives chloramphenicol, the more likely it is that he or she will develop aplastic anemia.

7. Which of the following drugs is rarely associated with the development of aplastic anemia?
   a. Chloramphenicol
   b. Phenylbutazone
   c. Aspirin
   d. Chemotherapeutic agents

8. Ionizing radiation causes aplastic anemia by which of the following mechanisms?
   a. A dose-dependent destruction of bone marrow stem cells
   b. An idiosyncratic delayed development of bone marrow aplasia
   c. Disruption of chemical bonds to form free radicals that damage bone marrow cells
   d. All of the above

9. What is the most common congenital disorder associated with aplastic anemia?
   a. Fanconi's anemia
   b. Thrombocytopenia-absent radius (TAR) syndrome
   c. Congenital dyserythropoietic anemia, type 1
   d. Diamond-Blackfan anemia

10. Which of the following is not seen in the peripheral blood of patients with aplastic anemia?
   a. Normochromic, normocytic anemia
   b. Increased reticulocyte count
   c. Relative lymphocytosis
   d. Decreased neutrophils

11. What is the appearance of the bone marrow biopsy in aplastic anemia?
   a. Hypercellular
   b. Normocellular
   c. Hypocellular
   d. Fibrotic

12. The differential diagnostic considerations for bone marrow hypoplasia does not include which of the following disorders?
   a. Severe malnutrition
   b. Myeloproliferative disorder
   c. Aplastic anemia
   d. Recent chemotherapy

13. What is the treatment of choice for severe aplastic anemia in patients who are under the age of 50?

   a. Multiple transfusions
   b. Androgens
   c. Bone marrow transplantation
   d. Erythropoietin therapy

14. What is the definition of pure red cell aplasia?
   a. Lack of hematopoietic precursors in the bone marrow
   b. Abnormal giant normoblasts in the bone marrow
   c. Lack of erythroid precursors with normal white blood cell and megakaryocytic precursors
   d. Dysplastic red cell precursors with normal white blood cell and megakaryocytic precursors

15. What features do the congenital dyserythropoietic anemias (CDAs) have in common?
   a. Anemia, microcytosis, erythroid hyperplasia, and abnormal erythroblasts
   b. Anemia, erythoid hyperplasia with abnormal erythroblasts, and indirect hyperbilirubinemia
   c. Anemia, lysis in acidified serum, and indirect hyperbilirubinemia
   d. Anemia, macrocytosis, erythroid hyperplasia with abnormal erythroblasts, and indirect hyperbilirubinemia

ANSWERS

1. **a** (p 135)
2. **c** (p 136)
3. **d** (p 136)
4. **b** (pp 137–138)
5. **d** (p 137)
6. **a** (p 137)
7. **c** (p 138, Table 8–3)
8. **d** (p 137)
9. **a** (pp 138–139)
10. **b** (p 139)
11. **c** (p 140)
12. **b** (p 139, Table 8–5)
13. **c** (p 141)
14. **c** (p 141)
15. **b** (p 142)

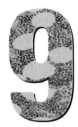

Introduction to Hemolytic Anemias: Intracorpuscular Defects

I—HEREDITARY DEFECTS OF THE RED CELL MEMBRANE

Stan Zail, MB, BCh, MD, FRCPath
Theresa L. Coetzer, PhD

Objectives

At the end of this chapter, the learner should be able to:

1 Define intracorpuscular and extracorpuscular red cell defects as related to hemolytic processes.
2 List laboratory tests that reflect increased red cell destruction.
3 Calculate a reticulocyte production index.
4 Name laboratory tests that help to classify the cause of red cell hemolysis.
5 Identify the red cell membrane abnormalities associated with hereditary spherocytosis.
6 Recognize abnormal laboratory results associated with hereditary spherocytosis.
7 Name the functional abnormalities affecting membrane skeleton proteins in hereditary elliptocytosis.
8 Recall laboratory findings associated with hereditary elliptocytosis.
9 Identify the abnormalities that cause the severe fragmentation and microspherocytosis characteristic of hereditary pyropoikilocytosis.
10 List rare disorders of membrane cation permeability.

CLASSIFICATION OF HEMOLYTIC ANEMIAS

A hemolytic state exists when the in vivo survival of the red cell is shortened. The presence of anemia in an individual patient is, however, dependent on the degree of hemolysis and the compensatory response of the erythroid elements of the bone marrow. Normal bone marrow is able to increase its output about sixfold to eightfold, so that anemia is not manifested until this capacity is exceeded, corresponding to a red cell life span of about 15 to 20 days or less. Anemia may, however, occur with more moderate shortening of the

146

red cell life span if there is an associated depression of bone marrow function, which may occur with certain systemic diseases or exposure to chemicals or drugs.

A useful classification of the hemolytic anemias entails their subdivision into those disorders associated with an intrinsic (intracorpuscular) defect of the red cell and those associated with an extrinsic (extracorpuscular) abnormality. Red cells from a patient with an intracorpuscular defect have a shortened survival in both the patient and in a normal recipient, whereas normal donor red cells survive normally in the patient. In contrast, normal red cells, when transfused into a patient with an extracorpuscular abnormality, are destroyed more rapidly. The patient's red cells, when transfused into a healthy recipient, have normal survival, provided they have not been irreversibly damaged. Hemolytic states have also traditionally been regarded as intravascular or extravascular; that is, sequestration occurs in reticuloendothelial tissue. However, vigorous extravascular hemolysis may often be associated with signs of hemoglobin release into the plasma such as hemoglobinemia and decreased haptoglobin levels. The distinction is still useful from a clinical standpoint because certain hemolytic states are associated with predominantly intravascular hemolysis (e.g., paroxysmal nocturnal hemoglobinuria and infections caused by *Clostridium* spp. or *Plasmodium falciparum*).

Hemolytic anemias may be classified as follows:
1. Intracorpuscular defects
   a. Hereditary defects
      (1) Defects in the red cell membrane
      (2) Enzyme defects
      (3) Hemoglobinopathies
      (4) Thalassemia syndromes
   b. Acquired defects
      (1) Paroxysmal nocturnal hemoglobinuria
2. Extracorpuscular defects
   a. Immune hemolytic anemias
   b. Infections
   c. Chemicals and toxins
   d. Physical agents
   e. Microangiopathic and macroangiopathic hemolytic anemias
   f. Splenic sequestration (hypersplenism)
   g. General systemic disorders (in which hemolysis is not the dominant feature of the anemia)

APPROACH TO DIAGNOSIS OF A HEMOLYTIC STATE

The approach to diagnosis of a hemolytic state initially involves establishing the fact that the rate of red cell destruction is increased and then determining the cause of hemolysis.

Establishing the Presence of Hemolysis

Diagnostic tests used to establish the presence of hemolysis rely on the fact that hemolysis is characterized by both increased cell destruction and increased production.

Tests Reflecting Increased Red Cell Destruction

The most frequently used tests in this category are the serum unconjugated (indirect) bilirubin and serum haptoglobin level determinations. The serum unconjugated bilirubin level seldom exceeds 3 to 4 mg/dL in uncomplicated hemolytic states and reflects the catabolism of heme derived from red cells phagocytized by the reticuloendothelial system (Fig. 9–1). The test is, however, relatively insensitive, as is the measurement of fecal stercobilinogen and urine urobilinogen that represents further stages in the disposition of unconjugated bilirubin by the liver (see Fig. 9–1). Because the unconjugated bilirubin is bound to albumin, it cannot pass the glomerular filter, and the jaundice is said to be "acholuric." On the other hand, a decreased serum haptoglobin level is a very sensitive test of both intravascular and extravascular hemolysis, and reflects the rapid clearance by the reticuloendothelial system of a complex formed between liberated hemoglobin and circulatory haptoglobin. Drawbacks to the use of serum haptoglobin levels are that low levels may occur in hepatocellular disease, reflecting decreased synthesis by the liver, and that some individuals, particularly in black populations, may have a genetically determined deficiency of haptoglobin. Increased synthesis of haptoglobin in acute inflammatory states or malignancy may also mask depletion of serum haptoglobin owing to hemolysis.

Other tests that reflect increased red cell destruction, particularly if it is primarily intravascular, are those that test for the presence of hemoglobinemia, hemoglobinuria, and hemosiderinuria. The assessment of hemoglobinemia requires stringent precautions in the prevention of hemolysis during blood collection. Once the hemoglobin-binding capacity of serum haptoglobin is exceeded, hemoglobin passes through the glomerulus as alpha-beta chain dimers and reassociates to α_2-β_2 tetramers in the tubule, where the hemoglobin is reabsorbed and degraded. The liberated iron is conserved as ferritin and hemosiderin. When the tubular reabsorptive capacity for hemoglobin is exceeded, hemoglobinuria ensues and is detectable either by spectroscopic examination or by commercially available dipsticks that detect heme. Staining of the urine sediment for iron (e.g., with Prussian blue) will detect the hemosiderin- and ferritin-containing renal tubular cells that are sloughed several days after a hemolytic episode. Some of the free plasma hemoglobin may be oxidized to methemoglobin with subsequent dissociation of ferri-heme, which combines with albumin to form methemalbumin. Methemalbumin can be detected spectroscopically by Schumm's test. This test is relatively insensitive and is seldom positive in mild hemolytic states. In routine practice, determination of red cell survival using ^{51}Cr-labeled red cells is seldom required to document an increased rate of red cell destruction. The fate of hemoglobin when processed intravascularly or extravascularly is shown diagrammatically in Figure 9–1.

Tests Reflecting Increased Red Cell Production

The compensatory bone marrow response to hemolysis results in the delivery of young red cells in the form

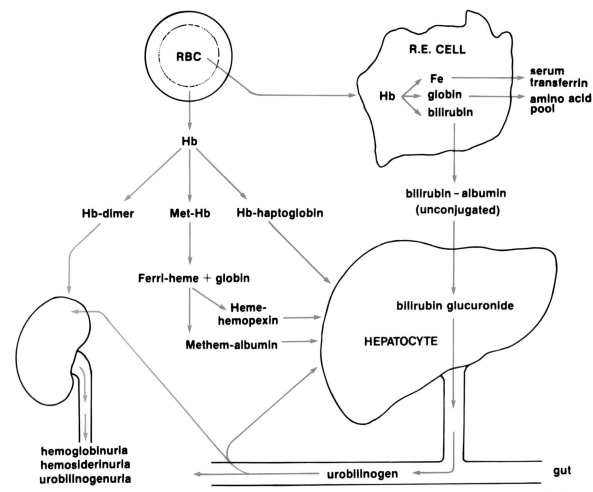

FIGURE 9-1   Diagrammatic representation of the disposition of hemoglobin after intravascular or extravascular destruction of red cells.

of reticulocytes into the circulation. These young cells contain RNA, which stains supravitally with dyes such as new methylene blue or brilliant cresyl blue. The normal reticulocyte count has a range of 0.2% to 2.0%. This reflects the fact that each day approximately 1% of the red cell mass is destroyed and replaced by young red cells from the bone marrow, since red cell survival is approximately 120 days. The reticulocyte count is always elevated in a hemolytic state in which there is a normal compensatory bone marrow response. However, a more accurate assessment of red cell production is required, since the percentage of reticulocytes may be "spuriously" elevated because the reticulocytes may be diluted into a lesser number of total circulating red cells. In addition, in response to the anemia, reticulocytes may leave the bone marrow prematurely and mature in the circulation for longer than the normal maturation time of one day, again leading to a falsely elevated reticulocyte count. These cells (so-called shift reticulocytes) are recognizable as large bluish-gray erythrocytes on Romanowsky stains.

The reticulocyte production index (RPI) corrects the hematocrit to a normal value of 45% and takes into account the maturation time of the reticulocyte at a particular hematocrit (approximately 1.0 day at a hematocrit of 45%, 1.5 days at 35%, 2.0 days at 25%, and 2.5 days at 15%).[1]

$$RPI = \frac{\% \text{ Reticulocytes}}{\text{Retic maturation time}} \times \frac{\text{Hematocrit}}{45}$$

For example, an RPI of 5.3 is calculated for a patient suspected of having a hemolytic state with the following indices: Hb 12.0 g/dL, hematocrit 36%, reticulocyte count 10%, shift cells present.

An RPI of greater than 2.5 to 3.0 is generally regarded as indicative of a hemolytic state, but it is very important to exclude the presence of hemorrhage in a particular patient, because this too may lead to an elevated RPI. Although the RPI is probably the single most useful test to detect a hemolytic state, a cautionary note is in order, because the test may not be sensitive enough to detect mild hemolytic states (see Chap. 31).

Establishing the Cause of Hemolysis

Once having documented the presence of hemolysis, the approach followed by Lux and Glader[2] in estab-

TABLE 9-1 Predominant Red Cell Morphology Commonly Associated with Nonimmune Hemolytic Disorders

Spherocytes
Hereditary spherocytosis
Acute oxidant injury (HMP shunt defects during hemolytic crisis, oxidant drugs, and chemicals)
Clostridium welchii septicemia
Severe burns, other red cell thermal injuries
Spider, bee, and snake venoms
Severe hypophosphatemia

Bizarre Poikilocytes
Red cell fragmentation syndrome (microangiopathic and macroangiopathic hemolytic anemias)
Hereditary elliptocytosis in neonates
Hereditary pyropoikilocytosis

Elliptocytes
Hereditary elliptocytosis
Thalassemias
Iron deficiency
Megaloblastic anemia

Stomatocytes
Hereditary stomatocytosis and related disorders
Stomatocytic elliptocytosis

Irreversibly Sickled Cells
Sickle cell anemia
Symptomatic sickle syndromes

Intraerythrocytic Parasites
Malaria
Babesiosis
Bartonellosis

Prominent Basophilic Stippling
Thalassemias
Unstable hemoglobins
Lead poisoning
Pyrimidine-5'-nucleotidase deficiency

Spiculated or Crenated Red Cells
Acute hepatic necrosis (spur cell anemia)
Uremia
Infantile pyknocytosis
Abetalipoproteinemia
McLeod blood group

Target Cells
Hemoglobins S, C, D, and E
Thalassemias
Hereditary xerocytosis

Nonspecific or Normal Morphology
Embden-Meyerhof pathway defects
HMP shunt defects
Adenosine deaminase hyperactivity with low red cell ATP
Unstable hemoglobins
Paroxysmal nocturnal hemoglobinuria
Dyserythropoietic anemias
Copper toxicity (Wilson's disease)
Cation permeability defects
Erythropoietic porphyria
Vitamin E deficiency
Hypersplenism

Source: Adapted from Lux and Glader.[2]

lishing the cause of hemolysis is pragmatic and logical and will be the technique followed in this chapter. The initial step consists of separating patients into Coombs test–positive (i.e., immunohemolytic anemias) and Coombs test–negative groups. The latter group is then further divided into "smear-positive" and "smear-negative" subgroups. It is fundamentally impotant to assess morphology in peripheral smears that are free of artifact. On the basis of the classification according to the predominant morphological criteria associated with a particular disease state (Table 9–1), it is possible to narrow considerably the differential diagnosis and then institute further appropriate tests to make a definitive diagnosis.

It is also worth emphasizing that many hemolytic states are associated with an underlying disease, as will become apparent in the ensuing chapters, and this should not be lost sight of in the assessment of the individual patient.

HEREDITARY DEFECTS OF THE RED CELL MEMBRANE

Red Cell Membrane Structure

An understanding of the etiology and pathophysiology of hemolytic states caused by defects of the red cell membrane requires some knowledge of the structure and biochemistry of the membrane. The ability of the red cell to deform and to subsequently regain its original biconcave disc shape is determined by three factors: (1) cell surface area to volume ratio; (2) the viscoelastic properties of the membrane, which depend on the structural and functional integrity of the membrane skeleton; and (3) the cytoplasmic viscosity, which is determined primarily by hemoglobin.

The structural organization of the red cell membrane and its underlying network of proteins has been reviewed in Chapter 3, and only some aspects of the membrane proteins implicated in the pathogenesis of hemolytic anemia will be emphasized here.

The red cell membrane *skeleton* is a loosely knit two-dimensional network consisting mainly of spectrin, actin, and protein 4.1.[3] Stretched skeletons that had been negatively stained and viewed by high-resolution electron microscopy[4] reveal a hexagonal lattice of predominantly spectrin tetramers with some hexamers joined together by junctional protein complexes (Fig. 9–2). These junctional complexes are composed of short F-actin filaments containing 12 to 14 β-actin monomers and protein 4.1, as well as the actin-binding proteins adducin, dematin (protein 4.9), and tropomyosin.[5] The skeleton is linked to the lipid bilayer by interactions with the integral membrane proteins band 3 and glycophorin C. The primary attachment occurs via a high-affinity interaction between band 3 and ankyrin, which in turns binds to spectrin.[6] Pallidin (protein 4.2) also participates in this complex.[7] Secondary attachment sites of lower affinity are provided by interactions between band 3 and protein 4.1,[8] as well as among glycophorin C, protein 4.1, and protein p55.[9] Spectrin and protein 4.1 also interact directly with the lipid bilayer.[3]

Red cell *spectrin* is an elongated flexible heterodimer

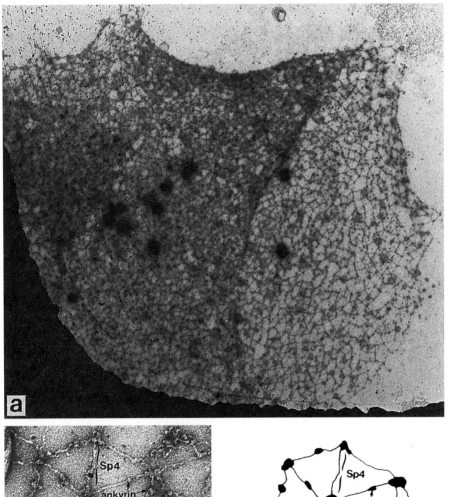

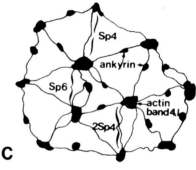

FIGURE 9-2 Transmission electron micrographs and drawing of negatively stained membrane skeletons. (*a*) An area of spread skeleton network; (*b*) and (*c*) the hexagonal lattice made up by spectrin tetramers (Sp4), hexamers (Sp6) or double tetramers (2Sp4). Crosslinking junctional complexes are thought to contain short F-actin filaments and protein 4.1. Globular ankyrin structures are bound to spectrin filaments about 80 nm from their distal ends. (From Liu et al,[4] with permission.)

composed of stoichiometric amounts of two structurally related, but functionally distinct, α and β polypeptides that are encoded by separate genes.[10–12] The two subunits are aligned side by side with an antiparallel arrangement of their N and C terminals. α Spectrin contains 22 tandem 106 amino acid repeats, known as a spectrin motif, whereas β spectrin has 17 repeats[11–13] (Fig. 9–3). Recent x-ray crystallography has verified the triple helical structure of this motif.[14] Spectrin can also be subdivided into structural domains (αI to αV and βI to βIV) that are resistant to mild proteolysis by trypsin.[15] In the head region of the molecule, $\alpha\beta$ spectrin dimers self-associate to form tetramers via an interaction between two helixes from the C-terminal repeat of the βI domain and a third helix from the N-terminal repeat of the αI domain.[16] Repeats 15 and 16 of β spectrin form the ankyrin-binding domain; the N terminal binds actin and protein 4.1 and the C terminal is phosphorylated.[10] An important aspect in the biogenesis of the membrane skeleton is that α spectrin is synthesized in about threefold excess over β spectrin[17] and undergoes slower degradation,[18] indicating that β spectrin is the rate-limiting component in spectrin assembly.

Red cell *band 3* (reviewed by Tanner[19]) is divided into two structurally and functionally distinct domains. The ±43-kd N-terminal cytoplasmic domain contains binding sites for several proteins, including ankyrin, protein 4.1, and pallidin. The ±52 kd C-terminal region has up to 14 transmembrane segments intercalated in the lipid bilayer that form the anion-exchange channel.

Ankyrin (reviewed by Peters and Lux[20]) is a pyramid-shaped protein that has an N-terminal 89-kd band 3

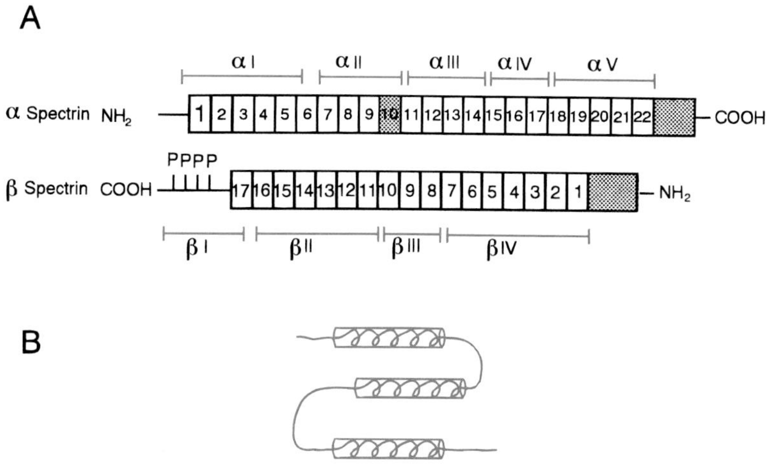

A

B

FIGURE 9-3 Schematic representation of spectrin structure. (*A*) The subunit of α and β spectrin showing the antiparallel arrangement of the N and C terminals; the homologous repeat units (open squares) and the trypsin-resistant domain structure are indicated above the α chain and below the β chain. α Spectrin has 5 domains (αI–αV) and 22 repeats. β Spectrin has 4 domains (βI–βIV) and 17 repeats. The hatched squares indicate nonhomologous regions. (*B*) Diagrammatic triple α helical structure of one of the spectrin repeats.

binding domain, formed by a series of repeats of 33 amino acids each. Spectrin binds to the central domain of ankyrin, whereas the C-terminal portion is a regulatory domain that is alternatively spliced.

Some properties of the red cell membrane proteins involved in hemolytic anemia are outlined in Table 9–2.

Classification

Ideally, the classification of hereditary defects of the red cell membrane should be based on the delineation of specific abnormalities of the membrane. The last few years have witnessed an explosive increase in knowledge in achieving this goal, particularly in the characterization of specific abnormalities of the membrane skeleton. At present, however, all patients with clinical and morphological evidence of a membrane defect cannot yet be categorized in this way, so that the classification used is still based on the prime morphological features of the disorder.

Four main groups are delineated:
1. Hereditary spherocytosis (HS)
2. Hereditary elliptocytosis (HE) and morphologically related disorders including hereditary pyropoikilocytosis (HPP), spherocytic HE, and Southeast Asian ovalocytosis (SAO).
3. Hereditary stomatocytosis
4. Hereditary xerocytosis

By far the most common and well-characterized groups of disorders are HS and HE, and this review will focus on these entities. The other inherited red cell abnormalities are rare and their etiology is less clear.

The currently accepted nomenclature for the membrane protein defects[21] utilizes an abbreviation of the mutant protein (e.g., Sp, Ank, Bd3, 4.1), followed by the name of the city or region of origin of the patient in whom the mutation was first described, for example, Sp$_{Cagliari}$. Superscripts are used for α-spectrin defects that impair dimer self-association and entail the spectrin abbreviation followed by a superscript designation

---

TABLE 9–2 **Properties of Selected Red Cell Membrane Proteins Implicated in Hemolytic Anemia**

Protein	SDS PAGE Band*	Mol Wt (kD)†	Gene Symbol	Chromosomal Localization	Diseases
Skeletal proteins					
α Spectrin	1	281	SPTA1	1q22 → q23	HS, HE, HPP
β Spectrin	2	246	SPTB	14q23 → q24.2	HS, HE, HPP
Protein 4.1	4.1	66	EL1	1p33 → p34.2	HE
Integral proteins					
Band 3	3	102	EPB3	17q21 → qter	HS, SAO
Stomatin	7	32	EPB72	9q34.1	HSt
Glycophorin C	PAS-2	14	GYPC	2q14→ q21	HE
Connecting proteins					
Ankyrin	2.1	206	Ank 1	8p11.2	HS
Pallidin	4.2	77	EPB42	15q15 → q21	HS, HE

*Proteins are separated by sodium dodecyl sulfate polyacrylamide gel electrophoresis (SDS PAGE) and stained with Coomassie blue or periodic acid-Schiff (PAS) reagent.
†Molecular weight is calculated from the amino acid sequence.
Abbreviations: HS = hereditary spherocytosis; HE = hereditary elliptocytosis; HPP = hereditary pyropoikilocytosis; HSt = hereditary stomatocytosis; SAO = Southeast Asian ovalocytosis.

of the tryptic domain that is altered and the size of the largest mutant tryptic fragment, for example, $Sp\alpha^{I/65}$. Truncated or elongated spectrin or 4.1 variants are designated by superscripts indicating the size of the mutant protein, for example, $Sp\beta^{220/218}$.

Hereditary Spherocytosis

Mode of Inheritance

Hereditary spherocytosis (HS) is the most common hereditary hemolytic anemia in Northern Europeans (Fig. 9–4). It occurs in other ethnic groups, but its prevalence is not known. In most cases (±75%), it follows a classic autosomal dominant pattern of inheritance, but in about a quarter of families both parents are clinically normal, suggesting autosomal recessive inheritance or decreased penetrance of a dominant gene or a new mutation.

Etiology and Pathophysiology

The fundamental expression of the membrane defect in HS is a loss of surface area of the red cell resulting in a decreased surface-to-volume ratio. This is manifested morphologically as spherocytosis, although it should be noted that the majority of HS cells are spherostomatocytic rather than truly spherocytic. Such cells tolerate less swelling than normal red cells and are osmotically fragile. The decrease in surface-to-volume ratio also makes the cells less deformable than normal. This has a particularly deleterious effect on their survival in the spleen and explains one of the hallmarks of HS, which is the excellent clinical response to splenectomy in most, but not all, cases. The exact pathogenesis of the loss of surface area of the HS cell is still an enigma. The defects thus far described are heterogeneous and involve deficiencies of spectrin, ankyrin, band 3, and pallidin, or very rarely, a dysfunctional band 3 or β spectrin. These proteins interact vertically to connect the membrane skeleton to the lipid bilayer. Table 9–3 summarizes these defects. A

TABLE 9–3 Defects of Red Cell Membrane Proteins in HS
Protein Deficiencies
Spectrin
Ankyrin
Spectrin and ankyrin
Band 3
Pallidin
Protein Dysfunction
β Spectrin–4.1 interaction
Band 3–pallidin interaction

more detailed discussion of the molecular pathogenesis of these abnormalities is given below.

Spectrin deficiency is a common underlying cause of HS. The number of spherocytes, the severity of the disease, and the response to splenectomy correlate closely with the degree of spectrin deficiency.[22] Autosomal recessive HS is usually associated with more severe spectrin loss and a poor response to splenectomy. The mutations causing spectrin deficiency have not yet been defined. Since α spectrin is synthesized in excess over β spectrin,[17] an α-spectrin mutation should only be manifested as spectrin deficiency in homozygotes. Heterozygotes, for example, asymptomatic carrier parents of recessively inherited HS, have normal amounts of membrane spectrin since there are still sufficient α chains to bind stoichiometrically to β spectrin. Since β spectrin is rate-limiting for heterodimer assembly during erythroid development,[17] a partial deficiency of β spectrin would be expected to manifest as a dominant trait with decreased membrane-bound spectrin. Functional β spectrin mutations, for example, $Sp_{Kissimmee}$, are rare and cause a decreased binding to protein 4.1 as well as mild spectrin deficiency.[23] A decreased spectrin content may also be a secondary phenomenon resulting from a primary defect in one of the proteins attaching β spectrin to the membrane, for example, ankyrin or band 3.

Ankyrin deficiency was first described in two cases of severe atypical HS[24] due to decreased mRNA production and synthesis of an unstable molecule.[25] The spectrin content of the membrane was also reduced to a similar extent (±50%) because of a lack of ankyrin binding sites. More recently, it has been shown that a primary ankyrin deficiency of varying degree is a common cause of dominant and recessively inherited HS.[26] Interstitial deletions of chromosome 8 involving the ankyrin gene (8p11.2),[27] as well as balanced translocations involving chromosome 8p11, have been reported in HS.[28] Several ankyrin mutations have been defined,[26] including a promoter point mutation; missense point mutations that alter the codon resulting in an amino acid substitution, for example $Ank_{Dusseldorf}$; or a nonsense mutation resulting in a stop codon, for example, $Ank_{Bovenden}$. Small deletions, such as $Ank_{Stuttgart}$, or insertions, such as $Ank_{Einbeck}$, change the reading frame of the gene, and such frameshift mutations create abnormal stop codons resulting in premature chain termination.[26] Ank_{Prague} is a lower-

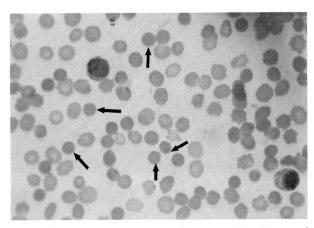

FIGURE 9–4 Photomicrograph of peripheral blood smear of patient with hereditary spherocytosis (HS). Note the microspherocytes [small condensed spherocytes with no central pallor (*arrows*)].

molecular-weight form of ankyrin, apparently resulting from abnormal splicing.[29] Interestingly, the ankyrin gene mutations have thus far been unique to each kindred.

A primary *band 3* deficiency has recently been associated with HS, especially in white subjects. The mutations thus far described include a 10-base-pair duplication, $Bd3_{Prague}$,[30] and a cluster of point mutations in several arginine codons in the C-terminal membrane domain.[31] The mutant band 3 is either not inserted into the membrane or is lost from the membrane as the cells mature in the circulation. Two HS patients have also been described with mutations in the cytoplasmic domain of band 3 that impair pallidin binding.[21]

Pallidin deficiency is rare in Europeans, but relatively common in the Japanese population, mainly because of a point mutation altering mRNA processing, $pallidin_{Nippon}$.[32] A single base deletion causing a frameshift, $pallidin_{Lisboa}$, has been documented in a non-Japanese subject.[33]

The primary membrane defects in HS, described above, involve postulated vertical interactions between the skeleton and the lipid bilayer.[34] The exact mechanism whereby these defects cause spherocyte formation is not known, but a postulated pathway of the pathophysiology of HS is summarized in Figure 9–5.[21,35] Spectrin- or band 3–deficient areas destabilize the membrane and allow the skeleton to be uncoupled from the lipid bilayer. This results in loss of portions of the bilayer in the form of microvesicles, which reduces the membrane surface area and decreases the surface-to-volume ratio. These cells are selectively trapped and "conditioned" in the spleen, where they progressively lose more surface area and are ultimately destroyed.

Clinical Manifestations

The classic presenting features of patients with HS are the triad of jaundice, anemia, and enlarged spleen, but many patients do not show all these signs. The age of presentation can vary from within a day or two after birth to old age, and sometimes HS may be diagnosed only during family studies or investigation for other reasons. About two thirds of HS patients present with a mild uncompensated hemolytic state manifesting with the aforementioned classic signs. Characteristically, the jaundice is said to be "acholuric," as unconjugated bilirubin cannot pass the glomerular filter. Many of these patients have pigment gallstones, presumably due to increased concentrations of bilirubin in the bile. About a quarter of HS patients have a mild hemolytic state that is compensated for, and such patients are not anemic and are usually asymptomatic. A minority of patients (about 10%) have a severe hemolytic anemia that may require blood transfusion. Aplastic crises, in which erythropoiesis is suppressed, leading to more pronounced anemia, occurs particularly in this group but may supervene in patients with milder forms of the disease. The usual cause of such crises is infection of erythropoietic precursors by parvovirus B19. An uncommon complication of prolonged hemolysis, which is not limited to HS, is chronic leg ulceration.

Clinical Laboratory Findings

Evidence of Hemolytic Process The laboratory features of extravascular hemolysis, outlined earlier, are usually apparent. Hyperbilirubinemia is found in about 50% of the patients, and haptoglobins are variably reduced. Classic features of intravascular hemolysis such as hemoglobinemia, hemoglobinuria, or hemosiderinuria do not occur. The reticulocyte production index is elevated above 2.5 in most cases (presplenectomy).

Red Cell Indices Anemia is usually mild. The mean level of hemoglobin in several series is about 12 to 13 g/dL, but individual cases may vary widely depending on the severity of hemolysis and the degree of compensation. The mean corpuscular volume (MCV) is usually within normal range both before and after splenectomy but can be low, normal, or high. The mean corpuscular hemoglobin (MCH) tends to parallel the MCV. Although the MCV is usually normal, because of the red cell's

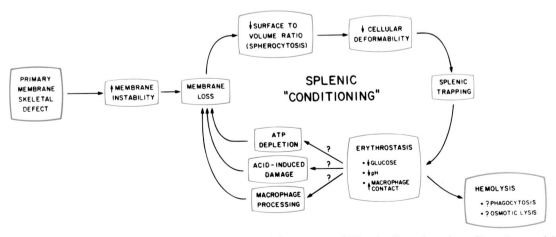

FIGURE 9–5 Postulated mechanisms of "conditioning" and destruction of HS red cells in the spleen. (From Lux and Glader,[2] with permission.)

spheroidal shape, the diameter of some cells is substantially decreased and these appear as dark, rounded microspherocytes on the peripheral smear. The mean corpuscular hemoglobin concentration (MCHC) is elevated (>36%) in about 50% of patients and probably reflects mild cellular dehydration, particularly of cells that have undergone splenic conditioning and that have low levels of cell water and potassium (see section in this chapter on etiology and pathophysiology).

Morphology of Peripheral Smear The morphological hallmark of HS is the spherocyte (see Fig. 9–4). Although in many instances the detection of these cells may present no difficulty, in some patients their detection may provoke argument even among experienced hematologists. It is particularly important to examine well-prepared smears free of any artifact. In typical cases, before splenectomy there may be varying degrees of polychromasia, poikilocytosis, and anisocytosis with many normal discoid cells, but the overriding impression is one of increased numbers of uniformly round cells (see Fig. 9–4). Some of the cells appear as microspherocytes, are dark and round, and lack central pallor. Pincered or mushoom-shaped cells are sometimes noted; these are often, but not exclusively, found in band 3–deficient subjects.

Special Laboratory Tests Osmotic Fragility Test (See Chap. 31.) This test is essentially a measure of the surface-to-volume ratio of the red cell. Red cells of patients with HS, because of their decreased surface area to volume ratio, have an increased osmotic fragility test. It is important to note that about 25% of HS patients have normal osmotic fragility of fresh red cells, particularly in the very group that is mildly affected and is difficult to diagnose on morphological grounds. Patients in the latter group, as well as patients with

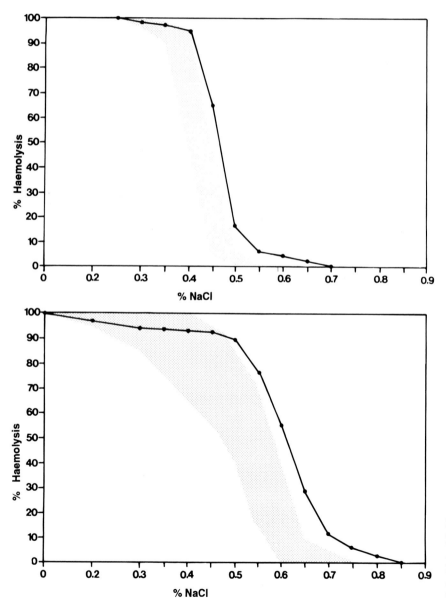

FIGURE 9–6 Osmotic fragility curves of fresh blood (*top*) and incubated blood (*bottom*) obtained from a patient with HS. The normal range is shown by dotted areas. Note the increased fragility of the HS red cells to osmotic lysis.

more typical cases, with very rare exceptions have abnormal osmotic fragility of red cells that have been stressed by prior sterile incubation for 24 hours. During the 24-hour incubation, because of relative membrane instability, HS cells have greater loss of membrane surface. A corollary of the use of the incubated osmotic fragility test is that if the test result is normal, it is highly unlikely that one is dealing with a patient with HS. Representative osmotic fragility curves for fresh and incubated normal and HS red cells are shown in Figure 9–6. It is important to note that increased osmotic fragility is independent of the cause of spheroidal cells (e.g., it may be found in autoimmune hemolytic anemia, burns, and so on) (see Chap. 31).

Autohemolysis Test This relatively sensitive test in the diagnosis of HS measures the structural and metabolic integrity of the HS red cell membrane under conditions of erythrostasis and relative lack of glucose, that is, sterile incubation of red cells in their own plasma for 48 hours at 37°C. The HS red cell leaks to sodium. To "keep its head above water," the cell utilizes ATP and glucose to drive the cation pump to a greater extent than normal. Associated with the increased activity of the pump, there is a greater turnover of membrane phospholipids and associated membrane fragmentation with a decrease in surface-to-volume ratio until the critical hemolytic volume is reached and autohemolysis occurs. The usual range of autohemolysis in HS cells is variable and is about 10% to 50%, compared with control values of 0.2% to 2.0%. However, a few patients show only minimally elevated autohemolysis or may even be within the normal range. In most HS patients, addition of glucose markedly diminishes autohemolysis but not usually to within the normal range of samples incubated with glucose (0% to 1.0%). A minority of patients show no correction of autohemolysis with glucose, a finding also obtained with many patients with spherocytosis associated with autoimmune hemolytic anemia. It should be noted that many laboratories do not use this test routinely (see Chap. 31 for the procedure).

Red Cell Membrane Studies The most common defect in HS involves a deficiency of one of the membrane proteins, and this may be documented by polyacrylamide gel electrophoresis of sodium dodecyl sulfate solubilized red cell membrane proteins (SDS PAGE).

Treatment From the foregoing discussion of the pathophysiology of the HS red cell and the central role of the spleen in "conditioning" such cells and ultimately leading to their destruction, it should not be surprising that splenectomy is functionally curative in most patients with this disease. In the relatively rare patients with severe spectrin deficiency (below 40% spectrin), clinical improvement occurs after splenectomy, but ongoing hemolysis and anemia may continue. In the usual case, although spherocytosis persists, "conditioned" microspherocytes are no longer seen and red cell life span is normal or very near normal. At one time, many authorities recommended splenectomy uniformly in all patients with HS because of the risks of biliary tract disease and the development of aplastic crises, but this view has been considerably tempered in recent years. Patients with mild, compensated cases of HS are usually not offered splenectomy

unless the previously mentioned complications intervene. An important consideration in infants and young children is the risk of postsplenectomy sepsis, particularly with *Streptococcus pneumoniae*, so that most authorities recommend deferment of splenectomy until about 6 years of age. In severe cases, however, splenectomy may have to be performed earlier; but in either event, treatment with pneumococcal vaccine is recommended, preferably starting before splenectomy. Younger children may also require prophylactic penicillin or other antibiotics after splenectomy, but the latter course is controversial. Failure of splenectomy is almost always associated with an accessory spleen not removed at surgery, or more rarely due to autotransplantation of splenic tissue in the peritoneal cavity, leading to splenosis.

CASE STUDY 1

A 40-year-old woman presented to her physician with an attack of acute cholecystitis. Physical examination revealed a palpable spleen in addition to the signs of acute cholecystitis. On investigation she was found to have numerous gallstones, and a routine blood count showed a mild, compensated hemolytic state: Hb, 13.8 g/dL; HCT, 38%; MCV, 80 fL; MCHC, 36%; reticulocyte count, 7%; shift cells present; RPI 3.9. The peripheral smear showed moderate numbers of spherocytes and a few microspherocytes. The Coombs test was negative. Unconjugated bilirubin was 2.5 mg/dL, and the conjugated bilirubin was 0.5 mg/dL. Haptoglobin concentration was less than 10 mg/dL (normal range: 25 to 180 mg/dL). Further investigation revealed that osmotic fragility of both fresh and incubated venous blood was increased. Autohemolysis was 25% after 48 hours' incubation, corrected to 3% in the presence of glucose. After the acute episode had settled, an elective cholecystectomy was performed. A diagnosis of hereditary spherocytosis was made and confirmed in a subsequent study of her family when two of her three children were found to have mild, compensated hemolytic states associated with spherocytosis. In view of the risk of recurrence of common bile duct calculi, an elective splenectomy was performed 6 months later, curing the hemolytic state.

Questions

1. Why was a Coombs test performed on this patient?
2. What type of hemolysis is occurring in this patient?
3. What is the surface-to-volume ratio of these red cells as indicated by the osmotic fragility test?
4. In what type of hemolytic anemia is the osmotic fragility uncorrected by glucose?
5. Which RBC indice is typically increased in HS?

Hereditary Elliptocytosis

Mode of Inheritance

Hereditary elliptocytosis (HE) is a group of disorders found in all ethnic groups, characterized by the presence of large numbers of elliptical red cells in the peripheral blood (Fig. 9–7). It has become clear over the past few years that this relatively common disorder is genetically, biochemically, and clinically heterogeneous. Most of the variants are inherited in an autosomal dominant fashion, including a morphologically and clinically distinct syndrome found in Southeast Asian and South African populations. Hereditary pyropoikilocytosis (HPP) is a recessively inherited, very severe form of HE.

Clinical Phenotypes

Three major clinical and morphological phenotypes have been delineated by Palek and Lux,[21,35] including common HE, spherocytic HE, and stomatocytic HE. *Common HE* is the most prevalent, especially in African populations. At least six clinical subtypes have been categorized. These range from an asymptomatic carrier state with normal red cell morphology to homozygous HE and HPP with severe hemolysis and bizarre poikilocytic and spherocytic morphology. Other common HE subtypes exhibit varying degrees of hemolysis, with the most frequently occurring clinical form of mild HE showing no or minimal hemolysis.

The second clinical category of HE is *spherocytic HE*, a relatively rare phenotypic hybrid of mild HE and HS, in which the clinical course resembles HS and responds well to splenectomy. Stomatocytic HE or *Southeast Asian ovalocytosis* (SAO) constitutes the third clinical phenotype. It is common in Melanesian and other Southeast Asian populations, in whom it has a selective protective effect against malaria. Recently it has also been described in a South African family.[36]

Common Hereditary Elliptocytosis

Etiology It is now well established that a defect in the red cell membrane skeleton exists in HE. A fundamental observation is that both red cell ghosts and membrane skeletons of HE subjects retain their elliptical shape and also show marked instability when subjected to mechanical stress. Several underlying molecular abnormalities involving skeletal protein deficiencies or defects have been defined, reflecting the

heterogeneity of this disorder (reviewed in Refs. 21 and 35). Table 9–4 summarizes these defects and a more detailed discussion of the underlying mutations is given below.

Spectrin mutations, specifically α-chain abnormalities that impair *spectrin dimer self-association,* are the most common. This functional defect is caused by a structural alteration that is detected by limited tryptic digestion of isolated spectrin. Most of these defects are located in the N-terminal αI domain of spectrin, and thus far nine cleavage defects have been defined, the most common being $\alpha^{I/74}$, $\alpha^{I/65}$, and $\alpha^{I/46}$.[37–42] Causative point mutations in the α-spectrin gene have been described in several kindred, resulting in an amino acid substitution close to the cleavage site.[43–46] This alters the conformation of the molecule, exposing new tryptic cleavage sites and decreasing the ability to form tetramers.

Abnormalities of *protein 4.1* have also been implicated in HE, especially in some North African and European populations. A partial or complete absence of protein 4.1 is the result of a deletion or point mutation inactivating the erythroid-specific translational start site in some kindred, for example, 4.1_{Madrid}.[47–49]

Hereditary Pyropoikilocytosis (HPP) This is an interesting, relatively rare, severe hemolytic disease now recognized as part of the HE group of disorders. The peripheral blood smear is characterized by microspherocytosis, micropoikilocytosis, fragments, and relatively few, if any, elliptocytes (Fig. 9–8). A hallmark of the condition is thermal instability of the red cells, which fragment at 45°C, in vitro, as opposed to 49°C for normal red cells.[50] HPP subjects are compound heterozygotes and all cases thus far investigated exhibit two genetic defects:

1. A mutant α or β spectrin that shows severe impairment of spectrin dimer self-association ($\text{Sp}\alpha^{I/74}$, $\text{Sp}\alpha^{I/46}$, and $\text{Sp}\alpha^{I/61}$).[51]
2. A partial spectrin deficiency, due either to an unstable elliptocytogenic mutant spectrin or to a decreased synthesis of α spectrin.[52] This presumably causes the characteristic microspherocytosis.

Pathophysiology of Common HE and HPP A hypothesis has been put forward by Palek[21,34] to explain the formation of elliptocytes, although the exact mechanism has not been proven. The different types of mo-

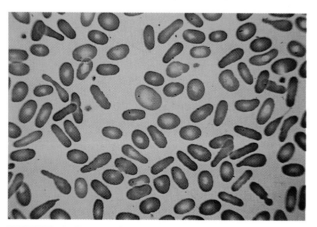

FIGURE 9–7 Hereditary elliptocytosis (HE, peripheral blood). Note the high percentage of elliptocytes or ovalocytes.

TABLE 9–4 **Defects of Red Cell Membrane Proteins in HE**
Protein Deficiencies
Protein 4.1
Glycophorin C
Spectrin (HPP)
Protein Dysfunction
Spectrin dimer self-association
α-Spectrin mutations
β-Spectrin mutations
Truncated α or β spectrin
Spectrin-ankyrin interaction
Protein 4.1–spectrin interaction
Band 3 (SAO)

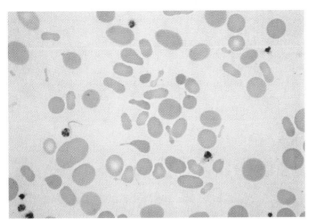

FIGURE 9-8 Hereditary pyropoikilocytosis (HPP, peripheral blood). Note the bizarre micropoikilocytosis, red cell budding, microspherocytes, and elliptocytes.

lecular defects in common HE usually involve horizontal interactions between proteins of the membrane skeleton (Fig. 9–9). Defective spectrin dimer self-association or protein 4.1 abnormalities weaken the skeleton and, under the influence of shear stress in the circulation, the cells become distorted and progressively lose their ability to regain their original disc shape, resulting in elliptocytes and poikilocytes.

In the case of HPP, the clinical severity and morphology are thought to be the result of a combination of horizontal and vertical defects. Spectrin self-association (horizontal defect) is severely impaired in HPP, which markedly decreases the strength and stability of the skeleton, resulting in poikilocytes and cell fragmentation. Spectrin deficiency impairs the vertical interaction of the skeleton with the lipid bilayer and results in microspherocytes as described for HS (see Fig. 9–9).

Southeast Asian Ovalocytosis

SAO, or stomatocytic HE, is very common in ethnic Southeast Asian populations. It is an asymptomatic condition characterized by rigid red cells with a unique spoon-shaped ovalocytic morphology that are resistant to invasion by malaria parasites.[53] The underlying molecular defect[54-56] involves band 3. The mutant band 3 is functionally abnormal and exhibits, for example, increased binding to ankyrin,[54] an inability to transport anions,[57] and markedly restricted lateral and rotational mobility in the membrane.[58] The pathophysiologic mechanism causing membrane rigidity and malaria resistance is not known. One speculative possibility is that conformational changes in the cytoplasmic domain of band 3 inhibit the mobility of the protein and may also enhance ankyrin binding and strengthen the membrane bilayer–skeleton interaction. This results in a rigid membrane that prevents parasite attachment and entry.

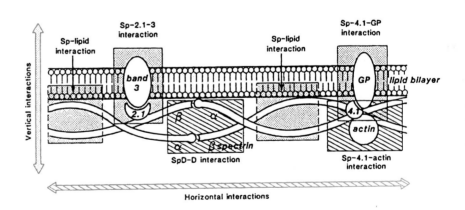

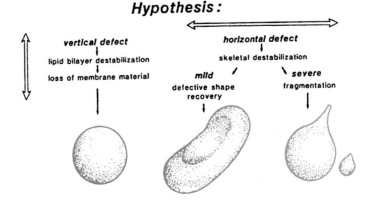

FIGURE 9-9 Pathophysiology of the red cell lesion in HS, HE, and HPP. The top section is a diagrammatic illustration of the vertical and horizontal interactions between the red cell membrane components. The bottom left-hand section illustrates a defect in a vertical interaction resulting in spherocytes and HS. The bottom right-hand section illustrates a defect in a horizontal interaction resulting in elliptocytes and poikilocytes (HE and HPP). (From Palek,[61] with permission.)

Clinical Laboratory Findings

Evidence of Hemolytic Process The usual picture in the most common variant (mild HE) is that of a very mild, compensated hemolytic anemia in which the only features may be a slight reticulocytosis and decreased haptoglobin levels. Many patients show no biochemical evidence of a hemolytic process. In the more severe cases, such as in spherocytic HE or in HE with infantile poikilocytosis, the usual features of extravascular hemolysis outlined earlier are found.

Morphology of Peripheral Smear The morphology of the peripheral smear obviously varies with the clinical phenotypes of HE. In the usual variant of mild HE with no hemolysis or a compensated hemolytic state, the red cells show prominent uniform elliptocytosis, the cells being elliptic rather than oval or egg-shaped (see Fig. 9–7). Usually more than 30% of the red cells are elliptocytic, but many patients have a higher proportion of elliptocytes, for example, more than 75%. Very elongated or rod-shaped cells are characteristic and often constitute more than 10% of the red cells. In patients with uncompensated hemolysis (mild HE with sporadic hemolysis), the red cells show more prominent poikilocytosis and a small proportion of elliptocytes may have budlike projections. The rare patients with homozygous HE or HPP (see Fig. 9–8) present with an even greater degree of poikilocytosis, as does the infant with mild HE and poikilocytosis of infancy. In such infants, there is prominent poikilocytosis, microspherocytosis, fragmentation, budding of red cells, and a variable degree of elliptocytosis (Fig. 9–10). By the time the infant reaches the age of 1 to 2 years, the morphology has changed to that characteristic of mild HE. In the neonatal period, the red cells show increased thermal sensitivity (which is also a characteristic of HPP), but the diagnosis is suggested by finding evidence of mild HE in one parent.

Red cell morphology in spherocytic HE is very variable, but the hallmarks are less prominent elliptocytosis with spherocytes and microspherocytes. The proportion of spherocytes and elliptocytes varies in different kindreds and even within the same kindred. Patients with stomatocytic HE or SAO have a characteristic red cell morphology. The elliptocytes are more rounded and have one or two transverse bars giving them the appearance of double stomatocytes.

Red Cell Indices

In the common variants of mild HE with compensated and uncompensated hemolysis, the MCV is usually normal or slightly elevated, the latter finding probably reflecting an associated reticulocytosis. MCH and MCHC are also usually within the normal range. In infants with HE and poikilocytosis, the MCV may be decreased and the MCHC is either normal or slightly elevated. In HPP, the MCV is always decreased and the MCHC is usually elevated.

Special Laboratory Tests

Osmotic Fragility and Autohemolysis The osmotic fragility and autohemolysis tests are useful additional tests in delineating some of the HE phenotypes. In patients with mild HE (compensated and uncompensated), both the preincubation and the postincubation osmotic fragility and autohemolysis results are normal. Rarely, patients with mild HE and uncompensated hemolysis may have increased autohemolysis corrected by glucose. However, in HPP preincubation and postincubation osmotic fragility is markedly increased and autohemolysis is increased and unaffected by glucose. Preincubation and postincubation osmotic fragility is uniformly increased in spherocytic HE and autohemolysis is characteristically increased but corrected by glucose. Children with HE and infantile poikilocytosis have increased osmotic fragility and

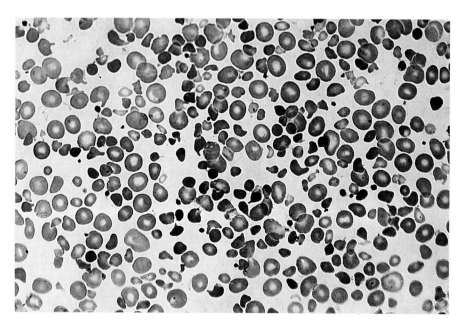

FIGURE 9–10 Photomicrograph of peripheral blood smear of a patient with mild HE and poikilocytosis of infancy. Note the bizarre poikilocytosis and fragmentation.

autohemolysis in the early neonatal period that revert to normal with the development of more prominent elliptocytosis.

Red Cell Membrane Studies   Red cell membrane protein deficiencies or size abnormalities may be detected by SDS PAGE and subsequent quantitation as described for HS.

Treatment

Patients with mild HE (compensated) have a benign disorder with no splenomegaly and require no therapeutic intervention. Those with HE and uncompensated hemolysis usually benefit from splenectomy, which is also uniformly beneficial to patients with spherocytic HE. Patients with HE and infantile poikilocytosis should be recognized and treated symptomatically, as they will improve spontaneously with the development of a picture indistinguishable from mild HE.

CASE STUDY 2

A 45-year-old woman presented to her physician complaining of malaise and tiredness on mild exertion. On physical examination, she was found to have slight scleral icterus and a two-finger splenomegaly. A blood count revealed the following: Hb, 11.0 g/dL; Hct, 32%; MCHC, 34.3%; MCV, 100 fL; reticulocyte count, 12.0%; shift cells on peripheral smear; and RPI, 5.7. The peripheral smear showed about 80% elliptocytes with some poikilocytosis consisting of a few fragmented cells and budding elliptocytes. Unconjugated bilirubin was 3.5 mg/dL, conjugated bilirubin 0.6 mg/dL, and haptoglobin 15 mg/dL (normal range 25 to 180 mg/dL). Preincubation and postincubation osmotic fragility and autohemolysis were within the normal range. Examination of her family showed striking elliptocytes with normal hemoglobin and reticulocyte count in her father and in one of her three children. A diagnosis of mild HE with sporadic hemolysis was made, and a good response to splenectomy was obtained.

Questions

1. How can the anemia presented here be classified?
2. What parameter(s) is/are suggestive of effective erythropoiesis?
3. Do the laboratory values presented here indicate hemolysis in this patient?
4. What is the significance of the RPI value?

DISORDERS OF MEMBRANE CATION PERMEABILITY

Hereditary Stomatocytosis (Hydrocytosis) and Hereditary Xerocytosis

This is a heterogeneous group of rare disorders characterized by alterations in the permeability of the red cell membrane to cations (reviewed in Ref. 59). Two main clinical and morphological syndromes have been

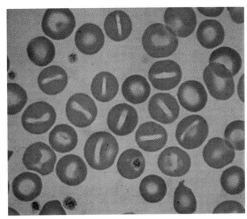

FIGURE 9–11 Hereditary stomatocytosis (peripheral blood). Note the high percentage of red cells with a central slit of pallor. (From Bell, A: Hematology. In Listen, Look and Learn. Health and Education Resources, Inc., Bethesda, MD, with permission.)

described and consist on one hand of hereditary stomatocytosis (hydrocytosis), in which the red cells are swollen (Fig. 9–11), and on the other hand of hereditary xerocytosis, in which the red cells are markedly dehydrated (see Fig. 9–12). A number of intermediate syndromes have been described, but these will not be considered here.

Modes of Inheritance

Most reported cases of hereditary stomatocytosis are inherited in autosomal dominant fashion, but some patients who have a more severe degree of hemolysis show autosomal recessive inheritance. Hereditary xerocytosis is inherited by autosomal dominant transmission.

Etiology and Pathophysiology

An important determinant of the water content of red cells is their total content of sodium and potassium. To maintain osmotic equilibrium water enters cells in which the total cation content is increased leading to swelling and hydrocyte formation. In contrast, a net

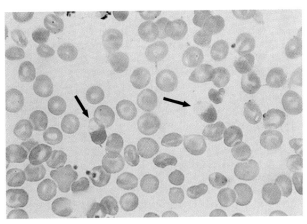

FIGURE 9–12 Hereditary xerocytosis (peripheral blood).

loss of cations results in a movement of water out of the cell with formation of dehydrated cells or xerocytes.

The basic abnormality of stomatocytic red cells is a marked increase in the passive permeability of sodium into the cell and of potassium out of the cell. The defect in sodium permeability is greater than that for potassium. Although the sodium-potassium pump is stimulated by the influx of sodium, it cannot cope with the influx, and the total cation content of the cell increases with resultant water influx and formation of hydrocytes. Recently a deficiency of one component of band 7 (protein 7.2, stomatin, see Table 9–2) has been reported in red cell membranes of a few such patients, although the DNA sequence is normal[60] How this relates to the permeability lesion is unknown. Because of the influx of water, stomatocytes have an increased volume with a decreased surface-to-volume ratio and the attendant consequences of decreased red cell deformability and susceptibility to splenic sequestration. Although splenectomy is predictably beneficial in most patients with hereditary stomatocytosis, paradoxically some patients with severe permeability defects do not have significant hemolysis, suggesting that other, still unknown factors may be important in the destruction of these cells.

Stomatocytes are also found in Rh null disease, a hemolytic anemia characterized by an absence of the Rh antigens. This disorder is clinically and biochemically heterogeneous, and the molecular pathophysiology is not completely understood.

Red cells from patients with hereditary xerocytosis have an increased efflux of potassium that is greater than the sodium influx. Although the influx of sodium leads to stimulation of the sodium-potassium pump, it is insufficient to correct the loss of potassium. Irreversible potassium and total cation loss occurs with resultant dehydration and formation of xerocytes that have an increased surface-to-volume ratio. These dehydrated cells, however, have an increased MCHC and presumably increased cell viscosity, which makes them less deformable and liable to sequestration in the reticuloendothelial system. The red cells are not specifically sequestrated in the spleen, so that splenectomy does not have a beneficial effect.

Clinical Laboratory Findings

Morphology of Peripheral Smear The characteristic morphological features of hereditary stomatocytosis are a tendency toward macrocytosis and the presence of increased numbers of stomatocytes on the peripheral smear. These are red cells with a central slit or stoma (see Fig. 9–11). On phase contrast or scanning electron microscopy, the cells have a bowllike appearance. In hereditary xerocytosis, there is an increase in the number of target cells reflecting the greater surface-to-volume ratio of these cells. Small spiculated red cells and cells with hemoglobin concentrated in one part of the cell are also features of hereditary xeroxytosis (see Fig. 9–12).

Red Cell Indices The MCV in both hereditary stomatocytosis and hereditary xerocytosis is elevated, despite the cellular dehydration in the latter condition. The MCHC is decreased in hereditary stomatocytosis and increased in hereditary xerocytosis.

Special Laboratory Tests Osmotic fragility is increased in hereditary stomatocytosis and reflects the decreased surface-to-volume ratio. Red cell sodium concentration is elevated and potassium concentration is decreased. Total monovalent cation content is increased. In contrast, red cells in hereditary xerocytosis have strikingly decreased osmotic fragility, reflecting the increased surface-to-volume ratio. Red cell potassium concentration is markedly decreased, sodium concentration may be normal or slightly increased, and total cation concentration is decreased.

Treatment

Most patients with hemolysis caused by hereditary stomatocytosis show a good response to splenectomy. However, patients with hereditary xerocytosis, as stated earlier, do not benefit from splenectomy, presumably because of more generalized sequestration of these cells.

CASE STUDY 3

A 6-year-old boy was noted by his mother to have slight scleral icterus and was referred for further investigation. He complained of some tiredness on exertion but was otherwise symptoms-free. Physical examination showed only a one-finger splenomegaly. A blood count showed the following: Hb, 10.8 g/dL; Hct, 29%; MCHC, 37%; MCV, 100 fL; reticulocyte count, 10%. Numerous target cells, some spiculated cells, and a few cells showing eccentric concentration of hemoglobin at one pole of the red cell were seen on the peripheral smear. The unconjugated bilirubin level was mildly elevated, and serum haptoglobin levels were decreased. There was no hemoglobinemia or hemosiderinuria. The osmotic fragility curve was strikingly decreased. Determination of red cell cation concentrations revealed a markedly decreased red cell potassium level of 65 mEq/L of RBCs (normal 90 to 104 mEq/L of RBCs) and a slightly elevated red cell sodium level of 15 mEq/L of RBCs (normal 5 to 12 mEq/L of RBCs). Similar findings were obtained in the child's father, who had previously been diagnosed at another center as having an "unusual" form of anemia. A diagnosis of hereditary xerocytosis was made. Splenectomy was not advised, and the child has remained with a hemoglobin level varying between 9.5 and 11.0 g/dL over the past 2 years.

Questions

1. How can this anemia be classified as indicated by the RBC indices?
2. What does the decreased osmotic fragility represent?
3. Why would a splenectomy not be beneficial in this case?
4. Why are these red cells (xerocytes) said to be dehydrated with regard to osmotic equilibrium?

REFERENCES

1. Hillman, RS and Finch, CA: Red Cell Manual, ed 7. FA Davis, Philadelphia, 1996.

2. Lux, SE and Glader, BE: Disorders of the red cell membrane. In Nathan, DG and Oski, FA (eds): Hematology of Infancy and Childhood, ed 2. WB Saunders, Philadelphia, 1981, p 456.
3. Liu, SC and Derick, LH: Molecular anatomy of the red blood cell membrane skeleton: Structure—function relationships. Semin Hematol 29:231, 1992.
4. Liu, SC, Derick, LH, and Palek, J: Visualization of the hexagonal lattice in the erythrocyte membrane skeleton. J Cell Biol 104:527, 1987.
5. Gilligan, DM and Bennett V: The junctional complex of the membrane skeleton. Semin Hematol 30:74, 1993.
6. Bennett, V and Stenbuck, PJ: The membrane attachment protein for spectrin is associated with band 3 in human erythrocyte membranes. Nature 280:468, 1979.
7. Cohen, CM, Dotimas, E, and Korsgren, C: Human erythrocyte membrane protein 4.2 (Pallidin). Semin Hematol 30:119, 1993.
8. Pasternack, GR, Anderson, RA, Leto, TL, and Marchesi VT: Interactions between protein 4.1 and band 3: An alternative binding site for an element of the membrane skeleton. J Biol Chem 260:3676, 1985.
9. Marfatia, SM, Lue, RA, Branton, D, and Chisti, AH: In vitro binding studies suggest a membrane-associated complex between erythroid p55, protein 4.1, and glycophorin C. J Biol Chem 269:8631, 1994.
10. Gallagher, PG and Forget, BG: Spectrin genes in health and disease. Semin Hematol 30:4, 1993.
11. Sahr, KE, Laurila, P, Kotula, L, et al: The complete cDNA and polypeptide sequences of human erythroid α spectrin. J Biol Chem 265:4434, 1990.
12. Winkelmann, JC, Chang, JG, Tse, WT, et al: Full length sequence of the cDNA for human erythroid β spectrin. J Biol Chem 265:11827, 1990.
13. Speicher, DW and Marchesi, VT: Erythrocyte spectrin is comprised of many homologous triple helical segments. Nature 311:177, 1984.
14. Yan, Y, Winograd, E, Viel, A, et al: Crystal structure of the repetitive segments of spectrin. Science 262:2027, 1993.
15. Speicher, DW, Morrow, JS, Knowles, WJ, and Marchesi, VT: A structural model of human spectrin: Alignment of chemical and functional domains. J Biol Chem 257:9093, 1982.
16. Speicher, DW, De Silva, TM, Speicher, KD, et al: Location of the human red cell spectrin tetramer binding site and detection of a related "closed" hairpin loop dimer using proteolytic footprinting. J Biol Chem 268:4227, 1993.
17. Hanspal, M and Palek, J: Biogenesis of normal and abnormal red blood cell membrane skeleton. Semin Hematol 29:305, 1992.
18. Woods, CM and Lazarides, E: Degradation of unassembled alpha and beta spectrin by distinct intracellular pathways: regulation of spectrin topogenesis by beta spectrin degradation. Cell 40:959, 1985.
19. Tanner, MJA: Molecular and cellular biology of the erythrocyte anion exchanger (AE1). Semin Hematol 30:34, 1993.
20. Peters, LL and Lux, SE: Ankyrins: Structure and function in normal cells and hereditary spherocytes. Semin Hematol 30:85, 1993.
21. Palek, J and Jarolim, P: Clinical expression and laboratory detection of red blood cell membrane mutations. Semin Hematol 30:249, 1993.
22. Agre, P, Asimos, A, Casella, JF, and McMillan, D: Inheritance pattern and clinical response to splenectomy as a reflection of erythrocyte spectrin deficiency in hereditary spherocytosis. N Engl J Med 315:1579, 1986.
23. Becker, PS, Tse, WT, Lux, SE, and Forget, B: β Spectrin Kissimmee: A spectrin variant associated with autosomal dominant hereditary spherocytosis and defective binding to protein 4.1. J Clin Invest 92:612, 1993.
24. Coetzer, TL, Lawler, J, Liu, SC, et al: Partial ankyrin and spectrin deficiency in severe atypical hereditary spherocytosis. N Engl J Med 318:230, 1988.
25. Hanspal, M, Yoon, SH, Yu, H, et al: Molecular basis of spectrin and ankyrin deficiencies in severe hereditary spherocytosis: Evidence implicating a primary defect of ankyrin. Blood 77:165, 1991.
26. Eber, SW, Lux, SE, Gonzalez, JM, et al: Discovery of 8 ankyrin mutations in hereditary spherocytosis (HS) indicate that ankyrin defects are a major cause of dominant and recessive HS. Blood 82 (Suppl 1):308a, 1993.
27. Lux, SE, Tse, WT, Menninger, JC, et al: Hereditary spherocytosis associated with deletion of the human ankyrin gene on chromosome 8. Nature 345:736, 1990.
28. Bass, EB, Smith, SW Jr, Stevenson, RE, and Rosse, WF: Further evidence for localization of the spherocytosis gene on chromosome 8. Ann Intern Med 99:192, 1983.
29. Jarolim, P, Rubin, HL, Brabec, V, et al: Abnormal alternative splicing of erythroid ankyrin mRNA in two kindred with hereditary spherocytosis (ankyrin Prague and ankyrin Rakovnik). Blood 82(suppl 1):5a, 1993.
30. Jarolim, P, Rubin, HL, Liu, SC, et al: Duplication of 10 nucleotides in the erythroid band 3 (AE1) gene in a kindred with hereditary spherocytosis and band 3 protein deficiency (Band 3 Prague). J Clin Invest 93:121, 1994.
31. Jarolim, P, Rubin, HL, Brabec, V, et al: Mutations of conserved arginines in the membrane domain of erythroid band 3 lead to a decrease in membrane-associated band 3 and to the phenotype of hereditary spherocytosis. Blood 85:634, 1995.
32. Bouhassira, EE, Schwartz, RS, Yawata, Y, et al: An alanine to threonine substitution in protein 4.2 cDNA associated with a Japanese form of hereditary hemolytic anemia (protein 4.2 Nippon). Blood 79:1846, 1992.
33. Hayette, S, Dhermy, D, dos Santos, ME, et al: A deletional frameshift mutation in protein 4.2 gene (allele 4.2 Lisboa) associated with hereditary hemolytic anemia. Blood 85:250, 1995.
34. Palek, J: Disorders of red cell membrane skeleton: An overview. In Kruckeberg, WL, Eaton, JW, Brewer, GJ, et al.: Erythrocyte Membranes 3: Recent Clinical and Experimental Advances. New York, Liss, 1984, p 177.
35. Becker, PS and Lux, SE: Disorders of the red cell membrane. In Nathan, DG and Oski, FA (eds): Hematology of Infancy and Childhood, ed 4. WB Saunders, Philadelphia, 1993, p 529.
36. Coetzer, TL, Beeton, L, van Zyl, D, et al: Southeast Asian ovalocytosis (SAO) in a South African kindred with hemolysis is not linked to the band 3 Memphis polymorphism. Blood 84(suppl 1):543a, 1994.
37. Coetzer, TL, Sahr, K, Prchal, J, et al: Four different mutations in codon 28 of α spectrin are associated with structurally and functionally abnormal spectrin α$^{I/74}$ in hereditary elliptocytosis. J Clin Invest 88:743, 1991.
38. Sahr, KE, Coetzer, TL, Moy, LS, et al: Spectrin Cagliari: An ala → gly substitution in helix 1 of β spectrin repeat 17 that severely disrupts the structure and self-association of the erythrocyte spectrin heterodimer. J Biol Chem 268:22656, 1993.
39. Tse, WT, Lecomte, M-C, Costa, FF, et al: Point mutation in the β-spectrin gene associated with α$^{I/74}$ hereditary elliptocytosis. Implications for the mechanism of spectrin dimer self-association. J Clin Invet 86:909, 1990.
40. Gallagher, PG, Tse, WT, Coetzer, T, et al: A common type of the spectrin αI 46-50a-kD peptide abnormality in hereditary elliptocytosis and pyropoikilocytosis is associated with a mutation distant from the proteolytic cleavage site. Evidence for the functional importance of the triple helical model of spectrin. J Clin Invest 89:892, 1992.
41. Hassoun, H, Coetzer, TL, Vassiliadis, JN, et al: A novel mobile element inserted in the α spectrin gene: Spectrin

Dayton. A truncated α spectrin associated with hereditary elliptocytosis. J Clin Invest 94:643, 1994.

42. Sahr, KE, Tobe, T, Scarpa, A, et al: Sequence and exon-intron organization of the DNA encoding the αI domain of human spectrin. Application to the study of mutations causing hereditary elliptocytosis. J Clin Invest 84:1243, 1989.

43. Yoon, S-H, Yu, H, Eber, S and Prchal, JT: Molecular defect of truncated β-spectrin associated with hereditary elliptocytosis. β Spectrin Gottingen. J Biol Chem 266:8490, 1991.

44. Kanazaki, A, Rabodonirina, M, Yawata, Y, et al. A deletion frameshift mutation of the β spectrin gene associated with elliptocytosis in spectrin Tokyo ($\beta^{220/216}$). Blood 80:2115, 1992.

45. Tse, WT, Gallagher, PG, Pothier, B, et al. An insertional frameshift mutation of the β-spectrin gene associated with elliptocytosis in spectrin Nice ($\beta^{220/216}$). Blood 78:517, 1991.

46. Zail, SS and Coetzer, TL: Defective binding of spectrin to ankyrin in a kindred with recessively inherited hereditary elliptocytosis. J Clin Invest 74:753, 1984.

47. Dalla Venezia, N, Gilsanz, F, Alloisio, N, et al: Homozygous 4.1 (−) hereditary elliptocytosis associated with a point mutation in the downstream initiation codon of protein 4.1 gene. J Clin Invest 90:1713, 1992.

48. Conboy, JG: Structure, function, and molecular genetics of erythroid membrane skeletal protein 4.1 in normal and abnormal red blood cells. Semin Hematol 30:58, 1993.

49. Cartron, J-P, Le Van Kim, C, and Colin, Y: Glycophorin C and related glycoproteins: structure, function and regulation. Semin Hematol 30:152, 1993.

50. Zarkowsky, HS, Mohandas, N, Speaker, C, and Shohet, SB. A congenital haemolytic anaemia with thermal sensitivity of the erythrocyte membrane. Br J Haematol 29:537, 1975.

51. Coetzer, TL, Lawler, J, Prchal, JT, and Palek, J: Molecular determinants of clinical expression of hereditary elliptocytosis and pyropoikilocytosis. Blood 70:766, 1987.

52. Coetzer, TL and Palek, J: Partial spectrin deficiency in hereditary pyropoikilocytosis. Blood 67:919, 1986.

53. Mohandas, N, Lie-Injo, LE, Friedman, M, and Mak, JW: Rigid membranes of Malayan ovalocytes: A likely genetic barrier against malaria. Blood 63:1385, 1984.

54. Liu, S-C, Zhai, S, Palek, J, et al: Molecular defect of the band 3 protein in Southeast Asian ovalocytosis. N Engl J Med 323:1530, 1990.

55. Tanner, MJA, Bruce, L, Martin, PG, et al: Melanesian hereditary ovalocytes have a deletion in red cell band 3. Blood 78:2785, 1991.

56. Jarolim, P, Palek, J, Amato, D, et al: Deletion in erythrocyte band 3 gene in malaria-resistant Southeast Asian ovalocytosis. Proc Natl Acad Sci USA 88:11022, 1991.

57. Schofield, AE, Reardon, DM and Tanner, MJA: Defective anion transport activity of the abnormal band 3 in hereditary ovalocytic red blood cells. Nature 355:836, 1992.

58. Mohandas, N, Winardi, R, Knowles, D, et al: Molecular basis for membrane rigidity of hereditary ovalocytosis. A novel mechanism involving the cytoplasmic domain of band 3. J Clin Invest 89:686, 1992.

59. Palek, J: Acanthocytosis, stomatocytosis and related disorders. In Williams, WJ, Beutler, E, Erslev, AJ, and Lichtman, MA (eds): Hematology, ed 4. McGraw-Hill, New York, 1990, p 582.

60. Lande, WM, Thiemann, PVW, and Mentzer, WC, Jr: Missing band 7 membrane protein in two patients with high Na, Low K erythrocytes. J Clin Invest 70:1273, 1982.

61. Palek, J: Hereditary elliptocytosis and related disorders. In Williams, WJ, Beutler, E, Erslev, AJ, and Lichtman, MA (eds): Hematology, ed 4. McGraw-Hill, New York, 1990, p 569.

QUESTIONS

1. What happens when normal donor red cells are transfused into a patient with an intracorpuscular red cell defect?
   a. Donor cells are destroyed
   b. Donor cells have normal survival
   c. Depends on the severity of the defect
   d. Depends on the severity of the anemia

2. Which of the following tests is not used to determine increased red cell destruction?
   a. Unconjugated (indirect) bilirubin
   b. Serum haptoglobin
   c. Shumm's test
   d. Reticulocyte count

3. An anemic patient investigated for a hemolytic state has the following laboratory findings: hemoglobin, 8 g/dL, hematocrit, 23%; reticulocyte count, 8%; shift cells on peripheral smear. What is the reticulocyte production index (RPI)?
   a. 8
   b. 4
   c. 2
   d. 1

4. What tests are useful in the classification of the cause of red cell hemolysis?
   a. Direct Coombs' test
   b. Indirect Coombs' test and hemoglobin level
   c. Reticulocyte count and hemoglobin electrophoresis
   d. Red cell enzyme studies and iron-binding capacity

5. Which of the following red cell membrane protein deficiencies do not cause hereditary spherocytosis?
   a. Ankyrin
   b. Protein 4.1
   c. Spectrin
   d. Pallidin
   e. Band 3

6. Which of the following laboratory tests would not be typical of hereditary spherocytosis?
   a. Increased osmotic fragility
   b. Spherocytes on peripheral smear
   c. Decreased MCHC
   d. Increased RPI

7. Which is the most frequent functional abnormality affecting membrane skeleton proteins in common hereditary elliptocytosis?
   a. Defective binding of spectrin to ankyrin
   b. Defective spectrin tetramer assembly
   c. Defective binding of ankyrin to protein 3
   d. Deficiency of protein 4.1

8. Which of the following abnormalities are thought to cause the severe fragmentation and microspherocytosis characteristic of hereditary pyropoikilocytosis?
   a. Subsceptibility of spectrin to thermal denaturation
   b. Defective membrane spectrin tetramer assembly and spectrin deficiency
   c. Unstable membrane lipids
   d. Membrane ankyrin deficiency

9. Which disorders are classified as disorders of membrane cation permeability?
   a. Hereditary stomatocytosis and hereditary xerocytosis
   b. Sideroblastic anemia and myelofibrosis

c. Autoimmune hemolytic anemia and microangiopathic hemolytic anemia

d. Ehlers-Danlos syndrome and Bernard-Soulier syndrome

ANSWERS

1. **b** (p 147)
2. **d** (p 147)

3. **c** (p 148)
4. **a** (p 149)
5. **b** (p 152 [Table 9–3])
6. **c** (pp 154–155)
7. **b** (p 156)
8. **b** (p 157)
9. **a** (p 159)

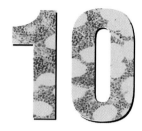

Introduction to Hemolytic Anemias: Intracorpuscular Defects

II—HEREDITARY ENZYME DEFICIENCIES

Sue J. Sim, MD

Sara McCarron, MD

Armand B. Glassman, MD

Objectives

At the end of this chapter, the learner should be able to:

1   Name the most common glycolytic enzyme deficiency associated with the hexose monophosphate shunt or pentose phosphate pathway.
2   Name the most common glycolytic enzyme deficiency associated with Embden-Meyerhof pathway.
3   Identify the particles associated with oxidative denaturation of hemoglobin.
4   List laboratory test results that would suggest a deficiency of G6PD.
5   Identify a laboratory test result that would indicate a PK deficiency.
6   Name the deficiency that causes hemoglobin to be oxidized from the ferrous to the ferric state.

HISTORY

In 1926, 72 plantation workers in Panama suffered acute hemolysis after receiving the antimalarial drug 8-aminoquinoline. Subsequent reports from widely scattered geographic locations added credence to the relationship of hemolysis, cyanosis, and methemoglobinemia to the ingestion of certain antimalarial drugs. In 1953 Dacie and his associates[1] evaluated apparently heterogeneous cases of congenital hemolytic anemias that had several common characteristics. There was no detectable abnormal hemoglobin, the antiglobulin test result was negative, and the osmotic fragility was normal. The term *hereditary nonspherocytic hemolytic anemia* (HNSHA) was used to describe the group, which was later found to be associated with red cell enzyme abnormalities. Biochemical and molecular studies rapidly advanced the further characterization of these anemias.

The most common anemia in this group is caused by deficiency of glucose-6-phosphate dehydrogenase (G6PD), an enzyme in the hexose monophosphate pathway. The second most frequent enzyme deficiency is that of pyruvate kinase (PK), an essential enzyme in the Embden-Meyerhof pathway. Many other enzyme deficiencies have also been identified. Laboratory testing is directed toward identification of the specific en-

This work was supported in part by the Olla S. Stribling Chair for Cancer Research.

zyme deficiency. Treatment is generally supportive, although experimental gene therapy may have a future role.

SPECIFIC ENZYMOPATHIES

Glucose-6-Phosphate Dehydrogenase Deficiency

G6PD deficiency, one of the most common genetic abnormalities known, is thought to affect over 400 million people worldwide. Carson and associates[2] identified the enzyme G6PD deficiency in 1956 in an individual who developed hemolytic anemia following the administration of the antimalarial drug primaquine (8-aminoquinoline). Yoshida[3] first purified the enzyme from human red cells in 1966. Further progress characterized the diverse variants of G6PD by sequencing of amino acids, cloning of cDNA, and sequencing of nucleotides.

More than 400 variants of G6PD enzyme have been described on the basis of biochemical and genetic analyses.[4-6] Recent advances in molecular biology have enabled classification of the variants into approximately 50 gene mutation groups.[6,7] Nearly all of these variants are the result of point mutations[8] that produce structurally abnormal and/or functionally defective enzymes.

Mode of Inheritance G6PD deficiency is transmitted by a mutant gene located on the X chromosome.[9] The gene encoding G6PD has been mapped specifically on Xq28 in humans.[10] The disorder is fully expressed in men (hemizygous) who inherit the mutant gene from their mothers, who are carriers. In women, full expression of the disorder occurs when two mutant genes (homozygous) are inherited. The heterozygous woman has a mosaic of one red blood cell population with normal enzyme activity and another with deficient enzyme activity.[11] The expression of G6PD deficiency varies markedly among heterozygotes, which is explained in part by the X-inactivation hypothesis.[12] In females, one of the two X chromosomes (maternally or paternally derived) becomes randomly inactivated in each cell of the early embryo. Thus, each somatic cell in a heterozygote expresses either one or the other Gd allele. The ratio of the two cell types may vary widely, not only in different individuals but also among different tissues, even within the same individual.[13]

Distribution of the mutant gene for G6PD deficiency is worldwide; however, the highest incidence occurs in the darkly pigmented racial and ethnic groups. In fact, most of the studies of G6PD variants have been done on samples from African Americans, people of Mediterranean ancestry, and Asians. Normally active G6PD, type Gd B, is the most common form of the enzyme in all populations and exists in 99% of whites in the United States. Another variety of the G6PD enzyme, Gd A+, is commonly found in Africans, has normal activity, but differs from Gd B by a single amino acid substitution that alters its electrophoretic mobility.[14] The Gd A+ variant is found in about 20% of African men.[15,16] Among African Americans who possess the Gd A+ gene, there is a reduced activity variety designated Gd A−, which can be demonstrated in 10% to 15% of the men. Approximately 20% of African-American women are heterozygous for the Gd A− gene. Gd A− is the prototype of the mild form of G6PD deficiency.

Among whites, G6PD Mediterranean (G6PD Med) is the most common variant, although the overall prevalence is low. Among Kurdish Jews, however, the incidence of G6PD Med may be as high as 50% to 60%. G6PD Med (also known as G6PD B−) is the prototype of a more severe enzyme deficiency associated with acute hemolytic anemia, including favism. The variant Gd Canton is more commonly found in native people of Southeast Asia and China. There is a high frequency of G6PD deficiency in Taiwan and southern China. Approximately 20% to 40% of neonatal jaundice in these areas is related to G6PD deficiency, whereas neonatal jaundice is rarely attributed to G6PD deficiency in the United States.[17] Table 10–1 lists the type of G6PD variant found in selected populations.

The variants have been generally designated by geographic names. With the use of modern techniques of molecular biology, these variants have been reclassified in terms of the exact sites of nucleotide substitutions. Using this nomenclature, Gd A+ would be designated as G6PD A^{376G} to indicate the presence of guanine at nucleotide 376.[18]

Pathogenesis

G6PD catalyzes the first step in the hexose monophosphate shunt (or pentose phosphate) aerobic glycolytic pathway. Oxidative catabolism of glucose is accompanied by reduction of NADP to NADPH (Fig. 10–1), which is subsequently required to reduce glutathione. Reduced glutathione (GSH) is an important source of reducing potential that protects hemoglobin from oxidative denaturation.

The activity of G6PD is highest in young erythrocytes and decreases with cell aging. Under normal conditions, the individual with G6PD deficiency compensates for the shortened life span of the erythrocytes by producing more early red cells (reticulocytosis). Oxidative stress, however, can lead to a mild to severe hemolytic episode. A deficiency of GSH results in oxidative destruction of certain erythrocyte components, including sulfhydryl groups of globin chains and the cell membrane.[19-21] In addition, more than 50 chemical agents may induce hemolysis in G6PD-deficient

Enzyme Type	Population Usually Associated
Gd B (normal)	All
Gd Med (also known as Gd B−)	Whites (Mediterranean area)
Gd A+	Africans (~16% of African Americans)
Gd A−	Africans
Gd Canton	Asians

TABLE 10–1 **Distribution of Some Common G6PD Variants**

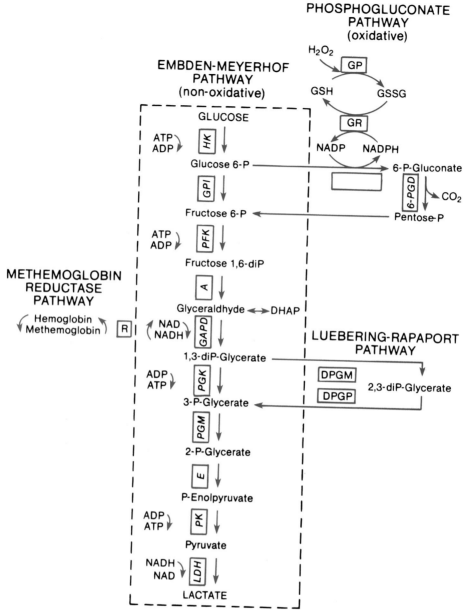

FIGURE 10–1 Red cell metabolic pathways. The nucleated red cell depends almost exclusively on the breakdown of glucose for energy requirements. The Embden-Meyerhof (nonoxidative or anaerobic) pathway is responsible for most of the glucose utilization and generation of ATP. In addition, this pathway plays an essential role in maintaining pyridine nucleotides in a reduced state to support methemoglobin reduction (the methemoglobin reductase pathway) and 2.3-diphosphoglycerate synthesis (the Luebering-Rapaport pathway). The phosphogluconate pathway couples oxidative metabolism with pyridine nucleotide and glutathione reduction. It serves to protect red cells from environmental oxidants. (From Hillman, RS and Finch, C: Red Cell Manual, ed. 5, FA Davis, Philadelphia, 1985, p 14, with permission.)

erythrocytes. Table 10–2 lists the drugs that have more commonly been reported to induce hemolysis in individuals with G6PD deficiency. The hemolytic episode results when G6PD-deficient erythrocytes fail to maintain adequate levels of GSH.[21,22] The resulting oxidation of hemoglobin leads to progressive precipitation of irreversibly denatured hemoglobin (Heinz bodies) (see Fig. 4–2, Chap. 4). The cells lack normal deformability when sulfhydryl groups are oxidized and consequently encounter difficulties passing through the microcir-

culation. Premature destruction of the cells results when they undergo intravascular lysis or are sequestered and destroyed in the liver or spleen. This early destruction may sometimes be detected in the peripheral blood smear with the formation of small condensed bite- or helmet-shaped red cells (Fig. 10–2).

Certain G6PD-deficient individuals also exhibit a sensitivity to the fava bean (favism) (Fig. 10–3). These individuals develop severe hemolysis after ingesting the fava bean or even after inhaling the plant's pollen.

TABLE 10–2 **Drugs and Chemicals Associated with Hemolytic Anemia in G6PD Deficiency**	
Acetanilide	Pamaquine
Chloramphenicol	Pentaquine
Dapsone	Phenylhydrazine
Daunorubicin	Primaquine
Doxorubicin	Sulfacetamide
Methylene blue	Sulfamethoxazole
Nalidixic acid	(Gantanol)
(Neg Gram)	Sulfanilamide
Naphthalene	Sulfapyridine
Niridazole (Ambilhar)	Thiazolesulfone
Nitrofurantoin	Toluidine blue
(Furadantoin)	Trinitrotoluene
	(TNT)

Source: Modified from Beutler,[4] p 1631.

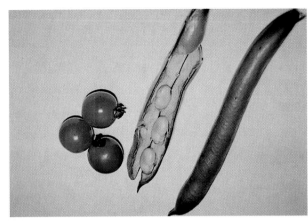

FIGURE 10–3 Fava beans. (Note: the tomatoes were added for color and contrast.)

Favism is found in some individuals with G6PD deficiency of the Mediterranean and Canton types. Divicine and Isouramil are the known active compounds that probably cause the favism.[20]

Clinical Manifestations

The majority of G6PD-deficient persons are asymptomatic most of the time and go through life without ever being aware of their genetic trait. G6PD enzyme activity of 20% of normal or even slightly less is sufficient for normal red cell function and survival under ordinary circumstances.

However, newborns with this intrinsic defect or people who take certain drugs or get infections may suffer various degrees of hemolysis from these challenges to the G6PD-deficient erythrocytes. Symptoms of the disorder are related to the severity of the hemolytic episode. Two to three days after the administration of the offending drug, the erythrocyte count decreases, along with the hemoglobin content. The anemia appears normochromic and normocytic and there is an increase in

reticulocytes. The patient may or may not experience back pain. Hemoglobinuria and jaundice may also be evidence of the hemolytic process. Table 10–3 compares the clinical features of the two most common variants.

The hemolytic episode in Gd A– is usually self-limiting. Young cells that are produced in response to the anemia have levels of G6PD that are nearly normal[23] and have better survival characteristics. Hemolysis associated with G6PD Med is more easily induced, usually more severe, and has been reported to result in death on occasion. Red blood cell transfusions may be indicated for hemolytic episodes in patients with G6PD Med.

Laboratory Testing

G6PD deficiency should be suspected after a clinical episode of acute hemolysis following administration of chemical or therapeutic agents known to cause the reaction in patients with the disorder. Laboratory changes of nonspecific type include a fall in hemoglobin (and hematocrit), hemoglobinuria (urine can turn brown to almost black secondary to presence of hemoglobin), Heinz bodies in the erythrocytes, evidence of hemolysis in the serum, elevated serum bilirubin levels, and markedly decreased or absent haptoglobin levels. Generally there are no significant alterations in leukocyte or platelet counts or function.

Laboratory investigation of hemolytic anemia when there is evidence (family history or drug sensitivity, or both) of G6PD deficiency may include several screening procedures. Oxidative denaturation of hemoglobin results in formation of Heinz bodies. These small particles of precipitated hemoglobin can be visualized by supravital staining using certain basic dyes such as crystal violet (see Fig. 4–2, Chap. 4). Heinz bodies will appear as small (1 to 4 μm) purple inclusions, usually on the cell periphery. They are not seen with Romanowsky stains such as Wright's stain. Although Heinz bodies may be seen in some other enzyme deficiencies, they are not seen in pyruvate kinase (PK) deficiency, which is the second most common RBC enzyme deficiency. Some unstable hemoglobins also form Heinz

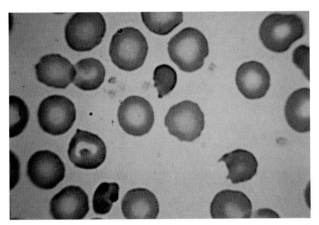

FIGURE 10–2 Peripheral blood smear from a patient with a G6PD deficiency. Note the small condensed "bite" or "helmet" cells.

TABLE 10–3 **Comparison of Clinical Features of Gd A⁻ and Gd Med (Gd B⁻)**		
Clinical Feature	**Gd A⁻**	**Gd Med**
Cells affected by defect	Aging erythrocytes	All erythrocytes
Hemolysis with drugs	Unusual	Common
Hemolysis with infection	Common	Common
Favism	No	Occasionally
Degree of hemolysis	Moderate	Severe
Transfusions required	No	Occasionally
Chronic hemolysis	No	No
Hemolytic disease of newborn	Rare	Occasionally

bodies after incubation of erythrocytes at 37°C for 48 hours.

Other test procedures that may be used to screen for G6PD deficiency include the methemoglobin reduction test[24] and the ascorbate-cyanide test.[25] In the methemoglobin reduction test, a simple and sensitive screening procedure, G6PD-deficient erythrocytes fail to reduce methemoglobin in the presence of methylene blue. The ascorbate-cyanide test, which measures perioxidative denaturation of hemoglobin, is not specific for G6PD deficiency, because it will yield moderately positive results if the patient has PK deficiency or certain hemoglobins are unstable.

The fluorescent spot test and the specific G6PD assay are positive only with G6PD deficiency.[26] When a mixture of glucose-6-phosphate, nicotinamide adenine denucleotide phosphate (NADP), saponin, and buffer is mixed with blood and placed on filter paper, G6PD converts the NADP to its reduced form, NADPH. When the filter paper is observed under fluorescent light, those erythrocytes that fail to convert NADP to NADPH (i.e., are deficient in G6PD) will lack fluorescence. The quantitative assay of G6PD is based on the measurement of the rate of reduction of NADP to NADPH measured at 340 nm.[27]

The diagnosis of G6PD deficiency during an acute hemolytic episode may be difficult. The deficiency may be obscured by the younger erythrocyte population (which has more G6PD) as the older G6PD-deficient erythrocytes are destroyed.

Pyruvate Kinase Deficiency

In 1960 De Gruchy and associates[28–29] reported that some patients with hereditary nonspherocytic hemolytic anemia (HNSHA) had elevated red blood cell concentrations of 2,3-diphosphoglycerate (2,3-DPG). This elevation suggested a block in anaerobic glycolysis further down the pathway (see Fig. 10–1). The enzyme was identified in 1961, when a severe deficiency of red blood cell PK was found in three patients with HNSHA.[30] PK catalyzes one of the reaction steps in the Embden-Meyerhof pathway of anaerobic glycolysis. Because mature red blood cells lack mitochondria, they are dependent on anaerobic glycolysis for the generation of adenosine 5′-triphosphate (ATP). The diminished capacity to generate ATP in PK-deficient red blood cells results in cell membrane fragility and a hemolytic anemia.

Since its discovery in 1961, more than 300 cases of PK deficiency have been reported, and many of these were cases of variant enzymes with different biochemical characteristics.[31,32] The nucleotide sequence of cDNA for the human PK gene and sequences of several of the mutations that cause HNSHA have been described.[33,34] PK deficiency is the most common enzymatic disease involving anaerobic glycolysis of the red blood cell. Together, G6PD deficiency and PK deficiency constitute most cases of HNSHA arising from red blood cell enzyme deficiencies.

Mode of Inheritance

PK deficiency is inherited as an autosomal recessive trait, but true homozygotes are rare and are restricted to children of consanguineous parents. The most common mode of inheritance is that of double heterozygosity, that is, when two mutant variants of the PK enzyme are simultaneously inherited from each parent.[32,35,36] To date, approximately 20 different mutations of the PK gene are known to produce a hemolytic anemia.[37] Thus, the clinical symptoms of PK deficiency are observed both in true homozygotes and in double heterozygotes for the PK gene. Both sexes appear to be affected equally.

There is increasing evidence that PK deficiency is worldwide in distribution, with most of the cases reported to date in Northern Europe, the United States, and Japan. Other cases have been reported in Australia, Canada, China, Costa Rica, Hong Kong, Italy, Mexico, the Near East, New Zealand, the Phillipines, Saudi Arabia, Spain, and Venezuela.[35,38–41]

The Pennsylvania Amish have a high frequency of PK deficiency, which has been traced back to a single immigrant couple. In affected families, consanguinity is common. Thus, the PK deficiency in the Amish population is the result of a true homozygote condition.[42]

Pathogenesis

PK deficiency results in a decreased capacity to generate ATP (see Fig. 10–1). The ATP-requiring membrane pumps that maintain the proper electrochemical gradients begin to fail with decreasing concentrations of ATP. This results in cell water loss with cell shrinkage, distortion of cell shape, and increased membrane rigidity.[43,44] These membrane abnormalities result in premature destruction of the red blood cells in the spleen and liver with consequent anemia. It has been shown that PK-deficient reticulocytes consume six to seven times more oxygen than normal reticulocytes.[44] In most cells, the drop in ATP regeneration because of a block in the glycolytic pathway would be compensated for by oxidative phosphorylation, but that capacity is lost in red blood cells as they mature and they lose mitochondria.

Clinical Manifestations

The severity of the hemolytic disease associated with PK deficiency varies from mild to severe, depending upon the properties of the mutant enzymes.[35,45,46] True homozygotes are anemic and jaundiced at birth and may require repeated transfusions during life. Less severely affected patients may come to clinical attention later in childhood or early adulthood because of anemia, jaundice, and/or an enlarged spleen. The hemolytic anemia is often more pronounced during periods of infection or other stresses. There is an increased incidence of pigmented gallstone formation with these patients, as is true with all chronic hemolytic disorders.

Interestingly, these patients may tolerate exercise to a greater degree than might be expected from the extent of their anemia. Red blood cell concentrations of 2,3-DPG are increased up to three times the normal levels in patients with PK deficiency because of the enzyme block (see Fig. 10–1).[35] The increase of 2,3-DPG decreases the affinity of O_2 to hemoglobin and consequently O_2 is more readily released to the tissues where it is needed. For this reason, transfusion therapy should be based upon the patient's tolerance of the anemia. Removal of the spleen benefits some patients because it increases the life span of the altered red blood cells.

Laboratory Testing

The peripheral blood smears of patients with PK deficiency typically show a normochromic, normocytic anemia with varying degrees of reticulocytosis. Accelerated erythropoiesis may result in polychromasia, poikilocytosis, anisocytosis, and nucleated red blood cells. Both the hemoglobin and the hematocrit levels are decreased from normal. The serum usually has a moderate increase in unconjugated bilirubin, and the haptoglobin level is decreased or absent.[46,47]

Several screening tests may be used to distinguish the nonspherocytic anemia of PK deficiency from the anemias of hereditary spherocytosis and the unstable hemoglobinopathies. These tests are nonspecific and serve only as a mechanism for classifying the type of anemia. Diagnosis is made on the basis of specific testing for the PK enzyme.

Screening tests may include the osmotic fragility test and the autohemolysis test (see Chap. 31), as well as the antiglobulin test and red blood cell survival tests. Erythrocytes that are PK-deficient will show osmotic fragility near normal when the test is performed on freshly drawn blood. If the blood is incubated, some patients exhibit an increase in osmotic fragility.[19] Sterile defibrinated blood is used to perform the test for autohemolysis. When normal erythrocytes are incubated in their own serum at 37°C, they will gradually lyse, showing up to 3.5% lysis after 48 hours. Erythrocytes from patients with nonspherocytic anemias, as well as those with hereditary spherocytosis, demonstrate an increased amount of autohemolysis. When glucose is added prior to incubation, erythrocytes from the patient with hereditary spherocytosis will show a normal amount of hemolysis. The addition of glucose does not correct the increased autohemolysis of PK-deficient erythrocytes (Fig. 10–4). The antiglobulin test in PK deficiency is negative and the red blood cell survival is decreased.

A fluorescence screening test, which is relatively simple and sensitive, is used for the diagnosis of PK deficiency. It is based on the following coupled enzyme assay:

$$PEP + ADP + Mg^{2+} \xrightarrow{\text{PK enzyme}} Pyruvate + ATP$$

$$Pyruvate + \underset{\text{(UV fluorescence)}}{NADH} + H^+ \xrightarrow{\text{LDH enzyme}}$$

$$Lactate + \underset{\text{(No fluorescence)}}{NAD^+}$$

and takes advantage of the fact that NADH fluoresces when it is illuminated with long-wave ultraviolet (UV) light, whereas NAD does not fluoresce. PEP, NADH, ADP, Mg^{2+}, and LDH are added to a patient sample of blood, which is spotted on filter paper and examined with a UV light. If the blood lacks PK enzyme, NADH

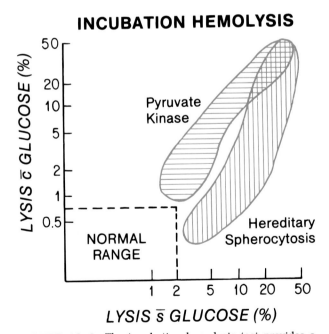

FIGURE 10–4 The incubation hemolysis test provides a further measure of cell resistance to hemolysis. Pyruvate kinase-deficient blood demonstrates an abnormal rate of hemolysis that is independent of the presence or absence of glucose in the incubation medium. In contrast, the blood from a patient with hereditary spherocytosis shows more marked hemolysis when glucose is absent. (From Hillman, RS and Finch, C: Red Cell Manual, ed. 5, FA Davis, Philadelphia, 1985, p 97, with permission.)

TABLE 10–4 **Laboratory Differentiation of Methemoglobinemia**			
Methemoglobinemia Resulting From	Methemoglobin Level	Enzyme Activity	Hemoglobin Electrophoresis
Hereditary enzyme deficiency	Increased	Decreased	Normal
Toxic substance exposure	Increased	Normal	Normal
Hemoglobin M disease	Increased	Normal	Abnormal

will not be oxidized and the fluorescence will persist for 45 minutes to an hour. If the blood is normal and has the PK enzyme, the fluorescence will disappear in 15 minutes, because NAD$^+$ does not fluoresce.[35,47] It should be noted that leukocytes contain a PK isoenzyme that will also catalyze the same reaction. Therefore, blood must be centrifuged and plasma and buffy coat removed prior to testing the erythrocytes. In addition, patients who have recently been transfused may have enough donor cells remaining in circulation to give erroneous test results.

Any abnormal fluorescence spot test should be followed with a confirmatory quantitative PK enzyme assay. This involves the same coupled reaction mechanism as above, but the conversion of NADH to NAD$^+$ is measured spectrophotometrically at 340 nm under standard conditions. Most PK-deficient individuals have 5% to 25% of normal activity.[35,47]

Methemoglobin Reductase Deficiency

Hemoglobin that is oxidized from the ferrous to the ferric state is called *methemoglobin*. Normally, about 1% of the circulating hemoglobin is in the form of methemoglobin. The balance between methemoglobin formation and reduction is maintained by the NADH–methemoglobin reductase (also called diaphorase) pathway. Methemoglobinemia may occur either when there is decreased enzyme activity or when production of methemoglobin exceeds the reducing capacity of the enzyme system. Hereditary deficiency of NADH–methemoglobin reductase results in increased levels of methemoglobin. This congenital deficiency is inherited as an autosomal recessive trait.[48] The heterozygote does not usually show signs of methemoglobinemia unless challenged with certain drugs.

The major clinical feature of methemoglobinemia is cyanosis. Because methemoglobin cannot carry oxygen, some patients exhibit symptoms similar to those of anemia, and some patients develop a compensatory mild polycythemia (see Chap. 21). The course of this disorder is generally benign, and patients are treated only for cosmetic reasons. In cases of severe cyanosis, methylene blue is administered intravenously to activate the NADH–methemoglobin reductase system.

In addition to the hereditary deficiency of NADH–methemoglobin reductase, methemoglobinemia may be caused by the hemoglobin M diseases or to acute reaction to various drugs or toxic substances. An abnormality in the globin structure of hemoglobin results in the hemoglobin M diseases (see Chap. 11).

The laboratory differentiation of the types of methemoglobinemia is shown in Table 10–4. Methemoglobin has a maximum absorbance band at 630 nm. The addition of cyanide causes the band to disappear, and the change in absorbance is directly proportional to the concentration of methemoglobin.[49] Methemoglobin is increased to varying degrees in all three disorders; enzyme activity is decreased only in hereditary NADH–methemoglobin reductase deficiency. Hemoglobin electrophoresis produces normal-appearing results in patients with methemoglobinemia except in the hemoglobin M diseases.

Other Enzyme Deficiencies

Except for the deficiencies of G6PD and PK, reports of hereditary enzyme deficiencies have been limited to a few rare cases. In a study of 350 cases of suspected enzyme-deficient hemolytic anemia, Beutler[50] reported 13.9% G6PD deficiencies and 9.9% PK deficiencies. Glucose phosphate isomerase (GPI) was the third most commonly identified enzyme deficiency (1.7%). Although there have been reports of other enzyme deficiencies (glycolytic and nonglycolytic), not all such deficiencies have been associated with hemolytic anemia.

Laboratory tests are available to assay many of the specific enzymes. Some of these tests may be available only through reference laboratories. Most laboratories, however, will be able to screen patients with a suspected hemolytic anemia caused by enzyme deficiency. The antiglobulin, erythrocyte survival, autohemolysis, osmotic fragility, and Heinz body tests can all be useful in distinguishing the enzyme deficiencies from hereditary spherocytosis and the unstable hemoglobinopathies.

CASE STUDY

A 26-year-old African-American man was referred to the clinical laboratory for investigation of reported hemoglobinuria. The patient had recently been diagnosed as having infectious mononucleosis. The following laboratory data were obtained:

RBC	$3.7 \times 10^{12}/L$
Hgb	11.0 g/dL
Hct	32%
MCV	86.0 fL
MCHC	34.0 g/dL
WBC	$9.5 \times 10^9/L$
Differential	
Segs	40%
Bands	3%
Lymphs	48% (many atypical)
Monos	7%
Eos	2%
Platelets	Adequate
Reticulocytes	14.5% (uncorrected)

The red blood cell (RBC) morphology was normochromic and normocytic. Polychromasia was noted. A slight poikilocytosis was also noted, with some red cells showing irregular protrusions. Upon further investigation, the anti-human-globulin test result was found to be negative. On the basis of the antiglobulin test, the hemolytic process was considered not to be the result of an immune reaction. A normal hemoglobin electrophoresis was reported.

The hematologist suggested that the patient return in 30 days for testing for erythrocyte enzyme deficiency. At that time the patient was found to have an erythrocyte G6PD activity of 15% of normal.

Hemolysis can be induced in G6PD-deficient individuals by infection with certain viral agents including the Epstein-Barr virus. Testing to confirm erythrocyte G6PD activity should be done after the patient has had sufficient time to recover from the hemolytic episode. Since the younger RBCs have higher G6PD content, spuriously elevated G6PD levels may be found during or immediately after the hemolytic episode.

Questions

1. What does the reticulocyte count in this patient represent?
2. Calculate the corrected reticulocyte count?
3. What type of G6PD correlates to this patient's familial background?
4. What RBC inclusion might also be found on the peripheral blood smear with supravital stains?
5. What further testing can be performed in diagnosing G6PD deficiency?
6. What type of hemolysis is present here?

REFERENCES

1. Dacie, JR, et al: Atypical congenital haemolytic anemia. Q J Med 22:79, 1953.
2. Carson, PE, et al: Enzymatic deficiency in primaquine-sensitive erythrocytes. Science 124:484, 1956.
3. Yoshida, A: Glucose-6-phosphate dehydrogenase of human erythrocytes. I. Purification and characterization of normal (B+) enzyme. J Biol Chem 241:4966, 1966.
4. Beutler, E and Yoshida, A: Genetic variation of glucose-6-phosphate dehydrogenase: A catalog and future prospects. Medicine 67:311, 1988.
5. Beutler, E: The genetics of glucose-6-phosphate dehydrogenase deficiency. Semin Hematol 27:137, 1990.
6. Hirono, A and Miwa, S: Human glucose-6-phosphate dehydrogenase: Structure and function of normal and variant enzymes. Haematologia 25:85, 1993.
7. Vulliamy, TJ, et al: Diverse point mutations in the human glucose-6-phosphate dehydrogenase gene cause enzyme deficiency and mild or severe hemolytic anemia. Proc Natl Acad Sci USA 85:5171, 1988.
8. Kletzien, RF, et al: Glucose-6-phosphate dehydrogenase: A "housekeeping" enzyme subject to tissue-specific regulation by hormones, nutrients, and oxidant stress. FASEB J 8:174, 1994.
9. Desorges, JF: Genetic implications of G-6-PD deficiency. N Engl J Med 294:1438, 1976.
10. Pai, GS, et al: Localization of loci for hypoxanthine phosphoriboxyltransferase and glucose-6-phosphate dehydrogenase and biochemical evidence of non-random x-chromosome expression from studies of a human x-autosome translocation. Proc Nat Acad Sci USA 77:2810, 1980.
11. Beutler, E, et al: The normal human female as a mosaic of x-chromosome activity: Studies using the gene for G-6-PD deficiency as a marker. Proc Nat Acad Sci, USA 48:9, 1962.
12. Beutler, E: Biochemical abnormalities associated with hemolytic states. In Weinstein, IM and Beutler, E (eds): Mechanisms of Anemia in Man. McGraw-Hill, New York, 1962, p 195.
13. Luzzatto, L: Glucose-6-phosphate dehydrogenase: Genetic and haematological aspects. Cell Biochem Funct 5:101, 1987.
14. Takizawa, T, et al: A single nucleotide base transition is the basis of the common human glucose-6-phosphate dehydrogenase variant A(+). Genomics 1:228, 1987.
15. Beutler, E: Glucose-6-phosphate dehydrogenase deficiency. N Engl J Med 324:169, 1991.
16. Beutler, E: The molecular biology of G6PD variants and other red cell enzyme defects. Annu Rev Med 43:47, 1992.
17. Chiu, DTY, et al: Molecular characterization of glucose-6-phosphate dehydrogenase (G6PD) deficiency in patients of Chinese descent and identification of new base substitution in the human G6PD gene. Blood 81:2150, 1993.
18. Beutler, E: Glucose-6-phosphosphate dehydrogenase: New prospectives. Blood 73:1397, 1989.
19. Beutler, E: Glucose-6-phosphate dehydrogenase deficiency. In Williams, WJ, et al (eds): Hematology, ed 2. McGraw-Hill, New York, 1977, p 466.
20. Arese, P and De Flora, A: Pathophysiology of hemolysis in glucose-6-phosphate dehydrogenase deficiency. Semin Hematol 27:1, 1990.
21. Johnson, RM, et al: Oxidant damage to erythrocyte membrane in glucose-6-phosphate dehydrogenase deficiency: Correlation with in vivo reduced glutathione concentration and membrane protein oxidation. Blood 83:1117, 1994.
22. Beutler E: Glucose-6-phosphate dehydrogenase deficiency. In Stanbury, JB, et al (eds): The Metabolic Basis of Inherited Disease. McGraw-Hill, New York, 1978, p 1430.
23. Beutler, E, Dern, RJ, and Alving AS: The hemolytic effect of primaquine. IV. The relationship of cell age to hemolysis. J Lab Clin Med 44:439, 1954.
24. Grewer, GJ, et al: The methemoglobin reduction test for primaquine-type sensitivity of erythrocytes: A simplified procedure for detecting a specific hypersusceptibility to drug hemolysis. JAMA 180:386, 1962.
25. Jacob, HS and Jandl, JH: A simple visual screening test for glucose-6-phosphate dehydrogenase deficiency employing ascorbate and cyanide. N Engl J Med 274:1162, 1966.
26. Beutler, E, et al: International committee for standardization in hematology: Recommended screening test for glucose-6-phosphate dehydrogenase (G-6-PD) deficiency. Br J Haematol 43:465, 1979.
27. Beutler, E: Red Cell Metabolism. A Manual of Biochemical Methods, ed 2. Grune & Stratton, New York, 1975.
28. De Gruchy, GC, et al: Non-spherocytic congenital hemolytic anemia. Blood: 1371, 1960.
29. Robinson, MA, et al: Red cell metabolism in non-spherocytic congenital haemolytic anaemia. Br J Haematol 7:327, 1961.
30. Valentine, WN, et al: A specific glycolytic enzyme defect (pyruvate kinase) in three subjects with congenital nonspherocytic hemolytic anemia. Trans Assoc Am Physicians 74:100, 1961.
31. Miwa, S and Fujii, H: Pyruvate kinase deficiency. Clin Biochem 23:155, 1990.

32. Miwa, S, et al: Concise review: Pyruvate kinase deficiency: Historical perspective and recent progress of molecular genetics. Am J Hematol 42:31, 1993.
33. Tani, K, et al: Human liver type pyruvate kinase: Complete amino acid sequence and the expression in mammalian cells. Proc Nat Acad Sci 85:1792, 1988.
34. Baronciani, L and Beutler, E: Analysis of pyruvate kinase-deficiency mutations that produce nonspherocytic hemolytic anemia. Proc Nat Acad Sci 90:4324, 1993.
35. Lukens, J: Hereditary hemolytic anemias associated with abnormalities of erythrocyte anaerobic glycolysis and nucleotide metabolism. In Lee, GR, et al (eds): Wintrobe's Clinical Hematology, ed 9. Lea & Febiger, Philadelphia, 1993, Chap. 34.
36. Lakomek, M, et al: Erythrocyte pyruvate kinase deficiency: A kinetic method for differentiation between heterozygosity and compound-heterozygosity. Am J Hematol 31:225, 1989.
37. Baronciani, L and Beutler, E: Prenatal diagnosis of pyruvate kinase deficiency. Blood 84:2354, 1994.
38. Feng, CS, et al: Prevalence of pyruvate kinase deficiency among the Chinese: Determination by the quantitative assay. Am J Hematol 43:271, 1993.
39. de Medicis, E, et al: Hereditary nonspherocytic hemolytic anemia due to pyruvate kinase deficiency: A prevalence study in Quebec, Canada. Hum Hered 42:179, 1992.
40. Fonella, A, et al: Iron status in red-cell pyruvate kinase deficiency: Study of Italian cases: Br J Haematol 83:485, 1993.
41. Wei, DC, et al: Hemozygous pyruvate kinase deficiency in Hong Kong ethnic minorities. J Paediatr Child Health, 28:334, 1992.
42. Kanno, G, et al: Molecular abnormality of erythrocyte pyruvate kinase deficiency in the Amish. Blood 83:2311, 1994.
43. Keith, AS: Pyruvate kinase deficiency and related disorders of red cell glycolysis. Am J Med 41:762, 1966.
44. Mentzer, WC, Jr, et al: Selective reticulocyte destruction in erythrocyte pyruvate kinase deficiency. J Clin Invest 50:688, 1971.
45. Lakomek, M, et al: Erythrocyte pyruvate kinase deficiency: Relations of residual enzyme activity, altered regulation of defective enzymes and concentrations of high energy phosphates with the severity of clinical manifestations. Eur J Haematol 49:82, 1992.
46. Rapaport, SI: Introduction to Hematology, ed 2d. JB Lippincott, 1987, Chaps. 6, 7.
47. Kjeldsberg, C, ed: Practical Diagnosis of Hematologic Disorders, rev ed. ASCP Press, Chicago, 1991, Chap. 9.
48. Jaffe, ER: Hereditary methemoglobinemias associated with abnormalities in the metabolism of erythrocytes. Am J Med 41:786, 1966.
49. Evelyn, KA and Malloy, HT: Micro determination of oxyhemoglobin, methemoglobin and sulfhemoglobin in a single sample of blood. J Biol Chem 126:655, 1938.
50. Beutler, E: Red cell enzyme defects as nondiseases and as diseases. Blood 54:1, 1979.

QUESTIONS

1. What is the most common glycolytic enzyme deficiency associated with the pentose phosphate pathway (aerobic pathway)?
   a. Pyruvate kinase deficiency
   b. Glucose-6-phosphate dehydrogenase deficiency
   c. Hexokinase deficiency
   d. Glutathione reductase deficiency

2. What is the most common glycolytic enzyme deficiency associated with Embden-Meyerhof pathway (anaerobic pathway)? (Use answer choices for question 1.)

3. Oxidative denaturation of hemoglobin results in formation of small particles that are visualized with supravital staining. What is the term for these particles?
   a. Basophilic stippling
   b. Howell-Jolly bodies
   c. Pappenheimer bodies
   d. Heinz bodies

4. In the evaluation of a patient for G6PD deficiency, which of the following test results would indicate a deficiency of the enzyme?
   a. Increased formation of Heinz bodies
   b. Lack of fluorescence in the fluorescent spot test
   c. Failure to reduce methemoglobin in the presence of methylene blue
   d. All of the above

5. Which laboratory test result would indicate a patient who is PK-deficient?
   a. Abnormal rate of hemolysis that is independent of the presence or absence of glucose in the incubation medium
   b. Lack of fluorescence in the fluorescent spot test
   c. A change in the indicator from red to yellow in the orthocresol red test
   d. Increase in osmotic fragility

6. What deficiency causes hemoglobin to be oxidized from the ferrous to the ferric state?
   a. G6PD deficiency
   b. PK deficiency
   c. NADH–methemoglobin reductase deficiency
   d. Lactate dehydrogenase deficiency

ANSWERS

1. **b** (p 164)
2. **a** (p 164)
3. **d** (p 167)
4. **d** (pp 167–168)
5. **a** (p 169)
6. **c** (p 170)

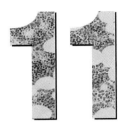

Hemolytic Anemias: Intracorpuscular Defects

III. THE HEMOGLOBINOPATHIES

Denise M. Harmening, PhD, MT(ASCP), CLS(NCA)

Objectives

At the end of this chapter, the learner should be able to:
1   Characterize hemoglobinopathies.
2   Define qualitative and quantitative hemoglobin defects.
3   Name the amino acid substitution found in sickle cell anemia.
4   List factors contributing to the sickling process.
5   Name and describe the three types of sickle cell anemia.
6   List tests useful in the laboratory diagnosis of sickle cell disease.
7   List characteristics for sickle cell trait.
8   Name the amino acid substitution found in hemoglobin C disease and list characteristics of
    the disease.
9   Identify the laboratory finding that helps provide a diagnosis of hemoglobin SC disease.
10   Identify causes of methemoglobinemia.

Hemoglobinopathies are defined in the broadest sense as conditions in which abnormal hemoglobins are synthesized. Greater than 625 hemoglobin variants have been described.[1] Most of these hemoglobin variants were discovered coincidentally and are of no clinical significance. However, approximately one third (200) of these variants represent hemoglobinopathies with clinically significant hemolytic anemia caused by the type of abnormal hemoglobin produced. The hemoglobinopathies are either inherited abnormalities or genetic mutations resulting in a defect in the structural integrity or function of the hemoglobin molecule.

More than 90% of the hemoglobin variants are single amino acid substitutions in the alpha (α), beta (β), delta (δ), or gamma (γ) globin chains as a result of a single-point mutation in one of the globin genes.[2] Hemoglobin variants are inherited as codominant traits according to classic mendelian genetics. For example,

173

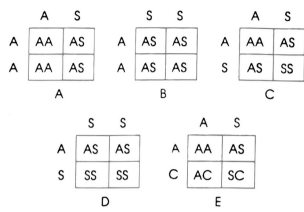

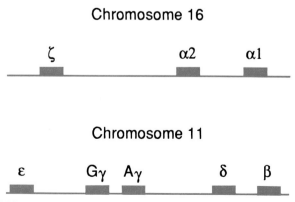

FIGURE 11-1 Inheritance of abnormal hemoglobins. (*A*) With one parent heterozygous for an abnormal hemoglobin, the offspring have a one-in-two chance of carrying the trait. (*B*) With one parent homozygous for an abnormal hemoglobin, all offspring will carry the trait because that parent can contribute only an abnormal gene. (*C*) With both parents heterozygous for the abnormality, the chances are one in four for normal, two in four for heterozygous, and one in four for homozygous. (*D*) With both parents carrying the same abnormal hemoglobin—one homozygous and one heterozygous—the offspring have a 50-50 chance of being either homozygous or heterozygous. (*E*) With parents carrying two different abnormal hemoglobins, offspring have a one-in-four chance of not inheriting an abnormality, a one-in-two chance of carrying the trait for one or the other abnormality, and a one-in-four chance of carrying both abnormalities in condominance.

when both parents carry one gene that codes for an abnormal hemoglobin (such as HbS), there is a 25% chance with each pregnancy that the infant will be homozygous (inheriting two genes for HbS), resulting in sickle cell anemia (Fig. 11–1, block C). A total of eight genes are inherited from each parent on two homologous chromosomes that code for polypeptide chains. The α and zeta (ζ) genes are located on chromosome 16, with two α and one ζ gene per chromosome. The β, δ, γ, and epsilon (ϵ) genes are located on chromosome 11, with one β, δ, ϵ, and two γ genes per chromosome (Fig. 11–2). The reader should refer to Chapter 3 for a review of normal hemoglobin structure. Table 11–1 re-

Chromosome 16

$$\zeta \qquad\qquad \alpha 2 \qquad \alpha 1$$

Chromosome 11

$$\epsilon \qquad G\gamma \; A\gamma \qquad \delta \quad \beta$$

FIGURE 11-2 Location of the globin genes on chromosomes 16 and 11.

Globin Chains	Hemoglobin	Normal (%)	Stage of Development
$\alpha_2\epsilon_2$	Gower 2		
$\zeta_2\epsilon_2$	Gower 1		Embryo
$\zeta_2\gamma_2$	Portland		
$\alpha_2{}^A\gamma_2$	F	50–85	
$\alpha_2{}^G\gamma_2$	F		Fetus
$\alpha_2\beta_2$	A	95–97	
$\alpha_2\delta_2$	A2	2	Adult

TABLE 11-1 Composition of Normal Physiologic Hemoglobins

views the composition of normal physiologic hemoglobins.

CLASSIFICATION

Classification of hemoglobinopathies is somewhat arbitrary. Hemoglobin disorders may be divided into two very broad categories: qualitative and quantitative hemoglobinopathies. In the qualitative category, hemoglobins are formed normally in structure ($\alpha_2\beta_2$) but differ in the sequence of the amino acids composing the globin chain. This category is the one usually referred to in the general discussion of hemoglobinopathies. Quantitative defects are those characterized by decreased production of hemoglobin with a decreased synthesis of one particular globin chain, which is commonly known as thalassemia (see Chap. 12).

A more inclusive method of classification allows division of the hemoglobinopathies into five major categories:

1. Abnormal hemoglobins without clinical significance
2. Aggregating hemoglobins (i.e., sickle cell anemia)
3. Unbalanced synthesis of hemoglobin (thalassemia)
4. Unstable hemoglobins
5. Hemoglobins with abnormal heme function

Table 11–2 summarizes this classification of hemoglobinopathies.

TABLE 11-2 Classification of Hemoglobinopathies

- Abnormal hemoglobins without clinical significance
- Aggregating hemoglobins (structural abnormalities with amino acid substitution *away* from the crevice of the heme, i.e., HbS, HbC)
- Unbalanced synthesis of hemoglobin (thalassemia)
- Unstable hemoglobins
- Hemoglobins with abnormal heme function (structural abnormalities with amino acid substitutions *near* the crevice of the heme)

HEMOGLOBINOPATHIES

The majority of hemoglobinopathies (hemoglobin variants) result from β-chain abnormalities. Many of these variants have no associated physiologic consequences. There also can be α-, γ-, and δ-chain abnormalities, but these conditions are usually clinically benign. Some individuals with β-chain abnormalities present with abnormal hemoglobins resulting in clinical disease. From the first description of a sickle cell by Herrick[3] in 1910, research efforts continue to define, understand, and treat these abnormalities associated with inherited abnormal hemoglobins.

Most hemoglobinopathies arise from a single amino acid substitution. For example, when valine substitutes for glutamic acid in the sixth position of the β chain, HbS is produced rather than HbA. When lysine replaces glutamic acid at position six of the β chain, HbC is produced. These changes truly represent a molecular alteration; a feature that was initially appreciated by Linus Pauling in the late 1940s when he won the Nobel prize for defining sickle cell anemia as a molecular disease.[4] The abnormality was demonstrated by electrophoresis to be located in the protein portion of the hemoglobin molecule.

Nomenclature

Investigators began naming the abnormal hemoglobins with capital letters, but with the end of the alphabet rapidly approaching, they changed to the use of names of places. A letter plus a place name indicates identical mobility on electrophoresis, but there are different substitutions. It should be noted, in general, that there is more than one abnormal hemoglobin with the same letter designation (i.e., $HbC_{Georgetown}$, HbC_{Harlem}, $HbG_{Philadelphia}$, $HbG_{San\ Jose}$, HbO_{Arab}, $HbO_{Indonesia}$).[5] The description of the variant can also involve identifying the chains and the substitution. For example, homozygous HbS is $\alpha_2\beta_2{}^s$ or $\alpha_2\beta_2{}^{6Val}$ or $\alpha_2\beta_2{}^{6Glu\text{-}Val}$. Hemoglobin $G_{Philadelphia}$, the most common α-chain variant in the black population, is written $\alpha_2{}^{G\ Phil}\beta_2$ or $\alpha_2{}^{68Lys}\beta_2$ or $\alpha_2{}^{68Asn\text{-}Lys}\beta_2$. Additionally, the exact helix of the secondary structure and the position in that helix can be indicated. For example, the designations would be $\alpha_2\beta_2{}^{6(A3)}$ for HbS and $\alpha_2{}^{68(E17)}\beta_2$ for $HbG_{Philadelphia}$.

Sickle Cell Anemia

Historic Overview

In 1910, a 20-year-old black student from the West Indies was described by Herrick[3] as suffering from a severe hemolytic anemia in which peculiarly elongated, "sickled" red cells were found on his peripheral blood smear. The classic hematologic features included not only the presence of sickle cells on the peripheral blood smear but also nucleated red cells indicative of a severe anemia, cardiac enlargement, icterus, and leukocytosis. The presence of target cells as well as a normocytic, normochromic anemia is also generally associated with hemoglobinopathies. Sickle cell anemia represents the most common type of severe hemoglobinopathy with an estimated prevalence in the United States of 1 in 375 African-American live births.[5] It is estimated to affect more than 50,000 Americans![5]

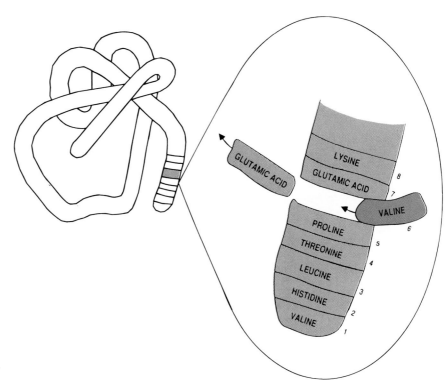

FIGURE 11–3 Amino acid substitution in hemoglobin S.

TABLE 11–3 **Sickle Cell Disease (a Group of Genetic Disorders Characterized by the Production of HbS)**

Disorder	Incidence in African-American Live Births	
Sickle cell anemia (HbSS)	1 in 375	(0.26%)
SC disease (HbSC)	1 in 835	(0.12%)
Sickle β-thalassemia	1 in 1,667	(0.06%)

Source: Sickle Cell Disease Guide Panel.[5]

Definition

The term *sickle cell disease* is used generically to describe a group of genetic disorders characterized by the production of the abnormal hemoglobin S (HbS).[5] Sickle cell anemia (SCA) is the most common type of sickle cell disease and represents the homozygous form, in which the individual inherits a double dose of the abnormal gene that codes for hemoglobin S. This type of hemoglobin differs from normal hemoglobin by the single amino acid substitution of valine for glutamic acid in the sixth position from the NH_2 terminal end of the β chain (Fig. 11–3). The structural formula for sickle cell anemia (HbSS) is $\alpha_2\beta_2^{6\text{Glu-Val}}$. The formula alternatively may be written as $\alpha_2\beta_2^S$ or $\alpha_2\beta_2^{6\text{Val}}$. The gene for hemoglobin S occurs with greatest frequency in tropical Africa, particularly Central Africa. In the United States, the birth incidence of the homozygous state (HbSS) is approximately 0.26% (1 in 375 African-American babies).[6] It is estimated that 8% to 10% of American blacks carry the trait (one gene) for hemoglobin S.

Although in the United States sickle cell disease is most commonly found in persons of African ancestry, it has also been found in individuals from the Caribbean, South and Central America, Mediterranean (Turkey, Greece), the Middle East, and India.[6] Table 11–3 lists the other common variants of sickle cell disease with their estimated incidence.

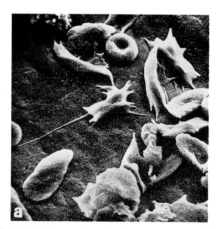

FIGURE 11–4 Scanning electron micrograph (SEM) of sickle cells. (From Bell, A: Hematology. In Listen, Look and Learn. Health and Education Resources, Inc., Bethesda, MD, with permission.)

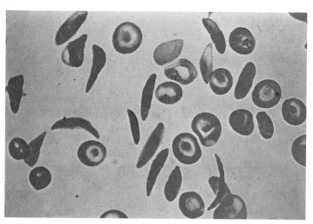

FIGURE 11–5 Sickle cell disease (peripheral blood). Note the sickle-shaped red cells and target cells. (From Bell, A: Hematology. In Listen, Look and Learn. Health and Education Resources, Inc., Bethesda, MD, with permission.)

Pathophysiology

Hemoglobin S is soluble and usually causes no problem when properly oxygenated. However, when the oxygen tension decreases, this single amino acid substitution in the β-globin chain of HbS polymerizes, forming tactoids or fluid polymers (Fig. 11–4). As these polymers realign, they cause the red cell to deform into the characteristic sickle shape (Fig. 11–5). The sickling process is dependent on the degree of oxygenation, pH, and dehydration of the patient. A decrease in oxygenation and pH as well as dehydration promotes sickling. Sickle cells in circulation increase the viscosity of the blood, which slows circulation, thereby increasing the time of exposure to a hypoxic environment, particularly in the small vasculature of the spleen. This then promotes further sickling. There are two types of sickle cells: reversible and irreversible. The sickling of the cell is reversible up to a point. However, repeated sickling eventually damages the red blood cell (RBC) membrane permanently. The formation of rigid sickle cells is likely to plug small blood vessels, further lowering the pH and oxygen tension and increasing the number of sickled cells, resulting in both acute and chronic tissue damage.[7] The tissue injury is secondary to the obstruction of blood flow and hypoxia produced by the abnormally shaped sickle red cells. This leads to hypoxia, painful crises, and infarction of organs. It should be noted that the presence of HbF and HbA in

TABLE 11–4 **Factors Affecting the Severity of HbS**

Amount of HbS	Vascular stasis
Other hemoglobins	Temperature
Thalassemia	pH
G6PD deficiency	Viscosity
Deoxygenation	MCHC
Amount of HbF	Dehydration

Abbreviations: G6PD = glucose-6-phosphate dehydrogenase; MCHC = mean corpuscular hemoglobin concentration.

RBCs with HbS modifies the degree or severity of the sickling.[8] Table 11–4 lists other factors affecting the severity of HbS.

Clinical Features

The hallmark features of sickle cell disease are chronic hemolytic anemia and vaso-occlusion resulting in ischemic tissue injury.[7] All tissues and organs within the body are at risk for damage as a result of the vascular obstruction produced by the sickled red cells. Organs at greatest risk include the spleen, kidney, and bone marrow, since in these organs blood flow is slow in the venous sinuses and there is a reduced oxygen tension and low pH.[9] In addition, the eye and head of the femur are also target sites for ischemic injury because of the limited terminal arterial blood supply to these areas.

Sickle cell anemia is usually diagnosed early in life, when the level of HbF declines. Hemoglobin SS typically presents as a severe chronic hemolytic anemia, with hemoglobin levels in the range of 6 to 8 g/dL. Characteristically, the patient demonstrates an asthenic physique and is mildly jaundiced (Fig. 11–6). Many complications are associated with the disease, with the major manifestations being "sickle crises." There are three types of crisis: aplastic, hemolytic, and painful (vaso-occlusive).[10]

An aplastic crisis is usually associated with infections, particularly to parvoviruses, which cause a temporary marrow aplasia reflected in a low reticulocyte count. The marrow is simply overworked as a result of the stress related to the continuous stimulus for production of new red cells. With an already shortened red cell life span, even a temporary decrease or arrest in red cell production causes a drastic anemia. During the evaluation of the febrile patient, a fall in the reticulocyte count can also indicate the onset of aplastic crises that require future monitoring of the hemoglobin level in the SCA patient. Aplastic crises usually spontaneously resolve within 5 to 10 days.[7]

A hemolytic crisis reflects an acute exacerbation of the anemia with a resulting fall in hemoglobin and hematocrit levels, an increased reticulocyte count, and jaundice.[10] Acute splenic sequestration is the cause, resulting in a decrease in hemoglobin and hematocrit level, which usually occurs in infants and young children between 5 months and 2 years of age.[7] Intrasplenic pooling of vast amounts of blood results in enlarged spleens of some children with SCA. The usual clinical features of a hemolytic crisis include sudden weakness, rapid pulse, faintness, pallor of the lips and mucous membranes, as well as abdominal fullness resulting from the enlarged spleen.[7] In contrast to this process, multiple infarctions and subsequent fibrosis lead to a process termed *autosplenectomy* in adult patients with SCA.

Vaso-occlusive or painful crisis is the hallmark of sickle cell anemia.[7] The crisis is usually associated with severe pain, caused by rigid sickle cells in the small blood vessels, resulting in tissue damage and necrosis. The decreased blood flow causes regional hypoxia and acidosis, further exacerbating the ischemic injury. A painful crisis usually lasts 4 to 6 days but sometimes persists for weeks.[7] Painful crisis can be precipitated by infection, fever, acidosis, dehydration, and exposure to extreme cold. Some patients have reported that even emotional states such as anxiety, stress, and depression may cause their painful crises.

Generally, three principles of therapy are applied in the management of painful crisis: adequate rehydration, pain relief using sufficient analgesics, and antibiotic therapy to treat any precipitating or underlying illness such as infection.[11] In severe cases, exchange transfusion may be necessary to reduce the hemoglobin S content in the blood of the patients with SCA. However, the mainstay of therapy for painful crisis is hydration (administration of fluid volumes) to correct fluid and electrolyte deficits in an attempt to maintain normal serum electrolyte concentrations.

Symptoms and clinical manifestations of SCA are many and varied. Table 11–5 lists the most prominent types of clinical manifestations associated with SCA. As mentioned previously, these clinical presentations represent the sequelae of repeated infarction. Table 11–6 provides a more comprehensive list, dividing the clinical features of SCA into hematologic and nonhematologic categories.

Infarction Infarcts can occur virtually anywhere in the body: in bones, joints, lungs, liver, kidneys, eye, central nervous system, and spleen.[7] In the lungs, pulmonary infarction from sickling in the pulmonary microvasculature produces the acute chest syndrome in SCA patients. It is a common cause of hospital admission and in some cases represents a medical emergency. The acute chest syndrome represents an acute illness characterized by fever, chest pain, prostration,

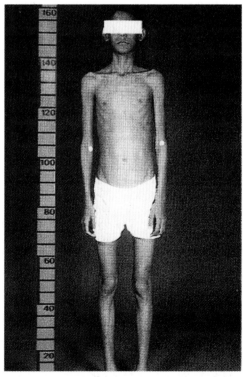

FIGURE 11–6 Asthenic physique with mild jaundice. (Reproduced with permission from Sandoz Pharmaceuticals Corporation.)

TABLE 11–5. **Clinical Manifestations of Sickle Cell Anemia**

Cutaneous manifestations (leg ulcers)
Cardiac enlargement
Joint and skeletal problems
Arthritis
Renal complications (renal papillary necrosis)
Bone marrow infarctions
Conjunctival vascular abnormalities
Gastrointestinal symptoms
Hepatomegaly
Autosplenectomy
Cholelithiasis
Priapism (persistent, painful penile erection)

and the presence of pulmonary infiltrates on the chest x-ray.[12] The syndrome in adults is characteristically a result of pulmonary infarction, although other causes such as bacterial or viral infection have been reported. This contrasts the acute chest syndrome in SCA children, which is usually caused by an infections agent. Pleuritic chest pain is the dominant symptom of acute chest syndrome in adults, whereas fever, cough, and tachypnea are often the only complaints in infants and young children who are affected.[7]

The most common cutaneous manifestation in SCA is the development of ulcers or sores on the lower leg (Fig. 11–7). Approximately 8% to 10% of patients develop leg ulcers, which are usually manifested between 10 and 50 years of age and are very difficult to resolve.[7]

In sickle cell disease, bones and joints are frequent sites of pathology, with musculoskeletal pain the most common symptom. There can be bone marrow hyperplasia, infection, or infarction. Infarction is also commonly responsible for the symptoms of the hand-foot syndrome observed in SCA. Dactylitis (the painful swelling of the hands and feet) occurs commonly in infants and young children with SCA and is observed exclusively in patients in that age group.[7] In many in-

TABLE 11–6 **Clinical Features of Sickle Cell Anemia by Category**

Hematologic
* Aplastic crisis
* Hemolytic crisis
* Vaso-occlusive crisis

Nonhematologic

* Abnormal growth	* Cardiopulmonary
* Bone and joint abnormalities	o Enlarged heart
o Pain	o Heart murmurs
o *Salmonella* infection	o Pulmonary infarction
o Hand-foot dactylitis	* Eye
* Genitourinary	o Retinal hemorrhage
o Renal papillary necrosis	* Central nervous system
o Priapism	* Leg ulcers
* Spleen and liver	* Risky pregnancy
o Autosplenectomy	
o Hepatomegaly	
o Jaundice	

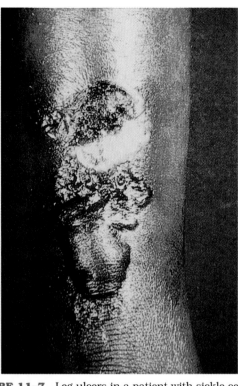

FIGURE 11–7 Leg ulcers in a patient with sickle cell anemia. (Reproduced with permission from Sandoz Pharmaceuticals Corporation.)

fants it is the first manifestation of the disease. The characteristic hand-foot syndrome develops later in life as a result of microinfarction of small bones of the hands and feet, which leads to unequal growth and bone deformities of the fingers and toes (Fig. 11–8). In addition, episodes of painful swollen joints and aseptic necrosis of the femoral head and other articulating bones are caused by the process of infarction.

Infections Serious bacterial infections remain a major cause of morbidity and mortality in patients with SCA. Table 11–7 lists the organisms implicated in causing infections in these patients.

The most significant cause of death during early childhood is the severe overwhelming septicemia and meningitis brought on by *Streptococcus pneumoniae*.[5] In SCA, splenic dysfunction develops during infancy and predisposes the infant to overwhelming infections from encapsulated bacteria, such as *S. pneumoniae* and *Haemophilus influenzae*.[5] After the first decade of life, anaerobic and enteric organisms become important pathogens, causing infections in adult patients with SCA. Repeated splenic infarcts result in autosplenectomy by the adult years. These patients then become more prone to serious infections with encapsulated organisms such as *S. pneumococcus* and *H. influenzae*.

In comparison to healthy individuals, infections in patients with SCA cause greater morbidity, disseminate more rapidly, and are more difficult to resolve. In particular, pyelonephritis recurs regularly in these patients, is difficult to treat, and is often associated with septicemia.[7] This infection results in a predisposition

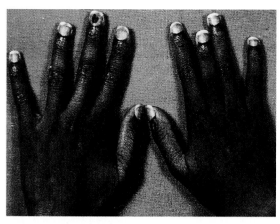 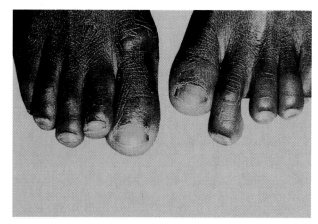

FIGURE 11-8 Hand-foot syndrome in a patient with sickle cell anemia. (Reproduced with permission from Sandoz Pharmaceuticals Corporation.)

to sickling in the renal papilla, ultimately causing renal papillary necrosis, which frequently develops along with the pyelonephritis (see section on sickle cell nephropathies).

Table 11-8 outlines the multiple factors responsible for the increased susceptibility to infection in patients with SCA.

The relationship between the incidence of the malarial parasite and the frequency of the abnormal hemoglobin S gene requires further explanation. Malaria, caused by a parasite of the *Plasmodium* species, is still a serious disease in tropical areas, with *Plasmodium falciparum* being responsible for the most life-threatening situations. Cells carrying HbS, when parasitized by *P. falciparum*, sickle more quickly than nonparasitized cells.[13] The sickling affects the cycle of the parasite in one of two ways: directly, by killing the parasite, or indirectly, by causing the parasitized sickle cells to be sequestered in the spleen. The fact that persons homozygous for the HbS gene often lack spleens by the time they reach adulthood (autosplenectomy or functional asplenia) may be one reason why malaria is exceptionally severe, and often fatal, in these cases.

Sickle Cell Nephropathies In the kidney, intravascular sickling occurs more rapidly than in any other organ because of deoxygenation of HbS in the acidic and hyperosmolar environment of this organ.

The combination of hypoxia, hypertonicity, and acidosis in the kidney leads to sickling, stasis, and ischemia of the renal medulla and papillary tip leading to progressive renal events. Eventually, over time, a number of sickle cell nephropathies develop. Hyposthenuria, the inability of the kidney to concentrate the urine, is the earliest and most common nephropathy in sickle cell disease, occurring usually in the first decade.[7] Progressive renal pathology occurs in patients with SCA as renal tubular dysfunction and atrophy present in the second decade of life. The third decade of life in SCA is characterized by interstitial nephritis, papillary necrosis, pyelonephritis, and the nephrotic syndrome, to name a few of the renal disorders that may develop. In the fourth decade and beyond, end-stage renal disease develops because of one or more of the sickle cell nephropathies, resulting in chronic renal failure.[7]

It should be noted that hyperuricemia and gross hematuria occur commonly in patients with SCA. Hyperuricemia occurs in approximately 15% of children and 40% of adults with SCA because of increased urate production associated with the accelerated erythropoietic rate and decreased renal clearance of urate.[7] Gross hematuria occurs commonly not only in SCA but also in sickle cell trait because of the sickling, stasis, ischemia, and extravasation of blood in the kidney.[14]

TABLE 11-7 **Organisms Implicated in Causing Infections in Patients with SCA**			
Bacterial	**Viral**	**Fungal**	**Parasitic**
Streptococcus pneumoniae	Rubeola	*Coccidioides immitis*	*Plasmodium* sp.
Haemophilus influenzae	Cytomegalovirus	*Histoplasma capsulatum*	
Neisseria meningitidis			
Mycoplasma pneumoniae			
Staphylococcus aureus			
Streptococcus pyogenes			
Mycobacterium tuberculosis			
Escherichia coli			
Salmonella species			

TABLE 11–8 Factors Responsible for the Increased Susceptibility of SCA Patients to Infections

- Reticuloendothelial blockage caused by increased hemolysis
- Stasis of sickled RBCs in the sinusoids of the liver and spleen
- Secondary splenic dysfunction
- Deficiency of nonantibody serum opsonic activity

Stroke Stroke occurs in 6% to 12% of patients with SCA.[7] Stroke represents an array of neurologic complications caused by an ischemic or hemorrhagic lesion in a specific cerebral vessel.[15] The neurologic manifestations may be focal (i.e., hemiparesis) or more generalized such as coma or seizure. Recurrent episodes of stroke cause progressively greater impairment and increased mortality. The most common cause of stroke in children is cerebral infarction.[7] With age, subarachnoid and intracerebral hemorrhage become increasingly common.

Infarction strokes recur in at least two thirds of SCA patients who are *not* chronically transfused. SCA patients with hemorrhagic stroke (intracerebral or subarachnoid hemorrhage) have a high mortality rate during the acute stage (as high as 50%).[7]

Sickle Cell Trait

In sickle cell trait, the heterozygous form of the disease, individuals inherit both a normal β-globin gene and a sickle-globin gene (β^s). As a result, individuals with sickle cell trait produce both normal HbA and HbS, with a predominance of HbA in an approximate ratio of 60:40.[14] Figure 11–9 is a peripheral smear from an individual with sickle cell trait. The structural formula is $\alpha_2\beta_1$, $\beta_1^{6glu-val}$. The frequency of this heterozygous condition in American blacks is approximately 8%.[6] Individuals with HbS trait are usually asymptomatic, but occasionally episodes of hematuria and hyposthenuria occur as a complication of sickle cell trait because of sickling in the kidney. Therefore, the potential for sickling exists, and the drastic lowering of pH

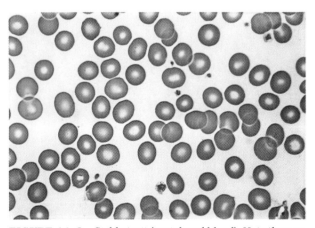

FIGURE 11–9 Sickle trait (peripheral blood). Note the normal-appearing smear.

or reduction in oxygen tension can precipitate a crisis. Causes of this include severe respiratory infections, air travel in unpressurized aircraft, anesthesia, and congestive heart failure. Even excessive exercise can lead to a significant buildup of lactic acid, resulting in sickling and subsequent infarction. Several deaths of American black soldiers with sickle cell trait have been reported as a result of rigorous basic training at altitudes greater than 4000 feet, which led to a buildup of lactic acid, following by acidosis and subsequent organ infarction.

Laboratory Diagnosis of Sickle Cell Anemia and Sickle Cell Trait

The following laboratory tests should be performed to diagnose sickle cell disease: the complete blood count (CBC), a reticulocyte count, evaluation of the peripheral smear, hemoglobin electrophoresis, and measurement of hemoglobins A_2 and F.[7]

The chronic anemia of HbSS typically is quite severe, with hemoglobin levels ranging between 6 and 8 g/dL. The RBC indices are normochromic and normocytic. The peripheral red blood picture can be striking with numerous target cells, fragmented red cells, polychromasia, nucleated red cells, and usually sickle cells (see Fig. 11–5). Siderotic granules and Howell-Jolly bodies may be seen in the red cells as a result of rapid RBC turnover and "stressed" erythropoiesis. An average reticulocyte count will be between 5% and 20%. The reticulocyte count, however, decreases during an aplastic crisis; a falling reticulocyte count may herald the onset of such a crisis. There may be a neutrophilic leukocytosis with a shift to the left and thrombocytosis. The bone marrow reflects a marked erythroid hyperplasia, except during an aplastic crisis.

In individuals with the trait, sickle cells are not present on the peripheral blood smear. On rare occasions, however, sickle cells may be observed in the peripheral blood smear during a crisis episode.

Laboratory Screening for Sickle Cell Disease According to the Clinical Practice Guideline on Sickle Cell Disease published by U.S. Department of Health and Human Services in April, 1993, all newborns, regardless of race or ethnic background, should be screened for the presence of HbS (Table 11–9).[5]

Newborn screening for sickle cell disease began in the United States in the early 1970s. The initial screening programs grew out of the recognition that SCA was associated with significant morbidity and mortality. Today newborn hemoglobinopathy screening is performed in more than 40 states, the District of Columbia, Puerto Rico, and the Virgin Islands.[5]

The first step most commonly used to characterize hemoglobin is electrophoresis. Cellulose acetate and isoelectric focusing (IEF) are the most commonly used electrophoretic methods.[5] Electrophoresis separates different hemoglobins by electrical charge.

The definitive test for HbS is a hemoglobin electrophoresis on cellulose acetate at alkaline pH, followed if necessary by electrophoresis on citrate agar at acid pH (Fig. 11–10). The patient with SCA produces no normal β chains; therefore, there will be no HbA on electrophoresis (unless the patient has been recently transfused). Hemoglobin S constitutes 80% or more of

TABLE 11–9 **Screening Methods**

Criteria	Cellulose Acetate Electrophoresis	Isoelectric Focusing	High-Performance Liquid Chromatography
Equipment cost	$2500	$4000	$30,000
Cost per test (consumables)	$0.15–0.25	$0.35–0.50	$0.10–1.75
Samples run per hour	200	72	5–20
Advantages	Semi-quantitative Simple to operate	Sharper bands	Automated Quantitative
Disadvantages	Densitometer for quantitation	Densitometer for quantitation	Complex to use

Note: Labor costs vary with number of samples per run.
Source: Sickle Cell Disease Guide Panel.[5]

hemoglobin with HbF ranging from 1% to 20%.[14] When HbF levels are higher than 20%, there is an improvement in the severity of the disease.[8] This is seen in newborns and in a combination of HbS with hereditary persistence of fetal hemoglobin (HPFH) (see Chap. 12). In SCA, the HbA_2 level may be slightly increased with a mean of 3.4%.[14] Hemoglobins with similar charges have similar migration patterns during electrophoresis, especially on cellulose acetate. Hemoglobins D and G both migrate to the same position as HbS at alkaline pH. HbE and HbO_{Arab} migrate in the same position as HbC. Citrate agar electrophoresis is very useful because it clearly separates HbS from HbG and D, and HbC from HbE and HbO_{Arab} at acid pH.

Citrate agar electrophoresis is rarely used as the primary electrophoretic method for screening, but it is used by many laboratories to confirm the presence of abnormal hemoglobins detected by other methods.[16] This practice of employing two laboratory methods is called a two-tier screening technique.[5] In sickle cell trait, hemoglobin electrophoresis at alkaline pH shows 60% HbA, 40% HbS, and usually elevated HbA_2 (mean 3.6%).[14] At acid pH, one band is present in the A position ($HbA + HbA_2$), while the other band migrates to the S position (see Fig. 11–10).

It should be noted that most hemoglobin variant traits, without coexistent conditions such as iron deficiency or thalassemia, have alkaline electrophoretic patterns with an approximate 60:40 ratio of normal to abnormal hemoglobin.

Two previously used screening tests should *not* be used for newborn screening. These are the sickle cell preparation using sodium metabisulfite and solubility tests using a concentrated phosphate buffer, a hemo-

lyzing agent, and sodium dithionate. These tube solubility tests either isolate HbS at an interface or cause the abnormal hemoglobin to precipitate (Fig. 11–11). Both tests depend on the concentration of HbS in the red cell or hemolysate.

The low level of S hemoglobin in cells of the neonate is believed to explain the unreliability of these tests during the newborn period. Although sickle cell disease should not be diagnosed from either a sickle cell preparation or solubility test because neither of these tests will reliably distinguish sickle cell trait from SCA, many hospitals still perform these tests on adult patients.[16] It is important to note that some rare hemoglobins also sickle, giving positive solubility tests. Table 11–10 lists some of the rare hemoglobins that sickle. Since HbS, G, and D all migrate in the same position on cellulose acetate electrophoresis, it is helpful to know that HbG and HbD do not give a positive tube solubility test.

Recent articles have advocated DNA analysis as an additional testing method for detection of the sickle cell gene.[17] However, presently, this method is both costly and limited in the number of genotypes that can be identified.

Treatment of Sickle Cell Anemia

With advances in the diagnosis, treatment, and prevention of complications, the life expectancy of individuals with sickle cell disease has improved. There is an 85% chance that infants with SCA will survive to age 20.[5]

The principal causes of death in infants with SCA include overwhelming infections with *S. pneumoniae*,

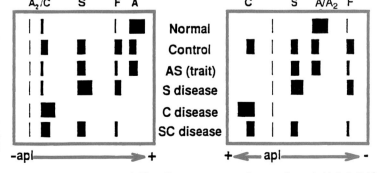

FIGURE 11–10 Electrophoretic patterns of hemoglobin on (A) cellulose acetate, run at pH 8.4, and (B) citrate agar, run at pH 6.0 to 6.5 (apl = point of application).

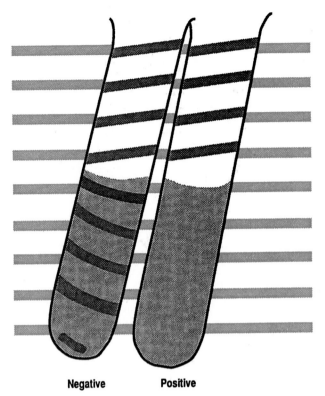

Negative   **Positive**

FIGURE 11–11 Tube solubility screening test for sickle cell anemia.

cerebral vascular accidents, and acute splenic sequestration crises.[5] Twice-daily administration of oral penicillin reduces both the morbidity and mortality from pneumococcal infection in SCA in infants.[5] In addition, administration of age-appropriate immunizations should be given, including pneumococcal, conjugated *H. influenzae*, and hepatitis B vaccines.[5]

A variety of drugs are being tested for their potential in ameliorating the effects of SCA. Ideally the best drug or drug combination would inhibit polymerization of the abnormal hemoglobin while having little effect on the oxygen affinity of the hemoglobin molecule. Many drugs seem to increase the oxygen affinity, which increases the hemoglobin and hematocrit and thus the viscosity of the blood. Because increased viscosity would have a detrimental effect on the sickling process, such drugs should be avoided.

The National Heart, Lung, and Blood Institute (NHLBI) announced in 1995 the treatment of daily administration of the drug hydroxyurea to reduce the fre-

quency of painful episodes or "crises" in patients with SCA.[18] Recurrent painful episodes are the most disabling feature of SCA.

Findings of a multicenter study of hydroxyurea in patients with SCA reported a 50% reduction in hospital admissions.[19] However, hydroxyurea may not be appropriate for all patients with SCA and patients need to know that this drug is *not* a cure.

Hydroxyurea has been the drug of choice to treat myeloproliferative disorders such as polycythemia vera (see Chap. 21). Why this drug works in SCA is not completely understood, but it is believed to induce the production of HbF in RBCs.[20,21] Increased levels of HbF in RBCs prevent the sickling, therefore preventing vaso-occlusion and painful crises.[22] Hydroxyurea, however, is a cytotoxic agent and has the potential to cause life-threatening cytopenia. Therefore, SCA patients using this drug must be carefully evaluated and monitored. This drug should not be used in patients who are likely to become pregnant or those unable to follow instructions regarding their treatment.

Because there is still no cure for HbSS, efforts must be made to try and keep the patients in as controlled a state as possible. A good diet, early treatment of infection, and avoidance of situations that could precipitate a crisis still represent the mainstay of traditional treatment.[11]

Blood transfusions may be required for acute situations and for prevention of certain complications of SCA; however, the number should be limited to avoid excessive blood viscosity. Although it is known that blood transfusions reduce the risk of recurrent strokes, chronic transfusions are associated with serious complications such as an increased risk for intracranial hemorrhage.[23] Exchange transfusions are beneficial in certain situations.[7] In SCA patients with higher hematocrits (20% or greater in children, 25% or above in adults) an exchange transfusion technique may be safer than a simple blood transfusion.[7] Table 11–11 lists the general considerations and indications for blood transfusions in SCA.

Pharmacologic therapeutic strategies are still currently being tested on a multicenter scale.[24–27] Table 11–12 lists the goals of these therapeutic approaches to the treatment of SCA. Table 11–13 lists various approaches to specific therapy with a specific drug.

Bone marrow transplantation is currently being investigated in the United States for the treatment of sickle cell anemia and may represent a potential cure.[28] A national trial of bone marrow transplantation has been conducted on selected SCA patients with severe symptoms of sickle-induced vasculopathy.[29] Although marrow transplantation has been recognized since the 1980s as a potential cure, the risks (high mortality) associated with this procedure created considerable caution for use as a treatment.[30] However, the risks appear sufficiently reduced in the 1990s and the long-term benefit of marrow transplantation is being investigated and compared to conventional supportive care and pharmacologic treatment such as hydroxyurea and transfusion therapy.[31] Initial studies have indicated that bone marrow transplantation is effective in SCA patients in reducing pain and morbidity from vaso-occlusive crises, improving osteonecrosis, and reversing reticuloendothelial dysfunction after

TABLE 11–10 Examples of Rare Hemoglobins That Sickle and Give a Positive Tube Solubility Test

HbC_{Harlem} ($HbC_{Georgetown}$)
$HbC_{Ziquinchor}$
$HbS_{Memphis}$
HbS_{Travis}
$Hb_{Alexandra}$
$Hb_{Porto-Alegre}$

TABLE 11-11   General Considerations and Indications for Blood Transfusion in Patients with SCA

Consideration	Indications
To improve the oxygen-carrying transport in red cells by simple transfusions	Severely anemic as reflected by dyspnea, postural hypotension, high-output cardiac failure, angina, or cerebral dysfunction Sudden fall in hemoglobin or hematocrit levels during acute splenic or hepatic sequestration crisis Hemoglobin level <5.0 g/dL or hematocrit of 15% in patients who exhibit fatigue and dyspnea along with erythroid hypoplasia or aplasia
To improve microvascular perfusion by decreasing the number of red cells containing HbS by partial exchange transfusion	Life-threatening events, such as cerebrovascular accidents including stroke and transient ischemic attacks (TIAs) Arterial hypoxia syndrome (fat embolization) Acute progressive lung disease Unresponsive acute priapism Eye surgery when performed under local anesthesia and in the nonanemic patient

Source: Charache, Lubin, and Reid.[7]

TABLE 11-12   Treatment of SCA: Goals of Therapeutic Approaches

Increase the production of fetal hemoglobin in the adult
Decrease microvascular entrapment of sickle cells
Modify the oxygen affinity or solubility of sickle hemoglobin
Change the volume of the sickle erythrocyte
Alter expression of the abnormal sickle gene

transplantation.[32,33] On a worldwide level, experience with bone marrow transplantation for SCA has been more limited.[34]

The future treatment of gene therapy for SCA as well as other hemoglobinopathies is also currently under investigation.[35–39] The success of gene therapy for hemoglobinopathies depends on the ability of researchers to isolate, enrich, and insert genes into hematopoietic pluripotential stem cells.[31]

Hemoglobin C (HbC) Disease and Trait

HbC disease is found almost exclusively in the black population. HbC differs from normal HbA by the single

TABLE 11-13   Effects of Approaches to Specific Therapy

Therapeutic Approach	Drugs	Effect
Inhibition of HbS polymerization	Urea Ethanol Peptides	Noncovalent hemoglobin modification
	Cyanate Pyridoxal Glyceraldehyde	Covalent hemoglobin modification
	DDAVP Cetiedil Hyponatremia	Erythrocyte modification (increase in red cell volume, decrease in 2,3-DPG)
	Hydroxyurea 5-Azacytidine	Genetic modification (increase in gamma gene globin expression, bone marrow transplantation)
Decreased erythrocyte microvascular entrapment	Nifedipine	Vasodilator

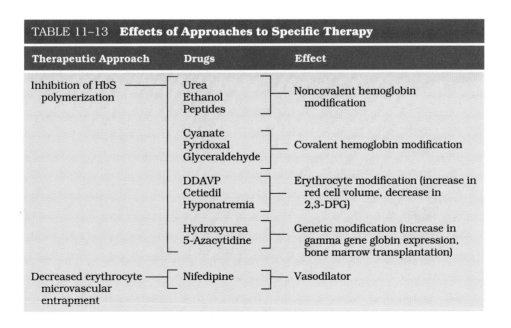

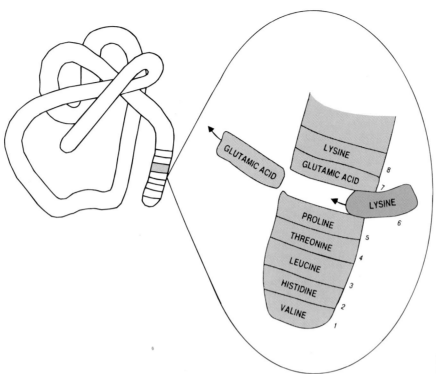

FIGURE 11–12 Amino acid substitution in hemoglobin C.

amino acid substitution of lysine for glutamic acid in the sixth position from the NH₂ terminal end of the β chain (Fig. 11–12). This represents the exact same substitution point as HbS but with a different amino acid. The structural formula for HbC, the presence of which is often referred to as HbC disease, is $\alpha_2\beta_2^{6Glu\text{-}Lys}$. Hemoglobin C is seen with great frequency in West Africa, particularly northern Ghana, where the incidence is 17% to 28%.[14] In the United States, only 0.02% of blacks have HbC disease.[14] The clinical manifestations are mild chronic hemolytic anemia with associated splenomegaly and abdominal discomfort. The red cell morphology is typically normocytic, normochromic, with numerous target cells (50% to 90%) and occasionally microspherocytes, fragmented cells, and folded cells (see Fig. 11–13). HbC crystals (Fig. 11–14) or "bar-of-gold" crystals occur more often in the red cells of individuals who have been splenectomized than in those whose spleen is intact. Figure 11–15 is a scanning electron micrograph (SEM) of HbC crystals. These crystals can be demonstrated in wet preparations by washing the red cells and then suspending them in a sodium citrate solution.[14] The reticulocyte count is slightly increased. Hemoglobin bands, at alkaline pH, are approximately 95% HbC plus A₂, less than 7% HbF, and no HbA. HbE, O$_{Arab}$, C, and A₂ all

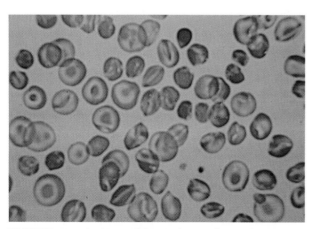

FIGURE 11–13 Hemoglobin C disease (pre-splenectomy). Note the numerous target and envelope forms.

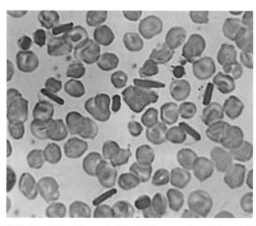

FIGURE 11–14 Hemoglobin C disease (peripheral blood). Note the particular crystals: "bar of gold" and numerous target cells (post-splenectomy). (From Bell, A: Hematology. In Listen, Look and Learn. Health and Education Resources, Inc., Bethesda, MD, with permission.)

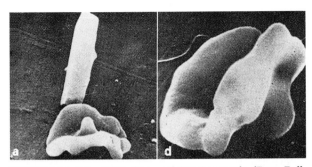

FIGURE 11–15 SEM of hemoglobin C crystals. (From Bell, A: Hematology. In Listen, Look and Learn. Health and Education Resources, Inc., Bethesda, MD, with permission.)

migrate to the same position at alkaline pH. HbC can be separated from these other hemoglobins at acid pH (see Fig. 11–10 and refer to Chapter 31 for other hemoglobin migration patterns).

HbC trait, $\alpha_2\beta_1^{6Glu-Lys}$, is present in 2% to 3% of American blacks, and these individuals are clinically asymptomatic.[14] The only significant finding on the peripheral blood smear is targeting. At alkaline pH, there is approximately 60% HbA and 40% HbC plus A_2.

Hemoglobin D (HbD) Disease and Trait

Hemoglobin D has several variants. The most common variant in American blacks is HbD$_{Punjab}$, which is synonymous with HbD$_{Los Angeles}$. Its frequency is less than 0.02%.[14] Both the homozygous ($\alpha_2\beta_2^{121Glu-Gln}$) and the heterozygous ($\alpha_2\beta_{1\beta1}^{121Glu-Gln}$) states are asymptomatic. The peripheral blood smear is unremarkable, except for a few target cells. Hemoglobin D migrates electrophoretically to the same position as HbS and HbG at alkaline pH but migrates with HbA at acid pH. HbD is a nonsickling soluble hemoglobin.

Hemoglobin E (HbE) Disease and Trait

HbE occurs with greatest frequency in Burma, Thailand, Cambodia, Laos, Malaysia, and Indonesia.[14] This variant is now prevalent in the United States because of the influx of refugees from Southeast Asia. The homozygous state ($\alpha_2\beta_2^{26Glu-Lys}$) presents with little or no anemia; target cells; and microcytic, hypochromic red cell indices. On alkaline electrophoresis, there is approximately 95% to 97% HbE + A_2 and the remainder is HbF. HbE migrates with HbC and HbO$_{Arab}$ at alkaline pH, but migrates with HbA at acid pH. HbE trait ($\alpha_2\beta_{1\beta1}^{26Glu-Lys}$) is asymptomatic clinically. There is microcytosis, target cells, and approximately 70% HbA and 30% HbE + A_2 on routine electrophoresis.[40] HbE is slightly *unstable* and there is an associated thalassemic component with this hemoglobin variant. This is responsible for the microcytosis, and the lower-than-expected quantified value of HbE in HbAE.[40]

It has been postulated that HbE may protect against malaria, because areas such as Thailand that are highly endemic for malaria also have a high incidence of the HbE gene. Some authors attribute this effect to the fact that the parasite *P. falciparum* multiplies more slowly in HbE red cells than in the HbAE or HbAA red cells.[14]

Hemoglobin O$_{Arab}$ (HbO$_{Arab}$) Disease and Trait

HbO$_{Arab}$ is a rare hemoglobin variant that occurs infrequently in black, Arab, and Sudanese populations. Homozygous O$_{Arab}$ ($\alpha_2\beta_2^{121Glu-Lys}$) exhibits a mild hemolytic anemia with slight splenomegaly and target cells on the peripheral blood smear. This hemoglobin migrates electrophoretically with HbC, HbE, and HbA$_2$ at alkaline pH but separates at acid pH migrating in the HbA position. In the heterozygous state of HbO$_{Arab}$ ($\alpha_2\beta_1\beta_1^{121Glu-Lys}$) the patient is asymptomatic.

Hemoglobin S with Other Abnormal Hemoglobins

As mentioned previously, sickle cell disease is a generic term for a group of genetic disorders that include SCA, hemoglobinopathies in which HbS is in association with another abnormal hemoglobins, and the sickle β-thalassemia syndromes.[5] This section will focus on defining the disorders which have HbS and another abnormal hemoglobin. Sickle β thalassemia will be briefly mentioned at the end of this section. Table 11–14 lists the common and uncommon forms of sickle cell disease.

Hemoglobin SC Disease (HbSC)

Hemoglobin SC disease ($\alpha_2\beta_1^{6Val}\beta_1^{6Glu-Lys}$) occurs when the gene for HbS is inherited from one parent and that for HbC from the other. About 0.12% of black Americans have SC disease.[5] Patients with HbSC disease are generally less anemic and experience a milder course than those with SCA. However, because of increased blood viscosity, this condition has a greater incidence of retinal hemorrhage, renal papillary necrosis, and necrosis of the femoral head.[39] Peripheral blood smear findings include target cells, folded red cells, and occasionally glove-shaped intracellular crystals (Fig. 11–16). The solubility test results are positive owing to the presence of HbS. Hemoglobin electrophoresis at alkaline pH separates HbS and HbC in approximately equal amounts (Fig. 11–17). HbF is usually less than 2% compared with average HbF levels of about 6% in SCA. Electrophoresis at acid pH will confirm the S and C hemoglobins (see Fig. 11–10). Table 11–15 compares the incidence of the most common hemoglobinopathies found in American blacks.

TABLE 11–14 Common and Uncommon Forms of Sickle Cell Disease

Common	Uncommon
(HbSS) sickle cell anemia	(HbSD) hemoglobin SD disease
(HbSC) sickle-HbC disease	(HbSO$_{Arab}$) hemoglobin SO$_{Arab}$
(HbSβ^+) sickle β^+-thalassemia	(HbSE) hemoglobin SE disease
(HbSβ^0) sickle β^0-thalassemia	(HbS/Lepore) hemoglobin S Lepore

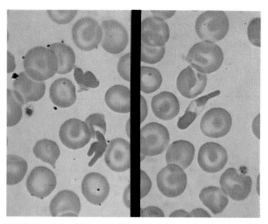

FIGURE 11-16 Hemoglobin SC disease (peripheral blood). Note the type of "Washington monument" crystals and target cells. (From Bell, A: Hematology. In Listen, Look and Learn. Health and Education Resources, Inc., Bethesda, MD, with permission.)

Hemoglobin SD Disease (HbSD)

The combination of HbS and HbD, although rare, presents an interesting diagnostic problem. Because these hemoglobins migrate together at alkaline pH, the electrophoretic pattern is similar to that of SCA. Solubility tests are positive. The clinical severity of HbSD disease, however, falls between that of SCA and sickle cell trait. Acid electrophoresis separates these two hemoglobins. HbS has its own migration point, whereas HbD will migrate with HbA in the same position. Refer to Chapter 31.

Hemoglobin SO$_{Arab}$ (HbSO$_{Arab}$)

The combination of HbS and HbO$_{Arab}$ can have a clinical presentation that is similar in severity to that of SCA. The anemia is severe, with typical sickle cells seen on the peripheral blood smear. This condition might initially be confused with HbSC on routine elec-

trophoresis; however, differentiation can be made with acid electrophoresis.

Hemoglobin S/β-Thalassemia Combination (HbS/β-thalassemia)

The severity of HbS combined with β-thalassemia depends on the degree of suppression of β-globin chain synthesis. HbS/β°-thalassemia is a severe condition that clinically resembles SCA; on the other hand, HbS/β⁺-thalassemia generally has a milder clinical presentation. The reader is referred to Chapter 12 for a detailed discussion of HbS/β-thalassemia and other hemoglobin variants that occur in combination with thalassemia.

Laboratory Diagnosis of HbS with Other Abnormal Hemoglobins

In cases where HbS is found in association with another abnormal hemoglobin, the diagnosis can be made in many instances from hemoglobin electrophoresis alone. However, there can be some difficulty in distinguishing between SCA and some of the sickle β-thalassemia syndromes such as HbS/β°-thalassemia, HbS/β⁺-thalassemia, HbSδ/β-thalassemia, and HbS in association with hereditary persistence of fetal hemoglobin syndrome (HbS HPFH).[7] In these cases, the electrophoresis demonstrates only HbS, HbF, and HbA$_2$. It is important to properly diagnose these disorders because the clinical manifestations and subsequent treatment are different. For example, HbS/β°-thalassemia is similar in severity to SCA. Patients with HbSδ/β-thalassemia have few symptoms; HbS/β⁺-thalassemia is a milder form and HbS HPFH is usually asymptomatic with no anemia. Measurement of HbF and HbA$_2$ may be helpful in distinguishing these conditions, since patients with HbSS, HbS/β°-thalassemia, HbSδ/β-thalassemia, and HbS HPFH all have similar electrophoretic patterns.[7] In HbS/β°-thalassemia, HbA$_2$ levels are greater than 3.5% and are low in patients with HbSδ/β-thalassemia and HbS HPFH.[7] Generally, HbF levels are higher in all the HbS/β-thalassemias in comparison to HbSS. Assessment of HbF in the parents may be indicated in cases where HbS HPFH is suspected.[7] Table 11-16 summarizes the clinical and hematologic findings in the common variants of sickle cell disease.

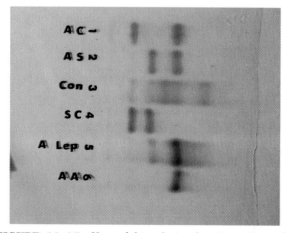

FIGURE 11-17 Hemoglobin electrophoretic patterns (1) Hemoglobin (Hb) A\C, (2) Hb A\S, (3) commercial control; (4) Hb S\C, (5) HbA\Lepore, and (6) Hb A\A normal control.

TABLE 11-15 **Incidence of Common Hemoglobinopathies in American Blacks**		
Condition	**Genotype**	**Incidence (All Ages)**
Hemoglobin C disease	$\alpha_2\beta^C\beta^C$	0.02% (1 in 4500)
Hemoglobin C trait	$\alpha_2\beta^A\beta^C$	3.0% (1 in 33)
Sickle cell anemia	$\alpha_2\beta^S\beta^S$	0.26% (1 in 375)
Sickle cell trait	$\alpha_2\beta^A\beta^S$	8.0% (1 in 13)
Sickle C disease	$\alpha_2\beta^S\beta^C$	0.12% (1 in 835)
Sickle β-thalassemia	$\alpha_2\beta^S\beta^O$	0.06% (1 in 1667)

TABLE 11–16   Clinical and Hematologic Findings in the Common Variants of Sickle Cell Disease after the Age of 5 Years

Disease Group	Clinical Severity	Hemoglobin Electrophoresis				Hematologic Values*			
		S (%)	F (%)	A_2 (%)	A (%)	Hb (g/dL)	Retic (%)	MCV (fL)	RBC Morphology
SS	Usually marked	>90	<10	<3.5	0	6–10	5–20	>80	Sickle cells nRBC Normochromic, normocytic Anisocytosis Poikilocytosis Target cells Howell-Jolly bodies
$S\beta°$ Thal	Marked to moderate	>80	<20	>3.5	0	6–10	5–20	<80	Sickle cells nRBC Hypochromic Microcytosis Anisocytosis Poikilocytosis Target cells
$S\beta+$ Thal	Mild to moderate	>60	<20	>3.5	20 (A)	9–12	5–10	<75	No sickle cells Hypochromic Microcytosis Anisocytosis Poikilocytosis Target cells
SC	Mild to moderate	50	<5	—	50 (C)	10–15	5–10	75–95	"Fat" sickle cells Anisocytosis Poikilocytosis Target cells
S HPFH	Asymptomatic	>70	>30	<2.5	—	12–14	1–2	<75	No sickle cells Anisocytosis Poikilocytosis Rare target cells

*Hematologic values are approximate.
Source: Charache, Lubin, and Reid.[7]
Abbreviations: SS = Sickle cell anemia; $S\beta°$Thal = Sickle beta no thalassemia; $S\beta+$Thal = Sickle beta plus thalassemia; S HPFH = HbS in association with the hereditary persistence of fetal hemoglobin syndrome; SC = Hemoglobin SC disease; nRBC = nucleated red blood cells.
There is a tremendous variability between disease groups and between individual patients of the same group, particularly with regard to clinical severity.

HEMOGLOBIN VARIANTS WITH ALTERED OXYGEN AFFINITY

High-affinity hemoglobins, which are inherited as autosomal dominant disorders, are seen in the heterozygous state. These hemoglobins bind oxygen more readily and release it less easily to the tissues. The result is tissue hypoxia, which stimulates increased erythropoietin production. This, in turn, causes a compensatory increase in red cell mass, with increases in red cell count and hemoglobin and hematocrit levels, producing erythrocytosis and congenital polycythemia. Other hematologic parameters are normal. There is a shift to the left in the oxygen dissociation curve, and a diagnosis is established by measuring P_{50} levels (Fig. 11–18). Individuals with these hemoglobin variants are asymptomatic.

Hemoglobins with decreased oxygen affinity release oxygen quite readily to the tissues. There is a shift to the right in the oxygen-dissociation curve (see Fig. 11–18). As more oxygen is released per gram of he-

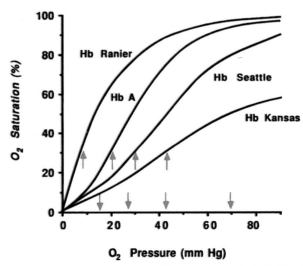

FIGURE 11–18 Oxygen equilibrium curve of whole blood from subjects with hemoglobin$_{Ranier,Seattle}$, and $_{Kansas}$ and from normal controls.

TABLE 11–17 **Hemoglobins Associated with Altered Oxygen Affinity**			
Increased O$_2$ Affinity and Polycythemia		**Decreased O$_2$ Affinity— May Have Mild Anemia or Cyanosis**	
Hb$_{Chesapeake}$	$\alpha_2{}^{92Leu}\beta_2$	Hb$_{Kansas}$	$\alpha_2{}^{102Thr}\beta_2$
HbJ$_{Cape\ Town}$	$\alpha_2{}^{92Gln}\beta_2$	Hb$_{Titusville}$	$\alpha_2{}^{94Asn}\beta_2$
Hb$_{Malmö}$	$\alpha_2\beta_2{}^{97Gln}$	Hb$_{Providence}$	$\alpha_2\beta_2{}^{82Asn,Asp}$
Hb$_{Yakima}$	$\alpha_2\beta_2{}^{99His}$	Hb$_{Agenogi}$	$\alpha_2\beta_2{}^{90Lys}$
Hb$_{Kempsey}$	$\alpha_2\beta_2{}^{99Asn}$	Hb$_{Beth\ Israel}$	$\alpha_2\beta_2{}^{102Ser}$
Hb$_{Ypsi\ (Ypsilanti)}$	$\alpha_2\beta_2{}^{99Tyr}$	Hb$_{Yoshizuka}$	$\alpha_2\beta_2{}^{108Asp}$
Hb$_{Hiroshima}$	$\alpha_2\beta_2{}^{146Asp}$	Hb$_{Seattle}$	$\alpha_2\beta_2{}^{70Asp}$
Hb$_{Rainier}$	$\alpha_2\beta_2{}^{145Cys}$		
Hb$_{Bethesda}$	$\alpha_2\beta_2{}^{145His}$		

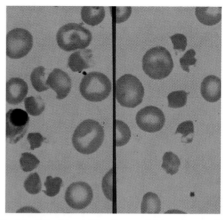

FIGURE 11–19 Unstable hemoglobin: hemoglobin$_{Zurich}$ (peripheral blood). (From Bell, A: Hematology. In Listen, Look and Learn. Health and Education Resources, Inc., Bethesda, MD, with permission.)

moglobin, erythropoietin concentrations fall. This can result in decreased hemoglobin concentration with the development of a mild anemia. There may also be mild cyanosis associated with a decreased oxygen saturation level. Hemoglobins with increased or decreased oxygen affinities are listed in Table 11–17. In cases of unexplained erythrocytosis or cyanosis, oxygen affinity studies may be helpful.

UNSTABLE HEMOGLOBINS

More than 180 unstable hemoglobins have been described, with fewer than 50% associated with a hemolytic disorder.[41,42] Unstable hemoglobins are hemoglobin variants in which amino acid substitutions or deletions have weakened the binding forces that maintain the structure of the molecule. The instability may cause hemoglobin to denature and precipitate in the red cells as Heinz bodies (see Fig. 4–2). Most unstable hemoglobin variants are inherited as autosomal dominant disorders.[41] However, absence of a positive family history is not always helpful, as new mutations are common. Many mutations producing unstable hemoglobinopathies are single amino acid substitutions in either the α, β, γ, or δ globin chains, which affect a few key areas of the hemoglobin structure. By far the majority of these substitutions are in the β-globin chain, followed by an α-chain substitution and only a few in γ or δ chains. Many of the unstable hemoglobins have high oxygen affinity and therefore may not cause anemia, making diagnosis in this group of patients particularly difficult. When anemia is present, the degree of hemolysis associated with an unstable hemoglobin varies considerably.[41] Some patients experience severe chronic hemolysis with jaundice and splenomegaly. However, most patients have a mild compensated condition and seek medical attention only after exacerbation of the hemolysis caused by infection and increased temperature or exposure to oxidative drugs.[41] Reticulocytosis is variable. Hypochromia may be apparent on the peripheral blood smear, and the mean red cell hemoglobin concentration (MCHC) can be low in some cases because the unstable hemoglobin may be denatured and "pitted" out of the cell by the

mononuclear phagocytic cells of the spleen. Figure 11–19 depicts erythrocytes in hemoglobin$_{Zurich}$, an unstable hemoglobin.

Hemoglobin electrophoresis is usually not a very helpful laboratory method to detect unstable hemoglobins; however, subtle indications of an abnormality may be observed.[41] These include an increased level of HbA$_2$, a common finding in unstable β-chain hemoglobins and the presence of minor electrophoretic components such as free α-globin chains indicative of an unstable β globin (Table 11–18).[41]

Most hospitals still perform the isopropanol precipitation or heat denaturation test for detection of unstable hemoglobins. Newer techniques such as isoelectric focusing can resolve many hemoglobin mutations with only a very slight alteration in their isoelectric point, and globin chain analysis can be performed by reversed phase HPLC (high-performance liquid chromatography).[41]

METHEMOGLOBINEMIA

Methemoglobinemia is a clinical condition associated with methemoglobin levels greater than 1% of the total hemoglobin.[43] Methemoglobin contains the oxidized ferric form of iron (Fe^{3+}) rather than ferrous form (Fe^{2+}). In this state, the molecule is unable to bind oxygen and results in cyanosis. The blood is chocolate-brown. Generally, there are three causes of methemoglobinemia:

1. Hemoglobin M variants (dominant inheritance)
2. NADH-diaphorase deficiency (recessive inheritance)
3. Toxic substance (acquired)

There are five variants of HbM (Table 11–19), which result from a single amino acid substitution in the globin chain that stabilizes iron in the ferric form. If the substitution occurs in the α chain, cyanosis is present at birth. Cyanosis does not occur with a β-chain substitution until approximately 6 months of age.[43] This

TABLE 11–18 Unstable Hemoglobins*

α-Chain Abnormalities		β-Chain Abnormalities		
Hb$_{Torina}$	$\alpha_2^{43Val}\beta_2$	Hb$_{Leiden}$	$\alpha_2\beta_2^{6or7}$	(Glu deleted)
Hb$_{L-Ferrara}$	$\alpha_2^{47Gly}\beta_2$	Hb$_{Sogn}$	$\alpha_2\beta_2^{14Arg}$	
Hb$_{Hasharon}$	$\alpha_2^{47His}\beta_2$	Hb$_{Freiburg}$	$\alpha_2\beta_2^{23}$	(Val deleted)
Hb$_{Ann\ Arbor}$	$\alpha_2^{80Arg}\beta_2$	Hb$_{Riverdale\ Bronx}$	$\alpha_2\beta_2^{24Arg}$	
Hb$_{Etobicoke}$	$\alpha_2^{84Arg}\beta_2$	Hb$_{Genova}$	$\alpha_2\beta_2^{28Pro}$	
Hb$_{Dakar}$	$\alpha_2^{112Gln}\beta_2$	Hb$_{Tacoma}$	$\alpha_2\beta_2^{30Ser}$	
Hb$_{Bibba}$	$\alpha_2^{136Pro}\beta_2$	Hb$_{Philly}$	$\alpha_2\beta_2^{35Phe}$	
		Hb$_{Louisville}$	$\alpha_2\beta_2^{42Leu}$	
		Hb$_{Hammersmith}$	$\alpha_2\beta_2^{42Ser}$	
		Hb$_{Zurich}$	$\alpha_2\beta_2^{63Arg}$	
		Hb$_{Toulouse}$	$\alpha_2\beta_2^{66Glu}$	
		Hb$_{Bristol}$	$\alpha_2\beta_2^{67Asp}$	
		Hb$_{Sydney}$	$\alpha_2\beta_2^{67Ala}$	
		Hb$_{Shepherd's\ Bush}$	$\alpha_2\beta_2^{74Asp}$	
		Hb$_{Seattle}$	$\alpha_2\beta_2^{70ASP}$	
		Hb$_{Boras}$	$\alpha_2\beta_2^{88Arg}$	
		Hb$_{Santa\ Ana}$	$\alpha_2\beta_2^{88Pro}$	
		Hb$_{Gun\ Hill}$	$\alpha_2\beta_2^{91-95}$	(5 a.a. deleted)
		Hb$_{Sabine}$	$\alpha_2\beta_2^{91Pro}$	
		Hb$_{Köln}$	$\alpha_2\beta_2^{98Met}$	
		Hb$_{Kansas}$	$\alpha_2\beta_2^{102Thr}$	
		Hb$_{Wein}$	$\alpha_2\beta_2^{130Asp}$	
		Hb$_{Olmsted}$	$\alpha_2\beta_2^{141Arg}$	

*Hemoglobins that may precipitate as Heinz bodies after splenectomy: congenital Heinz body hemolytic anemia. a.a. = amino acids

correlates with the switch from γ to β chains. The presumptive diagnosis of HbM is made from the absorption spectra of hemolysates, and hemoglobin electrophoresis on agar gel at pH 7.1.[43] Patients have obvious cyanosis but otherwise are generally asymptomatic. No specific treatment is indicated or possible.

The enzyme NADH-diaphorase reduces cytochrome b5, which converts the naturally occurring ferric iron back to the ferrous state. To confirm NADH-diaphorase deficiency, a quantitative enzyme assay is necessary. Although nearly all enzyme-deficient individuals are asymptomatic, some find their lifelong cyanosis to be a cosmetic hardship. The level of methemoglobin can be reduced with the administration of ascorbic acid or methylene blue.[43]

Acquired methemoglobinemia can occur in healthy individuals when drugs or other toxic substances oxidize hemoglobin in circulation. Patients who appear to be symptomatic from methemoglobinemia should be treated promptly with intravenous methylene blue.

TABLE 11–19 Hemoglobins Associated with Methemoglobinemia and Cyanosis

HbM$_{Boston}$	$\alpha_2^{58Tyr}\beta_2$
HbM$_{Iwate}$	$\alpha_2^{87Tyr}\beta_2$
HbM$_{Saskatoon}$	$\alpha_2\beta_2^{63Tyr}$
HbM$_{Milwaukee}$	$\alpha_2\beta_2^{67Glu}$
HbM$_{Hyde\ Park}$	$\alpha_2\beta_2^{92Tyr}$

GENERAL SUMMARY OF LABORATORY DIAGNOSIS

Hemoglobinopathies usually cannot be correctly diagnosed with a single laboratory procedure. It is usually necessary to correlate the results of a CBC and RBC indices with additional laboratory tests such as a reticulocyte count, peripheral smear evaluation, hemoglobin electrophoresis, and, if necessary, measurement of HbA$_2$ and HbF. Selected patient information such as age, gender, ethnic background, family history, and physical symptoms is helpful.

Most abnormal hemoglobins are associated with RBC indices that are normocytic and normochromic. Microcytosis and hypochromia are seen in some variants (e.g., HbE). Abnormal red cell morphology may or may not be noted on the peripheral blood smear, and reticulocyte counts are often elevated.

Screening tests include hemoglobin electrophoresis, isoelectric focusing (IEF), and HPLC.

Cellulose acetate electrophoresis at alkaline pH (see Fig. 11–10) is commonly performed first. Electrophoresis on citrate agar at acid pH can further differentiate abnormal hemoglobins. HbF quantitation should be done following the newborn period, when this hemoglobin is seen on cellulose acetate.

IEF, a type of sensitive electrophoresis, separates hemoglobins according to their isoelectric points. Superior IEF resolution differentiates some hemoglobins that migrate to the same electrophoretic point at alkaline and acid pH. On the initial patient visit, other laboratory tests should also be performed, including urinalysis; liver function tests; and urea, creatinine, and electrolyte measurements. In addition, a chest x-ray should be obtained.

CASE STUDY

A 13-year-old African-American girl was admitted to the hospital appearing acutely ill with fever and abdominal pain. On physical examination, an enlarged spleen was evident. Laboratory test results were as follows:

Hgb	5.0 g/dL
Hct	15%
RBC	$1.4 \times 10^{12}/L$
WBC	$2.2 \times 10^9/L$
Reticulocyte count	1%
Differential	
Segmented neutrophils	62%
Bands	12%
Lymphocytes	19%
Monocytes	4%
Eosinophils	2%
Basophils	1%
RBC indices	Normal
Platelet count	$400 \times 10^9/L$
Peripheral blood smear	(see Fig. 11–16)

Hemoglobin electrophoresis, alkaline pH, showed one band in the HbS position, and one band in the HbC position. The hemoglobins were quantified as 55% HbS and 45% HbC + A_2. HbS and HbC were confirmed by electrophoresis at acid pH.

Questions

1. Describe the morphological features of this peripheral blood smear.
2. In reviewing the electrophoretic data, what diagnosis is suggested?
3. Comment on crystal formation in this condition.
4. Discuss the clinical presentation of the patient. Is it consistent with HbSC disease?
5. This young girl's parents have no hematologic problems; therefore, for her to have HbSC disease, what would be their most likely genotypes?
6. The inheritance of structurally abnormal hemoglobins follows simple mendelian laws. With parents having the trait form of HbS and HbC, what would be the expected genotypes in each of four children?

Answers

1. Numerous target cells are present on the peripheral blood smear, along with some cells that appear to have shadows of precipitating intraerythrocytic crystals.
2. The data suggest a diagnosis of HbSC disease.
3. The crystals in HbSC disease appear to be only partially formed, or there may be more than one formation. The crystals in the red cells often are described as having a glove-shaped appearance with several "fingers" protruding.
4. Generally, HbSC disease has a milder presentation than SCA; however, this patient appears to be experiencing a severe episode of SC crisis. This is indicated by her acute illness, abdominal pain, and a decrease in hemoglobin and hemat-

ocrit levels without an increase in the reticulocyte count.
5. With no hematologic problems, one parent would be expected to have HbS trait (HbAS), while the other would most likely have HbC trait (HbAC).
6. The probability for offspring would be one child with HbAA, one with HbAS, one with HbAC, and one with HbSC.

REFERENCES

1. Huisman, TH: The structure and function of normal and abnormal haemoglobins. Baillieres Clin Hematol 6:1–30, 1993.
2. Steinberg, MH: Genetic modulation of sickle cell anemia. Proc Soc Exp Biol Med 209:1–13, 1995.
3. Herrick, JB: Peculiar elongated and sickle-shaped red corpuscles in a case of severe anemia. Arch Intern Med 6:517, 1910.
4. Pauling, L, et al: Sickle cell anemia, a molecular disease. Science 110:543, 1949.
5. Sickle Cell Disease Guideline Panel. Sickle Cell Disease: Screening, Diagnosis, Management, and Counseling in Newborns and Infants. Clinical Practice Guideline No. 6. AHCPR Pub. No 93-0562. Rockville, MD: Agency for Health Care Policy and Research, Public Health Service, U.S. Department of Health and Human Services. April, 1993.
6. Sickle Cell Disease: Guideline and Overview. Am J Hematol. 47:152–154, 1994.
7. Charache, S, Lubin, BL, and Reid, CD (eds): Management and Therapy of Sickle Cell Disease. U.S. Department of Health and Human Services, Public Health Service, National Institutes of Health. NIH Publication 91:2117, August, 1991.
8. Steinberg, MH: Sickle cell anemia and fetal hemoglobin. Am J Med Sci 308:259–265, 1994.
9. Bastian, HM: Hematologic disorders including sickle cell syndromes, hemophilia, and beta-thalassemia. Curr Op Rheumatol 7:70–72, 1995.
10. Embury, SH, Hebbel, RP, Mohandas, N, and Steinberg, MH: Sickle Cell Disease: Basic Principles and Clinical Practice. Raven Press, New York, 1994.
11. Piomelli, S: Sickle cell disease in the 1990s: The need for active and preventive intervention. Semin Hematol 28:227–232, 1991.
12. Platt, OS, Brambilla, DJ, Rosse, WF, Milner, PF, et al: Mortality in sickle cell disease. Life expectancy and risk factors for early death. N Engl J Med 13:331:1022–1023, 1994.
13. Shinar, E and Rachmilewitz, EA: Hemoglobinopathies and red cell membrane function. National Magen David Adom Blood Bank, National Blood Services. Tel hashomer, Israel 6:357–369, 1993.
14. Lee, GR: Wintrobes Clinical Hematology. Lea & Febiger, Philadelphia, 1993.
15. Hess, DC, Adams, RJ, and Nichols, FT: Sickle cell anemia and other hemoglobinopathies. Semin Neurol 11:314–328, December 1991.
16. Sandhaus, LM and Harvey, FG: Laboratory methods for the detection of hemoglobinopathies in the community hospital. Clin Lab Med 13:801–816, 1993.
17. Camaschella, C and Saglio, G: Recent advances in diagnosis of hemoglobinopathies. Critical Rev Oncol Hematol 14:89–105, 1993.
18. Clinical Alert from the National Heart, Lung, and Blood Institute (NHLB). January, 1995.
19. Charache, S and Terrin, ML: Effect of hydroxyurea on the frequency of painful crises in sickle cell anemia. N Engl J Med 18:1372–1374, 1995.

20. Adragna, NC, Fonseca, P and Lauf, PK: Hydroxyurea affects cell morphology, cation transport, and red blood cell adhesion in cultured vascular endothelial cells. Blood 83:553–560, 1994.
21. Ohene-Frempong, K, Honiuchi, K, Bulgarelli, W, et al: Hydroxyurea increase HbF production in children with sickle cell disease. Blood 82:472a, 1993.
22. The Multicenter Study of Hydroxyurea. Preventing pain in sickle cell anemia (HbSS) baseline data from patients in a hydroxyurea trial. Blood 82:356a, 1993.
23. Wang, WC, Kovnar, EH, Tonkin, IL, et al: High risk of recurrent strokes after discontinuance of five to twelve years of transfusion therapy in patients with sickle cell disease. J Pediatr 118:377–382, 1991.
24. Perrine, SP, Ginder, GD, Faller, DV, et al: A short-term trial of butyrate to stimulate fetal-globin-gene expression in the beta-globin disorders. N Engl J Med 328:81–86, 1993.
25. Sher, GD, Entsush, B, Ginder, G, et al: Intravenous infusions of arginine butyrate increases γ-globin mRNA expression and F-reticulocytes in patients (PTS) with homozygous β-thalassemia and sickle cell disease. Blood 82:312a, 1993.
26. Dover, GJ, Brisilow, S, Charache, S: Induction of fetal hemoglobin production in subjects with sickle cell anemia by oral sodium phenybutyrate. Blood 84:339–343, 1994.
27. Fibach, E, Prasanna, P, Rodgers, GP, Samid D: Enhanced fetal hemoglobin production by phenylacetate and 4-phenylbutyrate in erythroid precursors derived from normal donors and patients with sickle cell disease. Blood 82:2203–2206, 1993.
28. Johnson, FL, Mentzer, WC, Kalinyak, KA, et al: Bone marrow transplantation for sickle cell disease: The United States experience. Am J Pediatr Hematol Oncol 16:22–26, 1994.
29. Beutler, E and Sullivan, KM: Bone marrow transplantation for sickle cell disease. In Forman, SJ, Blume, KG, and Thomas, ED (eds): Bone Marrow Transplantation. Blackwell Boston, 1994, pp. 840–848.
30. Thomas ED: Marrow transplantation for non-malignant disorders. N Engl J Med 312:46–47, 1985.
31. Rodgers, GP, Olivieri, NF, Sullivan, K, and Kan, YW: Current and future strategies for the management of hemoglobinopathies and thalassemia. The Education Program of ASH. Nashville, TN, December 2–6, 1994.
32. Bernaudin, F, Hernigou, PH, Kuentz M, et al: Favorable evolution of sickle cell disease (SCD) related osteonecrosis after bone marrow transplantation (BMT). Blood 82:355a, 1993.
33. Ferster, A, Bujan, W, Corazza, F, et al: Bone marrow transplantation corrects the splenic reticuloendothelial dysfunction in sickle cell anemia. Blood 81:1102–1105, 1993.
34. Vermylen, C and Cornu, G: Bone marrow transplantation for sickle cell disease: The European experience. Am J Pediatr Hematol Oncol 16:22–26, 1994.
35. Walsh, CE, Liu, JM, Miller, JL, et al: Gene therapy for human hemoglobinopathies. Proc Soc Exp Biol Med 204:289–300, 1993.
36. Walsh, CE, Liu, JM, Xiao, X, et al: Regulated high level expression of a human gamma-globin gene introduced into erythroid cells by an adeno-associated virus vector. Proc Natl Acad Sci 89:7257–7261, 1992.
37. Mulligan, RC: The basis science of gene therapy. Science 260:926–932, 1993.
38. Kiem, HP, Darovsky, B, von Kalle, C, et al: Retrovirus-mediated gene transduction into canine peripheral blood repopulating cells. Blood 83:1467–1473, 1994.
39. Steinberg, MH: Genetic modulation of sickle cell anemia. Proc Soc Exp Biol Med 209(1):1–13, 1995.
40. Lubin, BH, Witkowska, HE, and Kleman, K: Laboratory diagnosis of hemoglobinopathies. Clin Biochem 24:363–374, 1991.
41. Williamson, D: The unstable hemoglobins. Blood Rev 7:146–163, 1993.
42. International Hemoglobin Information Center, Variants list. Hemoglobin 16:217–160, 1992.
43. Williams, WJ, Beutler, E, Erslev, AJ, et al: Hematology, ed 5. McGraw-Hill, New York, 1995.

QUESTIONS

1. Which of the following is not a characteristic of hemoglobinopathies?
   a. Conditions in which abnormal hemoglobins are synthesized
   b. Result from inherited abnormalities or genetic mutations
   c. All are manifested in clinically significant conditions
   d. Result in a defect in structural integrity of function of the hemoglobin molecule

2. Which of the following are used in the nomenclature system for abnormal hemoglobins?
   a. Capital letters
   b. Names of places
   c. Names of chains and substitutions
   d. All of the above

3. What is the amino acid substitution found in sickle cell anemia?
   a. Substitution of valine for glutamic acid in the sixth position from the NH_2 terminal beta chain
   b. Substitution of lysine for glutamic acid in the sixth position from the NH_2 terminal beta chain
   c. Substitution of lysine for glutamic acid in the 26th position from the NH_2 terminal beta chain
   d. Substitution of valine for glutamic acid in the 121st position from the NH_2 terminal beta chain

4. What factors contribute to the sickling of RBCs?
   a. Increase in pH and oxygenation
   b. Decrease in pH and oxygenation and dehydration
   c. Increase in pH and decrease in oxygenation
   d. Decrease in dehydration and increase in pH and oxygenation

5. Which of the following are crises associated with sickle cell anemia?
   a. Aplastic crisis with low reticulocyte count and infections
   b. Hemolytic crisis with splenic sequestration; decreased hemoglobin and hematocrit, increased reticulocyte count, and jaundice
   c. Vaso-occlusive/painful crises with severe pain, tissue damage, and necrosis
   d. All of the above

6. What are the therapeutic goals in the treatment of sickle cell anemia?
   a. Decrease microvascular entrapment of sickle cells or change the volume of RBCs
   b. Modify oxygen affinity or solubility of sickle hemoglobin
   c. Increase production of fetal hemoglobin
   d. All of the above

7. What is the amino acid substitution found in hemoglobin C disease?
   a. Substitution of valine for glutamic acid in the sixth position from the NH_2 terminal beta chain
   b. Substitution of lysine for glutamic acid in the sixth position from the NH_2 terminal beta chain

c. Substitution of lysine for glutamic acid in the 26th position from the NH$_2$ terminal beta chain

d. Substitution of valine for glutamic acid in the 121st position from the NH$_2$ terminal beta chain

8. Which of the following is not true for hemoglobin C disease?
   a. Mild anemia
   b. Numerous target cells
   c. Crystals in red cells
   d. Hemoglobin C can be separated from other hemoglobins at an alkaline pH

9. Which finding would be most useful in establishing a diagnosis of hemoglobin SC disease?
   a. Target cells and sickle cells on peripheral blood smear
   b. Severe anemia; increased reticulocyte count
   c. Hemoglobin electrophoresis at alkaline pH
   d. RBC indices

10. Which of the following is a cause of methemoglobinemia?
    a. Hemoglobin M variants

b. NADH-diaphorase deficiency

c. Toxic substances

d. All of the above

ANSWERS

1. **c** (pp 173–174)
2. **d** (p 175)
3. **a** (p 176)
4. **b** (p 176)
5. **d** (p 177)
6. **d** (p 183 [Table 11–12])
7. **b** (pp 183–184)
8. **d** (pp 184–185)
9. **c** (p 185)
10. **d** (p 188)

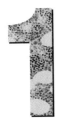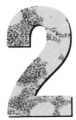

Hemolytic Anemias: Intracorpuscular Defects

IV. THALASSEMIA

Chantal Ricaud Harrison, MD

Objectives

At the end of this chapter, the learner should be able to:
 1 Name the hemoglobin defect of thalassemia.
 2 Describe the clinical expression of different gene combinations of alpha and beta thalassemia.
 3 Describe the condition known as hereditary persistence of fetal hemoglobin (HPFH).
 4 Name the most characteristic laboratory finding for the diagnosis of thalassemia.
 5 List red cell indices that help to distinguish thalassemia from iron deficiency.
 6 Describe the appearance of the peripheral smear in thalassemia.
 7 Explain the use of the Kleihauer-Betke acid elution test in the diagnosis of thalassemia.
 8 Name the test used as a population screening test for thalassemia carriers.
 9 List conditions in which quantitation of hemoglobin F is important.
 10 Describe the use of routine chemistries for differentiation of thalassemia from iron-deficiency anemia.

The thalassemia syndromes consist of a diverse group of inherited disorders that manifest themselves clinically as anemia of varying degrees. These disorders are the result of a defective production of the globin portion of the hemoglobin.

In 1925 Thomas B. Cooley and Pearl Lee described the first cases of severe thalassemia in several North American children of Mediterranean origin.[1] *Cooley's anemia* is still a commonly used term for this form of severe thalassemia, which is also termed *thalassemia major*. The name *thalassemia* was actually applied to these clinical syndromes a few years later. The term is derived from the Greek word *thalassa*, which means "sea," since at that time all of the cases described were from the Mediterranean coastal region. It is now well known that the distribution of thalassemia is

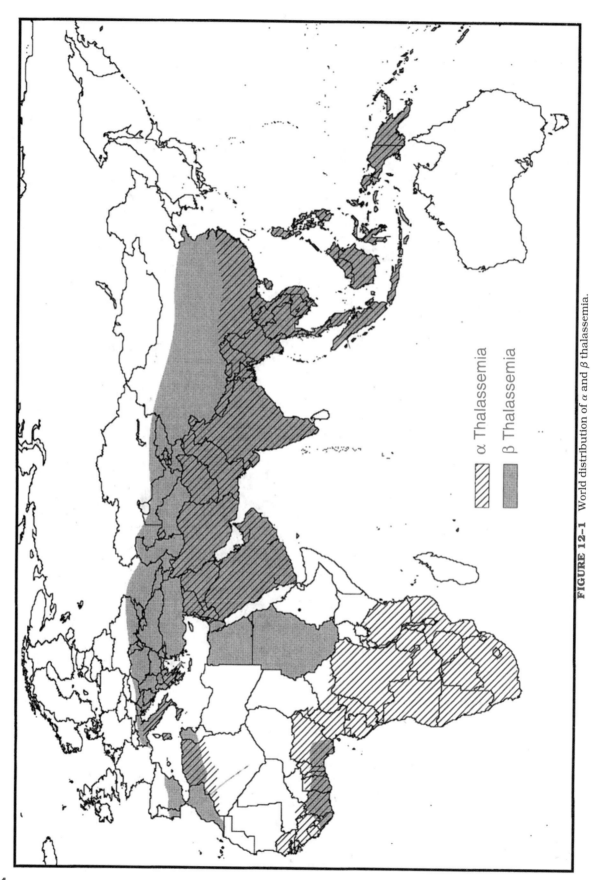

FIGURE 12–1 World distribution of α and β thalassemia.

α Thalassemia

β Thalassemia

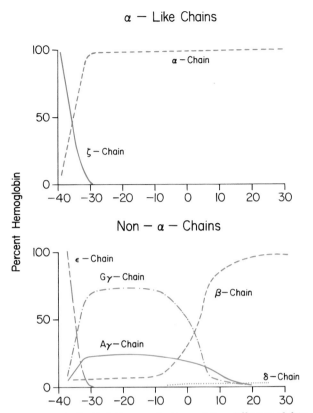

FIGURE 12-2 Relative production of the different globin chains from conception to 30 weeks after birth. (*Top*) ζ embryonic chain production has been almost totally replaced by α chain production around 12 weeks after conception. (*Bottom*) ϵ chain production runs parallel with zeta chain production. The β chain production stays at very low levels from 6 weeks after conception until it increases suddenly a few weeks before birth, while the γ chain production suddenly decreases. The δ chain production starts a few weeks before birth and stays low. The $G\gamma$ chain to $A\gamma$ chain production ratio is 3:1 before birth and gradually reverses to 2:3 during the first few months of life.

worldwide and not restricted to the Mediterranean Sea area. It was later realized that the original severe clinical disease described by Cooley was the result of a homozygous defect in hemoglobin production, whereas many milder cases described as *thalassemia minima* or *thalassemia minor* were manifestations of a heterozygous defect.

The thalassemia syndromes are often considered part of a larger category of hematologic disorders called hemoglobinopathies (disorders in hemoglobin synthesis or production). Hemoglobinopathies are further divided into two main categories. One group is the result of an inherited structural defect in one of the globin chains resulting in an abnormal hemoglobin (true hemoglobinopathies), which may have abnormal physical or physiologic properties. Examples of these structural abnormalities are hemoglobin S, hemoglobin C, hemoglobin E, and so on. The second group consists of the thalassemia syndromes, which are caused by an abnormality in the rate of synthesis of the globin chains. With a few minor exceptions, the globin chains

produced are structurally normal, but there is an imbalance in production of the two different types of chain, resulting in an absolute decrease in the amount of normal hemoglobin formed, as well as an excess production of one type of chain that may precipitate and induce hemolysis.

There are two major types of thalassemia: α thalassemia, which is caused by a defect in the rate of synthesis of alpha chains, and β thalassemia, caused by a defect in the rate of synthesis of β chains. The world distribution of thalassemia is summarized in Figure 12–1. The marked similarity in worldwide distribution of thalassemia with malignant malaria caused by *Plasmodium falciparum* has been attributed to the process of gene selection secondary to a protective effect against *P. falciparum* malaria brought about by the heterozygous state of thalassemia.[2]

Because the hemoglobin structural variants (such as hemoglobin S and hemoglobin C in West Africans and African-Americans or hemoglobin E in Southeast Asians) occur in the same population where α or β thalassemia is frequent, the two types of genetic defects may be found in the same person, resulting in variability of clinical expression of the two defects.

GENETICS OF HEMOGLOBIN SYNTHESIS

All normal human hemoglobins have a general tetrameric structure consisting of two alphalike (alpha or zeta, respectively, abbreviated as α or ζ) and two betalike (beta, delta, A-gamma, G-gamma, or epsilon, respectively, abbreviated as β, δ, $^A\gamma$, $^G\gamma$, and ϵ) chains (see Chap. 3). In the normal adult, most (95% to 97%) of the hemoglobin is $\alpha_2\beta_2$ (hemoglobin A) and a minor fraction (about 2.5%) is $\alpha_2\delta_2$ (hemoglobin A₂). A small amount of hemoglobin F (always less than 2%) may also be found. Figure 12–2 demonstrates the relative amount of the different globin chains produced from embryonic stage to early childhood. Table 12–1 lists the different normal hemoglobins found throughout human development, as well as the abnormal hemoglobins found in patients with thalassemia. The ζ and α globin genes are found on chromosome 16 and the

TABLE 12–1 **Composition of Hemoglobins Found in Normal Human Development and Abnormal Hemoglobins Found in Thalassemia**

Globin Chains	Hemoglobin	State
$\alpha_2\beta_2$	A	Adult
$\alpha_2\delta_2$	A₂	
$\alpha_2 A\gamma_2$	F	Fetus
$\alpha_2 G\gamma_2$	F	
$\alpha_2\epsilon_2$	Gower 2	↑
$\zeta_2\epsilon_2$	Gower 1	Embryo
$\zeta_2\gamma_2$	Portland	
β_4	H	α Thalassemia
γ_4	Bart's	
α_2 precipitate	—	β Thalassemia

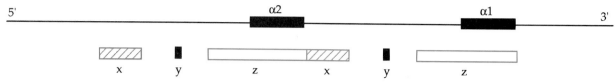

FIGURE 12-3   The areas of homology (x, y, and z) can lead to mispairing.

genes for ϵ, $^G\gamma$, $^A\gamma$, δ and β globins on chromosome 11. There are two closely linked genes, both active and coding for identical α-globin chains though at different levels of activity in the normal adult. The α_2-globin gene is expressed at two to three times the rate of the α_1-globin gene.[3] Detailed mapping of the DNA shows great similarity between the two α genes and between the two regions immediately upstream (5') of each α gene.[4] There are three areas of homology in DNA blocks called x, y, and z (Fig. 12–3) including or juxtaposed to the α genes. These homologous blocks render this area more susceptible to mispairing. Crossing over in this area of chromosome 16 may result in deletions of one α gene. Occasionally a chromosome with three α genes can be produced. This explains why most α thalassemias are the result of a gene deletion. On the other hand, most β thalassemias are the result of point mutation affecting the regulation of the rate of production of the β-globin chain. To better understand how this occurs, a short review of the biochemical progression from the original chromosomal deoxyribonucleic acid (DNA) to the final globin chain polypeptide is shown in Figure 12–4. The gene is represented by a length of chromosomal DNA, which consists of alternating coding and noncoding (or intervening) sequences. These are often referred to as *exons* and *introns*, respectively. Only the coding sequences (exons) contain the information that will be finally translated into the polypeptide chain. The exact role of the intervening sequences (introns) is not clear at present, although it is thought that they may be involved in the rate of progression of the synthetic process. The DNA is transcribed into a large ribonucleic acid (RNA) called heterogeneous nuclear RNA (HnRNA), which contains all the coding and noncoding sequences of the genes. This HnRNA is then processed into the messenger RNA (mRNA), which contains only the coding sequences and which diffuses into the cytoplasm to be translated by the ribosomes

into the final globin chain. Upstream of the coding portion of the gene (also called the 5' direction) are promoter areas crucial to the initiation of transcription and to the level and accuracy of the gene expression.

The genetic defect in β thalassemia is usually the result of a point mutation affecting: (1) one of the noncoding intervening sequences of the original globin-chain gene, producing inefficient splicing from HnRNA to mRNA, thereby decreasing the amount of mRNA produced; (2) the promoter area decreasing the rate of expression of the gene; (3) the termination of the gene that leads to the lengthening of the globin chain with additional amino acids, in which case the mRNA is unstable causing a reduction in globin synthesis; and (4) the creation of a stop codon leading to early termination of the globin-chain synthesis.[5] In all cases the final result is a decreased or absent production of the β-globin chain.

PATHOPHYSIOLOGY OF THALASSEMIA

Figure 12–5 illustrates the formation of the normal human hemoglobin from two identical globin chains coded by chromosome 11 and two identical globin chains coded by chromosome 16.

In thalassemia there is a defect in the rate of production of one of the globin chains, resulting in a decrease in the amount of normal physiologic hemoglobin produced, creating a microcytic, hypochromic anemia. There will also be an excess of globin chains produced by the unaffected genes. In the case of α thalassemia, the excess γ chains and β chains can form stable tetramers: hemoglobin Bart's (γ_4) and hemoglobin H (β_4), respectively. However, these hemoglobins are physiologically useless and precipitate in older red cells, causing a shortened red cell life span. In the case of β thalassemia, the excess α chains form α_2 precipitates, which cause hemolysis of the red cell precursors in the bone marrow, resulting in ineffective erythropoiesis.

Beta Thalassemia

In beta (β) thalassemia the disease will not manifest itself until the switch from γ-chain to β-chain synthesis has been completed. This usually occurs several months after birth. Thus, the clinical presentation of a patient with this disease usually occurs during the first year of life. There is often compensatory absolute or relative increase in production of γ chains and δ chains, resulting in an increased level of hemoglobin F and hemoglobin A_2. The genetic background for β thalassemia is very heterogeneous and over 90 different mutations have been described, but they may be

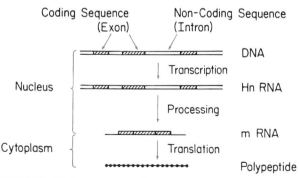

FIGURE 12-4   Diagram of the progression from gene to peptide. Hn = heterogeneous nuclear; m = messenger.

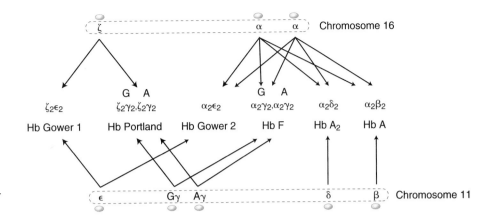

FIGURE 12-5 Formation of normal human hemoglobins.

broadly subdivided into β^0 and β^+ thalassemia. At the molecular level, there is heterogeneity in the basis for the genetic abnormality with a specific group of mutations commonly found in each geographic area.[6]

β^0 Thalassemia

This gene results in complete absence of production of β chains. This particular gene is commonly found in the Mediterranean area, particularly in northern Italy, Greece, Algeria, and Saudi Arabia. It is also common in Southeast Asia.

β^+ Thalassemia

The β^+-thalassemia gene produces a reduced number of β chains. There is heterogeneity in β^+ thalassemia, and at least three different groups of genes have been described. The type 1 β^+-thalassemia gene produces the least amount of β chains (about 10% of normal production) and is found throughout the Mediterranean region, the Middle East, the Indian subcontinent, and Southeast Asia. The type 2 β^+-thalassemia gene produces a greater amount of β chains (about 50% of normal production) and is characteristically found in the blacks of West Africa and North America. The type 3 β^+-thalassemia gene produces an even greater number of β chains and causes a much milder form of β thalassemia. It is found sporadically in Italy, Greece, and the Middle East.

Clinical Expression of the Different Gene Combinations

Homozygosity for the β^0 or β^+ thalassemia gene, or compound heterozygosity for the β^0 and β^+ genes, causes a severe form of thalassemia called *thalassemia major*. The only exception is perhaps the homozygous type 2 or type 3 β^+ thalassemia, which causes a milder form of thalassemia that has sometimes been called *thalassemia intermedia*. In thalassemia major, a severe hypochromic, microcytic anemia develops during the first year of life (Fig. 12–6). The hemoglobin level is usually below 7 g/dL and consists mostly of hemoglobin F and hemoglobin A₂. This severe chronic anemia starting so early in life is a strong stimulus for eryth-

ropoiesis. This causes marked expansion of the marrow space and characteristic skeletal changes of the skull, long bones, and hand bones. The skull radiographs show widening of the diploic space and demonstrate characteristic radiating striations giving typical "hair-on-end" appearance (Fig. 12–7). The marrow expansion of the facial bones produces a characteristic facial appearance with hypertrophy of the maxilla causing forward protrusion of the upper teeth and overbite, a relatively sunken nose, widely spaced eyes, and prominent cheek bones, resulting in a Mongoloid facies (Fig. 12–8). The long bones of the hands and feet have cortical thinning with porosity of the medullary space. These changes are not a specific feature of thalassemia and are found in other severe chronic congenital hemolytic anemias, but are most prominent in β thalassemia major. Without careful medical supervision and a therapeutic program including blood transfusions, iron chelation, and early treatment of infection, children with thalassemia major will have numerous complications, which include massive hepatosplenomegaly, recurrent infections, spontaneous

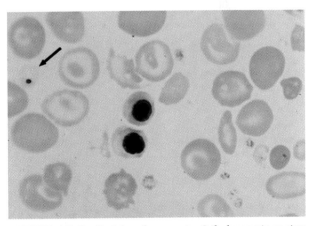

FIGURE 12-6 Peripheral smear in β-thalassemia major. Note the nucleated red cells, the Howell-Jolly body in the hypochromic microcyte (*arrow*), the numerous target cells, and the moderate anisocytosis and poikilocytosis (Wright's stain). (From Bell, A: Hematology. In Listen, Look and Learn. Health and Education Resources, Inc., Bethesda, MD, with permission.)

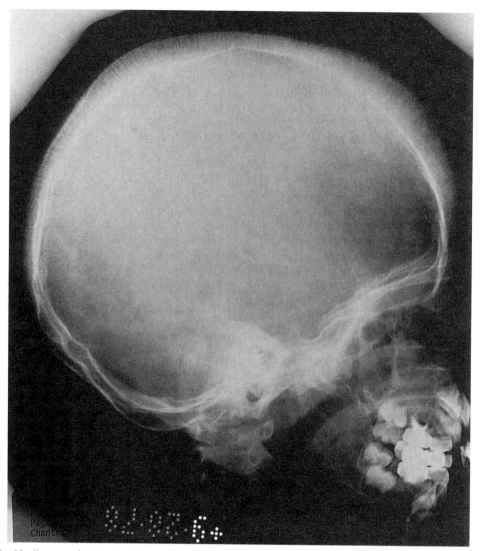

FIGURE 12-7   Skull x-ray of a 5-year-old child with homozygous β-thalassemia. Note the dilatation of the diploic space and the typical "hair-on-end" appearance caused by subperiosteal bone growth in radiating strations.

fractures, leg ulcers, dental and orthodontic problems, and compression syndromes caused by tumor masses from extramedullary hematopoiesis. If the condition is left untreated, these children will usually die in early childhood.

Heterozygosity for the β^0- or β^+-thalassemia gene causes a mild form of chronic hypochromic, microcytic anemia that has been called "thalassemia minor" (Fig. 12–9). Although the degree of anemia is variable with hemoglobin levels from 10.5 to 13.9 g/dL, it is impossible to determine whether the patient has the β^0 or β^+ gene on clinical grounds alone. In general, the levels of hemoglobin F and hemoglobin A_2 are mildly elevated. The patients are usually completely asymptomatic, although symptoms may occur under stressful situations, such as pregnancy. The patient with heterozygous β^+ type 3 thalassemia usually shows no clinical or laboratory evidence of anemia and has been called the silent carrier.

Alpha Thalassemia

In contrast to β thalassemia, alpha (α) thalassemia is usually manifested immediately at birth and even in utero, as the α genes are activated early in fetal life. Another characteristic of α thalassemia is that because each chromosome 16 carries two α genes, the total normal complement of α genes is 4. Thus, there will be a greater variety in severity of disease, as one, two, three, or four α genes may be affected in one patient.

Owing to the wide variety of genetic backgrounds and the difficulty in defining the heterozygous carrier state, there has been much confusion in the classification and nomenclature of α thalassemias. Much of this confusion is the result of the indiscriminate use of a phenotypic or genotypic classification without clear definition. We will use a genotypic classification that parallels the classification used for β thalassemia.

Another characteristic of α thalassemia is the fact

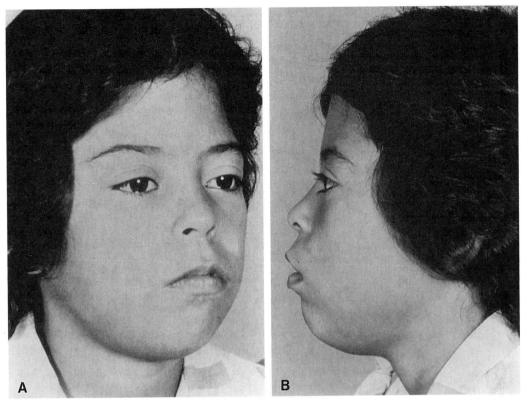

FIGURE 12–8 (*A*) Front face and (*B*) profile of an 11-year-old child with homozygous β-thalassemia who is receiving hypertransfusion. The characteristic facial changes are not as prominent as in an untransfused child but are still present. Note bossing of the skull, hypertrophy of the maxilla with prominent malar eminences, depression of the bridge of the nose, and mongoloid slant of the eyes.

that the decreased or absent α-chain production will result in excess γ chains during fetal life and at birth and in excess β chains later on. This will cause the formation of stable tetramers, such as γ_4 (hemoglobin Bart's) and β_4 (hemoglobin H), which can be detected by hemoglobin electrophoresis. These stable, nonfunctional tetramers precipitate in older red cells, forming

[figure]

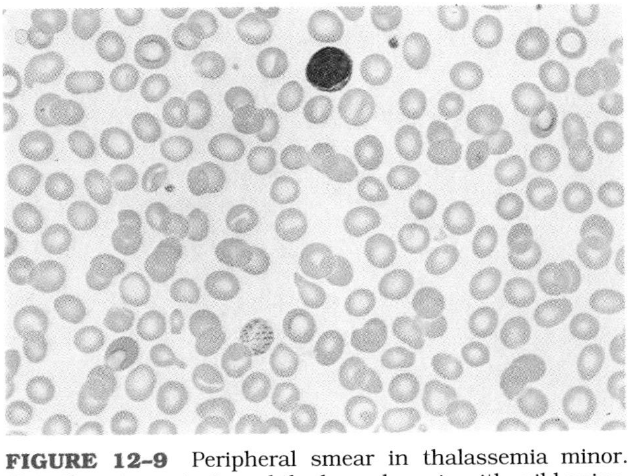

FIGURE 12–9 Peripheral smear in thalassemia minor. Note the microcytosis and the hypochromia with mild anisocytosis and poikilocytosis. A few target cells and basophilic stippling are present. (Wright's stain, magnification ×400)

inclusion bodies, and interfere with membrane function, which results in decreased red cell survival and may induce a hemolytic crisis during infectious episodes.

α^0 Thalassemia (α Thalassemia 1)

α^0 *Thalassemia* and *alpha thalassemia 1* have been used interchangeably in the past to describe a genetic determinant. However, because α thalassemia 1 has been also used to describe the phenotypic or clinical expression of a disease, α^0 thalassemia is the preferred term for the description of the genetic determinant. This gene results in complete absence of production of α chains. This means that both α genes on chromosome 16 are nonfunctional. Studies by DNA hybridization techniques have shown that the α^0 determinant is the result of α-gene deletions. In addition, they also demonstrated that there are at least nine major haplotypes resulting in α^0 thalassemia, depending on the amount of DNA that has been deleted from the chromosome. Each haplotype appears to be characteristic of a certain population in the world. α^0-Thalassemia genes are found frequently in Southeast Asia and less frequently in the Mediterranean area. They also occur sporadically in other parts of the world. This gene may be recognized in adults through the detection of small amounts of ζ-globin chain.[7]

α^+ Thalassemia (α Thalassemia 2)

Again α^+ *thalassemia* is the better term to describe the genetic determinant, because *alpha thalassemia 2* has been used to describe both the genetic determinant and a phenotypic expression. The α^+-thalassemia gene is characterized by a reduction in the output of α chains. This may be because of a deletion of a single α gene on chromosome 16, which leaves the other α gene intact and able to function. Other types of α^+-thalassemia genes are caused by nondeletion mutants that affect the regulation of the α-chain synthesis. This is similar to the situation in the β thalassemias. A third type of α^+-thalassemia genetic background is associated with α-globin structural mutants. Overall, a minimum of 20 major genetic defects resulting in the α^+-thalassemia gene have been defined. These different thalassemia genes result in different levels of α-chain output. For example, the nondeletion regulatory type of defect, also called $\alpha\alpha^T$ and found in Saudi Arabia, is more severe than the single-gene-deletion type of defect, also called $-\alpha$ and commonly found throughout the Mediterranean area, the Middle East area, the Indian subcontinent, Southeast Asia, Africa, and Malaysia.

Clinical Expression of the Different Gene Combinations

α Thalassemia can be divided into four clinical categories depending on the severity of the disease. The most severe expression of α thalassemia is the hemoglobin Bart's hydrops fetalis syndrome, which is caused by homozygosity of the α^0-thalassemia gene. This is a lethal disease, and infants with hemoglobin Bart's hydrops fetalis die either in utero or soon after birth. They produce no α chain, and the only hemoglobins found are hemoglobin Bart's (γ_4) and hemoglobin Portland ($\zeta_2\gamma_2$). Because hemoglobin Bart's is useless as an oxygen carrier, survival of the fetus into the third trimester or until birth is entirely the result of the presence of hemoglobin Portland. At birth, these infants are severely anemic and edematous, and demonstrate ascites, marked hepatomegaly, and splenomegaly. Significant morbidity and mortality can occur in the mothers, owing to obstetric complications. This condition is quite common in Southeast Asia and is found sporadically in the Mediterranean area.

The second most severe clinical expression of α thalassemia is hemoglobin H disease. In this entity, only one α gene out of four is functioning. This is usually the result of a double heterozygosity of an α^0-thalassemia gene with an α^+-thalassemia gene but is also found in Saudi Arabia as the result of homozygosity of the more severe form of the α^+-thalassemia gene—the nondeleted $\alpha\alpha^T$ gene. Clinically, hemoglobin H disease is characterized by a variable degree of microcytic, hypochromic anemia, which is somewhat intermediate between the clinical pictures of thalassemia minor and thalassemia major and has often been called thalassemia intermedia. The patients have a mild to moderate degree of anemia and may develop the physical and bony characteristics of thalassemia major, as well as splenomegaly and hepatomegaly. They will, however, survive into adulthood without blood transfusion and do not usually suffer from severe iron overload. The anemia usually becomes worse with infections, pregnancy, and folic acid deficiency states. Hemolytic crises may occur with infections. Adults with hemoglobin H disease will have from 5% to 40% hemoglobin H, with the remainder being mostly hemoglobin A with a small amount of hemoglobin A_2 and hemoglobin Bart's. Infants who later develop hemoglobin H disease usually have between 19% and 27% hemoglobin Bart's at birth, with the remainder composed of hemoglobin F and hemoglobin A. Hemoglobin H and hemoglobin Bart's can easily be identified by hemoglobin electrophoresis because they migrate anodally at pH 6.5 to 7.0. In addition, hemoglobin H shows a characteristic appearance of multiple ragged inclusions in many red cells after incubation with brilliant cresyl blue, the so-called golf-ball appearance (Fig. 12–10).

The α^0-thalassemia trait, also called α-*thalassemia 1 trait*, is caused by the defect of two of the four α genes. This is usually the result of heterozygosity for the α^0-thalassemia gene but could also be the result of homozygosity for the α^+-thalassemia gene. The condition is characterized by the presence at birth of 5% to 15% hemoglobin Bart's, which disappears with development and is not replaced by hemoglobin H. There is a minimal amount of anemia with slight hypochromia and microcytosis present. The MCV is usually between 70 and 75 fL. After hemoglobin Bart's disappears, the hemoglobin electrophoretic pattern becomes normal. This condition exists in 3% of African Americans and in children may be confused with iron deficiency.

The last category of α thalassemia is the α^+-thalassemia trait, also called α-*thalassemia 2 trait*. This is the result of a defect in one of the four alpha globin genes and is characterized by the presence of a very small amount (up to 2%) of hemoglobin Bart's at birth; after the disappearance of hemoglobin Bart's during development, no recognizable hematologic abnormality will be present, except for a borderline low MCV (78 to 80 fL). This condition is found in up to 30% of African Americans.

Table 12–2 summarizes the different genetic backgrounds associated with the four different clinical expressions of α thalassemia.

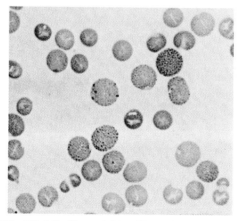

FIGURE 12–10 Hemoglobin H inclusions (supravital stain). (From Bell, A: Hematology. In Listen, Look and Learn. Health and Education Resources, Inc., Bethesda, MD, with permission.)

TABLE 12–2 **Genetic Background of α-Thalassemia Clinical Syndromes (Mating Combinations)**

CHROMOSOME →	NORMAL	α^+			α°
Genes ↓ →	$\alpha\alpha$	$-\alpha$	$\alpha^{CS}\alpha$	$\alpha\alpha^T$	—
$\alpha\alpha$	N	αthal 2	αthal 2	αthal 2	αthal 1
$-\alpha$	αthal 2	αthal 1	αthal 1	αthal 1	H
$\alpha^{CS}\alpha$	αthal 2	αthal 1	αthal 1	αthal 1	H
$\alpha\alpha^T$	αthal 2	αthal 1	αthal 1	H	H
—	αthal 1	H	H	H	Bart's

Abbreviations: $\alpha\alpha$ = normal haplotype; $-\alpha$ = deletion of one alpha gene: $\alpha^{CS}\alpha$ = Hb Constant Spring: $\alpha\alpha^T$ = nondeletion α-thalassemia gene; — = deletion of both α genes. (The clinical phenotype resulting from the combination of these haplotypes is found at the intersection of the corresponding column and row.) N = normal clinical phenotype; αthal 1 = α° trait, 5–15% Hb Bart's at birth, mild anemia; αthal 2 = $\alpha+$ trait, 0–2% Hb Bart's at birth, minimal hematologic changes; H = hemoglobin H disease; Bart's = hemoglobin Bart's hydrops fetalis.

Delta-Beta Thalassemias and Hemoglobin Lepore Syndrome

Delta-beta ($\delta\beta$) thalassemias are a diverse group of thalassemias characterized by a combined defect in δ- and β-chain synthesis. They can be described as demonstrating a normal level of hemoglobin A_2 and an unusually high level of hemoglobin F in the heterozygote, and absent hemoglobin A and A_2 in the homozygote. The $\delta\beta$ thalassemias can be subdivided into two groups according to the type of hemoglobin F produced. If both $^G\gamma$ and $^A\gamma$ chains are produced—that is, if both γ genes are active—this variety is then called $^G\gamma^A\gamma\delta\beta$ thalassemia. If only $^G\gamma$ chains are produced, which means that the $^A\gamma$ gene as well as the δ and the β genes are inactive, this variety is then called $^G\gamma\delta\beta$ thalassemia. Another syndrome of $\delta\beta$ chain abnormality involves the production of an abnormal hemoglobin. This abnormal hemoglobin, called hemoglobin Lepore after the name of the family in which it was first found, has been shown to be a fusion of the δ and β chains, which is the product of a fusion gene formed by an unequal crossing over.

Figure 12–11 indicates diagrammatically the production of hemoglobin Lepore by this unequal crossing over. At least three different hemoglobin Lepores have been described, varying in the exact location of the unequal crossing over.

All $\delta\beta$ thalassemias studied thus far have been shown to be the result of a deletion. They can be described at the genetic level as three different entities, depending on the amount of DNA lost: hemoglobin Lepore syndrome results from a partial deletion of the δ and β genes, $^G\gamma^A\gamma\delta\beta$ thalassemia from a complete deletion of the δ and β genes, and $^G\gamma\delta\beta$ thalassemia from a deletion of the $^A\gamma$ gene in addition to the deletion of the δ and β genes.

$\delta\beta$ thalassemias are less common than β thalassemias and have been found sporadically in Greeks, African Americans, Italians, and Arabs.

The γ-chain synthesis in $\delta\beta$ thalassemia is usually more efficient than in β thalassemia, and in general the former results in a milder clinical disease than the latter. Patients with homozygous $\delta\beta$ thalassemia have a mild to moderate degree of anemia and rarely required blood transfusion, except occasionally during times of stress such as infection or pregnancy. The clinical course is usually described as thalassemia intermedia. This is also true of the double heterozygous $\delta\beta$ and β thalassemia. However, the homozygous state for hemoglobin Lepore appears to be somewhat more severe and closer to the clinical state of homozygous β thalassemia. Most patients with homozygous hemoglobin Lepore are transfusion-dependent. Double heterozygosity for β thalassemia and hemoglobin Lepore also causes a clinical disorder similar to homozygous β thalassemia.

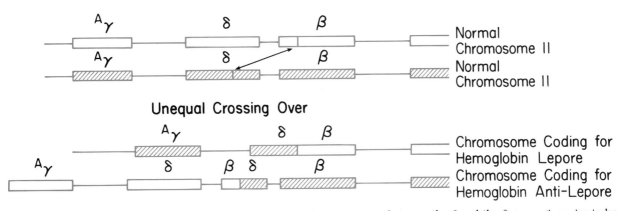

FIGURE 12–11 Hemoglobin Lepore formation. An abnormal crossing-over between the β and the δ genes gives rise to hemoglobin Lepore and to hemoglobin anti-Lepore.

Heterozygosity for $\delta\beta$ thalassemia and hemoglobin Lepore results in a mild form of anemia that is clinically described as thalassemia minor and is similar to the condition of patients with heterozygous β thalassemia.

Hereditary Persistence of Fetal Hemoglobin

Hereditary persistence of fetal hemoglobin (HPFH) consists of a group of conditions characterized by the persistence of fetal hemoglobin synthesis into adult life. These conditions can be classified into two different categories according to the distribution of hemoglobin F among the red cells. Fetal hemoglobin is more resistant than adult hemoglobin to elution at acid pH and can be demonstrated on a peripheral smear by the acid elution test of Kleihauer and Betke. Using this stain, the hereditary persistence of fetal hemoglobin conditions can be divided into a pancellular form, in which hemoglobin F is uniformly distributed among the red cells, and a heterocellular form, in which hemoglobin F is found in a small percentage of the cells only (Fig. 12–12). In the normal adult, cells containing hemoglobin F can occasionally be found, but the amount is always less than 2% and is usually less than 1%. These cells are called F cells.

Heterocellular HPFH appears to be an inherited condition in which the number of F cells is increased without concurrent abnormalities in δ- and β-chain production. Its most common form is the Swiss type, in which individuals have up to 3% hemoglobin F but are otherwise hematologically normal. At the DNA level, there appear to be no gross abnormalities of the δ and β genes.

On the other hand, pancellular HPFH appears to be a form of $\delta\beta$ thalassemia in which the γ genes were not switched off and are able to compensate fully for the lack of δ- and β-chain production. The most common form of pancellular HPFH is the African type, in which there is a deletion of the β- and δ-globin genes that is associated with synthesis of $^G\gamma$ and $^A\gamma$ chains, which almost compensates for the lack of production of δ and β chains. Hemoglobin F constitutes 100% of the hemoglobin in the homozygous state and 15% to 30% of the hemoglobin in the heterozygous state. The hemoglobin F is homogeneously distributed among the red cells and consists of a mixture of $^G\gamma$ and $^A\gamma$ chains. Clinically, the homozygotes demonstrate features of thalassemia minor and the heterozygotes will be hematologically normal.

Another form of pancellular HPFH is the Greek type, in which about 15% hemoglobin F is present in the heterozygous state. This hemoglobin F is also found uniformly distributed among the red cells but is only the $^A\gamma$ type. The homozygous state for this type of pancellular HPFH has not been described. In general, heterozygous or homozygous HPFH causes no significant clinical abnormalities.

Thalassemia Associated with Hemoglobin Variants

The molecular basis of the hemoglobinopathies can be broadly divided into two groups. In the first group, the genetic defect involves the synthesis of the β chain; this group includes β thalassemia, hemoglobin S, hemoglobin C, and hemoglobin E. In the second group, the genetic defect involves the α-chain synthesis; the α thalassemias are included in this group. Homozygosity or double heterozygosity for defective genes within the same group usually results in severe disease that is often lethal. Double heterozygosity with one gene from one group and a second gene from the other group usually shows no interaction, and a defective gene in one group may even result in a clinical improvement of the condition of a patient who is homozygous for a defective gene in the other group. Although thalassemia has been described in association with a large number of hemoglobin structural variants, we will only consider the interactions with the more common hemoglobin variants (i.e., β thalassemia with hemoglobin S, hemoglobin C, and hemoglobin E, and α thalassemia with hemoglobin S).

β Thalassemia with Hemoglobin S

This condition was first recognized in individuals who had inherited a single hemoglobin S gene and who demonstrated about 65% hemoglobin S and 35% hemoglobin A, which is the reverse of the proportions found in patients with sickle cell trait. This condition is the result of the inheritance of a hemoglobin S gene from one parent and a β-thalassemia gene from the other. β thalassemia with hemoglobin S (also called the β-thalassemia sickle cell syndrome) has been widely seen in Africa, the Mediterranean area, the Middle East, and the West Indies, as well as in African-Americans. There is great variety in the clinical severity of this syndrome, depending mostly on the type of β-thalassemia gene inherited. If the β-thalassemia gene is the β^0 type, no hemoglobin A will be produced and the clinical condition will be indistinguishable from classic sickle cell anemia, characterized by severe anemia presenting in early childhood and recurrent sickling crises. If the β-thalassemia gene is β^+ type 1, a small

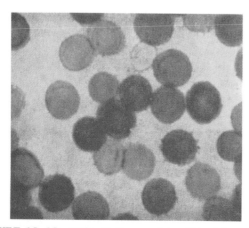

FIGURE 12–12 Betke-Kleihauer stain of blood from a patient with hereditary persistence of fetal hemoglobin (HPFH). Note that all the red cells stain red, owing to the varying amounts of hemoglobin F.

amount of hemoglobin A will be produced, possibly representing up to 15% of the total hemoglobin. Patients in this group have severe anemia with a hemoglobin level in the 7- to 8-g/dL range and experience less frequent and less severe sickling crises than those in the β^0 group. If the β-thalassemia gene is β^+ type 2, as found in most African Americans, a greater amount of hemoglobin A will be produced, representing up to 30% of the total hemoglobin. Patients in this group have a very mild anemia with hemoglobin in the 11-g/dL range and are usually asymptomatic, the condition being diagnosed later in life or during the course of a family study. These patients, as a rule, will not experience any sickling crisis except under the most severe hypoxic conditions.

β Thalassemia with Hemoglobin C

The β thalassemia with hemoglobin C syndrome demonstrates great variability in clinical and hematologic manifestations, which is directly related to the type of β-thalassemia gene that interacts with the hemoglobin C gene; however, the great majority of patients with this syndrome are West Africans and African Americans. In this racial group, the more common β thalassemia gene is β^+ type 2. In this case the β thalassemia with hemoglobin C syndrome will be characterized by a mild degree of usually asymptomatic anemia, in which the clinical and hematologic findings are very similar to those found in heterozygous beta thalassemia.

β Thalassemia with Hemoglobin E

Double heterozygosity for β thalassemia and hemoglobin E is unusual in that it results in a clinical disorder that is much more severe than homozygous hemoglobin E disease. Patients with this syndrome are distributed widely throughout the Far East. The condition follows a clinical course very similar to that of homozygous β thalassemia, with a very severe anemia occurring in early childhood and the development of the characteristic features of thalassemia major if the patient is not started on a regular blood transfusion program.

α Thalassemia with Sickle Cell Anemia

The occurrence of α thalassemia in conjunction with sickle cell anemia has a positive influence on the clinical expression of the disease. Patients with such a genetic background have an increased percentage of hemoglobin F, which is thought to result in a decreased severity of the sickling process. Of interest is the fact that the amount of hemoglobin F present is roughly proportional to the number of α genes affected. Patients with the α^0-thalassemia trait have an average of 16% hemoglobin F, and those with the α^+-thalassemia trait have an average of 8% hemoglobin F.[8]

CLINICAL COURSE AND THERAPY

The clinical course and therapy of patients with thalassemia can be broadly subdivided into three categories: thalassemia major, thalassemia intermedia, and thalassemia minor. A fourth category, termed thalassemia minima, is applied to healthy silent carriers who show no clinical symptoms and minimal to no hematologic abnormalities. Table 12–3 summarizes the different genetic backgrounds that result in each of these clinical outcomes.

By itself, as a single entity, stands hemoglobin Bart's hydrops fetalis, in which the affected infants are either stillborn or die within a few days after birth. For this condition, no therapy is available. The clinical significance of this entity is related more to the obstetric problems that may arise in the affected infants' mothers. Pregnancy is often complicated by toxemia, obstructed labor, and postpartum hemorrhage, which may result in severe morbidity and mortality. Clinical emphasis for this entity is in the prevention of the disease through early antenatal diagnosis, which should result in termination of pregnancy for the protection of the mother's health.

Thalassemia major is the most severe clinical expression of thalassemia and characteristically occurs in patients with homozygous β^0 or β^+ thalassemia or with double heterozygous β^0 and β^+ thalassemia, as well as in patients with homozygous hemoglobin Lepore, double heterozygous β thalassemia with hemo-

TABLE 12–3 **Genetic Background of the Different Clinical Courses of Thalassemia**			
Major	**Intermedia**	**Minor**	**Minima**
Homozygous β^0 thal	Homozygous β^0 or β^+ thal or double heterozygous	Heterozygous β^0 thal	Heterozygous β^+ thal (type 3)
Homozygous β^+ thal (type 1)	β^0/β^+ thal in association with α thal	Heterozygous β^+ thal (type 1 or type 2)	
Double heterozygous β^0/β^+ thal	Homozygous β^+ thal (type 2 or type 3)	Heterozygous $\delta\beta$ thal	
Homozygous Hb Lepore (some)	Homozygous Hb Lepore (some)	Heterozygous Hb Lepore	
Double heterozygous Hb Lepore/β^0 or β^+ thal	Double heterozygous $\delta\beta$ thal/β thal	Double heterozygous β thal/HPFH	Homozygous HPFH
Double heterozygous HbE/β^0 or β^+ thal	Double heterozygous Hb Lepore/$\delta\beta$ thal		Heterozygous HPFH
	Hemoglobin H disease	α Thalassemia 1	α Thalassemia 2

globin Lepore, and double heterozygous β thalassemia with hemoglobin E.

Untreated thalassemia major usually presents within the first year of life with failure to thrive, pallor, a variable degree of jaundice, and abdominal enlargement, with hemoglobin levels from 4 to 8 g/dL. These patients' survival is dependent on a lifelong blood transfusion program. It is now clear that a high transfusion program (hypertransfusion) that maintains the hemoglobin level at 11.5 g/dL on the average is better than an intermittent program that allows the hemoglobin level to drop to a point when the child is severely symptomatic. Hypertransfusion allows for better development, suppresses ineffective erythropoiesis (thus preventing the serious bony deformities), and provides for an overall better quality of life. This, however, draws on considerable blood resources and may not be available in the very countries where thalassemia major is a main public health concern.

In the presence of splenomegaly, splenectomy plays a clear role in decreasing the blood transfusion requirement. However, it should preferably not be performed until the child has reached at least 5 years of age, to decrease the risk of overwhelming infection—particularly of pneumococcal origin.

With regular blood transfusion, these children will survive but will develop severe iron overload owing to increased iron absorption and to the loading of iron from the blood transfusions. This iron overload results in hemochromatosis, and these patients die in their second or third decade, usually of cardiac failure. In the meantime, they will have developed multiple organ damage, with lack of pubertal development probably because of iron toxicity to the pituitary gland, cirrhosis of the liver (which may be the result of either hemochromatosis or posttransfusion hepatitis), and diabetes caused by iron toxicity to the pancreas. This iron overload may be improved with the early introduction of iron chelation therapy. Recent assessment of iron chelation therapy with deferoxamine seems to indicate that an adequate iron balance can be achieved and that longer survival will be attained.[9]

Alternate modes of therapy for thalassemia major in the future may be found in the areas of bone marrow transplantation,[10] genetic engineering, and pharmacologic manipulations such as hydroxyurea or azacitinidine that may induce the "switching back on" of the γ-globin gene.[11,12] The current optimal therapy for thalassemia major relies on intensive use of a fairly sophisticated level of health care that cannot be achieved in most of the countries where thalassemia major is a serious problem without shunting the major thrust of the health resources in that direction.

Another approach to this problem at the health planning level is to decrease the number of births of infants with thalassemia major. This has been successful in certain countries, particularly Cyprus, with the implementation of mass population screening for the detection of heterozygous carriers, genetic counseling, and antenatal diagnosis for couples at risk. Recent developments in antenatal diagnosis, using DNA hybridization techniques in association with chronic villi sampling, enable physicians to make a diagnosis during the first trimester of pregnancy, thus making early termination of pregnancy much more widely available and acceptable.

Thalassemia intermedia covers a broad spectrum of clinical expression of thalassemia, bridging the gap between the severe, lethal form of thalassemia major and the mild, often asymptomatic anemic state of thalassemia minor. The definition of thalassemia intermedia is relative, since the clinical state of patients in this group varies from a mild disability to severe incapacitation without transfusion. Thalassemia intermedia could be defined as a form of thalassemia in which patients have variable degrees of symptomatic anemia, jaundice, splenomegaly, and many of the complications of thalassemia major, but survive into adulthood without a large blood transfusion requirement.

The genetic background of thalassemia intermedia is also extremely varied. It includes patients with homozygosity for the less severe forms of the β-thalassemia gene (such as β^+ type 2 and β^+ type 3 thalassemia), homozygous δβ thalassemia, double heterozygous δβ thalassemia with β thalassemia, hemoglobin H disease, and patients who are homozygous for β thalassemia but who have also inherited a gene for α thalassemia or who have the ability to synthesize the γ chains more efficiently. The exact definition of the genetic background of a patient with thalassemia intermedia requires a careful and extensive family study.

Patients with thalassemia intermedia usually present at a somewhat older age—usually after the age of 2—and with a slightly higher level of hemoglobin (between 6 and 10 g/dL) than patients with thalassemia major. There is great overlap between the two conditions at presentation; however, it is very important to differentiate between them. The only therapy for thalassemia major is regular blood transfusion in conjunction with iron chelation. The management of thalassemia intermedia involves mostly supportive therapy with only occasional blood transfusion under special circumstances.

The serum bilirubin level is significantly more elevated in patients with thalassemia intermedia than in those with thalassemia major. Patients with thalassemia intermedia may develop the severe bony deformities and compression syndromes caused by marrow hyperplasia and extramedullary erythropoiesis characteristic of thalassemia major. They are susceptible to frequent, sometimes severe infections, and gallbladder problems from the formation of gallstones. These children usually have an acceptable level of growth and development (although puberty may be delayed by a few years), and will reach adulthood if infections are controlled and if they enjoy good nutrition with particular emphasis on prevention of folic acid deficiency. They usually develop splenomegaly and may become transfusion-dependent if severe hypersplenism occurs. This usually requires splenectomy. Children with thalassemia intermedia may develop iron overload because of increased gastrointestinal absorption, but this is a much slower process than that experienced by patients with thalassemia major, and the complications from iron overload occur much later in life. Women with thalassemia intermedia may get pregnant and will require blood transfusions as well as folic acid supplementation throughout the pregnancy.

Thalassemia minor is a clinical entity in which the

genetic defects of thalassemia are expressed as a mild microcytic, hypochromic anemia, usually in the 9- to 11-g/dL range, and is asymptomatic except during periods of stress such as pregnancy, infection, or folic acid deficiency. Most patients with thalassemia minor are heterozygous for the β^+-thalassemia gene, the β^0-thalassemia gene, or the α^0-thalassemia gene. The genetic background of thalassemia minor also includes heterzygosity for hemoglobin Lepore and for $\delta\beta$ thalassemia. Patients with thalassemia minor are usually diagnosed incidental to a family study of an index case with thalassemia major or by population screening. They usually require no therapy if they maintain good nutrition. It is important that they not be misdiagnosed as having iron-deficiency anemia.

BLOOD TRANSFUSION IN THALASSEMIA

The three main concerns that need to be addressed regarding patients with thalassemia major who will be on a regular blood transfusion program are: (1) the development of iron overload, (2) the development of alloimmunization, and (3) the risk of transfusion-transmitted diseases. The problem of iron overload can be approached from two directions—by increasing the iron excretion or by decreasing the amount of iron transfused. This latter option can be performed by increasing the length of survival of the transfused red cells, which requires selection of the younger red cells (also called neocytes) for transfusion. Young red cells and reticulocytes have a lower specific gravity than old red cells, and by using a differential centrifugation technique, the blood unit can be separated so that the upper layer of cells is collected. These red cells have a longer life expectancy and can decrease the transfusion requirement of a patient by lengthening the interval of the blood transfusion schedule.

Alloimmunization is a recurrent problem of all chronically transfused patients. These patients often develop antibodies to white cell as well as to red cell antigens. Antibodies to white cell antigens cause febrile nonhemolytic transfusion reactions that are unpleasant. These reactions can be avoided by routinely transfusing leukocyte-reduced red cells. Alloimmunization to red cell antigens is a more serious problem, since this can cause acute or delayed hemolytic transfusion reactions and may seriously affect the availability of compatible blood. It is a good idea to obtain a complete phenotype of the patient's red cells before embarking on a regular transfusion program.

Transfusion-transmitted diseases are a common complication in multitransfused patients. Patients with thalassemia major often develop hepatitis. This risk has been significantly decreased in many areas of the world with the recent introduction of testing for hepatitis C. Some patients may develop a chronic form of hepatitis that, in conjunction with the iron toxicity of iron overload, may damage the liver severely and result in cirrhosis of the liver.

LABORATORY DIAGNOSIS OF THALASSEMIA

The hallmark of thalassemia is the finding of a microcytic, hypochromic anemia. Although more sophisticated laboratory procedures are needed to define exactly the type of thalassemia, the original diagnosis of thalassemia can be made or strongly suspected on the basis of the results of routine hematology procedures.

Routine Hematology Procedures

Automated Blood Cell Analyzer (see Chap. 32)

The thalassemias in general are characterized by a decrease in Hb, Hct, MCV, and MCH in conjunction with a normal-to-increased RBC, a normal to mildly decreased MCHC, and a normal red cell distribution width (RDW). The only exception is thalassemia major, in which the degree of anisocytosis is such that the RDW is increased. The decrease in MCV is usually striking and disproportionate to the decrease in Hb and Hct. This fact, in conjunction with the relatively high RBC and the normal RDW, offers a useful discrimination index between heterozygous α or β thalassemia and iron deficiency.[13] In iron deficiency, the RDW is increased and the decrease in MCV is less striking and only observed when the anemia is more severe. In heterozygous thalassemia, the MCH is usually below 22 pg and the MCV below 70 fL, whereas the hemoglobin level is in the 9- to 11-g/dL range.

Peripheral Smear Examination

The careful examination of a well-prepared peripheral smear is essential to the diagnosis of thalassemia.

Wright's Stain   In homozygous β and double heterozygous non-α thalassemia, the peripheral smear demonstrates extreme anisocytosis and poikilocytosis with bizarre shapes, target cells, ovalocytes, and large number of nucleated red cells (see Fig. 12–6). There is marked hypochromia and microcytosis. In heterozygous β thalassemia, the cells are hypochromic and microcytic with a mild to moderate degree of anisocytosis and poikilocytosis. Target cells are frequent, and basophilic stippling is often seen. The peripheral smear of a patient with the sickle cell thalassemia syndrome can be differentiated from that of a patient with pure sickle cell anemia by the presence of hypochromia, microcytosis, numerous target cells, and only an occasional sickled cell.

In hemoglobin H disease, the peripheral smear will demonstrate hypochromia with microcytosis, target cells, and mild to moderate anisopoikilocytosis. Patients with heterozygous α^0 thalassemia usually demonstrate a mild hypochromia and microcytosis, whereas those with heterozygous α^+ thalassemia usually have a perfectly normal peripheral smear.

Supravital Stains   The reticulocyte count is usually elevated up to 10% in hemoglobin H disease and up to 5% in homozygous β thalassemia but is disproportionately low in relation to the degree of anemia in the latter condition.

In hemoglobin H disease, incubation of the red cells with brilliant cresyl blue stain will cause in vitro precipitation of hemoglobin H owing to the redox action of the dye. This results in a characteristic appearance of most of the red cells, which will display multiple discrete inclusions, the appearance of which has often been compared to that of a golf ball (see Fig. 12–10).

Occasionally, and after extensive searching, such cells containing hemoglobin H inclusions can be found in the α^0-thalassemia carrier.

In splenectomized patients with homozygous β thalassemia or hemoglobin H disease, incubation of the blood with methylviolet stain can demonstrate Heinz body–like inclusions, which represent in vivo precipitation of the abnormal hemoglobin.

Acid Elution Stain (see Chap. 31) The acid elution technique originally described by Kleihauer and Betke is based on the fact that an acid pH of about 3.3, hemoglobin A is eluted from an air-dried, alcohol-fixed blood smear, whereas hemoglobin F is resistant to elution. A controlled preparation containing a mixture of adult and cord cells must also be stained and examined in parallel to check the quality of the technique, as this technique is very sensitive to many variables.

This stain is very useful in demonstrating the distribution of hemoglobin F and can be used to differentiate between pancellular and heterocellular HPFH. It is also useful in differentiating heterozygous $\delta\beta$ thalassemia from heterozygous pancellular HPFH, since the former usually has a heterocellular distribution of hemoglobin F.

Osmotic Fragility (see Chap. 31)

The red cells of patients with homozygous or heterozygous β thalassemia, hemoglobin H disease, and α^0-thalassemia trait have a decreased osmotic fragility. This fact is not very useful for diagnostic purposes in a specific patient, but it is the basis of a simple, inexpensive method of screening for the thalassemia carrier state in large populations.

Hemoglobin Electrophoresis

Hemoglobin electrophoresis plays an important role in the diagnosis of thalassemia by allowing the detection of increased levels of hemoglobin A_2 and hemoglobin F as well as the presence of abnormal hemoglobins, such as hemoglobin H, hemoglobin Bart's, hemoglobin Lepore, hemoglobin Constant Spring, or other structurally abnormal hemoglobins that can be found in association with thalassemia (hemoglobin S, hemoglobin C, hemoglobin E). Table 12–4 contains a summary of

the different patterns of the hemoglobins present in the non-α-thalassemia syndromes.

Routine hemoglobin electrophoresis to confirm the diagnosis of thalassemia is done at an alkaline pH around 8.4 on cellulose acetate or starch gel. At that pH, the hemoglobins will migrate from the most cathodal to the most anodal in the following order: first hemoglobin Constant Spring; then hemoglobins A_2, C, and E migrate in the same band; next hemoglobins S and Lepore, again in the same band; next hemoglobin F followed by hemoglobin A; then hemoglobin Bart's; and last, hemoglobin H. The different patterns of migration of the different hemoglobins is illustrated in Figure 12–13. Cellulose acetate or starch gel electrophoresis can be done at low to neutral pH to detect hemoglobin H and hemoglobin Bart's easily, as they migrate anodally (i.e., in opposite direction of other hemoglobins) at this pH.

Cellulose Acetate

Cellulose acetate electrophoresis is becoming more popular and has replaced starch gel electrophoresis in many laboratories, owing to its simple, rapid method. It uses a smaller sample than starch gel electrophoresis, and minor components such as hemoglobin Constant Spring and small amounts of hemoglobin A_2 may be overlooked. Small amounts of hemoglobin A in the presence of mostly hemoglobin F also can be difficult to detect.

Other Gels

Starch gel electrophoresis is a little more cumbersome and time-consuming. The results of the starch gel electrophoresis are similar to those of the cellulose acetate procedure.

Citrate agar gel electrophoresis, which is performed at an acid pH between 5.9 and 6.2, has a minor role in the diagnosis of the thalassemias.

Hemoglobin Quantitation

Although an experienced observer can detect an increased level in hemoglobin A_2 or hemoglobin F on cellulose acetate or starch gel electrophoresis, actual

TABLE 12–4 **Hemoglobins A, A_2, and F Levels in the Different Non-α Thalassemias**			
	HbA (%)	HbA$_2$ (%)	HbF (%)
Homozygous β^0 thal	0	2–5	95–98
Homozygous β^+ or double heterozygous β^+/β^0 thal	5–35	2–5	60–95
Homozygous $\delta\beta$ thal	0	0	100
Homozygous Hb Lepore	0	0	75 (25% Hb Lepore)
Heterozygous β thal	90–95	3.5–7	2–5
Heterozygous $\delta\beta$ thal	80–92	1–2.5	5–20
Heterozygous Hb Lepore	75–85	2	1–6 (7–15% Hb Lepore)
Homozygous HPFH	0	0	100
Heterozygous HPFH (African type)	65–85	1–2.5	15–35
Heterozygous HPFH (Greek type)	75–85	1.5–2.5	15–25
Normal	97.5	2.5	0.2–1

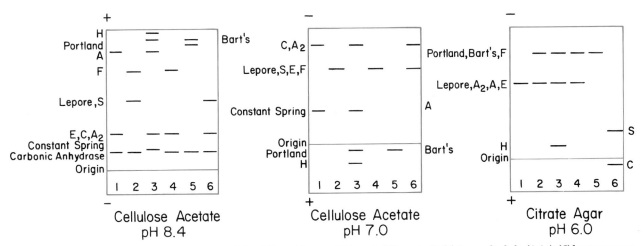

FIGURE 12–13 Diagram of the migration of the different hemoglobins at different pH. (*1*) Normal adult. (A A$_2$); (*2*) homozygous Hb Lepore (F, Lepore); (*3*) HbH/Constant Spring disease $\alpha^{CS}\alpha$/—(Constant Spring, A$_2$, A, Bart's H); (*4*) double heterozygous HbE/β-thalassemia (E,F); (*5*) Hb Bart's hydrops fetalis syndrome (Portland, Bart's); (*6*) HbS/C disease (S, C).

quantitation is necessary to establish definitively the diagnosis of thalassemia.

Hemoglobin A$_2$ Quantitation

The elevation of hemoglobin A$_2$ is an excellent tool for the detection of a heterozygote carrier of β thalassemia. It is characteristic of heterozygous β thalassemia and specific with no overlap values between heterozygous carriers and normal individuals. The level of hemoglobin A$_2$ ranges between 3.5% and 7% in heterozygous β thalassemia, whereas normal values are always below 3.5%. A few rare variants of β thalassemia with normal A$_2$, which are called normal A$_2$ β thalassemia, do exist, and can be distinguished only in the carrier state from heterozygous α thalassemia by globin-chain synthesis. Also, in an iron-deficient patient with β thalassemia minor, hemoglobin A$_2$ may be reduced to normal levels. The percent of hemoglobin A$_2$ can be quantified by elution following cellulose acetate electrophoresis, microcolumn chromatography, or high-performance liquid chromatography.[14]

Hemoglobin F Quantitation

The hemoglobin F levels are useful in the definition of the type of thalassemia involved, and a summary of the levels of hemoglobin F corresponding to the different types of thalassemia can be found in Table 12–4. The hemoglobin F level is normally below 2%. Approximately half of the β-thalassemia carriers have a mildly elevated level of hemoglobin F—usually below 5%.

Routine Chemistry

The indirect bilirubin level is elevated in thalassemia major and intermedia, ranging from 1 to 6 mg/dL. It is characteristically more elevated in thalassemia intermedia than in thalassemia major.

The assessment of the iron status of the patient by the determination of the serum iron level, total iron-binding capacity (TIBC), and serum ferritin level is useful in the differentiation of a thalassemia carrier from a patient with iron-deficiency anemia, as well as in the assessment of the iron load in a patient with thalassemia major or intermedia. The serum iron and the serum ferritin levels are low and the TIBC increased in patients with iron deficiency. These values are normal in patients with thalassemia minor, unless they have concurrent iron deficiency. Patients with thalassemia major who have been transfused have increased levels of serum iron that will approach 100% saturation of the TIBC. The serum ferritin level is elevated and indicates the amount of iron deposited in the tissues.

DIFFERENTIAL DIAGNOSIS OF MICROCYTIC, HYPOCHROMIC ANEMIA

The differential diagnosis of microcytic, hypochromic anemia includes iron deficiency, α thalassemia, β thalassemia, anemia of chronic disease, hemoglobin E disease, sideroblastic anemia, and lead poisoning. The evaluation of the clinical history, the hemoglobin level, and the red cell indices (in particular MCV and MCH) usually narrow down the diagnosis. The sometimes difficult differential between the thalassemia carrier and iron deficiency can be done by evaluating the serum iron and ferritin levels and the TIBC. A markedly elevated free erythrocyte protoporphyrin (FEP) will identify a child with lead poisoning. Cellulose acetate electrophoresis will usually allow differentiation between a β-thalassemia carrier, an α-thalassemia carrier, or the presence of hemoglobin E. The differentiation between these diseases is summarized in Table 12–5.

CASE STUDY

A 25-year-old man of Chinese extraction is being evaluated because he was found to be anemic when he attempted to donate blood. He otherwise has no complaints; he is active in sports and feels healthy. A complete blood count gives the following results: The RBC is 5.76 million, the Hb is 10.4 g/dL, the

TABLE 12–5.	**Differential Diagnosis of Microcytic Hypochromic Anemia**					
	RDW	Serum Iron	TIBC	Serum Ferritin	FEP	A$_2$ Level
Iron deficiency	↑	↓	↑	↓	↑	nl
α Thalassemia	nl	nl	nl	nl	nl	nl
β Thalassemia	nl	nl	nl	nl	nl	↑
Hemoglobin E disease	nl	nl	nl	nl	nl	nl
Anemia of chronic disease	nl	↓	↓	↑	↑	nl
Sideroblastic anemia	↑	↑	nl	↑	↓	nl
Lead poisoning	nl	nl	nl	nl	↑	nl

Abbreviations: RDW = red cell volume distribution width; TIBC = total iron-binding capacity; FEP = free erythrocyte protoporphyrin; nl = normal.

Hct is 35.9%, the MCV is 62 fL, the MCH is 18.1 pg, the MCHC is 29%, and the RDW is 13.5%. The peripheral blood smear shows hypochromic, microcytic erythrocytes with a mild anisocytosis; occasional target cells but no basophilic stippling can be found.

The serum iron is 95 mg/dL (normal 60 to 150 mg/dL), the TIBC is 305 mg/dL (normal 260 to 360 mg/dL), and the ferritin level is 175 μg/dL (normal 30 to 300 μg/dL). Cellulose acetate electrophoresis shows an increased amount of hemoglobins F and A$_2$, which are quantitated to 4.5% and 5%, respectively.

Questions

1. What are the diagnoses that you entertain at this time?
2. What laboratory tests do you think are most useful to diagnose the cause of his anemia?
3. What is your diagnosis now, and what is the significance of this diagnosis for this patient?

Answers

1. On clinical history alone, the possibilities of anemia of chronic disease and lead poisoning can be ruled out in a healthy young man. We are left with the possibility of iron deficiency, a β-thalassemia carrier, an α-thalassemia carrier, sideroblastic anemia, and hemoglobin E disease (which should be considered in a person of Chinese extraction).
2. A serum iron level, TIBC, serum ferritin level, and cellulose acetate electrophoresis are appropriate tests that may differentiate among these conditions.
3. Sideroblastic anemia and iron deficiency can be ruled out by the normal iron level, TIBC, and ferritin level. Although hemoglobin E migrates in the same area as hemoglobin A$_2$, on cellulose acetate electrophoresis, a patient with heterozygous or homozygous hemoglobin E would have a much larger amount of hemoglobin in that band; thus, hemoglobin E disease is ruled out. An α-thalassemia carrier would have a normal hemoglobin electrophoresis pattern; therefore, the diagnosis in this patient is heterozygous β thalassemia. Making the diagnosis of β-thalassemia heterozygosity in this patient is important for two reasons. First, the patient must be reassured that this level of hemoglobin and hematocrit is normal for him, and he should not be placed on iron therapy, which could be harmful. Second, the patient needs to be educated regarding the possibility of his having a child with a severe congenital anemia and its therapeutic implications if he marries someone who is a carrier of β thalassemia, hemoglobin E, or hemoglobin S. His spouse should be screened for the presence of these genes and genetic counseling such as antenatal diagnosis offered if she in fact is a carrier.

REFERENCES

1. Cooley, TB and Lee, P: A series of cases with splenomegaly in children with anemia and peculiar bone changes. Trans Am Ped Soc 37:29, 1925.
2. Nagel, RL and Roth, EF: Malaria and red cell genetic defects. Blood 74:1213, 1989.
3. Liebhaber SA, Cash, FE, and Ballas, SK: Human α-globin gene expression. The dominant role of the α2-locus in mRNA and protein synthesis. J Biol Chem 261:15327, 1986.
4. Liebhaber, SA, Goossens, M, and Kan, YW: Homology and concerted evolution at the α1 and α2 loci of human α-globin. Nature 290:26, 1981.
5. Huisman, TH: The beta- and delta-thalassemia repository. Hemoglobin 16:237, 1992.
6. Huisman, THJ: Frequencies of common β-thalassemia alleles among different populations: Variations in clinical severity. Br J Haematol 75:454, 1990.
7. Tang, WT, et al: Immunocytological test to detect adult carriers of (—^{SER}/) deletional α-thalassemia. Lancet 342:1145, 1993.
8. Emburg, SH, et al: Concurrent sickle-cell anemia and α-thalassemia. Effect on severity of anemia. N Engl J Med 306:270, 1982.
9. Brittenham, GM, et al: Efficacy of deferoxamine in preventing complications of iron overload in patients with thalassemia major. N Engl J Med 331:567, 1994.
10. Lucarelli, G, et al: Marrow transplantation in patients with thalassemia responsive to iron chelation therapy. N Engl J Med 329:840, 1993.
11. Goldberg, MA, et al: Treatment of sickle cell anemia with hydroxyurea and erythropoietin. N Engl J Med 323:366, 1990.
12. Lowrey, CH and Nienhuis, AW: Brief report: Treatment with azacitidine of patients with end-stage β-thalassemia. N Engl J Med 329:845, 1993.
13. Johnson, CS, Tegos, C, and Bentler, E: Thalassemia minor: Routine erythrocyte measurements and differentiation from iron deficiency. Am J Clin Pathol 80:31, 1982.
14. Tan, GB, et al: Evaluation of high performance liquid chromatography for routine estimation of haemoglobins A$_2$ and F. J Clin Pathol 46:852, 1993.

BIBLIOGRAPHY

Bunn, HF and Forget, BG: Hemoglobin: Molecular, Genetic and Clinical Aspects. WB Saunders, Philadelphia, 1986.

Fosburg, MT and Nathan, DG: Treatment of Cooley's anemia. Blood 76:435, 1990.

Higgs, DR, et al: A review of the molecular genetics of the human α-globin gene cluster. Blood 73:1018, 1989.

Kazazian, HH: The thalassemia syndromes: Molecular basis and prenatal diagnosis in 1990. Semin Hematol 27:209, 1990.

Modall, B and Berdoukas, V: The Clinical Approach to Thalassemia. Grune & Stratton, New York, 1984.

Orkin, SH: Disorders of hemoglobin synthesis: The thalassemias. In Stamatoyannopoulos, G, et al (eds): The Molecular Basis of Blood Diseases. WB Saunders, Philadelphia, 1987, p 106.

Steinberg, MH: Review: Thalassemia: Molecular pathology and management. Am J Med Sci 296:308, 1988.

Weatherall, DJ, et al: The Hemoglobinopathies. In Scriver, CR, et al (eds). The Metabolic Basis of Inherited Diseases. McGraw-Hill, New York, 1989, p 2281.

Weatherall, DJ (ed): The Thalassemias. Methods in Hematology. Churchill-Livingstone, New York, 1983.

Weatherall, DJ, and Clegg, JB: The Thalassemia Syndromes. Blackwell Scientific Publications, Boston, 1981.

WHO Working Group: Community Control of Hereditary Anemias: Memorandum from a WHO meeting. Bull WHO 61:63, 1983.

WHO Working Group: Hereditary Anemias: Genetic Basis, Clinical Features, Diagnosis and Treatment. Bull WHO 60:643, 1982.

QUESTIONS

1. What is the hemoglobin defect found in thalassemia syndromes?
   a. Abnormal incorporation of iron molecule
   b. Defective production of the globin portion
   c. Excessive production of porphyrins
   d. Amino acid substitution

2. What type of globin chains and hemoglobin are characteristics of α thalassemia?
   a. Two α chains and two β chains (HbA)
   b. Two α chains and two δ chains (HbA$_2$)
   c. Four β chains (HbH) or four γ chains (HbBart's)
   d. Two α chains and two γ chains (HbF)

3. Which type of thalassemia has primarily hemoglobin Bart's and shows the following clinical expressions: infants die in utero or soon after birth; severe anemia, marked hepatomegaly and splenomegaly, and ascites?
   a. Homozygous α thalassemia
   b. Homozygous β thalassemia
   c. Thalassemia minor
   d. α-Thalassemia trait

4. What is the term for the clinical course of homozygous thalassemias caused by defects in δ- and β-chain synthesis?
   a. Thalassemia minor
   b. Thalassemia major
   c. Thalassemia trait
   d. Thalassemia intermedia

5. Hereditary persistence of fetal hemoglobin (HPFH) is characterized by the persistence of fetal hemoglobin into adult life. What are the clinical manifestations of this condition?
   a. Chronic anemia with skeletal abnormalities caused by excessive erythropoiesis
   b. Asymptomatic except during pregnancy or stressful situations
   c. Hydrops fetalis syndrome
   d. No significant abnormalities for heterozygous; minor symptoms for homozygous

6. What is the clinical manifestation of α thalassemia with sickle cell anemia?
   a. Severe, life-threatening anemia
   b. Relatively asymptomatic until placed in an oxygen-deprived environment
   c. Less severe than sickle cell anemia alone
   d. Skeletal abnormality, but milder anemia than sickle cell anemia

7. What is the primary risk to thalassemia major patients who are on a high-transfusion (hypertransfusion) program?
   a. Hyperviscosity of the blood
   b. Iron overload
   c. Citrate toxicity
   d. Electrolyte imbalance

8. What routine hematologic finding is indicative of thalassemia?
   a. Microcytic, hypochromic anemia
   b. Macrocytic, hypochromic anemia
   c. Normocytic, normochromic anemia
   d. Macrocytic, normochromic anemia

9. How can iron deficiency be distinguished from heterozygous α or β thalassemia?
   a. RDW will be decreased in heterozygous thalassemia with increased MCH and MCV with Hgb in 10- to 14-g/dL range; iron deficiency with increased RDW, MCH, and MCV
   b. RDW normal in heterozygous thalassemia with decreased MCH and MCV with Hgb in 9- to 11-g/dL range; RDW increased in iron deficiency with decreased MCV and MCH only with severe anemia
   c. RDW increased in heterozygous thalassemia with decreased MCH and MCV with Hgb in 5- to 9-g/dL range; RDW normal in iron deficiency with normal MCV and MCH
   d. RDW, MCH, and MCV normal in heterozygous thalassemia; RDW, MCH, and MCV all increased in iron deficiency

10. Which of the following cells might not be found in a patient with homozygous β thalassemia?
   a. Target cells
   b. Ovalocytes
   c. Sickle cells
   d. Nucleated red cells

11. Which test is useful in demonstrating the distribution of hemoglobin F and in differentiating pancellular HPFH, heterocellular HPFH, and heterozygous $\delta\beta$ thalassemia?
   a. Osmotic fragility
   b. Betke-Kleihauer acid elution test
   c. Serum ferritin level
   d. Complete blood count

12. Which of the following findings would be indicative of heterozygous β thalassemia?
   a. Hemoglobin A$_2$ level 3.5% to 7%
   b. Hemoglobin F level below 2%
   c. Hemoglobin A level 65% to 85%
   d. Hemoglobin A$_2$ level below 3.5%

ANSWERS

1. **b** (p 193)
2. **c** (p 196)
3. **a** (p 200)
4. **d** (p 201)
5. **d** (p 202)
6. **c** (p 203)
7. **b** (p 205)
8. **a** (p 205)
9. **b** (p 205)
10. **c** (p 205)
11. **b** (p 206)
12. **a** (p 207)

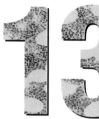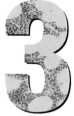

Hemolytic Anemias: Intracorpuscular Defects

V. PAROXYSMAL NOCTURNAL HEMOGLOBINURIA

Kathryn A. Grenier, MT(ASCP), CLT(CA)

Objectives

At the end of this chapter, the learner should be able to:
1 Define *paroxysmal nocturnal hemoglobinuria.*
2 Describe the red cell abnormality associated with paroxysmal nocturnal hemoglobinuria.
3 Describe the three types of paroxysmal nocturnal hemoglobinuria.
4 List clinical features of paroxysmal nocturnal hemoglobinuria.
5 List laboratory findings characteristic of paroxysmal nocturnal hemoglobinuria.
6 Describe the sugar water test.
7 Describe the Ham's test (sucrose hemolysis test).
8 List therapies for treatment of paroxysmal nocturnal hemoglobinuria.

DEFINITION AND HISTORY

Paroxysmal nocturnal hemoglobinuria (PNH) is an acquired hemolytic anemia with an insidious onset, resulting in a chronic hemolytic state. In this disorder, the red cell membrane is abnormal, causing the red cells to be highly sensitive to the hemolytic action of complement.[1] The membrane defect present in the blood cells is a disorder arising at the level of the multipotential stem cell. Frequently associated with the chronic hemolysis are leukopenia, thrombocytopenia, hemosiderinuria, and hemoglobinuria.

In 1866, William Gull published the first case of PNH.[2] He described an anemic patient with "hematuria" that varied throughout the day but was the worst in the morning. He recognized that the urinary pigment was the result of some breakdown product of the red cells. Other clinical investigators have confirmed that hematuria was most pronounced in the morning,[3] described the presence of "perpetual hemosiderinuria,"[4,5] and demonstrated that PNH red cells underwent lysis when the serum and cells were exposed to carbonic acid.[6]

In 1930, Thomas H. Ham described in detail the acidified serum lysis test (Ham's test).[7,8] Ham also demonstrated that some patients with PNH, presenting with chronic hemolysis, had positive acidified serum lysis test results but did not have hemoglobinuria.

Although PNH is fairly rare, much progress and research have increased our understanding of the mech-

211

anism of hemolysis, the role of complement, and causes of the defects.

ETIOLOGY AND PATHOPHYSIOLOGY

PNH is an acquired intracorpuscular defect caused by an abnormality in the hematopoietic cell membranes. This abnormality causes the cells, especially the erythrocytes, to be more sensitive than normal to lytic action of complement (Fig. 13–1). This defect is associated with an abnormal clone of hematopoietic stem cells, probably resulting from a mutagenic event that is passed on to its progeny.[9] This defect may occur during the course of bone marrow hypoplasia or recovery from an aplastic episode,[10] although it has also occurred without evidence of marrow hypoplasia.

The membrane defect in PNH is caused by at least nine missing cell surface proteins that comprise complement regulating proteins, membrane enzymes, and immune function proteins (Table 13–1). These proteins are normally bound to the cell surface by a glycosylphosphatidylinositol (GPI) anchor. In PNH, the GPI anchor is not synthesized by the cells. Deficiency of the complement regulatory protein's decay-accelerating factor (DAF), homologous restriction factor (HRF), or C8-binding protein and the membrane inhibitor of reactive lysis (MIRL) play the largest role in the complement sensitivity that is seen in PNH.[11–13] DAF is an integral membrane protein that accelerates the spontaneous decay of the C3 convertase enzyme for the classic and alternate complement activation pathways. The role of the MIRL protein is to regulate the effectiveness of the complement unit, C5bC9, the com-

TABLE 13–1 **Proteins Absent from the Cell Membranes in PNH**
Complement-Regulating Proteins
Decay accelerating factor (DAF)
Membrane inhibitor of reactive lysis (MIRL)
Homologous restriction factor (HRF) or C8 binding protein
Membrane Enzymes
Erythrocyte acetylcholinesterase
Leukocyte alkaline phosphatase
Lymphocyte 5'-ectonucleotidase
Immune Function Proteins
Lymphocyte function antigen 3 (LFA-3)
Neutrophil Fcγ III receptor (CD16)
Monocyte antigen (CD14)

Source: Adapted from Handin, Lux, and Stossel,[24] p 370.

plement membrane attack complex. Homologous restriction factor (HRF) or C8-binding protein may regulate the activation of the terminal complex of complement. HRF is a membrane regulatory protein that inhibits complement-mediated lysis by the C5b-9 complex (membrane attack unit) by binding C8.[12–15] The importance of HRF in the regulation of complement activation is still in question.

The deficiency of DAF, MIRL, and HRF expression is the molecular explanation for the underlying clonal abnormality that affects granulocytes, monocytes, and platelets as well as the erythrocytes in patients with PNH.[11,12,14] Studies of the affected erythrocytes also

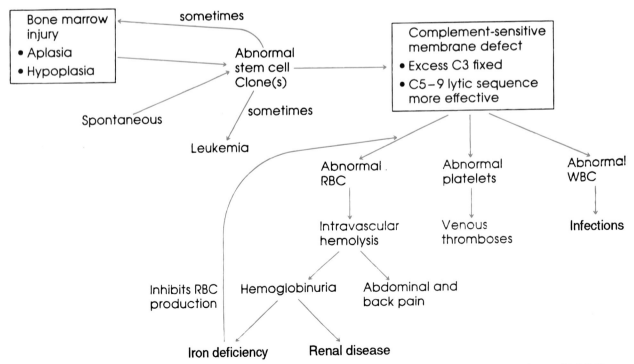

FIGURE 13–1 Pathophysiology of paroxysmal nocturnal hemoglobinuria (PNH) (From Beck, WS: Hematology, ed 3. MIT Press, Cambridge, 1982, with permission.)

show the following abnormalities: decreased or missing membrane acetylcholinesterase,[16,17] altered membrane lipids,[18] increased sensitivity to peroxidation,[19] and craters and pits of the erythrocyte membrane as demonstrated by electron microscopy.[20]

Complement has a major role in the pathogenesis of PNH and will be discussed in detail at the end of this chapter. The PNH erythrocytes have been classified into three categories based on their interaction with complement. In PNH, the erythrocytes react abnormally with complement components C3 and C5 to C9. In PNH I, erythrocytes react normally with complement and are thought to represent residual normal cells because they are similar to normal erythrocytes in all respects.[21] The PNH II erythrocytes have moderate sensitivity to complement component C3 and are three to five times more sensitive to lysis by complement than are normal erythrocytes.[22] PNH II erythrocytes appear to be deficient in the complement regulatory protein DAF only.[11] PNH III erythrocytes are the cells most sensitive to complement, being 15 to 25 times more sensitive to complement component C3 than normal erythrocytes; in addition to binding increased amounts of C3, they also have increased sensitivity to the terminal complement component, C5 to C9.[23] PNH III erythrocytes are deficient in both DAF and HRF membrane proteins.[11]

Patients with PNH usually have variable combinations of the three different types of PNH erythrocytes. Eighty percent of all patients with PNH have the combination of PNH I and PNH II cells, whereas the other 20% have variable combinations of PNH I, PNH II, and PNH III cells.[23] The degree of hemolysis depends on the proportion of abnormal cells and the severity of the cellular membrane defects. The proportion of abnormal cells varies from patient to patient, and the intensity of the clinical symptoms is related to the percentage of PNH III cells present.

CLINICAL FEATURES

Diverse clinical presentations of PNH are common. The disease occurs most often in middle-aged adults, but occasionally occurs in children and elderly persons. Both genders are equally affected. Most patients with PNH present with symptoms of anemia, which may be mild to severe and are the result of the chronic hemolysis.

The classic presentation of hemoglobinuria as a result of significant intravascular hemolysis is most noticeable in the patient's first morning urine specimen. The cause of this sleep-induced hemolysis was thought to be related to an increased retention of CO_2, or a slight drop in blood pH. However, current research indicates that it is related to the increased susceptibility of the red cell membrane to complement activation.[24] Up to 25% of patients present with this classic symptom,[23] however, irregular episodes of intravascular hemolysis with hemoglobinuria may be triggered by infections (most commonly viruses), surgery, menstruation, administration of iron, and a variety of drugs.

In contrast to hemoglobinuria, hemosiderinuria is present in most patients. Recurrent hemolysis results

in loss of body iron into the urine. This iron is derived from plasma hemoglobin that is absorbed and catabolized in the renal tubules. Iron-laden tubular cells appear in the urine and can be stained for hemosiderin. Prolonged loss of iron can lead to iron-deficiency anemia, which may mask the diagnosis of PNH.

Patients commonly present with infections, abdominal pain, headaches, and back pain, symptoms thought to be caused by intravascular thrombi. One of the major complications of PNH is the formation of venous thromboses of the hepatic, abdominal, cerebral, or subdermal veins. Formation of these thrombi may be attributed to the activation of complement-sensitive platelets by the complement component C3.[10,25] Also, during the thrombotic episodes, features of disseminated intravascular coagulation (DIC) may appear (see Chap. 29).

Aplastic anemia may precede or coexist with PNH. In such cases, pancytopenia and marrow hypoplasia are present. Complement-sensitive erythrocytes occur transiently and in small numbers in certain patients with aplastic anemia. In a few patients, complement-sensitive erythrocytes are increased in number and persist, making these rare cases of aplastic anemia indistinguishable from PNH.

DIAGNOSIS OF PNH

The diagnosis of PNH depends on the detection of complement-sensitive erythrocytes in the peripheral blood.[10] The diagnosis is difficult if based solely on clinical features and evaluation of the bone marrow and peripheral blood smears. PNH should be included in the differential diagnosis of patients with the following disorders: (1) hemolytic anemia of unknown origin, (2) pancytopenia associated with a hypoplastic or aplastic bone marrow, (3) iron deficiency of unknown origin, and (4) unexplained episodic hemoglobinuria.[26] PNH must also be differentiated from other causes of chronic hemolytic anemia (both inherited and acquired), congenital dyserythropoiesis type II, or hereditary erythroblast multinuclearity with positive acidified serum test (HEMPAS), and paroxysmal cold hemoglobinuria.[1]

Laboratory Evaluation

Characteristic laboratory findings in PNH are anemia, leukopenia, and thrombocytopenia.[27] The anemia may be mild to severe, depending on the number and type of PNH erythrocytes present. Hemoglobin levels may vary from normal to less than 6 g/dL. No characteristic red blood cell morphological abnormalities are observed in the peripheral blood; in fact, patients most commonly present with a normocytic, normochromic anemia. Slight macrocytosis and polychromasia caused by increased numbers of reticulocytes in the peripheral blood may be seen (Fig. 13–2). This reticulocytosis is a compensatory mechanism for the hemolytic process, and although the reticulocyte count is usually elevated (5.0% to 10.0%), the absolute reticulocyte count may be low with respect to the degree of anemia present. This discrepancy is attributed

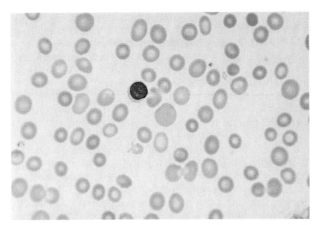

FIGURE 13-2 Peripheral blood smear from a patient with PNH. (Magnification ×600.)

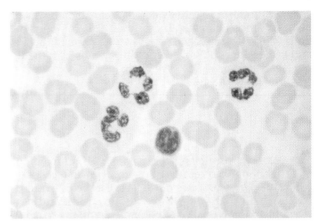

FIGURE 13-3 Leukocyte alkaline phosphatase (LAP) stain of peripheral blood showing little or no activity in chronic myelocytic leukemia (CML).

to the presence of iron deficiency or to the bone marrow stem cell defect itself.[28] With associated iron deficiency, the erythrocytes appear microcytic and hypochromic. During an exacerbation of hemolysis, nucleated red blood cells may be seen in the peripheral blood smear. Spherocytes, although present in other types of hemolytic anemias, are generally not seen. Schistocytes or fragmented red blood cells are occasionally seen with acute hemolysis and may suggest the presence of an intravascular thrombosis.[23]

Also present in PNH erythrocytes is decreased membrane acetylcholinesterase, a finding that is most apparent in the reticulocytes.[10,16] The severity of the decrease in acetylcholinesterase activity parallels the severity of the disease.

Granulocytes, like the red cells, have the same membrane defects that render them more sensitive to the lytic action of complement and to antibodies.[29] When observed by light microscopy and with routine staining, they appear to have no characteristic morphological abnormality. Leukopenia, primarily caused by a decrease in granulocytes, is often observed. The granulocytes have decreased leukocyte alkaline phosphatase (LAP) activity ranging from zero to low normal (Fig. 13-3). The LAP score can aid in distinguishing PNH from aplastic anemia because in the latter the LAP score is normal to elevated.

Platelet counts vary in PNH. Moderate thrombocytopenia is present, with counts ranging from 50.0 to 100.0×10^9/L. The platelets have the same membrane defect as the erythrocytes and granulocytes. Although decreased in number, the platelets have a normal function and life span.

Because almost all patients with PNH have hemosiderin in their urine, testing for urinary hemosiderin will aid in confirming the diagnosis. A random urine sample is centrifuged and the sediment stained with potassium ferrocyanide (Prussian blue), which will detect the presence of hemosiderin. If present, the hemosiderin granules will stain blue.

Hemoglobinuria, when present, must be differentiated from hematuria. This may be accomplished by performing a routine urinalysis with microscopic examination looking for the absence of intact red cells and the presence of a positive blood result on the dipstick. Hemoglobinuria can lead to the formation of hemoglobin casts in the renal tubules and eventually cause renal failure.

Other laboratory procedures that aid in diagnosing PNH are nonspecific tests for intravascular and extravascular hemolysis, including indirect bilirubin (increased), plasma hemoglobin (increased), haptoglobin (decreased), and Coombs test (negative).

As expected, the bone marrow shows erythroid hyperplasia (Fig. 13-4). This is the result of increased erythropoiesis subsequent to chronic hemolysis. The increased erythropoiesis is usually normoblastic, although some megaloblastic changes may be noted. Occasionally, a hypoplastic or even aplastic marrow is seen. The bone marrow usually reveals adequate numbers of myeloid and platelet precursors, except after an aplastic episode when the myeloid and platelet precursors are decreased. Bone marrow iron stains often reveal decreased iron stores.

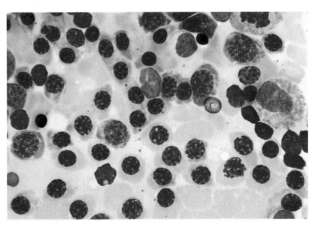

FIGURE 13-4 Bone marrow aspirate smear from a patient with paroxysmal nocturnal hemoglobinuria demonstrating erythroid hyperplasia. (Magnification ×500.)

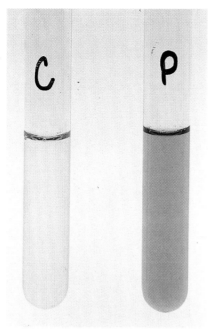

FIGURE 13-5   Sugar water test. The tube on the left represents the control (*C*), and the tube on the right represents the patient (*P*) with a positive sugar water test. Ten to 80% hemolysis is seen in PNH.

Diagnostic Tests

Sugar Water Test (Sucrose Hemolysis Test)

The sugar water test (Fig. 13–5) is used as a screening procedure when the diagnosis of PNH is considered. The sucrose provides a medium of low ionic strength that promotes the binding of complement, especially C3, to the red cell membranes. The low-ionic-strength solution used in the sugar water test activates complement via the classic or alternate pathway. The complement-sensitive PNH red cells are lysed, whereas normal cells will be unaffected.

Ten to 80 percent red cell lysis is seen in PNH (Fig. 13–5). Less than 5% red cell lysis is usually considered negative for PNH. A small amount of lysis (less than 5%) has been observed in patients with megaloblastic anemia, autoimmune hemolytic anemia, and leukemia. False-negative results occasionally occur if the serum lacks complement or if an unbuffered sucrose solution is used (see Chap. 31).

However, a definitive diagnosis of PNH depends on the results obtained with Ham's test.

Ham's Test (Acidified Serum Lysis Test)

Ham's test, or the acidified serum lysis test, is used to confirm the diagnosis of PNH (Fig. 13–6). Serum is acidified, which activates complement via the alternate pathway and enhances the binding of C3 to the cell membrane. The PNH erythrocytes lyse because they are deficient in the membrane proteins DAF, MIRL, and HRF, rendering them more sensitive to lysis by complement. Normal erythrocytes will be unaffected.

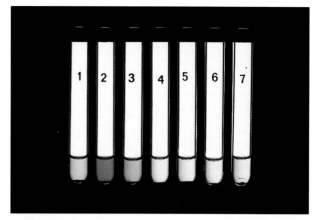

FIGURE 13-6   Ham's test. Positive results occur in patient with PNH. A positive test is reported when hemolysis occurs in tube number 1, containing fresh normal serum and patient cells; tube number 2, containing acidified normal serum and patient cells; and tube number 3, containing acidified patient serum and patient cells.

In order to confirm a positive Ham's test result, the following characteristics must be demonstrated: (1) Hemolysis occurs with the patient's cells and not with control cells, and (2) hemolysis is enhanced by acidified serum and does not occur with the heat-inactivated serum[28] (heating serum to 56°C for 30 minutes inactivates complement activity). For an outline of the Ham's test procedure and interpretation of results, refer to Table 13–2. This test is specific for PNH when it is shown that the patient's own serum is capable of lysing his or her own cells.[30]

A positive Ham's test result will be seen in the rare disorder called congenital dyserythropoietic anemia (CDA) type II, or HEMPAS. In this disorder, lysis does not occur with the patient's own serum; lysis in this case is the result of an unusual red cell antigen that reacts with IgM, a complement-activating antibody present in many normal sera.[23] The sugar water test for this disorder will also yield a negative result. Spherocytes also lyse in acidified serum because of the decreased pH; therefore, they will lyse in the tube containing the complement-inactivated serum.[23]

THERAPY

No specific therapeutic regimen is employed in the treatment of PNH. Treatment is usually directed toward the complications that arise from infections, anemia, and thromboses. In uncomplicated mild cases, therapy is not needed.

In patients with severe iron-deficiency anemia, iron therapy is usually given, either orally or parenterally. However, patients may experience hemolytic episodes after iron therapy. Iron therapy causes an increase in the production of normal as well as abnormal erythrocytes. Oral administration of iron produces less hemolysis, but the iron loss as hemosiderin may be so great that the oral doses cannot compensate for the iron deficiency present.[31]

TABLE 13–2 **Acidified Serum Lysis Test**							
	1	2	3	4	5	6	7
Fresh normal serum	0.5 mL	0.5 mL			0.5 mL	0.5 mL	
Patient's serum			0.5 mL				
Heat-inactivated normal serum				0.5 mL			0.5 mL
0.2 N HCl		0.05 mL	0.05 mL	0.05 mL		0.05 mL	0.05 mL
50% patient's red cells	0.05 mL	0.05 mL	0.05 mL	0.05 mL			
50% normal red cells					0.05 mL	0.05 mL	0.05 mL
Pattern of lysis in positive test	Trace	+++	++	—	—	—	—

Source: Adapted from Dacie and Lewis,[27] and Nelson, D: Clinical Diagnosis and Management by Laboratory Methods, ed 17. WB Saunders, Philadelphia, 1984, p 673.

In the severely anemic patient, blood transfusions are required; however, stored whole blood or packed red cells may cause an exacerbation of hemolysis. This hemolysis is thought to be the result of infusion of activated complement components; therefore, it is best to use washed or frozen deglycerolized red blood cells. Transfusions cause an increase in the red cell mass and hemoglobin level, and at the same time cause a temporary decrease in the production of the abnormal erythrocytes.

Hemolytic episodes associated with PNH may be controlled with the use of adrenocorticosteroids. Patients with any degree of bone marrow hypoplasia respond best to therapy with androgens. The androgens have a stimulatory effect on erythropoiesis and are thought to inhibit complement activation. Although androgens may be helpful, one must consider the possible side effects. Prednisone, a corticosteroid, has been used with success in suppression of hemolytic episodes. High doses of prednisone have proven the most beneficial but are associated with various side effects. However, moderate to high doses given on alternate days significantly decrease the side effects.[31]

Anticoagulant therapy is indicated in patients who are prone to the formation of venous thromboses or in whom a known life-threatening thrombosis exists. Heparin is the anticoagulant of choice in treating thromboses, but it can precipitate a hemolytic crisis. Administered in low doses, heparin can activate complement and thereby increase the probability of a hemolytic crisis.[32] However, when administered in high doses, heparin has been effective in the treatment of thromboses and has been shown to inactivate complement, thereby diminishing the chance of a hemolytic crisis.[32]

Certain patients with PNH have such severe bone marrow hypoplasia that a bone marrow transplant may be indicated. Transplants have been reported successful in severe cases. After the transplant, the abnormal clone of cells may be eliminated and replaced by a normal cell population.

CLINICAL COURSE AND PROGNOSIS

PNH is a chronic disease. Patients have survived 20 to 43 years after diagnosis, although the average survival is 10 years.[27] The most common cause of death is thromboembolism. Patients with bone marrow hypoplasia often die from infections or hemorrhage.[19] In a few patients, the disease may decrease in severity or completely disappear with time. Some patients have complete clinical remissions with persisting laboratory abnormalities. Occasionally, acute myelogenous leukemia develops in patients with PNH.[33,34] When PNH transforms to acute leukemia, the abnormal complement-sensitive population of erythrocytes disappears.[27] PNH has also been classified as a preleukemic or myelodysplastic syndrome.[35]

ROLE OF COMPLEMENT

Complement is a group of serum proteins that interact with each other to bring about, among other events, complement-dependent cell-mediated lysis. Complement can be activated by two different routes, the classic or the alternate (properdin pathway).

Classic Pathway

Activation of the classic pathway is initiated by immune complexes containing IgG (IgG 1, IgG 2, IgG 3) or IgM (see Fig. 13–7). The first complement component, C1, consists of three subunits, C1q, C1r, C1s, as well as calcium (recognition unit). C1q initiates the complement cascade by interacting with the Fc (crystallizable fragment) portion of the immunoglobin (Fig. 13–7). C1q then causes the activation of C1r, which then activates C1s. (A bar across the top of a complement component denotes its active form.) C4 is the second complement protein to be activated. This occurs when C1s cleaves C4 into its activated components; C4a, which remains in the plasma; and C4b, a small portion of which attaches to the cell membrane with the rest remaining in the plasma, inactivated. C2 attaches to C4b in the presence of magnesium and is then cleaved by C1s into the a and b subunits. C2a combines with C4b and forms the enzyme C3 convertase (C4b2a), and C2b is released into the plasma.

Amplification of complement activity occurs now with the action of C3 convertase on C3. This enzyme (C4b2a) cleaves C3 into its active components, C3a and C3b, and is able to cleave hundreds of C3 mole-

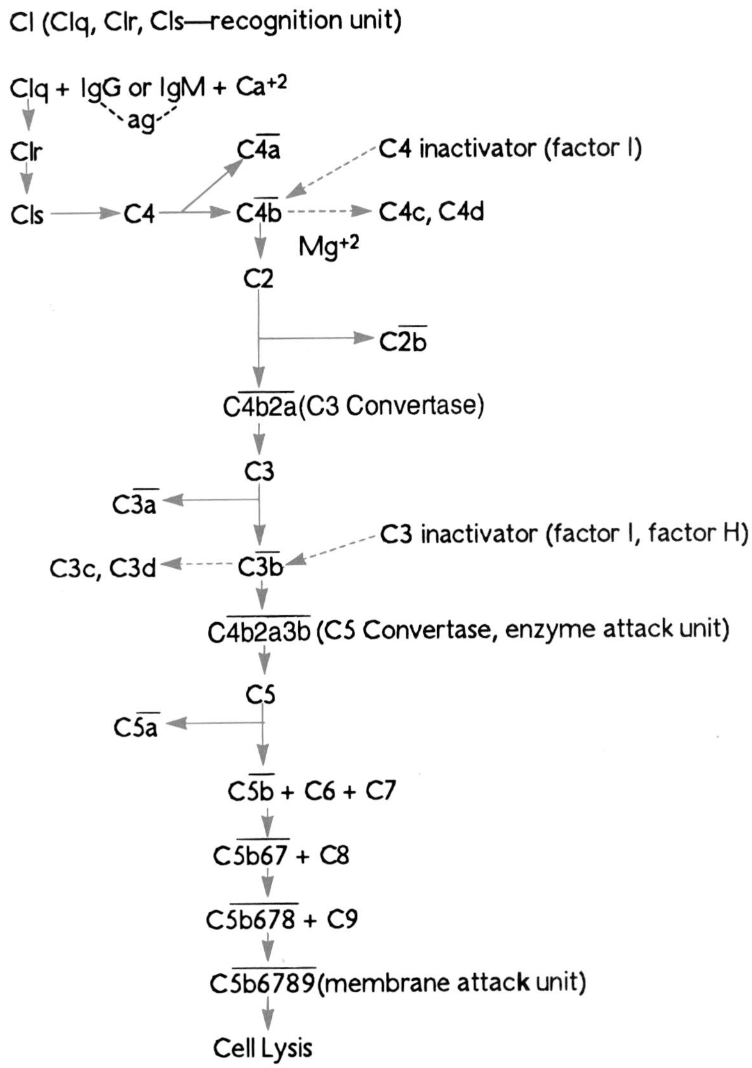

CI (CIq, CIr, CIs—recognition unit)

CIq + IgG or IgM + Ca^{+2}
　　　　＼・ag・／
CIr　　　　　　　　　　C$\overline{4a}$　　　　← C4 inactivator (factor I)

CIs ⟶ C4 ⟶ C$\overline{4b}$ - - - - ► C4c, C4d
　　　　　　　　　▼　　Mg^{+2}
　　　　　　　　　C2
　　　　　　　　　　　　　► C$\overline{2b}$

C$\overline{4b2a}$(C3 Convertase)
　　　　　　　▼
　　　　　　　C3
C$\overline{3a}$ ◄
　　　　　　　▼
　　　　　　　　　　　　- - - C3 inactivator (factor I, factor H)
C3c, C3d ◄- - - - C$\overline{3b}$ ◄

C$\overline{4b2a3b}$ (C5 Convertase, enzyme attack unit)
　　　　　　　▼
　　　　　　　C5
C$\overline{5a}$ ◄
　　　　　　　▼
　　　　C$\overline{5b}$ + C6 + C7
　　　　　　　▼
　　　　C$\overline{5b67}$ + C8
　　　　　　　▼
　　　　C$\overline{5b678}$ + C9
　　　　　　　▼
　　　　C$\overline{5b6789}$(membrane attack unit)
　　　　　　　▼
　　　　　Cell Lysis

FIGURE 13-7 Classical pathway of complement activation.

cules. C3a is released into the plasma and acts as an anaphylatoxin. C3b binds to the cell membrane and combines with C4b2a to form another enzyme, C5 convertase (C4b2a3b). Some of the C3b molecules attached to other sites on the cell are inactivated (C3bi), or are cleaved by C3 inactivator to C3c, which is released into the plasma, and to C3d, an inactive subunit that remains attached to the cell. The components C4, C3, C2 are referred to as the *enzyme activation unit.*

C5 convertase (C4b2a3b) cleaves C5 into the components C5a, which is released into the plasma and acts as an anaphylatoxin and a chemotactic agent, and C5b, which binds C6 and C7 to the cell membrane. Membrane-bound C5b67 causes binding of C8, resulting in immediate ion flux into the cell. The C5b678 complex can bind up to six C9 molecules, together forming the membrane attack unit, C5b6789, which causes cell lysis and accelerated movement of ions into the cell. With binding of C9, cell lysis results (see Fig. 13–7).

Complement activity is regulated by certain inhibitors (C1s inhibitor, C3b inactivator, C4 inactivator) and by the instability of certain components (C4b2a, and C4b2a3b).[36]

Alternate (Properdin) Pathway

The alternate, or properdin, pathway of complement activation also results in cell lysis but by a different mechanism and group of proteins. The alternate pathway bypasses the complement components C1, C2, and C4 and enters at C3. This pathway consists of a distinct group of proteins: complement component C3; factor B, which is enzymatically cleaved into fragments Bb (biologically active) and Ba; factor D, which cleaves factor B; properdin (P), a serum protein that stabilizes the C3bBb complex; and factor H (C3b inactivator accelerator), which aids in controlling activation of the alternate pathway (Fig. 13–8).[37]

The alternate pathway may be triggered by certain micro-organisms, polysaccharides, liposaccharides, aggregates of IgA, and cells or particles even in the absence of specific antibody.

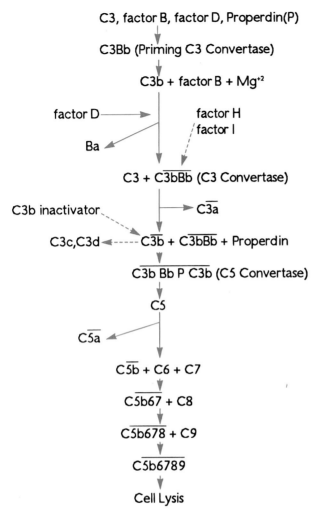

FIGURE 13-8 Alternate pathway of complement activation.

CASE STUDY

A 43-year-old man presented to his physician with complaints of lower back pain, fatigue, easy bruising, and a sudden onset of dark urine on arising in the morning. Laboratory studies and a bone marrow aspirate were then ordered by his physician, and they disclosed the following:

1. Complete Blood Cell Count (CBC)

HCT	28%
WBC	$3.3 \times 10^9/L$
Platelet count	$76 \times 10^9/L$
Retic	5.1%
Corrected Retic	3.2%

Differential:

Segmented neutrophils	34%
Lymphocytes	64%
Monocytes	2%
NRBC	1/100 WBC

1+ Poikilocytosis
2+ Anisocytosis
2+ Polychromasia

Figure 13-2 shows the peripheral blood smear from this patient.

2. The chemistry profile was normal except for an increased lactic dehydrogenase (LDH) value, (780 IU/L) and bilirubin (Total 2.9 mg/dL, direct 0.4 mg/dL).
3. A urinalysis was performed and was positive for hemoglobin.
4. The bone marrow aspirate revealed a hypercellular marrow with relative erythroid hyperplasia. There were adequate numbers of myeloid and platelet precursors (see Fig. 13-4).

Further studies were performed after initial tests were completed.

5. Urinary Hemosiderin: Positive
6. Sugar water test: Positive (12%)
7. Ham's test: Positive

Diagnosis: *Paroxysmal nocturnal hemoglobinuria*

Questions

1. What type of hemolysis is evident in this patient?
2. What abnormal RBC morphology is present in Figure 13-4?
3. Given the NRBC count, is a corrected WBC count needed?
4. How would you classify the M:E ratio in Figure 13-4?
5. If the granulocytes in this patient were scored for LAP activity, what would you expect the result to be?

REFERENCES

1. Williams, WJ, Beutler, E, Erslev, AJ, et al: Hematology, ed 2. McGraw-Hill, New York, 1977, p 560.
2. Gull, WP: A case of intermittent hematuria, with remarks. Guys Hosp Rep 12:381, 1866.
3. Strubing, P: Paroxysmale Hamoglobinurie. Dtsch Med Wschr 8:1, 1882.
4. Marchiafava, E: Anemia emolitica con emosiderinuria perpitua. Policlinico (sez med) 18:241, 1931.
5. Micheli, F: Anemia (splenomegalia) emolitica con emoglobinuria-emosiderinuria tipo Marchiafava. Hematologica 12:101–123, 1931.
6. Hijmas van den Bergh, AA: Ictere hemolytique avec crises hemoglobinuriques. Fragilite globulaire Rev Med 31:63, 1911.
7. Ham, TH and Dingle, JH: Studies on destruction of red blood cells—II. Chronic hemolytic anemia with paroxysmal nocturnal hemoglobinuria—Certain immunological aspects of the hemolytic mechanism with special reference to serum complement. J Clin Invest 18:657, 1939.
8. Ham, TH: Chronic hemolytic anemia with paroxysmal nocturnal hemoglobinuria—A study of the mechanism of hemolysis in relation to acid base equilibrium. N Engl J Med 217:915, 1937.
9. Rosse, WF: Phosphatidylinositol-linked proteins and paroxysmal nocturnal hemoglobinuria. Blood 75:1595–1601, 1990.
10. Beck, WS: Hematology, ed 3. Massachusetts Institute of Technology Press, Cambridge, MA, 1982, p 211.
11. Nicholson-Weller, A, Spicer, DB, and Austen, KF: Deficiency of the complement regulatory protein, 'decay accelerating factor' on membranes of granulocytes, monocytes and platelets in Paroxysmal Nocturnal Hemoglobinuria. N Engl J Med 312:1091–1097, 1985.
12. Rosse, WF: Paroxysmal nocturnal hemoglobinuria and

decay accelerating factor. Annu Rev Med 41:431–436, 1990.

13. Zalman, LS, Wood, LM, Frank, MM, et al: Deficiency of the homologous factor in paroxysmal nocturnal hemoglobinuria. J Exp Med 165:572–577, 1987.

14. Eichner, ER, Spivak, JL, Sims, PJ, and Selby, GB: Hematology—1989, Education program. The Anemias; Paroxysmal Nocturnal Hemoglobinuria. American Society of Hematology, 1989, pp 3–4.

15. Schonermark S, Rauterberg EW, Shin ML, Loke S, et al: Homologous species restriction in lysis of human erythrocytes: a membrane derived protein with C8-binding capacity functions as an inhibitor. J Immunol 136:1772, 1986.

16. Chow, FL, Telen, MJ, and Rosse, WF: The acetylcholinesterase defect in paroxysmal nocturnal hemoglobinuria: Evidence that the enzyme is absent from the cell membrane. Blood 66:940, 1986.

17. Metz, J, Bradow, BA, Lewis, SM, et al: Acetylcholinesterase activity of the erythrocytes in paroxysmal nocturnal hemoglobinuria in relation to the severity of the disease. Br J Haematol 6:372, 1960.

18. Mengal, CE, Kann, HE, Meriwether, WD, et al: Studies of paroxysmal nocturnal hemoglobinuria erythrocytes: Increased lysis and lipid peroxide formation by hydrogen peroxide. J Clin Invest 46:1715, 1967.

19. Mengal, CE, Ebbert, L, Stickney, D, et al: Biochemistry of PNH cells; nature of the membrane defect. Ser Haematol 5:88, 1972.

20. Lewis, SM, Lambertenghi, G, Ferrone, S, et al: Electron microscope study of PNH red cells and AET-treated normal cells (PNH-like). J Clin Pathol 24:667, 1971.

21. Rosse, WF and Adams, JP: The membrane abnormalities in paroxysmal nocturnal hemoglobinuria. Prog Clin Biol Res 30:457, 1979.

22. Dacie, JV: Paroxysmal nocturnal hemoglobinuria. Sangre 25:890, 1980.

23. Wintrobe, ME, Lee, GR, Boggs, DR, et al (eds): Clinical Hematology, ed 8. Lea & Febiger, Philadelphia, 312:978, 1981.

24. Handin, RI, Lux, SE, and Stossel, TP: Blood: Principles and Practice of Hematology. JB Lippincott, Philadelphia, 1995.

25. Rosse, WF: Paroxysmal nocturnal hemoglobinuria in aplastic anemia. Clin Haematol 7:541, 1978.

26. Sun, NC: Hematology—An Atlas and Diagnostic Guide, ed 1. WB Saunders, Philadelphia, 1983, p 90.

27. Dacie, JV and Lewis, SM: Paroxysmal nocturnal hemoglobinuria, clinical manifestations, hematology and nature of the disease. Ser Haematol 5:3, 1972.

28. Kjeldsberg, C, Beutler, E, Bell, C, et al: Hematologic Disease, Practical Diagnosis, ed 2. ASCP Press, Chicago, 1989, p 162.

29. Okuda, K, et al: Membrane expression of decay accelerating factor on neutrophils from normal individuals and patients with paroxysmal nocturnal hemoglobinuria. Blood 75:1186–1191, 1990.

30. Hoffbrand, AV and Lewis, SM: Post Graduate Hematology, ed 2. Appleton-Century-Crofts, New York, 1981, p 232.

31. Rosse, WF: Treatment of paroxysmal nocturnal hemoglobinuria. Blood 60:20, 1982.

32. Logue, GL: Effects of heparin on complement activation and lysis of paroxysmal nocturnal hemoglobinuria red cells. Blood 50:239, 1977.

33. Cowell, DE, Pasquale, DN, and Dekker, P: Paroxysmal nocturnal hemoglobinuria terminating as acute leukemia. Cancer 43:1914, 1979.

34. Krause, JR: Paroxysmal nocturnal hemoglobinuria and acute nonlymphoblastic leukemia. Cancer 51:2078, 1983.

35. Rosse, WF: Paroxysmal nocturnal hemoglobinuria—present status and future prospects. West J Med 132:219, 1980.

36. Muller, LE, Ludke, HR, Peacock, JE, and Tomar RH: Manual of Laboratory Immunology, ed 2. Lea & Febiger, Philadelphia 1991, Chap. 6, pp 120–141.

37. Fearson, DT and Austen, KF: The alternate pathway of complement—A system of host resistance to microbial infections. N Engl J Med 303:259, 1980.

BIBLIOGRAPHY

Dacie, JV and Lewis, SM: Paroxysmal nocturnal hemoglobinuria, clinical manifestations, hematology and nature of the disease. Ser Haematol 5:3, 1972.

Forman, K, Sokol, RJ, Hewitt, S, et al: Paroxysmal nocturnal hemoglobinuria—A clinicopathological study of 26 cases. Acta Haematol 71:217, 1984.

Goetz, O and Muller-Eberhard, HJ: The alternate pathway of complement activation. Adv Immunol 24:1, 1976.

Griscelli-Bennaceur, A, Gluckman, E, Scrobohaci, ML, Jonveaux, P, et al: Aplastic anemia and paroxysmal nocturnal hemoglobinuria: Search for a Pathogenic Link. Blood 85:1354–1363, 1995.

Hartman, RC and Jenkins, DE, Jr: The "sugar water" test for paroxysmal nocturnal hemoglobinuria. N Engl J Med 275:155, 1966.

Hartman RC, Jenkins DE, Jr, and Arnold, AB: Diagnostic specificity of sucrose hemolysis test for paroxysmal nocturnal hemoglobinuria. Blood 35:462, 1970.

Holguin, MH, Wilcox, LA, Bernshaw, NJ, et al: Relationship between membrane inhibitor of reactive lysis and the erythrocyte phenotypes of paroxysmal nocturnal hematuria. J Clin Invest 1989;84:1387.

Kinoshita, T, Medof, ME, Silbor, R, and Nussenzweig V: Distribution of decay accelerating factor in the peripheral blood of normal individuals and patients with paroxysmal nocturnal hemoglobinuria. J Exp Med 162:75, 1985.

Muller-Eberhard, HJ: Complement. Ann Rev Biochem 44:697, 1975.

Nakakuma, H, Nagakura, S, Iwamoto, N, Kawaguchi, T, et al: Paroxysmal nocturnal hemoglobinuria clone in bone marrow of patients with pancytopenia. Blood 85:1371–1376, 1995.

Rosse, WF: Paroxysmal nocturnal hemoglobinuria. In Handin, RI, Stossel, TP, and Lux, SE (eds): Blood: Principles and Practice of Hematology. JB Lippincott, Philadelphia, 1995, pp 367–376.

Rosse, WF: Paroxysmal nocturnal hemoglobinuria—present status and future prospects. West J Med 132:219, 1980.

Selvaraj, P, Dustin, ML, Silber, R, et al: Deficiency of lymphocyte function-associated antigens 3 (LFA-3) in paroxysmal nocturnal hemoglobinuria: functional correlates and evidence for a phosphatidylinositol membrane anchor. J Exp Med 166:1011, 1987.

Terstappen, LWMM, Nguyen, M, Lazarus, H, and Medof, ME: Expression of the DAF (CD55) and CD59 antigens during normal hematopoietic cell differentiation. Leukocyte Biol 52:652–660, 1992.

QUESTIONS

1. Which statement best describes paroxysmal nocturnal hemoglobinuria?
   a. Acquired hemolytic anemia associated with cellular membrane abnormalities
   b. Congenital hemolytic anemia associated with the inflammatory response
   c. Acquired or congenital hemolytic anemia associated with enzyme deficiencies

d. Hemolytic anemia of unknown origin associated with auto-antibodies

2. What causes the red cell defect of PNH?
   a. Rare red cell antigens
   b. Deficiency of decay-accelerating factor (DAF), membrane inhibitor of reactive lysis (MIRL), and homologous restriction factor (HRF), complement regulatory proteins.
   c. Excessive amounts of complement components C5 to C9.
   d. G6PD enzyme deficiency.

3. Which type of PNH erythrocyte is most sensitive to lysis by complement?
   a. PNH I
   b. PNH II
   c. PNH III
   d. PNH I and PNH II equally sensitive

4. Which list is the most complete for clinical features of PNH?
   a. Hemoglobinuria, hemosiderinuria, abdominal pain, headaches, and back pain
   b. Weakness, fatigue, hepatosplenomegaly, back pain
   c. Recurrent infections, skin ulcers, spontaneous fractures, dental problems
   d. Persistent bacterial infections, jaundice, kernicterus, and weight loss

5. What nonspecific laboratory findings are characteristic for PNH?
   a. Microcytic, hypochromic anemia; leukocytosis; thrombocytosis; decreased indirect bilirubin
   b. Macrocytic, hypochromic anemia; leukopenia with decreased lymphocytes; normal to elevated LAP; thrombocytopenia; increased haptoglobin
   c. Normocytic, hypochromic anemia; leukopenia with decreased neutrophils; thrombocytosis with giant platelets; decreased plasma hemoglobin
   d. Normocytic, normochromic anemia; leukopenia with decreased granulocytes; low LAP; thrombocytopenia; urine hemosiderin

6. Which of the following is a correct description of the sugar water test (sucrose hemolysis test)?

a. PNH cells are lysed by complement after exposure to low-ionic-strength sugar water.
b. PNH cells are lysed by antibody and complement after heating to 56°C in sugar water solution (5%).
c. Patient's serum is acidified to enhance complement binding and lysis of patient cells.
d. Patient's serum is heat-inactivated and treated with HCl; complement is added; patient cell lysis occurs.

7. What is a correct description of Ham's test (acidified serum lysis test)?
   a. PNH cells are lysed by complement after exposure to low-ionic-strength sugar water.
   b. PNH cells are lysed by antibody and complement after heating to 56°C in sugar water solution (5%).
   c. Patient's serum is acidified to enhance complement binding and lysis of patient cells.
   d. Patient's serum is heat-inactivated and treated with HCl; complement is added; patient cell lysis occurs.

8. Which of the following is not usually a treatment for PNH?
   a. Anticoagulant therapy
   b. Blood transfusion/marrow transplant
   c. Adrenocorticosteroids
   d. Immunosuppressive therapy

ANSWERS

1. **a** (p 211)
2. **b** (p 212)
3. **c** (p 213)
4. **a** (p 213)
5. **d** (pp 213–214)
6. **a** (p 215)
7. **c** (p 215)
8. **d** (p 216)

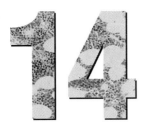

Hemolytic Anemias: Extracorpuscular Defects

VI. IMMUNE AND NONIMMUNE HEMOLYTIC ANEMIA

Suzy L. Nicol, MT(ASCP)SBB
Denise M. Harmening, PhD, MT(ASCP), CLS(NCA)
Ralph Green, BAppSci(MLS), FAIMS

Objectives

Upon completion of this chapter, the learner should be able to:
1 List mechanisms of immune hemolysis.
2 Define alloimmune hemolytic anemia.
3 Characterize immediate hemolytic transfusion reactions.
4 Characterize delayed hemolytic transfusion reactions.
5 Describe the causes of hemolytic disease of the newborn.
6 Define autoimmune hemolytic anemia.
7 Characterize warm autoimmune hemolytic anemia.
8 List features of cold agglutinin syndrome.
9 Describe the principle of the Donath-Landsteiner test used for paroxysmal cold hemoglobinuria.
10 List mechanisms for drug-induced immune hemolytic anemia.

IMMUNE HEMOLYTIC ANEMIA

Mechanisms of Immune Hemolysis

Intravascular Hemolysis

Intravascular hemolysis, as the name implies, occurs within the vascular system and results from activation of the *classic complement* pathway via immunoglobulin G (IgG) or IgM antibodies (see Chaps. 22 and 13 for an explanation of immunoglobulins and complement, respectively). Intravascular hemolysis occurs when antibodies that bind to antigenic determinants on red cells activate complement to completion (i.e., lysis). This occurs only when the activation process is intense enough to overwhelm the natural regulatory process that inactivates complement. IgM is a very efficient activator of complement because of its pentameric structure. A single molecule of IgM is capable of initiating complement activation by the classic pathway.[1,2] The ability of IgG antibodies to activate complement is dependent on several factors: (1) The IgG subclass IgG3 is the most efficient at activating complement, followed by IgG1, then IgG2. IgG4 is not capable of complement activation.[3] The biologic properties of the IgG subclasses are summarized in Table 14–1. (2) The number and location of IgG molecules on the red cell surface. At least two IgG molecules must be in close enough proximity to allow crosslinking of complement receptors, which initiates complement activation.[1,3] (3) The physical location of the red cell antigens influences the binding of IgG. (4) The ability of the immunoglobulin to remain attached to the red cell surface (avidity) is important as well.

Antibody-Dependent Cellular Cytotoxicity Another possible mechanism of direct (intravascular) lysis of immunoglobulin-coated red cells is *antibody-dependent cellular cytotoxicity* (ADCC). Many white cell lines [macrophages/monocytes, neutrophils, and natural killer lymphocytes (NK cells)] have receptors on their membranes that bind immunoglobulins and complement degradation products.[4] The cells with such receptors are collectively referred to as *effector cells*. The effector cell receptors specific for IgG1 and/or IgG3 are called Fc receptors (FcR). They are called FcR because they bind the Fc (fragment, constant) of these immunoglobulins (see Chap. 22 for a review of immunoglobulin structure). The effector cells also have receptors for complement degradation products, C3b and iC3b. These receptors are called CR1 and CR3, respectively (see Chap. 13 for a review of complement activation). ADCC results when the immunoprotein (IgG3, IgG1, C3b, or iC3b) is bound to its respective FcR (or CR) of the effector cell. This interaction will cause the release of lytic enzymes.[5,6] It should be noted that not all IgG1 and IgG3 immunoglobulins are capable of mediating lysis.[7] The role of complement receptors in ADCC is not well established. It is very likely that complement degradation products work synergistically with IgG3 and/or IgG1 to enhance ADCC.[5]

Laboratory Findings Hemoglobin is released into the blood when red cells are destroyed intravascularly. This condition of free hemoglobin liberation in the blood is called *hemoglobinemia*. Free hemoglobin is filtered through the kidneys, resulting in *hemoglobinuria* (free hemoglobin in the urine). Hemoglobinuria may be confused with hematuria (intact red cells in the urine), especially when the urine is red. It is important to distinguish between the two because hemoglobinuria is an indicator of hemolysis, whereas hematuria is not related to hemolysis. Microscopic examination of the urine may be helpful in differentiating the presence of intact red cells from hemoglobin.

Within hours of intravascular hemolysis, *haptoglobin* is depleted. As little as 5 mL of lysed red cells can bind all of the available haptoglobin. However, haptoglobin, which is synthesized in the liver, can return to normal levels within 24 hours (see Chap. 3 under red cell senescence). Because haptoglobin is an acute phase reactant protein, concentrations may vary considerably depending on several factors, such as underlying disease processes. Consequently, care must be taken when interpreting haptoglobin levels as an indicator of hemolysis. It is advisable to have a "baseline" haptoglobin level to compare to the haptoglobin level following suspected hemolysis. See Figure 14–1 for the sequence of laboratory findings.

Other laboratory findings that may be associated with intravascular hemolysis include elevated *serum bilirubin* level (primarily indirect); elevated *lactate dehydrogenase* (LDH) levels, an enzyme of red cell metabolism; and possible *reticulocytosis*. Table 14–2 summarizes the laboratory findings. (For a review of hemoglobin catabolism, see Chap. 3, Erythrocyte Senescence.)

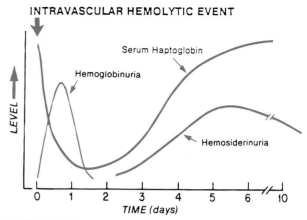

INTRAVASCULAR HEMOLYTIC EVENT

FIGURE 14–1 Indicators of acute intravascular hemolysis. Within a few hours of an acute hemolytic event, free hemoglobin is cleared from plasma and the serum haptoglobin falls to undetectable levels; hemoglobinuria ceases soon after. If no further hemolysis occurs, the serum haptoglobin level recovers, and methemalbumin disappears within several days. The urinary hemosiderin can provide more lasting evidence of the hemolytic event.

Extravascular Hemolysis

Extravascular hemolysis is the phagocytosis of red cells by fixed phagocytes within the *reticuloendothelial system* (RES). The two major organs of the RES are the *spleen* and the *liver*. In the red pulp region of the spleen, macrophages with Fc receptors (see ADCC above) line the splenic cords. Antibody-coated red cells interact with the Fc receptors, resulting in complete or partial phagocytosis. In the case of partial phagocytosis, part of the red cell membrane is removed. If the cell

TABLE 14–1 Biologic Properties of IgG Isotypes				
Characteristic	**IgG1**	**IgG2**	**IgG3**	**IgG4**
% Total serum IgG	65–70	23–28	4–7	3–4
Complement fixation (classic pathway)	Yes	Yes	Yes	No
Binding to macrophage Fc receptors	Yes	No	Yes	No
Placental transfer	Yes	Yes	Yes	Yes
Biologic half-life (days)	21	21	7–8	21

TABLE 14–2	**Mechanisms of Immune Hemolysis**	
	Intravascular	**Extravascular**
Mechanism	IgM or IgG3, IgG1, IgG2 (two IgG molecules within close proximity of each other) activate complement to completion Antibody dependent cellular cytotoxicity (ADCC)	IgM and/or IgG sensitization with/without iC3b (inactivated complement) Cell-mediated phagocytosis
Organ	Occurs within blood vessels	Spleen: IgG alone or IgG + iC3b coated cells Liver: iC3b alone or IgG + iC3b coated cells
Laboratory findings	Hemoglobinemia Hemoglobinuria Serum haptoglobin: decreased Indirect bilirubin: elevated Lactate dehydrogenase (LDH): elevated	Spherocytosis Serum haptoglobin: decreased Indirect bilirubin: elevated Positive direct antiglobulin test

membrane is able to repair itself, a dense, sphere-shaped, red cell called a *spherocyte* is formed. Spherocytes lack deformability and become physically trapped in the spleen; those that do escape the spleen can be seen in the peripheral blood, and their presence is indicative of immune-mediated hemolysis (Fig. 14–2).

As previously mentioned, both IgG and IgM antibodies are capable of activating complement. However, the activation process does not always go to completion (C1 through C9). In most cases complement activation will be stopped by an inhibitory factor (control mechanism) at the C3b stage. C3b is cleaved to form iC3b. If activation is stopped, iC3b is further broken down into C3dg, which will remain attached to the red cell membrane.[6]

Red cells coated with IgG1 or IgG3 are preferentially removed in the spleen[6] rather than the liver because blood passing through the spleen becomes hemoconcentrated altering the ratio between free IgG in the plasma and cell-bound IgG. Free IgG can bind to Fc receptors blocking their ability to bind the IgG that is attached to red cells. The condition of hemoconcentration in the spleen shifts the ratio of free IgG to red cell–bound IgG in favor of the red cell–bound IgG. The activated form of complement (C3b) or its inactivated form (iC3b) is not present in the free form in plasma; therefore the hemoconcentration of blood in the spleen does not contribute significantly to the destruction of complement-coated red cells.[5] However, cells coated with both IgG and C3b/iC3b are phagocytized more efficiently in the spleen than if they are sensitized by IgG alone.[5]

The liver has the largest concentration of macrophages with receptors specific for immune complexes, thus the liver is the major site of removal for red cells coated with complement or heavily coated with IgG.[2,6] There is very little removal of red cells coated with small amounts of IgG in the liver because of the high concentration of free IgG located there. Cells sensitized with both IgG and iC3b/C3d will be removed in the liver and the spleen.

Laboratory Findings Spherocytes or *spherocytosis* may be seen on the peripheral blood smear when extravascular hemolysis has occurred. *Serum bilirubin* levels (indirect) may be elevated and *urobilinogen* concentration may be increased in urine and stool specimens (see Chap. 3 for a review of hemoglobin catabolism). The *direct antiglobulin test* (DAT) may be positive, as well as the *indirect antiglobulin test* (antibody screening test). See Table 14–2 for a summary of laboratory findings. Table 14–3 lists the factors that influence immune hemolysis.

Classification of Immune Hemolytic Anemias

Numerous classifications of immune hemolytic anemias have been proposed; however, three broad categories are usually used:

1. *Alloimmune*: Patient produces alloantibodies to foreign red cell antigens introduced through transfusions, pregnancy, or organ transplantation.

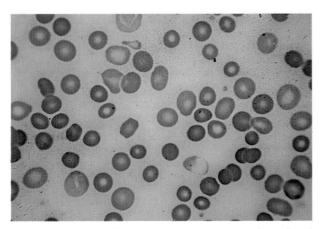

FIGURE 14–2 Autoimmune hemolytic anemia (peripheral blood). Note spherocytes and polychromasia.

TABLE 14–3 Factors Influencing the Presence and Extent of Immune Hemolysis

Antibody
Immunoglobulin class and subclass
Concentration
Avidity
Thermal reactivity (determined by the nature of the predominant noncovalent bonds formed at the time of the antigen antibody reaction)

Antigen
Number and density
Cellular distribution
Presence of soluble antigen

Complement
Concentration of complement factors
Concentration and activity of regulating factors

Reticuloendothelial System
Activity of phagocytic cells (influenced by underlying disease processes, generation and activity of lymphokines and interleukins, and any concurrent drug therapy)

2. *Autoimmune*: Control mechanism for autoreactive antibodies is lost and antibodies directed against the patient's own red cells develop.
3. *Drug-induced*: Patient produces antibodies directed at a particular drug, its metabolites, or red cells coated with the drug.

Alloimmune Hemolytic Anemia

Alloimmunization is the process in which the immune system of an individual is stimulated by a foreign antigen and produces the corresponding antibody. The antibody produced by this immune response is termed an *alloantibody*. The antibody coats the foreign red cells introduced into the circulation, resulting in shortened red cell survival. Alloantibody production may result from: (1) transfusion of blood (exposure to foreign donor red cell antigens), (2) pregnancy (foreign antigens on fetal cells released into the maternal circulation), and (3) organ transplantation (exposure to foreign antigens on "passenger cells" that may be released into the recipient).

Alloimmune hemolytic anemia is usually associated with blood transfusions. An antibody present in the recipient is directed against a foreign red cell antigen located on the transfused cells. Basically there are two types of transfusion reactions, acute hemolytic and delayed hemolytic.

Acute Hemolytic Transfusion Reactions

Hemolytic transfusion reactions (HTRs) are characterized by acute *intravascular* hemolysis and are associated with the ABO blood group antibodies. The immunoglobulins associated with the ABO blood group are IgM or both IgM and IgG. In individuals who have both types (IgM and IgG), the majority of antibody is IgM with a minor amount of IgG.[8] Ordinarily, an individual possesses antibodies directed toward the A or B antigens absent from their own red cells. As stated above, IgM antibodies are efficient activators of complement, which results in immediate destruction of the transfused cells.

Symptoms of acute HTRs are variable. Typical symptoms are fever, shaking, chills, and pain or burning sensation along the infusion site. Other symptoms include nausea, vomiting, lower back pain, hypotension, and chest pain. See Table 14–4 for a list of clinical features. An incoherent, unconscious, or anesthetized patient cannot verbalize his or her symptoms and therefore is at risk of receiving more than one unit of incompatible blood.

The laboratory findings in HTR are those associated with intravascular hemolysis (see Table 14–2).

The treatment of HTR focuses on prompt termination of the transfusion. As stated in the discussion of intravascular hemolysis, free hemoglobin is filtered through the kidneys. Red cell stroma can clog and damage renal glomeruli, thus fluids are administered intravenously to maintain renal function.

Delayed Hemolytic Transfusion Reactions

Delayed HTRs (DHTRs) are associated with antibodies to blood groups other than the ABO blood group. Antibodies implicated in DHTR are usually IgG, which may activate complement, causing sensitization of the red cells with C3 but seldom leading to intravascular hemolysis. DHTRs are the most common type of transfusion reactions. They are caused by an anamnestic or secondary response to the transfused red cells. This occurs in previously immunized patients whose alloantibody level (after the initial stimulation) had dropped to serologically undetectable levels. As a result, the initial antibody screening and compatibility tests on the patient's pretransfusion sample are negative. Once re-exposed (transfused) to the foreign red cell antigen, an anamnestic response is mounted by the recipient. The titer rises and antibody may be detected in the posttransfusion sample as early as 48 hours after the transfusion. This type of reaction is termed *delayed* because it takes time for the patient to produce sufficient antibody to destroy the transfused cells. Characteristically, the reaction may occur anywhere from 2 to 10 days following transfusion.[9]

The symptoms of DHTR are usually mild and nonspecific; therefore it may not be recognized by clinicians.[10] Symptoms include mild fever, mild jaundice, and an unexpected fall in hemoglobin (or conversely, lack of expected rise in hemoglobin after transfusion).

Laboratory findings are those associated with extravascular hemolysis, but most cases are subclinical

TABLE 14–4 Clinical Features of Acute Hemolytic Transfusion Reactions

Fever	Hemoglobinuria
Chills	Shock
Chest pains	Generalized bleeding
Hypotension	Oliguria
Nausea	Anuria
Flushing	Back pain
Dyspnea	Pain at infusion site

TABLE 14–5 **Antibodies Most Commonly Implicated in DHTR**	
Antibody	**Blood Group System**
Anti-Jk^a	Kidd
Anti-K	Kell
Anti-c̄	Rh
Anti-E	Rh
Anti-Fy^a	Duffy
Anti-Jk^b	Kidd
Anti-C	Rh
Anti-e	Rh

TABLE 14–7 **Frequency of Types of HDN**	
ABO HDN	65%
Rh HDN	33%
Other	2%

and only discovered serologically (by DAT, antibody screening, and compatibility tests).[10]

Treatment is rarely necessary, and investigation focuses on accurately identifying the antibody to ensure blood for future transfusions will be negative for the foreign antigen that corresponds to the patient's antibody. Table 14–5 lists the antibodies most commonly implicated in DHTRs and Table 14–6 summarizes the laboratory findings.

Hemolytic Disease of the Newborn

Hemolytic disease of the newborn (HDN) is an immune hemolytic disorder caused by maternal and fetal blood group incompatibility (maternal IgG antibodies destroy antigen-containing fetal red cells). The transport mechanism for maternal immunoglobulins is selective in that only IgG antibodies can cross the placenta.

Pregnant women can become immunized to foreign fetal red cell antigens when an exchange of fetal blood occurs during pregnancy and at delivery [*fetal-maternal hemorrhage* (FMH)]. The amount of whole blood exchanged is normally only 1 mL. There is some evidence that as little as 0.03 mL of red cells can stimulate an immune response.[11,12] Thus, it is possible to become immunized from miscarriages and abortions. Blood transfusions can also stimulate an immune response as mentioned above in alloimmune hemolytic anemia. If a pregnant woman has been previously immunized to a foreign red cell antigen, and that antigen is present on the red cells of the fetus, the exchange of blood that occurs early in the pregnancy will be sufficient to stimulate an anamnestic response in the mother. The mother can produce increasing amounts of antibody directed against the fetal red cells.[13] The fetal red cells will become coated with maternal antibodies and destroyed by extravascular hemolysis. Responding to this increased red cell destruction, fetal hematopoietic tissue increases erythrocyte production. The fetal bone marrow may not be able to keep up with the increased need for red cells and *extramedullary hematopoiesis* occurs, causing liver and splenic enlargement. The fetus may not be able to compensate for the hemolysis, and an anemia characterized by increased numbers of erythroblasts may result. Hence, the term *erythroblastosis fetalis* has been used to describe HDN. There are two major forms of HDN; HDN associated with ABO and that associated with Rh(D) or other blood groups. Table 14–7 lists the frequencies of the various types of HDN. Table 14–8 compares ABO and Rh(D) HDN. For further information, see Harmening, DM: *Modern Blood Banking and Transfusion Practices, Third Edition.* F. A. Davis, Philadelphia, 1994.

Autoimmune Hemolytic Anemia

Autoimmune hemolytic anemia (AIHA) represents an abnormality within the immune system whereby the ability for self-recognition of an individual's own red cell antigens is lost. Recent experiments support that recognition of self occurs during embryogenesis by inactivation of autoreactive B and T lymphocytes. Under certain conditions (e.g., bacterial or viral infections), these autoreactive B and T lymphocytes escape the mechanism for tolerance of self.[14] As a result, patients produce antibodies that bind to their own red cells (autoantibody). AIHA can be broadly divided into warm or cold types. The warm type (WAIHA) is the most common, accounting for approximately 70% of all cases.[15,16] This type involves autoantibodies whose serologic reactivity is optimal at 37°C. Cold AIHA involves autoantibodies whose optimal serologic reactivity oc-

TABLE 14–6 **Differential Diagnosis of Hemolytic Anemia**		
Parameter/Analyte	**Extravascular**	**Intravascular**
Serial Hgb and Hct	Decreased	Decreased
Reticulocyte count*	>1%	>1%
RBC morphology	Spherocytes	
Serum bilirubin (indirect)	Increased	Increased
Serum haptoglobin†	Decreased‡	Decreased
Serum LDH (isoenzyme LDH1)	Increased‡	Increased
Hemoglobinemia	Absent	Present
Hemoglobinuria	Absent	Present

*May not show increase immediately.
†Important to compare with a prehemolysis "baseline" value.
‡More likely to be present with intravascular hemolysis.

TABLE 14–8   Comparison of ABO and Rh HDN

	ABO	Rh
Severity	Mild	Severe
Child affected	First-born (40–50% of cases)	Usually second or subsequent births (first-born: 5% of cases)
Blood groups	Mother: O	Mother: Rh negative
	Child: A or B	Child: Rh positive
Anemia	Uncommon, mild	Severe
Stillbirths/hydrops fetalis	Rare	Frequent
Jaundice	Mild	Severe
Spherocytes on peripheral blood smear	Usually present	None
Direct Coombs' test result	Negative or weakly positive	Positive
Maternal antibodies	Inconsistent, inconclusive	Always present
Antenatal diagnosis	Unnecessary	Necessary
Treatment (dependent on severity)	Phototherapy (common)	Exchange transfusion (common newborn treatment)
	Exchange transfusion (rare)	Intrauterine (common antenatal treatment)
Types of antibody	IgG (immune)	IgG (immune)
Prophylaxis	None	RhIG
		Antenatal RhIG

curs at 4°C but also react at temperatures between 25° and 31°C. Two types of cold AIHA have been described: (1) cold agglutinin syndrome and (2) paroxysmal cold hemoglobinuria (PCH).

Some drugs may induce the formation of autoantibodies that may be difficult to distinguish from other cases of AIHA. Drug-induced immune hemolytic anemia is the third type of AIHA, representing approximately 12% of cases in various studies.[16] Table 14–9 lists the frequency of the various types of AIHA.

"Coombs-Negative" AIHA

Occasionally the DAT result is repeatedly negative in a patient who has clear evidence of hemolysis with no other apparent cause. These patients represent a small group who are referred to as having DAT-negative AIHA.[17] More sensitive techniques for the detection of IgG and/or C3d on red cells have shown that many of the patients have increased levels of these immunoproteins on their cells. The routine laboratory DAT can detect immunoglobulin sensitization of as little as 200 molecules of IgG per red cell.[16] More sensitive techniques are capable of detecting as few as 20 IgG molecules.[18] When interpreting DAT results, it is important to remember that a positive DAT is not indicative of immune hemolysis, but if hemolysis is present or suspected, it could be because of immune mechanisms. The DAT result can be positive in up to 8% of hospitalized patients who have no signs or symptoms of hemolysis.[15,16] In most of these patients the positive result was caused by complement sensitization, prob-

ably secondary to the disease process from which the patient was suffering.

Warm Autoimmune Hemolytic Anemia

The incidence of WAIHA in the community is very rare (1 in 80,000),[19,20] with a slightly higher frequency of the disease in women than in men.[19] Most individuals who develop WAIHA are over 40 years of age.[16]

WAIHA may be idiopathic, with no underlying disease process, or it may be secondary to a pathologic disorder. Table 14–10 lists the disorders reported to be associated with WAIHA. Signs and symptoms usually do not appear until a significant anemia has developed. Pallor, weakness, dizziness, dyspnea, jaundice, and unexplained fever occasionally are presenting complaints. Hemolysis is usually extravascular and occurs predominantly in the spleen. The degree of hemolysis can be acute (hemoglobin less than 70 g/L) or mild. The onset of WAIHA is usually insidious and may be precipitated by a variety of factors such as infection, trauma, surgery, pregnancy, or psychologic stress.

TABLE 14–10   Disorders Reported to Be Frequently Associated with WAIHA

Reticuloendothelial neoplasms such as chronic lymphocytic leukemia, Hodgkin's disease, non-Hodgkin's lymphomas, thymomas
Collagen disease such as systemic lupus erythematosus, scleroderma, rheumatoid arthritis
Infectious diseases such as viral syndromes in childhood
Immunologic diseases such as hypogammaglobulinemia, dysglobulinemia, and other immune-deficiency syndromes
Gastrointestinal diseases such as ulcerative colitis
Benign tumors such as ovarian dermoid cysts

Source: Modified from Petz, LD and Garratty G (eds): Acquired Immune Hemolytic Anemias: Churchill Livingstone, New York, 1980, p 32, with permission.

TABLE 14–9   Percentage of Reported Cases of AIHA

Warm AIHA	70%
Cold agglutinin syndrome	16%
Paroxysmal cold hemoglobinuria	1–2%
Drug-induced	12%

Serologic Evaluation Evaluation with a polyspecific antiglobulin reagent reveals a positive DAT. On further analysis with monospecific antiglobulin reagents, the DAT result is positive for both IgG and C3d in 67% of all cases. The remainder are positive with IgG (20%) or C3d (13%) alone.[2]

The serum of a patient with WAIHA will usually demonstrate evidence of free autoantibody at low titer (e.g., weak reactivity). In 80% of the cases the immunoglobulin is IgG alone or together with IgA, IgM, and/or C3.[16] Complement proteins act synergistically with immunoglobulins to cause red cell hemolysis. In fact, the severity of hemolysis is correlated with the presence of complement in addition to IgG.[21,22] Although it is not performed in routine diagnostic testing, the presence of IgA and/or IgM may be found in addition to IgG if appropriate antisera is used.[16] WAIHA can present several difficult problems in serologic testing. The serologic problems of WAIHA are twofold:

1. The patient's red cells are strongly coated with autoantibody, which interferes with phenotyping.
2. Autoantibody present in the serum may mask an underlying alloantibody.

Autoantibody Specificity The autoantibodies produced in WAIHA usually react with all cells tested. Serologic studies have suggested that some autoantibodies are directed at Rh blood group antigens because of their lack of reactivity (apparent compatibility) with Rh_{null} cells, which lack all Rh blood group antigens.[14] Further analysis of these autoantibodies with apparent Rh specificity have demonstrated that the reactivity was directed at a red cell membrane protein (which is also lacking in Rh_{null} cells).[23] On rare occasions, other specificities have also been reported.[2,14,16]

Laboratory Diagnosis The blood smear can display classic signs of extravascular hemolysis: polychromasia reflecting reticulocytosis (see Fig. 14–2), spherocytosis, and red cell fragmentation. In rare occasions, WAIHA is associated with reticulocytopenia. Reticulocytopenia at the time of intense hemolysis is associated with a high patient mortality rate.

Evidence of hemolysis can be seen on laboratory analysis; bilirubin (particularly the unconjugated indirect fraction) and urinary urobilinogen may be elevated. In severe cases, depleted serum haptoglobin, hemoglobinemia, hemoglobinuria, and increased lactate dehydrogenase (LDH) may be demonstrated.

Treatment The prognosis for patients with WAIHA is generally poor. Therapy is usually aimed at treating the primary disease if one is present. Measures to support cardiovascular function are important in patients who are severely anemic. Transfusion is usually avoided, if possible, because this may only accelerate the hemolysis instead of ameliorating the anemia. However, transfusion should be used in life-threatening situations.

Because all donor blood will invariably be incompatible, it is general practice to use donor blood that is least reactive in the crossmatch and that is antigen-negative for any clinically significant alloantibodies that may be present in the patient's serum. Blood is transfused slowly, in small volumes (100 mL), and the patient is observed closely for any adverse reactions.[24] Some hematologists advocate the use of phenotypically similar blood irrespective of its degree of incompatibility in the crossmatch. The rationale for this approach is that patients with autoimmune antibodies may be more likely to produce alloimmune antibodies, which can be masked by the autoantibodies. A recent study indicates that the incidence of alloimmunization or adverse hemolytic transfusion reactions in patients with WAIHA is no greater than the incidence found in other multitransfused patient populations.[25]

Three forms of treatment are generally used, depending on the severity of the disorder: corticosteroid administration, splenectomy, and immunosuppressive drugs. Corticosteroids such as prednisone produce their effect by several proposed mechanisms: (1) reduction of antibody synthesis,[26] (2) altered antibody avidity,[26] and (3) depression of macrophage activity,[27] which reduces the clearance of antibody-coated red cells.[16] Splenectomy would be considered only after corticosteroid therapy has failed. Immunosuppressive drugs are the absolute last approach in the management of WAIHA.

Normal Cold Autoagglutinins

Cold-reacting autoantibodies (autoagglutinins) are present in all normal human sera.[28–30] The specificity of these cold autoantibodies includes anti-I, anti-H, and anti-IH. Practically all adults have the I and H antigens present on their red cells. Generally, most examples of anti-I, anti-H, and anti-IH have no clinical significance, and most of these autoantibodies are often too weak to be detected by routine serologic testing. This is primarily because of their low concentration in

TABLE 14–11	**Comparison of Characteristics of Normal and Pathologic Cold Autoantibody**	
Characteristic	**Benign**	**Pathologic**
Thermal amplitude	<22°C	Broad: up to 32°C
Spontaneous autoagglutination	None	Significant degree which disperses on warming to 37°C
Titer	<64 at 4°C	>1000 at 4°C
Albumin enhancement	None	Reactivity enhanced
Clonality of antibody	Polyclonal	Idiopathic = monoclonal Secondary to infection = polyclonal
Clinical significance	None	Causes cold AIHA
Usual antibody specificity	Anti-I	Anti-I
Direct antiglobulin test (DAT)	Negative or weak positive with polyspecific antiglobulin reagent	2 to 3+ with polyspecific antiglobulin reagent

the serum and their narrow thermal range (4° to 22°C).[29] Table 14–11 compares the characteristics of normal cold autoantibodies found in healthy adults with those of pathologic cold autoantibodies. The benign autoagglutinins differ in many ways from the pathologic cold autoagglutinins that produce cold agglutinin syndrome (or cold AIHA). The fundamental characteristic that differentiates benign autoagglutinins from pathologic autoagglutinins is the thermal range. Pathologic cold autoagglutinins react at or above 30°C.[31]

Pathologic Cold Autoantibodies

Pathologic cold antibodies can be divided into (1) idiopathic cold agglutinin syndrome (idiopathic CAS), (2) cold agglutinin syndrome secondary to infection (secondary CAS), and (3) paroxysmal cold hemoglobinuria (PCH).

Cold Agglutinin Syndrome (Idiopathic CAS) Cold agglutinin syndrome, also called cold hemagglutinin disease (CHD) or idiopathic cold AIHA, represents approximately 16% of the cases of AIHA.[16] CAS occurs predominantly in older individuals, with a peak incidence after 50 years of age,[16] and equally affects both men and women. Although the disease is often called idiopathic, a careful evaluation of the patient may reveal the presence of a lymphoproliferative disorder.[14] Because of this association, it is prudent to investigate patients for possible malignancy when they present with a pathologic cold autoantibody and no other obvious cause, such as infection.

CAS is a hemolytic anemia produced by a cold autoantibody that optimally reacts at 4°C, but also reacts at temperatures greater than 30°C (i.e., wide thermal range).[16,32,33] The antibody is usually an IgM immunoglobulin, which quite efficiently activates complement.[28] Antibody specificity in this disorder is almost always anti-I,[28–30] less commonly anti-i, and rarely anti-Pr.[30]

Cold hemagglutinin disease is rarely severe and usually seasonal, as the cold winter months often precipitate the signs and symptoms of a chronic hemolytic anemia. Acrocyanosis of the hands, feet, ears, and nose is frequently the patient's main complaint, along with a sense of numbness in the extremities when exposed to the cold. These symptoms occur because the cold autoantibody agglutinates the individual's red cells in the capillaries of the skin, causing local blood stasis.[28] During cold weather, the temperature of an individual's skin and exposed extremities can fall to as low as 28°C, activating the cold autoantibody. This activated cold antibody agglutinates red cells and fixes complement as the erythrocytes flow through the capillaries of the skin. When the erythrocytes return to the body core (where the temperature is 37°C), the cold agglutinin elutes off the red cells, leaving activated complement behind. Hemolysis occurs from the completion of the complement cascade or by removal of red cells sensitized with C3b/iC3b by macrophages in the liver (see the previous section on intravascular hemolysis for a review). If any red cells coated with C3b/iC3b escape destruction in the liver, their complement proteins are further degraded to C3d, for which there are no receptors on macrophages.[5] The patient's DAT result will be positive with monospecific anti-C3d antiglobulin reagents.

This hemolytic episode is not associated with fever, chills, or acute renal insufficiency, characteristic of patients with PCH (see below). Hemoglobinemia and, less frequently, hemoglobinuria may be detected after exposure to the cold. Patients also display weakness, pallor, and weight loss, which are characteristic symptoms of chronic anemia. CAS usually remains quite stable, and when it does progress, it is insidious in intensity. Other clinical features of cold hemagglutinin disease include jaundice and Raynaud's phenomenon[28] (symptoms of cold intolerance, such as pain and a bluish tinge in the fingertips and toes, owing to vasospasm).

Laboratory Findings Most patients with CAS present with reticulocytosis and a positive DAT result (C3d only). In some cases autoagglutination of anticoagulated whole blood samples occurs as the blood cools to room temperature. As a result of this autoagglutination, performance of blood counts and preparation of blood smears may be difficult.

The tendency for spontaneous autoagglutination of red cells from these patients dictates that serum samples must be maintained and separated at 37°C to obtain accurate results for the antibody titer and thermal amplitude studies.[34] Similarly, samples for the determination of DAT results must be collected into ethylenediamine tetra-acetic acid (EDTA) to inhibit any in vitro attachment of complement to the cells following collection.

A simple serum screening procedure can be performed by testing the patient serum's ability to agglutinate normal saline-suspended red cells at 20°C and 4°C. If this test result is positive, further steps must be taken to determine the titer and thermal amplitude of the cold autoantibody; if negative, the diagnosis of cold hemagglutinin disease is unlikely.[32]

The peripheral blood smear in patients with cold hemagglutinin disease may show rouleaux (red cells appear stacked on top of one another like a roll of coins), autoagglutination (physical clumping of cells), polychromasia, and/or a mild to moderate anisocytosis and poikilocytosis (Fig. 14–3). Table 14–12 sum-

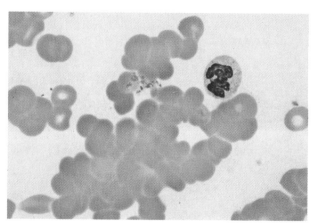

FIGURE 14–3 Cold hemagglutinin disease (peripheral blood). Note the autoagglutination of red cells, polychromasia, anisocytosis, and poikilocytosis.

TABLE 14–12 Clinical Criteria for the Diagnosis of Cold Agglutinin Syndrome

- Clinical signs of an acquired hemolytic anemia, with a history (which may or may not be present) of acrocyanosis and hemoglobinuria upon exposure to cold
- A positive DAT result using polyspecific antisera
- A positive DAT result using monospecific C3 antisera
- A negative DAT result using monospecific IgG antisera
- The presence of reactivity in the patient's serum owing to a cold autoantibody
- A cold agglutinin titer of 1000 or greater in saline at 4°C with visible autoagglutination of anticoagulated blood at room temperature

marizes the clinical criteria for diagnosis of cold hemagglutinin disease.

CAS Secondary to Infections Cold hemagglutinin disease can also occur as a transient disorder that is secondary to infections. Episodes of cold autoimmune hemolytic anemia often occur following upper respiratory infections. Approximately 50% of patients suffering from pneumonia caused by *Mycoplasma pneumoniae* have elevated titers (>64) of cold autoagglutinins.[16,32,33] Secondary CAS develops in the second or third week of the patient's illness, and a rapid onset of hemolysis with symptoms of pallor and jaundice is usually found. Resolution of the episode usually occurs in 2 to 3 weeks because the hemolysis is self-limiting.[28] The offending cold autoantibody is an IgM immunoglobulin with characteristic *anti-I* specificity. Very high titers of the cold autoagglutinnin are seen almost exclusively in patients with mycoplasma pneumonia. It has been reported that the cold agglutinin produced in this infection is an immunologic response to the mycoplasmal antigens and these antibodies cross-react with the red cell I antigen.[35,36]

Both the antibodies produced in CAS and CAS secondary to mycoplasma pneumonia have anti-I specificity. They differ in that the autoantibody in CAS is invariably monoclonal (IgM kappa light chain)[37] whereas the autoantibody in the disease secondary to infection is polyclonal (IgM with both kappa and lambda light chain types).[38] The monoclonality of the autoantibody in CHD suggests a possible underlying lymphoproliferative disorder.

Infectious Mononucleosis (IM) IM may also be associated with a hemolytic anemia caused by a cold autoagglutinin. Many studies have reported an association of *anti-i* production in infectious mononucleosis. The percentages of patients with IM who developed anti-i varies from 8%,[39] 50%,[40] to 68%.[41] The antibody is usually a low-titer IgM cold agglutinin with a narrow thermal range. A small number (1%) of these patients who develop anti-i produce a high-titer IgM cold agglutinin with a wide thermal range[42] that causes in vivo hemolysis. Acute illness with sore throat and high fever, followed by weakness, anemia, and jaundice, is characteristic of infectious mononucleosis. For a review of infectious mononucleosis, see Chapter 17. Table 14–13 lists the cold autoantibody specificity most commonly found in the various infections that cause secondary cold hemagglutinin disease.

Treatment Treatment of CAS, secondary CAS, and the anemia associated with IM is the same. Most patients require no treatment and are instructed to avoid the cold, keep warm, or move to a milder climate. One ingenious doctor contacted the National Aeronautics and Space Administration (NASA) for an environmentally controlled space suit so that his patient would not have to remain inside during the acute phase of the disease.[43]

Transfusion is rarely required. If blood is needed, the blood should be ABO/Rh compatible and lack any antigens for which the patient has an alloantibody. Blood should be warmed using a blood warmer and transfused slowly with constant monitoring of the patient for adverse reactions.[28]

Paroxysmal Cold Hemoglobinuria

PCH is the least common type of AIHA, with an incidence of only 1% to 7%.[16] It occurs almost exclusively in children in association with viral disorders such as measles, mumps, chickenpox, infectious mononucleosis, and the ill-defined flu syndrome.[44]

Originally, PCH was described in association with syphilis, in which an autoantibody was formed in response to the *Treponema pallidum* organism, the causative agent of the disease.[45] However, with the discovery and use of antibiotics, PCH is no longer a commonly reported disorder related to syphilis.

Red cell destruction is the result of a cold-reacting IgG autoantibody termed an *autohemolysin*. This autohemolysin binds to the patient's red cells at lower temperatures and fixes complement. Hemolysis occurs when the red cells return to the body core (where the temperature rises to 37°C) and the sensitized cells undergo complement-mediated intravascular hemolysis.[44] This autoagglutinin only attaches to red cells at cooler temperatures and then activates complement in warmer temperatures. The antibody is an autoagglutinin with biphasic activity. Thus the antibody produced in PCH is called a *biphasic hemolysin*. The specificity of this antibody is *anti-P*.[29]

As the name implies, paroxysmal or intermittent episodes of hemoglobinuria occur upon exposure to the cold. These acute attacks maybe characterized by a sudden onset of fever, shaking chills, malaise, abdominal cramps, and back pains.[44] All the signs of intravascular hemolysis are evident, including hemoglobinemia, hemoglobinuria, and bilirubinemia (see Fig. 14–1). This results in a severe and rapidly progressive anemia. Polychromasia, nucleated red blood cells, and poikilocytosis are demonstrated in the peripheral blood smear. The symptoms of fever, chills, pain, and hemoglobinuria may resolve in a few hours or persist for days. Splenomegaly, hyperbilirubinemia, and renal

TABLE 14–13 Secondary Cold AIHA

Type of Infection	Cold Autoantibody Specificity
Mycoplasma pneumonia	Anti-I
Infectious mononucleosis	Anti-i
Lymphoproliferative disorder	Anti-I, i, or Pr

insufficiency may also develop. Table 14–14 compares and contrasts PCH versus cold agglutinin syndrome.

Donath-Landsteiner Test There is one classic diagnostic test for PCH. This test was developed by the two doctors for whom the test is named. A blood sample drawn from the patient is split into two aliquots maintained at different temperatures. One aliquot, used as the control, is kept at 37°C for 60 minutes. The other aliquot is cooled at 4°C for 30 minutes and is then incubated at 37°C for another 30 minutes. Both samples are then centrifuged and observed for hemolysis. A positive test result is hemolysis in the sample placed at 4°C and then at 37°C and no hemolysis in the control sample. Table 14–15 summarizes the Donath-Landsteiner test.

Treatment Protection from cold exposure is the only useful therapy. The hemolysis usually terminates spontaneously following resolution of the infectious process.[46] If anemia is severe, transfusions may be required. The same transfusion protocol as in CAS applies. Table 14–16 reviews and compares characteristics of warm and cold autoimmune hemolytic anemias.

Mixed Autoimmune Hemolytic Anemia

In recent years, a number of reports have drawn attention to the occurrence of mixed AIHA, in which patients exhibit autoantibodies having the characteristics of both warm and cold autoantibodies.[47–49] Patients with mixed-type AIHA usually present with an extremely acute condition.[50] This situation of both warm and cold autoantibodies is not to be unexpected when one realizes that a number of the lymphoproliferative and collagen diseases may be associated with either form of autoantibody.[2,50] See Table 14–10 for a review of associated disorders.

Drug-Induced Immune Hemolytic Anemia

The administration of drugs may lead to the development of a wide variety of hematologic abnormalities, including immune hemolytic anemia. Drug-induced immune hemolytic anemia represents approximately 12% of cases in various studies.[16,51] Historically, three

TABLE 14–15	**Donath-Landsteiner Test**	
	Whole Blood Control	Whole Blood Test
Procedure		
1. 30 min	37°C	4°C
2. 30 min	37°C	37°C
3. Centrifuge and observe		
Results		
Positive	No hemolysis	Hemolysis
Negative	No hemolysis	No hemolysis
Inconclusive	Hemolysis	Hemolysis

mechanisms have been described that lead to the development of drug-induced immune hemolytic anemia, as well as a fourth mechanism that leads to the development of a positive DAT but is not associated with hemolysis. Sufficient new data have emerged to perhaps reclassify these mechanisms. Nevertheless, it is instructive to review the traditional mechanisms.

Methyldopa-Induced (Autoimmune) Mechanism

Autoimmune reaction induced by methyldopa represents the most common drug-induced immune hemolytic anemia, accounting for approximately 70% of all cases.[52] The drugs implicated in this response include methyldopa and related drugs (Aldomet, L-dopa)[53] that are prescribed for the treatment of hypertension. Drug-induced AIHA by this mechanism is difficult to diagnose because it mimics WAIHA. There are several hypotheses for this drug-related anemia; however, the exact mechanism is still unknown. A positive DAT develops in approximately 12% to 15% of the patients receiving Aldomet (alphamethyldopa) and 1% to 3% of these patients go on to develop AIHA. The antibodies produced by patients suffering from this disorder react weakly with all cells tested, or demonstrate specificities similar to those found in WAIHA. Hemolysis is extravascular and the DAT result is strongly positive with anti-IgG, and negative with anti-C3. Pa-

TABLE 14–14	**Comparison of PCH and Cold Agglutinin Syndrome**	
	PCH	**Cold Agglutinin Syndrome**
Patient population	Children or young adults	Elderly or middle-aged
Pathogenesis	Following viral infection	Idiopathic, lymphoproliferative disorder following *Mycoplasma pneumoniae* infection
Clinical features	Hemoglobinuria: acute attacks upon exposure to cold (symptoms resolve in hours or days)	Acrocyanosis, autoagglutination of blood at room temperature
Severity of hemolysis	Acute and rapid	Chronic and rarely severe
Hemolysis	Intravascular	Extravascular, intravascular
Autoantibody	IgG (anti-P specificity) (biphasic hemolysin)	IgM (anti-I/i) (monophasic)
DAT	3+ (polyspecific Coombs' sera)/neg IgG/3–4+ C3 monospecific Coombs' sera	3+ (polyspecific Coombs' sera)/neg IgG/3–4+ C3 monospecific Coombs' sera
Thermal range	Moderate (<20°C)	High (up to 30–31°C)
Titer (4°C)	Moderate (<64)	High (>1000)
Donath-Landsteiner test	Positive	Negative
Treatment	Supportive (disorder terminates when underlying illness resolves)	Avoid the cold

TABLE 14–16	**Comparison of Warm and Cold Autoimmune Hemolytic Anemias**	
	WAIHA	**Cold AIHA**
Optimal reactivity	>32°C	<30°C
Immunoglobin class	IgG	IgM (exception: PCH-IgG)
Complement activation	May bind complement	Binds complement
Hemolysis	Usually extravascular (no cell lysis)	Usually intravascular (cell lysis)
Frequency	70–75% of cases	16% of cases (PCH: 1–2%)
Specificity	Frequently Rh	Ii system (PCH: anti-P)

tients may continue to have a positive DAT result for up to 2 years after discontinuation of the drug.

Drug Adsorption Mechanism

The second most common mechanism of drug-induced hemolytic anemia is that of drug adsorption. The drugs implicated in this response include the penicillins, the cephalosporins, and the streptomycins.[52] This mechanism requires two components (Fig. 14–4). First, the drug is nonspecifically adsorbed to the patient's red cells and remains firmly attached. Second, once adsorbed, the drug must be able to elicit an antibody response. The drug antibody is usually IgG and will react only with drug-treated red cells. Large doses of intravenous penicillin (10 million units daily) are needed to produce an immune response.[16] Approximately 3% of patients on high-dose intravenous penicillin develop drug antibodies causing a positive DAT, but only 5% of these patients have actual clinical hemolysis.[16]

Laboratory findings include signs of extravascular hemolysis. The disorder develops over a period of 7 to 10 days. The DAT results are strongly positive with anti-IgG and negative with anti-C3.

Immune Complex Mechanism

The third type of drug-induced hemolytic anemia is caused by the immune complex mechanism. The most common drugs involved in this response include quinidine and phenacetin.[52] Table 14–17 lists other drugs associated with the immune complex mechanism. The patient responds to these drugs by producing an antibody (IgG and/or IgM) against the drug that binds to the drug, forming an antibody-drug immune complex (Fig. 14–5). The antibody-drug complex then adsorbs onto the patient's red cells and complement is activated. The antibody-drug immune complex is merely adsorbed onto the red cell membrane (not bound to it) and easily disassociates, leaving activated complement behind. Only a small amount of the drug is necessary to produce this response.

Laboratory findings include evidence of intravascular hemolysis with hemoglobinemia and hemoglobinuria. The DAT result is positive with complement components only, since the immune complex has disassociated. In vitro agglutination reactions are generally observed during serologic testing only when the drug is added to the patient's serum and test red cell mixture.[54]

Membrane Modification Mechanism (Protein Adsorption)

As the name implies, the drug modifies the red cell membrane so that normal plasma proteins are nonspecifically adsorbed onto the patient's red cells (Fig. 14–6). Cephalosporins are the drugs implicated in this response.[55] The red cells become coated with numerous plasma proteins such as albumin, fibrinogen, and globulins. Approximately 3% of patients receiving the drug develop a positive DAT result because of the nonspecific protein adsorption by the red cells. Hemolytic anemia has not been reported in association with this mechanism of drug-induced positive DAT.

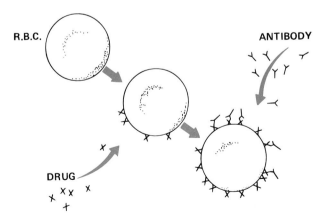

FIGURE 14–4 Drug absorption mechanism. (From Petz, LD and Garratty, G (eds): Acquired Immune Hemolytic Anemias. Churchill Livingstone, New York, 1980, with permission.)

TABLE 14–17	**Drugs Implicated in Immune Complex, or "Innocent Bystander," Mechanism**
Quinidine	Insecticides
Quinine	Dipyrone
Phenacetin	Anhistine
Stibophen	Antazoline
p-Aminosalicylic acid	Chlorpromazine
Sulfonamides	Aminopyrine
Thiazide	Isoniazid

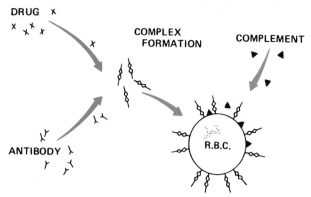

FIGURE 14-5 Immune complex mechanism. (From Petz, LD and Garratty, G (eds): Acquired Immune Hemolytic Anemias. Churchill Livingstone, New York, 1980, with permission.)

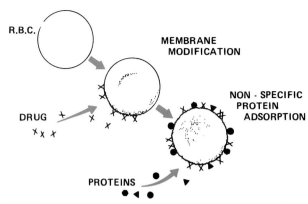

FIGURE 14-6 Membrane modification mechanism. (From Petz, LD and Garratty, G (eds): Acquired Immune Hemolytic Anemias. Churchill Livingstone, New York, 1980, with permission.)

The above classification used for the drug-induced immune hemolytic anemias provides a convenient mechanistic approach as to how drugs may be incriminated in immune hemolysis. Recent reports have demonstrated immune hemolytic anemia from certain drugs with more than one mechanism. More recently, it has been suggested that only a single mechanism may be responsible for all drug-related immune hemolysis (unifying theory).[54] Table 14-18 compares the four mechanisms of drug-related anemia. Table 14-19 contrasts the antibody characteristics of the various types of autoimmune hemolytic anemias.

TABLE 14-18	**Mechanisms Leading to Development of Drug-Related Antibodies**				
Mechanism	**Prototype Drugs**	**Immunoglobulin Class**	**DAT**	**Biologic Results**	**Frequency of Hemolysis**
Immune complex formation (innocent bystander)	Quinidine Phenacetin	IgM or IgG	Positive (often to complement fragments only; however, IgG may be present)	Eluate often negative	Small doses of drug may cause acute intravascular hemolysis with hemoglobinemia and hemoglobinuria; renal failure is common
Drug adsorption	Penicillins Cephalosporins Streptomycin	IgG	Positive (strongly) due to IgG sensitization	Eluate often negative	3–4% of patients on large doses (10 million units) daily of penicillin, which is one of the most common causes of drug induced immune hemolysis, usually extravascular in nature
Membrane modification (nonimmunologic protein adsorption)	Cephalosporins	Numerous plasma proteins (nonimmunological sensitization)	Positive due to a variety of serum proteins	Eluate negative	No hemolysis; however, 3% of patients receiving the drug develop a +DAT
Autoimmunity	Methyldopa (Aldomet)	IgG	Strongly positive (due to IgG sensitization)	Eluate positive (warm autoantibody identical to antibody found in WAIHA)	0.8% develop a hemolytic anemia that mimics a WAIHA (depends on the dose of the drug); 15% of patients receiving Aldomet develop a +DAT

TABLE 14-19 Summary of Antibody Characteristics in AIHA				
	Warm Reactive Autoantibody	**Cold Reactive Autoantibody**	**PCH**	**Drug-Related Autoantibody**
Immunoglobulin characteristics	Polyclonal IgG, IgM, and IgA may also be present; rarely IgA alone	Polyclonal IgM-infection Monoclonal kappa chain IgM in cold agglutinin disease	Polyclonal IgG	Polyclonal IgG
Complement activation	Variable	Always	Always	Depends on mechanism of drug, antibody, and RBC interaction
Thermal reactivity	20°C–37°C; optimum 37°C	4°C–32°C occasionally to 37°C; optimum 4°C	4°C–20°C; biphasic hemolysin	20°C–37°C; optimum 37°C
Titer of free antibody	Low (<32) May only be detectable using enzyme treated cells	High (>1000 at 4°C)	Moderate to low (<64)	Depends on mechanism of drug, antibody and RBC interaction
Reactivity of eluate with antibody screening cells	Usually panreactive	Nonreactive	Nonreactive	Panreactive with Aldomet type antibody. Nonreactive in all other circumstances
Most common specificity	Anti-Rh precursor -common Rh -LW -En^a/Wr^b -U	-I -i -Pr	Anti-P	Anti-e–like; Aldomet, antidrug
Site of RBC destruction	Predominantly spleen with some liver involvement	Predominantly liver, rarely intravascular	Intravascular	Intravascular and spleen

NONIMMUNE HEMOLYTIC ANEMIA

Acquired nonimmune hemolytic anemias represent a diverse group of conditions that lead to the shortened survival of red cells by various mechanisms. Often a number of mechanisms will be operative at the same time, for example, malaria leads to mechanical destruction of red cells, and in addition immunologic factors also play a role in shorten red cell survival. Classifications may be made along either causative or mechanistic lines. Table 14–20 provides a classification incorporating both approaches.

Intracellular Infections

Malaria

Malaria is the most common protozoal infection in humans. It has a high incidence in the tropical and subtropical regions of the world, accounting for a fair percentage of the anemia in those regions. It has been estimated that more than 400 million people suffer from the disease, which results in the deaths of more than 1.5 million persons annually. Most fatalities occur in nonimmune children; those who survive a childhood infection invariably suffer from an ongoing debilitating disease. Over the last 20 years, control measures have significantly reduced the incidence of the disease, but recently the incidence of the disease has risen to epidemic proportions. The increased in-

cidence of infections has resulted from: (1) the organism becoming resistant to many of the antimalarial drugs (e.g., chloroquine), and (2) the mosquito vector having become resistant to insecticides. There are four species of malaria that can infect humans: *Plasmodium vivax*, *P. falciparum*, *P. ovale*, and *P. malariae*. *P. vivax* and *P. falciparum* are responsible for most infections in humans. In the case of *P. falciparum*, the disease can have a very rapid and often fatal course. *P. malariae* and *P. ovale* infections are uncommon. *P. ovale* infections are confined to certain areas of Africa.

The number of patients presenting with malaria is also increasing in countries such as the United States, Europe, and Australia because of increased travel to endemic tropical and subtropical regions.

Life Cycle The malarial parasite has a complex life cycle. The insect vector is the *Anopheles* mosquito, of which numerous species can transmit the parasite. Figure 14–7 illustrates the malarial life cycle.

Clinical Presentation Typically, patients seek medical attention as a result of the often violent rigors, fever, and profuse sweating that accompany the periodic rupture of infected red cells. Early in the infection, these episodes may not show classic periodicity, which can be helpful in determining the species of parasite with which the patient is infected. It is not uncommon for an individual to be infected with multiple species. In that case, periodicity may not be evident. Nausea, vomiting, and diarrhea may be present. Patients frequently complain of headache, fatigue, and varying de-

TABLE 14–20	**Classification of Nonimmune Acquired Hemolytic Anemias**	
Cause	**Examples**	**Mechanisms**
Infections		
Intracellular	Malaria	Physical disruption and immune
	Babesiosis	Physical disruption
Extracellular	Bartonella	Direct action on RBC membrane and RES sequestration
	Clostridia	Enzymatic action on RBC membrane
	Bacterial sepsis: meningococcal, pneumococcal	Physical disruption secondary to DIC
	Viral	Unknown
Mechanical		
Macroangiopathic	Cardiac prosthesis	Physical disruption because of shear stress
	March hemoglobinuria	Physical disruption
Microangiopathic	Hemolytic uremic syndrome (HUS)	Physical disruption
	Thrombotic thrombocytopenic purpura (TTP)	Physical disruption
Chemicals and physical agents		
Oxidative agents	Dapsone at high dosage	Direct oxidation of RBC membrane components
Nonoxidative agents	Lead	Alteration of RBC membrane components
	Venoms	Possible direct effect on RBC membrane by enzymes
Osmotic effect	Water (drowning or water irrigation during surgery)	Osmotic lysis
	Burns	Localized dehydration
Acquired membrane disorders	Vitamin E deficiency; abetalipoproteinemia	RBC membrane oxidation; lack of membrane deformability
	Liver disease	Lipid abnormalities of RBC membrane lead to decrease in deformability
	Renal disease	Retained metabolic products cause membrane changes leading to a decrease in deformability
Hypersplenism		Sequestration of normal cells

grees of arthralgia and myalgia. Quite often these symptoms are attributed to a viral infection that could be fatal. It is always advisable to inquire if the patient has been overseas, and which countries have been visited.

Splenomegaly is present in 40% to 50% of patients with acute malaria. It is present in virtually all patients with chronic malaria, accounting for the high incidence of splenomegaly in the tropics.[56]

Laboratory Diagnosis Anemia associated with *Plasmodium* is normochromic and normocytic. Leukocytopenia is present in many cases, as is thrombocytopenia (particularly in individuals with *P. falciparum* infections). Diagnosis of malaria is made by examination of a peripheral blood smear. Blood should be taken just prior to the onset of fever because the parasitemia is greatest at this time. However, this is possible only when periodicity of the infection is present. Examination of an unfixed Giemsa- or Wright-stained blood smear (thick preparation) is performed to ascertain the presence of malarial parasites. Staining is usually performed at a pH of 7.2 to enhance the blue staining of the parasites' cytoplasm. Determination of the species of parasite may be made on this smear if schizonts are present (by the number of merozoites within the schizont). If only trophozoites are present, the examination of a thin blood smear is nec-

essary. Often more than one parasite is present in a single cell (Fig. 14–8). *P. falciparum* gametocytes have a characteristic sausage or crescent shape, assisting in the identification. Occasionally it is possible to see irregular purple inclusions called *Maurer's dots* in the red cell cytoplasm; these are probably breakdown products of hemoglobin. *P. vivax* gametocytes are round, ameboid forms that expand and distort the red cell. Bluish purple inclusions called *Schüffner's dots* are often seen in red cells infected with *P. vivax* and *P. ovale* (Fig. 14–9). Table 14–21 summarizes the features of the different malarial parasites infecting humans.

Immunoassays are being introduced to help screen large numbers of patients for the presence of infection. Flow cytometry has also been used with some success to show the presence of malarial parasites in red cells.

Babesiosis

Infection by *Babesia microti* represents a zoonotic infection, as humans are not natural hosts for the parasite. The disease is carried by ticks (*Ixodes* species) and normally infects cattle, deer, and rodents.[57] The disease is usually tick-borne in humans, but has apparently also been transmitted by blood transfusion.[58,59] Infection tends to be self-limiting, although

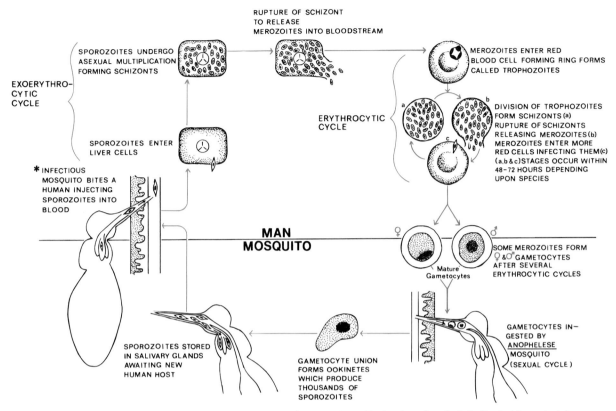

FIGURE 14-7   Malarial life cycle in humans and mosquitoes. Beginning of cycle is indicated by asterisk.

in splenectomized patients it can follow an acute course and be fatal. Patients usually present with a history of malaise, headache, and fever, sometimes associated with vomiting and diarrhea. In splenectomized patients this condition can progress to rigors and acute intravascular hemolysis with associated hemoglobinemia, hemoglobinuria, jaundice, and renal failure.

Laboratory Diagnosis   Diagnosis of the disease is made by examination of the peripheral blood, where parasites very similar to *P. falciparum* are seen in the red cells (Fig. 14–10). A history of possible exposure to ticks and a lack of recent travel to areas where malaria is endemic is helpful to diagnosis correctly. Serologic tests for antibodies to *Babesia* have been described.[60]

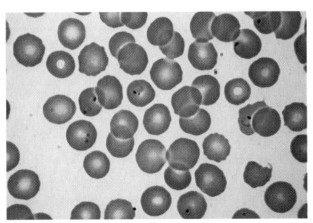

FIGURE 14-8   Ringed forms of *Plasmodium falciparum* in red blood cells (RBCs). Note that the same RBCs may be infected with more than one ring.

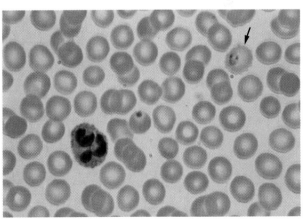

FIGURE 14-9   Late stages of *Plasmodium vivax* malaria, Schüffer's dots. Note and contrast the platelet on the RBC (*center*) and the ring form of malaria toward the periphery (*arrow*).

TABLE 14–21	**Characteristics of Malarial Parasites Infecting Humans**			
	P. falciparum	*P. vivax*	*P. malariae*	*P. ovale*
Incubation period (days)	6–10	10–12	13–16	10–12
Asexual life cycle (h)	48	48	72	48
RBCs infected	All	Reticulocytes	Senescent	Reticulocytes
Secondary exoerythrocytic development	No	Yes	Yes	Yes
Duration of relapses in untreated patients	Not applicable	3–5 yr	up to 40 yr	3–5 years
Level of parasitemia	50–60%	2–5%	2–3%	2–3%
Ring form	Small, delicate, may have two chromatin dots, often an edge of RBC	Large irregular, poor outline One chromatin dot	Large thick, prominent chromatin dot	Large irregular, poor outline One chromatin dot
	Maurer's dots	Schüffner's dots		Schüffner's dots
Schizonts	Rarely seen in peripheral blood 8–32 merozoites	Large, about same size as RBC 12–25 merozoites	Small "daisy-head" 6–16 merozoites	Irregular arrangement 4–16 merozoites
Gametocytes	Crescent or sausage shape	Round and expand RBC	Round, same size as RBC	

Extracellular Infections

Bartonellosis (Oroya Fever)

This disease is restricted to northern areas of South America including Peru, Ecuador, and Columbia. The name Oroya fever derives from the city of Oroya in the Peruvian Andes, where many railroad construction workers were affected by the disease in the late 1800s. It is also referred to as Carrion's disease,[61] named after the medical student who died as a result of a self-experiment designed to determine the nature of the infection.

Bartonellosis has a high fatality rate in nonimmune patients and is caused by the organism *Bartonella bacilliformis*. Infection is transmitted by the sandfly (*Phlebotomus*), and there does not appear to be any intermediate host. The organisms adhere to the red cell surface and appear as gram-negative rods in the acute phase of the disease. In the recovery phase they assume a coccoid appearance.

The disease has two clinical phases. The first is the hemolytic phase (Oroya fever), which may not occur in all patients. When it does occur, there is a rapid onset with marked intravascular hemolysis. Red cells are also sequestered in the spleen and liver.[62] The anemia can be quite severe and blood smears show many nucleated red cells and a reticulocytosis.[62] Antibiotic therapy including penicillin, streptomycin, and tetracyclines is effective in treating patients in this stage of the infection.[56] The second stage of the disease (verruca peruviana) is nonhematologic and involves the development of verrucous nodes (warty tumors) over the patients face and extremities.

Infection by Clostridium perfringens (welchii)

This organism is a gram-positive, spore-forming bacillus that is responsible for the development of gas gangrene. Infections with this organism are generally located in deep tissues where anaerobic conditions required for the organism's survival exist. The organism is normally present in the environment and may infect tissues exposed by trauma and surgical procedures. There is a high incidence of the infection in septic abortions.[63] The organism is responsible for extensive tissue damage because of the release of enzymes and toxins. Septicemia from *C. perfringens* may produce an acute intravascular hemolytic process resulting from the release of an *alpha toxin* or *lecithinase*. This process, combined with phospholipases and possibly proteinases, also produced by the organism, acts on the red cell membrane to cause its destruction.[64] Hemolysis is often severe, with marked hemoglobinemia and hemoglobinuria. Acute renal failure may develop quite

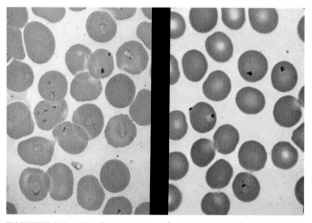

FIGURE 14–10 Comparison of parasitemia of malaria (*left*) and babesiosis (*right*).

TABLE 14-22 Organisms Associated with Hemolytic Anemia			
Bacteria	**Viruses**	**Protozoa**	**Fungi**
Bartonella bacilliformis	Coxsackie	*Babesia microti*	*Aspergillus*
Clostridium perfringens	Cytomegalovirus	*B. divergens*	
Escherichia coli	Epstein-Barr	*Plasmodium falciparum*	
Haemophilus influenzae	Herpes simplex	*P. malariae*	
Mycobacteria tuberculosis	Influenza A	*P. ovale*	
Mycoplasma pneumoniae	Rubeola	*P. vivax*	
Neisseria meningitidis	Varicella	*Toxoplasma*	
Salmonella sp.			
Shigella sp.			
Streptococcus sp.			
Vibrio cholera			
Yersinia enterocolitica			

rapidly, and prognosis is generally poor.[65] Microspherocytes are a common finding in the peripheral blood smear. Leukocytosis with a shift to the left and thrombocytopenia is present in most cases.

Improvements in the maintenance of aseptic conditions during and following surgery and the decrease in criminal abortions have caused this form of hemolytic anemia to become quite uncommon.

Table 14–22 lists the organisms that have been associated with hemolytic anemia.

Mechanical Etiologies

The passage of red cells through the vascular system subjects the cell to a wide range of environmental conditions. As red cells travel around the body, shear forces are highly variable and are influenced by: (1) the surface conditions of the vessel, (2) the size of the vessel lumen, (3) the rate at which the cell is moving, and (4) the number of other cells present at the same time. Other environmental conditions the cell must contend with in its travels include changes in pH, electrolytes, and protein concentration. The result of this mechan-

ical rupturing of the cell membrane is intravascular hemolysis accompanied by the presence of red cell fragments or schistocytes (Fig. 14–11).

Cardiac Prosthesis

Historically, hemolytic anemia associated with prosthetic heart valves was a complication of cardiac corrective surgery.[66]

The severity of the anemia is highly variable in patients with heart valve prostheses. Mild, compensated hemolysis is common; overt anemia is unusual, and rarely is the anemia severe enough to require transfusion.[66]

The peripheral blood smear shows many fragmented cells, helmet cells, and occasional spherocytes (Fig. 14–12). The reticulocyte count is usually elevated.[66] Leukocytes are usually normal and platelets are often reduced owing to their interaction with the abnormal surface.[67] Decreased haptoglobin, mild hemoglobinemia, mild hemosiderinuria,[68] and occasionally hemoglobinuria are present (depending on the amount of red cell destruction).

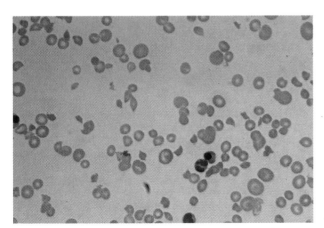

FIGURE 14-11 Peripheral blood showing red cell fragmentation with thrombocytopenia and nucleated RBCs from a case of thrombotic thrombocytopenia purpura (TTP). (Magnification ×40)

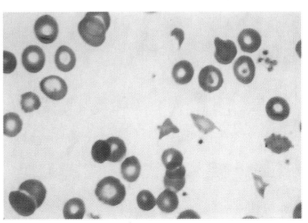

FIGURE 14-12 RBC fragmentation in microangiopathic hemolysis from a patient with prosthetic cardiac valve (mechanical hemolysis); note the presence of schistocytes.

Treatment of cardiac hemolysis can range from supportive therapy, which may include iron supplementation and transfusion,[69] to correcting the faulty valve or vessel surgically.

March Hemoglobinuria

This form of hemolytic anemia was first described in the late 1800s in a young German soldier who demonstrated frank hemoglobinuria following a field marching exercise.[70] The anemia has been described in individuals involved in strenuous and sustained physical activity.[71] Similar traumatic red cell destruction has been reported in a practitioner of karate[72] and a conga drum player.[73] The cause of the anemia is complex, involving: (1) direct physical disruption of red cells as they flow through the capillaries of the feet or hands, (2) iron loss in sweat, and (3) adaption to right-shifted oxygen dissociation curve.[74]

The blood picture of patients with march hemoglobinuria usually demonstrates a normal hemoglobin, although there may be an increase in the reticulocyte count. Hemoglobinemia and hemoglobinuria are episodic and present only following exercise. This obvious association with exercise is helpful in distinguishing the hemoglobinuria from other causes (such as PNH). Fragmented red cells are not a feature of the condition.

Treatment is merely wearing cushion-sole shoes or running on a softer surfaces.

Microangiopathic Hemolytic Anemia

Microangiopathic hemolytic anemia (MAHA) refers to a group of clinical disorders characterized by fragmentation of the red cells intravascularly. The hemolytic process involves fragmentation of red cells as they pass through abnormal arterioles.[75] Most often, the abnormalities in the microcirculation are caused by the deposition of fibrin strands resulting from intravascular activation of the coagulation system (see Chap. 29). The degree of hemolysis correlates with the amount of thrombosis present.[76] In addition to the intravascular destruction of the red cells, the fragments produced lack deformability, leading to an increase in extravascular hemolysis.

The manifestations are most prominent in two related clinical entities: hemolytic uremic syndrome (HUS) and thrombotic thrombocytopenic purpura (TTP). Refer to Chapter 27.

Oxidative Hemolysis

Oxidative stress on the red cell may affect either the globin chains or the heme group of the hemoglobin molecule. Most oxidizing agents affect the hemoglobin molecule by denaturing the globin chains producing either *Heinz bodies* or by oxidizing the heme group to produce *methemoglobinemia* (see Chap. 10).

Nonoxidative Hemolysis

Arsenic Continued exposure to arsenic gas gives rise to intravascular hemolysis with anemia and hemoglobinuria.[77] Marked methemalbumin formation

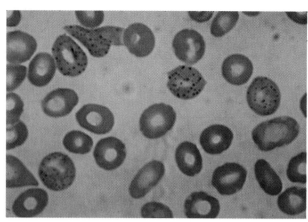

FIGURE 14-13 Peripheral blood from a patient with lead poisoning. Note the normocytic hypochromic red cells with the classic punctate basophilic stippling.

causes the serum of affected patients to turn a characteristic brown.

Lead The anemia that is produced by lead exposure is caused by decreased synthesis and not by direct hemolysis (see Chap. 6).[78] The red cells of patients exposed to lead have a shortened red cell survival.[79] Lead poisoning is usually a problem of young children who have been eating materials painted with lead-based paints. Children who are affected by lead poisoning may show a normocytic, hypochromic blood picture, with classic punctate *basophilic stippling* (Fig. 14-13).

Copper Very high levels of copper ions have been associated with suicide attempts in which copper sulfate solution is ingested[80] and with Wilson's disease.[81] The hemolytic process is unknown, although it has been shown that high levels of copper ions can affect a number of intracellular enzymes (e.g., pyruvate kinase and hexokinase).[82] The anemia may be associated with the presence of spherocytes.

Venoms A number of venoms, particularly those from some spiders, contain potent enzymes capable of directly acting on the red cell membrane to produce lysis of the cell. Bee stings may produce a hemolytic process in some people. Snake venoms, although hemolytic in vitro, rarely cause hemolysis in vivo.

Osmotic Effects

Burns Patients who have suffered severe burns over more than 15% of their body generally show evidence of intravascular hemolysis.[83] The hemolytic process is thought to be caused by the direct effect of the heat on the red cells in the affected area. Red cells that are heated to temperatures in excess of 49°C undergo changes including fragmentation, budding, and microspherocyte formation; blood collected within 24 hours of such heating will show evidence of these changes (Fig. 14-14). Because the cells are osmotically and mechanically fragile, they are rapidly removed from the circulation, and blood collected after that time is often normal in appearance.

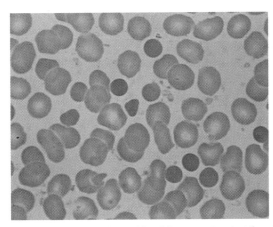

FIGURE 14–14 Peripheral blood from a patient with extensive burns. Note typical microspherocytes and membranous fragments. (From Bell, A: Hematology. In Listen, Look and Learn. Health and Education Resources, Inc., Bethesda, MD, with permission.)

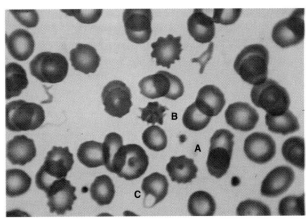

FIGURE 14–17 Renal disease (peripheral blood). Note presence of (A) burr cells, (B) thorn cell, and (C) blister cell. (From Bell, A: Hematology. In Listen, Look and Learn. Health and Education Resources, Inc., Bethesda, MD, with permission.)

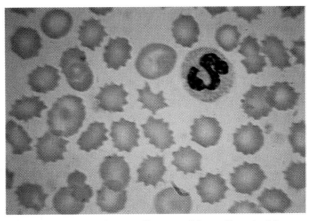

FIGURE 14–15 "Spur-cell anemia" (acanthocytosis) associated with severe liver disease.

Acquired Membrane Disorders

A number of mechanisms can be implicated in producing changes to red cell membranes, which can result in the shortened lifespan of the cell. Any change that compromises the cell's deformability or its resistance to oxidative stress can potentially contribute to a hemolytic process. For example, spur-cell anemia, observed primarily in patients with alcoholic cirrhosis, is a condition in which the red cells assume a characteristic shape with a number of fine fingerlike spike protrusions (Fig. 14–15). Lipid disorders can also result in loss of red cell deformability. A congenital red cell abnormality seen in a β-lipoproteinemia may contribute to the diagnosis of the condition as the cells assume the classic shape of acanthocytes (Fig. 14–16). In end-stage renal disease, many of the cells take on the appearance of burr cells, or echinocytes (Fig. 14–17), which have numerous small spines over their entire surface. Other conditions in which echinocytes are seen include pyruvate kinase deficiency and bleeding states associated with peptic ulcers.

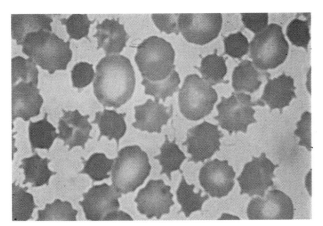

FIGURE 14–16 Acanthocytosis from a patient with abetalipoproteinemia. (From Hyun, BH, Ashton, JK, and Dolan, K: Practical Hematology. A Laboratory Guide with Accompanying Filmstrip. WB Saunders, Philadelphia, 1975, with permission.)

CASE STUDY 1

A 26-year-old white woman diagnosed with rheumatoid arthritis came into the emergency room with complaints of weakness and shortness of breath. Laboratory findings revealed that the patient was severely anemic. She had received many red cell transfusions over the past 8 years, but had not received any transfusions in over a year. The peripheral blood smear demonstrated a mild spherocytosis. The cross-match and antibody screen tests were weakly positive at the antiglobulin phase. On further testing, the patient's direct antiglobulin test (DAT) was also weakly positive with IgG immunoglobulin coating her red cells. The effort to obtain compatible blood for transfusion was complicated because the patient's serum reacted weakly with all cells tested.

Questions

1. What is the most likely diagnosis?
2. What other laboratory tests should be requested to aid in the diagnosis?
3. What is the treatment for this patient?

Answers

1. WAIHA
2. Reticulocyte count, indirect bilirubin, and serum haptoglobin
3. Steroids

CASE STUDY 2

A 38-year-old man was diagnosed with pneumonia 3 weeks previously. He returned to the hospital because he was experiencing severe weakness and shortness of breath on slight exertion. The patient was pale and jaundiced. Laboratory findings revealed severe anemia. The peripheral blood smear demonstrated marked aggregation of erythrocytes. The cross-match and antibody screen tests were both strongly positive at the room temperature phase (20°C). On further testing, the patient's direct antiglobulin test (DAT) was also strongly positive with complement proteins. The Donath-Landsteiner test was negative. Thermal amplitude studies revealed immunoglobulin reactivity up to 34°C.

Questions

1. What is the most likely diagnosis?
2. What other laboratory tests should be requested to aid in the diagnosis?
3. What is the treatment for this patient?

Answers

1. Cold hemagglutinin disease (CHD) secondary to pneumonia infection
2. Reticulocyte count, indirect bilirubin, and serum haptoglobin
3. Keep patient warm until primary infection subsides

CASE STUDY 3

A 50-year-old African-American man complained of headaches, fatigue, and general malaise over the past 2 weeks. The patient then developed a high fever followed by severe chills that persisted for approximately a day. The fever and chills subsided and the patient thought he was getting better until last night, when he experienced another bout of fever and chills. Laboratory findings revealed that the patient was anemic and slightly leukocytopenic. The laboratory noted that odd, blue, "crescent-moon" inclusions were seen in approximately 10% of his red cells. On further testing, the direct antiglobulin test (DAT) was negative. The cross-match and antibody screening tests were also negative.

Questions

1. What is the most likely diagnosis?
2. What other laboratory tests should be requested to aid in the diagnosis?
3. What is the treatment for this patient?

Answers

1. *P. falciparum*
2. Thin smear preparation
3. Quinine sulfate, 650 mg three times a day

REFERENCES

1. Frank, MM: Mechanisms of cell destruction in immuno-hemolytic anemia. In Bell, CA: (ed): Laboratory Management of Hemolysis. AABB, Arlington, VA, 1979.
2. Garratty, G: Autoimmune hemolytic anemia. In Garratty, G (ed): Immunobiology of Transfusion Medicine. Marcel Dekker, New York, 1994.
3. Devine, DV: Complement. In Anderson, KC and Ness, PM (eds): Scientific basis of transfusion medicine: Implications for clinical practice. WB Saunders, Philadelphia, 1994.
4. Garratty, G: Factors affecting the pathogenicity of red cell auto and alloantibodies. In Nance, SJ (ed): Immune destruction of red blood cells. AABB, Arlington, VA, 1989.
5. Żupańska, B: Cellular immunoassays and their use for predicting the clinical significance of antibodies. In Garratty, G (ed): Immunobiology of Transfusion Medicine. Marcel Dekker, New York, 1994.
6. Anderson, DR and Kelton, JG: Mechanisms of intravascular and extravascular cell destruction. In Nance, SJ (ed): Immune Destruction of Red Blood Cells. AABB, Arlington, VA, 1989.
7. Rozsnyay, X, Sarmay, G, Walker, M, et al: Distinctive role of IgG1 and IgG3 isotypes in FcγR-mediated function. Immunology 66:491.
8. Walker, RH (ed): Technical Manual, ed 11. AABB, Bethesda, MD, 1993.
9. Mollison, PL, Engelfriet, CP, and Contreras, M: Blood Transfusions in Clinical Medicine, ed 9. Blackwell Scientific, Oxford, 1993.
10. Ness, PM, Shirey, RS, and Thoman, SK: The differentiation of delayed serologic and delayed hemolytic transfusion reactions: incidence, long-term serologic findings, and clinical significance. Transfusion 30:688, 1990.
11. Mollison, PL: Some aspects of Rh hemolytic disease and its prevention. In Garratty, G (ed): Hemolytic Disease of the Newborn. AABB, Arlington, VA, 1984.
12. Jakobowicz, R, Williams, L, and Silberman, F: Immunization of Rh negative volunteers by repeated injections of very small amounts of Rh positive blood. Vox Sang 23:376, 1972.
13. Keith, LG and Berger, GS: The risk of Rh immunization associated with abortion, spontaneous and induced. In Frigoletto, FD, Jewett, JF, and Konugres, AA (eds): Rh Hemolytic Disease New Strategy for Eradication. GK Hall, Boston, 1982.
14. Siegel, DL and Silberstein, LE: Red blood cell autoantibodies. In Anderson, KC and Ness, PM (eds): Scientific basis of transfusion medicine: Implications for Clinical Practice. WB Saunders, Philadelphia, 1994.
15. Dacie, JV and Worlledge, SM: Auto-immune hemolytic anemias. Prog Hematol 6:82, 1969.
16. Petz, LD and Garratty, G: Acquired immune hemolytic anemias. Churchill Livingstone, New York, 1980.
17. Gilliand, BC, Baxter, E, and Evans, RS: Red cell antibodies in acquired hemolytic anemia with negative antiglobulin serum tests. N Engl J Med 285:252, 1971.
18. Rowe, GL and Davies, H: A study using an enzyme linked antiglobulin test on patients with a positive direct antiglobulin test (abstr). Book of Abstracts from the ISBT/AABB Joint Congress. AABB, Arlington, VA 1990, p 87.
19. Pirofsky, B: Autoimmunization and the autoimmune hemolytic anemias. Williams & Wilkins, Baltimore, 1969, p 63.

20. Bottiger, LE and Westerholm, B: Acquired haemolytic anaemia. Acta Med Scand 193:223, 1973.
21. Hsu, TCS, Rosenfield, RE, Burkart, P, et al: Instrumented PVP-augmented antiglobulin tests. Vox Sang 26:305, 1974.
22. Sokol, RJ, Hewitt, S, Booker, DJ, and Bailey, A: Red cell autoantibodies, multiple immunoglobulin classes and autoimmune hemolysis. Transfusion 30:417, 1990.
23. Victoria, EJ, Pierce, SW, Branks MJ, and Masouredis, SP: IgG red blood cell autoantibodies in autoimmune hemolytic anemia bind to epitopes on red cell membrane band 3 glycoprotein. J Lab Clin Med 115:74, 1990.
24. Kruskall, M: Clinical management of transfusions to patients with red cell antibodies. In Nance, SJ (ed): Immune Destruction of Red Blood Cells. AABB, Arlington, VA 1989.
25. Salama, A, Berghöfer, H, and Mueller-Eckhardt, C: Red blood cell transfusion in warm-type autoimmune haemolytic anaemia. Lancet 340:1515, 1992.
26. Rosse, JF: Quantitative immunology of immune hemolytic anemia. II. The relationship of cell-bound antibody to hemolysis and the effect of treatment. J Clin Invest 50:734, 1971.
27. Kay, NE and Douglas, SD: Monocyte-erythrocyte interaction in vitro in immune hemolytic anemias. Blood 50:889, 1977.
28. Beck, ML: The I blood group collection. In Moulds, JM and Woods, LL (eds): Blood Groups: P, I, Sdᵃ and Pr. AABB, Arlington, VA, 1991.
29. Issitt, PD: Applied Blood Group Serology, ed 3. Montgomery Scientific, Miami, 1985.
30. Issitt, PD: Cold-reacting autoantibodies outside the I and P blood groups. In Moulds, JM and Woods, LL (eds): Blood Groups: P, I, Sdᵃ and Pr. AABB, Arlington, VA, 1991.
31. Garratty, G, Petz, LD, and Hoops, JK: The correlation of cold agglutinin titrations in saline and albumin with haemolytic anaemia. Br J Haematol 35:587, 1977.
32. Mougey, R: Cold autoimmune hemolytic anemia: A review of clinical and laboratory considerations. Immunohematology 1:1, 1984.
33. Judd, WJ: Investigation and management of immune hemolysis—autoantibodies and drugs. In Wallace, ME and Lievitt, JS (eds): Current Applications and Interpretation of the Direct Antiglobulin Test. AABB, Arlington, VA, 1988.
34. Shirey, RS and Barrasso, C: Cold agglutinins. Continuing education slide presentation. Organon Teknika, Durham, NC, 1993.
35. Janney, FA, Lee, LT, and Howe, C: Cold hemagglutinin cross = reactivity with *Mycoplasma pneumoniae*. Infect Immun 22:29, 1978.
36. Costea, N, Yakulis, VJ, and Heller, P: Inhibition of cold agglutinins (anti-I) by *M. pneumoniae* antigens. Proc Soc Exp Biol (NY) 139:476, 1972.
37. Capra, JP, Kehoe, JM, Williams, RC, et al: Light chain sequences of human IgM cold agglutinins. Proc Nat Acad Sci (Wash) 69:40, 1972.
38. Harbo, M and Lind, K: Light chain type of transiently occurring cold haemagglutinins. Scand J Haematol 3:269, 1966.
39. Jenkins, WJ, Koster, HG, Marsh, WL, Carter, RL: Infectious mononucleosis: An unsuspected source of anti-i. Br J Haematol 11:480, 1965.
40. Wolledge, SM and Dacie, JV: Haemolytic and other anaemias in infectious mononucleosis. In Carter, HG and Penman, RL (eds): Infectious mononucleosis. Blackwell Scientific, Oxford, 1969.
41. Rosenfield, RE, Schmidt, PJ, Calvo, RC, and McGinniss, MH: Anti-i, a frequent cold agglutinin in infectious mononucleosis. Vox Sang 10:631, 1965.
42. Horwitz, CA, Moulds, J, Henle, W, et al: Cold agglutinins in infectious mononucleosis and heterophile-antibody-negative mononucleosis like syndromes. Blood 50:195, 1977.
43. Bell, WR, et al: Cold agglutinin hemolytic anemia: management with an environmental suit. Ann Intern Med 106:243, 1987.
44. Anstall, HB and Blaylock, RC: The P blood group system: biochemistry, genetics and clinical significance. In Moulds, JM and Woods, LL (eds): Blood groups: P, I, Sdᵃ and Pr. AABB, Arlington, VA, 1991.
45. Donath, J and Landsteiner, K: Über kälte häemoglobinurie. Ergbn Hyg Bakt 7:184, 1925.
46. Levine, P, Celano, MJ, and Falkowski, F: The specificity of the antibody in paroxysmal cold hemoglobinuria (PCH). Transfusion 3:278, 1963.
47. McCann, EL, Shirey, RS, Kickler, TS, and Ness PM: IgM autoagglutinins in warm autoimmune hemolytic anemia: A poor prognostic feature. Acta Haematol 88:120, 1992.
48. Shirey, RS, Kickler, TS, Bell WR, Little B, et al: Fatal immune hemolytic anemia and hepatic failure associated with a warm-reacting IgM autoantibody. Vox Sang 52:219, 1987.
49. Sokol, RJ, Hewitt, S, and Stamps, BK: Autoimmune haemolysis: An 18 year study of 865 cases referred to a regional transfusion center. Br Med J 282:2023, 1981.
50. Shulman, IA, Branch, DR, Nelson, JM, et al: Autoimmune hemolytic anemia with both cold and warm autoantibodies. JAMA 253:1746, 1985.
51. Worlledge, SM: Immune drug induced haemolytic anaemias. In Girdwood RH (ed): Blood Disorders Due to Drugs and Other Agents. Excerpta Medica, Amsterdam, 1973.
52. Garratty, G, and Petz, LD: Drug-induced immune hemolytic anemia. Am J Med 58:398, 1975.
53. Carstairs, KC, Breckenridge, A, Dollery, CT, and Worlledge, SM: Incidence of a positive direct Coombs test in patients on α-methyldopa. Lancet 2:133, 1966.
54. Garratty, G: Review: Immune hemolytic anemia and/or positive direct antiglobulin tests caused by drugs. Immunohematology 12:41, 1994.
55. Jamin, D, Demers, J, Shulman, I, et al: An explanation for nonimmunologic adsorption of proteins onto red blood cells. Blood 67:993, 1986.
56. Buetler, E: Hemolytic anemia due to infections with micro-organisms. In Beutler, E, Lichtman, MA, Coller, BS, and Kipps, TJ (eds): Williams Hematology, ed 5. McGraw-Hill, New York, 1995.
57. Ruebush, TK, II, Cassaday, PB, Marsh, HJ, et al: Human babesiosis on Nantucket island. Ann Intern Med 86:6, 1977.
58. Jacoby, GA, Hunt, JV, Kosinski, KS, et al: Treatment of transfusion-transmitted babesiosis by exchange transfusion. N Engl J Med 303:1098, 1980.
59. Smith, RP, Evans, AT, Popovsky, M, et al: Transfusion-acquired babesiosis and failure of antibiotic treatment. JAMA 256:2726, 1986.
60. Chisholm, ES, Sulzer, AJ, and Ruebush, TK, II: Indirect immunofluorescence test for human Babesia microti infection: Antigenic specificity. Am J Trop Med Hyg 35:921, 1985.
61. Ricketts, WE: *Bartonella bacilliformis* anemia (Oroya fever). A study of thirty cases. Blood 3:1025, 1948.
62. Reynafarje, C and Ramos, J: The hemolytic anemia of bartonellosis. Blood 17:562, 1961.
63. Clancy, MT and O'Brian, S: Fatal *Clostridium welchii* septicaemia following acute cholecystitis. Br J Surg 62:518, 1975.
64. Simpkins, H, Kahlenberg, A, Rosenberg, A, et al: Structural and compositional changes in the red cell membrane during *Clostridium welchii* infection. Br J Haematol 21:173, 1971.
65. Mahn, H and Dantuono, LM: Postabortal septicotoxemia

due to *Clostridium welchii.* J Obstet Gynecol 70:604, 1955.

66. Erslev, AJ: Traumatic cardiac hemolytic anemia. In Beutler, E, Lichtman, MA, Coller, BS, and Kipps, TJ (eds): Williams Hematology, ed 5. McGraw-Hill, New York, 1995.

67. Harker, LA and Slichter, SJ: Studies of platelet and fibrinogen kinetics in patients with prosthetic heart valves. N Engl J Med 283:1302, 1970.

68. Slater, SD, Rahman, M, and Lindsay, RM: Renal function in chronic intravascular haemolysis associated with prosthetic cardiac valves. Clin Sci 44:511, 1973.

69. Kornowski, R, Schwartz, D, Jaffe, A, et al: Erythropoietin therapy obviates the need for recurrent transfusion in a patient with severe hemolysis due to prosthetic valves. Chest 102:315, 1992.

70. Fleischer, R: Über eine neute form von hämoglobinurie beim menschen. Berlin Klin Wochenschr 18:691, 1881.

71. Gilligan, DR, Altschule, MD, and Katersky, EM: Psychologic intravascular hemolysis of exercise: Hemoglobinemia and hemoglobinuria following cross-country runs. J Clin Invest 22:859, 1943.

72. Streeton, JA: Traumatic hemoglobinuria caused by karate exercises. Lancet 2:191, 1967.

73. Furie, B and Penn, AS: Pigmenturia from conga drumming: Hemoglobinuria and myoglobinuria. Ann Intern Med 80:727, 1974.

74. Erslev, AJ: March hemoglobinuria and sports anemia. In Beutler, E, Lichtman, MA, Coller, BS, and Kipps, TJ (eds): Williams Hematology, ed 5. McGraw-Hill, New York, 1995.

75. Bull, BS, Rubenberg, ML, Dacie, JF, and Brain, MC: Microangiopathic haemolytic anaemia: Mechanisms of red cell fragmentation: In vitro studies. Br J Haematol 14:643, 1968.

76. Rubenberg, ML, Regoeczi, E, Bull, BS, et al: Microangiopathic haemolytic anaemia: The experimental production of haemolysis and red cell fragmentation by defibrination in vivo. Br J Haematol 14:627, 1968.

77. Jenkins, GC, Ind, JE, Kazantzis, G, and Owen, R: Arsenic poisoning: Massive haemolysis with minimal impairment of renal function. Br Med J 2:78, 1965.

78. Beutler, E: Hemolytic anemia due to chemical and physical agents. In Beutler, E, Lichtman, MA, Coller, BS, Kipps, TJ (eds): Williams Hematology, ed 5. McGraw-Hill, New York, 1995.

79. Waldron, HA: The anemia of lead poisoning: A review. Br J Ind Med 23:83, 1966.

80. Klein, WJ, Jr, Metz, EN, and Price, AR: Acute copper intoxication: A hazard of hemodialysis. Arch Intern Med 129:578, 1972.

81. Hansen, PB: Wilson's disease presenting with severe haemolytic anaemia. Ugeskr Laeger 150:1229, 1988.

82. Boulard, M, Blume, K, and Beutler, E: The effect of copper on red cell enzyme activities. J Clin Invest 51:459, 1972.

83. Shen, SC, Ham, TH, and Fleming, EM: Studies on the destruction of red blood cells. III. Mechanism and complications of hemoglobinuria in patients with thermal burns: Spherocytosis and increased osmotic fragility of red blood cells. N Engl J Med 229:701, 1943.

84. Wagner, HN, Jr, Razzak, MA, Gaertner, RA, et al: Removal of erythrocytes from the circulation. Arch Intern Med 110:90, 1962.

QUESTIONS

1. What are the mechanisms of immune hemolysis?
   a. IgG or IgM antibodies that activate the classic complement pathway
   b. Antibody-dependent cellular cytotoxicity (ADCC) mediated by NK cells, monocytes/macrophages, and granulocytes
   c. Complement and phagocytic cells in a reaction of immune adherence
   d. All of the above

2. What is the process in which the immune system produces antibodies to foreign red cell antigens introduced into their circulation through transfusion, pregnancy, or organ transplantation?
   a. Alloimmune hemolytic anemia
   b. Autoimmune hemolytic anemia
   c. Drug-induced immune hemolytic anemia
   d. None of the above

3. Which finding is not characteristic for immediate hemolytic transfusion reactions?
   a. Acute intravascular hemolysis
   b. Most commonly caused by ABO IgM complement-activating antibodies
   c. Increase in plasma haptoglobin
   d. Hemoglobinemia, hemoglobinuria, and hemosiderinuria

4. Which is true concerning delayed hemolytic transfusion reactions?
   a. Antibodies are not demonstrable in patient serum until 10 to 14 days after transfusion.
   b. Antibodies are usually IgG formed from a secondary response.
   c. Hemoglobinemia and hemoglobinuria are present.
   d. Findings include a negative direct antiglobulin test result and antibody screen.

5. What causes hemolytic disease of the newborn (HDN)?
   a. Maternal IgG antibodies, formed as a result of a previous blood exposure and/or pregnancy, cross the placenta and attach to fetal cells.
   b. Fetal IgG antibodies cross the placenta and attach to maternal red cells.
   c. Maternal IgM antibodies, formed as a result of a previous blood exposure and/or pregnancy, cross the placenta and attach to fetal cells.
   d. Fetal IgM antibodies attach to fetal red cells and cross the placenta to enter the mother's circulation.

6. Which of the following is not a hematologic finding for HDN?
   a. Mild to severe anemia
   b. Microcytosis and hypochromia
   c. Reticulocytosis
   d. Spherocytes and nucleated RBCs

7. What immune system abnormality results in the loss of self-recognition for an individual's own red cell antigens?
   a. Alloimmune hemolytic anemia
   b. Autoimmune hemolytic anemia
   c. Drug-induced immune hemolytic anemia
   d. None of the above

8. Which is not a characteristic of warm autoimmune hemolytic anemia?
   a. Variable anemia
   b. Reticulocytosis and spherocytosis
   c. Positive result for Donath-Landsteiner test
   d. DAT result usually positive for both IgG and C3d

9. What are features of cold agglutinin syndrome?
   a. Usually an IgM antibody
   b. Reticulocytosis and positive DAT result
   c. Tendency for spontaneous autoagglutination of RBC samples
   d. All of the above

10. What is the principle of the Donath-Landsteiner test?
   a. Antibody binds red cells at 37°C and causes lysis at 4°C.
   b. Antibody binds red cells at 4°C and causes lysis at 37°C.
   c. Antibody binds red cells at 4°C or 37°C and causes immediate lysis.
   d. Antibody binds red cells at 4°C or 37°C but causes lysis only at 4°C.

11. Which of the following is a proposed mechanism for drug-induced immune hemolytic anemia?
   a. Immune complex
   b. Drug adsorption (hapten)
   c. Membrane modification
   d. All of the above

12. What are causes for nonimmune hemolytic anemia?
   a. Infections
   b. Mechanical, chemical, and physical agents
   c. Acquired membrane disorders
   d. All of the above

13. How is laboratory diagnosis made for malarial infection?
   a. Examination of peripheral blood smear
   b. Recovery of the organism
   c. Measuring hepatic enzymes
   d. Skin testing

14. Which of the following organisms are associated with hemolytic anemia?
   a. *Mycoplasma pneumoniae*
   b. Epstein-Barr virus
   c. *Babesia microti*
   d. All of the above

ANSWERS

1. **d** (pp 221–222)
2. **a** (p 223)
3. **c** (p 224)
4. **b** (p 224)
5. **a** (p 225)
6. **b** (p 225)
7. **b** (p 225)
8. **c** (pp 226–227)
9. **d** (p 228)
10. **b** (p 230)
11. **d** (pp 230–232)
12. **d** (pp 233–239)
13. **a** (p 234)
14. **d** (pp 229–237); Table 14-22 (p 237)

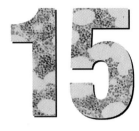

Anemia Associated with Systemic, Nonhematologic Disorders

Carmen J. Julius, MD
Sandra Gwaltney-Krause, MA, MT(ASCP)

Objectives

At the end of this chapter, the learner should be able to:

1 Describe the anemia of inflammation.
2 List the many causes of the anemia of inflammation.
3 Identify laboratory findings characteristic of the anemia of inflammation.
4 List the cytokines important in inducing the anemia of inflammation.
5 Describe the treatment for anemia of inflammation.
6 List the three categories of causes of the anemia associated with malignancy and some causes under each category.
7 Name the major cause of the anemia associated with renal disease and renal failure.
8 Discuss the many causes of the anemia associated with liver disease.
9 Describe the characteristics of the red blood cells in anemia associated with liver disease.
10 Describe the etiology of the anemia associated with alcoholism.

Anemias produced by inflammation and systemic diseases are perhaps the most common hematologic abnormalities encountered in the laboratory. It is important for the clinician and the medical technologist to recognize the characteristics of these anemias in patients with systemic diseases and to understand the hematologic assays that can differentiate them from other causes of anemia. Anemia without other clinical symptoms at the initial evaluation of a patient may be the first indication of a systemic disease (e.g., an occult malignancy). Likewise, a sudden change in the complete blood count (CBC) of a patient who has been diagnosed with an inflammatory or systemic disease may indicate a new complication.

Many disease entities are outlined below. All have a common theme that forms the basis of this chapter, that is, the effects of systemic disorders (i.e., nonhematologic disorders) on bone marrow and red blood cell production.

ANEMIA ASSOCIATED WITH CHRONIC DISORDERS AND INFLAMMATION

Anemia associated with chronic disorders (ACD) is the term formerly used to describe the anemia associated with chronic infections and other states of chronic inflammation. Because these disorders are common, this is one of the most frequently encountered anemias.[1] Recent research has demonstrated a mechanism involved in the inflammatory response to tissue injury, rendering the term ACD obsolete. *Anemia of inflammation* (AOI) has been suggested as a more appropriate term because it more definitely describes the mechanism of the disorder.[2,3] Therefore, this term is used throughout this chapter.

The Inflammatory Response and Body Defense Mechanisms

The General Inflammatory Response (First Line of Defense)

Inflammation is one of the body's responses to tissue injury from physical agents, foreign organisms, and immune reactions in the host. Inflammatory and hemostatic responses occur simultaneously to control any damage at the injured area (see Chaps. 29 and 30). The coagulation cascade and the complement, fibrinolytic, and kinin systems interact to modulate inflammation (see Chaps. 26, 29, and 30).

During the inflammatory process, complement can be activated directly by microorganisms via the alternative pathway or the antibody-induced classical pathway. The presence of C3a, C5a, and other chemotaxins attracts phagocytes to the site of injury, where they recognize and phagocytize foreign substances or organisms. Neutrophilic granulocytes, monocytes, and macrophages possess receptors for complement that can induce exocytosis of granules containing proteolytic enzymes, free ion radicals, and other inflammatory metabolites and endocytosis of complement-coated foreign substances.

Inflammation will persist as long as injury and damage persist. When the source of inflammation is persistent and the condition is chronic, mediators from the humoral and cell-mediated immune responses contribute to the onset of anemia (Fig. 15–1). Table 15–1 lists the functions of the various types of T-cell lymphocytes in cell-mediated immunity.

Etiology and Pathophysiology

Evidence does not uphold one single cause for AOI, but rather several overlapping mechanisms, all induced by the inflammatory process. Possible causes include: (1) decreased red blood cell (RBC) life span, (2) impaired iron metabolism from faulty iron release from RE stores, (3) decreased erythropoietin levels, and (4) suppression of erythropoiesis by cytokines from activated macrophages and lymphocytes because of the underlying disease and inflammation. Each of these possibilities contributes to AOI.[4] Table 15–2 lists the cytokines that contribute to inflammation and Table 15–3 summarizes the functions of macrophages.

Decreased Red Blood Cell Survival and Life Span

Decreased life span of RBCs is seen in patients with AOI.[4] Mean survival of RBCs in some cases is 90 days, compared with 120 days in healthy persons.[4] The mechanism for this decrease is unclear, but it may be because of the extracorpuscular effects of activated macrophage-monocytes of the RE system.[5,6] These cells have increased phagocytic capabilities in patients with inflammatory processes and may be responsible for the shortened erythrocyte survival.

Reticuloendothelial Iron Block

Anemia from RE iron block is another possible contributor to AOI. Although there is a decrease in intestinal iron absorption[4] and impaired iron reutilization by the hepatocytes in these patients,[4] there is an abundance of iron transported to the RE system stores.[7] Iron in the RE system stores normally and is available to the plasma by both slow and quick release mechanisms.[8] In AOI, there is increased apoferritin synthesis.[9] Surplus apoferritin binds a larger amount of iron entering the cell.[9] Therefore, the rapid release mechanism or pool of iron is markedly decreased.

Macrophages of the RE system demonstrate large coarse aggregates of iron despite the low serum iron. The iron appears trapped within the RE system and is unable to be fully utilized in erythropoiesis. Ferritin is increased because of the increased RE system iron stores (see Chap. 6). This results in the paradoxic ferrokinetics typical of AOI (i.e., a sideropenic or functionally iron-deficient state). The resulting hypoferremia sets off a "domino effect" of decreased transferrin saturation, which limits the supply of iron to the marrow and increases the amount of free erythrocyte protoporphyrin (FEP)—that is, a porphyrin ring without iron.[6] Thus there is decreased heme production.

Decreased Erythropoietin Levels

One of the controversies regarding AOI is whether or not patients have an ineffective level of erythropoietin (EPO). The EPO levels in anemic patients with chronic inflammatory disorders are elevated when compared with levels from patients with a normal hematocrit.[4,10] Still others have demonstrated that this response is blunted relative to the anemia seen in control patients with uncomplicated iron-deficiency anemia.[11–14] From this information it appears that the patient attempts to counteract the anemia with increased EPO production by the kidneys, but that the response is not adequate for compensation of the anemia. The response of the bone marrow to EPO is much less than expected for the amount of EPO secreted.[15] This is most likely the major problem and perhaps one of the major reasons for AOI.[16]

Suppression of Erythropoiesis and the Role of Cytokines

One of the newest keys to understanding anemia of inflammation is the suppressor-inhibitor effects of erythropoiesis by IL-1, TNF-α, and interferon gamma (IFN-γ).[16] Sera from patients with chronic inflammatory disorders (e.g., rheumatoid arthritis, systemic lupus erythematous, and juvenile chronic arthritis) have been shown to inhibit erythropoiesis in vitro.[17,18] The inhibition of early erythrocytic progenitors, burst-forming unit–erythroid (BFU-E) and colony-forming unit–erythroid (CFU-E), corresponds with the severity of the anemia and indicators of inflammation such as the presence of acute phase reactants. Research now

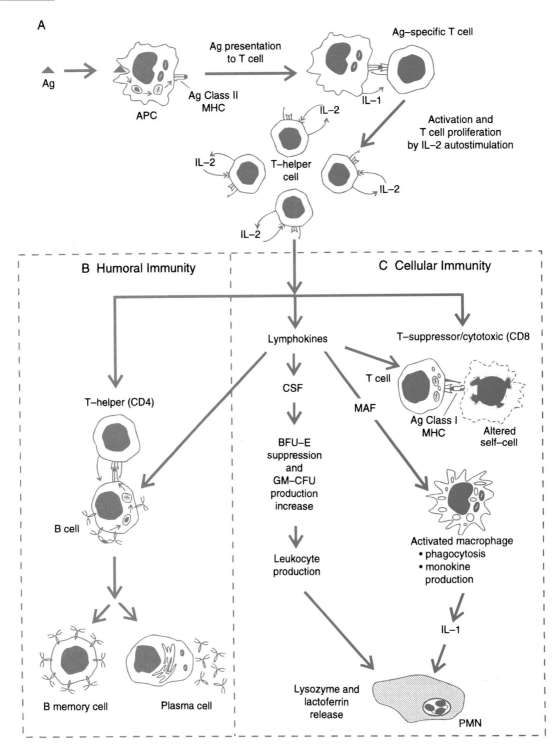

FIGURE 15-1 The mechanism of humoral and cellular immunity. (*A*) The antigen phagocytized by the APC is digested and small antigenic fragments or epitopes are associated with the class II MHC and presented to a T cell with a receptor specific for the antigen. Formation of the antigen-receptor complex between the two cells and IL-1 secreted by the APC provide the signals for the T cell to be activated and secrete IL-2 for its autostimulation and proliferation to effector T-helper cells. (*B*) Humoral immunity. The T-helper effector cell (CD4) and some of its lymphokines provide the necessary signals for the B cell with the same antigen specificity to be activated and proliferate to B memory and antibody-producing plasma cells. (*C*) Cellular immunity. Some of the lymphokines from the activated CD4 cells and the complex formed between antigens associated with class I MHC on altered self-cell and T-cytotoxic cell (CD8) receptors cause the activation of the CD8 cells, which mediate the cytotoxic killing of the altered self-cells. Some of the other lymphokines produced also play significant roles in hematopoiesis and activation of phagocytic cells. Ag = antigen, APC = antigen-presenting cell, MHC = major histocompatibility complex, IL-1 = interleukin 1, IL-2 = interleukin 2, CSF = colony-stimulating factor, BFU-E = Burst-forming units–erythroid, GM–CFU = granulocyte/macrophage–colony-forming units, PMN = polymorphonuclear neutrophils, MAF = macrophage-activating factor.

TABLE 15–1   Thymus-Derived Lymphocytes

Helper (inducer) T cells
Aid B-cell maturation in bone marrow
Supply activating (permissive) signals to B cells
Activate the generation of different antibody classes
Activate effector T cells

Effector T cells
Two types, producing delayed hypersensitivity and
    cytotoxic effects. Responsible for:
1. Immunologic surveillance for malignant cells
2. Eradication of established viral and fungal infection
3. Eradication of intracellular bacterial infection
4. Destruction of parasites

Suppressor (immunoregulatory) T cells
Control inflammation produced by T cells
Control antibody production
Balance ratio of immunoglobulin classes
Block activation of T- and B-cell clones reactive to "self"

Source: From Dwyer, JM: The Cell-Mediated Immune System. Cutter Biologicals, Emeryville, CA, 1982, p 3, with permission.

indicates that cytokines may be the key signal regulating hematopoiesis in inflammatory disease states.[16]

IL-1 has been examined for its potential hematopoietic suppressive capabilities because of its mediation of various facets of the acute phase reaction. There is also a close correlation between the severity of anemia and the severity of inflammatory activity.

Evidence also suggests that TNF-α, another cytokine from activated macrophages, may be involved in the pathogenesis of AOI.[19] Very low concentrations of TNF-α were shown to inhibit erythroid progenitor growth in normal bone marrow cultures. This was demonstrated at concentrations similar to those found in affected patients.[16]

It is becoming increasingly evident that what was originally regarded by early investigators as a "simple anemia" is far from simple. The effect of monokines and lymphokines on granulocyte, macrophage, and other hematopoietic progenitor cells appears to be responsible for AOI. Indeed, mechanisms responsible for host protection against infection and tissue injury be-

TABLE 15–2   Cytokines That Contribute to Inflammation

Cytokine	Target Cell	Activity
IL-1	T cells, B cells, macrophages and tissue cells	Lymphocyte activation, macrophage activation, acute phase reaction
IL-2	T lymphocytes	Stimulates proliferation of activated T cells
IL-3 (multilineage colony-stimulating factor)	Stem cells	Stimulates differentiation of bone marrow stem cells
IL-4 (B-cell growth factor)	B lymphocytes	B-cell proliferation
IL-5	B lymphocytes eosinophils, precursor cells	B-cell growth and differentiation, eosinophil differentiation
IL-6	B lymphocytes, hepatocytes	Stimulates antibody production and acute phase reactants
Migration inhibition factor (MIF)	Macrophages	Inhibits migration
Macrophage activation factor (MAF)	Macrophages	Activates macrophages and enhances their functions
Leukocyte chemotaxis factor (LCF)	Phagocytes	Promotes chemotaxis to site of injury
Leukocyte inhibition factor (LIF)	Phagocytes	Inhibits migration
GM-CSF	Stem cells	Stimulates differentiation of granulocyte-monocyte precursor cells
M-CSF	Stem cells	Stimulates differentiation of monocytes
G-CSF	Stem cells	Stimulates differentiation of granulocytes
Interferon gamma (INF-γ)	Macrophages	Activates macrophages for cytotoxic functions; induces MHC II molecules on APCs
Tumor necrosis factor—alpha (TNF-α)	Macrophages, granulocytes	Activates macrophages, granulocytes and cytotoxic cells

Abbreviations: MHC = major histocompatibility complex; GM-CSF = granulocyte/macrophase–colony-stimulating factor; M-CSF = monocyte–colony-stimulating factor; G-CSF = granulocyte–colony-stimulating factor

TABLE 15–3 **Macrophage Functions**

Production of IL-1
Fever
Neutrophil activation
Release of acute-phase reactants
Lymphocyte activation and proliferation
  Lymphokine production
  Antibody production

Antigen Processing and Presentation

Tumor Destruction
Production of TNF
Cytotoxic action
Toxic factors

Phagocytic Activities
Fc and C3 receptors
Microcidal and bacteriostatic activities
Protection from parasites
Removal of particulate substances and damaged cells
Lymphokine receptors (MAF, MIF)

Inflammation and Tissue Alterations
Fibroblast activation
  Collagenase synthesis
Synthesis and secretion of factors
Lysozyme, plasminogen activators, elastase, complement
  components

Abbreviations: TNF = tumor necrosis factor; MAF = macrophage-activating factor; MIF = Macrophage inhibitory factor

come detrimental to the host indirectly. Although the exact mechanism is still being researched, IL-1 and TNF-α (products of activated macrophages) have emerged as key pathogenic factors.[15] Synergy among many cytokines has also been postulated.[4,20] Theoretically, any disease that involves tissue injury and inflammation can, over a period of 1 to 2 months, result in anemia.

Characteristics

Anemia of inflammation is a hypoproliferative, mild anemia that is usually normocytic and normochromic. There is very little reticulocytosis for the severity or degree of anemia. It may be hypochromic if the disease increases in severity.

Anemia of inflammation is characterized by a normal or low mean corpuscular hemoglobin concentration (MCHC), mean corpuscular volume (MCV), low serum iron level, a decreased total iron-binding capacity

(TIBC), and a low iron-transferrin saturation, despite normal to increased iron stores in RE cells. The fact that iron stores can be elevated in bone marrow aspirates in AOI is helpful in differentiating this anemia from iron-deficiency anemia. Indeed, bone marrow iron stores are increased, yet red blood cell iron is decreased. Sideroblast (iron-laden nucleated RBC precursors) counts approach 0%. Normal range is at least 15 to 20% of all nucleated RBC precursors. This is in contrast to iron-deficiency anemia, in which both storage and sideroblast iron are markedly decreased or absent.

Serum ferritin levels are usually increased in AOI—another useful aid in differentiating it from iron-deficiency anemia (Table 15–4). Transferrin saturation generally falls between 5% and 16%. Free erythrocyte protoporphyrins are elevated because no iron is available to the red cell precursors for incorporation into the porphyrin ring. Thus the RBC cannot complete production of the heme moiety for production of the hemoglobin molecule.

Slight decreases can be seen in hematocrit (Hct), hemoglobin (Hgb), MCV, and MCHC, with a corresponding increase in RBC distribution width (RDW).[21] The anemia can become fully developed within 1 to 2 months after the onset of the illness or inflammatory stimulus and usually worsens if the underlying disease becomes aggravated or more severe.

Several other biochemical changes occur in patients with anemia of inflammation. Acute-phase reactants appear in the serum, including fibrinogen, C-reactive protein, amyloid A protein, ceruloplasmin, haptoglobin, and C3.[3] The increase in fibrinogen contributes to the accelerated erythrocyte sedimentation rate (ESR) seen in patients with infections and chronic inflammatory conditions. Some have called the persistent acute phase response of AOI a "chronic" acute phase response.[3] If vitamin B_{12}, folate, or iron deficiency also occurs during AOI (because of loss or decreased intake), it can change the parameters of the otherwise normocytic, normochromic anemia. Macrocytosis and megaloblastosis are present with vitamin B_{12}–folate deficiency, whereas microcytosis is seen in iron deficiency (see Chaps. 6 and 7). This is true in any subcategory of anemia associated with systemic disorders.

Treatment

The degree of anemia seen in patients with AOI correlates with the severity of the inflammatory disease. Severity of inflammation is usually measured by ESR

TABLE 15–4 **Comparison of AOI with Iron-Deficiency Anemia**			
	Normal	**AOI**	**IDA**
Serum iron (μg/dL)	50–150	↓	↓
TIBC (μg/dL)	300–360	↓	↑
Ferritin (μg/dL)	20–250	↑	↓
Transferrin saturation (%)	20–45	↓	↓
FEPs (μg/dL of RBCs)	15–80	↑	↑
RE marrow iron deposits	2–3+	↑	↓
Sideroblasts (%)	40–60	↓	↓
Reticulocytes (%)	0.5–2.0	↓	↓

Abbreviations: IDA = iron-deficiency anemia; FEPs = free erythrocyte protoporphyrins

and the presence of other acute-phase reactants. The anemia seen with inflammatory processes is generally mild and usually does not require intervention. When the underlying disorder is treated, the CBC (hemogram) results return to normal. If the inflammatory process is treated with long-term anti-inflammatory medications, acute-phase reactants decrease, Hgb levels increase, and Epo levels decrease to normal level.[10] When an inflammatory disorder becomes exacerbated, or remains severe for a long time, the anemia is more severe and may necessitate treatment.

Despite the low serum iron levels, there is not a true iron deficiency. Instead, it is a lack of iron availability. Treatment of this anemia with iron is ineffective and, in some cases, can actually be harmful. An excess of iron could increase the virulence of an infecting organism and exacerbate an underlying infection. Transfusion may be another possibility, depending on the Hgb and Hct levels in a given patient.[4] In patients with severe anemia and no sign of remission in their disease, this may be a viable alternative, but only after a proper evaluation of body iron stores—possibly including a bone marrow evaluation—has taken place.

In the past few years, recombinant human erythropoietin (rHuEpo) has offered a new treatment alternative. Clinical trials have indicated that rHuEpo may improve erythropoiesis in most patients with anemia of renal failure.[22] More recently, rHuEpo has been approved by the Food and Drug Administration (FDA) to treat the severe anemia in acquired immunodeficiency syndrome (AIDS) patients receiving azidothymidine (AZT) and in patients with rheumatoid arthritis.[23] Although AOI is not entirely caused by an Epo deficiency, high concentrations of this hormone were able to counteract the suppressive effects of IL-1.[4,24]

ANEMIA ASSOCIATED WITH INFECTION

Anemia is frequently seen with chronic infections. In essence, it is a subset of AOI. It is usually brought on by inflammatory mediators. It too is a sideropenic anemia, that is to say, a "functional" iron deficiency. It can develop gradually and will remain until the infection is

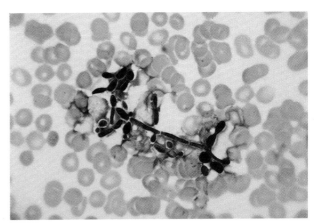

FIGURE 15-3 Candidemia, peripheral blood. *Candida albicans* is seen in the peripheral blood in hyphae, pseudohyphae, and yeast forms. Note that some of the organism has broken out of the cytoplasm of disintegrating monocytes, of which nuclear remnants are still visible.

successfully treated. Although most infections can now be treated effectively with antibiotic therapy, a number of chronic infections still remain that can produce anemia.

Bacterial, Fungal, and Viral Infection

In general, any bacterium or fungus that is capable of persisting for more than 2 weeks can cause anemia. Figures 15–2 through 15–5 are examples of AOI. The severity of the anemia correlates with the intensity of fever and thus the presence of inflammatory products (acute-phase reactants). Some examples of infections and causative agents giving rise to this form of anemia are listed in Table 15–5. All of these infections tend to be chronic and may result in weight loss and inflammation. Other lingering infections such as leprosy, typhoid fever, tularemia, brucellosis, and Lyme disease can also produce this type of anemia.[25]

Anemia may also result from infection with organisms and various induced processes such as hemorrhage caused by toxins and parasite invasion (see Figs. 14–9 and 14–10), virus-induced autoimmune hemo-

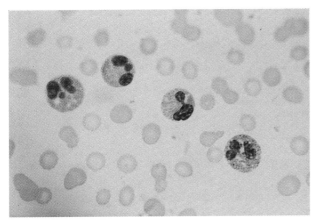

FIGURE 15-2 Anemia of infection (AOI). Peripheral blood of a patient with septicemia (bacterial infection in the blood). Note the increase in neutrophils with vacuolization and toxic granulation.

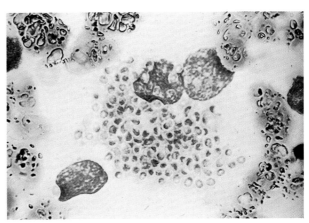

FIGURE 15-4 Histoplasma capsulatum (peripheral blood).

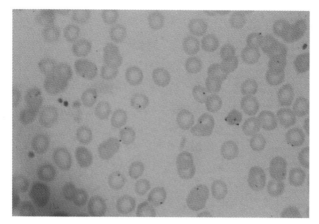

FIGURE 15–5   Malaria infection—plasmodium species (peripheral blood).

lytic anemias (see Chap. 14), and virus-induced aplastic anemias[26] (see Chap. 8).

Parvovirus B19 is an interesting virus in that it has specific tropism for erythroid precursors.[27] Infection with this parvovirus can cause bone marrow erythroid hypoplasia[28] and absolute reticulocytopenia[29]—in essence an RBC aplastic "crisis."[30,31]

Viral Infection: Human Immunodeficiency Virus Infection and the Acquired Immunodeficiency Syndrome

Viral infections are usually not associated with AOI and are caused by many different mechanisms. One notable exception is the anemia associated with human immunodeficiency virus (HIV) infection and AIDS. HIV infection is a devastating condition caused by direct destruction of CD4 T lymphocytes (helper-inducer cells) by HIV. By reducing the CD4 T-cell count, the HIV renders the host immunocompromised and susceptible to many opportunistic pathogens. Most HIV-infected patients may develop pancytopenia or one or more of the cytopenias during the course of the disease.[32]

Anemia develops early and becomes more severe as the disease progresses. Approximately 75% of patients with AIDS are anemic.[33] Anemia has been noted in preliminary findings of HIV-infected individuals before secondary infections ensue and medications are started.[32] Infections with *Mycobacterium avium, M. intracellulare,* herpes simplex virus, *Pneumocystis carinii,* and cytomegalovirus (CMV) contribute to the state of chronic infection and chronic inflammation.[33,34] The anemia associated with HIV infection can be worsened by a concurrent condition such as one or more opportunistic infections as HIV infection persists and progresses.

Pathophysiology and Characteristics

The hematologic picture seen in HIV-positive patients is a normocytic, hypoproliferative anemia with a decreased reticulocyte count. Bone marrow aspirates demonstrate dysplastic features,[32,34–36] an increase in marrow reticulin, and progressive aplasia. The direct infection of bone marrow cells has been implicated as the main pathogenic factor in the thrombocytopenia of HIV infection.[37,38] A direct effect on RBC precursors has also been postulated.[34] Decreased production of RBCs can be attributed to several possible mechanisms:

1. There is a suppression of erythropoiesis caused by an increase in cytokine production (similar to AOI).
2. Bone marrow histiocytes have been observed phagocytizing RBCs and white blood cells (WBCs).
3. HIV antibodies circulate through the bone marrow and destroy altered precursor RBCs.

TABLE 15–5 Examples of Chronic Bacterial and Fungal Infections That Commonly Cause Anemia	
Infection	**Common Causative Agents**
Chronic meningitis	*Mycobacterium tuberculosis, Cryptococcus neoformans, Coccidioides immitis*
Malignant otitis externa	*Pseudomonas aeruginosa*
Empyema	Anaerobic bacteria, *Staphylococcus aureus,* aerobic gram-negative bacilli
Cavitary pulmonary disease	*M. tuberculosis, Histoplasma capsulatum, Nocardia asteroides, Actinomyces israeli,* anaerobic bacteria, *Aspergillus niger, Blastomyces dermatitidis, Pseudomonas pseudomallei*
Endocarditis	Staphylococci and streptococci, *Candida albicans*
Intra-abdominal abscess (hepatic, splenic, renal, and so on)	Anaerobic bacteria, streptococci, aerobic gram-negative bacilli
Chronic peritonitis	*M. tuberculosis*
Chronic osteomyelitis	*Staphylococcus aureus,* anaerobic bacteria, aerobic gram-negative bacilli, *Blastomyces dermatitidis*
Chronic arthritis	*M. tuberculosis*

Source: From Strausbaugh, LJ: Hematologic Manifestations of Bacterial and Fungal Infections. In Bagby, GC (ed): Hematologic Aspects of Systemic Disease, Hematol Oncol Clin North Am, WB Saunders, Philadelphia, 1987

Because of the already documented effects of IL-1 and TNF-α on erythropoiesis, current theory suggests that the inflammatory process is predominantly responsible for the anemia associated with AIDS. The normocytic, normochromic anemia is thus similar to AOI but can be slightly more severe in degree. Indeed, AIDS patients demonstrate an RE system iron blockade[32] and iron studies similar to AOI.[35] For the most part, the anemia of HIV infection and AIDS is a subset of AOI.

Treatment

Treatment in HIV infection includes antibiotics (prophylactic or with infections), supportive care, and azidothymidine (AZT) therapy if applicable. Anemia in the HIV-positive patient can be exacerbated by the use of AZT. AZT inhibits HIV replication and has helped to prolong life in many AIDS patients. Anemia and granulocytopenia are the major adverse effects associated with AZT.[39] Patients with less advanced infection at the initiation of AZT are less likely to develop severe anemia and granulocytopenia.

AZT therapy can cause a macrocytosis that can somewhat change the features of the anemia of AIDS.[40] It does this because it is a deoxyribonucleotide synthesis inhibitor acting at a similar point in the deoxyribonucleic acid (DNA) synthetic pathway as would a vitamin B_{12} or folate deficiency. It has also been associated with a worsening of the RE system iron blockade seen in HIV infection and AIDS.[32] Just like in any AOI, when the hematologic picture changes, one should suspect complicating factors. In AZT treatment this means the emergence of macrocytosis in an otherwise normocytic, normochromic AOI.[40]

When AZT therapy is stopped, increases in Hct and reticulocyte counts are observed. To treat this severe anemia, AZT therapy often must be discontinued or its dosage reduced. Recently the FDA has approved the use of rHuEpo to treat severe anemia in patients with AIDS.[22,41,42] Recombinant erythropoietin may reduce or eliminate the need for red cell transfusions in AIDS patients receiving AZT therapy.

ANEMIA ASSOCIATED WITH CONNECTIVE TISSUE (COLLAGEN) DISORDERS

All of the chronic, systemic connective tissue (collagen) disorders have the ability to produce AOI because they are, by nature, inflammatory diseases. Indeed, the anemia of connective tissue disorders is a subset of AOI. Anemia is the most common hematologic abnormality seen in patients with rheumatoid arthritis (RA), systemic lupus erythematosus (SLE), mixed connective tissue disease (MCTD), scleroderma, dermatomyositis, and Sjögren's syndrome.[43] Figure 15–6 shows a lupus erythematosus (LE) cell from a patient with active SLE.

Etiology and Pathophysiology

As in all other types of AOI, there is a direct correlation among acute-phase reactants, disease severity, and the presence or absence of anemia.[44] Production of altered transferrin molecules has been demonstrated in RA with anemia.[45] This could lead to different affinity for iron in these altered transferrin molecules. Furthermore, some authors have reported decreased serum Epo levels in patients with RA,[46] as well as decreased marrow response to Epo.[47] This is in addition to suppression of marrow by cytokines, lactoferrin release, [48] and iron binding similar to AOI[47] and acute-phase reactant inhibition of transferrin iron uptake.[49] Indeed, there are many mechanisms that cause AOI in RA.[47] In SLE, serum inhibitors against myeloid and erythroid colony formation have been found.[50,51]

Other factors may complicate the picture of this anemia. Iron-deficiency anemia may develop from gastrointestinal blood loss from the ingestion of aspirin or other anti-inflammatory drugs. Gastrointestinal blood loss can occur as a consequence of ulcer disease, which may represent "stress ulcers" from disease activity or ulcers in response to medication administered for the primary disease.

Some collagen diseases (e.g., SLE, RA, and sclero-

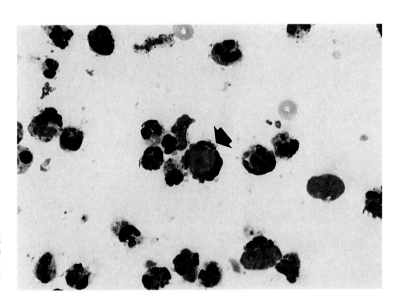

FIGURE 15–6 Pleural fluid from an individual with systemic lupus erythematosus (SLE). The predominant cell is a polymorphonuclear leukocyte (PMN). A PMN that has phagocytized nuclear material (LE cell) is seen (*arrow*).

derma) are also associated with the production of autoantibodies (see warm autoimmune hemolytic anemia in Chap. 14). This can lead to a spherocytic and microcytic anemia in addition to or as opposed to the normocytic anemia of AOI, which is typical of an otherwise uncomplicated collagen disorder.

Renal disease is yet another complication of certain disorders such as SLE. The development of chronic renal disease, superimposed on the AOI, can change the hematologic picture (see Anemia Associated with Renal Disease and Renal Failure).

Characteristics

These patients exhibit the laboratory features typical of AOI. The anemia is usually normocytic, normochromic, and mild, and its severity reflects the activity and severity of the primary disease process. The reticulocyte count is depressed or low. Bone marrow findings are nonspecific in regard to myeloid, erythroid, and megakaryocytic cell lines.[52] Plasmacytosis is commonly seen. This most likely represents a response to chronic antigen stimulation in the background of these chronic autoimmune disorders.[52]

Treatment

The AOI seen in collagen disorders is treated similarly to the other disorders in this category. If the underlying disease can be treated effectively to decrease the inflammatory process, the anemia should improve. Severe disease is associated with a more profound anemia. As stated earlier, the anemia, like other AOIs, is refractory to iron therapy.[4]

The use of rHuEpo has become an attractive alternative to transfusion to increase hematopoiesis in the anemic patient. Use has been seen in and approved for individuals with RA.[53,54]

ANEMIA ASSOCIATED WITH MALIGNANCY

Hematologic abnormalities are very common in patients with both hematologic and nonhematologic malignancies (Fig. 15–7). Their type and their presence or

TABLE 15–6 **Mechanisms of Anemia in Malignancy**
1. Direct Effects
Replacement of marrow by malignant cells
Primary hematologic malignancy
Ineffective erythroid production
Qualitative reduction in erythropoiesis
Metastatic marrow infiltration
Quantitative reduction in erythropoiesis
Replacement of marrow by fibrosis
Acute and chronic blood loss
2. Indirect Effects
"Anemia of malignant disease"
Anemia of associated organ failure (e.g., renal, hepatic)
Malnutrition and vitamin deficiency
Microangiopathic hemolytic anemia
Immune hemolytic anemia
3. Treatment-Associated Anemia
Immediate
Chemotherapy
Radiation therapy
Late
Secondary myelodysplasia or leukemia
Idiopathic
?Depleted marrow reserve
Microangiopathic hemolytic anemia (postmitomycin)

absence depend on a multitude of factors, including the type of cancer, the site or sites involved by the malignancy in the body, the patient's therapy protocol, and the extent of the primary disease's involvement of the hematopoietic tissues (bone marrow) (Table 15–6). Anemia is not an uncommon presenting symptom of an otherwise occult malignancy. It can be caused by decreased RBC production, increased red blood cell destruction, and the toxic effects of the treatment of the malignancy.

Etiology and Pathophysiology
Direct Effects

When the bone marrow is infiltrated by a malignant tumor (myelophthisis), it can lead to anemia (myelo-

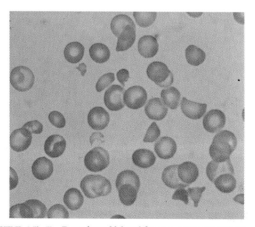

FIGURE 15–7 Peripheral blood from a patient with disseminated carcinoma. Note presence of schistocytes and helmet cells. (From Bell, A: Hematology. In Listen, Look and Learn. Health and Education Resources, Inc., Bethesda, MD, with permission.)

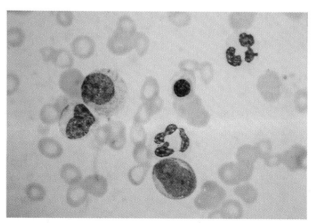

FIGURE 15–8 Leukoerythroblastosis, a peripheral blood picture that often accompanies marrow infiltration by tumors (myelophthisic anemia). Note the presence of immature red and white cells.

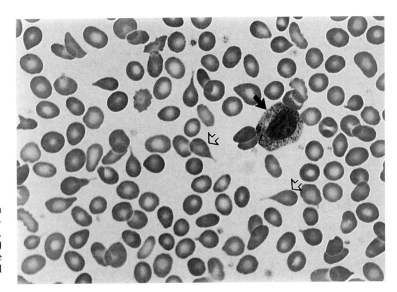

FIGURE 15–9 Peripheral blood smear from an individual with myelophthisic anemia. Note left-shifted granulocyte precursors (*solid arrow*). Teardrop-shaped red blood cells (*open arrows*) are indicative of marrow fibrosis in this type of leukoerythroblastic reaction. Nucleated red blood cell precursors were seen in other fields.

phthisic anemia). Leukoerythroblastosis (the presence of both immature WBC and RBC precursors) can frequently be seen on the peripheral blood smear (Fig. 15–8). Although leukoerythroblastosis can be seen in reactive and congenital conditions in approximately one-third of cases,[55] it is because of the myelophthisis in the balance of cases. Indeed, most individuals would reserve the term leukoerythroblastosis for the myelophthisic variant only. The term leukoerythroblastosis most often refers to marrow fibrosis.

Leukoerythroblastosis with "teardrop" RBCs is often a clue to marrow infiltration by the tumor and associated bone marrow fibrosis (Fig. 15–9) as opposed to a reactive process that usually demonstrates leukoerythroblastosis and normal RBC morphology (Fig. 15–10). Marrow fibrosis for any reason can lead to "teardrop" RBCs and leukoerythroblastosis. This includes metastatic tumor to the bone marrow. Marrow invasion can occur with solid tumors, particularly oat cell carcinoma; carcinoma of the lung; breast carcinoma; prostate cancer; and, in some instances, lymphoma.[56] Extensive marrow invasion can eventually lead to pan-

cytopenia. The anemia usually improves, but only if there is a response to treatment for the malignancy.

Blood loss can be another major cause of anemia in patients with malignancies. Chronic blood loss will result in a hypochromic anemia more consistent with iron-deficiency anemia. Renal cell carcinoma and transitional cell carcinoma are two tumors that produce significant blood loss through hematuria.[56] Metastatic mucin-producing tumors (e.g., adenocarcinoma of stomach and adenocarcinoma of the prostate) can be associated with chronic or acute disseminated intravascular coagulation (DIC), which can be associated with bleeding (blood loss) or nonimmune RBC hemolysis (see Chap. 29). Metastatic carcinoma with high cell "turnover" or death and significant release of tissue factor can lead to activation of the coagulation system, depletion of platelets and coagulation factors, and bleeding tendencies. Microangiopathic hemolytic anemia is one of the more common sources of the hemolytic anemia seen in widespread disseminated carcinoma. Again, this is a result of activation of the coagulation system. This leads to fibrin deposition in

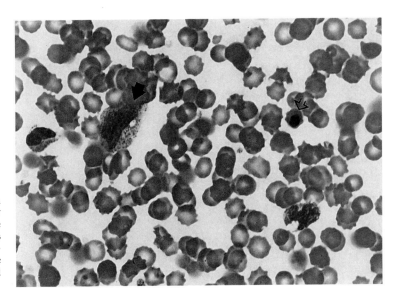

FIGURE 15–10 Peripheral blood smear from a neonate with leukoerythroblastosis caused by severe blood loss associated with birth (a reactive condition). Left-shifted granulocyte precursors (*solid arrow*) and nucleated red blood cell precursors (*open arrow*) are seen. Although some "burr" cells are seen, no teardrop-shaped red blood cells are identified.

small blood vessels causing mechanical "shear-induced" trauma to the red cells as they pass through the vessel (see Chap. 29). Schistocytes, fragmented cells, and helmet cells can be seen on the peripheral blood smear.

Indirect Effects

Malignant tumors elicit a chronic inflammatory response that is not related to necrosis or infection. The production and release of IL-1 and TNF-α by macrophages is responsible for the inflammatory process seen in malignancies. The consequence of the process is the alteration of normal red cell production, resulting in anemia. In other words, any malignant neoplasm that persists for more than a few weeks may result in the AOI.

The anemia seen in malignancies is similar to other AOIs in that there is a correlation between the degree of anemia and the extent of the underlying disease. Epo levels and response are blunted, and bone marrow is impaired in its response to endogenous Epo.[57,58] Severe anemia is usually seen in patients with metastatic cancer. The development of this type of anemia does not require or imply the invasion of the bone marrow by the tumor.

Treatment-Associated Anemia

Transient pancytopenia is expected in any patient undergoing aggressive treatment for hematologic or nonhematologic malignancies. Most combination chemotherapy protocols use one or more of the alkylating agents, which are directly toxic to rapidly dividing cells. When given frequently by intervals, alkylating agents can cause a dramatic decrease in the peripheral blood cell counts. Radiation therapy can also be toxic to bone marrow stem cells. The sequence of recovery in *bone marrow* is quite variable. Both erythroid and granulocytic regeneration usually precede megakaryocyte regeneration.[59] The half-life of red blood cells is considerably longer than the half-lives of the other two cell lines; therefore, red blood cell recovery in the peripheral blood lags behind white blood cell and platelet recovery. In addition, persistent anemia can result because of the *need for* and potential concurrent *deficiencies of* much-needed nutrients (e.g., folate, vitamin B_{12}).

Characteristics

The anemia of malignancy is usually a normocytic, normochromic, mild one. As stated above, many other processes can occur to change the severity or morphology of the anemia. The most important changes would be leukoerythroblastosis with "teardrop" RBCs indicating marrow fibrosis and a poor prognosis because of metastasis. Another change would be schistocytes indicating DIC and, most likely, widely disseminated carcinoma.

Treatment

In most cases, the anemia associated with malignancy is AOI. It is mild and requires little treatment.

ANEMIA ASSOCIATED WITH RENAL DISEASE AND RENAL FAILURE

Renal disease is associated with a wide variety of hematologic abnormalities. These include anemia, abnormal platelet function, abnormal WBC function[60] and coagulopathy. The latter two are usually due to the effects of uremia on platelet function and coagulation factor function. Anemia is a well-documented feature of acute and chronic renal failure.

Etiology and Pathophysiology

The major cause of the anemia of renal failure is decreased production of erythropoietin by damaged kidneys. The serum Epo level in patients with renal failure is usually in the same range as normal nonanemic patients. It can be slightly elevated, but the elevation is blunted when compared with the response in anemic, nonuremic patients.[61] Some renal diseases (renal cell carcinoma and polycystic kidney disease) are usually associated with erythrocytosis because of increased Epo production and release from the neoplastic or altered renal tissue. However, that is not always the case, as some patients may develop anemia (Table 15–7).

Inhibitory properties on erythropoiesis have been demonstrated in the plasma of patients with chronic renal failure, but identity of the inhibitor is unclear.[62]

Mild hemolysis and decreased red cell survival also contribute to this anemia. Hemolysis is in part caused by acquired defects in the erythrocyte membrane sodium-potassium ATPase and pentose phosphate shunt. The latter defect leaves the cell susceptible to oxidants (sulfonamides and dialysis tapwater) and can induce Heinz body (degraded Hgb) formation and hemolysis. Hypersplenism in patients on chronic hemodialysis also contributes to shortened red cell survival.

Coagulopathy develops in some patients with renal failure (see Chap. 29).

Iron-deficiency anemia may develop in patients with renal failure because of blood loss during dialysis. Oc-

---

TABLE 15–7 Mechanisms Involved in Anemia of Renal Disease

Hypoproliferative Anemia
↓ Erthropoietin - ↓ Erythroid committed precursors
Suppressive effects of uremic toxins on erythroid
 precursors
Folate deficiency (hemodialysis)

Hemolytic Anemia
Unfavorable chemical environment
Uremic toxins

Dilutional Anemia
Abnormal fluid retention

Blood Loss Anemia
Gastrointestinal bleeding
Blood drawn for laboratory tests
Hemodialysis
Chronic iron deficiency

Hypersplenism
Chronic renal dialysis associated splenomegaly

cult gastrointestinal blood loss from "stress" ulcers or uremic bleeding because of poor platelet function can also account for chronic iron loss.

Characteristics

In general, patients with renal failure are anemic primarily because of an inadequate quantity of circulating Epo and suppression of bone marrow response to the anemia. In most cases, the anemia is hypoproliferative, normocytic, and normochromic. Electrolyte disturbances as part of uremia can lead to the development of "burr" cells (Fig. 15–11). Renal failure patients with severe metabolic or electrolyte derangements (increasing creatinine and blood urea nitrogen [BUN] paralleling worsening disease) demonstrate these anomalies in peripheral blood smears of freshly drawn samples.

There is usually good compensation for the degree and severity of anemia. Other characteristics, including schistocytes and microcytes, can be seen because the anemia may evolve into other forms as a result of disease-related complications (e.g., DIC or iron loss because of chronic blood loss).

Treatment

Until the advent of rHuEpo there was no completely satisfactory treatment of the anemia associated with renal disease. Most patients treated with rHuEpo are able to become transfusion-independent.[63] Anemia and morbidity are reduced with rHuEpo therapy.[64–66] Major side effects have included iron deficiency (treated with iron supplements)[67–70] and an increase in blood pressure that can be treated with antihypertensive medications.[71]

Recombinant Epo has been used in dialysis and predialysis patients with renal disease with good efficacy.[72,73]

ANEMIA ASSOCIATED WITH LIVER DISEASE

A wide array of hematologic disorders is encountered in patients with liver disease. The morphology and degree of anemia, however, differ somewhat depending on the nature, acuity, or chronicity of the liver disease and on other associated effects (Table 15–8). Most cases of anemia associated with liver disease are seen in cases of chronic liver disease.

Etiology and Pathophysiology

In chronic liver disease, the anemia may appear marked but does not correlate with the degree of hepatocellular failure or severity of disease. Target cells and acanthocytes may be seen on the peripheral blood smear and are considered a consequence of the altered lipid production (Fig. 15–12) (see also Chap. 3). Macrocytosis can also be seen. Hemolytic anemia may occur with the presence of macrocytes and acanthocytes ("spur cells") because of the RBC membrane's rigidity or lack of permeability.[74]

A microcytic, hypochromic anemia may develop as a result of acute or, usually, chronic blood loss. Patients with liver disease or liver failure because of end-stage cirrhosis have decreased synthetic capacity for the production of coagulation factors—especially the vitamin K–dependent factors (see Chaps. 26 and 28). This may be a cause of chronic blood loss or severe bleeding associated with hemostatic challenges (i.e., surgery). Patients may also have hypersplenism. Hypersplenism is found in 15% to 20% of patients with cirrhosis and advanced liver disease.[75] This can be a cause of platelet sequestration leading to thrombocytopenia and chronic bleeding tendencies—especially gastrointestinal and mucosal surface bleeding. Hypersplenism can also lead to decreased red cell survival as abnormal RBCs are trapped in this major RE organ.

Characteristics

Macrocytosis can be seen in patients with cirrhosis, obstructive jaundice, and other types of liver disease. These macrocytes are round, slightly flattened RBCs with a slight increase in size and volume. The RBC MCV in liver disease is usually between 100 and 110

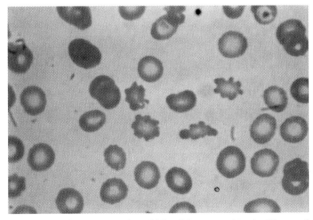

FIGURE 15–11 Peripheral blood from a patient with renal disease. Note the burr cells. (From Bell, A: Hematology. In Listen, Look and Learn. Health and Education Resources, Inc., Bethesda, MD, with permission.)

TABLE 15–8 **Mechanisms of Anemia in Liver Disease**
Direct Effects
Toxic effects of ethanol
Vacuolization of marrow hematopoietic precursor cells
Decreased marrow cellularity
Megaloblastic changes unassociated with folate deficiency
Acute and chronic blood loss
Gastrointestinal bleeding (alcoholism)
Liver disease—associated coagulopathies
Viral suppression of erythropoiesis
Indirect Effects
Dilutional anemia
Hypersplenism, erythrocyte sequestration
Hemolytic anemia
Spur-cell anemia (acanthocytosis)
RE macrophage activity
Malnutrition
Protein, folate, iron, and vitamin deficiencies
Anemia of inflammation

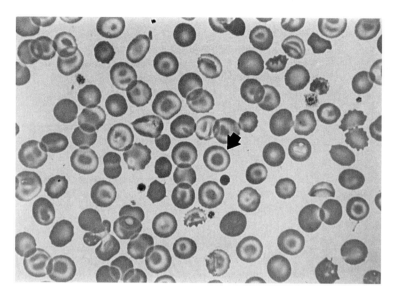

FIGURE 15-12 Peripheral blood smear from an individual with liver disease. Target cells (*solid arrow*) are caused by altered lipid metabolism with subsequent effects on red cell membrane.

femtoliters (fL). These macrocytes are not, however, the macro-ovalocytes seen in megaloblastic anemia (see Fig. 7–4, Chap. 7). Bone marrow examination shows macronormoblastic RBC precursors but *no* megaloblastic changes such as giant band forms, or hypersegmented neutrophils typical of a true megaloblastic anemia. The survival of these red cells is decreased owing to increased membrane lipids and lack of good deformability. This type of macrocytosis does not respond to vitamin B_{12} or folate therapy, and usually resolves only after improvement in liver function.

Megaloblastic macrocytes caused by folate deficiency may be seen in some patients with liver disease. This is caused by poor nutrition, usually as a result of chronic alcohol intake. Chronic alcohol intake is a significant cause of end-stage liver disease.

The anemia of chronic liver failure is often complicated by portal hypertension, hypersplenism, and increased plasma volume seen in splenomegaly. RBC mass is "pooled" in the venous system, sequestered in the spleen, or diluted in an increased plasma volume. These factors can yield a falsely decreased hematocrit, which may cause difficulty in evaluating the anemia. Therefore, anemia associated with chronic liver disease is initially considered normocytic, normochromic with variable RBC morphology and variable numbers of macrocytes, but it can be complicated by the simultaneous effects of iron deficiency (from blood loss) or folate deficiency (from poor dietary habits). Reticulocytosis is present depending upon the degree of anemia. Serum ferritin is increased reflecting a "chronic" acute-phase response. Decreased plasma iron may represent an element of AOI.

Treatment

Correction of dietary deficiencies (lack of iron or folate) can help the anemia. However, resolution of the liver disease corrects the macrocytosis, acanthocytosis, and anemia. In most instances, advanced liver dis-

ease and hypersplenism are present and irreversible. In these cases, dietary supplementation (iron, vitamin B_{12}, and folate) can be efficacious in preventing hematologic sequelae; however, bizarre red cell morphology and low-grade anemia may persist.

ANEMIA ASSOCIATED WITH ALCOHOLISM

One of the most common forms of liver disease is the result of chronic alcohol ingestion (Table 15-8). One of the widest arrays of hematologic abnormalities occurs in complications of acute and chronic alcoholism.

Etiology and Pathophysiology

Ethanol has direct toxic effects on precursor cells, marrow cellularity, and red cell morphology.[76–78] Vacuolization of erythroblasts in the bone marrow can be observed in alcoholic patients.[72–78] Heavy and prolonged alcohol abuse will also result in decreased bone marrow cellularity.[78] Alcohol and its metabolites are suppressants of hematopoietic–progenitor cell production.[76,78]

Macrocytosis is very common in chronic alcoholics and may not be caused by megaloblastic anemia.[79] In alcoholics who are not malnourished or have mild liver disease, there is still a macrocytosis that is not accompanied by any megaloblastic changes in the bone marrow or neutrophilic hypersegmentation in the peripheral blood. The mechanism of macrocytosis in alcoholism is unknown.[78]

Characteristics

The anemia associated with alcoholism is usually macrocytic. This change in cell size will remain until the patient stops consuming ethanol. The MCV remains elevated for 1 to 4 months afterward.[80] The ane-

TABLE 15–9 Endocrine Disorders/Diseases[81–83]

Endocrine Disorder/Disease	Type of Anemia	Pathogenesis (cause of)	Treatment
Pituitary dysfunction	N/N	Hypopituitarism	Exogenous replacement of thyroid hormone Androgens and/or estrogens Administration of corticosteroids
Adrenal insufficiency	N/N	Idiopathic (unknown cause)	Exogenous source of corticosteroids
Addison's disease		Destructive autoantibodies directed against parenchymal cells of the organs (autoimmune)	
Thyroid disease	N/N Mild macrocytic	Hyperthyroidism Hypothyroidism	Exogenous thyroid hormone
Hypogonadism	N/N	Defective internal secretion of the gonads	Androgens

N/N = Normocytic/normochromic

mia of liver disease may be present if advanced liver damage or disease is present.

Iron deficiency because of chronic blood loss (i.e., gastrointestinal bleeding such as bleeding from esophageal varices formed as a consequence of cirrhosis) or poor nutrition may also be present with folate deficiency, demonstrating a dimorphic blood picture on the peripheral blood smear. In this case, the MCV may be normal, but it will be a result of the average of two widely disparate "peaks" representing two populations of RBCs. Evaluation of the MCV histogram from an automated hematology instrument will demonstrate this fact. The RDW will be increased. This can also serve as a clue to the presence of these two nutritional deficiencies when they occur simultaneously.

"Spur cell" anemia because of acanthocytosis is mostly associated with severe alcoholic liver disease.[74] Spur cells have an increase in cholesterol, which decreases the deformability of the cell as it passes through the spleen.

Treatment

Treatment of the underlying liver disease is essential to the reversal of the anemia. Abstinence from alcohol will reverse the direct toxic effects on the bone marrow, and in a few months the MCV and RBC morphology should return to normal.

ANEMIA ASSOCIATED WITH ENDOCRINE DISEASE AND DISORDERS

The spectrum of endocrine diseases is wide, and their effect on metabolism is far-reaching and varied. Many hormones are involved in the regulation of hematopoiesis. Diseases of the pituitary, adrenal, thyroid glands, and gonads are most often involved in the development of anemia (Table 15–9).[81–83]

SUMMARY

The subject matter in this chapter is both wide and diverse. However, the anemias discussed in this chapter have a common theme. They are associated with systemic diseases. As a group, they are probably the most frequently encountered of the anemias. All of the diseases discussed can lead to an anemia that is secondary to or associated with the mechanisms causing the underlying disease state. Some of these disorders are linked by dysfunction or abnormalities in ferrokinetics and the mechanism of inflammation.

The anemia seen in these diseases is normochromic and normocytic. Other complicating factors can induce anisocytosis or poikilocytosis, which changes the characteristics of the RBC and the anemia.

These anemias are treated differently from other forms of anemia. The primary disease state deserves the most attention because it is the correction of this state that usually allows for the correction of the anemia. It should be noted that not every systemic disease demonstrates anemia.

This chapter discusses the characteristic features of the anemias associated with many systemic, nonhematologic disorders. Anemia may be the first sign of a previously undetected systemic disease. Changing RBC parameters may indicate new, complicating factors in an otherwise stable anemia associated with a systemic disease.

These are anemias with which the healthcare worker should be familiar due to their frequency in all patient groups seeking medical care.

CASE STUDY 1

A 22-year-old woman was admitted from the emergency department for tests. She had fever, dysuria, and lower back pain. Immediate laboratory results revealed the following.

Urinalysis	CBC
4+ urine protein	WBC: 11.8×10^9/L
1+ hemoglobin	RBC: 2.9×10^{12}/L
Many bacteria	Hgb: 8.3 g/dL
Moderate blood	Hct: 25%
Moderate WBCs	MCV: 88 fL
Casts: Few hyaline, few	MCH: 29 pg
granular	MCHC: 300 g/L or 30%
Chemistry:	RDW: 14.7%
BUN: 113 mg/dL	1+ aniso
Creatinine: 7.7 mg/dL	1+ poik
	1+ crenated RBCs

Blood cultures were drawn and eventually produced coagulase-negative *Staphylococcus*. Blood was still present in her urine after 2 days, and bleeding was noted from intravenous infusion sites. Coagulation tests were ordered before the patient was to go to surgery for kidney biopsy.

Platelet count: 296×10^9/L
PT: 11.7 s (control: 10.0–12.9 s)
APTT: 32 s (control: 23–35 s)
Bleeding time: >20 s
FDP: >40 μg/mL

APTT is activated partial thromboplastin time; FDP means fibrin/fibrinogen degradation products.

This patient was suffering from bacterial sepsis and renal failure. The admitting CBC demonstrated a mild anemia with some created red cell morphology typical of renal disease. The patient had received several units of packed red cells with no noticeable difference in her hematocrit. The anemia could be the product of several mechanisms. First, there was blood loss from her abnormal platelets (see Chap. 26) and from the DIC that she later developed. Her presenting anemia was most likely a result of the anemia of inflammation. Chronic and acute infections can produce this form of anemia. The anemia of renal disease was also present in this patient and was seen in conjunction with other causes of anemia.

Questions

1. Classify the anemia with regard to RBC indices.
2. Explain the significance of the RDW value in this case.
3. List the laboratory parameters in this case that coincide with anemia associated with renal disease.
4. What is the major cause of renal failure associated with anemia?
5. Why would chronic iron loss be a concern in this patient?

CASE STUDY 2

A 42-year-old woman presented to her physician with pain in both of her wrists and in the proximal joints in both of her hands. She had also recently begun experiencing right knee pain. Her laboratory results revealed the following:

WBC: 10.0×10^9/L
Hgb: 8.5 g/dL
Hct: 25%
MCV: 90 fL
RDW: 12.5% (normal 11–14%)
Erythrocyte sedimentation rate (ESR): 100 mm/h (normal 0–10 mm/h)
Rheumatoid Factor: Positive

Questions

1. What is the patient's diagnosis?
2. Give a reason for the increase in erythrocyte sedimentation rate (ESR).
3. Why was she anemic?

The patient's physician placed her on enteric-coated aspirin to protect her gastric lining for 3 months. She then reported no pain in her joints, wrists, or hands. Her ESR remained at 10 mm/h and her Hgb remained at 8.5 g/dL. Her physician decided to continue her on enteric-coated aspirin, since she had completed her course of iron supplements. She still reported feeling tired. Her physician also decided to start her on erythropoietin (rHuEpo) in an attempt to correct the anemia. After 4 weeks of rHuEpo therapy, the patient's Hgb was 12.8 g/dL and the hematocrit was 38%.

Her laboratory values were:
WBC: 10.0×10^9/L
Hgb: 12.8 g/dL
Hct: 0.38 L/L (or 38%)
MCV: 90 fL
RDW: 12.5 (normal, 11–14)

CASE STUDY 3

A 29-year-old woman with cholecystitis (inflammation of the gallbladder) was taken to elective surgery, where she underwent a cholecystectomy. Her preoperative laboratory values revealed:
WBC: 10.0×10^9/L
Hgb: 1.25 g/dL
Hct: 38%
Plt: 150×10^9/L

She was transported to the recovery room where, over 2 hours, her blood pressure was noted to be unstable. She was also noted to have a distended, tender abdomen. Laboratory tests revealed:
WBC: 10.0×10^9/L
Hgb: 1.24 g/dL
Hct: 38%
Plt: 150×10^9/L

She was given 3 to 4 L of 0.9% saline, which stabilized her blood pressure enough to allow her to be transferred back to surgery. Laboratory tests revealed:
WBC: 6.0×10^9/L
Hgb: 7.5 g/dL
Hct: 20%
Plt: 100×10^9/L

The evening shift medical technologist noted a significant change in the patient's hemoglobin level over the course of 1 to 2 hours in the recovery room by the use of a delta check (i.e, a significant change in laboratory value). The technologist called the recovery room to report the now lower value and to ask about proper specimen collection. The call was transferred to the operating room, where the patient was now undergoing an emergency laparotomy. The technologist reported the value to the physician (surgeon), who explained that the patient's abdomen was now full of blood (approximately 2 L) because of a damaged artery that was not "tied off" during surgery. The surgeon had just sutured the artery and was closing the abdominal wound after evacuating and suctioning the blood from the cavity.

Questions

1. Why was the patient's hemoglobin level normal when she had a distended abdomen full of blood?
2. What caused the hemoglobin value to decrease?
3. What other tests would be abnormal in this patient?

References

1. Krantz, SB: Pathogenesis and treatment of the anemia of chronic disease. Am J Med Sci 307:353, 1994.
2. Schilling, RF: Anemia of chronic disease: A misnomer (editorial). Ann Intern Med 115:572, 1991.
3. Kushner, I: Letter to the Editor. Ann Intern Med 116:521, 1992.
4. Damon, LE: Anemias of chronic disease in the aged: Diagnosis and treatment. Geriatrics 47:47, 1992.
5. Cartwright, GE: The anemia of chronic disorders. Semin Hematol 3:351, 1966.
6. Cartwright, GE and Lee, GR: The anemia of chronic disorders. Br J Haematol 21:147, 1971.
7. Denz, H, Fuchs, D, and Wachter, H: Altered iron metabolism and the anemia of chronic disease: A role of immune activation. (letter to the editor) Blood 79:2797, 1992.
8. Hlet, G, Cook, JD, and Finch, CA: Storage iron kinetics. VII. A biologic model for reticuloendothelial iron transport. J Clin Invest 53:1527, 1974.
9. Kurnick, MJE, Ward, HP, and Pickett, JC: Mechanism of the anemia of chronic disorders. Correlation of hematocrit value with albumin, vitamin B_{12}, transferrin and iron stores. Arch Intern Med 130:323, 1972.
10. Birgegard, G, Hallgren, R, and Caro, J: Serum erythropoietin in rheumatoid arthritis and other inflammatory arthritides: Relationship to anaemia and the effect of anti-inflammatory treatment. Br J Haematol 65:479, 1987.
11. Baer, AN, et al: Blunted erythropoietin response to anaemia in rheuamtoid arthritis. Br J Haematol 66:559, 1987.
12. Hochberg, MC, et al: Serum immunoreactive erythropoietin in rheumatoid arthritis: Impaired response to anemia. Arthritis Rheum 31;1318, 1988.
13. Ward HP, Mirnick, JE, and Pisarczyk, MJ: Serum levels of erythropoietin in anemias associated with chronic infection, malignancy, and primary hematopoietic disease. J Clin Invest 50:332, 1971.
14. Pavlovic-Kentera, V, et al: Erythropoietin in patients with anaemia in rheumatoid arthritis. Scand J Haematol 23:141, 1979.
15. Greendyke, RM, Sharma, K, and Gifford, FR: Serum levels of erythropoietin and selected other cytokines in patients with anemia of chronic disease. Am J Clin Pathol 101:338, 1994.
16. Means, RT and Krantz, SB: Progress in understanding the pathogenesis of the anemia of chronic disease. Blood 80:1639, 1992.
17. Dainiak, N, et al: Humoral suppression of erythropoiesis in systemic lupus erythematosus (SLE) and rheumatoid arthritis (RA). Am J Med 69:537, 1980.
18. Prouse, PJ, et al: Anaemia in juvenile chronic arthritis: Serum inhibition of normal erythropoiesis in vitro. Ann Rheum Dis 46:127, 1987.
19. Roodman, GD: Mechanisms of erythroid suppression in the anemia of chronic disease. Blood Cells 13:171, 1987.
20. Degliantoni, G, et al: Natural killer (NK) cell-derived hematopoietic colony-inhibiting activity and NK cytotoxic factor. Relationship with tumor necrosis factor and synergism with immune interferon. J Exp Med 162:1512, 1985.
21. Baynes, RD, et al: Hematologic and iron-related measurements in rheumatoid arthritis. Am J Clin Pathol 87:196, 1987.
22. Winnearls, CG: Treatment of anaemia in haemodialysis patients with recombinant erythropoietin. Nephron (suppl 1)51:26, 1989.
23. Zanjani, ED and Ascensao, JL: Erythropoietin. Transfusion 29:46, 1989.
24. Means RI, et al: Treatment of the anemia of rheumatoid arthritis with recombinant human erythropoietin: Clinical and in vitro studies. Arthritis Rheum 32:638, 1989.
25. Strausbaugh, LJ: Hematologic abnormalities in patients with bacterial and fungal infection. In Bagby, GC (ed): Hematologic Aspects of Systemic Disease. Hematol Oncol Clin North Am 1:186, 1987.
26. Sandberg, T, Lindquist, O, and Norkrans, G: Fatal aplastic anaemia associated with non-A, non-B hepatitis. Scand J Infect Dis 16:403, 1984.
27. Luban, NLC: Human parvoviruses: Implications for transfusion medicine. Transfusion 34:821, 1994.
28. Pattison, JR, et al: Parvovirus infections and hypoplastic crisis in sickle-cell anaemia. Lancet 1:664, 1981.
29. Kelleher, JF, et al: Human serum "parvovirus": A specific cause of aplastic crisis in children with hereditary spherocytosis. J Pediatr 102:720, 1983.
30. Mortimer, PP: Hypothesis: the aplastic crisis of hereditary spherocytosis is due to a single transmissible agent. J Clin Pathol 36:445, 1983.
31. Serjeant, GR, et al: Outbreak of aplastic crises with sickle cell anemia associated with parvovirus-like agent. Lancet 2:595, 1981.
32. Harris, CE, et al: Peripheral blood and bone marrow findings in patients with acquired immune deficiency syndrome. Pathology 22:206, 1990.
33. Spivak, JL, et al: Hematologic abnormalities in the acquired immune deficiency syndrome. Am J Med 77:224, 1984.
34. Kaloutsi, V, et al: Comparison of bone marrow and hematologic findings in patients with human immunodeficiency virus infection and those with myelodysplastic syndromes and infectious diseases. Am J Clin Pathol 101:123, 1994.
35. Castella, A, et al: The bone marrow in AIDS: A histologic, hematologic, and microbiologic study. Am J Clin Pathol 84:425, 1985.
36. Schneider, DR and Picker, LJ: Myelodysplasia in the acquired immune deficiency syndrome. Am J Clin Pathol 84:144, 1985.
37. Oksenhendler, E and Seligman, M: HIV-related thrombocytopenia. Immunodef Rev 2:221, 1990.
38. Glassman, AB: Thrombocytopenia: proposed mechanisms and treatment in human immunodeficiency virus infection. Ann Clin Lab Sci 19:319, 1989.
39. Fischl, MA, et al: Prolonged Zidovudine therapy in pa-

tients with AIDS and advanced AIDS-related complex. JAMA 262:2405, 1989.

40. Scates, S and Glaspy, J: The macrocytic anemias. Lab Med 21:736, 1990.

41. Glaspy, JA and Chap, L: The clinical application of recombinant erythropoietin in the HIV-infected patient. In Spivak, JL (ed): Hematol Oncol Clin North Am 8:945, 1994.

42. Phair, JP, et al: Recombinant human erythropoietin treatment: Investigational new drug protocol for the anemia of the acquired immunodeficiency syndrome. Overall results. Arch Intern Med 153:2669, 1993.

43. Richert-Boe, KE: Hematologic complications of rheumatic disease. In Bagby, GC (ed): Hematologic Aspects of Systemic Disease. Hematol Oncol Clin North Am 1:301, 1987.

44. Vreugdenhil, G, et al: Tumor necrosis factor alpha is associated with disease activity and the degree of anemia in patients with rheumatoid arthritis. Eur J Clin Invest 22:488, 1992.

45. Feelders, RA, et al: Transferrin microheterogeneity in rheumatoid arthritis. Relation with disease activity and anemia of chronic disease. Rheumatol Int 12:195, 1992.

46. Remacha, AF, et al: Erythroid abnormalities in rheumatoid arthritis: The role of erythropoietin. J Rheumatol 19:1687, 1992.

47. Baer, AN, Dessypris, EN, and Krantz, SB: The pathogenesis of anemia in rheumatoid arthritis: A clinical and laboratory analysis. Semin Arthritis Rheum 19:209, 1990.

48. Van Snick, JL, Masson, PL, and Heremans, JF: The involvement of lactoferrin in the hyposideremia of acute inflammation. J Exp Med 140:1068, 1974.

49. Graziadei, I, et al: The acute-phase protein alpha 1-antitrypsin inhibits growth and proliferation of human early erythroid progenitor cells (burst-forming units-erythroid) and of human erythroleukemic cells (K562) in vitro by interfering with transferrin iron uptake. Blood 83:260, 1994.

50. Fitchen, JJ, et al: Serum inhibitors of hematopoiesis in a patient with aplastic anemia and systemic lupus erythematosus: Recovery after exchange plasmapheresis. Am J Med 66:537, 1979.

51. Lam, SK and Quah, TC: Anemia in systemic lupus erythematosus. J Singapore Paediatr Soc 32:132, 1990.

52. Rosenthal, NS and Farhi, DC: Bone marrow findings in connective tissue disease. Am J Clin Pathol 92:650, 1989.

53. Pincus, T, et al: Multicenter study of recombinant human erythropoietin in correction of anemia in rheumatoid arthritis. Am J Med 89:161, 1990.

54. Salvarani, C, et al: Recombinant human erythropoietin therapy in patients with rheumatoid arthritis with the anemia of chronic disease. J Rheumatol 18:1168, 1991.

55. Weick, JK, Hagedorn, AB, and Linman, JW: Leukoerythroblastosis: Diagnostic and prognostic significance. Mayo Clin Proc 49:110, 1974.

56. Dutcher, JP: Hematologic abnormalities in patients with nonhematologic malignancies. In Bagby, GC (ed): Hematologic Aspects of Systemic Disease. Hematol Oncol Clin North Am 1:281, 1987.

57. Dowieko, JP and Goldberg, MA: Erythropoietin therapy in cancer patients. Oncology 5:31, 1991.

58. Spivak, JL: Cancer-related anemia: Its causes and characteristics. Semin Oncol 21:3, 1994.

59. Foucar, K: Effects of therapy, transplantation and detection of minimal residual disease. In Foucar, K: Bone Marrow Pathology. American Society of Clinical Pathologist Press, Chicago, 1995.

60. Zachee, P, Vermylen, J, and Boogaerts, MA: Hematologic aspects of end-stage renal failure. Ann Hematol 69:33, 1994.

61. Eschbach, JW and Adamson, JW: Anemia of end-stage renal disease (ESRD). Kidney Int 28:1, 1985.

62. Hocking, WG: Hematologic abnormalities in patients with renal diseases. In Bagby, GC (ed): Hematologic Aspects of Systemic Disease. Hematol Oncol Clin North Am 1:231, 1987.

63. Horl, WH: Erythropoietin and renal anemia. Biotechnology Therapeutics 2:213, 1991.

64. Navarro, M, et al: Anemia of chronic renal failure: treatment with erythropoietin. Child Nephrol Urol 11:146, 1991.

65. Watson, AJ, et al: Treatment of the anemia of chronic renal failure with subcutaneous recombinant human erythropoietin. Am J Med 89:432, 1990.

66. Eschbach, JW, et al: Correction of the anemia of end-stage renal disease with recombinant human erythropoietin: Results of a combined phase I and phase II clinical trial. N Engl J Med 316:73, 1987.

67. Sanders, HN, et al: Nutritional implications of recombinant human erythropoietin therapy in renal disease. J Am Diabet Assoc 94:1023, 1994.

68. Cermak, J: Iron stores in patients with chronic kidney failure treated with recombinant human erythropoietin. Vnitrni Lekarstvi (Czech) 40:174, 1994.

69. York, S: Current perspectives: iron management during therapy with recombinant human erythropoietin. Ann J 20:645, 1993.

70. Humphries, OE: Anemia of renal failure. Use of erythropoietin. In Wheby, MS (ed): Anemia. Med Clin North Am 76:711, 1992.

71. Johnson, CA and Chester, MI: Pathophysiology and treatment of the anemia of renal failure. Clin Pharm 7:117, 1988.

72. Macdougall, IC: Treatment of renal anemia with recombinant human erythropoietin. Curr Opin Nephrol Hypertension 1:210, 1992.

73. Kulzer, P, et al: Effectiveness and safety of recombinant human erythropoietin (r-HuEPO) in the treatment of anemia of chronic renal failure in non dialysis patients. European Multicentre Study Group. Int J Artif Organs 17:195, 1994.

74. Cooper, RA: Hemolytic syndromes and red cell membrane abnormalities in liver disease. Semin Hematol 17:103, 1980.

75. Klipstein, FA and Lindenbaum, J: Folate deficiency in chronic liver disease. Blood 25:443, 1965.

76. Meagher, RC, Sieber, F, and Spivak, JL: Suppression of hematopoietic-progenitor-cell proliferation by ethanol and acetaldehyde. N Engl J Med 307:845, 1982.

77. McCurdy, PR and Rath CE: Vacuolated nucleated bone marrow cells in alcoholism. Semin Hematol 17:100, 1980.

78. Chanarin, I: Haemopoiesis and alcohol. Br Med Bull 38:81, 1982.

79. Seppa, K, Laippala, P, and Saarni, M: Macrocytosis as a consequence of alcohol abuse among patients in general practice. Alcoholism 15:871, 1991.

80. Lindenbaum, J: Hematologic complications of alcohol abuse. Semin Liver Dis 7:169, 1987.

81. DeLellis, RA: Chapter 25. The Endocrine System. In Cotran, RS, Kumar, V, and Robbins, SL (eds): Robbins Pathologic Basis of Disease, ed 5. WB Saunders, Philadelphia, 1994, pp 1113–1171.

82. Colon-Otero, G, Menke, D, and Hook, CC: A practical approach to the differential diagnosis and evaluation of the adult patient with macrocytic anemia. Med Clin North Am 76:581, 1992.

83. Nomura, S, et al: Case report: Hypothyroidism as a possible cause of an acquired reversible hemolytic anemia. Am J Med Sci 302:23, 1991.

BIBLIOGRAPHY

Chisholm, M: Haematologic disorders in liver disease. In Wright, R, et al: Liver and Biliary Disease, Pathophysiology, Diagnosis, Management. WB Saunders, Philadelphia, 1985, p 189.

Erslev, AJ: Anemia of Endocrine Disorders. In Williams, WJ (ed): Hematology, ed 3. McGraw-Hill, New York, 1983, p 425.

Fantone, JC and Ward, PA: Mechanisms of Inflammation. In Cohen, AS and Bennett, JC (eds): Rhematology and Immunology, ed 2. Harcourt Brace Jovanovich, New York, 1986, p 403.

Jandl, JH: Blood. Little, Brown, Boston, 1987.

Luksenburg, H: Anemia associated with other disorders: Infection, renal disease, liver disease, endocrine disease, connective tissue disease, and malignancies. In Pittiglio, DH and Sacher, RA (eds): Clinical Hematology and Fundamentals of Hemostasis. FA Davis, Philadelphia, 1987, p 172.

Rapaport, SI: Introduction to Hematology. JB Lippincott, Philadelphia, 1987.

Savage, D and Lindenbaum, J: Anemia in alcoholics. Medicine 65:322, 1986.

Smith, HR and Chess, L: Cellular Basis of the immune response. In Cohen, AS and Bennett, JC (eds): Rheumatology and Immunology, ed 2. Harcourt Brace Jovanovich, New York, 1986, p 396.

Wiggins, RC, Fantone, J, Phan, SH: Mechanisms of Vascular Injury. In Tisher, CC and Brenner, BM (eds): Renal Pathology with Clinical and Functional Correlations. JB Lippincott, Philadelphia, 1989, p 975.

ACKNOWLEDGMENTS

The authors thank R. Sosolik, MD, for excellent photography in the preparation of the figures for this chapter and Penelope Martin for secretarial assistance.

QUESTIONS

1. Which of the following lists of laboratory findings would be most characteristic of the anemia of inflammation?
   a. Normocytic, hypochromic red blood cell; high serum iron level; increased TIBC; decreased ferritin levels; decreases in hemoglobin and hematocrit.
   b. Normocytic, normochromic red blood cell; low serum iron level; decreased TIBC; increased ferritin levels; decreases in hemoglobin and hematocrit.
   c. Microcytic, hypochromic red blood cell; normal serum iron level; decreased TIBC; normal ferritin levels; decreases in hemoglobin and hematocrit.
   d. Macrocytic, normochromic red blood cell; low serum iron level; decreased TIBC; decreased ferritin levels; decreases in hemoglobin and hematocrit.

2. Which of the following are causes for the anemia of inflammation?
   a. Increased destruction of red blood cells
   b. Impaired iron metabolism
   c. Suppression of erythropoiesis by cytokines
   d. All of the above

3. What are the main immune processes responsible for reducing hematopoiesis and inducing nutritional immunity?
   a. Cytokines from macrophages and lymphokines
   b. Antibodies from B lymphocytes
   c. Erythropoietin from kidney
   d. Hepatocellular factors from liver

4. What is the treatment for anemia of inflammation?
   a. Blood transfusion
   b. Iron therapy
   c. Treatment of the inflammation
   d. Human recombinant IL-1

5. Which are causes of anemia not associated with inflammation?
   a. Malignancy and neoplastic processes
   b. Connective tissue disorders
   c. Bacterial and fungal infections
   d. Endocrine, kidney, and liver disease

6. Leukoerythroblastosis with teardrop-shaped red blood cells is indicative of:
   a. Bone marrow fibrosis
   b. Bone marrow stress
   c. Abnormal lipid metabolism
   d. Renal disease

7. Macrocytosis in liver disease is caused by all of the following except:
   a. Abnormal lipid metabolism
   b. Direct effects of alcohol
   c. Iron deficiency
   d. Vitamin B_{12} and folate deficiency

8. What are the typical hematologic findings associated with anemia from endocrine dysfunction?
   a. Mild normocytic, normochromic anemia
   b. Anemia, abnormal platelets, and coagulopathy
   c. Target cells, macrocytes, and acanthocytes
   d. Marked anisocytosis and poikilocytosis, and dysfunctional leukocytes

9. What is the primary cause of anemia associated with renal disorders and renal failure?
   a. Blood loss from dialysis
   b. Decreased erythropoietin production
   c. Hemolytic processes
   d. Vitamin B_{12} and folate deficiencies

10. What is the typical appearance of anemia associated with liver disease?
    a. Normal red blood cell morphology
    b. Hypochromic, microcytic
    c. Macrocytic, normoblastic
    d. Macrocytic, megaloblastic

Answers:

1. **b** (p 248)
2. **d** (pp 245–248)
3. **a** (p 247)
4. **c** (pp 248–249)
5. **d** (pp 254–257)
6. **a** (p 254)
7. **c** (p 256)
8. **a** (p 257) (Table 15–9)
9. **b** (p 255)
10. **c** (pp 255–256)

Part III

WHITE BLOOD
CELL DISORDERS

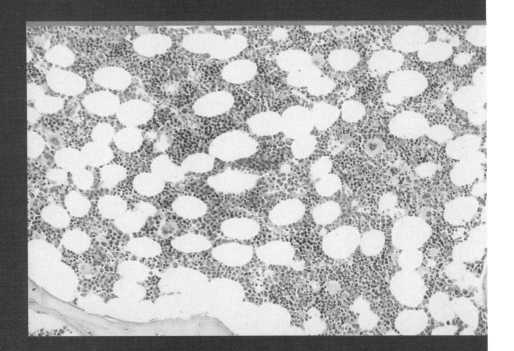

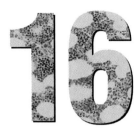

16

Cell Biology and Disorders of Neutrophils

Deirdre E. DeSantis, MS, MT(ASCP)SBB
Ronald G. Strauss, MD

Objectives

At the end of this chapter, the learner should be able to:
1. Identify the enzymatic contents of primary, secondary, and tertiary granules.
2. Characterize the changes in neutrophil count and morphology that develop in response to infections.
3. Define the three modes of neutrophilic migration.
4. Describe the changes in migration pattern that occur in a neutrophil as a result of chemoattractant stimulation.
5. Characterize the sequence of events that occur during phagocytosis.
6. Briefly discuss the biochemical pathway for the respiratory burst and active oxidative agents.
7. Briefly describe the organisms most commonly implicated causing infections in neutropenic patients.
8. Describe the classic clinical features of Chédiak-Higashi syndrome and the associated changes in neutrophil morphology.
9. Describe the inheritance of and molecular basis for chronic granulomatous disease.
10. Compare and contrast three white cell anomalies in regard to morphology.

CELL BIOLOGY OF NEUTROPHILS

Three major types of white blood cells (leukocytes) are noted in peripheral blood: lymphocytes, monocytes, and granulocytes. The function of all three white cell types is integral to host defense. Although the role of each type of white cell is quite different, all three function interdependently to maintain balance in the immune system. The lymphocytes may be subdivided into three broad categories designated as T, B, and null lymphocytes. Lymphocytes interact with phagocytes and antigen-presenting cells to regulate and mediate antibody production. Monocytes are phagocytes that enter tissues and differentiate into a variety of macrophages; they also serve as antigen-presenting cells. Granulocytes may be divided into three subsets (neutrophils, eosinophils, and basophils), based on morphology by light and electron microscopy, on the staining characteristics, and on contents of cytoplasmic granules. Neutrophils are the most numerous leukocytes found in peripheral blood, accounting for 50% to 70% of all circulating white blood cells in the adult. Like monocytes, neutrophils function as phagocytes that are capable of ameboid movement into the tissues

265

to engulf and destroy bacteria or fungus; they are the first phagocytic cells to mobilize at a site of infection. Neutrophils also play a role in mediating inflammatory processes. This chapter will focus exclusively on the neutrophil.

Production, Circulating Kinetics, and Morphology

All hematopoietic cells arise from a common, self-sustaining pool of pluripotent stem cells in the bone marrow. The pluripotent stem cells give rise to multipotential stem cells that become committed to differentiate into one of the following major cell lines: granulocyte-monocyte, erythrocyte, megakaryocyte, or lymphocyte. Human hematopoietic factors modulate the clonal expansion, differentiation, and maturation of stem cells, and regulate the activity of mature cells.[1-3] Alternately referred to as colony-stimulating factors (CSFs), these glycoproteins stimulate a specific cell line or a combination of cell lines (see Chap. 1). In particular, granulocyte–colony-stimulating factor (G-CSF) and granulocyte-macrophage–colony-stimulating factor (GM-CSF) target the expansion and maturation of cells committed to the neutrophil lineage. Granulocyte-CSF has also been described to enhance the microbial activity required for efficient phagocytosis in mature neutrophils. Other factors, such as interleukin-3, interact synergistically with CSFs to influence the production and function of neutrophils and monocytes; however, the interrelationship is incompletely defined.[4-8]

Myelopoiesis is the proliferation and maturation of the neutrophil cell line. Once committed to the neutrophil (or myelocyte) cell line, the precursors progress in an orderly sequence through five stages of development that include the myeloblast, promyelocyte, myelocyte, metamyelocyte, and band. The early stages (myeloblast, promyelocyte, and myelocyte) are marked by proliferation, whereas the later nondividing stages (metamyelocyte, band, and mature polymorphonuclear neutrophil) are noted for maturation and storage in a compartment of the bone marrow referred to as the marrow reserve. See Figure 1–17, which represents the proliferation and maturation stages of the neutrophil. Nondividing myeloid cells mature in and are stored by the bone marrow reserve in adults and by the liver and spleen of neonates until their release into the peripheral blood.[7] As the neutrophils mature, the cell size decreases while cell mobility and deformability increase.[7,9]

Mature neutrophils (or polymorphonuclear leukocytes) are easily recognized on blood smears prepared with Wright's stain by their dense multilobed nucleus and pink to tan cytoplasm that is peppered with pink and purple granules. Two types of cytoplasmic granules, primary (azurophilic or nonspecific) and secondary (specific), are present in the mature neutrophil, although only the secondary granules are visible with light microscopy. Most recently, a third type of granule (tertiary) has been identified using electron microscopy.[7,8] The contents of the primary, secondary, and tertiary granules are enzymes, most of which are involved in the killing and digestion of bacteria and fungi (Table 16–1).

TABLE 16–1 **Abridged Listing of the Contents of Neutrophil Granules**
• Primary granules
○ Lysozyme
○ Myeloperoxidase
○ Acid phosphatase
○ Elastase
○ Defensins
○ Cathepsin G
• Secondary granules
○ Lysozyme
○ Collagenase
○ Lactoferrin
○ B_{12}-binding protein
○ NADPH oxidase
○ Cytochrome b
• Tertiary granules
○ Plasminogen activator
○ Alkaline phosphatase
○ Gelatinase

Neutrophils are among the most mobile cell lines in humans.[9] Once in the bloodstream, mature neutrophils are equally divided into marginating and circulating pools, between which there is a constant exchange of cells.[7,8,10] The marginating pool consists of cells adhering to vessel endothelium within the vascular spaces. Marginating cells are described as rolling along vessel endothelium in search of an area of injury or inflammation where, by diapedesis, they enter the tissues for action.[7,8] Neutrophils in the circulating pool leave the blood in a random fashion after a half-life of approximately 7 hours and do not return to the bloodstream from tissues. Little is known of the kinetics of neutrophils after having entered the tissues; they are believed to remain in the tissues for 2 to 5 days, and if they are not used there in an inflammatory process, they die or are destroyed by other phagocytic cells. The bone marrow quickly replaces the neutrophils that have exited from the bloodstream with cells from the bone marrow reserve.

Neutrophil Counts in Bone Marrow and Peripheral Blood

Variations in the number and morphology of leukocytes in the bloodstream and bone marrow have long been used as clinical guides for the diagnosis of many diseases. These variations may reflect the response of normal leukocytes to an underlying disease, or may indicate a primary disorder intrinsic to leukocytes, such as leukemia. A thorough knowledge of established normal values and morphological characteristics of all cellular elements is important for recognizing and interpreting unexpected findings.

Marrow Counts

Although leukocytes are generally regarded as residents of peripheral circulation, the blood serves as a route of transportation from sites of production in the bone marrow to sites of function in the tissues. Granulocytes, lymphocytes, and monocytes are formed in the bone marrow for release into the bloodstream. In

TABLE 16-2	Percentages of Precursor Cell Types in the Bone Marrow				
Cell Type	Birth	1 mo	3 mo	12 mo	Adult
Erythrocytes	7–21	3–12	8–19	4–12	18–30
Granulocytes	54–72	27–33	25–50	25–44	50–70
early:late	1:12	1:9	1:9	1:10	1:5
Lymphocytes	8–20	35–55	32–56	32–58	3–17
Plasma cells	0	0	0	0–1	0–2

addition, lymphocytes proliferate in extramedullary lymphoid tissue such as the thymus. Values for the various cell types, as determined by differential cell counting of bone marrow samples from healthy individuals, are presented in Table 16-2.

Values are fairly constant except during infancy, when they vary according to age.[8] Erythrocyte precursors decrease shortly after birth and remain sparse until active erythropoiesis resumes during the second to third month of life. The percentage of myelocytic precursors (predominately neutrophils) falls precipitously during the first month of life because of a decrease in mature forms. Values are stable during infancy and increase during later childhood to adult levels. The number of lymphocytes increases dramatically during the first month of life, and this cell becomes the most numerous in the marrow throughout infancy. Plasma cells are virtually absent until approximately 6 months of age. In older children and adults, myelocytic precursors outnumber erythroid precursors about 4:1 in the bone marrow, with the postmitotic neutrophil forms (metamyelocytes, bands, and polymorphonuclear neutrophils) predominating to form the storage pool. During bacterial infections, the myeloid:erythrocyte ratio (M:E) may increase further owing to increased granulocyte production.

Blood Counts

Complete blood cell counting (the CBC) is accomplished routinely by automated methods on electronic analyzers based on electrical impedance and laser technologies. These whole-blood analyzers determine white cell, red cell, and platelet counts in addition to differentiating leukocytes according to the percentage of granulocytes, lymphocytes, and monocytes present. White blood cell counts vary considerably with age; the established normal range for white cell counts is provided in Table 16-3. Generally, only mature, nondividing leukocytes are present in the peripheral blood of healthy persons. In the myelocytic series, primarily mature polymorphonuclear neutrophils and a few band forms are expected. Because of the high number of cells evaluated by automated instruments, an occasional immature form may be noted; a single unexpected leukocyte should not be interpreted as abnormal unless other clinical or laboratory findings suggest the presence of disease.

A wide range in expected white blood cell number exists at birth in healthy infants with the neutrophil presenting as the predominant cell.[11,12] Although not apparent on Table 16-3, significant changes in the differential white blood cell count occur during the first

few days of life. At birth, the mean neutrophil count is about 8.0×10^9/L. This count rises rapidly to a peak value of about 13×10^9/L at 12 hours of age but then drops to a mean of about 5.0×10^9/L by 72 hours of age. Thereafter, the neutrophil count slowly decreases so that the lymphocyte becomes the predominant cell by the age of 2 to 3 weeks (4.0×10^9/L). During the first few days of life, an increased number of slightly immature neutrophils such as metamyelocytes and bands may be observed transiently in circulation. This early release of metamyelocytes and bands from the bone marrow reserve into the bloodstream is referred to as a *shift to the left*.

In neonatal populations, the activity of neutrophils has been shown to be diminished.[7] Studies have revealed decreases in neutrophil mobility, deformability, and adherence in healthy neonates, whereas stressed neonates have exhibited decreased phagocytic and bacteriocidal activity.[7] Accordingly, the compromised activity of neutrophils in the neonate may predispose this population to septicemia and should be considered if the expected shift to the left persists and is accompanied by a relatively low white blood cell count ($<3.0 \times 10^9$/L with 70% neutrophils with immature forms such as metamyelocytes and bands).[7,13] Newborns are particularly likely to develop severe neutropenia during bacterial infections because of depletion of the neutrophil storage pool in the bone marrow.[7,14]

A diurnal variation of neutrophil counts has been observed in adults but not in infants. Significantly higher values in the afternoon than in the morning are noted. In adults, white blood cell counts vary according to gender in that total leukocyte counts are slightly higher in women than in men owing to a significantly higher neutrophil number.[15] This phenomenon is apparently related to differences in sex hormones.[16] No gender-based difference in white cell count has been noted during childhood. Additionally, the mean total leukocyte and neutrophil counts in healthy African-American children are lower than counts in age-

TABLE 16-3	Range of Blood Leukocyte Counts (Absolute Number × 10⁹/L)			
Cell Type	Birth	6 mo	4 yr	Adult
Total leukocytes	4–40	5–24	5–15	4–11
Neutrophils	2–20	0.5–10	1.5–7.5	1.5–7.5
Lymphocytes	1–9	1.5–22	1.5–8.5	1–4.5
Monocytes	0–2	0–2.5	0–1	0–1
Eosinophils	0–1.5	0–2.5	0–1	0–0.5
Basophils	0–0.3	0–0.4	0–0.2	0–0.2

matched white children, although no racial differences are apparent in lymphocyte, monocyte, eosinophil, and basophil counts.[7,17]

Response to Infections

Neutrophils play a central role in removing infectious or inflammatory agents that challenge host immunity. Within minutes, neutrophils are stimulated to migrate from circulation through junctions between endothelial cells to the site of infection or inflammation. The classic response to infectious and inflammatory processes is an increase in the relative number of neutrophils known as neutrophilia. The accelerated release of neutrophils from the bone marrow reserve will be accompanied by a shift to the left, which may be defined as an increased number of metamyelocyte and band forms observed in the circulating pool. The increase in circulating neutrophil number and immaturity may similarly be observed in the early stages of neoplastic conditions such as chronic myelocytic leukemia (CML) as well as in myeloproliferative disorders. The major distinction is that the myelocytic precursors released during infectious response are more limited to the metamyelocyte and band, whereas in neoplastic processes, earlier precursor cells such as myelocytes, promyelocytes, and blasts are also present. The cytochemical staining technique, leukocyte alkaline phosphatase, is useful for differentiating neutrophilic response to infection (leukemoid reaction) from CML (see Chap. 33). No method can predict the source of inflammation with complete accuracy, particularly whether or not a bacterial infection is present. A number of reports have emphasized the lack of specificity and pitfalls of overinterpreting leukocyte counts.[18–20]

The kinetics of circulating neutrophils vary greatly depending on the type, duration, and intensity of the infection.[21] The immediate response to infection is transient neutropenia resulting from increased margination and accelerated delivery of neutrophils to the infected site. Within an hour, neutrophils are released from the bone marrow reserve into the bloodstream. In the early phases of infection, the circulating half-life of neutrophils is shortened and cell turnover is accelerated. Later, the circulating half-life returns to normal. Expansion of the proliferation, maturation, circulating, and marginating pools of neutrophils is accomplished by the following mechanisms:

1. More pluripotent stem cells are committed to the granulocyte differentiation pathway.
2. The generation (cell cycle) time of myelocytes is shortened.
3. Myelocytes undergo an extra division (thus, the proliferative pool of precursors may be expanded independently of an increased input of pluripotent stem cells).
4. The overall transit time through the bone marrow is accelerated.

In addition to changes in neutrophil number, alterations in neutrophil morphology may be observed in the forms of toxic granulation, Döhle bodies, and cytoplasmic vacuolization (Figs. 16–1 to 16–3). Toxic granulation is frequently associated with severe infection in which the cytoplasmic granules enlarge and take on darker-staining properties than normal. Toxic

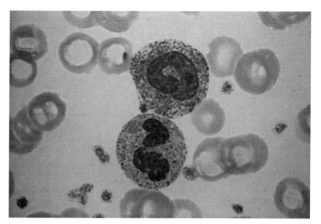

FIGURE 16–1 Toxic granulation (peripheral blood). Note the prominent dark-staining granules.

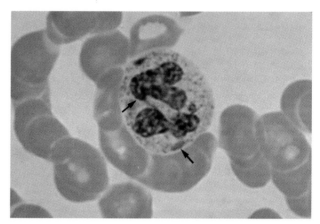

FIGURE 16–2 Dohle bodies (*arrows*). Note the large bluish bodies in the periphery of the cytoplasm.

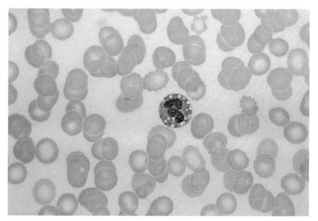

FIGURE 16–3 Vacuolated neutrophils suggesting the presence of infection or a severe inflammation.

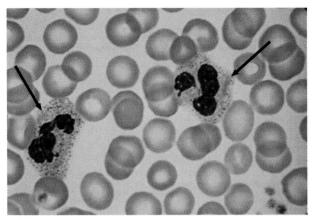

FIGURE 16–4 May-Hegglin anomaly. Note the Dohle body present in each neutrophil (arrows). Not shown in the slide but associated with May-Hegglin anomaly is the presence of giant platelets. (From Dutcher, T: Hematology. In Listen, Look and Learn. Health and Education Resources, Inc., Bethesda, MD, with permission.)

TABLE 16–4 **Qualitative and Quantitative Neutrophil Changes Noted in Responses to Infection**
Neutrophilia
Shift to the left
Toxic granulation
Döhle bodies
Vacuolization

granulation may be accompanied by the presence of pale blue inclusions in the periphery of the cytoplasm, which are referred to as Döhle bodies. They consist of a few strands of rough endoplasmic reticulum that have aggregated.[8,22] Döhle bodies are similar, but not identical, to the inclusions found in the hereditary leukocyte and platelet disorder known as the May-Hegglin anomaly (Fig. 16–4). Lastly, in response to infection, the cytoplasm may become vacuolated and, occasionally, contain ingested microorganisms. Although these features suggest the presence of infection, their presence holds little diagnostic value, since all may appear during bacterial and viral infection, pregnancy, massive trauma, drug reactions, and other toxic states.[8] All three morphological features are commonly observed, with toxic granulation reported as the most common morphological change in response to bacterial infection, followed by Döhle bodies and cytoplas-

mic vacuolization.[8] Table 16–4 summarizes the possible quantitative and qualitative changes in neutrophils during infection.

The function of circulating neutrophils, as well as their number and appearance, may be affected by infection. Both enhanced and impaired functions have been reported when compared with normal values in studies performed during infections.[23,24] Although a number of exceptions exist, it is generally accepted that mild infections enhance neutrophil functions,[25,26] whereas neutrophil functions are impaired during severe infections. The role that these acquired functional abnormalities play in the course of infections is unknown. When investigating patients for qualitative neutrophil defects, remember that abnormalities of function may be the consequence, not necessarily the cause, of infections.

Neutrophil Function

The main function of the neutrophil is the internalization of microorganisms for destruction, referred to as phagocytosis. Once bacteria infiltrate the tissues, neutrophils are stimulated for immediate action. For the purpose of discussion, phagocytosis is described as occurring in three distinct phases: migration and diapedesis; opsonization and recognition; and ingestion, killing, and digestion (Fig. 16–5).

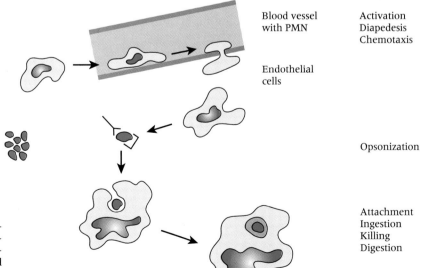

Blood vessel with PMN

Endothelial cells

Activation
Diapedesis
Chemotaxis

Opsonization

Attachment
Ingestion
Killing
Digestion

FIGURE 16–5 The phases of neutrophilic phagocytosis, which include activation, diapedesis, chemotaxis, opsonization, ingestion, killing, and digestion. (From Abramson, JS and Wheeler, JG,[7] p 110, with permission.)

TABLE 16–5 **Chemical Factors That Signal Neutrophil Activation**	
Chemoattractants	**Source**
N-formyl oligopeptides	Bacteria
C5a, C3b, and C3bi factors	Complement
Interleukin-8	Monocyte
Leukotriene B$_4$	Membrane phospholipid
Platelet activating factor	Neutrophils, basophils, macrophages

Migration and Diapedesis

As previously mentioned, neutrophils in the marginating pool roll along vessel endothelium in a random and nondirectional pattern until a site of injury or infection is encountered. Bacteria and sites of inflammation in the host send out signals in the form of chemoattractants (Table 16–5) that stimulate changes in morphology and migration pattern.[7–9,27,28] A re-engineering of the plasma membrane occurs in which the polymerization of actin filaments transforms the neutrophil shape from smooth and round to ruffled and flat with pseudopods (Fig. 16–6).[7–9] Under the stimulus of chemoattractants, the activated neutrophil migrates in a repetitive, wavelike motion to the site of infection. The process of directional migration (or locomotion) under the guidance of chemoattractants is known as *chemotaxis*. The chemoattractant forms a concentration gradient with the neutrophil migrating toward the area of highest concentration.[7,9] During chemotaxis, the neutrophil adheres to endothelial receptors and, by diapedesis, penetrates through narrow junctions between endothelial cells into the tissues. In diapedesis, the neutrophil is briefly retained by the vascular basement membrane, but then enters the tissues by passing through small openings in this membrane. This process is dependent on energy or adenosine triphosphate (ATP) production from glucose, requires calcium and magnesium, and is enhanced by the presence of chemotactic factors. Concurrent with the chemical stimulus, the rate of neutrophil migration may be accelerated by a process known as *chemokinesis*. Because neutrophils are the first phagocytes to migrate to the site of infection, the lag time between microorganism invasion and timely neutrophil migration is crucial for limiting the spread of infection and perhaps even preventing infection.[7] Animal studies of chemokinesis indicate that the optimum time for neutrophil migration and mobilization to the site of infection ranges from 2 to 4 hours.[7] Little is understood about the interrelationship of the three modes of neutrophil migration (Table 16–6); however, all are believed to contribute to the efficient mobilization of neutrophils to the site of injury.[7]

The first step in the process of neutrophil chemotaxis is the binding of chemoattractant molecules to specific receptors located on the plasma membrane of the neutrophil.[7–9,29] In addition to chemotaxis, the binding of chemoattractant and neutrophil receptor initiates other cellular events, which include neutrophil aggregation, secretion of the contents of cytoplasmic granules, and an increase in oxidative metabolism. Shortly thereafter, a number of dramatic biochemical events, referred to as signal transduction, occur, which mediate and amplify cellular events including chemotaxis.[27–29] Within seconds of chemotactic factor binding, the neutrophil membrane becomes more fluid, the concentration of cyclic adenosine monophosphate doubles, the electrical charge of the cell changes, and calcium is mobilized from the neutrophil membrane into the cytosol. All of these are believed to contribute to sustained directed motility of the neutrophil during chemotaxis.[7]

Many humoral and cellular factors have been described to promote chemotaxis, and several processes have been described to suppress neutrophil migration.[8,30–34] A suppression of neutrophil migration is necessary to immobilize activated neutrophils at the localized site of inflammation. These same suppressive mechanisms may protect normal tissues by limiting the inflammatory response.

Opsonization and Recognition

Migrating neutrophils cannot efficiently recognize and attach to most microorganisms. A mechanism referred to as opsonization facilitates recognition and attachment by marking the organism for ingestion. The term opsonization is of Greek origin and literally means "to prepare for dining."[8] Although chemotaxis is taking place, circulating immunoglobulin and activated complement components coat the surface of the bacteria. The marked bacterium, referred to as an opsonin, may be readily recognized and ingested by the neutrophil. Ingestion will not take place without the presence of membrane-bound immunoglobulin.[7] Furthermore, the recruitment of activated complement components enhances the opsonic potential of the immunoglobulin molecule. The plasma membrane of the

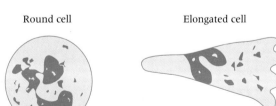

Round cell   Elongated cell

FIGURE 16–6 The change in shape of the neutrophil from smooth and round to ruffled and flat with pseudopods is caused by stimulation of chemoattractants. (Adapted from Kaplan, S and Brams, CA: Advance Testing for Neutrophil Function, 7(1), 1995, p 8.)

TABLE 16–6 **Three Modes of Neutrophil Migration**	
Mode of Migration	**Characteristics**
Random migration	Nondirectional
Chemokinesis	Nondirectional acceleration of migration speed
Chemotaxis	Directional

neutrophil carries receptors for the Fc fragment of the IgG molecule and activated complement only. Accordingly, the proteins that most effectively mark bacteria for recognition and attachment are IgG_1, IgG_3, C3b, and C3bi.[7,9,35]

Phagocytosis: Ingestion, Killing, and Digestion

The ingestion of the opsonized microbe begins as soon as the binding of membrane surface receptor of the neutrophil and microbe is complete. Depolarization of the neutrophil surface charge and rearrangement of membrane phospholipid and actin filaments occur near the binding site.[7-9] Membrane pseudopods extend around and envelop the microbe, forming an isolated vacuole known as a phagosome within the neutrophil cytoplasm. Simultaneously, cytoplasmic granules migrate to and fuse with the membrane of the phagosome, forming a phagolysosome (Fig. 16–7). Once fusion is accomplished, the cytoplasmic granules undergo degranulation, whereby their contents are released into the phagolysosome. The ingested organism is exposed to the lytic activity of granular enzymes within the phagolysosome, which leads to eventual killing and digestion. Ingestion, degranulation, and digestion require energy (ATP) that is generated via glucose phosphorylation by anaerobic glycolysis.[8,36-38]

Microorganism destruction (killing) may be accomplished by oxygen-dependent and non-oxygen-dependent mechanisms. An alteration in pH and the release of lysosomal and proteolytic enzymes into the phagolysosome represent the non-oxygen-dependent mode of killing the internalized particle. The lytic enzymes possess bactericidal activity, which is directed at cleaving segments of the bacterial cell wall. Alternately, oxygen-dependent killing involves the release of NADPH (nicotinamide adenine denucleotide phosphate) oxidase, which mediates the production of active oxygen metabolites such as superoxide and hydrogen peroxide during a process known as a respiratory burst. These active oxygen metabolites are capable of injuring microorganisms.

Studies performed in vitro suggest an orderly se-quence of events for phagolysosome formation.[39-41] The degranulation of secondary granules precedes that of the primary granules. In rat and human models, the timing of degranulation has been correlated with changes of pH in the internal environment of the phagolysosome. The contents of the secondary granules have been released into the phagolysosome within 30 seconds of particle ingestion, at which time the pH ranges between 6.5 and 7.4. Within the following 3 minutes, enzymes from the primary granules, such as myeloperoxidase, are released into the phagolysosome, at which time the pH steadily begins to fall to about 4.0. The timing of sequential degranulation and pH changes appears to be well coordinated, since the contents of secondary granules function optimally at a neutral pH and the contents of the primary granules function optimally in an acid range.[7,8,39-42]

Biochemistry of Phagocytosis

As noted, the energy required for ingestion, degranulation, and digestion is generated by the metabolism of glucose by anaerobic glycolysis. In addition to the consumption of glucose, neutrophil activity is associated with an increase in oxygen utilization referred to as the respiratory burst. The burst of consumed oxygen is converted to active oxygen metabolites such as superoxide anion and hydrogen peroxide, hydroxyl radical (OH•) and singlet oxygen ($^1O_2$), all of which are capable of microbe injury.[43-45] The best-understood pathway is the production of hydrogen peroxide. The activated neutrophil releases the enzyme NADPH oxidase into the phagolysosome, where it converts oxygen to superoxide anion ($•O_{2-}$), which is further reduced to hydrogen peroxide (H_2O_2). The enzymatic reaction is represented by the following:

$$NADPH + 2O_2 \rightarrow NADP^+ + 2O_{2-} + H^+$$
$$2O_{2-} + 2H^+ \rightarrow H_2O_2 + O_2$$

There is more discussion of the biochemical nature of NADPH later in this chapter. Many microorganisms possess enzymes that deactivate superoxide anion and hydrogen peroxide; therefore, the bactericidal and fun-

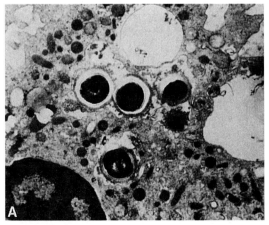
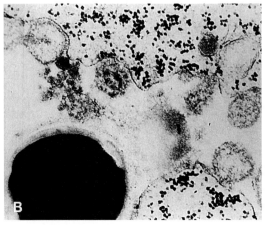

FIGURE 16–7   Electron microscopy of phagolysosome formation. (A) Staphylococci lie within phagcocytic vesicles limited by sacs formed from inverted pieces of the neutrophil membrane. Cytoplasmic granules are approaching the phagocytic vesicles. (B) Higher magnification shows degranulation with the discharge of granule contents into the vicinity of the staphylococcus.

TABLE 16–7 Inflammatory Diseases Associated with Neutrophil-Mediated Tissue Injury

Adult respiratory distress syndrome
Myocardial infarction
Rheumatoid arthritis
Inflammatory bowel disease
Emphysema
Glomerulonephritis
Gout

gicidal potential of these agents is limited.[7,8,45,46] The interaction of superoxide anion and hydrogen peroxide with other products of phagocytosis such as myeloperoxidase or lactoferrin may result in agents with more potent toxic activity. The myeloperoxidase–hydrogen peroxide–halide system is one example of an interaction that generates a potent toxic microbicidal agent.[7,8,45] Myeloperoxidase (MPO) is present in the primary granules and is delivered to the phagolysosome by degranulation. In the presence of a halide such as chloride, MPO catalyzes the formation of hypochlorous acid, which is the active ingredient in household bleach.[7,8,45] Bacteria are easily killed by hypochlorous acid and other reactive substances produced by this system. Another biochemical interaction that results in a potent bactericidal agent is the chelation of iron with superoxide and hydrogen peroxide to form an iron-oxygen complex and hydroxyl radicals. The secondary granules provide lactoferrin, which potentiates the iron-oxygen complex activity.[7,8]

Neutrophils possess antioxidant mechanisms that protect against injury to host tissue by the potent products of phagocytosis.[46,47] The enzyme superoxide dismutase is present in human neutrophils and is capable of converting superoxide anion to hydrogen peroxide. The hydrogen peroxide molecules are rapidly metabolized to form water by cytoplasmic glutathione peroxidase and catalase. Vitamin E and ascorbic acid also play antioxidant roles. Such protective mechanisms are reported to be necessary for restricting the activity of phagocytic agent against the phagolysosome. The release of granular contents and active oxygen metabolites is generally limited to the internal environment of the phagolysosome.[8] The release of these phagocytic agents into extracellular fluids during phagocytosis has been implicated as a cause of tissue injury in a number of inflammatory conditions (Table 16–7).

DISORDERS OF NEUTROPHILS

Disorders in the neutrophil cell line predispose an individual to recurrent bacterial infections that are resistant to treatment. Neutrophil disorders are classified as quantitative and qualitative, reflecting changes in neutrophil number and function, respectively. Quantitative disorders present as a decrease in the absolute neutrophil number and are referred to as neutropenia. Inadequate neutrophil number limits the po-

tential for effective mobilization and killing at the site of microbial invasion. Alternately, qualitative disorders are marked by neutrophil dysfunction because of impaired migration or altered bactericidal activity. As noted, phagocytosis occurs in a complex sequence of events ranging from activation, migration, and diapedesis to the recognition, ingestion, and killing of an opsonized particle. A deficiency or dysfunction in any one or a combination of these processes modifies neutrophil function. The remainder of this chapter will address quantitative and qualitative disorders of the neutrophil, the consequences of these disorders to the patient, and current modes of therapy.

Quantitative Disorders—The Neutropenias

Neutropenia is defined as an absolute decrease in the number of circulating neutrophils. This condition may be suspected in patients presenting with neutrophil counts of less than 1.5×10^9/L. The low neutrophil count, however, is not the sole indicator of neutrophilic disorder and should be correlated with clinical and laboratory findings. The normal level of circulating neutrophils varies with age and race, and refers to mature polymorphonuclear and band forms only. As previously noted, healthy infants may exhibit neutrophil numbers between 0.5 and 1.0×10^9/L. Epidemiologic data indicate that healthy individuals of African, Jordanian, Arab, and Yemenite Jewish heritage may exhibit neutrophil levels of 0.5 to 1.5×10^9/L without signs of disturbed granulocytic activity.[7,8,48]

Recurrent bacterial infections are the hallmark of persistent neutropenia[49]; the clinical pattern is usually related to the neutrophil count. Neutropenia may be mild with counts ranging from 1.0 to 1.5×10^9/L, moderate with counts ranging from 0.5 to 1.0×10^9/L, or severe with counts less than 0.5×1.0^9/L.[7,8] Severe and repeated infections are not of concern if the neutrophil count is maintained between 1.0 and 1.5×10^9/L. Life-threatening infections are not generally observed until the blood count falls below 0.2×10^9/L. The immune system of the neutropenic patient is believed to compensate for the neutrophil deficit by producing an increased number of circulating monocytes and accelerating humoral and cell-mediated activities.[8] The infections are usually well controlled if the neutrophil count increases transiently in response to the stress of infection.

Infections in the neutropenic patient are most commonly caused by endogenous normal flora such as *Staphylococcus aureus* and gram-negative enteric organisms; nosocomial infections caused by organisms such as *Pseudomonas* species are noted also. Mixed bacterial infections are not unusual. Although neutropenia increases host susceptibility to bacterial infection, the risk of viral, fungal, and parasitic infection is not heightened.[7,8] Most infections in the neutropenic individual occur in the cutaneous and soft tissues and typically manifest as cellulitis, furuncles, and abscesses. The major concern for these infections is the spread of the organism from the localized site into the bloodstream, resulting in a superinfection such as septicemia.

Neutropenic disorders are described to be acquired or congenital. Persistent cases of neutropenia are generally attributed to an intrinsic problem of the hematopoietic system, whereas transient conditions are linked to factors extrinsic to the bone marrow.[8] The absolute reduction in the circulating number of neutrophils may be attributed to one or a combination of the following mechanisms:

1. Decreased production by the bone marrow
2. Impaired release from the marrow into the blood
3. Increased destruction
4. Maldistribution resulting in pseudoneutropenia

The mechanism responsible for neutropenia may not be easily determined, since a limited number of sensitive testing methods are available clinically. Presumptive diagnosis may be made by evaluating bone marrow production through bone marrow biopsy, and neutrophil release from the marrow reserve and distribution in circulating and marginating pools through steroid stimulation and mobilization studies.[8,50] Identification of the cause is important for selecting appropriate therapy, monitoring prognosis, and counseling family members in congenital cases.

Acquired Neutropenias

Most acquired neutropenias occur as transient conditions because of factors extrinsic to the bone marrow; they may be associated with concomitant viral infection, alloantibody or autoantibody activity, reticuloendothelial sequestration, and the ingestion of certain drugs (Table 16–8). Neutropenia may be acquired as a secondary condition to processes such as aplastic anemia, malignancy of the bone marrow, and dietary B_{12} and folate deficiency.

Infection Viral infections are recognized as the most common cause of acquired neutropenia in children. Viruses implicated in inducing neutropenia include influenza A and B, rubella, rubeola, herpes virus family, hepatitis A and B, and respiratory syncytial virus (RSV). The accompanying neutropenia appears within 24 to 48 hours of viral infection onset and may persist for the period of acute viremia.[8] In particular, children under the age of 6 years experience neutropenia with a relative lymphocytosis during viral infections. A significant reduction in circulating neutrophil number has been observed in nonviral infections with mycobacterium, rickettsia, and histoplasma. In addition to affecting neutrophil number, many organisms have been demonstrated to inhibit efficient neutrophil function. *Bordetella pertussis* is an example of a bacterium that has been shown to survive phagocytosis by inhibiting the fusion of the phagosome with cytoplasmic granules.[7]

TABLE 16–8 **Factors Associated with Acquired Neutropenia**
Infection—especially viral
Autoantibodies
Alloantibodies
Reticuloendothelial sequestration
Drug ingestion
Secondary to underlying disease

Autoimmune Neutropenia Acquired neutropenia in the absence of disease has frequently been described as idiopathic. Recent evidence links some of these cases to drug ingestion and others to autoimmune processes such as Sjögren's syndrome, systemic lupus erythematosus, and rheumatoid arthritis. Autoantibodies directed against neutrophils have been detected in the serum of some patients with neutropenia of idiopathic origin. Anti-neutrophil antibodies may be of the IgG, IgM, or IgA immunoglobulin class; many are directed against neutrophil-specific antigens such as NA2, ND1, and NE1. No causal relationship has been established between the presence of autoantibody and reduced neutrophil number; however, survival studies utilizing radiolabeling techniques demonstrate that neutrophils opsonized by autoantibody exhibit a shortened half-life in circulation.[8] Immune neutropenia is an uncommon occurrence in adults, but is identified in infants and children with increased frequency because of improved techniques in identifying neutrophil-specific antibodies. Many instances of chronic benign neutropenia during childhood appear to be caused by anti-neutrophil antibodies.[51–52] Both clinical and laboratory findings are nonspecific and variable; antibody in patient serum directed against antigen on patient neutrophils must be demonstrated before an irrefutable pathogenic relationship may be established. Treatment includes antibiotics for specific bacterial infections and prednisone to limit the autoimmune response.

Isoimmune Neonatal Neutropenia Isoimmune (alloimmune) neonatal neutropenia has been characterized in infants with severe neutropenia to be analogous to Rh isoimmune hemolytic anemia.[52] The neutropenia occurs after maternal sensitization to neutrophil antigens carried by the fetus. The antigens are shared by the fetus and the father, but are absent in the mother. During pregnancy, anti-neutrophil antibody production is stimulated in the maternal immune system and these IgG antibodies cross the placenta and destroy fetal neutrophils. The anti-neutrophil antibodies are directed against neutrophil-specific antigens such as NA1, NA2, and NB1 and nonneutrophil-specific HLA antigens that are shared by neutrophils and other nucleated cells. Isoimmune neutropenia may be encountered in approximately 3% of all live births;[8] the condition is common in the firstborn child. Severe neutropenia may be present for up to 6 to 8 weeks of age or until the anti-neutrophil antibodies are cleared from neonatal circulation. After this time, the neutrophil count returns to the normal range expected for this age group. The transient neutropenia may be accompanied by cutaneous infections and infrequently progress into respiratory infection and life-threatening sepsis.[8] Therapy is usually supportive and consists of antibiotics when infections occur. If life-threatening sepsis arises, plasma exchange may be undertaken to remove maternal antibody from neonatal circulation. Follow-up therapy would include the administration of neutrophil concentrates that lack the antigen corresponding to maternal antibody.

Drug-Induced Neutropenia Pharmacologic compounds are recognized to cause disorders in neutrophil number and function.[7,8] Although the effect of drugs on neutrophil number is described as "idiosyn-

TABLE 16–9 **Drugs Associated with Causing Neutropenia**	
Drug Class	**Drug Prototype**
Antibiotics	Penicillin
	Chloramphenicol
Anti-inflammatory	Ibuprofen
Anticonvulsants	Phenytoin
Antithyroid	Propylthiouracil
Cardiovascular	Procainamide
Hypoglycemic	Chlorpropamide
Tranquilizer	Phenothiazine

cratic," the reduction in number may be dramatic, with levels falling to less than 0.2×10^9/L.[8] Drug-induced neutropenia is observed more frequently in women and in older populations.[8] For most drugs, the pharmacologic target for therapeutic action is not the neutrophil, so the resulting neutropenia is a consequence of the drug therapy (Table 16–9). A number of antimicrobial agents, such as penicillin and sulfonamide, provide clinical benefit by treating infection; at the same time, these drugs cause a transient neutropenic state. Other drugs are administered to specifically inhibit cellular response in inflammatory conditions such as rheumatoid arthritis and adult respiratory distress syndrome, since the tissue injury associated with these conditions is mediated by the neutrophil.[7] Corticosteroids and anti-inflammatory agents like ibuprofen are examples. Whether directly or circumstantially affecting the neutrophil, drugs influence the white cell through direct toxic action, by inducing autoimmune anti-neutrophil antibodies, or by disturbing neutrophil metabolism and phagocytic function. The drug-induced neutropenia may appear suddenly 1 to 2 weeks after drug ingestion. Fever and chills often develop. As soon as neutropenia is noted, the best course of action is to discontinue the administration of all nonessential drugs.[8]

Congenital Neutropenias

Congenital neutropenias occur as persistent or intermittent disorders arising from an inherited abnormality in cells of the myeloid line or those involving hematopoietic regulation; the defect is intrinsic to the bone marrow microenvironment (Table 16–10). Congenital disorders are not caused by factors extrinsic to the bone marrow such as infection, drug ingestion, or autoantibodies.

TABLE 16–10 **Disorders of Congenital Neutropenia**
1. Chronic benign neutropenia
2. Severe congenital neutropenia (Kostman's)
3. Myelokathexis
4. Cyclic neutropenia
5. Reticular dysgenesis
6. Fanconi's anemia
7. Dyskeratosis congenita
8. Shwachman-Diamond syndrome

Severe Congenital Neutropenia Severe congenital neutropenia (SCN) is a rare autosomal recessive disorder with chronic neutrophil counts of less than 0.2×10^9/L. Approximately 300 to 400 individuals in the United States are affected by this disorder.[7] Alternately known as Kostman's agranulocytosis, the condition is observed during the first few months of infancy. The severity and chronicity of infection result in a profound mortality rate, with 50% of all patients dying by the age of 7 months.[7] Clinical features of SCN include fever, subcutaneous abscesses, pneumonia, and urinary tract infections that progress into fatal sepsis or visceral abscess regardless of antibiotic therapy. Monocytosis and eosinophilia are also observed. Evaluation of the bone marrow reveals an absence of metamyelocytes, bands, and mature neutrophils that is attributed to a maturational arrest of myeloid cell production at the promyelocyte stage. Morphologically, the promyelocytes demonstrate cytoplasmic vacuolization and abnormal nuclei.[7,54] Myeloid cell death occurs in the bone marrow after this stage.[55] Bone marrow transplantation has been reported to be the only mode of treatment with potential success. Recent in vivo clinical trials with recombinant colony-stimulating factors (CSFs) hold the promise of improving the unfavorable prognosis.[7,8,56] The administration of granulocyte-CSFs (G-CSFs) has been shown to stimulate normal patterns of myelocytic differentiation and maturation with a significant rise in mature neutrophil number. SCN patients demonstrate normal to slightly elevated levels of G-CSF in the serum, indicating that the cause of the disorder is linked to a dysfunction in patient response to native G-CSF.[7,8]

Chronic Benign Neutropenia Chronic benign neutropenia is a heterogeneous group of disorders associated with neutrophil counts that fluctuate from 0.2 to 2.0×10^9/L. Accordingly, the risk of infection correlates with the degree of neutropenia. The clinical course is generally benign, with mild infections of the cutaneous tissues. Periods of remission, in which the neutrophil count is restored to normal, may continue for years. Bone marrow biopsy provides a variable picture with normal to decreased cellularity with a depleted storage compartment during periods of neutropenic exacerbation.[7,8] Bacterial infections may develop with increased frequency, but are usually well contained, since neutrophil number transiently rebounds in response to stress infection.[8] The autosomal dominant inheritance of moderate neutropenia by individuals of African, Yemenite Jewish, and Jordanian heritage may be included in this category. No treatment is indicated since the course of this group of disorders is generally uneventful.

Cyclic Neutropenia Cyclic neutropenia is a rare neutropenic condition that is noted for cyclic fluctuations in the neutrophil count. In humans, the cycles average 21 days, with periods of severe neutropenia for 3 to 10 days. The period of lowest neutrophil number is referred to as the *nadir*.[7,8] During the nadir, patients experience recurrent fever, oral ulcers, lymphadenopathy, skin infections, and, occasionally, more severe infections. As the neutrophil count returns to normal, the symptoms disappear. Seventy percent of all cases are congenital and are inherited in an ausotomal dominant pattern. In most cases, other cellular elements such as monocytes, eosinophils, and thrombocytes demonstrate cyclic variations that are asynchronous with the neutrophil cycle.[7,8] Most patients have a relatively long life span; as patients grow older, the cycles become less frequent and are replaced by a chronic mild neutropenia. Ten percent of all cases result in death from superinfection during the nadir. *Clostridium perfringens* has been isolated in a number of the fatal cases.[8] Although the cause of cyclic neutropenia remains unclear, many believe that the defect lies in a regulatory mechanism of hematopoiesis.[60,61] A canine form of the disorder is seen in gray collie dogs and has been subject to considerable study. The gray collie dogs have served as models for studying cyclic neutropenia and the findings support the concept of a stem cell defect because the disease is cured by marrow transplantation from healthy littermates. Moreover, the disease is produced in normal, healthy dogs transplanted with marrow from affected ones. Treatment with G-CSF has proven beneficial in increasing the absolute neutrophil number throughout the cycle, in shortening the duration of neutropenia, and in decreasing the frequency of cycles.[7]

Other rare causes of congenital neutropenia or pancytopenia are dyskeratosis congenita, Fanconi's anemia, myelokathexis, reticular dysgenesis, and Shwachman-Diamond syndrome. Additional diseases in which neutropenia and neutrophil dysfunction occur jointly, such as Chédiak-Higashi syndrome, are discussed later in this chapter.

Qualitative Disorders

Disorders of neutrophil function are characterized by bacterial infections that are caused by disturbances in neutrophil function. Neutropenia is often seen accompanying qualitative disorders of the neutrophil. The qualitative disorders will be presented according to the major defect expressed, although it is recognized that multiple abnormalities (including neutropenia) may be detected in some patients (Table 16–11).

Chemotaxis

Although these conditions are collectively referred to as chemotaxis disorders, it must be remembered that neutrophils are capable of three major types of migration: chemoattractant-directed movement known as *chemotaxis*, nondirectional random mobility, and chemoattractant-accelerated random mobility known as *chemokinesis*. Detecting an abnormality in one type of migration does not guarantee defects in the other types. Moreover, in vitro assays of neutrophil migration may not always correlate with in vivo studies. Finally, the basis for abnormal mobilization may be related to an intrinsic defect of the neutrophil or to an extrinsic imbalance in signal transduction or chemoattractants. Selected disorders of chemotaxis are listed in Table 16–12. The listing is not intended to be all-inclusive because new conditions continue to be reported. Disorders are grouped according to the most accepted pathogenetic mechanism, although it is realized that multiple mechanisms may be involved.

Cytoplasmic Granules

Myeloperoxidase Deficiency   Myeloperoxidase (MPO) deficiency is reported to be the most common congenital neutrophil disorder, with complete deficiency noted in 1 out of 4000 individuals and partial deficiency being seen in 1 out of 2000 individuals.[8] The disorder was believed to be rare, since most patients are not predisposed to more frequent bacterial infections and the clinical course is benign to mild.[65] Recent advances in flow cytometry have led to the identification of an increasing number of cases. Histochemical techniques have served as a more routine approach for recognizing MPO deficiency. MPO deficiency may be acquired or congenital with the latter being inherited in an autosomal recessive pattern.[65] MPO is present in the primary granules. During normal phagocytosis,

---

TABLE 16–11   Classes of Qualitative Neutrophil Disorders and Related Conditions

* Chemotaxis
  o Lazy leukocyte syndrome
  o Monosomy
* Cytoplasmic granules
  o Myeloperoxidase deficiency
  o Chédiak-Higashi syndrome
* Biochemical disturbance of respiratory burst
  o Chronic granulomatous disease
  o Glucose-6-phosphate dehydrogenase deficiency
  o Glutathione deficiency

TABLE 16–12   Selected Disorders of Neutrophil Chemotaxis with Selected References

Intrinsic Neutrophil Defects
Lazy leukocyte syndrome
Monosomy
Burns
Congenital ichthyosis
Chédiak-Higashi disease
Newborns
Actin dysfunction
Glycoprotein deficiency
Immotile cilia syndrome
Glycogenosis IB

Cell-directed inhibitors
Cancer
Surgical patients

Chemotactic factor-directed inhibitors
Anergy (various causes)
Cytomegalovirus
Liver cirrhosis
Acute lymphoblastic leukemia
Sepsis

Undefined mechanisms
Influenza A virus
Marrow transplant recipients
Hyperimmunoglobulin E
Uremia
Hemophilia
Peridontitis
Milk intolerance

this enzyme mediates the conversion of superoxide anion and hydrogen peroxide to more toxic killing agents such as hypochlorous acid. MPO patients demonstrate abnormal killing with an exaggerated respiratory burst and prolonged, but normal antimicrobial activity.[66,67] The diminished MPO-dependent bactericidal activity seems to be partially offset by this generalized increase in respiratory burst. MPO patients are unable to demonstrate effective killing of *Candida* and *Aspergilus* species, which may result in severe infection (see Fig. 15–3). In congenital MPO deficiency, neutrophils and monocytes lack MPO, whereas eosinophils contain normal levels.[67,68] The consequences of MPO deficiency are usually mild. Problems arise in patients with underlying diseases, such as diabetes mellitus, which further challenge the immune system and may lead to the development of disseminated candidiasis.[7,8]

Chédiak-Higashi Syndrome Chédiak-Higashi syndrome (CHS) is an autosomal recessive condition characterized by partial albinism of the cutaneous and ocular tissues, recurrent bacterial infections of cutaneous and soft tissues, mild bleeding tendencies, and the presence of giant lysosomal granules in leukocytes and platelets (Figs. 16–8 and 16–9).[69,70] Neurologic complications may also be noted. Nearly 200 cases of Chédiak-Higashi syndrome have been reported in the United States.[8] These patients usually die as a result of infection during early childhood. Cases surviving early childhood progress into an accelerated phase manifested by pancytopenia, organomegaly, and the spread of localized infections, which typically leads to death. *Staphylococcus aureus* accounts for 70% of all infections.[7]

CHS patients present with moderate neutropenia with counts ranging from 0.5 to 2.0 × 10^9/L.[8] Intramedullary destruction and splenic sequestration are implicated in causing the neutropenia. Aside from the neutropenia, the associated dysfunction in phagocytic activity is attributed to depressed chemotaxis and delayed degranulation, which slow the process of killing ingested bacteria. The disturbance of degranulation

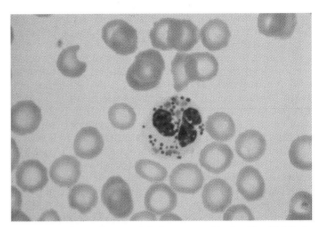

FIGURE 16–9 Neutrophil from a patient with Chédiak-Higashi syndrome. The cytoplasm is filled with strikingly large primary (azurophilic) granules. (From Dutcher, T: In Listen, Look and Learn. Hematology. Health and Education Resources, Inc., Bethesda, MD, with permission.)

may be ascribed to interference from the giant lysosomal granules.[69,70] These abnormal granules develop during early myelopoiesis because of an initial aggregation of primary granules followed by fusion with the secondary granules (see Fig. 16–8). The enzymatic contents of both granule types are found in the giant granules with the exception of elastase and cathepsin G.[8] The giant lysosomal granules are more evident in cells of the bone marrow than in circulating white cells. Monocytes, lymphocytes, melanocytes, and platelets may exhibit similar morphologic features. Platelets in CHS have been shown to be deficient in ADP and serotonin.

Management of CHS before the onset of the accelerated phase includes prophylactic antimicrobial therapy and high daily doses of ascorbic acid.[8] In the case of infection, aggressive intravenous treatment is required. The Epstein-Barr virus (EBV) is postulated to trigger the onset of the accelerated phase of CHS, so immunization to EBV may be beneficial.[8] Bone marrow transplantation holds the only hope for cure and optimally should be performed before the onset of the accelerated phase.[8]

Biochemical Disturbance of the Respiratory Burst

Phagocytosis and killing of bacteria are made possible by an increase in oxygen consumption. As previously noted, the respiratory burst is responsible for producing active oxygen metabolites with potent antimicrobial properties. The activated neutrophil releases the enzyme NADPH oxidase, which reduces oxygen to superoxide and other toxic oxygen species. NADPH oxidase is composed of four known oxidase subunits referred to as phagocyte oxidase subunits or *phox*.[8] The interaction of these four subunits results in the formation of the active oxygen metabolites during the burst.[7,8] Each *phox* subunit may be identified as a glycoprotein (gp) or a protein (p) and by its weight in kilodaltons. Two of the subunits, gp91-*phox* and p22-*phox*, are located in the plasma membrane and

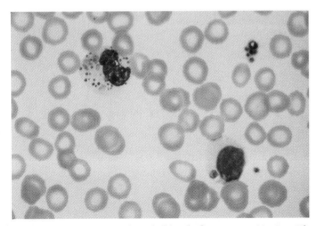

FIGURE 16–8 Peripheral blood from a patient with Chédiak-Higashi syndrome. (*Right*) Lymphocyte. (*Left*) Neutrophil. (From Dutcher, T: Hematology. In Listen, Look and Learn. Health and Education Resources, Inc., Bethesda, MD, with permission.)

specific granules. Together these subunits form the enzyme cytochrome b. The other two subunits include p47-*phox* and p67-*phox*, which are residents of the cytosol. Stimulation of NADPH oxidase leads to the migration of the cytosol subunits (p47-*phox* and p67-*phox*) to the plasma membrane. With the help of secondary mediators, the four subunits (gp91-*phox*, p22-*phox*, p47-*phox*, and p67-*phox*) are assembled into the active oxidant superoxide.[7,8] Other pathways interact with superoxide to yield more potent antimicrobial agents. NADPH and other potent products of phagocytosis must be regulated to prevent injury to host tissues. Antioxidants such as superoxide dismutase, catalase, and glutathione peroxidase work to restrict oxygen metabolite activity to the phagolysosome through rapid metabolism and neutralization.

Any biochemical disturbance in the complex pathway of the respiratory burst may induce neutrophil dysfunction. For the purposes of discussion, the biochemical defects most frequently associated with respiratory burst impairment will be addressed.

Chronic Granulomatous Disease Chronic granulomatous disease (CGD) is a familial, heterogeneous disorder of the neutrophil that may be chronic or intermittent. CGD is noted in 1 out of every 500,000 individuals who exhibit recurrent bacterial and fungal infections, generally during the first 12 months of life.[8] The congenital abnormality is associated with a failure in the activation of the respiratory burst, which results in little or no superoxide production.[71-73] The characteristic clinical picture of these patients is lymphadenitis; deep tissue infections such as osteomyelitis, visceral and hepatic abscesses, recurrent pulmonary infections, organomegaly, and infected eczematoid rash. CGD patients exhibit neutrophilia rather than neutropenia. The hallmark of CGD is the formation during chronic inflammatory reactions of granulomas that keep the organisms localized; the granulomas may cause obstructions of the gastrointestinal tract. *Staphylococcus aureus, Aspergillus,* and enteric organisms are most frequently implicated in causing infection. Catalase-positive organisms are especially successful in chronically colonizing in the CGD patient, since the catalase enzyme is capable of neutralizing hydrogen peroxide.[7] Cultures taken from the granulomas are often negative. CGD may be inherited as a sex-linked recessive or autosomal recessive trait. The first cases were observed in boys presenting with severe bacterial infections by the first year of life, and most of these patients died of septicemia or chronic pulmonary disease in early childhood. However, much clinical experience has been gained since the description of this disease, and it is now clear that the disease may be more heterogeneous and may not be recognized until early adulthood. Furthermore, CGD may develop in girls, demonstrating the autosomal recessive mode of inheritance.

Several mutations in the subunits of NAPDH oxidase have been described to disable respiratory burst activity (Table 16–13). In many cases, an absence in cytochrome b has been noted as a result of deficiencies in plasma membrane–derived gp91-*phox* or p22-*phox*.[7,8,74] Both subunits are required for normal expression of cytochrome b. The classic X-linked form and a rare subset of autosomal recessive cases dem-

TABLE 16–13 **Molecular Basis of Chronic Granulomatous Disease**		
Cytochrome b Subunit Affected	Mode of Inheritance	Neutrophil Structure Involved
p47-*phox*	Autosomal	Cytosol
p67-*phox*	Autosomal	Cytosol
gp91-*phox*	X-linked	Plasma membrane
p22-*phox*	Autosomal	Plasma membrane

onstrate an absence of cytochrome b. Alternately, most autosomal recessive cases reveal deficiencies in cytosol-derived p47-*phox* and p67-*phox*, whereas cytochrome b levels are normal.[7,8] In both scenarios, the failure to reduce oxygen to reactive molecules is responsible for the microbicidal defect in NADPH oxidase.[71-73] The ingestion of bacteria, degranulation, and phagolysosome formation are normal.

Diagnosis may be established by demonstrating a bactericidal defect caused by the absence of the oxidative burst by means of a nitroblue tetrazolium test (NBT), a luminol-enhanced assay, or by measuring respiratory burst activity with flow cytometry.[7] The X-linked recessive inheritance may be confirmed by studying the family history. Indicators of CGD include the presence of disease in male members of the maternal family and by the intermediate to low activity of neutrophils from the mothers and sisters of affected boys. In most cases, these female relatives are clinically well, but may occasionally present with an increased susceptibility to infections or a syndrome resembling systemic lupus erythematosus. CGD is the best understood disorder of neutrophils. Accordingly, progress has been made in modalities of treatment and the prognosis is improving. Aggressive prophylactic antibiotic therapy should be initiated as soon as a diagnosis is made. Gamma interferon is showing promise in limiting the frequency of infections; granulocyte transfusions are useful in poor responders.[7,8] Bone marrow transplantation is reserved for severe cases.[7,8]

Other patients have been reported with clinical problems similar to chronic granulomatous disease. These disorders may have additional atypical features such as impaired chemotaxis, low serum concentration of IgA, progressive loss of cellular immunity, and bactericidal defects selective for only single bacteria. *Familial lipochrome pigmentation of histiocytes* is such a disorder, characterized by hypergammaglobulinemia, recurrent infections (particularly pulmonary), arthritis, splenomegaly, neutrophil metabolic abnormalities, and pigment-containing macrophages. *Glucose-6-phosphate dehydrogenase (G6PD)* is the enzyme regulating the flow of glucose into the hexose monophosphate shunt, and neutrophil function is abnormal only when enzyme activity is severely deficient. A syndrome similar to CGD of childhood has been reported in both congenital and acquired G6PD deficiency.[75] *Glutathione peroxidase* is one component of the antioxidant mechanism responsible for protecting against injury to host tissue by the potent products of phagocytosis. A deficiency in glutathione peroxidase is considered by some[76] to produce a variant of CGD. *Glu-*

tathione reductase deficiency is characterized by hemolysis and a variety of neutrophil defects that are not associated with clinical infections.[77]

White Blood Cell Anomalies

Several abnormalities in neutrophil morphology are observed in patients without the involvement of infection, neutrophil dysfunction, or altered neutrophil number. Such abnormalities in neutrophil morphology are collectively referred to as white blood cell anomalies. Hypersegmentation and hyposegmentation of the nucleus are white cell anomalies that reflect the number of segmented lobes demonstrated in the mature neutrophil. *Hypersegmentation* is described in larger-than-normal neutrophils with six or more nuclear lobes present (see Chap. 7). A similar hypersegmentation of eosinophils has been reported with four or more nuclear lobes present. Hypersegmentation in the granulocytes may be an indicator of megaloblastic anemia or of a benign autosomal dominant condition known as hereditary constitutional hypersegmentation of neutrophils.

Alternately, *hyposegmentation* of the nucleus is characteristic of *Pelger-Huët anomaly*, in which the nucleus is found to be bilobed or to have no lobulation whatsoever.[78] In addition, nuclear chromatin is exceptionally coarse and condensed. In the heterozygous state, predominantly bilobed neutrophil forms are present that may be described as having a "dumbbell" or "pince-nez" appearance with two symmetric lobes being joined by a filament. In the homozygous state, no segmentation is evident and the nucleus takes on a round or oval shape (Fig. 16–10). "True" Pelger-Huët anomaly is inherited in an autosomal-dominant manner and is reported to be a benign familial condition observed in 1 out of 6000 individuals.[8] Acquired Pelger-Huët anomaly may be induced by drug ingestion or secondary to conditions such as leukemia. Acquired forms may often be referred to as pseudo-Pelger-Huët, in which 10% of the neutrophils may be trilobed. Care must be taken to distinguish Pelger-Huët cells from a

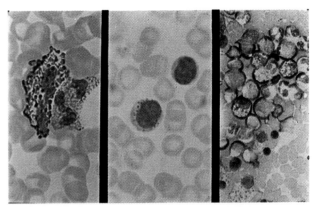

FIGURE 16–11 Alder-Reilly anomaly. (*Left and middle*) Note azurophilic granulation in cells from peripheral blood. (*Right*) Bone marrow. (From Hyun, BH, Ashton, JK, and Dolan, K: Practical Hematology. A Laboratory Guide with Accompanying Filmstrip. WB Saunders, Philadelphia, 1975, with permission.)

"shift to the left" in which an increase in metamyelocytes and bands is observed during severe infection. Generally, the nuclear chromatin is more condensed and coarse in Pelger-Huët neutrophils than in bands and metamyelocytes. Furthermore, in Pelger-Huët anomaly, greater than 70% to 90% of all neutrophils are affected.

Morphological changes may also be noted in the neutrophilic cytoplasm. The presence of prominent, dark-staining, coarse cytoplasmic granules in neutrophils, eosinophils, basophils, monocytes, and occasionally lymphocytes is known as *Alder's anomaly* or Alder-Reilly inclusions (Fig. 16–11). In some patients, only one cell type may be affected. These cytoplasmic inclusions are composed of precipitated mucopolysaccharide and are seen in association with inherited disorders of mucopolysaccharidosis such as Hunter's and Hurler's syndromes. These prominent granules are similar to those in toxic granulation except that they are larger, stain positive with metachromatic stains, and are a permanent morphological characteristic of the neutrophils.

Toxic granulation is a transient change in morphology caused by infectious or toxic agents. Granulocytes in the hereditary *May-Hegglin anomaly* have larger blue-staining cytoplasmic inclusions that resemble Döhle bodies (see Fig. 16–4). Under electron microscopy, these neutrophils are shown to have large granule-free areas in the cytoplasm that contain fibrils of ribonucleic acid.[79] Occasionally these Döhle-like inclusions may be seen in lymphocytes and monocytes. In addition to this morphological feature of the neutrophil, thrombocytopenia is reported along with giant platelets (see Chap. 26).

CASE STUDY 1

History of Present Illness A 3-year-old boy was admitted with a diagnosis of liver abscess after ultrasound examination. He had been ill with many

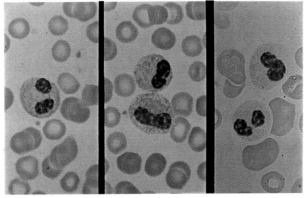

FIGURE 16–10 Pelger-Huët anomaly. Peripheral blood. (From Hyun, BH, Ashton, JK, and Dolan, K: Practical Hematology. A Laboratory Guide with Accompanying Filmstrip. WB Saunders, Philadelphia, 1975, with permission.)

infections since the age of 1 month. Types of infections included recurrent episodes of pneumonia and ear infection, perirectal abscess, osteomyelitis of the metacarpals, suppurative lymphadenitis, and mastoiditis. Organisms that were recovered from these sites of infection were *Staphylococcus aureus* and *Aspergillus*. Despite these episodes of infection, he experienced normal growth and development. The family medical history was remarkable in that an older brother and a cousin (the son of a maternal aunt) had suffered similar chronic infections, and one had died of chronic pneumonia caused by a gram-positive organism.

Physical Examination He appeared to be generally well. The skin was covered with scattered areas of crusted scabs described as an infected eczematoid rash. A Gram's stain of the rash revealed gram-positive cocci in clusters (*Staphylococcus*). Lymph nodes and liver were enlarged.

Laboratory Data The hemoglobin level was determined to be 9 g/dL, and the erythrocyte morphology was normal with slight hypochromia. The total white blood cell count was 33×10^9/L (28×10^9/L neutrophils). The neutrophils contained moderate toxic granulation and vacuoles. The platelet count was 427×10^9/L. Concentrations of serum immunoglobulins and complement components were all increased moderately.

Neutrophilia was consistently found on several occasions when earlier laboratory data were reviewed. Neutropenia was never documented. Studies of neutrophil migration and phagocytosis were normal. Oxidative metabolism in response to neutrophil stimulation was completely absent. Specifically, there was no postphagocytic increase in oxygen consumption; superoxide anion and hydrogen peroxide were not formed. Finally, neutrophils were unable to oxidize and kill *Staphylococcus* that had been phagocytized. Neutrophils from the mother were studied and on some assays performed at about 50% of normal capacity.

Discussion This patient exhibits characteristic features of the X-linked recessive form of chronic granulomatous disease of childhood, with severe and persistent infections caused by *Staphylococcus* organisms. Anemia and persistent neutrophilia are seen even when these patients are relatively free of infection. Neutrophils from these children are numerous, migrate normally, are capable of phagocytosis, and form phagocytic vesicles. The neutrophils of these patients, however, are unable to kill the phagocytized micro-organisms since they are unable to generate active oxygen metabolites such as superoxide anion and hydrogen peroxide. In some families, the X-linked nature of the inheritance pattern may be established by finding disease in male members of the maternal family and finding moderate defects in the mother.

CASE STUDY 2

History of Present Illness A 12-year-old girl was admitted with lobar pneumonia. She was perfectly well until 2 days before admission, when she developed fever and a cough. Over the previous 18 hours, her temperature had remained at approximately 104°F, and the cough was increasing in intensity. On one occasion, a sputum sample contained a few flecks of blood. In the past, she had experienced only the usual number of minor respiratory infections. She had no history of serious illness. Approximately 6 hours before admission, she began to breathe rapidly and her lips appeared blue.

Physical Examination She was acutely ill. Her temperature remained at 104°F; she was listless and slightly cyanotic. The patient exhibited shortness of breath and sweating, and complained of fatigue and muscle ache.

Laboratory Data The hemoglobin level was determined to be 14 g/dL. The total white blood cell count was 35×10^9/L (30×10^9/L neutrophils). Bands, metamyelocytes, and myelocytes were noted. The neutrophils contained marked toxic granulation; Döhle bodies and vacuoles were also noted. Many neutrophils contained tiny purple bodies that appeared to be gram-positive diplococci. Blood culture subsequently grew *Streptococcus pneumoniae*.

Discussion This child with lobar pneumonia exhibits the typical picture of a neutrophilic, leukemoid reaction to a bacterial infection. Both the absolute and relative neutrophil count were elevated with a marked increase in immature forms (bands, metamyelocytes, and myelocytes). Moreover, the alterations of neutrophil cytoplasm (toxic granulation, Döhle bodies and vacuoles) were characteristic of stress leukopoiesis. The presence of intracellular micro-organisms confirmed that this leukemoid reaction was caused by a bacterial infection. None of the other features are indicative of one specific condition. Additional causes that should be considered include hypersensitivity drug reactions, burns, and other inflammatory diseases such as rheumatoid arthritis.

Acknowledgment The coauthor acknowledges receipt of Transfusion Medicine Academic Award K07 HL01426 and Research Career Development Award K04 HD00255 from the National Institutes of Health.

REFERENCES

1. Brennan, JK, et al: Chemical mediators of granulopoieses: A review. Exp Hematol 8:441, 1980.
2. Quesenberry, PJ and Grosh, WW: A Surgeon's Guide to Hematopoietic Growth Factors. Ortho Biotech, CoMedica Inc., New York, 1992.
3. William, ME and Quesenberry, PJ: Hematopoietic growth factors. In Stass, SA (ed): Hematologic Pathology. Marcel Dekker, New York, 1991.
4. Miller, AM, et al: Modulation of granulopoiesis: Opposing roles of prostaglandins F and E. J Lab Clin Med 92:983, 1978.
5. Verma, DS, et al: Human leukocyte interferon preparation blocks granulopoietic differentiation. Blood 54:1423, 1979.
6. Broxmeyer, HE, et al: Specificity and modulation of the action of lactoferrin, a negative feedback regulator of myelopoiesis. Blood 55:324, 1980.

7. Abramson, JS, and Wheeler, JG: The Natural Immune System—The Neutrphil. Oxford University Press, Oxford, 1993.

8. Nathan, DG and Oski, FA: Hematology of Infancy and Childhood, ed 4. W B Saunders, Philadelphia, 1993, pp 882–951.

9. Krause, KH and Lew, D: Bacterial toxins and neutrophil activation. Semin Hematol 25:2, 1988.

10. Cartwright, GE, Athens, JW, and Wintrobe, MM: The kinetics of granulopoiesis in normal man. Blood 24:780, 1964.

11. Rosse, C, et al: Bone marrow cell populations of normal infants: The predominance of lymphocytes. J Lab Clin Med 89:1225, 1977.

12. Manroe, BL, et al: The neonatal blood count in health and disease: I. Reference values for neutrophilic cells. J Pediatr 95:89, 1979.

13. Christensen, RD, Bradley, PP, and Rothstein, G: The leukocyte left shift in clinical and experimental neonatal sepsis. J Pediatr 98:101, 1981.

14. Christensen, RD, et al: Granulocyte transfusion in neonates with bacterial infection, neutropenia, and depletion of mature marrow neutrophils. Pediatrics 70:1, 1982.

15. Bain, BJ and England, JM: Normal haematological values: Sex difference in neutrophil count. Br Med J 877:306, 1975.

16. Bain, BJ and England, JM: Variations in leucocyte count during menstrual cycle. Br Med J 2:473, 1975.

17. Caramihai, E, et al: Leukocyte count differences in healthy white and black children 1 to 4 years of age. Pediatrics 86:252, 1975.

18. Wright, PF, et al: Patterns of illness in the highly febrile young child: Epidemiologic, clinical and laboratory correlates. Pediatrics 67:694, 1981.

19. Morens, DM: WBC count and differential. Am J Dis Child 133:25, 1979.

20. Christensen, RD and Rothstein, G: Pitfalls in the interpretation of leukocyte counts of newborn infants. Am J Clin Pathol 72:608, 1979.

21. Walker, RI and Willemze, R: Neutrophil kinetics and the regulation of granulopoiesis. Rev Infect Dis 2:282, 1980.

22. Cawley, JC and Hayhoe, FGJ: The inclusions of the May-Hegglin anomaly and Döhle bodies in infection: An ultrastructural comparison. Br J Haematol 22:491, 1971.

23. McCall, C, et al: Functional characteristics of human toxic neutrophils. J Infect Dis 124:68, 1971.

24. McCall, CE, et al: Human toxic neutrophils: III. Metabolic characteristics. J Infect Dis 127:26, 1973.

25. Hill, HR, et al: Hyperactivity of neutrophil leukotactic responses during active bacterial infection. J Clin Invest 53:996, 1974.

26. van Epps, DE and Garcia, ML: Enhancement of neutrophil function as a result of prior exposure to chemotactic factor. J Clin Invest 66:167, 1980.

27. Becker, EL: Chemotaxis. J Allergy Clin Immunol 66:97, 1980.

28. O'Flaherty, IT and Ward, PA: Chemotactic factors and the neutrophil. Semin Hematol 16:163, 1979.

29. Schiffman, E: Leukocyte chemotaxis. Ann Rev Physiol 44:553, 1982.

30. Nelson, RD, et al: Chemotactic deactivation of human neutrophils: Possible relationship to stimulation of oxidative metabolism. Infect Immunol 23:283, 1979.

31. Gallin, JI and Wright, DG: Role of secretory events in modulating human neutrophil chemotaxis. J Clin Invest 62:1364, 1978.

32. Goetzl, EJ, et al: Specific inhibition of the polymorphonuclear leukocyte chemotactic response to hydroxy-fatty acid metabolites of arachidonic acid by methyl ester derivatives. J Clin Invest 63:1181, 1979.

33. Brozna, JP, et al: Chemotactic factor inactivators of human granulocytes. J Clin Invest 60:1280, 1977.

34. Ginsburg, I and Quie, PG: Modulation or human polymorphonuclear leukocyte chemotaxis by leukocyte extracts, bacterial products, inflammatory exudates, and polyelectrolytes. Inflammation 4;301, 1980.

35. Scribner, DJ and Farhney, D: Neutrophil receptors for IgG and complement: Their roles in the attachment and ingestion phases of phagocytosis. J Immunol 116:892, 1976.

36. Weissman, G, Smolen, JE, and Korchak, HM: Release of inflammatory mediators from stimulated neutrophils. N Engl J Med 303:27, 1980.

37. Ignarro, LJ, Lint TF, and George, WJ: Hormonal control of lysosomal enzyme release from human neutrophils. J Exp Med 139:1395, 1974.

38. Bainton, DF: Sequential degranulation of the two types of polymorphonuclear leukocyte granules during phagocytosis of microorganisms. J Cell Biol 58:24, 1973.

39. Jensen, MS and Bainton, DF: Temporal changes in pH within the phagocytic vacuole of the polymorphonuclear neutrophilic leukocyte. J Cell Biol 56:379, 1973.

40. Jacques, YV and Bainton, DF: Changes in pH within the phagocytic vacuoles of human neutrophils and monocytes. Lab Invest 39:179, 1978.

41. Weisdorf, DJ, Craddock, PR, and Jacob, HS: Glycogenolysis versus glucose transport in human granulocytes: Differential activation in phagocytosis and chemotaxis. Blood 60:888, 1982.

42. Badior, BM: Oxygen-dependent microbial killing by phagocytes. N Engl J Med 298:659, 1978.

43. DeChatelet, LR: Initiation of the respiration burst in human polymorphonuclear neutrophils: A critical review. J Reticuloendothel Soc 24:73, 1978.

44. Klebanoff, SJ: Antimicrobial mechanisms in neutrophilic polymorphonuclear leukocytes. Semin Hematol 12:117, 1975.

45. Stenson, WF and Parker, CW: Metabolism of arachidonic acid in ionophore-stimulated neutrophils. J Clin Invest 64:1457, 1979.

46. Rister, M and Baehner RL: The alteration of superoxide dismutase, catalase, glutathione peroxidase and NAD(P)H cytochrome C reductase in guinea pig polymorphonuclear leukocytes and alveolar macrophages during hyperoxia. J Clin Invest 58:1174, 1976.

47. Higgins, CP, et al: Polymorphonuclear leukocyte species differs in the disposal of hydrogen peroxide (H_2O_2). Proc Soc Exp Biol Med 158:478, 1978.

48. Shoenfeld, Y, et al: The mechanism of benign hereditary neutropenia. Arch Intern Med 142:797, 1987.

49. Howard, MW, Strauss, RG, and Johnston, RG, Jr: Infections in patients with neutropenia. Am J Dis Child 131:788, 1977.

50. Dale, DC, et al: Comparison of agents producing neutrophilic leukocytosis in man: Hydrocortisone, prednisone, endotoxin and etiocholanolone. J Clin Invest 56:808, 1975.

51. Conway, LT, et al: Natural history of primary autoimmune neutropenia in infancy. Pediatrics 79:728, 1987.

52. Lalezari, R and Radel, E: Neutrophil-specific antigens: Immunology and clinical significance. Semin Hematol 11:281, 1974.

53. Kostmann, R: Infantile genetic agranulocytosis. Acta Paediatr Scand 64:362, 1975.

54. Zucker-Franklin, D, L'Esperance, P, and Good, RA: Congenital neutropenia: An intrinsic cell defect demonstrated by electron microscopy of soft agar colonies. Blood 49:425, 1977.

55. Amato, D, Freedman, MH, and Saunders, EF: Granulopoiesis in severe congenital neutropenia. Blood 47:531, 1976.

56. Bonilla, MA, et al: Effects of recombinant colony-stimulating factor on neutropenia in patients with congenital agranulocytosis. N Engl J Med 320:1574, 1989.

57. Pincus, SH, Boxer, LA, and Stossel, TP: Chronic neutropenia in childhood: Analysis of 16 cases and a review of the literature. Am J Med 61:849, 1976.

58. Krill, CE Jr, Smith, HD, and Mauer, AM: Chronic idiopathic granulocytopenia. N Engl J Med 270:699, 1964.

59. Bohinjec, J: Myelokathexis: Chronic neutropenia with hyperplastic bone marrow and hypersegmented neutrophils in two siblings. Blut 42:191, 1980.

60. Andrews, RB, et al: Some immunological and haematological aspects of human cyclic neutropenia. Scand J Haematol 27:97, 1979.

61. Guerry, D, IV, et al: Periodic hematopoiesis in human cyclic neutropenia. J Clin Invest 52:3220, 1973.

62. Beard, MEJ, et al: Fanconi's anaemia. Q J Med 42:403, 1973.

63. Inoue, S, et al: Dyskeratosis congenita with pancytopenia (another constitutional anemia). Am J Dis Child 126:389, 1973.

64. Shwachman, H, et al: The syndrome of pancreatic insufficiency and bone marrow dysfunction. J Pediatr 65:645, 1965.

65. Cappelletti, P and Lippi, U: Hereditary myeloperoxidase deficiency: A rare condition? Diagnostic possibilities of a differential white cell autoanalyzer (Hemalog-D). Haematologica 68:736, 1983.

66. Nauseef, WM, Root, RK and Malech, HL: Biochemical and immunologic analysis of hereditary myeloperoxidase deficiency. J Clin Invest 71:1297, 1983.

67. Kitahara, M, et al: Hereditary myeloperoxidase deficiency. Blood 57:888, 1981.

68. Rosen, H and Klebanoff, SJ: Chemiluminescence and superoxide production by myeloperoxidase-deficient leukocytes. J Clin Invest 58:50, 1976.

69. Root, RK, Rosenthal, AS, and Balestra, DJ: Abnormal bactericidal metabolic, and lysosomal functions of Chédiak-Higashi syndrome leukocytes. J Clin Invest 51:649, 1972.

70. Oliver, JM: Cell biology of leukocyte abnormalities: Membrane and cytoskeletal function in normal and defective cells: A review. Am J Pathol 93:221, 1978.

71. Tauber, AI, et al: Chronic granulomatous disease: A syndrome of phagocyte oxidase deficiencies. Medicine 62:286, 1983.

72. Segal, AW: The electron transport chain of the microbial oxidase of phagocytic cells and its involvement in the molecular pathology of chronic granulomatosis disease. J Clin Invest 83:1785, 1989.

73. Galin, JI, et al: Recent advances in chronic granulomatous disease. Ann Intern Med 99:657, 1983.

74. Parkos, CA, et al: Absence of both the 91KD and 22KD sub-units of human neutrophil cytochrome b in two genetic forms of chronic granulomatous disease. Blood 73:1416, 1989.

75. Cooper, MR, et al: Complete deficiency of leukocyte glucose-6-phosphate dehydrogenase and defective bactericidal activity. J Clin Invest 51:769, 1972.

76. Holmes, B, et al: Chronic granulomatous disease in females. A deficiency of leukocyte glutathione peroxidase. N Engl J Med 283:217, 1970.

77. Roos, D, et al: Protection of phagocytic leukocytes by endogenous glutathione: Studies in a family with glutathione reductase deficiency. Blood 53:851, 1979.

78. Johnson, CA, et al: Functional and metabolic studies of polymorphonuclear leukocytes in the congenital Pelger-Huët anomaly. Blood 55:466, 1980.

79. Cawley, JC and Hayhoe, FGJ: The inclusions of the May-Hegglin anomaly and Döhle bodies of infection: An ultrastructional comparison. Br J Haematol 22:491, 1972.

QUESTIONS

1. The enzymatic contents of primary (azurophilic) granules include:
   a. NADPH oxidase and lactoferrin
   b. Cytochrome b and collagenase
   c. Myeloperoxidase and lysozyme
   d. Alkaline phosphatase and gelatinase

2. Directional migration toward a gradient stimulated by a chemoattractant is referred to as:
   a. Chemotaxis
   b. Random mobility
   c. Opsonization
   d. Chemokinesis

3. The marking of an invading microbe with IgG and complement to facilitate recognition is referred to as:
   a. Chemokinesis
   b. Opsonization
   c. Phagolysosome fusion
   d. Signal transduction

4. Which sequence reflects the *correct* order for phagocytosis?
   a. Release of cytoplasmic granules; binding of particle; ingestion; fusion of phagolysosome
   b. Ingestion; binding of particles; fusion of phagolysosome; release of cytoplasmic granules
   c. Binding of particle; ingestion; fusion of phagolysosome; release of cytoplasmic granules
   d. Fusion of phagolysosome; binding of particle; release of cytoplasmic granules; ingestion

5. In oxygen-dependent killing, the enzyme responsible for mediating the production of active oxygen metabolites during the respiratory burst is:
   a. Myeloperoxidase
   b. Lysozyme
   c. Lactoferrin
   d. NADPH oxidase

6. The two most important biochemical products of the respiratory burst that are involved with particle digestion during active phagocytosis are:
   a. Lactoferrin and gelatinase
   b. Superoxide dismutase and catalase
   c. Glutathione peroxidase and copper-zinc enzymes
   d. Superoxide anion and hydrogen peroxide

7. The morphological characteristic(s) associated with Chédiak-Higashi syndrome is/are:
   a. Giant lysosomal granules
   b. Hypersegmented agranular neutrophils with vacuolization
   c. Prominent dark-staining granules and pyknotic nuclei
   d. Pale blue inclusions in cytoplasm of neutrophils and giant platelets

8. The defect in chronic granulomatous disease is attributed to:
   a. Delayed degranulation caused by interference from aggregated lysosomal granules
   b. Deficiency in myeloperoxidase enzyme
   c. Deficiency or defect in cytochrome b
   d. Arrested maturation of neutrophils at the promyelocyte stage

9. Identify the disease characteristic(s) associated with Chédiak-Higashi syndrome:

a. Partial albinism and mild bleeding tendencies
b. Recurrent viral superinfections and candidiasis
c. Hypopigmentation of skin and chronic swollen lymph nodes
d. Periodic pneumonia that may result in lesions called pneumatoceles

10. Pelger-Huët anomaly may be characterized by:
a. Large neutrophils with hypersegmentation of the nucleus with more than six lobes
b. Dark-staining, coarse granules in cytoplasm of neutrophils, eosinophils, basophils, and monocytes
c. Pale blue inclusions of the cytoplasm of neutrophils and giant platelets
d. Hyposegmentation of nucleus with most neutrophils bilobed or monolobed

ANSWERS

1. **c** (p 266) (Table 16–1)
2. **a** (p 270)
3. **b** (p 270)
4. **c** (p 271)
5. **d** (pp 271)
6. **d** (p 271, 276)
7. **a** (p 276)
8. **c** (p 277)
9. **a** (p 276)
10. **d** (p 278)

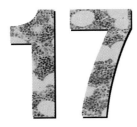

Reactive Lymphocytosis and Infectious Mononucleosis

Joe Marty, MS, MT(ASCP)

Objectives

At the end of this chapter, the learner should be able to:
1 Define lymphocytosis.
2 List several disorders that present with lymphocytosis.
3 Distinguish between absolute and relative lymphocytosis.
4 Distinguish between benign and malignant lymphocytosis.
5 Recognize morphological features of infectious mononucleosis and other reactive lymphocytoses.
6 List clinical features of infectious mononucleosis.
7 Utilize laboratory results for distinguishing infectious mononucleosis from other lymphocytoses.

DEFINITION OF LYMPHOCYTOSIS

Lymphocytosis is present when there is an excess of lymphocytes in the peripheral blood. Absolute lymphocyte counts decrease with age. In infants and young children, greater than 10.0×10^9 lymphocytes per liter represents lymphocytosis. In adults, greater than 4.0×10^9 lymphocytes per liter is defined as lymphocytosis. The absolute lymphocyte count is determined by multiplying the percent of lymphocytes (obtained from the peripheral blood differential) times the total leukocyte count (obtained from the complete blood count [CBC]).

Relative lymphocytosis refers to an increase in the percentage of lymphocytes when the absolute lymphocyte count is within normal range. This may occur when other hematopoietic elements are decreased, that is, in neutropenia, in which lymphocytes are not affected.

The term *reactive* lymphocytes is used to describe transformed or benign lymphocytes. The term *atypical* should *not* be used interchangeably with reactive because, in pathology, atypical is used to describe malignant-appearing cells. Other terms that have been used to describe the spectrum of reactive lymphocytes include immunocytes, transformed lymphocytes, immunoblasts, plasmacytoid lymphocytes, Turk and Downey cells. Reactive lymphocytes occur in normal patients, but usually account for less than 10% of the total lymphocytes present. In order to maintain consistency with laboratory reporting, each laboratory should have criteria and normal ranges for reactive lymphocytes in its procedure manual. Control slides with reactive lymphocytes should be reviewed on a regular basis with the staff to ensure uniformity in the reporting of reactive lymphocytes.

LYMPHOCYTE MORPHOLOGY

Reactive lymphocytes and normal lymphocytes (Table 17–1) vary in size, shape, and immunophenotypic markers (polyclonal). The cells do *not* originate from one precursor cell or clone. In contrast, lymphocytes in malignant disorders are similar in size, shape, (monomorphous), and immunophenotype because they originate from the same malignant clone (monoclonal). Lymphomas may vary in size depending on the particular malignancy. However, for any one malignancy, the size and appearance tend to be constant.

Reactive lymphocytes range in size from 9 to 30 μm. (Figure 17–1 illustrates the size variation that can be seen with reactive lymphocytes.) Resting small lymphocytes tend to be much smaller than reactive lymphocytes, range in size from 8 to 12 μm, and are similar in size to the upper right lymphocyte in Figure 17–1 (small arrow).

The ratio of the nuclear area to the visible cytoplasmic rim (N:C ratio) varies with reactive lymphocytes. One of the most important features in distinguishing reactive lymphocytes is the abundant amount of cytoplasm present when compared to smaller resting lymphocytes. Resting small lymphocytes have relatively little cytoplasm, whereas reactive lymphocytes have moderate amounts of cytoplasm. In Figure 17–1, three lymphocytes are present. In the center of the field is a large reactive lymphocyte with abundant cytoplasm (large arrow). The cytoplasm is usually pale blue with occasional azurophilic granules. A significant morphological feature of reactive lymphocytes is the uneven staining of the cytoplasm. With reactive lymphocytes, peripheral portions of the cytoplasm often stain darker blue than areas of the cytoplasm closer to the nucleus. Also, the cytoplasmic border is usually round, but it may be indented, as might be visualized by looking down at a ballerina's skirt.

The nucleus in reactive lymphocytes may be round, indented, or lobulated (Fig. 17–2). In reactive conditions, the appearance of the nuclear chromatin in the

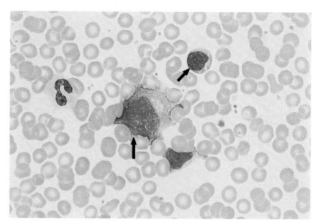

FIGURE 17–1 Three lymphocytes are present, one with abundant cytoplasm (low N:C ratio) and two with moderate amounts of cytoplasm from a patient with infectious mononucleosis. Note the variation in chromatin coarseness. The larger reactive or reactive-appearing lymphocyte has prominent cytoplasm indentations (*center arrow*).

lymphocyte population is variable and not monotonous. Generally, the nuclear chromatin is coarse or clumped and prominent clumping or coarseness of the chromatin similar to plasma cells may occur. Figure 17–3 illustrates a small "plasmacytoid" lymphocyte with prominent chromatin clumping, perinuclear halo, and an eccentric nucleus similar in appearance to a plasma cell. The nucleus in resting small lymphocytes is round and less variable. The chromatin may vary in coarseness, but not to the extent seen with reactive lymphocytes.

Nucleoli may be present in reactive lymphocytes. Such reactive lymphocytes can be differentiated from lymphoblasts or myeloblasts by having more abundant cytoplasm and a clumped chromatin pattern. Figure 17–4 illustrates a reactive lymphocyte with a prominent nucleolus, often referred to as an *immunoblast*, which is a descriptive morphological term and has no bearing on the lymphocyte type. Nucleoli are not present in resting small lymphocytes.

TABLE 17–1	**Lymphocyte Morphologies**	
	Reactive Lymphocyte	**Resting Small Lymphocyte***
Size	Large (9–30 μm)	Small (8–12 μm)
N:C Ratio[†]	Low to moderate	High to moderate
Cytoplasm	Abundant	Scant
	Colorless to dark blue	Colorless to light blue
Nucleus	Round to irregular	Round
Chromatin	Coarse to moderately fine[‡]	Coarse
Nucleoli	Absent to distinct	Absent
Typing	Polyclonal	Polyclonal

*Normal peripheral blood may contain a few medium-sized natural killer cells that are larger than resting small lymphocytes but smaller than large reactive lymphocytes.
[†]The N:C ratio is the ratio of the nuclear area to the visible cytoplasmic rim.
[‡]The chromatin is not as fine as that seen in blast cells.

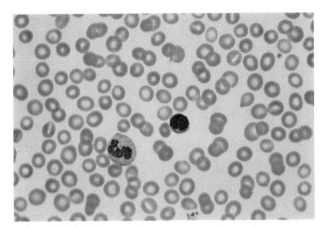

FIGURE 17-2   Lymphocyte with nuclear indentation.

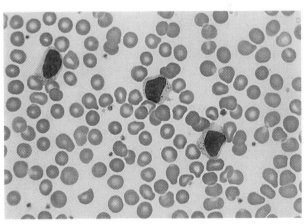

FIGURE 17-4   A large reactive lymphocyte with a prominent nucleolus (Immunoblast).

A few granules may be seen in the cytoplasm of lymphocytes (Fig. 17–5). These granules are azurophilic, appear lilac or purple, and are larger than the fine pink secondary granules present in neutrophils. When there are many lymphocytes with azurophilic granules and abundant cytoplasm, "large granular lymphocytosis" must be considered (Fig. 17–6). In contrast, the cytoplasm of monocytes contains many small granules and has a "ground-glass" appearance. Auer rods are *never* seen in lymphocytes.

In order to make a correct morphological evaluation, blood smears need to be made from a fingerstick or fresh tube of blood anticoagulated with EDTA. The cells need to be well stained, and the observer should look at areas of the smear that are neither too thick nor too thin. Improper pH of the Wright's stain buffer makes it difficult to evaluate nuclear and cytoplasmic features by altering the staining characteristics of these structures.

Morphological criteria alone usually enable one to distinguish reactive lymphocytosis from malignant disorders. When there is ambiguity, clinical history, cell typing, and serological findings will help. If nec-

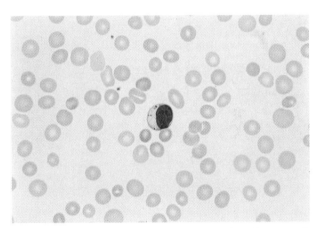

FIGURE 17-5   A small, mature-appearing lymphocyte with azurophilic granules.

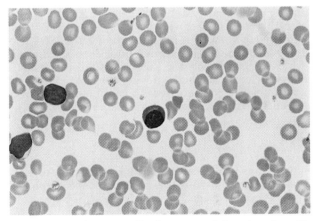

FIGURE 17-3   A small plasmacytoid lymphocyte with coarse chromatin and an eccentric nucleus.

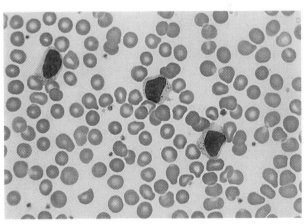

FIGURE 17-6   Reactive-appearing lymphocytes with prominent granulation from a patient with large granular lymphocytosis.

TABLE 17–2 Causes of Reactive Lymphocytosis

Viral
Adenovirus
Chickenpox
Cytomegalovirus
EBV (infectious mononucleosis)
Hepatitis
Herpes simplex
Herpes zoster
Human immunodeficiency virus (HIV)
Influenza
Paramyxovirus (mumps)
Rubella (measles)

Bacterial
Brucellosis
Paratyphoid fever
Pertussis (whooping cough)
Tuberculosis
Typhoid fever

Drug reactions
During recovery from acute infections (especially in children)

Miscellaneous
Acute infectious lymphocytosis
Allergic reactions
Autoimmune diseases
Hyperthyroidism
Malnutrition
Rickets
Syphilis
Toxoplasmosis

TABLE 17–3 Malignant Conditions That May Be Confused with Reactive Lymphocytosis

Acute Lymphocytic Leukemias
L-1
L-2
L-3

Acute Myelocytic Leukemias
M-3m
M-5a

Chronic Leukemias
Chronic lymphocytic leukemia (CLL)
Hairy-cell leukemia
Lymphocytosis of large granular lymphocytes
Prolymphocytic leukemia

Leukemic Phase of Lymphoma
Follicular lymphoma (typically small cleaved cell)
Mantle cell lymphoma
Other non-Hodgkin's lymphomas (e.g., large cell)

Miscellaneous
Adult T-cell leukemia/lymphoma (ATL/L)
Mycosis fungoides, Sézary syndrome
Plasma cell leukemia

essary, a bone marrow or lymph node biopsy may lead to the correct diagnosis. The most common causes of reactive lymphocytosis are shown in Table 17–2. Malignant conditions that may be confused with reactive lymphocytosis are listed in Table 17–3.

CAUSES OF REACTIVE LYMPHOCYTOSIS

Infectious Mononucleosis

History

In 1907, Turk described clinical symptoms in several patients who probably suffered from infectious mononucleosis caused by Epstein-Barr virus (EBV) infection.[1] Reactive lymphocyte morphology and clinical symptoms were correlated in 1920 by Sprunt who named the syndrome "infectious mononucleosis."[2] Downey, in 1923, described in further detail the unusual lymphocyte morphology associated with infectious mononucleosis.[3] Although morphology is still important, Downey's descriptive terminology of morphology is seldom used today. Infectious mononucleosis is an historical term. We now know that the large mononuclear cells originally described in infectious mononucleosis are lymphocytes and *not* monocytes.

In 1932 Paul noticed that sera from patients with infectious mononucleosis contained antibodies against sheep erythrocytes.[4] This discovery was the basis for the Monospot test (Ortho Pharmaceuticals). This contemporary test is the most popular and simplest method available for measuring IgM heterophil antibodies. Heterophil antibodies are antibodies that also react with cells of other species. (In particular, the IgM antibodies react with sheep and horse erythrocytes. The antibodies are not absorbed by guinea pig kidney in the Monospot test, and thus, if present, agglutinate horse erythrocytes.)

The DNA virus responsible for infectious mononucleosis was first observed in lymphoblasts cultured from patients with Burkitt's lymphoma[5] (see Chap. 23). This virus is now known as the Epstein-Barr virus (EBV). Convincing evidence that EBV was the causative agent for infectious mononucleosis was provided by Henle in 1967 by a chance observation.[6] He was able to establish a lymphocyte cell line from the blood of a laboratory worker who was infected with EBV and managed to show by serological studies that EBV was responsible for infectious mononucleosis. Additional evidence supporting the role of EBV in infectious mononucleosis has been provided by the detection of EBV nucleic acid sequences in lymphoid tissue from patients with infectious mononucleosis.[7,8]

Clinical Manifestations

Infectious mononucleosis is more commonly present in young individuals, the peak incidence being at about 20 years of age. The virus enters the body orally through the lymphoid tissue in the pharynx and infects B lymphocytes. The most consistent initial symptoms are sore throat, dysphagia, general malaise, and fatigue. The severity of the sore throat pain leads to difficulty in swallowing and anorexia. Other symptoms include fever, headache, sweating, and chills. Occasionally, individuals may have an autoimmune hemolytic anemia because of antibodies formed to the i red cell antigen (see Chap. 14).

Multiple organ involvement with related symptoms may be present in infectious mononucleosis. Enlargement of the anterior cervical lymph nodes is another physical finding during the first week. After a week or two, the swelling usually subsides. The nodes are firm but *not* tender or warm. At least one half of patients demonstrate a palpable spleen during the course of infection and, rarely, splenic rupture may occur. Hypersplenism may lead to mild anemia and/or thrombocytopenia. Hepatomegaly may be detected in up to 25% of patients with infectious mononucleosis. Liver enzymes and bilirubin levels may be elevated because of the liver involvement.

Infectious mononucleosis is uncommon in older adults and therefore the differential diagnosis of lymphocytosis is influenced by the age of the patient. For example, in a 50-year-old person with increasing numbers of benign-looking lymphocytes, the diagnosis of chronic lymphocytic leukemia (CLL) is more likely than infectious mononucleosis; however, in a child or young adult, CLL is extremely rare.

Differential Diagnosis

The differential diagnosis for infectious mononucleosis includes a variety of entities, listed in Tables 17–2 and 17–3. The differential may be narrowed considerably by evaluation of a blood smear and serologic findings. The skilled morphologist should be able to readily differentiate the reactive lymphocytes seen in infectious mononucleosis from malignant cells seen in leukemia or lymphoma. Cytomegalovirus, rubella, hepatitis, and other viral illnesses may have reactive lymphocytes and may require additional serological findings to distinguish them from EBV infection. Acute streptococcal pharyngitis, diphtheria, and other bacterial infections are identifiable by culture and the lymphocytes usually do not have the typical morphology seen in viral infections. Classical reactive lymphocytes and definitive serologic findings may not always be present, and therefore it may be difficult in some instances to distinguish between infectious mononucleosis and other processes. In those rare cases, additional studies, such as lymph node biopsy, may be necessary.

Treatment, Clinical Course, and Prognosis

Treatment of infectious mononucleosis is mostly symptomatic, with some patients requiring bedrest. Adrenocorticosteroids may be used for treatment in patients with anemia, thrombocytopenia, and neurologic complications. Antibiotics are not useful unless there are complications such as streptococcal pharyngitis. The fatality rate is approximately 1 per 3000 cases.[9] Complete recovery usually occurs within 2 months, and recurrences are extremely rare. It should be noted that not all children who have acquired immunity had a prior history or clinical symptoms of infectious mononucleosis. EBV infections in immunocompromised patients may be life-threatening. In view of the increasing incidence of patients with immunodeficiencies, the morbidity rate is likely to increase.

Cytomegalovirus Infection

Cytomegalovirus (CMV) belongs to the herpesvirus family and is endemic worldwide. The virus may be transmitted by oral, respiratory, and sexual means or by blood transfusion and organ transplantation. Patients with CMV infection may have a recurrence or reactivation of a latent infection such as seen in herpes simplex infection, or may be reinfected with a different CMV strain. CMV infection is the most common cause of heterophil-negative infectious mononucleosis. The diagnosis is made by demonstrating the presence of IgM antibodies to CMV or by shell vial tissue cultures.

Clinical Manifestations

In most immunocompetent individuals, CMV infection is usually asymptomatic. The clinical manifestations reflect the organ(s) of involvement. When CMV infection occurs in previously healthy individuals, the symptoms mimic EBV infection. Symptoms include fever, sore throat, splenomegaly, lymphadenopathy, and myalgia. Morphological changes in lymphocytes are indistinguishable from those seen in EBV infection. Because of liver involvement, mild to moderate elevation of liver function tests is common.

In immunocompromised individuals, CMV infection can be life-threatening. Since CMV infection is endemic, parenterally acquired infection from transfusions is a concern, especially with the increase in the numbers of individuals who are immunocompromised from chemotherapy, immunosuppressive drugs, or HIV infection.

Other Viral Infections

Any viral infection has the potential to elicit an immune response resulting in absolute lymphocytosis. Besides infectious mononucleosis, lymphocytes that appear "stimulated" or reactive may be seen in CMV and infectious hepatitis. CMV infection is the most frequent cause of a heterophil-negative (Monospot) mononucleosis-like syndrome. With a negative Monospot test, other viral infections, for example, rubella, human immunodeficiency virus (HIV),[10,11] herpesvirus-6,[12] and the adenoviruses should be considered.

Bacterial Infections

Lymphocytosis in bacterial infections occurs more commonly in chronic infections and during the recovery period following acute infections. The organisms most often responsible include *Brucella, Mycobacterium tuberculosis*, and spirochetes. Marked lymphocytosis with mature-appearing lymphocytes is seen in children with pertussis (whooping cough), in which absolute lymphocyte counts exceeding 50×10^9 cells per liter may be seen in 4% of the patients.[13] Morphologically, these cells appear similar to those seen in CLL and small lymphocytic lymphoma. In pertussis, immunologic marker studies reveal that the lymphocytes are predominantly helper T cells.[14] Prominent lymphadenopathy, which may be present in lymphoma or EBV infection, is also unusual in children with pertussis or infectious lymphocytosis.

Malignant Conditions

Table 17–3 lists malignant disorders that may be confused with reactive lymphocytosis. In general, the malignant cells in leukemia and lymphomas are monotonous in appearance and therefore are morphologically different from the reactive lymphocytes seen in benign conditions. Malignant cells in leukemias and lymphomas are monoclonal when immunophenotypically analyzed.

The morphology of lymphoblasts seen in acute lymphoblastic leukemia is different from that of reactive lymphocytes. Acute lymphoblastic leukemia is morphologically classified as L-1, L-2, or L-3, depending on the morphology of the cells (see Chap. 18). In contrast to reactive lymphocytes, blast cells in L-2 leukemia have fine chromatin and prominent nucleoli (arrow, Fig. 17–7). The cells in L-1 leukemia are monotonous in appearance and do not have as much cytoplasm as do reactive lymphocytes (Fig. 17–8). The N:C ratio is much higher in L-1 leukemia cells than in reactive lymphocytes. In L-3 leukemias (Fig. 17–9), abundant cytoplasmic vacuoles are present that are lacking in reactive lymphocytes. The cells present in prolymphocytic leukemia may also be confused with reactive lymphocytes. Figure 17–10 shows the prominent, usually single, nucleoli that are present in prolymphocytic leukemia. Reactive lymphocytes have more abundant cytoplasm and less prominent nucleoli than prolymphocytes.

Severe cytopenias that occur in acute leukemias are infrequent in benign lymphocytosis. With anemia or

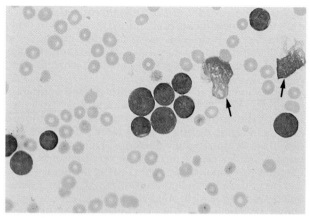

FIGURE 17–8 L-1 leukemia. These L-1 lymphoblasts have a high N:C ratio (scant cytoplasm), fine chromatin, and indistinct nucleoli. Except for the fine chromatin, note the similarity to mature lymphocytes. These cells should not be confused with reactive lymphocytes! Note the large "smudge cells" (arrows).

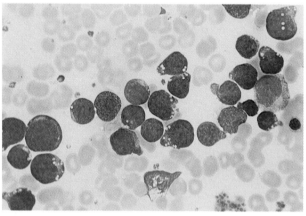

FIGURE 17–9 L-3 leukemia. Note the abundant cytoplasmic vacuoles and clumped chromatin.

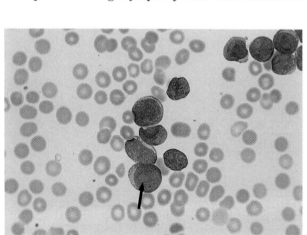

FIGURE 17–7 L-2 leukemia. The L-2 lymphoblasts have fine chromatin with a moderate amount of cytoplasm and nucleoli. Note the single prominent nucleolus in one of the lymphoblasts.

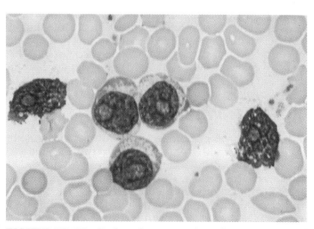

FIGURE 17–10 Prolymphocytes with moderate amounts of cytoplasm and prominent nucleoli.

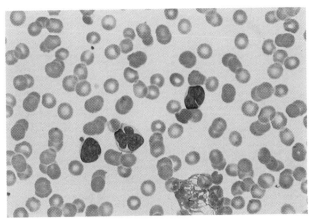

FIGURE 17–11 Lymphocytes from a patient with follicular small cleaved-cell lymphoma. Note the prominent nuclear clefting.

severe thrombocytopenia, the diagnosis of leukemia must be considered.

Patients with lymphoma may have a leukemic phase with circulating malignant cells. Except for the large-cell lymphomas, circulating lymphoma cells may easily be distinguished from reactive lymphocytes. Figure 17–11 shows the nuclear clefting seen in the leukemic phase of follicular small-cleaved-cell lymphoma. Fortunately, in large-cell lymphoma, malignant cells in the peripheral blood are rare. Prominent generalized lymphadenopathy is unusual in infectious mononucleosis but may occur in non-Hodgkin's lymphoma and Hodgkin's disease.

Miscellaneous Disorders

A poorly described entity with marked lymphocytosis called *infectious lymphocytosis* may occur in children. Its cause is unknown, but it is thought to be viral. The lymphocytes appear mature and are very similar to the lymphocytes seen in pertussis and CLL. Cleaved or convoluted nuclei are present.[15] Counts as high as 117×10^9 cells per liter have been reported,[16] and eosinophilia may be present.

Toxoplasma gondii is a protozoan infection that causes milder lymphocytosis than that seen in infectious mononucleosis. In toxoplasmosis, the lymph nodes are enlarged and have characteristic histologic features including reactive germinal centers and clusters of histiocytes. Patients are febrile and, rarely, there may be splenomegaly. In contrast to infectious mononucleosis, in this infection sore throat is not a prominent feature. Serologic tests are used to confirm the diagnosis.

Recently a disorder termed *chronic mononucleosis syndrome* was thought to be an unusual presentation of infectious mononucleosis. This disorder is now called *chronic fatigue syndrome*. It resembles infectious mononucleosis but differs in that patients have a prolonged course with chronic fatigue as the chief complaint. Its exact etiology is unknown.[17]

Relative lymphocytosis may occur in thyrotoxicosis and other disorders associated with neutropenia.

LABORATORY EXAMINATION

A variety of laboratory procedures may help in the correct diagnosis of patients with absolute lymphocytosis. A complete blood count (CBC), serology, and microbiologic culture are often performed. Of these procedures, the CBC with differential and serologic studies are the most useful.

Proper evaluation of the peripheral blood smear is crucial for the correct differential diagnosis in patients with absolute lymphocytosis. Especially in infectious mononucleosis, reactive lymphocytes are prominent and should easily be identified by the experienced observer. Figure 17–1 shows a reactive lymphocyte with abundant cytoplasm (low N:C ratio) and indented cytoplasmic borders (large arrow). The less experienced observer may mistake these unusual-appearing reactive lymphocytes for monocytes or blasts. However, as seen in Figure 17–12, monocytes typically have linear condensation of chromatin, whereas blasts (see Fig. 17–7) have chromatin strands that are more fine and evenly dispersed.

The lymphoblasts in L-2 leukemia or monoblasts in M-5a leukemia, a category of acute myelocytic leukemia, may also be mistaken for reactive lymphocytes. Figure 17–13 illustrates M-5a, monoblastic leukemia. Monoblasts have a low N:C ratio but fine chromatin is present as well as prominent nucleoli. Figure 17–7 shows the fine chromatin and prominent nucleoli (arrow) present in an L-2 lymphoblast. With reactive lymphocytes, a careful review of the cell morphology will reveal that, overall, the chromatin is not fine enough for the cells to be classified as blasts and that the overall morphology is variable and *not* monotonous as seen in leukemias.

Serologic tests play a critical role in establishing the diagnosis in patients with absolute lymphocytosis. In

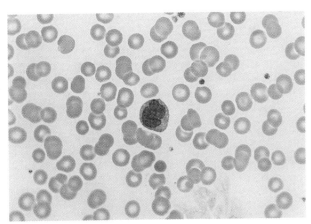

FIGURE 17–12 This monocyte has very fine granular cytoplasm, cerebriform nucleus, linear condensation of chromatin, and no nucleolus.

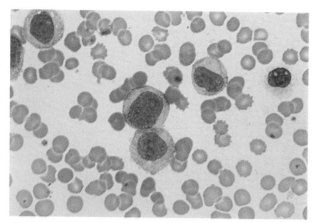

FIGURE 17–13 M-5a leukemia. These monoblasts have abundant cytoplasm (low N:C ratio), fine chromatin with some chromatin clumping, and prominent nucleoli.

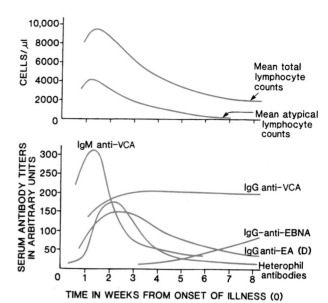

FIGURE 17–14 Time-course relationship between heterophil antibodies, various anti-Epstein-Barr virus antibodies, and the mean total and reactive lymphocyte counts. VCA = viral capsid antigen, EBNA = Epstein-Barr nuclear antigen, EA = early antigen, D = diffuse component. (From Lee, RG et al: Wintrobe's Clinical Hematology, ed 9, p 1658. Lea & Febiger, Philadelphia, 1993, with permission.)

the proper clinical setting, a positive Monospot (heterophil antibody) test with reactive lymphocytes in the peripheral blood (see Fig. 17–1) is diagnostic of infectious mononucleosis. A variety of antibodies formed by humoral responses may be measured when it is necessary to further elucidate the etiology of lymphocytosis in difficult cases or in cases where the Monospot test is negative (Table 17–4).

In the first week of viral infections, IgM antibodies are formed against viral capsid antigens. During the second week, as the immunologic response matures, IgG antibodies are formed. Figure 17–14 illustrates the pattern of the immunologic response and lymphocytosis that can be expected in patients with infectious mononucleosis. A rise in titer should be demonstrated by comparing acute and convalescent sera. Also, by using enzyme-linked immunosorbentassay (ELISA) techniques, antibodies to CMV and hepatitis can be measured. Finally, viral cultures may be performed.

The Monospot test is most frequently used for detection of infectious mononucleosis because the rise in titer of heterophil antibodies parallels the rise in titer of the more specific EBV antibodies. The Monospot test is much quicker, easier to use, and less expensive than

measuring viral-specific antibodies. If the Monospot test is initially negative, it should be repeated in 1 week if infectious mononucleosis is suspected. Serum may be analyzed for antibodies to specific EBV antigens; antibodies to CMV and hepatitis may be measured and viral cultures may be performed. Figure 17–15 diagrams some of the possible testing strategies.

In cases in which malignancy is being considered, lymphocytes may be further characterized by immunophenotyping. With leukemias and lymphomas, typing usually reveals a monoclonal cell population. Although it is the B cell that is infected by the EBV, most of the reactive lymphocytes in infectious mononucleosis are polyclonal T cells.

TABLE 17–4 Summary of Antibody Tests Useful in the Infectious Mononucleosis Differential Diagnosis

Antigen	Test Used	Description	Clinical Significance
Heterophil	Monospot	Antibodies to a variety of antigens	Appears late in the first week; detected with Monospot test; transient
EBV-VCA(IgM)	ELISA	IgM antibody to viral capsid antigen	Detectable in first week of infection; earliest detectable antibody; declines rapidly after second week
EBV-VCA(IgG)	ELISA	IgG antibody to viral capsid antigen	Detectable approximately 7 days after exposure; levels persist for life; responsible for immunity
EBNA	ELISA	Antibody to EBV nuclear antigen	Appears late in first month of infection and persists for life; may indicate past infection
EBV-EA	ELISA	Antibody to EBV early antigen complex	Seen in <5% of normal, healthy subjects; may indicate EBV-carrier state

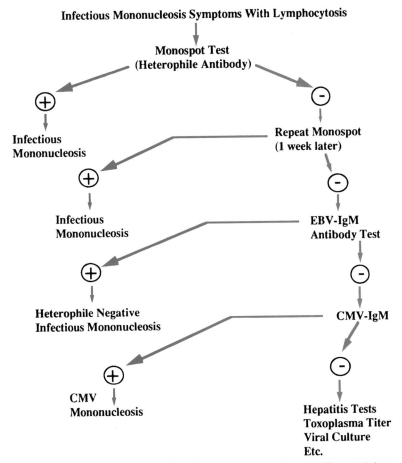

FIGURE 17-15 Testing strategies for infectious mononucleosis differential diagnosis.

CASE STUDY

A 13-year-old girl went to her physician because of sore throat, general malaise, and fever. On questioning, she explained that she had been feeling fatigued for about a week with some nausea and difficulty in drinking fluids. Physical examination revealed bilateral enlarged, firm cervical lymph nodes, mild splenomegaly, and hepatomegaly.

The laboratory data revealed a WBC of $15.0 \times 10^9/L$ hematocrit of 42%, platelets count at $12.5 \times 10^9/L$, and reticulocytes at 2.0%. A differential count of the peripheral blood revealed 65% lymphocytes, 25% granulocytes, and 10% monocytes. The differential report noted that 36% of the lymphocytes were reactive (see Fig. 17–1). Chemistry results showed that liver enzymes and bilirubin levels were slightly increased. No other abnormalities were noted.

After the physical examination, additional laboratory work was ordered. The throat culture for streptococci was negative. A Monospot test was then performed and found to be positive. No further laboratory work was ordered. After a few days of rest at home, the patient was allowed to return to school. No further problems were noted.

Questions

1. What is the differential diagnosis?
2. If the Monospot test was negative, what further testing should be done?
3. Why were the liver enzymes and bilirubin levels slightly elevated?

Answers

1. The differential diagnosis in this case includes EBV, infectious mononucleosis, viral pharyngitis, diphtheria, and streptococcal pharyngitis. The clinical history and clinical presentation are *not* consistent with other infections or malignancy. If the Monospot test had been negative, the differential diagnosis would need to be expanded.
2. With a negative Monospot test, further testing should first include an ELISA for EBV-VCA (IgM) and possibly a repeat Monospot in a week. If infectious mononucleosis as a diagnosis is ruled out, other laboratory procedures need to be performed. These would include further cultures, serological tests, and possibly lymph node and bone marrow biopsies.

3. Up to 25% of individuals with infectious mono-nucleosis may have liver involvement.

REFERENCES

1. Turk, W: Septische Erkrankhungen bei Verkummerung des Granulozylensystems. Wien Klin Wochenschr 20:157, 1907.
2. Sprunt, TP and Evans, FA: Mononuclear leukocytosis in reaction to acute infections ("infectious mononucleosis"). Bull Johns Hopkins Hosp 31:410, 1920.
3. Downey, H and McKinlay, CA: Acute lymphadenosis compared with acute lymphatic leukemia. Arch Intern Med 32:82, 1923.
4. Paul, JR and Bunnell, WW: The presence of heterophile antibodies in infectious mononucleosis. Am J Med Sci 183:90, 1932.
5. Epstein, MA, Achong, BG, and Barr, YM: Virus particles in cultured lymphoblasts from Burkitt's lymphoma. Lancet 1:702, 1964.
6. Henle, G, Henle, W, and Diehl, V: Relation of Burkitt's tumor-associated herpes-type virus to infectious mononucleosis. Proc Natl Acad Sci USA 59:94, 1968.
7. Weiss, LM and Movahed, LA: In situ demonstration of EBV genomes in viral-associated B cell lymphoprolifera-tions. Am J Pathol 134:651, 1989.
8. Young, L, Alfieri, C, Hennessy, K, et al: Expression of Ep-stein-Barr virus transformation-associated genes in tis-sues of patients with EBV lymphoproliferative disease. N Engl J Med 321:1080, 1989.
9. Penman, HG: Fatal infectious mononucleosis: A critical review. J Clin Pathol 23:765, 1970.
10. Buchanan, JG, Goldwater, PN, and Somerfield, SD: Mononucleosis-like-syndrome associated with acute AIDS retrovirus infection. NZ Med J 99:405, 1986.
11. Steeper, TA, Horowitz, CA, and Hanson, M, et al: Heter-ophil-negative mononucleosis-like illnesses with reactive lymphocytosis in patients undergoing seroconversions to the human immunodeficiency virus. Am J Clin Pathol 90:169, 1988.
12. Steeper, TA, Horowitz, CA, Ablaski, DV, et al: The spec-trum of clinical and laboratory findings resulting from human herpesvirus-6 (HHV-6) in patients with mono-nucleosis-like illnesses not resulting from Epstein-Barr virus or cytomegalovirus. Am J Clin Pathol 93:776, 1990.
13. Lagergren, JE: The white blood cell count and the eryth-rocyte sedimentation rate in pertussis. Acta Paediatr 52:405, 1963.
14. De Martino, M, Rossi, ME, Muccioli, AT, et al: Preferential increase of a T-cell subset as a cause of lymphocytosis in children with whooping cough. Boll Ist Sieroter Milan 63:479, 1984.
15. Kubic, VL, Kubic, PT, and Brunning, RD: The morpho-logic and immunophenotypic assessment of the lympho-cytosis accompanying *Bordetella pertussis* infection. Am J Clin Pathol 95:809, 1991.
16. Ryder, RJW: Acute infectious lymphocytosis. Am J Dis Child 110:299, 1965.
17. Koo, D: Chronic fatigue syndrome: A critical appraisal of the role of Epstein-Barr virus. West J Med 150:590, 1989.

QUESTIONS

1. Reactive lymphocytes may best be distinguished from blasts by the presence of which of the following morphological fea-tures?
   a. Prominent nucleoli
   b. Fine chromatin
   c. Heterogeneous cell population
   d. High N:C ratio

2. Which of the following antigens is detectable first by ELISA?
   a. EBNA
   b. EBV-VCA (IgM)
   c. EBV-VCA (IgG)
   d. Heterophil

3. Which of the following is *not* true regarding reactive lympho-cytosis?
   a. Clonal cell population
   b. Low N:C ratio
   c. Coarse chromatin
   d. Heterogeneous cell population

4. What is the most frequent cause of a heterophil (Monospot) negative mononucleosis-like syndrome?
   a. Human immunodeficiency virus
   b. Cytomegalovirus
   c. Hepatitis B
   d. *Toxoplasma gondii*

5. Which of the following conditions show(s) reactive lympho-cytes?
   a. Infectious mononucleosis
   b. Cytomegalovirus
   c. Hepatitis B
   d. All of the above

6. Absolute lymphocytosis is best described as:
   a. Greater than 70% lymphocytes on differential
   b. Presence of nucleoli in lymphocytes
   c. Monoclonal population of lymphocytes
   d. Greater than 4.0×10^9 lymphocytes per liter in an adult

7. Which of the following features are seen in reactive lympho-cytes?
   a. Low N:C ratio
   b. Blue cytoplasm
   c. Indented cytoplasmic borders
   d. All of the above

8. Which of the following clinical manifestations would be un-expected in infectious mononucleosis?
   a. Weight loss
   b. Sore throat
   c. Fatigue
   d. Fever

9. Malignant lymphomas may best be differentiated from infec-tious mononucleosis by which of the following features?
   a. Clonality
   b. Monotony
   c. Pattern of lymphadenopathy
   d. All of the above

10. Infectious mononucleosis is caused by which of the following?
    a. Heterophil virus
    b. *Bordetella pertussis*
    c. EBV
    d. None of the above

ANSWERS

1. **c** (p 288)
2. **b** (p 290) (Table 17–1)
3. **a** (pp 284–286)
4. **b** (p 287)

5. **d** (p 287)
6. **d** (p 283)
7. **d** (p 284)
8. **a** (pp 286–287)
9. **d** (pp 288–289)
10. **c** (p 286)

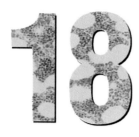

Introduction to Leukemia and the Acute Leukemias

Mary L. Perkins, MS, MT(ASCP)SH
J. Michael Odell, MD
Rita M. Braziel, MD

Objectives

At the end of this chapter, the learner should be able to:
1 Define leukemia.
2 Describe the classification of leukemias.
3 Name risk factors for leukemia.
4 Differentiate between acute myeloid leukemia and acute lymphoblastic leukemia.
5 Distinguish among types M0 through M7 of acute myeloid leukemia.
6 Distinguish among types L1 through L3 of acute lymphoblastic leukemia.
7 Distinguish among immunologic subtypes of acute lymphoblastic leukemia, including precursor B-cell, B-cell, and T-cell.

INTRODUCTION TO LEUKEMIA

Definition

Leukemia is a malignant disease of hematopoietic tissue characterized by replacement of normal bone marrow elements with abnormal (neoplastic) blood cells. These leukemic cells are frequently (but not always) present in the peripheral blood and commonly invade reticuloendothelial tissue, including the spleen, liver, and lymph nodes. They may also invade other tissues, infiltrating any organ of the body. If left untreated, leukemia eventually causes death.

Historic Perspective

The initial description of leukemia as a clinical entity was made by Bennett in Scotland and Virchow in Germany who independently published their findings in 1845.[1,2] Several cases of leukemia were reported in the literature prior to this; however, it was Bennett and Virchow who recognized the significance of their observations and attempted to define the disease.[3] They described a series of autopsy studies of victims of a progressive chronic disorder of unknown origin, in which enlarged spleens and purulent-appearing blood were found. The blood, when examined microscopically, revealed an astounding increase in "colorless" corpuscles. Bennett initially suggested that the marked increase in white blood cells was the result of an inflammatory process. Virchow chose the term *weisses blut* (white blood), which was later translated into Greek as "leukemia." He proposed that leukemia was caused by a neoplastic proliferation, or hyperplasia, of white blood cells. The ensuing debate between Bennett and Virchow continued for several years, but eventually even Bennett rejected inflammation as the cause of leukemia.

Virchow continued his study of leukemia and defined two groups characterized predominantly by either splenic or nodal involvement.[4] Today these groups are recognized as chronic myelocytic leukemia and chronic lymphocytic leukemia, respectively.

In 1857 Friedreich gave a classic account of a rapidly progressive form of leukemia,[5] to which the term *acute* was applied by Epstein in 1889.[6] Further classification was made possible in 1877 by Ehrlich's discovery of a triacid stain that permitted the morphological characterization of blood cells. It was readily shown that acute leukemia was associated with primitive cells, whereas chronic leukemia was associated with mature, well-differentiated cells.

At the turn of the century, Naegeli described the myeloblast and divided the acute leukemias into myeloblastic and lymphoblastic forms.[7] A decade later, Shilling described a monoblastic variant. Thus, the main morphological variants of acute and chronic leukemia were well established by 1930.[8] Since that time, classification of leukemia has been refined, and clinically distinct subgroups have been characterized. Today the clinical laboratory plays an important role in the diagnosis and classification of leukemia. The standard morphological analysis of leukemia is now augmented by cytochemical, cytogenetic, immunologic, and molecular techniques. Together these methods are used to delineate specific categories of leukemia for which distinct treatment protocols are used.

Certainly the most significant application of the biologic understanding of leukemia has been in the area of treatment. Complex therapeutic protocols using cytotoxic drugs, radiation, and, in some cases, bone marrow transplantation have improved the survival of many patients with leukemia and especially those with acute forms. This is most notable for children with acute lymphoblastic leukemia (ALL). Before the 1960s, childhood ALL was universally fatal, but with modern combined regimens over 50% of children with ALL achieve long-term remission and are potentially cured.[9,10]

Classification

Leukemia is classified according to cell type—with regard to both cell maturity and cell lineage. Cell maturity is used to distinguish between acute and chronic forms of leukemia. When the malignant cells are immature (stem cells, blasts, or "pro" forms) the leukemia is classified as acute; when the cells are predominantly mature, it is described as chronic. In general, these two groups correspond to a rapid (acute) or slow (chronic) clinical course. Leukemias are further defined according to cell lineage as lymphoid or myeloid. The term *myeloid* (*myelo*, Greek for "marrow"; *eidos*, "form") encompasses granulocytic, monocytic, megakaryocytic, and erythrocytic leukemias. Thus, utilizing cell maturity and cell lineage, leukemia is divided into four broad categories: acute lymphoblastic (ALL); acute myeloid (AML, also termed acute nonlymphoblastic leukemia or ANLL); chronic lymphocytic (CLL); and chronic myelocytic (CML). These groups are further defined by specific cell type, as outlined in Table 18–1. For example, ALL is either B- or T-cell derived, and AML is subdivided into acute myeloid, promyelocytic, myelomonocytic, monocytic, erythroleukemic, and megakaryoblastic forms, as currently reflected in the French-American-British (FAB) classification. The term *myeloid* is used in this chapter, although various synonyms have been applied to the acute nonlymphoblastic leukemias, such as *myelogenous*, *myeloblastic*, and *granulocytic*.

Etiology and Risk Factors

The origin of leukemia at the genetic level in most cases appears to be related to mutation and altered expression of oncogenes and tumor suppressor genes.[11] Most oncogenes regulate cell proliferation and differentiation. Abnormal oncogene or tumor suppressor gene expression induced by translocation and genetic fusion or mutation often results in unregulated cellular proliferation. Although the events that lead to this are not entirely understood, a number of host and environmental factors have been identified that are associated with increased risk of leukemic transformation.

Host Factors

Heredity Leukemia does not appear to be inherited, although some individuals have an increased predisposition for acquiring it. An identical twin of a patient with acute leukemia possesses a markedly increased relative risk of developing leukemia. There is also an increased incidence of leukemia, although less dramatic, in other family members of leukemic patients.[12]

Congenital Chromosomal Abnormalities Leukemia occurs with increased frequency in patients with congenital disorders that have an inherited tendency for chromosomal fragility (e.g., Bloom's syndrome and Fanconi's anemia) or with an abnormal chromosome constitution (e.g., Down's syndrome, Klinefelter's syndrome, and Turner's syndrome). An 18- to 20-fold increased incidence of acute leukemia is seen in children with Down's syndrome.[13]

Immunodeficiency An unusually high incidence of lymphoproliferative disease (lymphoid leukemia and lymphoma) has been noted in patients with hereditary immunodeficiency states, such as ataxia-telangiectasia and sex-linked agammaglobulinemia. It has recently been suggested that patients with ataxia-telangiectasia possess a defect that interferes with T- and B-lymphocyte gene rearrangement.[14]

Chronic Marrow Dysfunction Patients with chronic marrow dysfunction syndromes have an increased risk of acute leukemic transformation. Examples include the myelodysplastic syndromes, my-

TABLE 18–1	Classification of Leukemia			
Type of Leukemia	**Abbreviation**	**FAB***	**Alternate Names**	
Acute Myeloid				
Acute myeloblastic leukemia	AML		Acute nonlymphoblastic (ANLL)	
without morphological or cytochemical maturation		M0		
with minimal morphological and cytochemical maturation		M1		
with maturation		M2		
Acute promyelocytic leukemia	APL	M3	Hypergranular promyelocytic	
Acute myelomonocytic leukemia	AMML	M4	Naegeli-type leukemia	
Acute monocytic leukemia	AMoL	M5	Schilling-type leukemia	
Erythroleukemia	AEL	M6	Di Guglielmo's syndrome, erythremic myelosis	
Acute megakaryoblastic leukemia	AMegL	M7		
Acute Lymphoblastic	ALL			
Early pre-B-cell ALL		L1, L2	Common ALL	
Pre-B-cell ALL		L1, L2	Common ALL	
B-cell ALL		L3	Burkitt's leukemia	
T-cell ALL		L1, L2		
Chronic Myeloid				
Chronic myelogenous leukemia	CML		Chronic granulocytic leukemia	
Chronic eosinophilic leukemia	CEL			
Chronic basophilic leukemia	CBL			
Chronic Lymphoid				
Chronic lymphocytic leukemia	CLL			
B-cell CLL				
T-cell CLL				
Prolymphocytic leukemia	PLL			
Hairy cell leukemia	HCL		Leukemic reticuloendotheliosis	
Plasma cell leukemia			Multiple myeloma, leukemic phase	
Sézary syndrome			Mycosis fungoides, leukemic phase	

*French-American-British classification of acute leukemia.

eloproliferative disorders, aplastic anemia, and paroxysmal nocturnal hemoglobinuria. Secondary AML following chemotherapy in adults is often associated with chromosome 11q23 abnormalities.

Environmental Factors

Ionizing Radiation Leukemia is associated with exposure to ionizing radiation; this fact is dramatically illustrated in data collected in populations exposed to the use of nuclear weapons in Hiroshima and Nagasaki (Fig. 18–1). The occurrence of leukemia in this population is many times that of individuals not exposed to ionizing radiation, and it is highest in survivors with the greatest exposure.[15] Both acute and chronic forms of leukemia including AML, ALL, and CML, were reported. The role of exposure to electromagnetic radiation in causation of leukemia is controversial.[16,17]

Chemicals and Drugs A variety of chemicals and drugs have been associated with development of leukemia. In humans, benzene is the most frequently documented chemical toxin.[18] Pharmacologic agents include chloramphenicol and phenylbutazone. Certain cytotoxic chemotherapeutic agents, especially alkylating drugs, are also associated with leukemic transformation, and the risk in patients receiving alkylating agents is increased by the use of therapeutic radiation. This has been noted particularly in patients treated with combined chemoradiotherapy for Hodgkin's disease.

Viruses The human T-cell leukemia-lymphoma virus–I (HTLV-I) has been implicated as the causative agent of adult T-cell leukemia-lymphoma (ATL). This rare form of leukemia has a mature helper-inducer T-cell phenotype. ATL is endemic to southwestern Japan, the Caribbean basin, Africa, the southeastern United States, and several other geographic regions.[19] Another related virus, HTLV-II, has been isolated from patients with atypical hairy-cell leukemia (a chronic lymphoid leukemia).[20] The Epstein-Barr virus has been linked to African Burkitt's lymphoma.[21,22]

Incidence

The overall incidence of leukemia in the United States is 8 to 10 new cases per 100,000 individuals per year. In 1994, approximately 28,600 new cases were reported, about 50% acute and 50% chronic.[23] Leukemia strikes more adults than children (10:1) and has a slightly increased incidence in males compared to females (1–2:1).

Acute leukemia occurs at all ages, but ALL (acute lymphoblastic leukemia) is more common in children and AML (acute myeloid leukemia) is more common in adults. Of childhood leukemias, 75% are classified as ALL, whereas nearly 80% of all AMLs occur in adults.

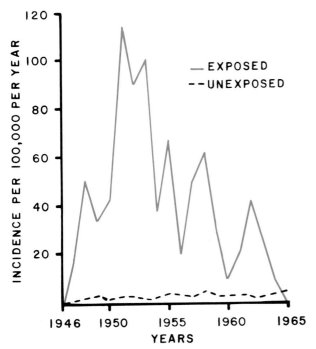

FIGURE 18–1 Leukemia incidence in Hiroshima, 1946–1965, in individuals exposed and nonexposed to atomic radiation. (From Gunz, FW, in Wintrobe, MM (ed): Blood, Pure and Eloquent. McGraw-Hill, New York, 1980, p. 528, with permission.)

Chronic leukemia is generally considered a disease of adults. CLL (chronic lymphocytic leukemia) is extremely rare in children and is unusual before the age of 40. CML (chronic myelocytic leukemia) may be seen at any age, but its peak incidence is between 30 and 50 years of age; the disease is rare in children, but a distinct juvenile variant is recognized (JCML).

Comparison of Acute and Chronic Leukemia

The clinical and laboratory features of acute and chronic leukemia differ in a number of respects, as summarized in Table 18–2. Patients with acute leukemia usually present with a sudden onset of symptoms, and if left untreated, the disease runs a rapidly fatal course of 6 months or less. In contrast, patients

TABLE 18–2 **Comparison of Acute and Chronic Leukemia**		
	Acute	**Chronic**
Age	All ages	Adults
Clinical onset	Sudden	Insidious
Course (untreated)	<6 months	2–6 years
Leukemic cells	Immature	Mature
Anemia	Mild to severe	Mild
Thrombocytopenia	Mild to severe	Mild
WBC	Variable	Increased
Organomegaly	Mild	Prominent

with chronic leukemia tend to have an insidious onset and a more indolent clinical course, usually lasting 2 to 6 years.

Patients with acute and chronic leukemia also show differences in their hematologic parameters. In general, bone marrow failure and its sequelae are much more prominent in the initial presentation of acute leukemia than in that of the chronic form. Anemia is consistently observed in the acute leukemic patient, although its severity is variable. Thrombocytopenia is common. The white blood cell count may be markedly elevated with numerous blasts; it may be normal or, in some cases, even decreased. Typically the various normal circulating white blood cells are diminished in number. In chronic leukemic patients, anemia is often mild at presentation. The platelet count is usually normal, but it may actually be increased in CML. Chronic leukemias almost always present with elevated white blood cell counts, which are often strikingly high.

Both acute and chronic leukemic patients can display enlargement of the spleen, liver, or lymph nodes, but this is more consistently seen in patients with chronic leukemia, in whom organomegaly tends to be more prominent and can occasionally be massive.

INTRODUCTION TO ACUTE LEUKEMIA

Clinical Features

Most patients with acute leukemia display a clinically abrupt onset of signs and symptoms of only a few weeks' duration. Patients often seek medical attention because of weakness, bleeding abnormalities, or flu-like symptoms. These abnormalities reflect the failure of the bone marrow to produce adequate numbers of normal cells and are caused by the proliferation and accumulation of leukemic cells in the marrow. Leukemic replacement eventually results in marrow failure and the resultant life-threatening complications of anemia, thrombocytopenia, granulocytopenia, and their sequelae. Anemia, the most consistent presenting feature, is associated with fatigue, malaise, and pallor. Hemorrhagic complications related to thrombocytopenia and in some cases to disseminated intravascular coagulation (DIC) are also common. These may be mild and restricted to easy bruising, petechiae, and mucosal bleeding; or they may be more severe, involving gastrointestinal tract, genitourinary tract, or central nervous system hemorrhage. Infections result from severe granulocytopenia. Bacterial infections are common (e.g., *Staphylococcus*, *Pseudomonas*, *Escherichia coli*, and *Klebsiella*), but fungal infections (e.g., *Candida* and *Aspergillus*) also occur. Viral infections are less frequent.[24]

Infiltration of other tissues, especially organs that play a role in fetal hematopoeisis, is often manifested by hepatospenomegaly or lymphadenopathy, particularly in acute lymphoblastic and acute monoblastic leukemia (AMoL); these are less frequently observed in the other acute nonlymphoblastic leukemias. A mediastinal mass caused by thymic involvement is a hallmark of T-cell ALL. Gingival hypertrophy and oral lesions are primarily seen in AMoL. Bone or joint pain, caused by pressure of the expanding leukemic cell population in the marrow cavity, commonly accom-

TABLE 18–3 Clinical Features of Acute Leukemia

Pathogenesis	Clinical Manifestation
Bone Marrow Failure	
Anemia	Fatigue, malaise, pallor
Thrombocytopenia	Bruising, bleeding
Granulocytopenia	Fever, infections
Organ Infiltration	
Marrow expansion	Bone or joint pain
Spleen	Splenomegaly
Liver	Hepatomegaly
Lymph nodes	Lymphadenopathy
Central nervous system	Neurologic symptoms
Gums, mouth	Gingival hypertrophy, oral lesions

panies the acute leukemias. Leukemic infiltration of the central nervous system, an ominous feature infrequently observed at initial presentation, is associated with signs and symptoms of increased intracranial pressure (nausea, vomiting, headache, papilledema) or cranial nerve palsies. These clinical features and their relationship to pathophysiology are summarized in Table 18–3.

Of all cases of AML, 5% to 10% are preceded by a recognizable "preleukemic" (myelodysplastic) syndrome. The myelodysplastic syndromes (MDS) are more common in patients over the age of 50 years and are associated with unexplained and persistent anemia, leukopenia, thrombocytopenia, and monocytosis, alone or in combination. The myelodysplastic syndromes are discussed in more detail in Chapter 19.

Laboratory Evaluation of Acute Leukemia

When acute leukemia is suspected, a series of laboratory tests is required to confirm the diagnosis and to classify the disease. The distinction between AML and ALL is particularly important; major features of this are outlined in Table 18–4.

Preliminary evaluation should include a complete blood count (CBC), platelet count, white cell differential, and peripheral blood smear examination. Anemia, which may be mild to severe and is usually normochromic and normocytic, is the most consistent finding. Typically, the platelets are decreased, although they may be normal in number. The white blood cell count is highly variable, ranging from decreased to markedly elevated. The blood smear usually reveals blasts or other immature cells, but they may be rare or absent ("aleukemic" leukemia). Circulating nucleated red blood cells are occasionally seen. Myelodysplastic features are sometimes present, including pseudo-Pelger-Huét cells and hypogranular neutrophils. These are more common in elderly patients with acute myeloid leukemia.

Once the diagnosis of leukemia is suggested by the clinical history, physical examination, and CBC and peripheral blood smear findings, a bone marrow aspirate and biopsy is usually obtained. Morphological examination of the bone marrow is often essential for establishing the diagnosis. The most widely accepted classification system, called the French-American-British (FAB) system, requires a blast count of 30% in bone marrow aspirate smears for confirmation of the diagnosis of acute leukemia.[25,26] Well-prepared smears of bone marrow aspirate material are generally the specimen of choice for classification of leukemia by morphological and cytochemical criteria.

A systematic approach to the classification of leukemia begins with a review of cellular morphology, which provides important clues about cell lineage and guides further studies required to make a definitive diagnosis. Morphological evaluation should be followed by cytochemical staining and immunologic cell marker studies. A battery of cytochemical stains that define granulocytic and monocytic differentiation is used to distinguish ALL from AML. When positive, these stud-

TABLE 18–4 Comparison of Acute Myeloblastic and Acute Lymphoblastic Leukemia

Factor	AML	ALL
Age	Common in adults, rare in children	Common in children, rare in adults
Blood	Anemia, neutropenia, thrombocytopenia; myeloblasts and promyelocytes	Anemia, neutropenia, thrombocytopenia; lymphoblasts and prolymphocytes
Morphology	Medium-to-large blasts, more cytoplasm than lymphoblasts, cytoplasmic granules, Auer rods; fine nuclear chromatin and distinct nucleoli	Small or medium blasts, scarce cytoplasm, no granules; fine nuclear chromatin and indistinct nucleoli
Cytochemistry	Positive peroxidase and Sudan black; negative TdT	Negative peroxidase and Sudan black; positive TdT
Extramedullary and focal disease	Common in spleen and liver; less common in lymph nodes and CNS	Common in lymph nodes, spleen, liver, CNS, and gonads

Abbreviations: AML = acute myeloblastic leukemia; ALL = acute lymphoblastic leukemia; TdT = terminal deoxynucleotidyl transferase; CNS = central nervous system

Source: Reproduced with permission from Kjeldsberg, CR (ed): Practical Diagnosis of Hematologic Disorders. ASCP Press, Chicago, 1989, p 349.

TABLE 18–5 **Morphologic Features to Differentiate Acute Myeloblastic Leukemia from Acute Lymphoblastic Leukemia**		
	AML Myeloblast*	**ALL Lymphoblast***
Blast size	Large	Small
Cytoplasm	Moderate	Scant
Chromatin	Fine, lacy	Dense
Nucleoli	Prominent (usually more than 2)	Indistinct (usually 2 or less)
Auer rods	Present in 50–60%	Never present

*These are general features. The morphology may vary considerably.
Source: Reproduced with permission from Kjeldsberg, CR (ed): Practical Diagnosis of Hematologic Disorders. ASCP Press, Chicago, 1989, p 374

ies exclude ALL and permit subclassification of AML. A marker useful in initial evaluation is the nuclear enzyme terminal deoxynucleotidyl transferase (TdT), which is present in most cases of ALL and is less commonly expressed in AML. Other immunologic cell marker studies are routinely used for further subclassification of acute leukemia, particularly in ALL.

Other laboratory studies used to evaluate acute leukemia include chromosome analysis, electron microscopy, molecular genetic studies, and DNA flow cytometry. Chromosome analysis is a valuable tool in identifying prognostically important subgroups of patients, and providing baseline data that may be useful in monitoring patients.[27] Electron microscopy is infrequently utilized, except in evaluation of poorly differentiated leukemia or acute megakaryoblastic leukemia. Molecular diagnostic studies are playing an emerging role in primary diagnosis and detection of minimal residual disease, and DNA flow cytometry yields prognostically useful information, particularly in patients with ALL.

The purpose and principles of these laboratory methods are discussed below; detailed procedures are outlined in Chapters 24 and 35.

Specimens

At the outset, care must be taken to ensure that an adequate specimen is obtained and that it is properly handled. Lack of technical excellence may obscure or complicate an otherwise straightforward diagnosis; an inadequate or improperly handled specimen is a common cause of diagnostic error.

At some institutions, evaluation of the peripheral blood cell morphology is performed on nonanticoagulated finger-stick smears. Anticoagulant etheylenediamine tetra-acetic acid (EDTA) causes subtle morphological artifacts of nucleated cells and platelets. A specimen left in EDTA for over 30 minutes may show artifactual vacuolation of monocytes and neutrophils, nuclear shape changes and swelling, as well as degranulation of platelets.[28,29]

Before a bone marrow specimen is collected, arrangements for special studies including cytochemistry and immunophenotyping should be made, and any special handling procedures should be noted; such procedures are also important to cytogenetic and ultrastructural studies. During the bone marrow procedure, the aspirate is collected first and smears made

immediately to avoid clotting. As the aspirate smears are pulled, the presence of bone marrow spicules should be confirmed. If spicules are not present, another aspiration may be necessary. For immunophenotyping or cytogenetic studies, the marrow aspirate is anticoagulated by aspirating directly into a syringe coated with heparin. After sufficient aspirate material is collected, the biopsy is obtained. The biopsy should be used, before fixation, to make touch preps by gently touching or rolling the biopsy along a glass slide. The biopsy should be blotted prior to making the touch preps; excess blood will obscure morphological detail. Touch preps are especially important when the aspirate produces a "dry" tap. Further details of the bone marrow procedure are discussed in Chapter 2.

Evaluation of Morphology

Cellular morphology is evaluated on a Romanowsky- (Wright-Giemsa-) stained blood or bone marrow smear in carefully chosen areas in which cells are not distorted by overcrowding. In the hands of an experienced morphologist, the cell type may be correctly identified; however, additional testing is always necessary to confirm the diagnosis.

Several cytologic features (outlined in Table 18–5) are helpful in distinguishing lymphoblasts from myeloblasts. These include the size of the blast, amount of cytoplasm, nuclear chromatin pattern, and the presence of nucleoli. The typical myeloblast (Fig. 18–2) is a

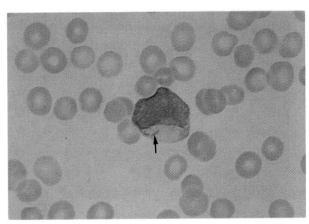

FIGURE 18–2   Myeloblast (note the Auer rod).

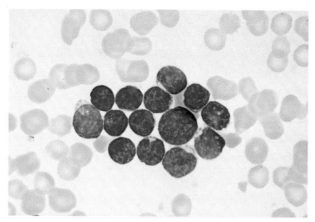

FIGURE 18–3 Lymphoblasts (peripheral blood).

large cell (15 to 20 μm in diameter) with a moderate amount of cytoplasm. Its nucleus has a fine reticulated chromatin pattern and multiple distinct nucleoli are often present. The typical lymphoblast (Fig. 18–3) is a smaller cell with scant cytoplasm. The nuclear chromatin often appears more dense than in the myeloblast, and nucleoli are usually indistinct when present. For a review of morphological descriptions of the blast stage, see Chapter 1.

Granulocytic differentiation is suggested by the presence of azurophilic granules. A very helpful morphological feature is the Auer rod, whose presence excludes ALL. Auer rods are cytoplasmic inclusions resulting from an abnormal fusion of primary granules and are pathognomonic for a myeloproliferative process, particularly AML (and rarely CML in myeloid blast crisis)[30]; they have also been described in myelodysplastic syndromes in transformation to AML.[31] On Romanowsky-stained smears, Auer rods appear as pink- or purple-staining rods or splinter-shaped inclusions (see Fig. 18–2). They are present in up to 60% of patients with AML,[32] but it may take a long careful review of the blood or marrow smear to find them; given their diagnostic importance, this search is well worth the effort. In acute promyelocytic leukemia, Auer rods are easy to find, some cells having "bundles" of cigar-shaped rods.

Cytochemistry

Special stains are used to identify chemical components of cells such as enzymes or lipids. These cytochemical stains are an important aid in the classification of acute leukemia because they identify cellular components that are associated with specific cell lines. For example, a positive myeloperoxidase or Sudan black B stain indicates myeloid differentiation, and a positive nonspecific esterase stain indicates monocytic differentiation. When any of these stains are positive, lymphoid origin is ruled out, with rare exceptions. Thus, the cytochemical stains help distinguish between ALL and AML. They are also used to subclassify AML.

The cytochemical reactions are performed by applying staining techniques to peripheral blood smears, bone marrow smears, or touch preps. Fresh preparations are preferred, especially for enzyme reactions. Control smears can be fixed in the appropriate fixative, allowed to air dry, and stored at −20°C for future staining. Caution should be taken when interpreting cytochemical stains. It is the leukemic cell population whose identity (cell lineage) is in question; therefore a positive reaction is determined by finding positive staining in the leukemic blasts rather than in mature cells. Table 18–6 summarizes the cytochemical reactions that are useful in the classification of acute leukemia. The cytochemical stain procedures are discussed in Chapter 33.

Myeloperoxidase Peroxidase is present in the primary granules of myeloid cells. These granules first appear in the early promyelocyte (late blast) and persist through subsequent stages of cell maturation.

TABLE 18–6 **Summary of Cytochemical Reactions Useful in Diagnosing Acute Leukemia**

Special Stain	Site of Action	Cells Stained	Comment
Myeloperoxidase	Mainly primary granules; Auer rods	Late myeloblasts, granulocytes; monocytes less intensely	Valuable in that the primary granules are not always visible; separates AML (+) from ALL (−)
Sudan black B	Phospholipids: membrane of 1° and 2° granules	Late myeloblasts, granulocytes; monocytes less intensely	Parallels peroxidase, but smears do not need to be fresh
Specific esterase (Naphthol AS-D Chloroacetate)	Cytoplasm	Neutrophilic granulocytes; mast cells	Parallels peroxidase, but less sensitive; useful on paraffin-embedded tissues
Nonspecific esterase Alpha-naphthyl acetate (ANAE) and butyrate	Cytoplasm	Monocytes; focal staining in T cells; ANAE also + in megakaryocytes	Useful for determining degree of monocytic differentiation; separates mono (+) from myelo (−) blasts
Periodic acid-Schiff	Glycogen and related substances	Lymphocytes; granulocytes; megakaryocytes	Helpful in supporting diagnosis of erythroleukemia

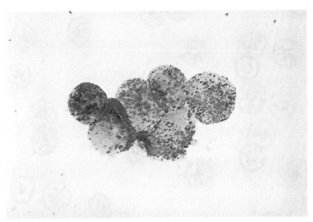

FIGURE 18–4 Myeloperoxidase positivity in acute promyelocytic leukemia.

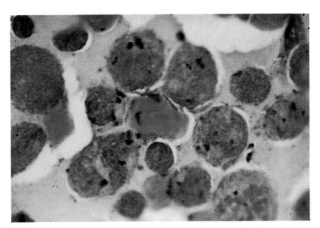

FIGURE 18–6 Specific esterase naphtol AS-D chloracetate positivity in AML (M2).

Monocytes have variable staining with peroxidase and are most often only weakly positive (Fig. 18–4). This enzyme is not present in lymphocytes or their precursors and is therefore useful in differentiating AML from ALL. It is more specific for granulocytic differentiation than the Sudan black B stain.

Effort should be made to use fresh smears when staining for peroxidase because the enzyme is labile.

Sudan Black B Phospholipids, neutral fats, and sterols are stained by Sudan black B (SBB) (Fig. 18–5). Phospholipids occur both in primary and secondary granules of granulocytic cells and to a lesser extent in monocytic lysozomal granules.

The SBB is the most sensitive stain for granulocytic precursors with a staining pattern that generally parallels the myeloperoxidase stain. As with the peroxidase stain, the SBB is used to differentiate AML from ALL. Positivity seldom occurs in lymphoid cells, but rare cases of SBB-positive ALL are observed.[33] The SBB stain, whose reactivity does not diminish with time, is particularly useful for specimens that are not fresh.

Specific Esterase (Naphthol AS-D Chloroacetate) The specific esterase stain (Fig. 18–6) roughly parallels

the peroxidase and Sudan black B stains, although it is not sensitive, and it is negative in eosinophils and monocytes. Its most important use is in demonstrating myeloid differentiation in paraffin-embedded tissue sections.

Smears or hydrated paraffin tissue sections are incubated in a buffered solution containing the substrate naphthol AS-D chloroacetate and a diazo salt (pararosaniline). The esterase enzyme is present within neutrophils, basophils, and mast cells.

Nonspecific Esterase (Alpha-Naphthyl Acetate or Butyrate) The nonspecific esterase (NSE) stain is used to identify monocytic cells (Fig. 18–7). It is diffusely positive in these cells and negative in granulocytic cells. Lymphoid cells are negative, except for T lymphocytes, which can demonstrate a focal staining pattern.

Different substrates are available for use in the NSE stain. Alpha-naphthyl butyrate is the most specific for monocyte differentiation, while alpha-naphthyl acetate is more sensitive. Both are positive in monocytes and their precursors as well as in macrophages. The alpha-naphthyl acetate, but not the butyrate, is also

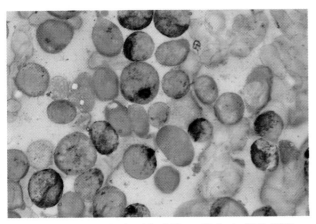

FIGURE 18–5 Sudan black B positivity in AML (M2).

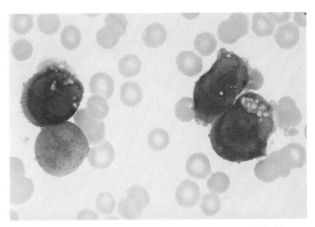

FIGURE 18–7 Nonspecific esterase (alpha-naphthyl butyrate) positivity in acute monocytic leukemia (M5).

positive in megakaryocytes and platelets. Another substrate, naphthol AS-D acetate (NASDA), is less specific and stains both monocytes and granulocytes. NASDA must be used in conjunction with a sodium fluoride inhibition step, which renders monocytic cells negative and thus differentiates them from granulocytic cells, which remain positive. Although NASDA is no longer routinely used, its staining pattern gave the "nonspecific" esterase its name.

Periodic Acid-Schiff The periodic acid-Schiff (PAS) reaction stains for glycogen and related compounds, including mucoproteins, glycoproteins, glycolipids, and polysaccharides. Lymphocytes, granulocytes, monocytes, and megakaryocytes may be positive, having either a diffuse or sometimes a granular staining pattern. Normal erythroid precursors are negative.

The PAS reaction is not very useful for characterizing acute leukemia. The typical block positivity (Fig. 18–8) associated with lymphoblastic leukemia may also occur in acute myeloid leukemia, especially the acute monocytic type.[34,35] Burkitt's type ALL (L3) is negative. The PAS stain should not be used to distinguish AML from ALL.

The PAS reaction may sometimes be helpful in supporting the diagnosis of erythroleukemia, where strong PAS positivity may be present in normoblasts. When present, this feature is helpful for differentiating erythroleukemia from pernicious anemia, in which the PAS reaction is negative except in rare cases. Normoblasts may also be positive in iron deficiency, thalassemia, severe hemolytic anemias, and some of the myelodysplastic syndromes.

Immunologic Marker Studies

A number of immunologic methods have proven to be indispensable to the diagnosis and classification of acute leukemia, especially of ALL. Antibodies are used to detect markers associated with cell lineage and maturation stage. Depending on the location of these cell markers (cell surface, cytoplasm, or nucleus) different methods are used to detect them. The following paragraphs briefly introduce the immunologic cell marker procedures. Their usefulness in the evaluation of acute

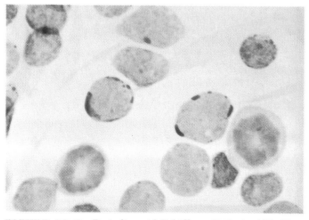

FIGURE 18-8 Periodic acid-Schiff positivity in ALL. Note the "block" staining pattern.

leukemia is discussed in the individual sections on AML and ALL.

Cell Surface Markers Cell surface markers are proteins on the cell membrane that can be detected with immunologic reagents. Different proteins are expressed at different stages of maturation; some are present early in development, whereas others do not appear until much later. Still other proteins may appear, disappear, then reappear at a later stage of development. This unique expression of proteins enables them to be used as markers of both cell lineage and maturation stage.

Although some surface markers can be detected with polyclonal antisera, many can only be detected with monoclonal antibodies. Table 18–7 lists some antibodies that are commonly used to evaluate leukemias and other lymphoproliferative and myeloproliferative disorders.

Surface marker studies are performed on cell suspensions derived either from bone marrow aspirates or peripheral blood. It is important to have fresh specimens with viable cells; nonviable cells lead to nonspecific staining, which may make interpretation impossible. An immunofluorescent method (direct or indirect) is used to stain the cells, and a flow cytometer is used to analyze them. (See Chap. 24 for a review of flow cytometry.) Figure 18–9 shows the surface staining pattern, as observed with a fluorescent microscope, that is typical of a strongly positive reaction.

Cytoplasmic Immunoglobulin The only cytoplasmic marker that is routinely used in the evaluation of acute leukemia is cytoplasmic immunoglobulin (μ heavy chain). It is a marker of pre-B cells. Cytoplasmic μ is usually detected by using a direct immunofluorescent procedure to stain cells on a glass slide. Fresh blood smears, bone marrow smears, touch preps, or cytocentrifuge preparations (cytopreps) may be used, but cytopreps of washed cell suspensions are preferred because they tend to produce lower background staining. Slides are fixed in acid alcohol, incubated with a fluorescein-conjugated antihuman IgM antiserum, and washed with buffered saline. A fluorescent microscope is used to determine if cytoplasmic staining is present. Pre-B cells are weakly to moderately positive.

Terminal Deoxynucleotidyl Transferase Terminal deoxynucleotidyl transferase (TdT) is a unique nuclear enzyme (DNA polymerase) present in stem cells and precursor B- and T-lymphoid cells.[36] High levels are found in most (90%) of the lymphoblastic leukemias, including both B- and T-lineage ALL. TdT, although not lineage-specific, provides information useful in the distinction of ALL from AML. Detectable levels of this enzyme have been noted in 5% to 10% of cases of AML,[37] although the level is usually lower than in lymphoblasts. TdT is also present in most cases of lymphoblastic lymphoma and in approximately one-third of cases of chronic myelocytic leukemia in blast crisis (CML-BC).[38] Its presence in cases of CML-BC is a predictor of the likelihood of a favorable response of the disease to treatment with vincristine and prednisone, drugs commonly employed in induction regimens for ALL.[39]

TdT can be detected by immunologic techniques (immunocytochemical or immunofluorescent) using fresh smears, touch preps, or cytopreps. When heparinized

TABLE 18–7 Monoclonal Antibodies Used for Study of Leukemia and Lymphoma		
Cluster Designation	Specific Antibodies	Major Hematopoietic Reactivity
CD1a	T6, Leu-6	Thymic and Langerhan's cells
CD2	T11, Leu-5	E-Rosette-forming T cells
CD3	T3, Leu-4	Mature T cells
CD4	T4, Leu-3	Helper-inducer T-cell subset
CD5	T1, Leu-1	Pan-T and some B-cells
CD7	Leu-9	Pan-T, early thymocytes
CD8	T8, Leu-2	Suppressor-cytotoxic T-cell subset
CD10	J5, CALLA	B-cell pre, some thym, grans and cALL
CD11b	Mo1, Leu-15	Monos and grans C3bi receptor
CD11c	Leu-M5	Monos, myeloid precursors but not grans
CD13	My 7	Most grans, monos
CD14	My 4, Leu-M3	Monos, minority of grans, and DRC
CD19	B4, Leu-12	B cells, early B-cell precursors
CD20	B1, Leu-16	B cells, midstage B-cell precursors
CD21	B2	C3d receptor on B cells and DRC
CD22	Leu-14	B cells
CD25	IL-2R1, IL2R	IL-2 receptor on T cells, activated T cells, and B cells
CD33	My 9	Myeloid progenitors
CD34	HPCA	Hematopoietic progenitor and stem cells
CD41	J15	Platelets and megakaryocytes (GPIIb/IIIa)
CD42b	AN51	Platelets and megakaryocytes (GPIb)
CD45	T200, HLe, LCA	Leukocytes
	Ia, HLA-DR	B cells, activated T cells and monocytes

Abbreviations: B cells (or B) = B lymphocytes; cALL = common ALL; CD = cluster designation; DRC = dendritic reticulum cells; grans (or G) = granulocytes; monos (or M) = monocytes; Pan = reactivity with many leukocyte populations; Plts (or P) = platelets; RS = Reed-Sternberg cells; T cell (or T) = T lymphocytes; Thym = thymocytes

specimens are to be studied, the sample must be washed to remove heparin, which causes false-negative staining. A positive reaction is indicated by a nuclear staining pattern (see Figure 18–10).

Cytogenetics

Cytogenetic analysis of leukemic cells is a critically important adjunct to the standard classification of acute leukemia. It is currently considered an essential component in the evaluation of the newly diagnosed leukemic patient, playing a major role in diagnosis, subclassification, selection of appropriate therapy, and monitoring the effects of therapy. A number of chromosomal abnormalities have been associated with distinct forms of leukemia (see following discussion of molecular genetics). Classic examples of this are the Philadelphia chromosome (t[9;22]) associated with

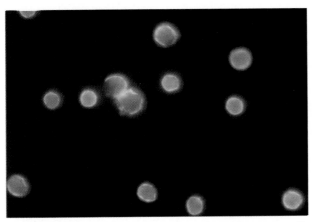

FIGURE 18–9 Surface immunoglobulin (sIg) positive cells in B-cell ALL (L3).

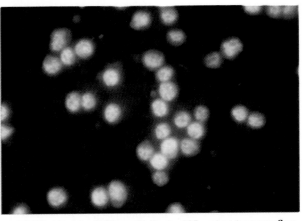

FIGURE 18–10 TdT positivity in ALL using immunofluorescence method.

CML, and the translocation t(15;17) consistently observed in acute promyelocytic leukemia. In addition to cytogenetic evaluation, flow cytometric analysis for DNA ploidy status may provide information useful to the evaluation of ALL.[40]

Cytogenetic studies are performed by evaluating chromosome metaphase preparations to detect numeric and structural karyotype (karyon, nucleus + typos, mark) abnormalities. Normal human cells have 46 chromosomes and are said to be diploid (*diplous*, "double," + *eidos*, "form"); that is, they have two haploid sets of chromosomes. An aneuploid population can be either hypodiploid or hyperdiploid, and can be identified as such by DNA flow cytometry as well as by cytogenetic examination.

Structural rearrangements include translocations, inversions, deletions, duplications, and isochromosomes. Of particular importance to the study of acute leukemia are the translocations that result from the movement of a DNA segment from one chromosome to another, and which are often associated with oncogene rearrangement, genetic fusion, and abnormal gene expression. Usually these result from a reciprocal interchange of portions of two nonhomologous chromosomes.

Chromosomal abnormalities (both numeric and structural) are found in the majority of patients with acute leukemia, and are seen in over 60% of patients with AML and over 65% of patients with ALL. The most common structural abnormalities are translocations. A number of these have been associated with distinct subgroups of AML or ALL with prognostic significance (see below). For example, patients with acute myelomonocytic leukemia (AML, M4) who exhibit an inversion or deletion of the long arm of chromosome 16 (inv [16q] or del [16q]) have a longer median survival than patients with other types of AML. Table 18–8 lists common cytogenetic abnormalities associated with acute leukemia.

Molecular Genetics

The molecular genetic basis for many of the acute leukemias has been elucidated in recent years. Extensive studies of the immunoglobulin and T-cell antigen receptor genes have been carried out, and other genes involved in many of the recurrent cytogenetic abnormalities described above have been cloned and characterized. DNA probes and PCR-based primers are available for rapid and precise detection of many specific cytogenetic abnormalities at the molecular level. Molecular diagnostic studies are primarily used to confirm the presence of a suspected chromosomal abnormality not detected by conventional cytogenetics, to analyze specimens that are not suitable for conventional cytogenetics, and to monitor minimal residual disease following therapy.

These methods permit detection of residual leukemic disease at extremely low levels, and clinical applications of these techniques are still being developed. The sensitivity of molecular techniques enables detection of leukemic subpopulations that are not identifi-

TABLE 18–8 Common Chromosome Abnormalities and Molecular Correlates Associated with Acute Leukemia[41–56]

Chromosome Abnormality	Associated Disorder	Involved Genes on Respective Chromosome	Detection Method
t(8;21)	AML with myelocytic maturation (M2) (associated with a favorable prognosis and good response to therapy)	ETO/AML1	Southern Blot RT-PCR
t(15;17)	Unique to APL (M3 & M3m) (associated with a favorable prognosis)	PML/RARα	RT-PCR
16q abnormality: inv(16) & del(16)	AMML with abnormal eosinophilia (M4E) (associated with a favorable prognosis)	CBFβ/MYH11	RT-PCR
t(9;11)	AMoL, especially poorly differentiated (M5a); also in other types of AML e.g. AMML (M4)	HRX	
t(9;22)	Most common in CML; occasionally found in AML and ALL (early pre-B, pre-B-cell, and T-cell phenotypes) (prognosis is fatal in ALL)	ABL/BCR	RT-PCR
t(4;11)	Mixed lineage leukemia with lymphoblastic (early pre-B) and monocytic features: common in infants	HRX/AF-4	RT-PCR
t(1;19)	ALL, pre-B-cell phenotype (30% incidence in this group) (associated with a very poor prognosis)	PBX1/E2A	RT-PCR
t(8;14), t(2;8) & t(8;22)	ALL, B-cell phenotype (Burkitt's leukemia): c-*myc* oncogene translocated to chromosome with Ig heavy or light-chain gene	c-MYC/IgH	
t(1;14)	ALL, T-cell phenotype (common thymocyte)	TAL 1/TCRD	

t = Translocation; inv = inversion; del = deletion; RT-PCR = reverse transcriptase polymerase chain reaction

able by conventional morphology or other methods; therefore, patients who are in clinical remission may be observed to possess minimal residual disease when PCR-based techniques are employed. The significance and clinical applications of this capability are not clearly defined at present. The molecular correlations of some of the most common chromosomal abnormalities in acute leukemia are listed in Table 18–8.[41–56]

Treatment of Acute Leukemia

Treatment of leukemia has two principal objectives: to eradicate the leukemic cell mass (cytoreduction) and to provide supportive care. Cures are infrequently realized, except in children with common ALL; however, induction of complete remission is a realistic goal for most patients with acute leukemia. Complete remission is defined as the absence of leukemia-related signs and symptoms, absence of demonstrable disease and return of marrow and blood granulocyte, platelet, and red cell values to normal ranges.

Three forms of antileukemic therapy are commonly used: cytoreductive chemotherapy, radiotherapy, and bone marrow transplantation. Chemotherapy is the mainstay of treatment, although bone marrow transplantation is being used more frequently. Radiotherapy is used as an adjunct to chemotherapy in patients who have localized tissue involvement that may be targeted with irradiation, and has been used for central nervous system (CNS) prophylaxis.

The treatment is administered in different phases including an induction and postremission phase. Induction therapy, the most intense phase of treatment, is designed to attain complete remission as quickly as possible; its success is the best predictor of long-term disease-free survival. The approach to postremission-phase treatment differs depending on the type of leukemia being treated. In children with ALL, post-remission therapy includes intensification, CNS prophylaxis, consolidation, and maintenance therapy. In patients with AML, postremission therapy is more controversial and contributes less to long-term survival.[24]

A number of different cytotoxic chemotherapeutic agents are used to treat acute leukemia. Their modes of action differ but, in general, they poison dividing cells, usually by blocking DNA or RNA synthesis. Combinations of drugs, each with different modes of action, are used. This approach helps to overcome leukemic cell drug resistance. Prednisone, vincristine, and asparaginase are used in most induction regimens for treatment of childhood ALL. CNS prophylaxis, an aspect of therapy given to prevent CNS relapse, has been essential to the improved survival of pediatric patients with ALL in recent decades. Patients with AML are usually treated with a combination of cytarabine and daunorubicin, among other agents. The drugs are given in dosages that have substantial marrow toxicity. The most common complications in patients undergoing chemotherapy arise from marrow hypoplasia and the resulting cytopenias. The use of hematopoietic growth factors such as GM-CSF (granulocyte-monocyte colony-stimulating factor) or G-CSF (granulocyte colony-stimulating factor) may potentially improve the status of supportive care in these patients.

Allogeneic bone marrow transplantation has emerged as an important treatment modality, especially for patients with AML, as well as ALL refractory to standard therapy. The patient's bone marrow is completely eradicated with intensive chemotherapy and total body radiation. This is followed by rescuing the patient with donor bone marrow cells that are collected from an HLA-compatible donor (or from the treated leukemic patient in complete remission, in the case of an autologous transplant) by repeated bone marrow aspirates. The donor cells are processed and then infused into the recipient intravenously. The infused cells travel to the recipient's "empty" marrow, where they engraft, multiply, and repopulate the marrow with healthy hematopoietic tissue. Engraftment takes 3 to 4 weeks, and hematologic values return to normal in 2 to 3 months.[24] The complications of bone marrow transplantation, including infections, hemorrhage, and graft-versus-host disease (GVHD), are numerous and can be fatal; it is not suitable therapy for all patients with leukemia. But for some, it offers a chance for long-term survival and a potential cure.

ACUTE MYELOID LEUKEMIA

FAB Classification of Acute Myeloid Leukemia

The need for uniform nomenclature and classification of acute leukemia prompted a group of French, American, and British hematologists to propose a new system in 1976.[57] This scheme, the FAB classification mentioned previously, has proven useful in standardizing the morphological classification of both acute myeloid and lymphoid leukemias. In the years since it was first introduced, the FAB cooperative group has made several modifications, striving to make the classification as objective and unambiguous as possible.[26] Although there are still some areas of ambiguity, the FAB system has gained wide acceptance.

The acute myeloid leukemias are divided into the following groups:

- M0: Myeloid without morphological or cytochemical maturation
- M1: Myeloid with minimal morphological and cytochemical maturation
- M2: Myeloid with maturation
- M3: Promyelocytic
- M4: Myelomonocytic
- M5: Monocytic (a) well and (b) poorly differentiated
- M6: Erythroid
- M7: Megakaryoblastic

These groups are defined according to the predominant cell type observed on Romanowsky- and cytochemically stained blood and bone marrow aspirate smears Table 18–9. Additional specialized studies are required to confirm the diagnosis of M0 (AML without morphological or cytochemical maturation) and M7 (acute megakaryocytic leukemia). A summary of the cytochemical reactions in each type of AML is found in Table 18–10.

AML, especially M6 type (erythroleukemia), is sometimes difficult to distinguish from certain myelodysplastic syndromes (refractory anemia with excess

TABLE 18–9	**FAB Classification of Acute Myeloblastic Leukemia**
Type	**Characteristics**
M0	*Myeloid without morphological or cytochemical maturation:* Morphologically undifferentiated leukemic blasts with myeloid immunophenotype
M1	*Myeloid with minimal morphologic and cytochemical maturation:* Marrow leukemia cells are primarily myeloblasts with no azurophilic granules
M2	*Myeloid with maturation:* Leukemia cells show prominent maturation beyond myeloblast stage
M3	*Promyelocytic:* Abnormal, hypergranular promyelocytes dominate; Auer rods easily found; increased incidence of DIC
M3m	*Microgranular variant of M3:* Indistinct granules; nucleus often reniform or bilobed; increased incidence of DIC
M4	*Myelomonocytic:* Both monocytic (monocytes and promonocytes) and myeloid differentiation (maturation beyond myeloblast stage)
M4E	*M4 with bone marrow eosinophilia:* Similar to M4 with marrow eosinophilia (abnormal and immature); associated with abnormal 16q karyotype
M5a	*Monocytic, poorly differentiated:* Monoblasts predominate, typically with abundant cytoplasm and single distinct nucleoli
M5b	*Monocytic, well differentiated:* Predominantly promonocytes in marrow and more pronounced maturation in blood
M6	*Erythroleukemia:* Dysplastic erythroblasts with multinucleation, cytoplasmic budding, vacuolation, and megaloblastoid changes
M7	*Megakaryoblastic:* Wide range of morphology, cytoplasmic projections sometimes present; electron microscopy or immunocytochemical stains necessary for diagnosis

blasts [RAEB] and RAEB in transformation). To address this problem, the FAB cooperative group proposed revised criteria for the classification of AML, including a stepwise evaluation of the bone marrow aspirate (Fig. 18–11).[26] A differential count is done of all nucleated cells (ANC) and of only nonerythroid cells (NEC). The ANC differential is used to determine the percentage of erythroblasts (all nucleated erythroid precursors): cases with more than 50% erythroblasts are further evaluated to differentiate between M6 (blasts ≥30% of NEC) and MDS (blasts <30% of NEC); cases with less than 50% erythroblasts are evaluated to differentiate between AML, types M1 to M5 (blasts ≥30% of ANC) and MDS (blasts <30% of ANC). The final classification of AML (M1 to M5) is based on characterization of the NEC fraction. The FAB subgroups are discussed in more detail later in this chapter.

The FAB classification system has largely failed to define groups of patients with AML that have distinct clinical outcomes. These patients generally have similar clinical courses regardless of their FAB subtype. Exceptions to this are AML with monocytic differentiation (M4 and M5b) who tend to have a lower rate of complete remission and a lower rate of survival,[32] and acute promyelocytic leukemia (M3), which is associated with a longer average survival rate.[58] Because of the limitations of morphological and cytochemical classification in prediction of biologic behavior in AML, immunologic and cytogenetic techniques are used to augment the FAB classification; these methods provide additional data that are useful in determining appropriate patient management.[59]

Surface Marker Analysis of Acute Myeloid Leukemia

The availablity of myeloid-specific monoclonal antibodies has permitted surface marker analysis of AML. The rationale for this is based on the notion that AML is a clonal disorder derived from a myeloid stem line, which displays the surface membrane antigens expressed in normal myeloid differentiation pathways.[60,61] A schematic representation of this is shown in Figure 18–12.

Although surface marker analysis does not play the critical role in AML classification that it currently plays in diagnosis of ALL, it provides useful information. These studies complement morphological and cytochemical evaluation; they can be used to distinguish

TABLE 18–10	**Cytochemical Reactions in Acute Myeloblastic Leukemia**							
	FAB Classification							
	M0	**M1**	**M2**	**M3**	**M4**	**M5**	**M6**	**M7**
Peroxidase or Sudan black	<3%	>3%	>50%	near 100%	20–80%	Variable	>3%	<3%
Nonspecific esterase	<3%	<20%	<20%	Variable	20–80%	>80%	Variable	Variable

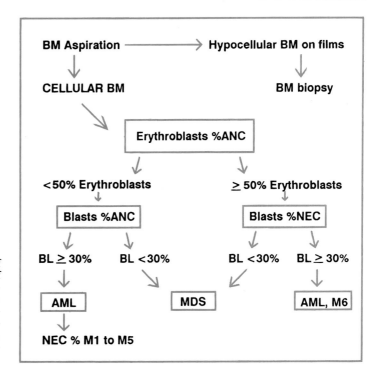

FIGURE 18–11 Suggested steps in the analysis of a bone marrow (BM) aspirate to reach a diagnosis of acute myeloid leukemia (AML) (M1 to M6) or myelodysplastic syndrome (MDS). BL = blast cells; ANC = all nucleated bone-marrow cells; NEC = nonerythroid cells, bone marrow cells excluding erythroblasts. (From Bennett, JM, Catovsky, D, Daniel, MT, et al: Ann Intern Med 103:626, 1985, with permission.)

AML from ALL, particularly when the leukemic cells are poorly differentiated, with negative or equivocal cytochemical stains (FAB M0 or M1). Expression of certain antigens may have prognostic significance. For example, Griffin and coworkers[62] showed that patients with AML whose leukemic cells express either CD13 or CD14 antigens have a lower rate of complete remission than patients whose cells lack these antigens. Expression of the progenitor cell antigen CD34 is a poor prognostic indicator in adult patients with AML.[63]

When surface marker analysis is performed to distinguish AML from ALL, it is important to choose a panel of markers that includes antibodies to several myeloid-associated antigens (e.g., CD33 [My9], CD13 [My7], CD14 [My4], CD41a [platelet GP IIb/IIIa]), as well as B- and T-lymphoid antigens. Multiple myeloid lineage-specific markers are necessary because no single marker defines all forms of AML.

The surface phenotypes expressed in cases of AML do not correlate well with the FAB classification. Although cases of AML with monocytic differentiation (M4 and M5) usually express monocyte-related surface markers (CD14), and cases of acute promyelocytic leukemia (M3) tend to express a promyelocytic phenotype (CD13 and CD33 positive, CD34 negative),[60] other AML subgroups exhibit widely variable phenotypes.

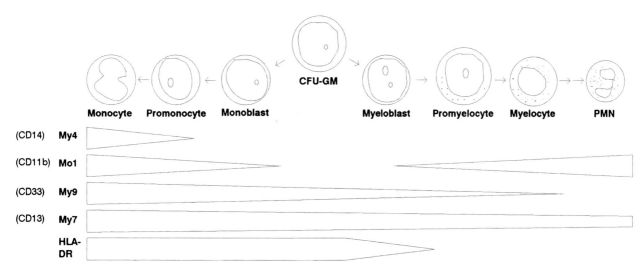

FIGURE 18–12 Distribution of myeloid and monocytic surface antigens. PMN = polymorphonuclear neutrophil; CFU–GM = colony-forming unit, granulocyte macrophage/monocyte.

Occasionally, mixed-lineage phenotypes are encountered, with coexpression of myeloid and lymphoid markers. These biphenotypic or bilineage leukemias may reflect origination of the malignant cell line from an early progenitor of both myeloid and lymphoid differentiation.

Acute Myeloid Leukemia Without Morphological or Cytochemical Maturation (M0)

Certain cases of acute nonlymphoblastic leukemia are encountered that show no definitive myeloid differentiation by conventional morphological and cytochemical analysis (minimally differentiated AML, FAB M0). These cases are characterized by the presence of primitive leukemic blasts showing no distinctive myeloid morphological features and lacking reactivity with the conventional battery of cytochemical stains (myeloperoxidase, Sudan black B, nonspecific esterase). However, they exhibit reactivity with at least one myeloid lineage-specific antigen (CD33, CD13, CD14) in the absence of lymphoid antigens. Such reactivity is required for classification as FAB M0. Lymphoid differentiation should be excluded by immunophenotyping. If a case fulfilling these criteria shows positivity for ultrastructural platelet peroxidase or platelet-specific antigens (CD41a, factor VIII), it is classified as acute megakaryoblastic leukemia (FAB M7).[64-66]

Acute Myeloid Leukemia with Minimal Morphologic and Cytochemical Maturation (M1)

The leukemic cells seen in cases of AML-M1 subtype are predominantly poorly differentiated myeloblasts (see Figs. 18–13 and 18–14). The nucleus typically has a fine lacy chromatin pattern and distinct nucleoli. The quantity of cytoplasm is usually moderate, although this varies. According to FAB criteria, less than 10% of the leukemic cells have azurophilic granules (primary granules) when observed on a Romanowsky-stained

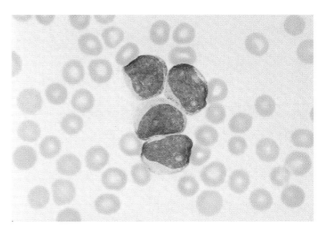

FIGURE 18–14 AML, M1, peripheral blood.

smear. The peroxidase or Sudan black reactions must demonstrate at least 3%, and less than 50% positivity in the leukemic population. The NSE reaction is positive in less than 20% of the cells. Auer rods, when present, are particularly helpful in distinguishing M1 from ALL (L2 variant).

Acute Myeloid Leukemia with Maturation (M2)

In cases of AML-M2 subtype, the leukemic marrow infiltrate resembles that of M1 except that evidence of maturation to or beyond the promyelocyte stage is present Figs. 18–15 to 18–17). Romanowsky-stained bone marrow smears show that promyelocytes make up greater than 10% of the immature cells. More than 50% of the leukemic cells are peroxidase or Sudan black positive. The NSE activity does not exceed 20%.

The acute myeloblastic leukemias (M1 and M2 combined) are the most common types of AML. Together, M1 and M2 account for approximately 50% of cases of AML.[64] Aside from their morphology and cytochemistry, they do not have unique features that set them

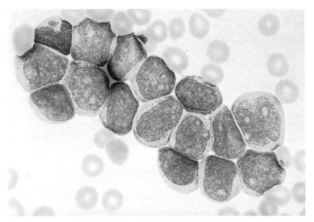

FIGURE 18–13 Acute myeloblastic leukemia (AML) without maturation, MI, bone marrow.

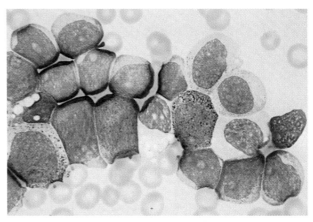

FIGURE 18–15 Acute myeloblastic leukemia with maturation, M2, bone marrow.

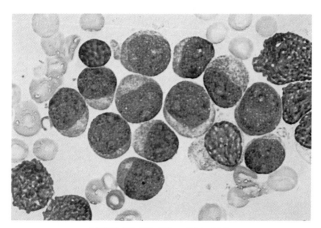

FIGURE 18-16 AML, M2.

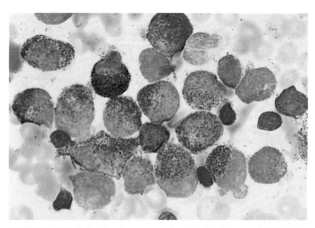

FIGURE 18-18 Acute promyelocytic leukemia, (APL) M3, bone marrow.

apart from other myeloid subgroups. Although a translocation of chromosomes 8 and 21 (t[8;21]) has been identified in approximately 18% of patients with AML, type M2,[67] this chromosome abnormality has also been found, although less frequently, in other FAB groups of AML. It is associated with the fusion gene ETO/AML1, the result of the fusion of the ETO gene on chromosome 8 with the AML1 gene on chromosome 21 (see Table 18-8).

Acute Promyelocytic Leukemia (M3)

The FAB classification defines acute promyelocytic leukemia (APL) solely by morphological criteria. The leukemic infiltrate is composed of abnormal promyelocytes with heavy granulation, sometimes obscuring the nucleus, and often abundant cytoplasm (Fig. 18-18). Auer rods are frequently seen, and some cells may contain bundles or stacks of Auer rods ("faggot cells"). The nucleus varies in size and shape and is often reniform (kidney-shaped) or bilobed. These cells are strongly positive with the peroxidase and Sudan black B stains (Fig. 18-19) and are usually negative with the NSE stain, but cases with positive NSE activity do occur.[68,69]

APL is associated with a high incidence of disseminated intravascular coagulation (DIC). The abnormal promyelocytes are rich in thromboplastic substances that, if released, trigger DIC. Most patients with APL present with hemorrhagic manifestations including petechiae, small ecchymoses, hematuria, and bleeding from venipuncture and bone marrow sites.[70] These presenting signs and symptoms may precede the diagnosis by several weeks. The most consistent coagulation abnormalities include a prolonged prothrombin time and thrombin time, elevated fibrin degradation products, and decreased amounts of plasma fibrinogen and factor V. Thrombocytopenia, which tends to be more severe than in other types of AML, is almost universally present. Schistocytes are sometimes evident on the peripheral blood smear. Because of the hemorrhagic complications associated with DIC, it is important to distinguish APL from other forms of AML. Anticoagulant therapy (heparin) is usually indicated in these cases and is most successful when initiated prior to antileukemic therapy.[70]

A unique feature of APL is the occurrence of a translocation involving chromosomes 15 and 17, t(15;17).

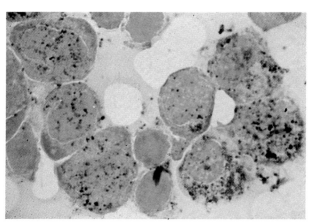

FIGURE 18-17 AML, M2 (myeloperoxidase stain).

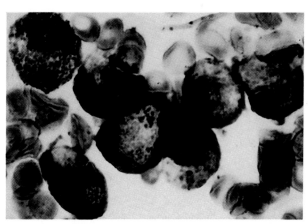

FIGURE 18-19 APL, M3 (Sudan black B stain).

This abnormality has not been reported in any other type of leukemia. It is associated with the hybrid gene PML/RARα, which forms the basis of a specifically targeted form of differentiation therapy, all trans-retinoic acid.[71-73]

A second form of APL is the microgranular variant (M3m).[74,75] The leukemic cells of M3m have primary granules that are not readily visible on Romanowsky-stained smears (Fig. 18–20). These granules can, however, be demonstrated with peroxidase and Sudan black staining or by transmission electron microscopy.[76] The disease, like typical APL, has a high incidence of DIC, and it is therefore important to recognize it for therapeutic considerations. Patients with the microgranular variant tend to have a higher WBC count than those patients with typical APL and may have a shorter survival.[32]

Morphologically, microgranular APL can be mistaken for acute myelomonocytic or monocytic leukemia. The leukemic cells appear monocytoid with prominent nuclear folding and abundant cytoplasm. The nucleus of most cells in the peripheral blood is reniform or bilobed. Granulation of these cells is scant or absent, although occasional cells with heavy granulation are almost always present. The bone marrow aspirate may reveal a morphological pattern that more closely resembles typical APL.[77]

The diagnosis of M3m can be confirmed with cytochemical studies including a peroxidase or Sudan black stain that are strongly positive. The NSE reaction is usually negative, but can be positive.[69] Cytogenetic studies of microgranular APL reveal the same abnormal karyotype [t(15;17)] that is found in the hypergranular form.

Acute Myelomonocytic Leukemia (M4)

Acute myelomonocytic leukemia (M4) is one of the most commonly diagnosed forms of AML, second only to the M2 group.[32] The leukemic cells of M4 are characterized by both granulocytic and monocytic differentiation (see Figs. 18–21 and 18–22). On a Romanowsky-stained smear it is usually easy to find cells with primary granules (granulocytic differentiation) as well

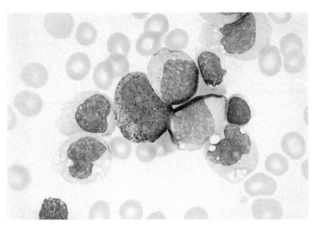

FIGURE 18–21 Acute myelomonocytic leukemia, AMML M4, bone marrow.

as cells with folded nuclei and moderate to abundant cytoplasm (monocytic differentiation). Both the peroxidase (or Sudan black) and NSE reactions are positive in 20% to 80% of the cells. When morphologic and cytochemical similarities make the distinction between M4 and M2 difficult, the diagnosis of M4 can be supported by finding a serum lysozyme level exceeding three times the normal level and a peripheral blood monocyte count of greater than $5 \times 10^9/L$.[26]

Some cases of M4 are associated with eosinophilia (usually 5% or more of the nonerythroid cells). The eosinophils appear immature and may have large basophilic staining granules. Unlike normal eosinophils, these cells stain positive with chloroacetate esterase (specific esterase) and with the PAS reaction. This M4 variant (M4Eo)[26] is closely associated with an abnormal chromosome 16 including either a deletion[78] or inversion of the long arm (16q).[79] Patients with the 16q abnormality and bone marrow eosinophilia have a longer median survival than patients with typical M4. The molecular genetic correlate is the hybrid gene CBFβ/MYH11.

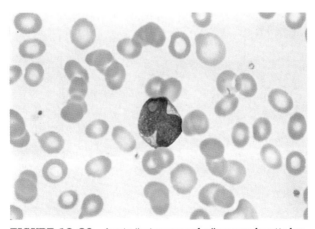

FIGURE 18–20 Acute "microgranular" promyelocytic leukemia, M3m, peripheral blood.

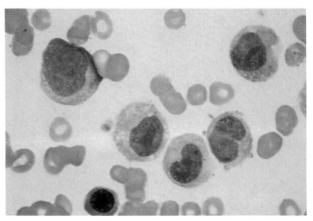

FIGURE 18–22 Acute myelomonocytic leukemia, M4, peripheral blood.

Acute Monocytic Leukemia (M5)

The FAB classification system divides acute monocytic leukemia (M5) into two subtypes: poorly differentiated (M5a) and well differentiated (M5b). M5a is characterized by a predominance of monoblasts, which typically are large with abundant cytoplasm and distinct nucleoli (Fig. 18–23). M5b is characterized by a spectrum of monocytic differentiation including promonocytes and monocytes. The peripheral blood usually has more monocytes than the bone marrow, in which the predominant cell is the promonocyte. This cell has abundant cytoplasm, its nucleus shows delicate folding or lobulation, and nucleoli may be seen (see Fig. 18–24). Both subtypes of M5 show greater than 80% positivity with the NSE stain. The peroxidase and Sudan black stains are negative or only weakly positive.

Acute monocytic leukemia (AMoL) has distinctive clinical manifestations associated with the monocyte's propensity to migrate to extramedullary sites. Skin and gum involvement (Fig. 18–25) is particularly characteristic. Lymphadenopathy frequently occurs, and sometimes the spleen and liver are markedly enlarged.[80] CNS involvement also has an increased incidence in these patients.[81,82]

The WBC count is frequently elevated in patients with AMoL; the median value of 60×10^9/L was reported in one study.[83] Markedly elevated leukocyte counts in AMoL patients have been shown to have a significant correlation with increased lysozyme levels, renal failure, and hypokalemia.[84] DIC is relatively common in patients with AMoL, especially following therapy, although hemorrhagic features are not as prominent as in patients with acute promyelocytic leukemia.

Serum and urine lysozyme levels (muramidase) are often elevated in cases of AML that have a significant monocytic component, including both AML types M4 and M5. Lysozyme is a hydrolytic enzyme found in mature monocytes and to a lesser extent in granulocytes. Serum and urine levels of this enzyme are elevated when there is rapid cell turnover. Such elevations are

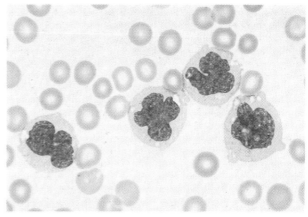

FIGURE 18–24 Acute monocytic leukemia, well-differentiated, M5b, peripheral blood.

most striking in the monocytic leukemias and are directly proportional to the amount of monocytic differentiation[85]; they are more elevated in cases of M5b than M5a. Those patients who have heavy urinary excretion of lysozyme may develop renal dysfunction resulting in hypokalemia, hypocalcemia, and azotemia.

Abnormalities involving the long arm of chromosome 11 (11q) have been found in about 35% of all M5 AMLs and in an even higher percentage of patients with M5a. The 11q abnormality appears to be particularly associated with children with M5a.[67]

Erythroleukemia (M6)

Acute erythroleukemia is characterized by an abnormal proliferation of erythroid and myeloid precursors. Patients with erythroleukemia have hypercellular bone marrows with marked erythroid hyperplasia (greater than 50% of ANC) associated with abnormal erythroid forms. Megaloblastoid changes can be seen in the erythroblasts along with other dysplastic features including bizarre multinucleation, markedly vacuolated cytoplasm of erythroblasts, and cytoplas-

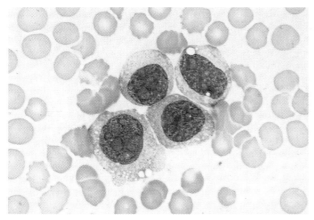

FIGURE 18–23 Acute monocytic leukemia (AMoL), poorly differentiated, M5a, peripheral blood.

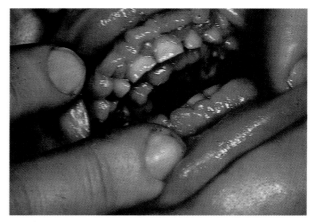

FIGURE 18–25 Gum hypertrophy: a clinical manifestation of acute leukemia.

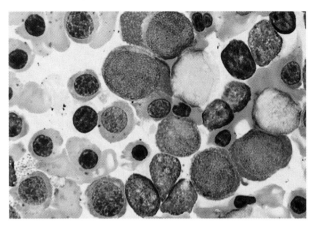

FIGURE 18–26 Erythroleukemia, M6, bone marrow.

mic budding (see Figs. 18–26 and 18–27). Cytoplasmic PAS positive staining in the neoplastic erythroblasts is consistent with the diagnosis of erythroleukemia, but is not absolutely specific, and negative staining does not rule it out. Myeloblasts and promyelocytes are present in increased numbers (greater than 30% of nonerythroid cells), and Auer rods may be seen. Abnormal megakaryocytes may also be present.

Erythroleukemia has three sequential morphologically defined phases in which the myeloid component varies. They are: (1) erythremic myelosis, in which abnormal erythroblasts predominate; (2) erythroleukemia, in which both erythroblasts and myeloblasts are increased; and (3) acute myeloid leukemia of the conventional type.[86] It is well recognized that many patients who are diagnosed with erythroleukemia will have their disease evolve into a leukemic stage indistinguishable from AML-M1, -M2, or -M4 type.[57]

Anemia is invariably present in patients with erythroleukemia, and is often more pronounced than in patients with other types of AML. Reticulocytopenia is common and is a result of ineffective erythropoiesis. Frequently the peripheral blood exhibits nucleated red blood cells (NRBCs) and myeloblasts, but it is possible

to see patients who are anerythremic (no NRBCs) or aleukemic (no blasts).

Caution must be taken when the diagnosis of erythroleukemia is considered. The possibility of megaloblastic anemia arising from either vitamin B_{12} or folic acid deficiency, congenital dyserythropoietic anemia, and the myelodysplastic syndromes must be excluded. These disorders may sometimes mimic erythroleukemia.

Acute Megakaryoblastic Leukemia (M7)

Acute megakaryoblastic leukemia (AMegL) is a relatively uncommon form of leukemia characterized by neoplastic proliferation of megakaryoblasts and atypical megakaryocytes. Recognition of this entity was aided by the use of platelet peroxidase (PPO) ultrastructural studies. PPO, which is distinct from myeloperoxidase, is specific for the megakaryocytic cell line.[87] This enzyme appears early in the differentiation of these cells and is localized in the nuclear membrane and endoplasmic reticulum.[88]

AMegL was not initially included in the FAB classification of AML because it could not be identified by conventional morphological and cytochemical studies; however, in 1985 increased recognition of this entity prompted the FAB cooperative group to add AMegL to the classification (M7).[89] M7 was the first subtype of AML to incorporate immunophenotype into criteria for diagnosis.

The blasts observed in AMegL display a wide range of morphology, from small cells with scant cytoplasm and dense chromatin to large cells with a moderate amount of cytoplasm and a fine reticulated chromatin pattern. Cytoplasmic projections are sometimes present (Fig. 18–28), and in some cases azurophilic granules resembling early granular megakaryocytes can be seen.[90] The presence of megakaryocytic fragments in the peripheral blood is also suggestive of AmegL.

Conventional cytochemistry can suggest the diagnosis of AMegL, but is not definitive. The myeloperoxidase and Sudan black reactions are negative, whereas acid phosphatase, PAS, and alpha-naphthyl acetate esterase (ANAE) are usually positive. The combination

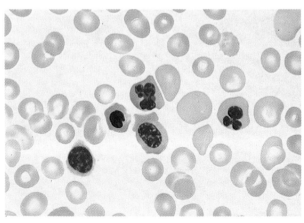

FIGURE 18–27 Erythroleukemia, M6, peripheral blood.

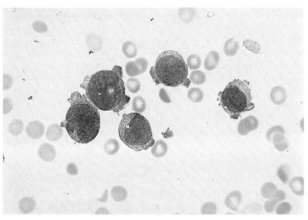

FIGURE 18–28 Acute megakaryoblastic leukemia, (AMegL) M7.

of a positive ANAE and a negative alpha-naphthyl butyrate esterase rules out monocytic leukemia and is highly suggestive of megakaryoblastic lineage.[91]

Electron microscopy for platelet peroxidase may be performed, but the diagnosis of AMegL is usually made by using an immunocytochemical demonstration of platelet-specific antigens. Antibodies against factor VIII–related antigen and platelet surface glycoprotein IIb/IIIa (fibrinogen receptor, CD41a) are the most sensitive and specific immunologic markers of AMegL.

AmegL may arise in the context of myelodysplasia or de novo. It has been observed as a transformation of existing hematologic disorders such as myelodysplastic syndromes, chronic myelocytic leukemia, and agnogenic myeloid metaplasia. AMegL has also been associated with acute myelofibrosis, which is characterized by diffuse marrow fibrosis, pancytopenia, and bone marrow megakaryoblast proliferation, but which usually lacks the splenomegaly and characteristic red cell morphological changes of chronic myelofibrosis. It has been suggested that acute myelofibrosis may be synonymous with AMegL, and may be related to neoplastic elaboration of platelet-derived growth factor (PDGF).[92]

CASE STUDY

A 42-year-old woman presented with a 2-month history of fatigue and weakness and a 2-week history of a sore throat. She reported a 15-pound weight loss over the last month or two. One week before admission, she started antibiotics for her sore throat, but she reported little improvement; she subsequently developed a peritonsillar abscess. On admission to the hospital, she was found to have an elevated WBC count with a large number of circulating blasts.

The physical examination of the patient showed an anxious, middle-aged woman whose vital signs were normal, aside from a slightly elevated temperature (37.6°C). Her right tonsil was enlarged and erythematous. She had no adenopathy and her liver and spleen were not palpable.

Laboratory studies were ordered and the following results were reported: hematocrit, 19.5%; hemoglobin, 6.3 g/dL; platelets, 64×10^9/L; and WBC count, 79.2×10^9/L. The differential included 80% blasts. Most of these cells were relatively large (15 to 20 μm) with a moderate amount of cytoplasm. The nuclei varied in shape from round or oval and some were indented or folded; most had several distinct small nucleoli. An occasional blast had azurophilic granules, but this was the exception. A bone marrow aspirate and biopsy were obtained, which both showed virtually total replacement of normal elements with sheets of poorly differentiated cells (Fig. 18–29). The biopsy was hypercellular, approaching 100% cellularity in some areas. The morphology of the aspirated cells was similar to those seen in the peripheral blood except that fewer of the cells had folded nuclei, and in general, the nucleocytoplasmic ratio was higher. Most of these cells showed very little differentiation though occasional

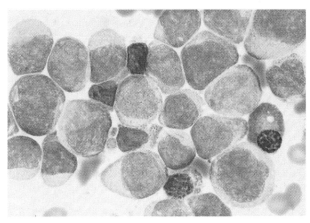

FIGURE 18–29   Case study bone marrow (AML).

cells with granulation were noted. Rare Auer rods were also observed. Cytochemical studies done on the aspirate smears were positive: the myeloperoxidase stain was positive in approximately 30% of the blasts and the NSE (alpha-naphthyl butyrate) was positive in occasional cells (less than 10%).

Diagnosis   Acute myeloid leukemia, FAB M1.

Follow-up   HLA matching was performed on the patient's brother and sister, but neither had a compatible tissue type. The possibility of a bone marrow transplantation was subsequently ruled out. The patient was placed on a standard protocol for acute myeloid leukemia. During her induction chemotherapy, she developed anemia, thrombocytopenia, and leukopenia. She required platelets and packed red blood cell transfusions. She also required broad-spectrum antibiotics for fever caused by neutropenia, although no specific pathogen could be identified. Three weeks after her induction chemotherapy, a repeat bone marrow showed no residual leukemia. She remained in complete remission for 11 months, but then relapsed. Attempts to induce a second remission were unsuccessful. She developed progressive hepatomegaly, jaundice, and persistent neutropenia. She also developed multiple infections and was unable to recover.

This case illustrates a typical course of acute myeloid leukemia. Although the patient was not cured, she did achieve and maintain a complete remission for nearly a full year.

Questions

1. Auer rods present in this patient rule out what other hematologic disorder?
2. How do the morphological characteristics presented here differ from a FAB M_0 classification?
3. What would you expect the myeloid-to-erythroid ratio to be in this case? (Refer to Fig. 18–29.)
4. What surface markers would be employed to differentiate this disorder from ALL?
5. Relate the development of multiple infections in this patient to the laboratory criteria provided.

ACUTE LYMPHOBLASTIC LEUKEMIA

FAB Classification of Acute Lymphoblastic Leukemia

The FAB classification system separates acute lymphoblastic leukemia (ALL) into three morphological groups (Table 18–11):
- L1: Small, uniform lymphoblasts
- L2: Large, pleomorphic lymphoblasts
- L3: Burkitt's type (vacuolated and deeply basophilic cytoplasm)

The morphology of these groups is evaluated on a bone marrow aspirate smear rather than peripheral blood. L1 ALL (Fig. 18–30) exhibits a uniform population of small blasts with scant cytoplasm, a homogeneous chromatin pattern, and inconspicuous nucleoli. The nuclear shape is regular, but occasional clefting may be present. L2 ALL (Figs. 18–31 and 18–32) is characterized by cellular heterogeneity. Some blasts may exhibit L1 features, whereas others are larger and have more abundant cytoplasm, a variable chromatin pattern and prominent nucleoli. Nuclear clefting and indentation are characteristic. This type may be difficult or impossible to distinguish morphologically from AML-M1. L3 ALL (Fig. 18–33) is composed of a uniform population of relatively large blasts that are characterized by moderate to abundant deeply basophilic, vacuolated cytoplasm. The nucleus has a round to oval contour without indentations. L3 ALL is referred to as "Burkitt's type" because its morphology is that seen in Burkitt's leukemia or lymphoma.

The distinction between L1 and L2 ALL is not always clear. Because of this, the FAB cooperative group proposed a simple scoring system based on cytologic features.[93] Other groups have modified this, assessing each case on a cell-by-cell basis to determine the percentage of L1 and L2 cells.[94,95] Individual L1 and L2 lymphoblasts can be differentiated most reliably by evaluating the nucleocytoplasmic ratio (high in L1, low in L2) and the absence (L1) or presence (L2) of nucleoli. Cases of "pure L1" ALL (>90% L1 blasts) have the best prognosis, cases of "pure L2" ALL (>50% L2 blasts) have a worse prognosis, and cases with mixed cell

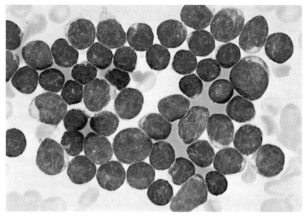

FIGURE 18–30 Acute lymphoblastic leukemia (ALL), L1, bone marrow.

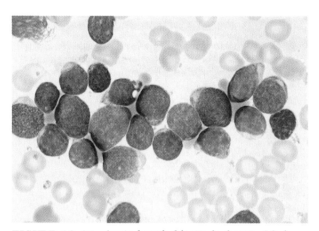

FIGURE 18–31 Acute lymphoblastic leukemia, L2, bone marrow.

TABLE 18–11	**FAB Classification of Acute Lymphoblastic Leukemia**		
Cytologic Features	**L1**	**L2**	**L3**
Cell size	Predominantly small	Large, heterogeneous	Large, homogeneous
Nuclear chromatin	Homogeneous in any one case	Heterogeneous	Finely stippled, and homogeneous
Nuclear shape	Regular, occasional clefting	Irregular, clefting and indentation common	Regular (round to oval)
Nucleoli*	Inconspicuous	One or more, often large	One or more, prominent
Cytoplasm*	Scanty	Variable; often moderately abundant	Moderately abundant, strongly basophilic
Cytoplasmic vacuolation	Variable	Variable	Prominent

*The most useful cytologic features in separating L1 from L2 lymphoblasts are quantity of cytoplasm and presence and prominence of nucleoli.
Source: Adapted from Bennett et al.[35]

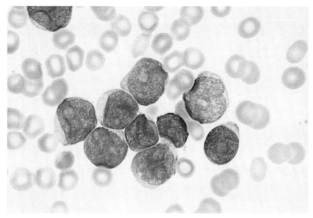

FIGURE 18–32 Acute lymphoblastic leukemia, L2, peripheral blood.

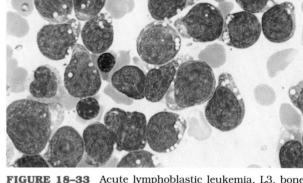

FIGURE 18–33 Acute lymphoblastic leukemia, L3, bone marrow.

types have an intermediate prognosis. L3 morphology is associated with the worst prognosis.[96] Regardless of the morphological classification described here, immunologic and cytogenetic techniques serve a critical function in determining modern therapeutic approaches to ALL.

Immunologic Classification of Acute Lymphoblastic Anemia

The immunologic classification of ALL is based on the stages of lymphocyte development, whose phenotypes are summarized in Table 18–12. Lymphoblasts are phenotyped using monoclonal antibodies (refer to Table 18–7). The nuclear enzyme TdT, which is found in immature lymphoid cells (both B and T lineage), is also utilized.

To appreciate fully the immunologic classification of ALL and other lymphoproliferative disorders (e.g., CLL, lymphoma, and multiple myeloma), it is important to understand lymphocyte ontogeny. These processes result from clonal proliferation of lymphoid cells—cells that have been "frozen" at a given stage of maturation, retaining some features of their normally differentiated counterparts. In the case of ALL, the malignant clone is arrested at an early stage of lymphocytic differentiation.

Lymphocyte Ontogeny

Lymphocytes originate from pluripotent stem cells (see Fig. 1–57) that are present in the yolk sac, fetal liver, spleen, and bone marrow. At birth and into adulthood, the stem cells are normally found only in the bone marrow, where they respond to specific growth factors (hormonelike substances) that trigger their commitment toward B- or T-lymphocyte differentiation. The microenvironment of these developing cells plays a critical role in their maturation: B cells develop in the bone marrow (bursa-equivalent tissue), whereas T cells develop in the thymus (from committed stem cells that have migrated there). Lymphocyte maturation in these organs is antigen-independent. After the lymphocytes have matured, they migrate to the peripheral lymphoid organs, including the lymph nodes, spleen, and other lymphoid tissues. In these organs, the lymphocytes remain in a resting state until they are stimulated to undergo antigen-dependent development.

B-Lymphocyte Development Early B-cell maturation (antigen-independent) is divided into three stages: early pre-B cell, pre-B cell, and mature B cell (Fig. 18–34). These stages are identified by their expression of TdT, surface markers (HLA-DR, CD10 [CALLA], CD19, CD20), and immunoglobulin (cyto-

	HLA-DR	CD19 (Pan-B)	CD10 (CALLA)	Cμ	sIg	(Pan-T)	CD7 TdT	FAB
TABLE 18–12 Immunologic Classification of Acute Lymphoblastic Leukemia								
Precursor B-cell	+	+	–	–	–	–	+	L1, L2
Early pre-B-cell	+	+	+	–	–	–	+	L1, L2
Pre-B-cell	+	+	+	+	–	–	+	L1, L2
B-cell	+	+	–/+	–	+	–	–	L3
T-cell	–	–	–/+	–	–	+	+	L1, L2
"Null" cell*	+	–	–	–	–	–	+	L1, L2

*Immunoglobulin gene rearrangement studies have shown that most of these are precursor B-cell ALLs.
Abbreviations: CALLA = common ALL antigen; Cμ = cytoplasmic mu; sIg = surface immunoglobulin; TdT = terminal deoxynucleotidyl transferase; FAB = French-American-British classification.

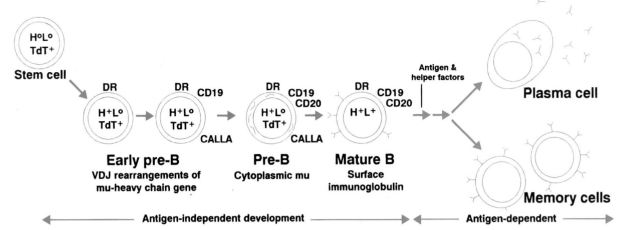

FIGURE 18–34 B-cell development. Heavy chain (H) and light chain (L) are designated as H°, L° if in embryonic form, and H+, L+ if rearranged.

plasmic or surface Ig). The early pre-B cell is TdT-positive and expresses HLA-DR, CD19, and usually CALLA (CD10). HLA-DR, a histocompatibility-related antigen, is expressed first, followed by CD19 and then CD10. CD19 is the most sensitive and specific surface marker for early B cells. During this stage, the immunoglobulin genes begin to undergo structural rearrangement (see below), followed by the production of cytoplasmic μ heavy chain. The presence of cytoplasmic μ distinguishes the pre-B cell from its predecessor, which otherwise has a similar phenotype. As the cell continues to mature, immunoglobulin light chains are produced and IgM is assembled and inserted into the plasma membrane. This surface Ig (sIg) is the hallmark

of the mature B cell that no longer expresses TdT. Each B cell expresses only one type of Ig light chain (kappa or lambda), a feature that is extremely helpful in identifying monoclonal proliferations of mature B cells.

Immunoglobulin genes are rearranged in a unique process that is normally limited to cells committed to B-cell differentiation. The Ig genes are composed of discontinuous segments of minigene families that, when productively rearranged, encode for the heavy chain and the kappa or lambda light chains (Fig. 18–35). Both IgM and IgD are expressed on the surface of the majority of mature B cells.

After maturation in the bone marrow, B cells circulate through the blood to the peripheral lymphoid or-

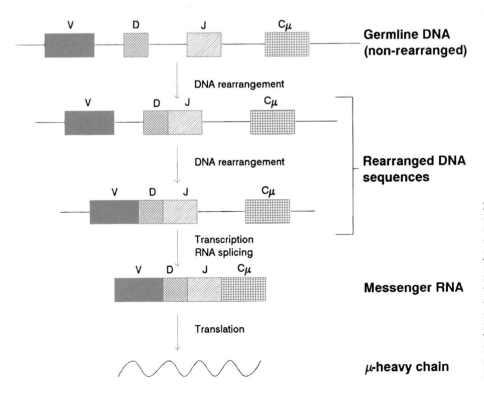

FIGURE 18–35 Schematic of immunoglobulin μ-heavy chain gene rearrangement. The variable (V), diversity (D), and joining (J) regions of germline DNA are linked through rearrangement and loss of intervening sequences. The VDJ complex, more intervening sequences, and a constant (Cμ) region are then transcribed. The resulting RNA is spliced, linking the VDJ and Cμ regions and creating a template for the Ig μ-heavy chain.

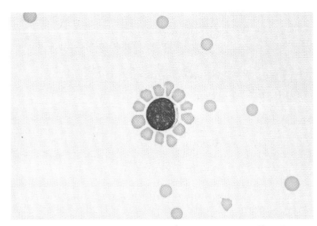

FIGURE 18–36 E-rosette formation in T-cell ALL.

gans, where they remain in a resting state until stimulated by specific antigens to undergo further development. Activated B cells undergo clonal expansion, producing daughter cells that retain the same antibody idiotype (antigen-binding region). Some

daughter cells become memory cells and regain the small mature B-cell morphology and phenotype, whereas others continue development toward a short-lived antibody secreting cell—the plasma cell. During this final development, the Ig heavy chain may undergo another isotype switch, to IgG, IgA, or IgE. The plasma cell produces large quantities of Ig and is characterized by a high concentration of cytoplasmic Ig. It does not express sIg, CD19, or CD20, although other antigens are sometimes expressed (e.g., PCA-1, PC-1).

T-Lymphocyte Development In the past, T cells were identified by incubating lymphocytes with sheep red blood cells and observing for E-rosette formation (Fig. 18–36). Now, with the availability of monoclonal antibodies, T cells are identified and subclassified using immunologic reagents. T-cell development (antigen-independent) in the thymus is divided into three main stages: stage I, early thymocyte; stage II, common thymocyte; and stage III, mature thymocyte. Stages I and II occur in the thymic cortex and the last stage occurs in the thymic medulla. Like early B cells, thymocytes express TdT and unique surface markers (Fig. 18–37). CD7, which is present on early thymocytes, is one of the earliest T-cell markers to be ex-

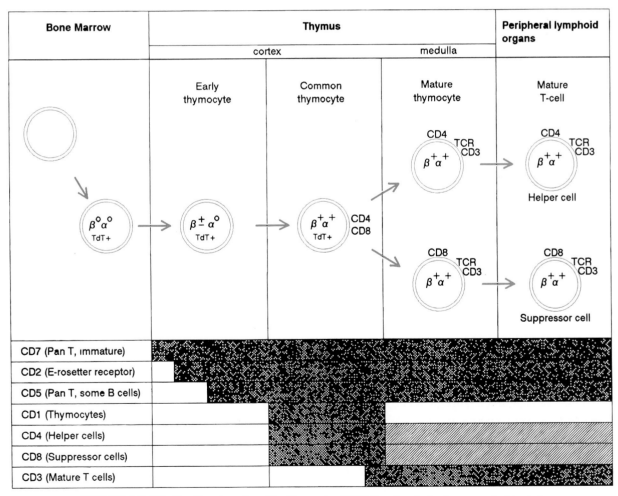

FIGURE 18–37 T-cell maturation. T-cell receptor (TCR) β and α chain genes are designated as $\beta°$, $\alpha°$ if in embryonic form, and $\beta+$, $\alpha+$ if rearranged.

pressed; it is also the most sensitive marker for T-cell ALL.[97] Its expression is followed by that of CD2 and CD5. As the thymocytes move into stage II of thymic development, they express CD1, a marker of common thymocytes, plus both CD4 and CD8. CD3 is the next marker to be expressed; it is usually absent or only weakly expressed at stage II, but it is fully expressed in the mature thymocyte (stage III). At this stage, CD1 and CD4 or CD8 are lost, giving the mature thymocyte a helper (CD4+) or suppressor (CD8+) phenotype.

During thymic maturation, the T cell synthesizes an antigen-receptor molecule called the T-cell receptor (TCR), which is closely associated with the CD3 molecule on the plasma membrane. Two TCR isotypes have been discovered, TCR-$\alpha\beta$ and TCR-$\gamma\delta$. The genes that encode for the α, β, γ, and δ polypeptides undergo rearrangement in a manner that parallels Ig gene rearrangements in the B cell. The TCR β gene (on chromosome 7) rearrangements precede TCR α (on chromosome 14) rearrangements. Less is known about the γ and δ genes or about the function of the TCR-$\gamma\delta$; but it is clear that rearrangement of the γ gene precedes that of the α and β genes.[98] The majority of mature T cells express the TCR-$\alpha\beta$ isotype.

Childhood Acute Lymphoblastic Leukemia versus Adult Acute Lymphoblastic Leukemia

The incidence of ALL differs markedly with age. For this reason and because of the generally poorer prognosis in adults, ALL may be considered in the broad context of childhood and adult ALL. The childhood group generally consists of patients who present with ALL at 15 years of age or earlier.

L1 morphology occurs most frequently in the pediatric age group, whereas the L2 type tends to be seen in adults. The incidence of L3 ALL does not differ significantly in children and adults.

B- and T-lineage ALLs occur at similar rates in children and adults, but differences in phenotypes are observed. For example, cases of childhood T-cell ALL rarely express HLA-DR, but this marker is expressed in a large percentage of adults with T-cell ALL.[99] A relatively high proportion of adults with early pre-B-cell ALL do not express CD10 (formerly termed *null cell* ALL).

Prognostic indicators are especially important in cases of childhood ALL. Most of these patients are able to achieve a complete remission and many are potentially cured. Unfortunately some children relapse, and some of these eventually succumb to their disease. The therapy used to achieve a cure has potentially toxic effects that are a special concern in growing children. To select those patients who will have an optimal response to less aggressive therapy, investigators have identified prognostic factors and defined clinical risk categories. These allow the type and intensity of therapy to be focused to each child's level of clinical risk of relapse and death.[100] Indicators of a poor prognosis include older age (>13 years), a high WBC count (>20 × 10^9/L), T-cell or mature B-cell phenotypes, L2 and L3 morphology, and structural chromosome abnormalities. Children with an early pre-B-cell phenotype,

with hyperdiploid lymphoblasts (>50 chromosomes) and a low WBC count, and without a structural chromosome abnormality have a very good prognosis.[40,101]

Precursor B-Cell Acute Lymphoblastic Leukemia (Early Pre-B and Pre-B)

Precursor B-cell ALL, including both early pre-B and pre-B cell types, is the most frequently encountered form of lymphoblastic leukemia. It is predominantly seen in the pediatric age group, although it may occur at any age. Its peak incidence is between the ages of 3 and 5 years and it is characterized in most childhood cases by L1 morphology. In adults, L2 morphology is more common. Early pre-B-cell ALL expresses HLA-DR and CD19. Pre-B-cell ALL has the same surface phenotype but also expresses cytoplasmic μ. Most of these precursor B-cell leukemias have CALLA (CD10) on their surface and are referred to as *common ALL.* Some of these, particularly pre-B-cell ALL, also express CD20, a pan-B-cell marker that first appears during the midstage of B-cell development.

Patients with precursor B-cell ALL usually present with disease predominantly localized to the blood and bone marrow. Prominent splenomegaly, hepatomegaly, and lymphadenopathy are infrequently seen at presentation. It is also uncommon for these patients to exhibit a markedly elevated white blood count (greater than 100 × 10^9/L).

In children, pre-B-cell ALL (cytoplasmic μ present) is associated with a poorer outcome than early pre-B ALL (cytoplasmic μ absent). Both groups have a high rate of achieving complete remission; however, patients with pre-B-cell ALL appear to have a shorter duration of remission.[102] Twenty to thirty percent of these patients have a translocation of chromosome 1 and 19 (t[1;19]).[103] This rearrangement is not generally found in cases of early pre-B-cell ALL. In adults, approximately 30% of pre-B-cell ALL is associated with the Philadelphia chromosome (t[9;22]).

B-Cell Acute Lymphoblastic Leukemia (Burkitt's Leukemia and Lymphoma)

B-cell ALL is a homogeneous group that accounts for only a small portion (2% to 5%) of all cases of ALL. It is the only phenotype that can be reliably predicted on the basis of morphology alone; L3 morphology is consistently observed, with a mature B-cell phenotype characterized by a high concentration of surface immunoglobulin (usually sIgM) and monoclonal light-chain restriction. CD19, CD20, and HLA-DR are positive; TdT is negative, and most cases do not express CD10. It is likely that these cells are derived from a transformed or stimulated B cell.[104] Virtually all cases have a characteristic translocation involving a rearrangement of the c-myc oncogene on chromosome 8 with the immunoglobulin heavy-chain gene on chromosome 14 or the light-chain genes on chromosomes 2 or 22 (t[8;14], t[2;8], or t[8;22]).[105,106]

The lymphoblasts found in cases of B-cell ALL are indistinguishable by cytologic, cytochemical, and immunologic criteria from tumor cells found in cases of Burkitt's lymphoma.[107] It is likely that B-cell ALL represents a leukemic phase of Burkitt's lymphoma (non-African type).

The prognosis for patients with B-cell ALL is poor. They respond poorly to current chemotherapy regimens and rarely achieve remission.[108]

T-Cell Acute Lymphoblastic Leukemia

T-cell markers are found in approximately 15% to 25% of all patients with ALL. These cases can be categorized into one of the three stages of thymocyte development.[109] CD7 is the most reliable marker of T-cell ALL, but CD2 and CD5 are also expressed in many cases. CD4 and CD8 are occasionally coexpressed and may be accompanied by the presence of CD3; approximately 10% express CALLA. The blasts of T-cell ALL are TdT-positive and are associated with both L1 and L2 morphology.

Patients with T-cell ALL often present with a mediastinal mass, a high WBC count (greater than 100×10^9/L in 50% of cases), hepatosplenomegaly, and early meningeal involvement. Males are affected more often than females, and the disease occurs more often in older children. These patients generally have a poorer prognosis than those with common ALL. Features that most consistently correlate with a better response to therapy include a low WBC count, younger age (≥ 15 years), and L1 morphology. There is also some evidence that certain surface markers may be associated with a better (CD5) or worse (CD3) prognosis.[110,111]

When patients present with a mediastinal mass, it may be difficult to distinguish T-cell ALL from lymphoblastic lymphoma. The cytologic features of this type of lymphoma are similar to those of ALL, although the lymphoma is generally associated with a more mature immunophenotype.[112] After a variable time, patients with lymphoblastic lymphoma almost always develop bone marrow involvement, which renders their condition indistinguishable from T-cell ALL. This distinction is generally based on clinical criteria. Patients who first present with prominent marrow and peripheral blood involvement are usually diagnosed with T-cell ALL.

Acute Leukemia, Unclassified and of Mixed Lineage

With the advent of immunophenotyping and other forms of biologic assessment of acute leukemia, subsets of acute leukemia not following clear lineage definition are being described more frequently. A significant number of patients with otherwise typical AML or ALL are found to have features of both cell types with use of immunologic, molecular, or biochemical techniques.[113] The lymphoid and myeloid antigens may be coexpressed by a single population of leukemic cells, or there may be biphasic populations with distinct lineage-specific phenotypes.[65] A sequential transformation may occur from one cell lineage to another. B- and T-cell antigen receptor gene rearrangements are more common in TdT-positive AML; AML with immunoglobulin or T-cell receptor gene rearrangements is more likely to express lymphoid and stem cell antigens.[114] The significance of these forms of mixed-lineage expression are unclear at present. Studies on the prognostic significance of lymphoid antigen expression in AML have yielded conflicting results.[115,116] Currently, mixed-lineage leukemias are treated on the basis of traditional morphological and cytochemical criteria. and as AML if the morphology and cytochemistry suggest undifferentiated leukemia.[65]

CASE STUDY

A 4-year-old boy first presented to his family doctor with a 3-week history of fatigue, weakness, and a persistent sore throat. On physical examination, he had a palpable spleen but no evidence of lymphadenopathy. He appeared pale and had multiple bruises over his lower extremities. A CBC, platelet count, and differential were done, with the following results:

CBC:

WBC	2.40×10^9/L	MCV	87.0 fL
RBC	2.41×10^{12}/L	MCH	29.0 pg
Hct	21.0%	MCHC	33.3 g/dL
Hgb	7.0 g/dL	Platelets	6.7×10^9/L

Differential:

3%	PMN
97%	Blasts

A bone marrow examination was performed and revealed sheets of small blasts having scant cytoplasm and indistinct nucleoli (see Fig. 18–30). Cytochemical and cell marker studies of the bone marrow aspirate gave the following results:

Cytochemistry:

Peroxidase—negative
NSE—negative

TdT: Strongly positive

Surface Markers:

CD3	Negative	CD10	100%
CD5	Negative	CD19	98%
CD7	Negative	CD20	Negative

Cytoplasmic μ: Negative

Diagnosis Acute lymphoblastic leukemia, common ALL (early pre-B; L1 type)

Follow-up This patient was placed on a protocol for ALL, to which he responded very well. His physical examination 2 months after induction chemotherapy was unremarkable except for some hair loss. His CBC was entirely normal, although his WBC count was low-normal. A bone marrow examination at this time was also normal. He was continued on therapy, including one reintensification phase followed by maintenance therapy. Eight years later, he is free of any signs of leukemia and is living a normal life.

Questions

1. What information presented in this case history coincides with a good prognosis?
2. The surface marker CD7 is found in what specific cell type?
3. Describe the significance of cytochemistry in this case in determination of a diagnosis.
4. What other type of ALL is of B-cell origin?

REFERENCES

1. Bennett, JH: Two cases of disease and enlargement of the spleen in which death took place from the presence of purulent matter in the blood. Edinburgh Med Surg J 64:413, 1845.
2. Virchow, R: Weisses Blut. Froiep's Notizen, 36:151, 1845.
3. Gunz, FW: The dread leukemias and the lymphomas: Their nature and their prospects. In Wintrobe, MM (ed): Blood, Pure and Eloquent: A Story of Discovery, of People and of Ideas. McGraw-Hill, New York, 1980, p 511.
4. Virchow, R: Die farblosen Blutkorperchen. In Gesammelte Abhandlungen sur Wissen schaftlichen Medizin. Meidinger, Frankfurt, 1856.
5. Friedrich, N: Ein neuer fall von leukamie. Arch Pathol Anat 12:37, 1857.
6. Epstein, W: Ueber die acute Leukamia und Pseudoleukamie. Dtsch Arch Klin Med 44:343, 1889.
7. Naegeli, O: Über rothes Knockenmark und Myeloblasten. Dtsch Med Wochenschr 26:287, 1900.
8. Forkner, CE: Leukemia and Allied Disorder. Macmillan, New York, 1938, p 5.
9. Smithson, WA, Gilchrist, GS, and Burgert, EO: Childhood acute lymphocytic leukemia. CA-A Cancer J Clin 30:158, 1980.
10. Pinkel, D: Curing children of leukemia. Cancer 60:1683, 1987.
11. Westin, EH, Wong-Staal, F, Gallo, RC: Retroviruses and Onc genes in human leukemias and lymphomas. In Bloomfield, CD (ed): Chronic and Acute Leukemias in Adults. Martinus Nijhoff, Boston, 1985.
12. Gunz, FW, Gunz, JP, Veale, AMO, et al: Familial leukaemia: A study of 909 families. Scand J Haematol 15:117, 1975.
13. Evans, KIK and Stewart, JK: Down's syndrome and leukemia. Lancet 2:1322, 1972.
14. Carbonari, M, Cherchi, M, Paganelli, R, et al: Relative increase of T cells expressing the gamma/delta rather than the alpha/beta receptor in ataxia-telangiectasia. N Engl J Med 322:73, 1990.
15. Bizzozzero, OJ, Johnson, KG, and Cicco, A: Radiation-related leukemia in Hiroshima and Nagasaki, 1946-64. I. Distribution, incidence and appearance in time. N Engl J Med 274:1095, 1966.
16. Bates, MN: Extremely low frequency electromagnetic fields and cancer. The epidemiologic evidence. Environ Health Persp 95:147, 1991.
17. Sahl JD, et al: Cohort and nested case-control studies of hematopoietic cancers and brain cancer among electric utility workers. Epidemiology 4:104, 1993.
18. Forni, A and Vigliani, EC: Chemical leukemogenesis in man. Semin Haematol 7:211, 1974.
19. Blattner, WA, Blayney, DW, Robert-Guroff, M, et al: Epidemiology of human T-cell leukemia/lymphoma virus. J Infect Dis 147:406, 1983.
20. Rosenblatt, JD, Chen, ISY, and Golde, DW: HTLV-II and human lymphoproliferative disorders. Clin Lab Med 8:85, 1988.
21. de-The, G, Geser, A, Day, NE, et al: Epidemiological evidence for causal relationship between Epstein-Barr virus and Burkitt's lymphomas from Ugandan prospective study. Nature 274:756, 2978.
22. Geser, A, de-The, G, Lenoir, G, et al: Final case reporting from the Ugandan prospective study of the relationship between EBV and Burkitt's lymphoma. Int J Cancer 29:397, 1982.
23. Cancer Facts & Figures—1994. American Cancer Society, Atlanta, GA.
24. Gale, RP (ed): Leukemia Therapy. Blackwell Scientific, Boston, 1986.
25. Bennett, JM, Catovsky, D, Daniel, MT, et al: Proposals for the classification of myelodysplastic syndromes. Br J Haematol 51:189, 1982.
26. Bennett, JM, Catovsky, D, Daniel, MT, et al: Proposed revised criteria for the classification of acute myeloid leukemia. Ann Intern Med 103:626, 1985.
27. Yunis, JJ: Should refined chromosomal analysis be used routinely in acute leukemias and myelodysplastic syndrome? N Engl J Med 315:322, 1986.
28. Shafer, JA: Blood and marrow morphology in acute leukemia patients receiving chemotherapy: A photo-essay. Am J Med Technol 49:77, 1983.
29. Shafer, JA: Artifactual alterations in phagocytes in the blood smear. Am J Med Technol 48:507, 1982.
30. Wintrobe, MM (ed): Clinical Hematology, ed 8. Lea & Febiger, Philadelphia, 1981, p 1493.
31. Seigneurin, D and Audhuy, B: Auer rods in refractory anemia with excess blasts: Presence and significance. Am J Clin Pathol 80:359, 1983.
32. Stanley, M, McKenna, RW, Ellinger, G, et al: Classification of 358 cases AML by FAB criteria: Analysis of clinical and morphologic features. In Bloomfield, CD (ed): Chronic and Acute Leukemias in Adults. Martinus Nijhoff, Boston, 1985, pp 147–178.
33. Stass, SA, Pui, SM, Rovigatti, U, et al: Sudan black B positive acute lymphoblastic leukemia. Br J Haematol 57:413, 1984.
34. Hayhoe, FGJ and Quaglino, D: Haematological Cytochemistry. Churchill Livingstone, Edinburgh, 1980, pp 130, 243, 265.
35. Bennett, JM and Reed, CE: Acute leukemia cytochemical profile: Diagnostic and clinical implications. Blood Cells 1:101, 1975.
36. Bearman, RM, Winberg, CD, Maslow, WC, et al: Terminal deoxynucleotidyl transferase activity in neoplastic and non-neoplastic hematopoietic cells. Am J Clin Pathol 75:794, 1981.
37. Casoli, C, Bonati, A, and Starcich, B: Ph1-positive acute myelocytic leukemia with high TdT levels. Cancer 52:1210, 1983.
38. Kung, PC, Long, JC, McCaffrey, RP, et al: TdT in the diagnosis of leukemia and malignant lymphoma. Am J Med 64:788, 1978.
39. Marks, SM, Baltimore, D, and McCaffrey, R: Terminal transferase as a predictor of initial responsiveness to vincristine and prednisone in blastic chronic myelogenous leukemia. A cooperative study. N Engl J Med 298:812, 1978.
40. Look, AT: The emerging genetics of acute lymphoblastic leukemia: Clinical and biologic implications. Semin Oncol 12:92, 1985.
41. Borowitz, MJ et al: Predictability of the t(1;19)(q23;p13) from surface antigen phenotype: Implications for screening cases of childhood ALL for molecular analysis: A Pediatric Oncology Group study. Blood 82:1086, 1993.

42. Crist, WM, et al: Poor prognosis of children with pre-B acute lymphoblastic leukemia is associated with the t(1;19)(q23;913). A Pediatric Oncology Group study. Blood 76:117, 1990.

43. Nourse, J, et al: Chromosomal translocation t(1;19) results in synthesis of a homeobox fusion mRAN that codes for a potential chimeric transcription factor. Cell 60:535, 1990.

44. Izraeli, S, et al: Detection and clinical relevance of genetic abnormalities in pediatric ALL: A comparison between cytogenetic and PCR analyses. Leukemia 7:671, 1993.

45. Downing, JR, et al: An AML-1-ETO fusion transcript is consistently detected by RNA-based polymerase chain reaction in AML containing the (8;21)(9q22;q22) translocation. Blood 81:2860, 1993.

46. Maseki, N, et al: The 8;21 chromosome translocation in AML is always detectable by molecular analysis using AML1. Blood 81:1573, 1993.

47. Nucifora, G, et al: Detection of DNA rearrangements in the AML1 and ETO loci and an AML-1/ETO fusion mRNA in patients with t(8;21) AML. Blood 81:883, 1993.

48. Nucifora, G, et al: Persistence of the 8;21 translocation in patients with AML type M2 in long term remission. Blood 82:712, 1993.

49. Crist, W, et al: Philadelphia chromosome positive acute lymphoblastic leukemia: clinical and cytogenetic characteristics and treatment outcome. A Pediatric Oncology Group Study. Blood 76:489, 1990.

50. Hunger, SP, et al: HRX involvement in de novo and secondary leukemias with diverse 11q23 abnormalities. Blood 81:3197, 1993.

51. Thirman, MJ, et al: Rearrangement of the MLL gene in ALL and AML with 11q23 chromosomal translocations. N Engl J Med 329:909, 1993.

52. Hilden, JM, et al: Heterogeneity in MLL/AF4 fusion messenger RNA detected by PCR in t(4;11) acute leukemia. Cancer Res 53:3853, 1993.

53. Biondi, A, et al: RARA gene rearrangements as a genetic marker for diagnosis and monitoring in acute promyelocytic leukemia. Blood 77:1418, 1991.

54. Miller WH, et al: Detection of minimal residual disease in APL by a reverse-transcription PCR assay for the PML/RARA fusion mRNA. Blood 82:1689, 1993.

55. Liu, P, et al: Fusion between transcription factor CBFB/PEBP2B and a myosin heavy chain in acute myeloid leukemia. Science 261:1041, 1993.

56. Hebert, J, et al: Detection of minimal residual disease in acute myelomonocytic leukemia with abnormal marrow eosinophils by nested polymerase chain reaction with allele specific amplification. Blood 84:2291, 1994.

57. Bennett, JM, Catovsky, D, Daniel, MT, et al: Proposals for the classification of acute leukemia. Br J Haematol 33:451, 1976.

58. Cunningham, I, Gee, TS, Reich, LM, et al: Acute promyelocytic leukemia: Treatment results during a decade at Memorial Hospital. Blood 73:116, 1989.

59. Bloomfield, CD and Brunning, RD: FAB M7: Acute megakaryoblastic leukemia—beyond morphology (letter to editor). Ann Intern Med, 103:451, 1985.

60. Griffin, JD, Mayer, RJ, Weinstein, HJ, et al: Surface marker analysis of acute myeloblastic leukemia: Identification of differentiation-associated phenotypes. Blood 62:557, 1983.

61. Karen, DF (ed): Flow Cytometry in Clinical Diagnosis. ASCP Press, Chicago, 1989, pp 111, 114.

62. Griffin, JD, Davis, R, Nelson, DA, et al: Use of surface marker analysis to predict outcome of adult acute myeloblastic leukemia. Blood 68:1232, 1986.

63. Campos, L, et al: Surface marker expression in adult acute myeloid leukemia: correlations with initial characteristics, morphology and response to therapy. Br J Haematol 72:161, 1989.

64. Sultan, C, Deregnaucourt, J, Do, YW, et al: Distribution of 250 cases of acute myeloid leukemia according to the FAB classification and response to therapy. Br J Haematol 47:545, 1981.

65. Cheson, BD, et al: Report of the National Cancer Institute-Sponsored Workshop on definitions of diagnosis and response in acute myeloid leukemia. J Clin Oncol 8:813, 1990.

66. Bennett, JM, et al: Minimally differentiated AML (FAB M0). Br J Haematol 78:325, 1991.

67. Bitter, MA, Le Beau, MM, Rowley, JD, et al: Associations between morphology, karyotype, and clinical features in myeloid leukemias. Hum Pathol 18:211, 1987.

68. Liso, V, Troccoli, G, and Grande, M: Cytochemical study of acute promyelocytic leukemia: Blut 30:261, 1975.

69. Tomonaga, M, Yoshida, Y, Tagawa, M, et al: Cytochemistry of acute promyelocytic leukemia (M3): Leukemic promyelocytes exhibit heterogeneous patterns in cellular differentiation. Blood 66:350, 1985.

70. Gralnick, HR, and Sultan, C: Acute promyelocytic leukemia: Hemorrhagic manifestations and morphologic criteria. Br J Haematol 29:373, 1975.

71. Castaigne, S, et al: All-trans retinoic acid as a differentiation therapy for acute promyelocytic leukemia. Blood 76:263, 1990.

72. Warrell, RP, et al: Differentiation therapy of acute promyelocytic leukemia with tretinoin (all trans retinoic acid). N Engl J Med 324:1385, 1991.

73. Rowley, JD, Golomb, HM, and Dougherty, C: 15/17 translocation. A consistent chromosomal change in acute promyelocytic leukaemia. Lancet 1:549, 1977.

74. Sultan, C, Surender, KJ, and Imbert, M: Variant form of hypergranular promyelocytic leukemia. ASCP Check Sample 25:4, 1983.

75. Jones, ME and Saleem, A: Acute promyelocytic leukemia. A review of the literature. Am J Med 65:673, 1978.

76. Goulomb, HM, Rowley, JD, Vardiman, JW, et al: "Microgranular" acute promyelocytic leukemia: A distinct clinical, ultrastructural, and cytogenetic entity. Blood 55:253, 1980.

77. Bennett, JM, Catovsky, D, Daniel, MT, et al: Correspondence: A variant form of hypergranular promyelocytic leukemia (M3). Br J Haematol 44:169, 1980.

78. Arthur, DC and Bloomfield, CD: Partial deletion of the long arm of chromosome 16 and bone marrow eosinophilia in acute nonlymphocytic leukemia: a new association. Blood 61:994, 1983.

79. LeBeau, MM, Larson, RA, Bitter, MA, et al: Association of an inversion of chromosome 16 with abnormal marrow eosinophils in acute myelomonocytic leukemia. N Engl J Med 309:630, 1983.

80. Rundles, RW: Monocytic leukemia. In Williams, WE, Beutler, E, Erslev, AJ, et al (eds): Hematology. McGraw-Hill, New York, 1972, p 896.

81. Meyer, RJ, Ferreira, PPC, Cuttner, J, et al: Central nervous system involvement at presentation in acute granulocytic leukemia: A prospective cytocentrifuge study. Am J Med 68:691, 1980.

82. Petersen, BA and Bloomfield, CD: Asymptomatic central nervous system leukemia in adults with ANLL in extended remission. Proc Am Soc Clin Oncol 18:341, 1977.

83. Tobelem, G, Jacquillat, C, Chastang, C, et al: Acute monoblastic leukemia: A clinical and biologic study of 74 cases. Blood 55:71, 1980.

84. Cuttner, J, Conjalka, MS, Reilly, M, et al: Association of monocytic leukemia in patients with extreme leukocytosis. Am J Med 60:555, 1980.

85. Catovsky, D, Hoffbrand, AV, Ikoku, NB, et al: Signifi-

cance of cell differentiation in acute myeloid leukaemia. Blood Cells 1:201, 1975.

86. Pribilla, W: Erythramie und erythroleukamie. In Gross, R and Van de Loo, J (eds): Leukamie, Springer-Verlag, Berlin, 1972.

87. Breton-Gorius, J, Reyes, F, Duhamel, G, et al: Megakaryoblastic acute leukemia: Identification by the ultrastructural demonstration of platelet peroxidase. Blood 51:45, 1978.

88. Breton-Gorius, J and Reyes, F: Ultrastructure of human bone marrow cell maturation. Int Rev Cytol 46:251, 1976.

89. Bennett, JM, Catovsky, D, Daniel, MT, et al: Criteria for the diagnosis of acute leukemia of megakaryocyte lineage (M7). Ann Intern Med 103:460, 1985.

90. Mirchandani, I and Palutke, M: Acute megakaryoblastic leukemia. Cancer 50:2866, 1983.

91. Koike, T: Megakaryoblastic leukemia: The characterization and identification of megakaryoblasts. Blood 64:683, 1984.

92. Bain, BJ, Catovsky, D, O'Brien, M, et al: Megakaryoblastic leukemia presenting as acute myelofibrosis: A study of four cases with the platelet-peroxidase reaction. Blood 58:206, 1981.

93. Bennett, JM, Catovsky, D, Daniel, MT, et al: The morphologic classification of acute lymphoblastic leukemia: Concordance among observers and clinical correlations. Br J Haematol 47:533, 1981.

94. Miller, DR, Leikin, S, Albo, V: Intensive therapy and prognostic factors in acute lymphoblastic leukemia of childhood: CCG 141. In Neth, R, Gallo, RC, Graf, H (eds): Haematology and Blood Transfusion: Modern Trends in Human Leukemia IV. Springer-Verlag, Berlin, 1981.

95. Miller, DR, Krailo, M, Bleyer, WA, et al: Prognostic implications of blast cell morphology in childhood acute lymphoblastic leukemia: A report from the Children's Cancer Study Group. Cancer Treat Rep 69:1211, 1985.

96. Lilleyman, JS, et al: FAB morphological classification of childhood lymphoblastic leukemia and its clinical importance. J Clin Pathol 39:998, 1986.

97. Foon, KA and Todd, RF: Immunologic classification of leukemia and lymphoma. Blood 68:1, 1986.

98. Strominger, JL: Developmental biology of T cell receptors. Science 244:943, 1989.

99. Sobol, RE, Royston, I, LeBien, TW, et al: Adult acute lymphoblastic leukemia phenotypes defined by monoclonal antibodies. Blood 65:730, 1985.

100. Weinberg, KI and Siegel, SE: Acute lymphoblastic leukemia in children, in Gale, RP (ed): Leukemia Therapy. Blackwell Scientific, Boston, 1986, p 25.

101. Pui, CH, Raimondi, SC, Dodge, RK, et al: Prognostic importance of structural chromosomal abnormalities in children with hyperdiploid (>50 chromosomes) acute lymphoblastic leukemia. Blood 73:1963, 1989.

102. Crist, W, Boyett, J, Jackson, J, et al: Prognostic importance of the pre-B-cell immunophenotype and other presenting features in B-lineage childhood acute lymphoblastic leukemia: A Pediatric Oncology Group study. Blood 74:1252, 1989.

103. Carroll, AJ, Crist, WM, Parmley, RT, et al: Pre-B cell leukemia associated with chromosome translocation 1:19. Blood 63:721, 1984.

104. Brouet, JC and Seligmann, M: The immunologic classification of acute lymphoblastic leukemias. Cancer 42:817, 1978.

105. Taub, R, Kirsch, I, Morton, C, et al: Translocation of the c-myc gene into the immunoglobulin heavy chain locus in human Burkitt lymphoma and murine plasmacytoma cells. Proc Natl Acad Sci USA 79:7937, 1982.

106. Dalla-Favera, R, Martinotti, S, Gallo, RC, et al: Translocation and rearrangements of the c-myc oncogene locus in human undifferentiated B-cell lymphomas. Science 219:963, 1983.

107. Flandrin, G, Brouet, JC, Daniel, MT, et al: Acute leukemia with Burkitt's tumor cells: A study of six cases with special reference to lymphocyte surface markers. Blood 45:183, 1975.

108. Greaves, MF, Janossy, G, Peto, J, et al: Immunologically defined subclasses of acute lymphoblastic leukaemia in children: Their relationship to presentation features and prognosis. Br J Haematol 48:179, 1981.

109. Reinherz, EL, Kung, PC, Goldstein, G, et al: Discrete stages of human intrathymic differentiation. Analysis of normal thymocytes and leukemic lymphoblasts of T-cell lineage. Proc Natl Acad Sci USA 77:1588, 1980.

110. Pui, CH, Behm, FG, Singh, B, et al: Heterogeneity of presenting features and their relation to treatment outcome in 120 children with T-cell acute lymphoblastic leukemia. Blood 75:174, 1990.

111. Shuster, JJ, Falletta, JM, Jeanette, Pullen, D, et al: Prognostic factors in childhood T-cell acute lymphoblastic leukemia: A Pediatric Oncology Group Study Group. Blood 75:166, 1990.

112. Roper, M, Crist, WM, Metzgar, R, et al: Monoclonal antibody characterization of surface antigens in childhood T-cell lymphoid malignancies. Blood 61:830, 1983.

113. Del Vecchio, L, et al: Immunodiagnosis of acute leukemia displaying ectopic antigens: Proposal for a classification of promiscuous phenotypes. Am J Hematol 31:173, 1989.

114. Foa, R, et al: Rearrangements of immunoglobulin and T-cell receptor beta and gamma genes are associated with terminal deoxynucleotidyl transferase expression in acute myeloid leukemia. J Exp Med 165:879, 1987.

115. Smith, FO, et al: Expression of lymphoid-associated cell surface antigens by childhood acute myeloid leukemia cells lacks prognostic significance. Blood 79:2415, 1992.

116. Jensen, AW, et al: Solitary expression of CD7 among T-cell antigens in acute myeloid leukemia: Identification of a group of patients with similar T-cell receptor beta and delta rearrangements and course of disease suggestive of poor prognosis. Blood 78:1292, 1991.

QUESTIONS

1. A 4-year-old boy presents with bruising, fever, and coughing. His WBC is 15×10^9/L; Hct, 23%; and platelets, 53×10^9/L. A bone marrow aspirate is obtained that reveals sheets of immature cells. Cytochemical studies for peroxidase and NSE are negative; the TdT is positive. Surface marker studies are done that show the following phenotype: HLA-DR+; CD19+; CD10+; cytoplasmic $\mu-$; sIg−; CD7−. What is the diagnosis?
   a. B-cell ALL
   b. Early pre-B-cell ALL
   c. Pre-B-cell ALL
   d. T-cell ALL

2. The WBC is 50×10^9/L with 80% blasts, 15% segs, and 5% lymphs. The bone marrow reveals sheets of immature cells. Cytochemical studies of these show that they are peroxidase-positive (20%) and the nonspecific esterase is negative. What is the diagnosis?
   a. AML, M1 type
   b. AML, M2 type
   c. AML, M4 type
   d. AML, M5 type

3. The WBC is 15×10^9/L with 90% blasts, 6% segs, and 4% monos. The blasts are relatively large and have abundant cytoplasm. Over 90% of them are positive with the nonspecific esterase stain and an occasional blast is positive with the Sudan black. What is the diagnosis?
   a. AML, M2 type
   b. AML, M3 type
   c. AML, M4 type
   d. AML, M5 type

4. Cytochemical stains were performed on bone marrow smears from an acute leukemia patient. All blasts were TdT-negative. Most of the blasts showed varying amounts of Sudan black B positivity; 50% of them stained positive for nonspecific esterase. What type of leukemia is indicated?
   a. Acute myeloblastic leukemia
   b. Acute lymphoblastic leukemia
   c. Acute myelomonocytic leukemia
   d. Acute erythroleukemia

5. Bone marrow examination reveals a hypercellular marrow with lymphoblasts that react with antisera specific for CD7 and TdT; however, the lymphoblasts are negative for sIg (surface immunoglobulins), and CD10 (CALLA). The diagnosis is:
   a. ALL, B-cell type
   b. ALL, early pre-B-cell type
   c. ALL, pre-B-cell type
   d. ALL, T-cell type

6. A 49-year-old woman is admitted to the hospital for easy bruising and menorrhagia. She has evidence of disseminated intra-vascular coagulation. Her WBC was 3×10^9/L with 95% large atypical mononuclear cells. Many of these cells were packed with large purple-staining granules, some have multiple Auer rods and all are strongly peroxidase positive. What is the diagnosis?
   a. AML, M2 type
   b. AML, M3 type
   c. AML, M4 type
   d. AML, M5 type

7. A 21-year-old patient's bone marrow is classified morphologically by the FAB system as an L3 acute lymphoblastic leukemia. Which of the following results best support this diagnosis?
   a. Expression of CD19
   b. Presence of cytoplasmic μ
   c. Presence of surface immunoglobulin
   d. Nuclear TdT reactivity

ANSWERS

1. **b** (pp 315–317)
2. **a** (p 308)
3. **d** (p 311)
4. **c** (p 310)
5. **d** (p 319)
6. **b** (p 309–310)
7. **c** (p 315)

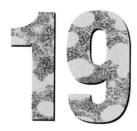

Myelodysplastic Syndromes

Giovanni D'Angelo, FCSLT
Martin Gyger, MD, FRCP(C)

Objectives

At the end of this chapter, the learner should be able to:
1 Give an overview of the clonal nature and stem cell origin of MDS.
2 Recognize the characteristic laboratory features of each subgroup of MDS.
3 List differential diagnostic criteria that are characteristic for each MDS subgroup.
4 Illustrate the complexity of RA diagnosis.
5 Distinguish RAEB and RAEB-t from AML.
6 Differentiate between primary and secondary MDS.
7 Characterize the diagnostic and pronostic values of cytogenetic studies.
8 Recognize the most important prognostic criteria for survival and leukemic transformation.
9 Summarize the most important clinical manifestations and causes of mortality.
10 Describe the therapeutic regimen that is most likely to achieve long-term survival.

Myelodysplastic syndromes (MDS) make up a group of more or less indolent clonal neoplastic hemopathies. The precise origin of the neoplastic clone has been at the center of an interesting debate over the past years. Indeed, although some argue that the cellular origin of MDS is a pluripotent stem cell with the ability to differentiate into all cell lineages, others favor the hypothesis that the myelodysplastic clone results from mutations affecting a pluripotent stem cell already committed or restricted to myeloid differentiation, thus excluding cells from the lymphoid lineages. This dilemma will be largely disussed in the first section of this chapter. The myelodysplastic syndromes occur predominantly in elderly people and, to a lesser extent, in children. Each type of MDS harbors to a variable extent morphological abnormalities in the peripheral blood and the bone marrow affecting one or several cell lineages. The anemia in patients with MDS is qualified as refractory in view of the fact that patients are not responsive to iron, folic acid, vitamin B_{12}, or any other hematinic therapies. Despite having normocellular or hypercellular bone marrows, patients with MDS paradoxically have less or more severe peripheral cytopenias. It is presumed that high intramedullary death of hematopoietic cells may be the biologic basis of this paradox. As opposed to acute myeloid leukemias, MDS have a subacute evolution with an invariably fatal outcome. Most patients die of infection or hemorrhage, but at least one third die of acute leukemic transformation. Terminologies and definitions for these groups of hematologic disorders have been numerous over the years and include preleukemic anemia,[1] preleukemic acute human leukemia,[2] chronic refractory anemia with sideroblasts,[3] smoldering leukemia,[4] preleukemic syndrome,[5] and refractory anemia with excess of myeloblasts.[6] In 1976, the French-American-British (FAB) Cooperative Group introduced the term *dysmyelopoietic syndrome*, and in 1982, the same group classified these syndromes into five distinct entities.[7,8] This classification can be considered a major contribution in the field of myelodysplastic disorders, because it enabled clinicians to establish their diagnosis more precociously and with more accuracy, and facilitated communication among workers. It also contributed to a better understanding of their evolution and finally as enlightened therapeutic decisions. Since the introduction of the FAB classification in 1982, we have witnessed major developments in the field of cytogenetics, such as its impact in relation to morphology and prognosis. We have also explored new areas related to the pathogenesis of MDS and the putative genes involved in their process. Finally, new hopes of curative therapy have come to light with the refinement of allogeneic marrow transplantation.

ETIOLOGY AND PATHOGENESIS

It is now well recognized that MDS are clonal hemopathies resulting in impaired hematopoiesis. On theoretical grounds, as shown in Fig. 19–1, two different types of stem cells may be involved in the clonal process: (1) A pluripotent stem cell with the capacities of both self-renewal and differentiation into all cell lineages (myeloid and lymphoid); this pluripotent stem cell is referred to as an *uncommitted pluripotent stem cell*. (2) A pluripotent stem cell that has lost its capacity for self-renewal and is already engaged specifically towards myeloid differentiation; this pluripotent stem cell is referred to as a *committed pluripotent stem cell*. The elucidation of the origin of the myelodysplastic clone is likely to improve our comprehension of the clinical aspects and pathogenesis of these neoplastic disorders.

Looking first at the nature of the blast cells in patients undergoing leukemic transformation during the course of their disease, one finds that in the vast majority of cases, blast cells display a myeloid or myelo-

Marrow Stem Cell Hierarchy

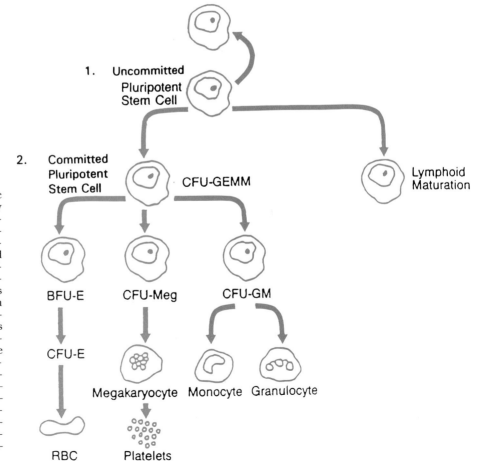

FIGURE 19–1 Schematic marrow stem cell hierarchy showing stem cells theoretically involved in the pathogenesis of myelodysplastic syndromes (MDS); uncommitted pluripotent stem cells with self-renewal and differentiation capacities into all cell lineages and committed stem cells with myeloid restricted differentiation capacity. Abbreviations used: CFU–GEMM = colony-forming unit — granulocyte erythrocyte - megakaryocyte - macrophage, BFU – E = burst-forming unit—erythroid, CFU–E = colony - forming unit—erythroid, CFU–Meg = colony - forming unit — megakaryocyte, CFU–GM = colony-forming unit — granulocyte-macrophage.

monocytic phenotype.[9] Although a hybrid phenotype (myeloid-lymphoid) can also be detected in rare cases,[10,11] acute leukemic transformation with a pure population of lymphoid cells is exceptional;[12,13] these blasts usually display an early B phenotype.[14] Thus, at first glance, by looking at the phenotypic nature of the blast cells involved in leukemic transformation, the overwhelming predominance of the myeloid phenotype theoretically points out the involvement of a committed pluripotent stem cell. The biologic characteristics of blast cells can also be scrutinized by more refined approaches such as molecular cytogenetics, X-linked inactivation assays, and the study of immunoglobulin and T-cell-receptor gene rearrangements. Although of great value, one must bear in mind that there are major discrepancies in the results of these various molecular-genetic approaches to the determination of clonality in MDS. Although molecular cytogenetics has consistently shown that myeloid cells are clonal while cells of lymphoid origin are polyclonal,[15-17] one cannot use these findings to conclude that the origin of the neoplastic clone in MDS is a myeloid-restricted progenitor. Indeed, MDS may be a multistep process in which cytogenetic changes occur as late events in an unstable myeloid-derived subclone. In favor of this hypothesis is the fact that some reports have described a clonal pattern of X-chromosome inactivation of both myeloid and lymphoid cells.[18-20] However, recent studies using highly purified cell fractions obtained by lineage-specific monoclonal antibodies and fluorescence-activated cell sorting have demonstrated that T lymphocytes, B lymphocytes, and NK cells were not involved in the clonal hematopoiesis.[21] Furthermore, deletion of DNA material on the long arm of chromosome 5 (5q-) is a frequent cytogenetic event in MDS (see Cytogenetics, later in this chapter). The recent use of highly polymorphic markers linked to the long arm of chromosome 5 has shown that myeloid but not lymphoid cells carry the abnormal interstitial deletion.[22] In view of the controversy surrounding the precise stem cell origin of MDS, it would seem wise to envisage MDS as a multistep process within a group of heterogeneous diseases; the question of clonality is still open to debate.

The exact molecular mechanisms involved in the genesis of the abnormal clone have not been clearly established. It is assumed, however, that secondary to a chemical, viral, and/or radiation insult, there is a disruption in the molecular mechanisms that govern cell proliferation, differentiation, and programmed cell

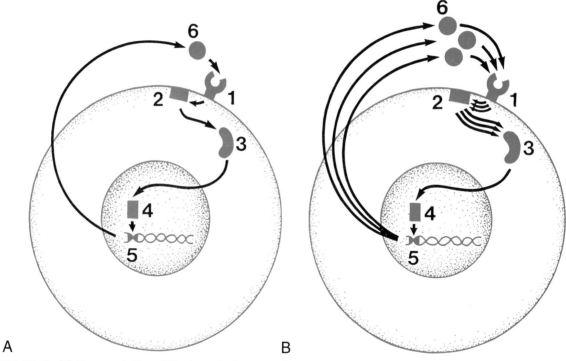

A   B

FIGURE 19-2 (*A*) Representation of the transduction signaling system that plays a central role in relaying signals from outside the cell to the nucleus. 1 = growth factor receptor; 2 = primary messenger with protein kinase activity; 3 = secondary messenger; 4 = intranuclear transcriptional factor; 5 = specific gene, the product of which may be a growth factor; or 6 = proteins involved as primary or secondary messengers. (*B*) Schematic demonstrating a disruption in the signal transduction system showing an increased production of a growth factor that transmits signals which may create an uncontrolled proliferation of the cell. Many genetic abnormalities such as mutations, chromosome deletions, translocations, and gene amplification may be responsible for such disruption in the signal transduction homeostasis.

death. These cellular events are under the control of pivotal genes that may be affected either by somatic mutations, chromosomal aberrations such as deletions, translocations, or amplifications leading to an MDS state. Two specific classes of genes may be involved in such a process: Those that harbor growth-promoting activity, so-called proto-oncogenes[23–25] and those that counterbalance growth-promoting proto-oncogenes, referred to as suppressor genes.[26–28] Crucial early mutations in any of these genes, followed by secondary events such as loss, gain, or structural rearrangements of chromosomes, are most likely responsible for the transition from a normal hematopoietic to a neoplastic MDS clone. For example, one of the genes that might be implicated in this process is the RAS gene. RAS protein plays a central role in relaying signals from the outside of the cell to the nucleus (the so-called signal transduction system, schematized in Fig. 19–2), and thus in the proliferation and differentiation synchrony of a specific hematopoietic progenitor.[29] Certain mutations in the RAS gene are likely to create a protein that is no longer susceptible to normal function, an event that might ultimately lead to myelodysplasia. Approximately 20% to 30% of patients with MDS harbor RAS mutations in their cells, and these are more frequent in patients undergoing leukemic transformation.[30] Furthermore, interstitial deletion of the long arm of chromosome 5 is among the most frequent chromosomal abnormality found in MDS.[31,32] Because this genetic abnormality leads to loss of DNA material, a tumor suppressor gene is presumed to be responsible for initiating or creating an abnormal myelodysplastic clone. Recent data showed that the interferon regulatory factor 1 (IRF-1) gene seems to be a strong candidate because it behaves like a tumor suppressor gene.[33,34] Other genes involved in cell proliferation are found on the long arm of chromosome 5, such as the granulocyte-macrophage colony-stimulating factor (GM-CSF) gene, interleukin-3, interleukin-4, interleukin-5, and the macrophage colony-stimulating factor gene.[35] None of these have been shown to be directly involved in the MDS process at this point in time.

The myelodysplastic hematopoiesis resulting from any gene disruption is characterized by a high degree of intramedullary death. This phenomenon, called apoptosis, is a gene-directed cellular self-destruction.[36,37] It has been recently shown that, although an end-stage karyorrhectic cell is easy to recognize under a light microscope, a large number of cells in myelodysplastic state are undergoing apoptosis, yet there may be only a few cells in the morphologically identifiable karyorrhectic stage.[38]

In summary, pivotal early mutations affecting genes involved in the control of cell proliferation and differentiation are likely to be responsible for the myelodysplastic state. Effective strategies for identifying mutant genes, growth factors, and molecules involved in the basic cell machinery are in progress, along with improved laboratory testing. Because MDS occurs mostly in elderly people, the role of prolonged exposure to environmental factors such as chemicals, radiations, or viruses should be investigated further.

MORPHOLOGICAL ABNORMALITIES IN PERIPHERAL BLOOD AND BONE MARROW

Definition of Specific Morphological Characteristics

At the laboratory level, the diagnosis of MDS is made by careful morphological study of blood and bone marrow smears using Wright-Giemsa stain and of bone marrow biopsy using hematoxylin-eosin and reticulin. The iron content of both marrow aspirate and biopsy specimens is revealed by the use of Prussian blue (Perl's iron stain[39]) and other special cytochemical stains. The distinctive criteria between each type of MDS relies mostly and essentially on the study of peripheral blood and bone marrow smears. MDS are most often suspected in patients presenting with anemia, which is usually normochromic, macrocytic, and refractory to all types of standard therapeutic approaches. A vast array of laboratory tools will help the physician in precisely diagnosing each type of MDS.[40–42]

Blasts

Some types of myelodysplastic syndromes are diagnosed according to the number of blasts in the bone marrow at initial diagnosis. There are two types of blasts according to FAB classification: Type I refers to a myeloblast of variable size, without any azurophilic granules or Auer rods (Fig. 19–3); type II refers to a myeloblast that is slightly larger and contains few azurophilic granules (1 to 20) (Fig. 19–4); in addition, Goasguen and associates[43] proposed a type III myeloblast containing more than 20 azurophilic granules with a basophilic cytoplasm and absence of the Golgi zone similar to type I and II myeloblasts.[43] All other mature cells with a greater number of granules and visible Golgi zone are classified as promyelocytes.

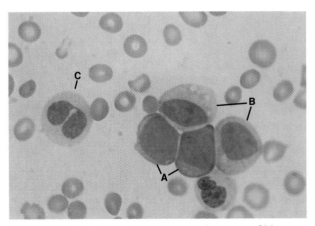

FIGURE 19–3 Refractory anemia with excess of blasts in transformation (RAEB-t) (bone marrow, ×1000 magnification). (*A*) Two blast cells. (*B*) Two immature granulocytes with some degree of hypogranularity and vacuolization. (*C*) Pelgeroid hypogranular neutrophil.

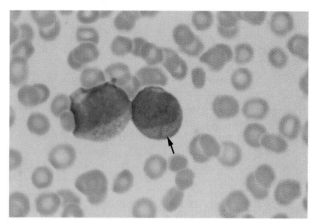

FIGURE 19–4 Two blasts with azurophilic rods, bone with an Auer rod (*arrow*). (Bone marrow, ×1000 magnification).

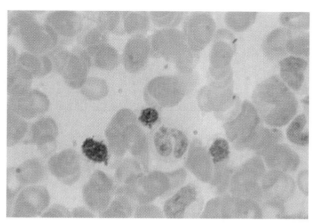

FIGURE 19–6 Prussian blue stain, bone marrow, ×1000 magnification. Three-ringed sideroblasts (sideroblasts type III).

Sideroblasts

Type I refers to normal sideroblasts containing one to four cytoplasmic granules. Approximately 15% to 50% of bone marrow erythroblasts are type I sideroblasts. Type II refers to abnormal sideroblasts; they harbor approximately 5 to 10 granules scattered throughout the cytoplasm. Type III is synonymous to ringed sideroblast, having more than 10 granules that cover at least a third of the nuclear rim or forming a complete ring around the nucleus.[44]

Lineage Dysplasia

Dyserythropoiesis

Peripheral Blood Anemia is present in at least 90% of cases and is most often macrocytic or normocytic with decreased number of reticulocytes. The morphological characteristics encountered are macrocytosis, anisopoikilocytosis, basophilic stippling, a dual red blood cell population (normochromic or hypochromic), Pappenheimer bodies, dacryocytes (teardrop cells), fragmented cells, elliptocytes, Howell-Jolly bodies, and acanthocytes.

Bone Marrow Erythroblasts harbor megaloblastoid changes such as dense chromatin or fine chromatin with asynchronous cytoplasm maturation, internuclear bridging, broad-based nuclear budding, binuclearity, multinuclearity, and increased pyknosis. Cytoplasmic abnormalities may include intense basophilia, Howell-Jolly bodies, and ghosted cytoplasms (Fig. 19–5). Using Perl's iron stain, abnormal sideroblasts type II and type III may be found (Fig. 19–6).

Dysgranulocytopoiesis

Peripheral Blood Neutropenia is found in almost 60% of patients and neutrophilia may be encountered occasionally. Neutrophils show variable degrees of hyposegmentation with abnormal chromatin (pseudo Pelger-Huet anomaly) or, rarely, atypical hypersegmentation. In the cytoplasm, one can find variable degrees of hypogranulation, occasionally persistent basophilic zones (pseudo Döhle bodies), and at times

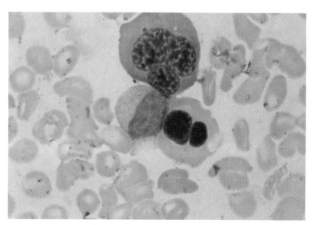

FIGURE 19–5 Wright-Giemsa stain, bone marrow, ×1000 magnification. Dysplastic multinucleated erythroblasts with asynchronous maturation (RAEB-t).

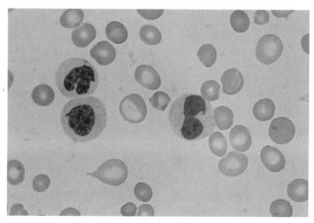

FIGURE 19–7 Refractory anemia with excess of blasts (RAEB) (peripheral blood, ×1000 magnification). Pseudo-Pelger-Huet anomaly, mononuclear Stodtmeister type.

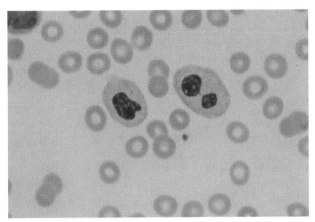

FIGURE 19-8 Bilobulated and monolobulated neutrophil (peripheral blood, ×1000 magnification).

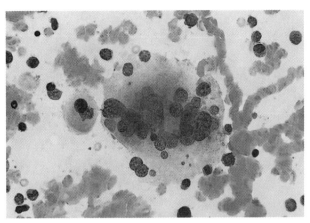

FIGURE 19-10 RAEB (bone marrow, ×1000 magnification). Large megakaryocyte with multilobulated nuclei, some of them distinctly detached and small in size.

hypergranulation with larger granules than usual. Combined nuclear and cytoplasmic dysplasia is detected in over 90% of cases (Figs. 19–7 and 19–8).

Bone Marrow The nuclei of neutrophils often show variable degrees of hyposegmentation such as bilobulation (pseudo Pelger-Huet) or monolobulation (pseudo Stodtmeister).[45] Other nuclear abnormalities include hypersegmentation, ringed formation, clumping of chromatin, and formation of chromatin sticks. According to the specific type of MDS, there may be numerous immature myeloid cells presenting an asynchronous maturation of the nucleus and cytoplasm. The cytoplasm is often hypogranular or completely degranulated with persistent basophilia at the rim of the cell. One can also observe hybrid myelomonocytic cells with specific staining properties for granulocytes (chloroesterase) and monocytes (α-naphtyl acetate or butyrate esterase). Vacuolated monocytes and/or myeloid precursors have also been observed in few cases.

Dysmegakaryocytopoiesis

Peripheral Blood Thrombocytopenia is present in almost 60% of patients and occasionally may be quite

severe (<20×10^9/L). Thrombocytosis is rare and usually associated with a specific chromosome abnormality (interstitial deletion of long arm of chromosome 5; this is fully discussed in the section entitled Laboratory Findings). A variable degree of morphological abnormalities such as gigantism, agranular platelets, platelets with giant granules, and in rare occasions micromegakaryocytes will be found. Phase contrast microscopy may also reveal platelet ballooning.[46]

Bone Marrow There are two characteristic morphological abnormalities of megakaryocytes in the bone marrow: (1) The presence of micromegakaryocytes (dwarf or mononuclear megakaryocytes). (2) Megakaryocytes with small nuclei detached from one another or separated by a thin strand of nuclear material (botryoid nuclei) and cytoplasmic hypogranularity. In rare cases, megakaryocytes show large cytoplasmic vacuoles (Figs. 19–9 and 19–10).

FAB CLASSIFICATION OF MYELODYSPLASTIC SYNDROMES[8,47]

MDS are classified into five distinct subgroups: refractory anemia (RA), refractory anemia with ringed sideroblasts (RARS), refractory anemia with excess of blasts (RAEB), refractory anemia with excess blasts in transformation (RAEB-t), and chronic myelomonocytic leukemia (CMML). The distinctive criteria between each subgroup of MDS rely essentially on the study of bone marrow aspirates stained with Wright-Giemsa and Prussian blue. The hematologic distinctive features of each MDS subgroup are summarized in Table 19–1.

Refractory Anemia

This type of MDS is by far the most difficult to recognize and diagnose. Indeed, the diagnosis rests mainly on the subjective identification of qualitative abnormalities according to the FAB classification, involving one or more bone marrow hematopoietic cell lineages, in a patient suspected or diagnosed as having

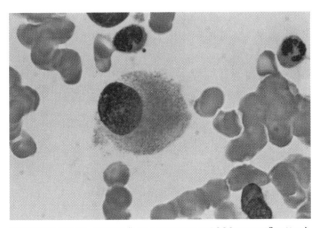

FIGURE 19-9 RAEB (bone marrow, ×1000 magnification). Monolobular (dwarf) megakaryocyte.

TABLE 19–1   Hematologic Features of MDS Subtypes

Type	Peripheral Blood	Bone Marrow	Dyshemopoiesis
RA	Blasts <1% Anemia, macrocytic, aregenerative Neutropenia and/or thrombocytopenia Occasionally abnormal neutrophils: pseudo Pelger-Huet and hypogranulation, few macro or giant platelets	Blasts <5% type I & II Hypercellular or normocellular* Ringed sideroblasts <15% Erythroid hyperplasia Some degree of dyserythropoiesis Dysgranulo and dysmegakaryopoiesis	+/+ + 1, 2, or 3 cell lineages
RARS	Blasts <1% Anemia, macrocytic, normocytic or Dimorphic (hypochromic, normochromic) Morphologic abnormalities can be similar to RA but not as common	Blasts <5% type I & II Hypercellular or normocellular Ringed sideroblasts >15% (15–90% of NRBC) Slight erythroid hyperplasia Dysgranulopoiesis-dysmegakaryopoiesis are not as common as in RA	+ 1 cell lineage Occasionally 2–3 cell lineages
RAEB	Blasts <5% Anemia, macrocytic or normocytic Cytopenia with hypogranular neutrophils, pseudo Pelger-Huet and other nuclear abnormalities. Macro or giant platelets may be present	Blasts 5–20% type I & II without Auer rods Hypercellular or normocellular* Ringed sideroblasts, variable Dyshemopoiesis of the three cell lineages with varying degrees of granulocytic or erythroid hyperplasia	+ + + All 3 cell lineages
RAEB-t	Blasts >5% With similar abnormalities as in RAEB	Blasts 20–30% type I & II or 5–20% with Auer rods Three lineage involvement as in RAEB	+ + + + All 3 cell lineages
CMML	Blasts <5% Monocytosis >1 × 10⁹/L With similar abnormalities as in other subgroups	Blasts 1–20% Hypercellular or normocellular* Monocytosis, promonocytes ≥20% Ringed sideroblasts, variable Many features of dysplasia as in other MDS	+ +/+ + + 2–3 cell lineages

*Hypocellular and marked fibrosis in 11% to 15%

RA. Anemia is present in more than 90% of patients. It is usually normochromic and macrocytic, but in some cases erythrocytes may be normocytic with a variable degree of morphological abnormalities that are usually more subtle than those found in other subgroups. Cytopenias are common, with the white blood cell count being less than 3.9×10^9/L and platelet count below 130×10^9/L. Morphological abnormalities such as dysgranulopoiesis or dysmegakaryopoiesis are more subtle than in other types of MDS. Bone marrow is usually normocellular or hypercellular. In rare cases, the marrow may be slightly hypocellular or may show a variable degree of fibrosis. Blast cells, types I and II, represent less than 5% of all nucleated cells, erythroid hyperplasia is relatively common with mild dyserythropoiesis, occasional ringed sideroblasts (less than 15% of nucleated red blood cells). Cytogenetic studies are crucial in the diagnosis of this peculiar type of myelodysplastic syndrome in view of the absence of quantitative criteria for its diagnosis. Indeed, the finding of a clonal chromosomal abnormality in such a setting confirms the diagnosis. Approximately 50% of patients have clonal chromosomal abnormalities. In the absence of clonal chromosomal abnormalities, establishment of its diagnosis, solely on the basis of single-lineage dysplasia, should be made with great caution. For example, iso-lated dyserythropoiesis seen on bone marrow smears may be a feature shared by a variety of hematologic disorders, including relatively benign diseases with no potential to progress to acute leukemia or with no relationship to MDS. When clonal markers cannot be identified, lineage dysplasia should be present in at least two cell lineages in order for a diagnosis of RA to be considered.

Refractory Anemia with Ringed Sideroblasts

RARS shares almost all the morphological features of RA with, however, a lesser degree of cell-lineage dysplastic change. Fortunately, the diagnosis rests also on a quantitative criterion, the presence of at least 15% ringed sideroblasts in the bone marrow (varying from 15% to 90% among nucleated red blood cells). Ringed sideroblasts are pathologic sideroblasts in which the usual migration of mitochondria from the nucleus toward the cytoplasm does not occur. As a result, they remain frozen around the nucleus, where insoluble iron conglomerate further contributes to their destruction. This feature, combined with the lineage dysplasia mentioned above, is sufficient to establish the diagnosis. Red blood cells are usually macrocytic or normocytic with dimorphic features (dual population of hypochromic and normochromic red blood cells). Leukopenia and thrombocytopenia are not as common as in refractory anemia (10% to 15% of cases).

Refractory Anemia with Excess of Blasts

In this type of MDS, the degree of lineage dysplasia is more significant. The anemia is macrocytic or normocytic with important morphological abnormalities such as ovalocytosis and dacryocytes, related to bone marrow dyserythropoiesis. On rare occasions, one can find a leukocytosis with an increased number of immature granulocytes. Although occasional blasts may be seen in the peripheral smear, the count is always below 5%. Dysgranulopoiesis with nuclear hyposegmentation (pseudo Pelger-Huet) and hypogranulation are frequent. Thrombocytopenia is a common feature, with giant size and hypogranular platelets. Bone marrow cellularity is normal or increased, with type I and type II myeloblasts ranging between 5% and 20%. Dys-

megakarycytopoiesis and dyserythropoiesis with ringed sideroblasts, although variable in number, can be significant.

Refractory Anemia with Excess Blasts in Transformation

This type of MDS is closely related to refractory anemia with excess blasts. The major difference lies with the number of blasts found in the bone marrow at initial diagnosis. In RAEB-t, the number of blasts ranges from 20% to 30%. In the peripheral blood, blasts are frequently above 5%. A number of cases exhibit Auer rods. The presence of Auer rods is diagnostic for refractory anemia with excess blasts in transformation, even if the number of blasts in the bone marrow is less than 20%. Acute myeloblastic leukemia, type M2, can mimic RAEB-t when the number of blasts is between 25–30%. The degree of lineage dysplasia in the bone

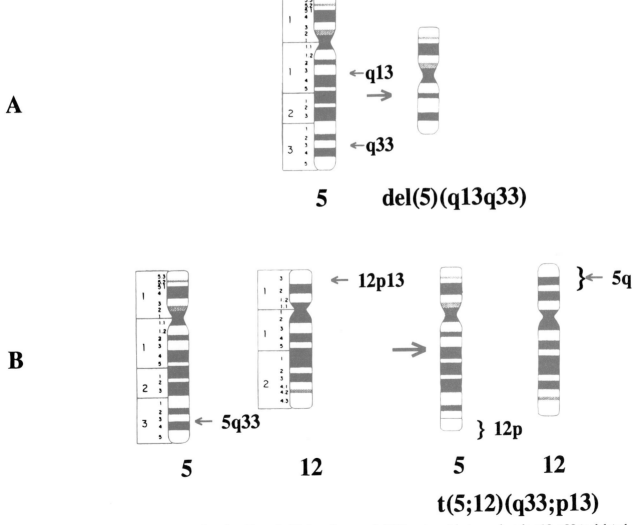

FIGURE 19–11 (*A*) Break points at bands q13 and q33 (*small arrows*). DNA segment between bands q13–q33 is deleted, resulting (*large arrow*) in a smaller chromosome 5. (*B*) Break points on chromosome 5, band q33 (*small arrow*) and on chromosome 12, band p13 (*small arrow*), followed by translocation of DNA (*large arrow*) between these two chromosomes.

marrow and the presence of a t(8;21), which is typical for a small proportion of AML type M2, helps to differentiate between these two entities.[48]

Chronic Myelomonocytic Leukemia (CMML)

This disease is controversial in regard to its classification as an MDS. In the blood and bone marrow, we observe the same morphological abnormalities as those found in the other types of MDS. However, on clinical grounds, this type of MDS is more closely related to chronic myeloproliferative disorders. Indeed, patients present often with splenomegaly or hepatomegaly. Also, occasionally white blood cell counts may be as high as 75×10^9/L, a picture closely resembling that of chronic myelogeneous leukemia (CML). In this situation, cytogenetics is the only means of distinguishing CMML from CML. Indeed, CML has a specific clonal marker, the Philadelphia chromosome → t(9; 22)(q34q11.2).[49] The bone marrow is usually hypercellular with monocytosis and blast cells varying between 1% and 20%. There are no specific chromosomal abnormalities in CMML as opposed to CML, except in rare cases with splenomegaly and eosinophilia, in which a recently new translocation has been reported: t(5;12)(q33;p13)[50] (Fig. 19–11). The diagnosis rests mainly on the presence of more than 1×10^9/L monocytes in the peripheral blood and the presence of at least 20% monocytic cells in the bone marrow. Lineage dysplasia in the peripheral blood and bone marrow is typical of other MDS.

In 1987, following a workshop held in Scottsdale, Arizona, new recommendations were issued proposing a new morphological, immunologic, and cytogenetic (MIC) working classification for MDS.[51] A major innovation in the MIC working classification was to underscore specific immunophenotypic and cytogenetic profiles ignored in the FAB classification, mostly specific cytogenetic characteristics that may be relevant in establishing prognosis within each type of MDS. Finally, it must be emphasized that the nomenclature of MDS in children is more confusing; several pediatric MDS have been reported that cannot be integrated in the FAB classification such as juvenile chronic myeloid leukemia (JCML), infantile monosomy 7 syndrome (IMo7), and MDS with eosinophilia. A modified FAB classification has thus been recently proposed for children with MDS.[52]

LABORATORY FINDINGS

Cytochemistry

Aberrant enzymatic activities, such as decreased myeloperoxydase, chloroesterase, alkaline phosphatase, and Sudan black B reaction in mature myeloid cells, as opposed to an increased activity in myeloid precursors, periodic acid-Schiff (PAS), positivity in erythroblasts, dual esterase in the myeloid, and monocytoid cells are often found in MDS. An increased number of RBCs with HbF (positive Kleihauer-Betke cytochemical reaction) is a common observation. Cytochemistry is of less diagnostic value in MDS with major qualitative and quantitative abnormalities such as

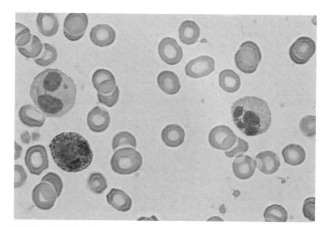

FIGURE 19–12 Peroxidase stain, peripheral blood, ×1000 magnification. Note one neutrophil with positive reaction and two negatives (RA).

RARS, RAEB, RAEB-t, and CMML. In RA, however, cytochemical studies in blood and bone marrow cells can contribute to a certain extent to a diagnosis. The frequency of cytochemical anomalies in RA patients from our observation and by others can be summarized as follows: in 20% to 78% of cases, neutrophil peroxidase shows reduced activity in most of the neutrophils (PMN) or an absence of activity in a small percentage; chloroesterase and LAP show decreased activity in mature neutrophils. LAP activity is increased in neutrophil precursors and 18% to 25% of erythroblasts will be positive for PAS; basophilic erythroblasts and proerythroblasts show granular and droplet reaction and more mature erythroblasts (polychromatophilic and orthochromatic) show a diffuse cytoplasmic reactivity. Occasionally, some erythrocytes (RBCs) also give a positive reaction of the homogeneous type (diffuse). Although no single cytoenzyme anomaly can be considered a specific early marker for leukemic transformation, a progressive deterioration of cytochemical enzymatic activities associated with morphological abnormalities can become indicators of impending leukemic phase. However, some of these changes in en-

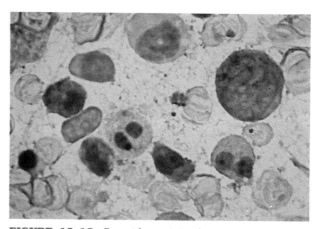

FIGURE 19–13 Peroxidase stain, bone marrow, ×1000 magnification: 2 pseudo-Pelger-Huët negative cells.

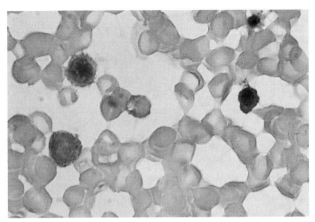

FIGURE 19–14 PAS stain, bone marrow, ×1000 magnification. Early erythroblast with positive large granules, late erythroblast with positive diffuse reaction. Also an erythrocyte with homogeneous diffuse reaction (RAEB).

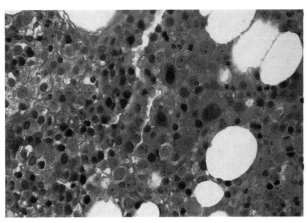

FIGURE 19–16 RAEB-t (bone marrow biopsy, H-E stain, ×400 magnification). Abnormal localization of immature precursors (ALIP) and monolobulated megakaryocytes.

zymatic activity must be interpreted with caution because infections, toxic bone marrow damage, and some congenital defective hematopoiesis may present similar cytochemical abnormalities[53–55] (Figs. 19–12 through 19–15).

Bone Marrow Histology

In patients with MDS, discrepancies between the cellularity estimate from biopsy specimens and that from aspirate smears occurs in up to 20% of cases. It is well accepted that the most accurate estimate of bone marrow cellularity is made from biopsy specimens. In addition to cellularity evaluation, bone marrow biopsy may be of great help in revealing typical histologic changes such as disruption of normal architecture with displacement of granulopoiesis, erythropoiesis, and megakaryocytopoiesis from their normal sites. Abnormal localization of immature precursors (ALIP), which are clusters or aggregates of myeloblasts and promyelocytes of usually three or more cells distant from the bone marrow trabeculae,

is also a feature of some MDS (Fig. 19–16). ALIP has been considered by some authors as an indicator of early leukemic transformation.[56] Bone marrow biopsy is especially relevant in the rare cases of MDS with severe myelofibrosis (10%)[57,58] (Fig. 19–17) or bone marrow hypoplasia.[59,60] Although dyserythropoiesis and dysgranulopoiesis are difficult to assess on bone marrow biopsy specimens, dysmegakaryocytopoiesis can be fairly estimated.

Immunology

Cells from peripheral blood, marrow aspirates, and triturated bone marrow biopsy specimens can be studied for specific cell surface antigen characterization by flow cytometry, and/or immunocytochemistry such as alkaline phosphatase antialkaline phosphatase methodology (APAAP). The increase of CD34+ cells (stem cell progenitors) in the bone marrow is of prognostic significance and usually correlates with impending leukemic transformation.[61–64] Blasts from patients evolving toward acceleration or transformation in any type of MDS may share antigens that are specific for

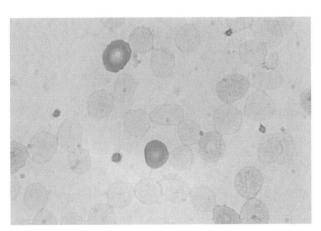

FIGURE 19–15 Kleihauer-Betke stain, peripheral blood, ×1000 magnification. The strongly stained RBCs contain Hb F; the faintly stained RBC is the result of elution Hb (RA).

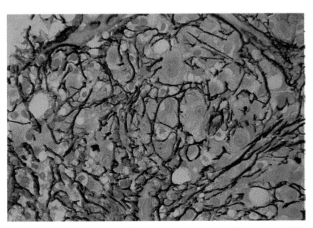

FIGURE 19–17 RAEB (bone marrow, reticulin stain, ×400 magnification). Severe fibrosis.

other cell lineages, mostly myeloid, monocytic, and lymphoid. In rare cases in which one finds a lymphoblastic proliferation, the immunophenotype pattern is consistently of the early B type (CD19+, CD10−, TdT+). RAEB and RAEB-t show higher myeloblastic and megakaryoblastic immunologic markers, whereas in RA, RARS, and CMML the granulomonocytic phenotype predominates. Hybrid lymphoid-myeloid cells or coexpression of granulomegakaryocytic antigens is also frequently observed in MDS, and one can also find rearrangements of the IgH and the TCR-γ and δ genes at the molecular level.

Patients with type I and II blasts expressing the H blood group antigen[65] have a poor prognosis as opposed to those expressing a pure myeloid phenotype. Expression of surface antigens from monocytes and granulocytes may vary considerably, with either loss or gain of specific and nonspecific antigens. Lymphopenia is frequently observed with a decrease in the number of CD4+ cells and slight increase of CD8+ cells.[66-68] It has been reported that an increased number of CD8+ cells at initial diagnosis in RA and RARS is associated with a decreased incidence of ANLL transformation. Although natural killer lymphocytes are decreased, antibody-dependent cellular cytotoxicity is conserved.

Fewer B-lymphocyte abnormalities have been reported. B-cell Epstein-Barr virus (EBV) receptors are decreased in number.[69] Immunoglobulin synthesis may be abnormally regulated. Hypergammaglobulinemia of polyclonal type can be observed in approximately 30% of patients with MDS, 12% with monoclonal gammopathy, and 13% with hypogammaglobulinemia. In patients with CMML, polyclonal hypergammaglobulinemia may be observed in more than 60% of cases.[70,71] Autoantibodies, in general, have been reported in 22% of all patients with MDS but in patients with CMML, it is more frequent (>50%). Platelet antibodies were present in 55% of those studied, erythrocyte autoantibodies were reported in 46%, and the direct antiglobulin test was positive in 8% of the IgG1 and C3d type.[72]

Cellular Dysfunctions

The genetic mutations or other abnormalities such as deletions, translocations, or gene amplification are responsible for a vast array of functional abnormalities within specific cell lineages.

Red Blood Cells

Several erythrocytic metabolic abnormalities may be encountered, the most frequent being pyruvate kinase deficiency and an increased level of fetal hemoglobin. Occasionally, one can find acquired hemoglobin H, increased i antigen, loss of ABO blood group antigens, demasking of Tn antigen, and sensitivity of RBC to complement (positive Ham-Dacie serum acid test and/or sugar water test).[73-76]

White Blood Cells

Abnormal granulocyte function is very frequently observed in most cases in relationship to decreased cytoplasmic granules and myeloperoxidase deficiency; alkaline phosphatase and esterase isoenzyme activities may also be decreased in granulocytes. Chemotaxis, adhesion, phagocytosis, and microbicidal capacity may be impaired.[77,78] These functional abnormalities are not necessarily related to hypogranulation. Indeed, abnormal phagocytosis, chemotaxis, or bactericidal activity in neutrophils have been closely associated to the loss of one chromosome 7 (monosomy 7) or the loss of a portion of the long arm of chromosome 7 (7q-). This specific dysfunction is associated with a high level of bacterial infection. In these situations, the gp130 molecule, produced by a gene located on chromosome 7, is secreted in inadequate amounts and is responsible for the major defect in chemotaxis and phagocytosis.[79]

Platelet

Platelet aggregation, adhesion, and other platelet functions are also frequently impaired in MDS.[80]

Culture Studies

A number of investigators have studied the in vitro growth patterns in MDS. Normally, there is a specific pattern of colonies in clusters that grow in culture from normal progenitor cells. Normal marrow cells pass through all stages of normal maturation to become morphologically recognizable mature cells. In vitro cultures of bone marrow cells from individuals with MDS have provided information about the nature of the pathophysiologic defect. In general, the ability of hematopoietic progenitor cells to form colonies is either reduced or absent.[81] The aberrant growth patterns are mostly observed in the more severe subgroups of MDS, such as RAEB and RAEB-t. Chronic myelomonocytic leukemia (CMML) is, however, a notable exception distinguished by increased colony growth.[82] Some investigators have tried to correlate in vitro growth patterns with the propensity to evolve to acute leukemia, dividing growth patterns into the leukemic type and the nonleukemic type. Given the lack of standardization and results that are often conflicting, there are no firm conclusions that can be made about growth patterns on either prognosis or leukemic potential in individual patients with MDS at this time. In vitro culture of bone marrow from patients with MDS is a valuable laboratory investigation that must be considered as an investigational complementary tool with cytogenetics and all the other laboratory tests mentioned previously.

Other laboratory findings such as increased muramidase both in serum and urine in CMML and increased serum ferritin and transferrin saturation may be abnormal in MDS.

Cytogenetics

The terminology and abbreviations used in describing chromosomes and their abnormalities are beyond the scope of this chapter. For detailed guidelines, the reader is referred to reference 83. Table 19–2 is a brief review adapted for the comprehension of this section. Figure 19–11 is a diagrammatic representation of the

TABLE 19–2 **Abbreviations and Terminology Used in Describing Chromosomes and Their Abnormalities**	
Abbreviation	**Significance**
p	Short arm of a chromosome
q	Long arm of a chromosome
p−, q−	Loss of chromosomal material from the short or long arm respectively
p+, q+	Addition of chromosomal material to the short and long arm respectively
del	Deletion of chromosomal material
t	Translocation of chromosomal material (DNA exchange between 2 chromosomes)
mar	Marker chromosome that is not fully characterized
+	Addition of a chromosome
−	Loss of a chromosome
Hypodiploid	Cells having fewer than 46 chromosomes
Hyperdiploid	Cells having more than 46 chromosomes
Complex karyotype	The presence of more than 2 chromosomal abnormalities in the same cell

Example. 47,XX,del(7)(q22),+8   The description order of chromosome abnormalities in a karyotype is the following: sex aberrations are specified first, followed by abnormalities of the autosomes listed in numerical order, irrespective of aberration type. In the example above, a breakpoint in the long arm of chromosome 7, at region (band) 22 (q22) has resulted in the loss (del) of chromosomal material → del(7)(q22); there is also a gain of 1 chromosome 8 → +8.

interstitial deletion of the long arm of chromosome 5→del(5)(q13q33) and translocation 5;12→t(5;12)(q33;p13).

Since the introduction of the FAB classification for MDS in 1982, cytogenetics has become one of the most informative laboratory tools in investigation and management. The nature and complexity of clonal chromosomal abnormalities have proved over time to be essential in the diagnosis and prognosis. Specific chromosome abnormalities documented in MDS constitute independent prognostic factors[84] and thus provide the opportunity to predict response to therapy and evolution. Furthermore, investigation of chromosome regions frequently affected in MDS has been a leading clue to the uncovery of basic molecular mechanisms involved in their pathogenesis.

Clonal cytogenetic abnormalities are detected in a range of 30% to 90% of patients with MDS.[85] Iterative cytogenetic studies will show that approximately 15% to 30% of patients with MDS have evidence of chromosome evolution, sometimes with concomitant leukemic transformation.[86] Most studies have shown that the frequency and nature of chromosome abnormalities vary with individual subtypes of MDS.[87–89] Thus, the lowest incidence of chromosome abnormalities is found in patients with RARS; deletion of DNA material along the long arm of chromosome 5 (5q−) is the most characteristic cytogenetic profile in patients with RA[31,32] (see Figs. 19–11 and 19–18). Patients with RAEB show a spectrum of chromosome abnormalities including 5q−, +8, 20q−, whereas those with RAEB-t harbor complex karyotypes with frequent involvement of −7[90,91] (Fig. 19–19). A small proportion of patients with CMLL harbor a specific translocation between chromosomes 5 and 12 → t(5;12)(q33;p13)[50] (see Fig. 19–11 for diagrammatic representation of this trans-

location). Finally, patients with secondary MDS are mostly characterized by an overrepresentation of −7, 5q− complex chromosome abnormalities and 12p−. Cytogenetic studies are of great diagnostic significance, mostly in patients with RA, because in this specific type of MDS the diagnosis rests mainly on the subjective identification of cell lineage qualitative abnormalities according to the FAB criteria. In this setting, the presence of nonrandom chromosome abnormalities remains the diagnostic hallmark of this MDS subtype.

Finally, in patients with RA, interstitial deletion of the long arm or chromosome 5 (see Figs. 19–11 and 19–18) is often found as the sole chromosome abnor-

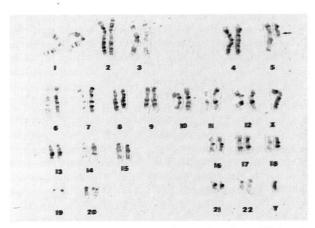

FIGURE 19–18 Karyotype with GTG banding, 450 bands resolution, showing the interstitial deletion of chromosome 5 → 46 XY, del (5)(q13q33) characteristically found in the 5q-syndrome.

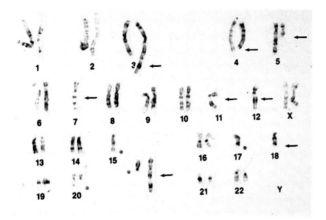

FIGURE 19-19 Karyotype GTG banding, resolution 450 bands, showing complex clonal abnormalities involving at least 8 chromosomes within the same cell, including del (5) (q13q33), -7, del (20)(q11.2).

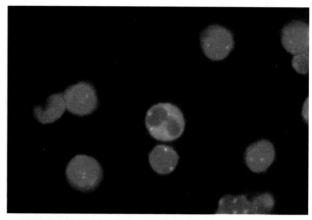

FIGURE 19-20 In situ hybridization showing +8 in a neutrophil and a normal lymphoid chromosome complement.

mality. In such instances, one finds typical clinical features such as female preponderance, age over 50, macrocytosis, normal or elevated platelet count, monolobular or dwarf megakaryocytes, and erythroid hypoplasia in the bone marrow. This entity is referred to as the 5q− syndrome. The clinical course in these patients is usually a predictable stable course with a low frequency of leukemic transformation.[31,32,92]

The risk of leukemic transformation has been demonstrated by several authors to be significantly related to the constitution of the karyotype in addition to the FAB type. In a recent study,[86] only 14% of patients with a normal karyotype displayed a leukemic transformation, whereas 42% of those with chromosome abnormalities did so. Monosomy 7 can be regarded as a genetic event with an unfavorable impact, whereas complex abnormalities (more than two clonal abnormalities within the same cell) are associated with the most serious outcome with a mean survival time ranging from 3 to 8 months.[84,86,93,94]

Sterotypic translocations such as t(8;21), t(15;17), and t(9;22), which are molecular events now recognized to be associated with specific hemopathies, are generally not found in MDS except those induced by chemotherapeutic regimens affecting topoisomerase II[95]. The presence of a t(9;22) (Philadelphia chromosome → Ph′) has very rarely been reported in MDS and should be considered exceptional.[95–97]

Finally, one must be aware that chromosome abnormalities are often difficult to characterize because of poor culture growth and contraction of chromosomes. Fortunately, it is now possible to use molecular probes that are complementary to specific DNA sequences located at various regions (the centromeric region, for instance) of all chromosome pairs. Under optimal conditions, these probes hybridize to complementary DNA in the genome. Fluorescent agents are used to reveal the hybridization. With this molecular approach (fluorescence in situ hybridization, FISH), the genome of a myelodysplastic cell can be scrutinized in its resting state (interphase).[15–17] An example is shown in Figure 19–20, in which a probe, complementary to the cen-

tromer of chromosome 8, has been chosen for hybridization on a peripheral blood film. The three yellow dots present in the nucleus of the neutrophil confirm the neoplastic nature of this cell. Note that lymphocytes in the neighborhood harbor a normal chromosome complement.

In summary, since the introduction of the FAB classification, cytogenetics has become a major investigative tool with a significant impact on diagnosis, prognosis, and the elucidation of the pathogenesis of the disease, and is being used routinely in most laboratories.

SECONDARY MYELODYSPLASTIC SYNDROMES

There are two types of MDS, primary and secondary. Primary (p-MDS) is de novo acquired, of unknown etiology. Secondary MDS (s-MDS) usually results from exposure to chemotherapy or chemoradiotherapy regimens, or to toxic agents.[98–100] Laboratory findings, clinical manifestations, and evolution closely resemble those of p-MDS, although s-MDS show a very high frequency of clonal chromosomal abnormalities and a higher tendency to early leukemic transformation, especially those with complex karyotypes.

An increasing number of patients have presented with s-MDS at hematologic and oncologic centers in recent years. For example, from 5% to 10% of patients undergoing autologous bone marrow transplantation with chemotherapy regimens with or without combined radiotherapy are prone to evolve to MDS.[101–103] Most of the cases of s-MDS are causally related to previous therapy with alkylating agents. In numerous studies, almost all alkylating agents in general use have been shown to be leukemogenic. Recently, other drugs used in transplant regimens, such as the epipodophylotoxins etoposide and tenoposide and adriamycin, have been shown to be leukemogenic if administered in combination with cysplatine, doxorubicin, or other alkylating agents.[104] In patients with MDS and a history of previous exposure to alkylating agents, cytogenetic studies usually show unbalanced aberrations, primarily −7, −5, 5q− and 7q−. Recently, an increasing number of patients with s-MDS have been observed to present balanced translocations. Studies now reveal that a vast majority of these patients have been previously exposed to cytostatic drugs such as epipodophylotoxins and the anthracyclines, targeting at DNA topoisomerase II, often in combination with other drugs, particularly alkylating agents. DNA topoisomerases are a class of enzymes important in various DNA transactions such as replication, transcription, and recombination.[105] Most of the balanced translocations involve band 11q23 and also band 21q22, including cases of t(9;11) and t(8;21). It thus seems that there might be two types of therapy-induced MDS, one in relationship with exposure to alkylating agents in which chromosomal aberrations are mostly numerical and one secondary to cytostatic agents targeting at DNA topisomerase II in which mostly balanced chromosome translocations are found.

The peripheral blood cytopenias and morphological anomalies are similar to the primary (de novo) disease. The bone marrow is hypocellular in one third of the patients or normal or hypercellular in the others. All these cell lineages show dysmyelopoietic changes.

CLINICAL MANIFESTATIONS

MDS are essentially disorders of elderly people, but may occur in young adults and occasionally in children. The incidence is estimated at 1 to 2 per 100,000 persons per year with a median age of 65 years.[106] It occurs more frequently in men, the male-female ratio ranging from 1.1:1 to 1.5:1.[107–109] There are no specific clinical manifestations in patients with MDS. Most commonly, the symptoms are those attributable to progressive bone marrow failure. According to the degree of bone marrow failure, patients will present clinical manifestations in relationship to the degree of anemia, neutropenia, or thrombocytopenia. Symptoms

related to cardiac failure such as severe dyspnea on exertion, infection, or hemorrhage are the main clinical manifestations of patients with MDS and severe bone marrow failure. In patients with RAEB and RAEB-t, these clinical manifestations may appear relatively early in the course of the disease. However, patients without excess blasts in the bone marrow may be asymptomatic for a long period of time. Fatigue and weakness are also clinical manifestations closely related to the degree of bone marrow failure and to the specific types of MDS. Rarely, patients may present features such as arthralgias, weight loss, fever, and cutaneous vasculitis.

Abnormal physical findings are not prominent or specific. The spleen may be palpable in 20% and the liver may be enlarged in approximately 10% of patients. Enlarged lymph nodes are not usually present. As opposed to the other types of MDS, in CMML, splenomegaly, hepatomegaly, lymphadenopathy, and nodular leukemic cutaneous infiltrates are more common.[110,111] It must be stressed, however, that the overall clinical picture of CMML is more closely related to myeloproliferative disorders such as CML, polycythemia vera, essential thrombocythemia, and primary myelofibrosis.

EVOLUTION AND PROGNOSIS

MDS usually progress to severe bone marrow failure, in which patients succumb from infections and/or bleeding and, less frequently from acute leukemic transformation in approximately 30% to 40% of cases (survival and leukemic progression for each subgroup of MDS are shown in Fig. 19–21). As stated earlier (see Etiology and Pathogenesis, pp. 325–327), blast crisis in MDS is characterized by an overwhelming majority of pure myeloid or myelomonocytoid phenotypes. Pure lymphoblastic transformation is a rare event even in the pediatric setting.[52] Although complete remissions can still be obtained with high-dose chemotherapy reg-

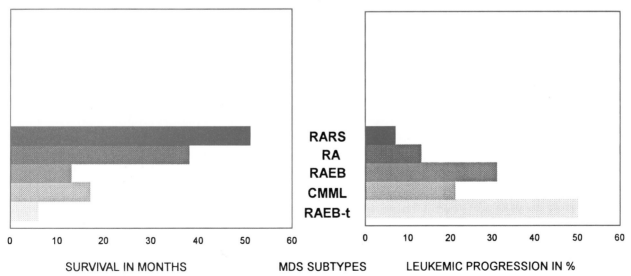

SURVIVAL IN MONTHS — MDS SUBTYPES — LEUKEMIC PROGRESSION IN %

RARS
RA
RAEB
CMML
RAEB-t

FIGURE 19–21 Survival and leukemic progression for each subgroup of MDS. Data pooled from several series with a total of 3554 patients.

imens in rare cases, acute leukemic transformation of MDS is usually fatal. Because MDS generally occur in the elderly population, a small proportion of patients die from unrelated neoplastic or non-neoplastic disorders. The evolution toward life-threatening bone marrow failure or leukemic transformation can be either gradual or abrupt. Initial assessment of the risk of early death was based on the FAB classification, in which most studies showed that patients could be classified as good or bad risks. Indeed, patients with RA were shown to have a median survival time of 50 months compared to a median survival time of 5 to 11 months for patients with RAEB, RAEB-t, and CMML.[112] It soon became obvious, however, that the FAB classification was of no avail in reflecting clinical heterogeneity within each subtype of MDS; other prognostic factors had to be looked for in conjunction with the FAB classification. The Valera (FAB)[113-118] and Bournemouth[114] scoring systems included risk factors related to qualitative and quantitative aspects of bone marrow and peripheral blood. The weakness of these systems was that the former did not consider the amount of blasts in the bone marrow as a risk factor for survival and/or acute leukemic transformation, and the latter gave an identical score for the percentage of blasts in the bone marrow and peripheral cytopenias. This was a major deficiency because the percentage of bone marrow blasts soon proved to be the most significant prognostic indicator in MDS.[115-121]

Other disease characteristics that may influence survival were investigated and integrated in new scoring systems,[115-118] as shown in Table 19–3. The nature of chromosome abnormalities became a strong prognostic indicator, independent of FAB subtype. As fully discussed in the section on cytogenetics, patients with monosomy 7 and complex karyotypes have much poorer median survival times. Another interesting observation was that patients with RA or RARS and abnormal localization of immature precursors in the bone marrow (ALIP), representing clusters of blasts, have a poor survival and a heightened risk of leukemic transformation.[56,118] Recently, the Bournemouth scoring system was modified and upgraded.[118] As shown in Table 19–3, it now includes most of the new biologic parameters that might influence evolution of

patients with MDS; patients are stratified into low-, intermediate-, and high-risk groups. Finally, pediatricians have identified a number of problems with definition and classification using the methods designed for adult MDS. Consequently, they have developed a pediatric scoring system including criteria such as fetal hemoglobin (HbF), platelets, and cytogenetics (FPC scoring system).[52]

The introduction of scoring systems proved useful for standardizing treatment strategies and also of informative value in therapeutic decision making. It must be stressed, however, that these scoring systems do not influence decision making for young patients eligible for allogeneic bone marrow transplantation, the only recognized treatment to significantly prolong survival and to be curative in a substantial proportion of patients. However, they may be of great value for patients with RA or RARS with median survival times of approximately 50 months. The nature of the karyotype and the presence or absence of ALIP should guide the clinician in decision making in regard to the timing of the transplantation. Finally, a number of molecular parameters that are not easily obtainable at the present time, such as the documentation of mutations in specific genes involved in the control of cell proliferation, may be of great value in the near future.

SPECIFIC DIAGNOSTIC PROBLEMS

CMML Because CMML may present with very high WBC counts and a significant number of immature myeloid cells in the peripheral blood, this disease entity may mimic CML. Cytogenetic studies are of major importance to distinguish between CMML and CML. The presence of t(9;22), which is diagnostic of CML, resolves the problem. When necessary, because 5% to 10% of patients with CML may not show t(9;22) with standard cytogenetic studies, molecular studies with either FISH or more sophisticated molecular techniques such as polymerase chain reaction may be necessary to identify t(9;22) in these patients. As stated earlier, rare cases of CMML harbor t(5;12).

RAEB-t/M2 FAB Myeloblastic Leukemia RAEB-t, as stated earlier, is defined by a blast count ranging between 20% and 30%. There is also a significant bi-

TABLE 19–3	**Clinical and Biological Parameters Included in Different Scoring Systems**						
Parameter	FAB	Bournemouth	Düsseldorf	Sanz	Goasguen	Bournemouth Modified	Pediatric
HEMOGLOBIN	−	+	+	−	+	+	−
NEUTROPHILS	+	+	−	−	−	+	−
PLATELETS	+	+	+	+	+	+	+
BM BLASTS	−	+	+	+	+	+	−
ALIP	−	−	−	−	−	+	−
CYTOGENETICS	−	−	−	−	−	+	+
DYSPLASIA	+	−	−	−	−	−	−
LDH	−	−	+	−	−	−	−
AGE	−	−	−	+	−	−	−
HbF	−	−	−	−	−	−	+
MEGAKARYOCYTES	+	−	−	−	−	−	−

Abbreviations: BM = Bone marrow; ALIP = abnormal localization of immature precursors; LDH = lactate dehydrogenase; HbF = fetal hemoglobin.

lineage or trilineage dysplasia in the bone marrow. M2 FAB type acute myeloblastic leukemia may present with blasts under 30% or close to 30%, which is the target percentage for the diagnosis of acute myeloid leukemia according to FAB classification criteria. It is often difficult for the clinician to distinguish between RAEB-t and M2 acute myeloid leukemia. This distinction is of major importance in view of the different therapeutic strategies undertaken for each of these diseases. The degree of lineage dysplasia and cytogenetic findings such as t(8;21), typical for M2 AML or monosomy 7, 7q−, monosomy 5, 5q−, which are most consistently found in MDS, may help in distinguishing between these two entities. Figure 19–22 depicts an algorithm according to the FAB criteria, which enables one to distinguish MDS from other types of AML.

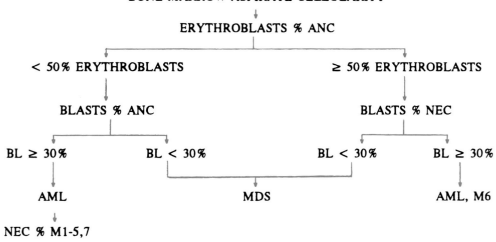

ANC = All nucleated cells
BL = Blast cells type I and II
NEC = Non erythroid cells
AML = Acute myeloid leukemia also known as acute nonlymphoblastic leukemia (ANLL)

When the erythroblasts (erythroid precursors) are ≥ 50% of ANC, the percentage of myeloblasts (type I, type II) from bone marrow smears is then calculated by excluding erythroblasts (% of NEC). If the result is < 30%, a diagnosis of MDS can be made. If BL ≥ 30%, the diagnosis is then AML, M6.

On the other hand, if the erythroblasts are < 50% of ANC, then the percentage of myeloblasts from bone marrow smears is calculated by including ANC. If BL < 30%, we are facing a MDS diagnosis. If BL ≥ 30%, then diagnoses of AML M1-M5 and M7 can be ascertained by excluding NEC.

Example: Erythroblasts 53%;   blasts 10%;   others 37%.
              10 of 47 is 21% total blasts excluding erythroblasts.
              We are thus dealing with a MDS.

Other Examples :	**Myeloblasts**	**Erythroblasts**	**Diagnosis**
	5 - 20%	< 50%	RAEB
	20 - 30%	< 50%	RAEB-t
	> 30%	< 50%	AML
	> 30%	> 50%	AML-M6

FIGURE 19–22   Algorithm according to FAB criteria proposed to distinguish MDS from different types of acute myeloid leukemia (AML).

Juvenile Chronic Myelomonocytic Leukemia Juvenile chronic myelomonocytic leukemia (JCMML) may also mimic chronic myeloid leukemia. Again, standard and molecular cytogenetic studies are of major importance in distinguishing between these two entities. In JCMML, many numerical changes, deletions, and translocations are found, mostly involving chromosomes 3, 5, 7, and 11, while t(9;22) →, the Philadelphia chromosome, is consistently absent.

Refractory Anemia As stated earlier, RA is the only MDS in which the diagnosis rests mainly on the subjective identification of qualitative abnormalities according to FAB, involving one or more bone marrow hematopoietic cell lineages. It is imperative in these cases that cytogenetic studies be undertaken in order to find clonal abnormalities that will confirm the diagnosis. In the absence of clonal abnormalities, one must be cautious in the interpretation of the degree of lineage dysplasia. Because isolated dyserythropoiesis on bone marrow smears is a feature shared by a variety of hematologic disorders with no relationship to MDS, dysplasia affecting at least two cell lineages is required in order to consider a diagnosis of RA.

MDS with Severe Myelofibrosis Rare cases of MDS show a dry tap on bone marrow aspiration. In these cases, bone marrow biopsy is essential to establish the diagnosis showing a marked increase in the marrow reticulin fibers.

Refractory Anemia with Ringed Sideroblasts One must be aware that zinc-induced sideroblastic anemia, alcohol intoxication, and hereditary sideroblastic anemia may mimic RARS.[122]

TREATMENT

MDS give rise to major therapeutic dilemmas[123] because the disease is not curable, except for patients eligible for an allogeneic bone marrow transplant program from matched-related or matched-unrelated donors.[124] Because the disease affects mostly elderly people and because very few patients are eligible for a bone marrow transplant, treatment is most often restricted to supportive measures such as blood component therapy and antibiotics. Because no generally effective therapy is available, most patients die in the preleukemic phase of the disease from infections or hemorrhage, both resulting from the profound cytopenias related to the malfunction of stem cells or from leukemic transformation.

Ideally, treatment should be directed at the total eradication of the neoplastic clone with restoration of normal hematopoiesis from all lineages. With the hope of achieving a cure, many patients have been treated with chemotherapy regimens used in acute myeloblastic leukemia. Unfortunately, this therapeutic approach has been of no avail.[125–127] Patients treated with therapy for acute myeloblastic leukemia have prolonged marrow aplasia and consequently a high mortality rate from infection and/or hemorrhage. Also, none of these patients have been cured of the disease. In view of the obvious failure of such a therapeutic approach, supportive measures such as blood component therapy and antibiotics have become the cornerstone of the treatment approach in MDS. Anemia often constitutes a major problem because most patients are elderly and suffer from neurologic and cardiovascular disorders. The severity of the anemia is often related to the subgroup of MDS (RA versus RAEB-t). As the disease progresses, red cell and platelet transfusion requirements are more often needed. Generally, these supportive measures are usually carried out on an outpatient basis and the ultimate goal of this treatment is to maintain the best quality of life, recognizing that cure is not possible.

During the course of MDS, precursor cell maturation becomes progressively impaired and culminates in a severe maturational block giving rise to profound potentially lethal cytopenias. It is thus no surprise that a vast array of differentiation-inducing agents such as retinoids, vitamin D analogs, glucocorticoids, interferons, hexamithylene-bisacetamide, low doses of cytosine arabinoside or 5-azacytidine, and hematopoietic growth factors have been used in clinical trials, either randomized or not.[128,129] The lesson that we have learned from all these trials is that inducing agents do not achieve a cure in MDS. Although some of these agents have resulted in minor improvement of peripheral cytopenias, others have accelerated the transformation of the disease into acute leukemia. Most of the cells that do differentiate bear functional and cytogenetic abnormalities from the clone from which it has differentiated.

Other agents such as those that modulate the immune system, such as corticosteroids and mostly interferon, have received some attention in the treatment of MDS. Interferon is a cytokine that possesses both antiproliferative and differentiation-inducing effects on normal and neoplastic cells. Also, interferon amplifies the cognitive phase of the immune response by increasing the expression of class I and class II major histocompatibility antigens on normal and neoplastic cells. Although interferon has proved effective in a few patients with chronic myelogenous leukemia, its profound myelosuppressive side effect in MDS and its inability to eradicate the malignant clone suggest that any schedule with interferon cannot be recommended for the treatment of patients with MDS.[130]

With the omnipresent failure of chemotherapy regimens or maturation-inducing agents, other cytokines classified as colony-stimulating factors (CSFs) or growth factors such as erythropoietin (Epo), granulocyte-macrophage colony-stimulating factor (GM-CSF), or granulocyte colony-stimulating factor (G-CSF) have been used in a number of clinical trials.[131] These factors have potent myelostimulatory effects. Treatment with these growth factors produces substantial increase in peripheral leukocyte counts but usually also exerts a stimulatory effect on the malignant clone, thus promoting transformation of MDS to overt AML. Except for anecdotal cases, patients treated with these growth factors do not enter into complete remission and cells promoted by these growth factors bear the functional, morphologic, and cytogenetical abnormalities of the initial malignant clone. Thus, CSFs may help to reduce the incidence of infections by increasing leukocyte counts, but on the other hand, they may accelerate the transformation to acute leukemia.

The only therapeutic approach recognized as inducing cures in MDS is allogeneic bone marrow transplantation.[122,132–134] Obviously, because the disease affects mostly elderly patients and also because matched related donors are found in approximately 30% of cases, very few patients can benefit from such a procedure. However, it is also possible to use matched unrelated donors. The chance of finding a matched unrelated donor worldwide for Caucasians is close to 60%. With the improvement of graft-versus-host disease (GVHD) prophylaxis and also the improvement in preventing cytomegalovirus disease, a cure can be obtained in 30% to 40% of cases. The mortality from GVHD is a major problem in the matched unrelated program. However, improvement in GVHD prophylaxis using T-cell-depleted marrows and many other approaches is encouraging.

CASE STUDY

N.B., a 78-year-old man, was admitted to the hospital with complaints of increasing weakness. Physical examination revealed pallor but no organomegaly. His medical history was uneventful.

The laboratory results were as follows:
for peripheral blood:

WBC	2.1×10^9/L
Hgb	8.5 g/dL
MCV	106 fL
RDW	24.5%
Plt	95×10^9/L

Blood smear showed 2% blasts, occasional pseudo-Pelger-Huet neutrophils with hypogranulation, occasional giant platelets, anisomacrocytosis, and occasional basophilic stippling. Bone marrow smear was hypercellular. Blast cells (type I and type II) constituted 23%, few blasts with Auer rods. Myeloid dysplasia was present with immature cells with an asynchronous maturation of the nucleus and cytoplasm. Pelgeroid cells with hypogranulation were seen. Erythroblasts (35%) with megaloblastoid changes and micromegakaryocytes (mononuclear) were present. Prussian blue stain showed 10% of ringed sideroblasts. Cytogenetic findings: complex karyotype including monosomy 7.

Diagnosis RAEB-t

Treatment Supportive therapy (transfusion)

Comments In this case, the diagnosis of RAEB-t can be reasonably confirmed on the basis of the percentage of bone marrow blasts being less than 30% and the presence of trilineage dysplasia. In this specific case, the presence of Auer rods did not help in the diagnosis. It must be emphasized that the presence of Auer rods would have been diagnostic of RAEB-t even if bone marrow blasts had been less than 20%. The presence of a complex karyotype and monosomy 7 are predictive of short survival and impending leukemic transformation. Elderly patients are not eligible for allogeneic bone marrow transplantation. In this case, supportive measures such as transfusions are the best therapeutic approach.

Questions

1. What is the relationship between the RDW result and observed red cell morphology?
2. Distinguish between type I and type II blasts in this case?
3. Which laboratory finding clearly distinguishes this MDS from AML M2?
4. Which laboratory finding presented here is common to both MDS and AML-M2?
5. What is the significance of Auer rods in this case?

REFERENCES

1. Hamilton-Paterson, JL: Preleukemic anemia. Acta Haematol 2:309, 1949.
2. Block, M, Jacobson, LW, and Belhard, WF: Preleukaemic acute human leukaemia. JAMA 151:1018, 1953.
3. Bjorkman, SE: Chronic refractory anemia with sideroblastic bone marrow. A study of four cases. Blood 11:250, 1956.
4. Rheingold, JJ, et al: Smouldering acute leukaemia. N Engl J Med 28:812, 1963.
5. Saarni, MI and Linman, JW: Preleukaemia. The hematological syndrome preceding acute leukemia. Am J Med 55:38, 1973.
6. Dreyfus, B: Preleukemic states. Blood Cells 2:33, 1976.
7. Bennett, JM, et al: Proposals for the classification of the acute leukaemias. Br J Haematol 33:451, 1976.
8. Bennett, JM, et al: Proposals for the classification of the myelodysplastic syndromes. Br J Haematol 51:189, 1982; Clin Haematol 15:909, 1986.
9. Tricot, G: The myelodysplastic syndromes: Different evolution patterns based on sequential morphological and cytogenetic investigations. Br J Haematol 59:659, 1985.
10. Komatsu, N: Simultaneous expression of lymphoid and myeloid phenotypes in acute leukemia arising from myelodysplastic syndrome. Am J Hematol 28:103, 1988.
11. San Miguel, JF: Myelodysplastic syndrome evolving to a mixt myeloid-lymphoid leukemia. Hematol Oncol 4:175, 1986.
12. Berneman, ZN: A myelodysplastic syndrome preceeding acute lymphoblastic leukemia. Br J Haematol 60:353, 1985.
13. Ascensao, JL: Lymphoblastic transformation of myelodysplastic syndrome. Am J Hematol 22:431, 1986.
14. San Miguel, JF: Acute leukemia after a primary myelodysplastic syndrome: Immunophenotypic, genotypic, and clinical characteristics. Blood 78:768, 1991.
15. Jenkins, RB, et al: Fluorescence in situ hybridization: A sensitive method for trisomy 8 detection in bone marrow specimens. Blood 79:3307, 1992.
16. Kibbelaar, RE, et al: Combined immunophenotyping and DNA in situ hybridization to study lineage involvement in patients with myelodysplastic syndromes. Blood 79:1823, 1992.
17. Anastasi, JF: Cytogenetic clonality in myelodysplastic syndromes studied with fluorescence in situ hybridization: Lineage, response to growth factor therapy, and clone expansion. Blood 81:1580, 1993.
18. Janssen, JWG, et al: Clonal analysis of myelodysplastic syndromes: evidence of multipotent stem cell origin. Blood 73:248, 1989.
19. Prchal, JT, et al: A common progenitor for human myeloid and lymphoid cells. Nature 274:590, 1978.
20. Culligan, DJ, et al: Clonal lymphocytes are detectable in only some cases of MDS. Br J Haematol 81:346, 1992.
21. van Kamp, J, et al: Clonal involvement of granulocytes and monocytes, but not of T and B lymphocytes and natural killer cells in patients with myelodysplasia: analysis by X-linked restriction fragment length polymorphisms and polymerase chain reaction of the phosphoglycerate kinase gene. Blood 80:1774, 1992.
22. Kroef, MJPL, et al: Myeloid but not lymphoid cells carry the 5q deletion: Polymerase chain reaction analysis of

loss of heterozygosity using mini-repeat sequences on highly purified cell fractions. Blood 81:1849, 1993.

23. Bishop, JM: Cellular oncogenes and retroviruses. Ann Rev Biochem 52:301, 1983.

24. Krontiris, TG: The emerging genetics of human cancer. N Engl J Med 309:404, 1983.

25. Willecke, K and Schafer, R: Human oncogenes. Hum Genet 66:132, 1984.

26. Weinberg, RA: Tumor suppressor genes. Science 254:1138, 1991.

27. Weinberg, RA: Oncogenes, antioncogenes, and the molecular bases of multistep carcinogenesis. Cancer Res 49:3713, 1989.

28. Sager, R: Tumor suppressor genes: The puzzle and the promise. Science 246:1406, 1989.

29. Bartram, CR: Molecular genetic aspects of myelodysplastic syndromes. Hematol Oncol Clin North Am 6:557, 1992.

30. Jacobs, A: Gene mutations in myelodysplasia. Leuk Res 16:47, 1992.

31. Boultwood, J, Lewis, S, and Wainscoat, JS: The 5q− syndrome. Blood 84:3253, 1994.

32. Pedersen, B, and Jensen, IM: Clinical and prognostic implications of chromosome 5q deletions: 96 high resolution studied patients. Leukemia 5:566, 1991.

33. Willman, CL et al: Deletion of *IRF-1*, mapping to chromosome 5q31.1, in human leukemia and preleukemic myelodysplasia. Science 259:968, 1993.

34. Harada, H, et al: Anti-oncogenic and oncogenic potential of interferon regulatory factors 1 and 2. Science 259:971, 1993.

35. Wasmuth, JJ, Bishop, DT, and Westbrook, CA: Report of the committee on the genetic construction of chromosome 5. Human Gene Mapping 11 (1991). Cytogenet Cell Genet 58:261, 1991.

36. Wyllie, A: Apoptosis. Br J Cancer 67:205, 1993.

37. Vaux, DL: Towards an understanding of the molecular mechanism of physiological cell death. Proc Natl Acad Sci USA 90:786, 1993.

38. Raza, A: Apoptosis in bone marrow biopsy sample involving stromal and hematopoietic cells in 50 patients with myelodysplastic syndromes. Blood 86:268, 1995.

39. Dacie, JV and Lewis, SM: Practical Haematology, ed 6. Edinbourgh, Churchill Livingstone, 1984, p 107.

40. Kouides, PA, and Bennett, JM: Morphology and classification of myelodysplastic syndromes. Hematol Oncol Clin North Am 6:485, 1992.

41. Hamblin, TJ and Oscier, DG: The myelodysplastic syndrome—A practical guide. Hematol Oncol 5:19, 1987.

42. Hast, R, et al: Diagnostic significance of dysplastic features of peripheral blood polymorphs in myelodysplastic syndromes. Leuk Res 13:173, 1989.

43. Goasguen, JE, et al: Prognostic implication and characterization of the blast cell population in the myelodysplastic syndrome. Leuk Res 15:1159, 1991.

44. Hast, R: Sideroblasts in myelodysplasia: Their nature and clinical significance. Scand J Haematol 36 (suppl 45):53, 1986.

45. Lindriz, EA: Pelger-Huet anomaly, the Stodmeister type. Atlas of Haematology, ed 2. Sandoz, 1994, p 82, Plate 143-B.

46. Jakobsen, P: Ballooning platelets in the myelodysplastic syndromes. Eur J Haematol 53:175, 1994.

47. Bennett, JM, et al: Proposed revised criteria for the classification of acute myeloid leukemia. Ann Intern Med 103:626, 1985.

48. Swirsky, DM, et al: 8;21 translocation in acute granulocytic leukaemia: Cytogenetical, cytochemical and clinical features. Br J Haematol 56:199, 1984.

49. Gale, RP, and Cannani, E: Review. The molecular biology of chronic myelogenous leukaemia. Br J Haematol 60:395, 1985.

50. Wlodarska, I: TEL gene is involved in myelodysplastic syndromes with either the typical t(5;12)(q33;p13) translocation or its variant t(10;12)(q24;p13). Blood 85:2848, 1995.

51. Recommendations for a morphologic, immunologic, and cytogenetic (MIC) working classification of the primary and therapy-related myelodysplastic disorders. Report of the Workshop held in Scottsdale, Arizona, February 23–25, 1987. Cancer Genet Cytogenet 32:1, 1988.

52. Passmore SJ: Pediatric myelodysplasia: A study of 68 children and a new prognostic scoring system. Blood 85:1742, 1995.

53. Schmalzl, F: The value of cytochemical investigations in the diagnosis of the myelodysplastic syndromes. In Schmalzl, F and Mufti, GJ (Eds): Myelodysplastic Syndromes. Springer-Verlag, Berlin, 1992, p 44.

54. De Pasquale, A and Quaglino, D: Enzyme cytochemical studies in myelodysplastic syndromes. In Schmalzl, F, and Mufti, GJ (eds): Myelodysplastic Syndromes. Springer-Verlag, 1992, p 51.

55. Seo, IS, Li, CY, and Yam, LT: Myelodysplastic syndrome: Diagnostic implications of cytochemical and immunocytochemical studies. Mayo Clin Proc 68:47, 1993.

56. Tricot, G, et al: Prognostic factors in the myelodysplastic syndromes: Importance of initial data on peripheral blood counts, bone marrow cytology, trephine biopsy and chromosomal analysis. Br J Haematol 60:10, 1984.

57. Delacretaz, F, et al: Histopathology of myelodysplastic syndromes: The FAB classification (proposals) applied to bone marrow biopsy. Am J Clin Pathol 87:180, 1987.

58. Rios, A, et al: Bone marrow biopsy in myelodysplastic syndromes: morphological characteristics and contribution to the study of prognostic factors. Br J Haematol 75:26, 1990.

59. Tricot, G, et al: Bone marrow histology in myelodysplastic syndromes. I. Histological findings in myelodysplastic syndromes and comparison with bone marrow smears. Br J Haematol 57:423, 1984.

60. Yoshida, Y, et al: Refractory myelodysplastic anaemias with hypocellular bone marrow. J Clin Pathol 41:763, 1988.

61. Soligo, DA, et al: CD34 immunohistochemistry of bone marrow biopsies: prognostic significance in primary myelodysplastic syndromes. Am J Hematol 46:9, 1994.

62. Sullivan, SA, et al: Circulating CD34+ cells: An adverse prognostic factor in the myelodysplastic syndromes. Am J Hematol 39:96, 1992.

63. Maciejewski, JP, et al: Phenotypic and functional analysis of bone marrow progenitor cell compartment in bone marrow failure. Br J Haematol 87:227, 1994.

64. Orazi, A, et al: Therapy-related myelodysplastic syndromes: FAB classification, bone marrow histology, and immunohistology in the prognostic assessment. Leukemia 7:838, 1993.

65. Koeller, U, et al: Immunological phenotyping of blood and bone marrow cells from patients with myelodysplastic syndromes. In Schmalzl, F and Mufti, GJ: Myelodysplastic syndromes. Springer-Verlag, Berlin, 1992, p 60.

66. Bynoe, AG, et al: Decreased T helper cells in the myelodysplastic syndromes. Br J Haematol 54:97, 1983.

67. Hokland, P, et al: Analysis of leukocyte differentiation antigens in blood and bone marrow from preleukemia (refractory anemia) patients using monoclonal antibodies. Blood 67:898, 1986.

68. Knox, SJ, et al: Studies of T-lymphocytes in preleukemic disorders and acute nonlymphocytic leukemia: In vitro radiosensitivity, mitogenic responsiveness, colony formation, and enumeration of lymphocytic subpopulations. Blood 61:449, 1983.

69. Anderson, RW, et al: Lymphocyte abnormalities in preleukemia. I. Decreased NK activity, anomalous immu-

noregulatory cell subsets and deficient EBV receptors. Leuk Res 7:389, 1983.

70. Economopoulos, T, et al: Immune abnormalities in myelodysplastic syndromes. J Clin Pathol 38:908, 1985.

71. Mufti, GJ, et al: Immunological abnormalities in myelodysplastic syndromes. I. Serum immunoglobulins and autoantibodies. Br J Haematol 63:143, 1986.

72. Sokol, RJ, et al: Erythrocyte autoantibodies, autoimmune haemolysis, and myelodysplastic syndromes. J Clin Pathol 42:1088, 1989.

73. Kahn, A: Abnormalities of erythrocyte enzymes in dyserythropoiesis and malignancies. Clin Haematol 10:123, 1976.

74. Newman, DR, Pierre, RV, and Linman, JW: Studies on the diagnostic significance of hemoglobin F levels. Mayo Clin Proc 48:199, 1973.

75. Salmon, C: Blood group changes in preleukemic states. Blood Cells 2:211, 1976.

76. Hauptman, GM, et al: False positive acidified serum test in a preleukemic dyserythropoiesis. Acta Haematol 59:73, 1978.

77. Martin, S, et al: Defective neutrophil function and microbicidal mechanisms in the myelodysplastic disorders. J Clin Pathol 36:1120, 1983.

78. Boogaerts, MA, et al: Blood neutrophil function in primary myelodysplastic syndromes. Br J Haematol 55:411, 1983.

79. Gyger, M, et al: Childhood monosomy 7 syndrome. Am J Hematol 13:329, 1982.

80. Lintula, R, et al: Platelet function in preleukaemia. Scand J Haematol 26:65, 1981.

81. Richert-Boe, KE, and Bagby, GC: In vitro hematopoiesis in myelodysplasia: liquid and soft-gel culture studies. Hematol Oncol Clin North Am 6:543, 1992.

82. Geissler, K, et al: Colony growth factors for chronic myelomonocytic leukemia cells. Blood 74:1472, 1989.

83. Karger, S (ed): Guidelines for Cancer Cytogenetics. Supplement to an International System for Human Cytogenetic Nomenclature (ISCN 1991).

84. Yunis, JJ, et al: Refined chromosome analysis as an independent prognostic indicator in de novo myelodysplastic syndromes. Blood 67:1721, 1986.

85. Heim, S, and Mitelman, F: Chromosome abnormalities in the myelodysplastic syndromes. Clin Haematol 15:1003, 1986.

86. Haase, D: Cytogenetic findings in 179 patients with myelodysplastic syndromes. Ann Hematol 70:171, 1995.

87. Jacobs, RH, et al: Prognostic implications of morphology and karyotype in primary myelodysplastic syndromes. Blood 67:1765, 1986.

88. Horiike, S, et al: Chromosome abnormalities and karyotypic evolution in 83 patients with myelodysplastic syndrome and predictive value for prognosis. Cancer 62:1129, 1988.

89. Yunis, JJ, et al: Refined chromosome study helps define prognostic subgroups in most patients with primary myelodysplastic syndrome and acute myelogenous leukemia.

90. Knapp, RH, Dewald, GW, and Pierre, RV: Cytogenetic studies in 174 consecutive patients with preleukemic or myelodysplastic syndromes. Mayo Clin Proc 60:507, 1985.

91. Musilova, J and Michalova, K: Chromosome study of 85 patients with myelodysplastic syndrome. Cancer Genet Cytogenet 33:39, 1988.

92. Mathew, P, et al: The 5q− syndrome: A single-institution study of 43 consecutive patients. Blood 81:1040, 1993.

93. Ayraud, N, et al: Cytogenetic study of 88 cases of refractory anemia. Cancer Genet Cytogenet 8:243, 1983.

94. Suciu, S: Results of chromosome studies and their relation to morphology, course and prognosis in 120 pa-

tients with de novo myelodysplastic syndrome. Cancer Genet Cytogenet 44:15, 1990.

95. Quesnel, B, et al: Therapy-related acute myeloid leukemia with t(8;21), inv(16), and t(8;16): A report on 25 cases and review of the literature. J Clin Oncol 11:2370, 1993.

96. Roth, DG: Chronic myelodysplastic syndrome (preleukemia) with Philadelphia chromosome. Blood 56:262, 1980.

97. Berrebi, A: Philadelphia chromosome in idiopathic acquired sideroblastic anemia. Acta Haematol 72:343, 1985.

98. Iurlo, A, et al: Cytogenetic and clinical investigations in 76 cases with therapy-related leukemia and myelodysplastic syndrome. Cancer Genet Cytogenet 43:227, 1989.

99. Pedersen-Bjergaard, J, et al: Therapy-related myelodysplasia and acute myeloid leukemia. Cytogenetic characteristics of 115 consecutive cases and risk in seven cohorts of patients treated intensively for malignant diseases in the Copenhagen series. Leukemia 7:1975, 1993.

100. LeBeau, MM, et al: Clinical and cytogenetic correlations in 63 patients with therapy-related myelodysplastic syndromes and acute nonlymphocyte leukemia: Further evidence of characteristic abnormalities of chromosomes no. 5 and 7. J Clin Oncol 4:325, 1986.

101. Stone, RM, et al: Myelodysplastic syndrome as a late complication following autologoues bone marrow transplantation for non-Hodgkin's lymphoma. J Clin Oncol 12:2535, 1994.

102. Miller, JS, et al: Myelodysplastic syndrome after autologous bone marrow transplantation: An additional late complication of curative cancer therapy. Blood 83:3780, 1994.

103. Darrington, DL, et al: Incidence and characterization of secondary myelodysplastic syndrome and acute myelogenous leukemia following high-dose chemoradiotherapy and autologous stem-cell transplantation for lymphoid malignancies. J Clin Oncol 12:2527, 1994.

104. Pedersen-Bjergaard, J, and Philip, P: Two different classes of therapy-related and de novo acute myeloid leukemia. Cancer Genet Cytogenet 55:119, 1991.

105. Liu, LF: DNA topoisomerase poisons as antitumor drugs. Annu Rev Biochem 58:351, 1989.

106. Galton, DAG: The myelodysplastic syndromes. Clin Lab Haematol 6:99, 1984.

107. Linman, JW, and Bagby, GC: The preleukemic syndrome (hemopoietic dysplasia). Cancer 42:854, 1978.

108. Aul, C, et al: Age-related incidence and other epidemiological aspects of myelodysplastic syndrome. Br J Haematol 82:385, 1992.

109. Oscier, D: Myelodysplastic syndromes. Ballieres Clin Haematol 1:389, 1987.

110. Copplestone, JA, et al: Monocytic skin infiltration in chronic myelomonocytic leukaemia. Clin Lab Haematol 8:115, 1986.

111. Da Silva, MAP, et al: Extramedullary disease in myelodysplastic syndromes. Am J Med 85:589, 1988.

112. Third MIC Cooperative Study Group: Recommendations for a morphologic, immunologic and cytogenetic (MIC) working classification of the primary and therapy-related myelodysplastic disorders. Cancer Genet Cytogenet 32:1, 1988.

113. Varela, BL, Chuang, C, and Bennett, JM: Modification in the classification of primary myelodysplastic syndromes: the addition of a scoring system. Haematol Oncol 3:55, 1985.

114. Mufti, GJ, et al: Myelodysplastic syndromes: a scoring system with prognostic significance. Br J Haematol 59:425, 1985.

115. Gyger, M, et al: Prognostic value of clonal chromosomal abnormalities in patients with primary myelodysplastic syndromes. Am J Hematol 28:13, 1988.

116. Coiffer, B, et al: Dysmyelopoietic syndromes. A search of prognostic factors in 193 patients. Cancer 52:83, 1983.

117. Mufti, GJ, and Galton, DAG: Myelodysplastic syndromes: Natural history and features of prognostic importance. Clin Haematol 15:953, 1986.

118. Mufti, GJ: A guide to risk assessment in the primary myelodysplastic syndrome. Hematol Oncol Clin North Am 6:587, 1992.

119. Aul, C: Primary myelodysplastic syndromes: Analysis of prognostic factors in 235 patients and proposals for an improved scoring system. Leukemia 6:52, 1992.

120. Sanz, GF: Two regression models and a scoring system for predicting survival and planning treatment in myelodysplastic syndromes: A multivariate analysis of prognostic factors in 370 patients. Blood 74:395, 1989.

121. Goasguen, JE: Prognostic factors of myelodysplastic syndromes-a simplified 3-D scoring system. Leukemia Research 14:255, 1990.

122. Fiske, DN, et al: Zinc-induced sideroblastic anemia: Report of a case, review of the literature, and description of the hematologic syndrome. Am J Hematol 46:147, 1994.

123. Cheson, BD: The myelodysplastic syndromes: Current approaches to therapy. Ann Intern Med 112:932, 1990.

124. Appelbaum, FR, et al: Bone marrow transplantation for patients with myelodysplasia. Pretreatment variables and outcome. Ann Intern Med 112:590, 1990.

125. Tricot, G, and Boogaerts, MA: The role of aggressive chemotherapy in the treatment of the myelodysplastic syndromes. Br J Haematol 63:477, 1986.

126. Fenaux, P, et al: Aggressive chemotherapy in adult primary myelodysplastic syndromes. Blut 57:297, 1988.

127. Martiat, P, et al: Intensive chemotherapy for acute non-lymphoblastic leukemia after primary myelodysplastic syndrome. Hematol Oncol 6:299, 1988.

128. List, AF, et al: Review article. The myelodysplastic syndromes: Biology and implications for management. J Clin Oncol 8:1424, 1990.

129. Kizaki, M, and Koeffler, HP: Differentiation-inducing agents in the treatment of myelodysplastic syndromes. Semin Oncol 19:95, 1992.

130. Aul, C, et al: Treatment of advanced myelodysplastic syndromes with recombinant interferon-alpha2b. Eur J Haematol 46:11, 1991.

131. Nagler, A, et al: Effects of recombinant human granulocyte colony stimulating factor and granulocyte-monocyte colony stimulating factor on in vitro hemopoiesis in the myelodysplastic syndromes. Leukemia 4:193, 1990.

132. Belanger, R, et al: Bone marrow transplantation for myelodysplastic syndromes. Br J Haematol 69:29, 1988.

133. Appelbaum, FR, et al: Bone marrow transplantation for patients with myelodysplasia: Pretreatment variables and outcome. Ann Intern Med 12:590, 1980.

134. Ratanatharathorn, V, et al: Busulfan-based regimens and allogeneic bone marrow transplantation in patients with myelodysplastic syndromes. Blood 81:2194, 1993.

BIBLIOGRAPHY

Knowles, DM (ed): Neoplastic Hematopathology, Williams & Wilkins, Baltimore, 1992.

Richard, Lee G, Bithell, TC, Foerster, J, et al (eds): Wintrobe's Clinical Hematology, ed 9. Vols I and II. Lea & Febiger, Philadelphia, 1993.

Hoffman, R, Benz, EJ, Shattil, SJ, et al (eds): Hematology, Basic Principles and Practice, ed 2. Churchill Livingstone, New York, 1995.

QUESTIONS

1. The type of anemia most commonly encountered in MDS is:
   a. Microcytic, hypochromic
   b. Normocytic, hypochromic
   c. Macrocytic, normochromic
   d. Dimorphic

2. All of the following are helpful morphological abnormalities in the diagnosis of MDS except:
   a. Vacuolated eosinophils
   b. Pseudo Pelger-Huet and hypogranulation
   c. Ringed sideroblasts
   d. Micromegakaryocytes, monolobular megakaryocytes

3. Which of the following parameters significantly helps in differentiating RAEB-t from AML M2?
   a. The percentage of bone marrow promyelocytes
   b. Immunophenotypic studies
   c. Degree of lineage dysplasia in the bone marrow
   d. Cytogenetic findings

4. Which of these cell surface antigens is of prognostic significance in MDS?
   a. CD19
   b. CD HLA-DR
   c. CD34
   d. CD33

5. The MDS subgroup with the most favorable evolution is:
   a. RAEB
   b. CMML
   c. RA
   d. RARS

6. Long-term survival and curability can be achieved in MDS with the following therapeutic approach:
   a. Chemoradiotherapy
   b. Allogeneic bone marrow transplantation
   c. Autologous bone marrow transplantation
   d. Growth factors

7. Which of the following agents may lead to secondary MDS?
   a. Hydrocortisone
   b. Colony-stimulating factors
   c. Irradiated blood components
   d. Agents targeting topoisomerase II

8. All of the following are most likely to affect prognosis in MDS except:
   a. Leukopenia
   b. Increased bone marrow myeloblasts
   c. ALIP
   d. Complex karyotype

9. In female patients with RA and elevated platelet counts, which chromosome abnormality is most often found?
   a. (5q−)
   b. t(8;21)
   c. (7q−)
   d. t(15;17)

10. Thirty to forty percent of MDS patients progress to acute leukemic transformation, in which the most frequent blast phenotype encountered is:
    a. Hybrid (myelolymphoid)
    b. Erythroid
    c. Myelomonocytoid
    d. Lymphoid

ANSWERS

1. **c** (p 327)
2. **a** (pp 327–329)
3. **a, d** (pp 331–333)
4. **c** (p 333)
5. **d** (p 337) (Fig. 19–21)
6. **b** (p 340)
7. **d** (p 337)
8. **a** (p 337–338)
9. **a** (p 336)
10. **c** (p 337)

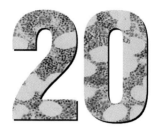

Chronic Leukemias

Laurel D. Holmer, MEd, MT(ASCP)SH

Objectives

At the end of this chapter, the learner should be able to:

1. List general features of chronic lymphocytic leukemia.
2. Name laboratory methods used to study lymphocytes in lymphoproliferative disorders.
3. List diagnostic criteria of chronic lymphocytic leukemia.
4. Describe treatment for chronic lymphocytic leukemia.
5. Explain differential diagnostic criteria that are used to characterize lymphocytic leukemias, lymphomas, and lymphoproliferative disorders.
6. List general features of chronic myelogenous leukemia.
7. Name laboratory features characteristic of chronic myelogenous leukemia.
8. Describe treatment for chronic myelogenous leukemia.
9. Explain differential diagnostic criteria that are used to characterize chronic myelogenous leukemia.
10. Evaluate case studies and pertinent laboratory data.

CHRONIC LYMPHOCYTIC LEUKEMIA

Chronic lymphocytic leukemia (CLL) is included in a general category of conditions known as the lymphoproliferative disorders (Table 20–1). CLL is the most common type of leukemia in older adults and is most frequently a neoplasm of B lymphocytes (B-CLL). A malignant proliferation of T lymphocytes (T-CLL) can occur, but this is less common. The hematologic ab-normalities of CLL are characterized by a peripheral blood and bone marrow lymphocytosis. Morphologically, the lymphocytes are small or slightly larger than normal lymphocytes and have a relatively mature, well-differentiated appearance with a hypercondensed, almost "soccer ball"-appearing nuclear chromatin pattern. Bare nuclei called smudge cells are common (Fig. 20–1). Morphological heterogeneity in CLL does exist and has been addressed by the French-American-British (FAB) group.[1]

TABLE 20-1	**The Lymphoproliferative**
Disorders	

Acute lymphoblastic leukemia (ALL)
Chronic lymphocytic leukemia (CLL)
Prolymphocytic leukemia
Non-Hodgkin's lymphomas
Hairy cell leukemia
Sézary syndrome
T-gamma lymphocytosis (large granular lymphocytosis [LGL])
Reactive lymphocytosis

The consequences of the accumulating lymphocyte mass in CLL include neutropenia, anemia, and thrombocytopenia. The normal bone marrow elements literally get crowded out by the excessive lymphoid production and the marrow space is packed with malignant lymphocytes. Lymphadenopathy, splenomegaly, or both may be present. In addition to the consequences of organ infiltration by malignant lymphocytes, altered humoral immunity in patients with CLL results from suppression of all classes of immunoglobulin, leading to hypogammaglobulinemia and a subsequent increase in susceptibility to infections. Another important complication of altered immunity that can develop in the CLL patient is autoimmune disease. The production of autoantibodies may lead to idiopathic thrombocytopenic purpura (Chap. 27) or autoimmune hemolytic anemia (Chap. 14) to further compromise the patient's hematologic status.

Patients with CLL are typically over 50 years of age at the time of diagnosis and frequently have a prolonged survival. Although some patients may die within a few years of diagnosis, more often they succumb to an unrelated disorder associated with elderly people. Generally, 50% of CLL patients will be alive 5

years after diagnosis, and 30% of patients can expect a survival of 10 years or more.

Etiology and Pathophysiology

To date, no specific etiologic agent or cause of CLL has been found. A possible viral cause continues to be investigated since the isolation of a type C retrovirus from the leukemic cells of patients with T-cell malignancies.[2–4] The finding of retroviral-like particles and reverse transcriptase activity in cultured cells of patients with B-derived CLL[5] supports a viral etiology of CLL, but additional studies are needed. Infection with human T-cell lymphotrophic virus type I (HTLV-1) has preceded the development of CLL in some patients.[6]

The pathophysiology of CLL is directly related to the accumulation of "long-lived," immunologically dysfunctional lymphocytes in the peripheral blood and bone marrow. Additional infiltration of the lymph nodes and spleen by the malignant lymphocytes occurs in 50% of patients, and cutaneous invasion occurs in 5% of patients.[7] As the bone marrow becomes more extensively infiltrated by the leukemic clone, marrow replacement results in anemia, thrombocytopenia, and neutropenia. Organ infiltration can lead to massive adenopathy with splenomegaly, hypersplenism, and subsequent peripheral cytopenias. An increased tendency for hemorrhage further contributes to anemia and compromises hemostasis.

Patients with CLL have significantly impaired immunologic activity. Hypogammaglobulinemia is found in approximately 50% of patients with CLL. The deficiency in immunoglobulin leads to infections with a variety of agents. Bacterial infections, especially of the respiratory tract, urinary tract, and skin, as well as viral infections such as herpes zoster and herpes simplex, are common and dramatically contribute to patient morbidity and mortality (Fig. 20–2). Autoimmunity is a phenomenon frequently seen in CLL with 15% to 35% of patients developing autoimmune hemolytic anemia at some time during the course of the disease.[7] Antibodies produced against red blood cells and detected with the direct antiglobulin (Coombs') test may precede, simultaneously occur with, or follow the development of CLL. Red cell aplasia is a rare occurrence.[8] Autoantibodies to platelets and neutrophils may also develop and lead to immune thrombocytopenic purpura (ITP) and neutropenia. The production of autoantibodies coupled with marrow crowding and hypersplenism can lead to strikingly low peripheral platelet and neutrophil counts. Although the leukemic clonal B cells from CLL patients often are the source of pathogenic autoantibodies that may react with antigens present on red blood cells and/or platelets, it is the nonmalignant polyclonal bystander B cells that have been shown to produce autoantibodies that contribute even more significantly to autoimmune disease.[9] Interestingly, the relatives of patients with CLL have also been shown to have an increased risk of autoimmune diseases. Immunoparesis in some patients may include the production of paraproteins. Bence-Jones paraproteinemia has been reported in up to 20% of patients with CLL,[10] and heavy-chain paraproteins, either IgM or IgG, can be detected. Figure 20–3 summarizes the pathophysiology of CLL.

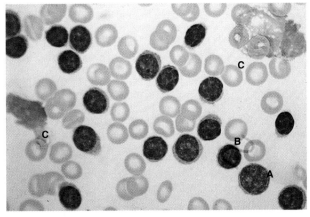

FIGURE 20-1 Photomicrograph of peripheral blood smear from a patient with chronic lymphocytic leukemia (CLL). Note the characteristic mature-appearing lymphocyte morphology with hypercondensed nuclear chromatin creating a "soccer ball" pattern. Two smudge cells are also seen. Note the lack of platelets in this thrombocytopenic patient. *A* denotes lymphoblasts; *B*, lymphocytes; and *C*, smudge cells.

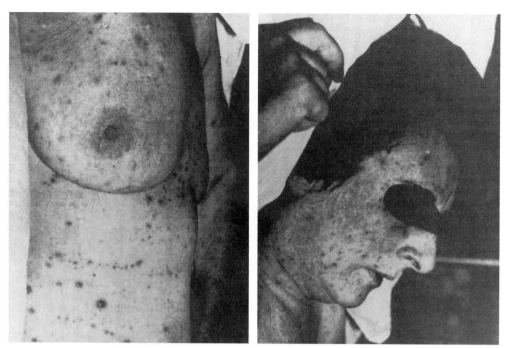

FIGURE 20–2 Severe generalized herpes zoster with a varicelliform rash in a patient with chronic lymphocytic leukemia. (From Henderson, ES: Diagnosis of leukemia. In Gunz, FW and Henderson, ES (eds): Leukemia, ed 4. Grune and Stratton, New York, 1983, p. 409, with permission.)

Immunologic Features and Methods for Studying Lymphocytes

In normal adult peripheral blood, 30% of the circulating lymphocytes have surface immunoglobulin (sIg) and are B cells, whereas 70% have no sIg and are T cells or null cells. Based on morphological features alone, it is not possible to distinguish B cells from T cells. When a lymphoproliferative process exists, it is important to be able to characterize the nature of the lymphocytes involved. A number of methods are available to study lymphocytes in lymphoproliferative disorders such as CLL and are listed in Table 20–2.

For the most part, the diagnosis of CLL can be done morphologically. A fairly straightforward immunologic characterization of the neoplasm as either B cell or T cell using the large number of monoclonal antibodies available for detecting differentiation antigens (cluster differentiation [CD] antigens) as shown in Table 20–3 confirms the diagnosis. Monoclonal antibodies are homogeneous populations of antibody molecules generally produced by somatic cell hybrids (hybridomas) between activated normal B cells and a plasmacytoma cell line. A list of presently accepted CD designations and some basic information concerning the molecules defined by these antibodies has been established by the Sixth International Workshop and Conference on Human Leukocyte Differentiation Antigens.[11] Use of monoclonal antibody technology is possible because as lymphocytes mature from pluripotent stem cells and migrate to lymphoid tissue, they acquire a variety of developmental markers that are helpful in identifying lymphocyte subpopulations.

Immunophenotypic marker expression and gene rearrangement during normal B-cell ontogeny is shown in Figure 20–4. The malignant B lymphocytes of CLL do not progress normally to the final stages of B-cell development, namely the plasma cells, but rather appear to be developmentally arrested at an earlier B-lymphocyte stage of differentiation. Studies have shown, however, that under certain in vitro conditions such as stimulation with phorbol ester, typical CLL cells can undergo transformation to more mature levels of B cell development.[12,13] The characteristic immunophenotype for B-CLL is expression of faint or low-density sIg with kappa or lambda light-chain B-cell-associated antigens (CD19, CD20, 79a), CD5, CD23, CD43, and faint CD11c. Of particular interest is the unique expression of CD5 in B-CLL. CD5 expression is normally seen on T lymphocytes and on most B cells of early ontogeny such as cord blood and fetal liver; however, normally only 20% of B cells in adult human peripheral blood express CD5. Although CD5− B-CLL does exist,[14] the propensity for CD5+ B-CLL has led to much speculation regarding this marker's functional role and its mechanisms of cell regulation. Study is ongoing to determine if differences in antigen expression and gene rearrangements are associated with variation in clinical course.[15–17]

As mentioned earlier, T-CLL is rare but can be distinguished from B-CLL on the basis of antigen differentiation. Immunophenotypic marker expression and

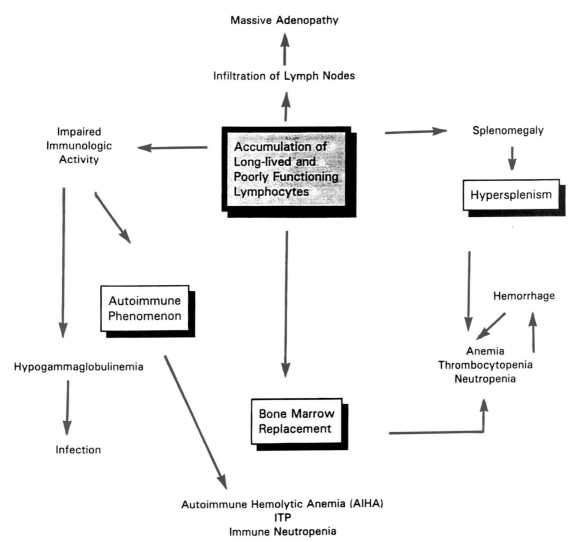

FIGURE 20-3 The pathophysiology of chronic lymphocytic leukemia. The three major processes that typically interact are marrow replacement by long-lived lymphocytes, hypersplenism, and autoimmunity. ITP = immune thrombocytopenic purpura.

gene rearrangement during normal T-cell ontogeny are shown in Figure 20–5.

The demonstration of sIg in B-CLL was mentioned earlier and is in fact the classical marker for B cells. The detection of a predominance of *either* kappa or lambda light chains by the B cells indicates monoclonality.[18] When conventional immunophenotypic techniques fail to reveal the nature of the lymphoid neoplasm, molecular probe technology using DNA probes can often contribute to the diagnosis and classification of malignancy by detecting gene rearrangements that occur in lymphocytes. On a molecular level, immunoglobulin (Ig) heavy and light chains are rearranged. The rearrangement of heavy-chain Ig genes occurs first and is followed by rearrangement of light-chain genes. The order of this rearrangement proceeds from mu to kappa to lambda, and is the earliest detectable commitment to B-cell development.[19] Monoclonality,

rather than polyclonality (the presence of a mixture of kappa- *and* lambda-bearing B lymphocytes) is a feature of many malignancies, including CLL; however, it is not, per se, indicative of malignancy. Analogous to Ig gene rearrangements in B cells is the ability of molecular probes to detect rearrangement patterns of the genes coding for the T-cell receptor (TCR), the antigen-specific surface molecule characteristic of T cells.[20] With the use of Ig and TCR gene probes to detect gene rearrangements at the molecular level, the unusual case of CLL that cannot be diagnosed and classified by morphology and cell markers can now be characterized. It must be stressed that it is extremely important that the final diagnosis of any lymphoproliferative disorder be made as a result of composite information from clinical data plus morphologic, histologic, and immunologic analysis.

Although CLL is generally characterized by an ele-

TABLE 20–2 Methods Used to Study Lymphocytes in Lymphoproliferative Disorders

Method	Marker Detected or Feature Demonstrated
Cytochemistry	Absence of peroxidase, Sudan black B, and esterase positivity in lymphoblasts
	Tartrate-resistant isozyme 5 of acid phosphatase (TRAP) in hairy cells
	Localized alpha-naphthol acetate esterase (ANAE) positivity in Golgi area of T cells, i.e. T-ALL, Sézary cell, T-CLL
Cytogenetics	Consistent chromosomal abnormalities such as t(8;14): B-cell ALL, Burkitt's lymphoma; t(14;18): follicular lymphoma; trisomy 12: CLL, WDLL; t(11;14): WDLL; t(4;11): ALL-L_2
Electron microscopy	Nuclear and cytoplasmic ultrastructure such as nuclear whorls in Sézary cells and ribosomal lamellar cytoplasmic aggregates in hairy cells
Immunofluorescence	Surface and cytoplasmic immunoglobulin on B cells
	TdT on pre-B cells and immature T cells
Immunoperoxidase	Various differentiation antigens on B
Flow Cytometry	Cells and/or T cells using monoclonal antibodies (see Table 20–3)
Molecular Probes	Rearrangements of the B-cell immunoglobulin (Ig) and T-cell receptor (TCR) genes
Rosette Formation	Sheep erythrocyte receptor on T cells

vated white blood cell count in which there are abundant lymphocytes to analyze, if the number of neoplastic cells is low, a technique for amplifying a specific segment of DNA called the *polymerase chain reaction* (PCR) can be applied to improve sensitivity. PCR methodology involves denaturation, primer annealing, and polymerization to yield millions of copies of the original scarce sequence of DNA.[21] This technique may be valuable for detecting minimal residual disease in patients who have previously been treated for CLL (or other leukemias or lymphomas) but currently lack histopathologic evidence of relapse.[22,23] The purpose of using PCR is to identify as early as possible those patients who will subsequently relapse but who currently have only

TABLE 20–3 Cluster Differentiation (CD) Markers and Proliferation

Markers (CD Designation)	Monoclonal Antibodies	Clinical Application
B Cells		
CD5	T1, T101, Leu1	B-CLL, some NHL, T lymphomas
CD9	BA-2 (p24)	Pre-B
CD10	J5, BA-3 (CALLA)	Lymph progenitor, CALL, some NHL
CD19	B4, Leu12	CALL, B-CLL, B-PLL, HCL
CD20	B1, Leu16	CALL, B-CLL, B-PLL, HCL
CD24	BA-1	Most B cells
CD22	B3, Leu14	Late B cells, hairy cells
CD25	TAC (IL-2 receptor)	HCL
T Cells		
CD1	T6	Some T-CLL, T-PLL, T-ALL
CD2	T11, Leu5, 9.6 (E rosette)	T-CLL, T-PLL, Sézary cells, LGL, ATLL
CD3	T3, Leu4	T-CLL, T-PLL, Sézary cells, IM
CD4	T4, Leu3	T-PLL, Sézary cells, IM, ATLL
CD5	T1, Leu1, 10.2	T-CLL, T-PLL, Sézary cells, ATLL
CD7	3A1, Leu9	T-PLL
CD8	T8, Leu2	T-CLL, some LGL, IM
CD25	Tac (IL-2 receptor)	ATLL
CD57	Leu7 (HNK1)	LGL

Abbreviations: B-CLL = B-lineage chronic lymphocytic leukemia; NHL = Non-Hodgkin's lymphoma; CALL = Common acute lymphocytic leukemia; B-PLL = B-lineage prolymphocytic leukemia; HCL = Hairy-cell leukemia; T-ALL = T-lineage acute lymphoblastic leukemia; LGL = Large granular lymphocytosis (T-gamma lymphocytosis); ATLL = Adult T-cell leukemia/lymphoma; IM = Infectious mononucleosis; HNK = Human natural killer.

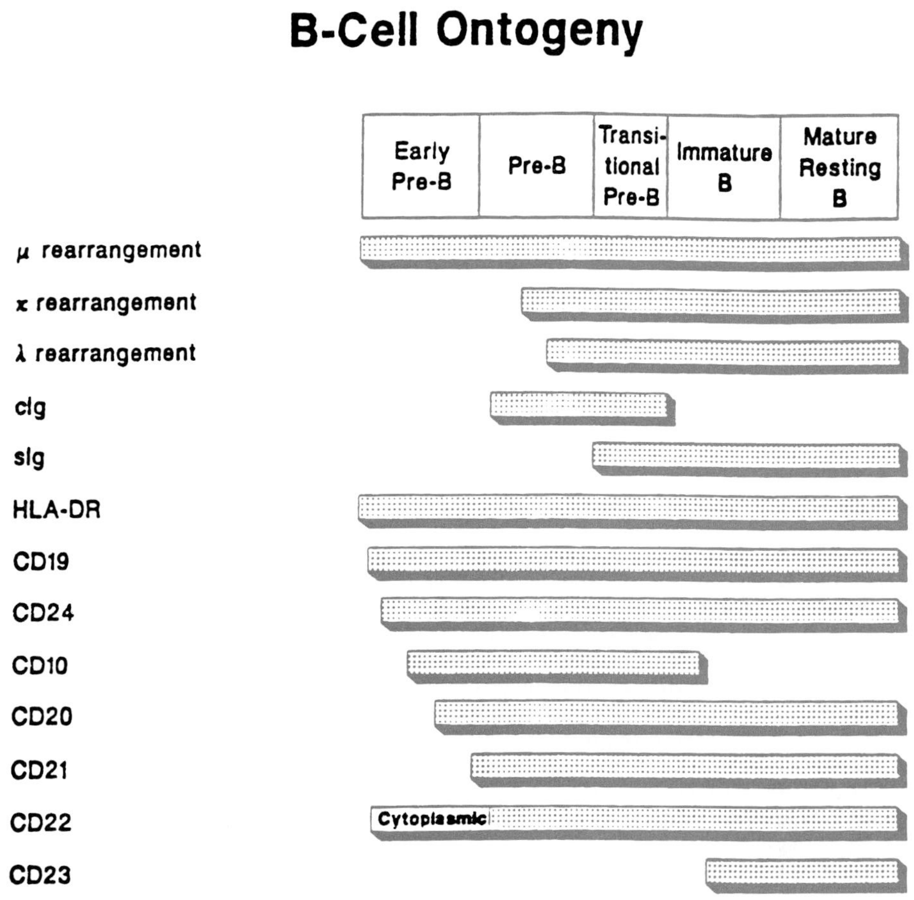

B-Cell Ontogeny

	Early Pre-B	Pre-B	Transitional Pre-B	Immature B	Mature Resting B
μ rearrangement					
ϰ rearrangement					
λ rearrangement					
cIg					
sIg					
HLA-DR					
CD19					
CD24					
CD10					
CD20					
CD21					
CD22	Cytoplasmic				
CD23					

FIGURE 20-4 Hypothetical schematic of marker expression and gene rearrangement during normal B-cell ontogeny. cIg = cytoplasmic immunoglobulin; sIg = surface immunoglobulin. (From Pui, CH et al: Clinical and biologic relevance of immunologic marker studies in childhood acute lymphoblastic leukemia. Blood 82:2, 1993, p. 344, with permission.)

T-Cell Ontogeny

	Prothymic Cell	Early Thymocyte	Intermediate Thymocyte	Mature Thymocyte	Circulating T-Cell
TCR δ rearrangement	?				
TCR γ rearrangement	?				
TCR β rearrangement	?				
TCR α rearrangement					
CD7					
CD5					
CD2					
CD1					
CD4					
CD8					
CD3	Cytoplasmic				
TCR (αβ or γδ)	Cytoplasmic				

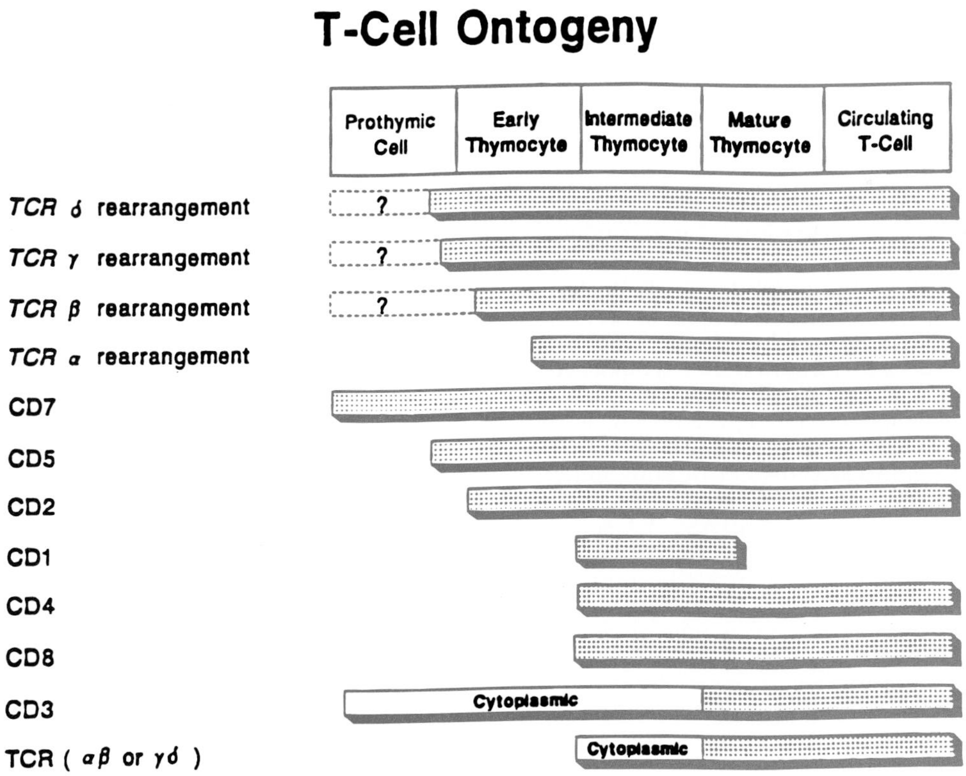

FIGURE 20-5 Hypothetical schematic of marker expression and gene rearrangement during T-cell ontogeny. TCR = T cell receptor. (From Pui, CH et al: Clinical and biologic relevance of immunologic marker studies in childhood acute lymphoblastic leukemia. Blood 82:2, 1993, p. 344, with permission.)

1% to 5% malignant cells present or have gene rearrangements present in malignant clones that require amplification in order to be detected.

Clinical Features

CLL occurs mainly in older adults, with 90% of all cases occurring in persons over age 50. CLL in patients under 40 years of age is rare; however, CLL in young adults has been described.[24] Like most other leukemias and myeloproliferative disorders, men are more likely to be affected than women, showing a 2:1 incidence. In contrast to the situation in acute leukemia, the signs and symptoms of CLL develop gradually, and the onset of the disease is difficult to pinpoint. In fact, it is not unusual for the disease to be accidentally discovered during the course of a routine visit to a physician. The duration of a relatively asymptomatic phase of CLL is extremely variable. Unexplained absolute and persistent lymphocytosis; cervical, supraclavicular, and/or axillary lymphadenopathy; and splenomegaly are the earliest signs of CLL. The clinical course is indolent, but as the disease progresses, chronic fatigue, recurrent or persistent infections, and easy bruising are the consequences of anemia, neutropenia, B-cell immunologic dysfunction, and thrombocytopenia. Hepatomegaly may accompany splenomegaly. Dermatologic manifestations such as nodular and diffuse skin infiltrations, erythroderma, exfoliative dermatitis, and secondary skin infections may occur. Leukemic lymphocytes may invade unusual locations such as the scalp, orbits, subconjunctivae, gums, pharynx, pleura and lung parenchyma, gastrointestinal tract, prostate, and gonads.[25] CLL has also been reported to occur simultaneously with acute myeloblastic leukemia (AML).[26] CLL is not usually considered curable with available therapy.

Laboratory Features

The requirements for the diagnosis of CLL have undergone revision since earlier criteria were established by Rai and colleagues[27] in 1975 and Binet and associates in 1981.[28,29] The International Workshop on Chronic Lymphocytic Leukemia recommends a minimum peripheral blood B-cell lymphocytosis of 5000/μL (5×10^9 cells/L) along with a 30% lymphocytosis of the bone marrow consisting of morphologically mature-appearing lymphocytes.[30] This guideline is similar to an earlier set of criteria established by the National Cancer Institute–sponsored working group to assist clinicians in clarifying a diagnosis when borderline disease features were encountered.[31] A new classification and terminology for the lymphocytic neoplasms, including CLL, have recently been proposed by the International Lymphoma Study Group.[32] Anemia, when it occurs, is usually normochromic, normocytic, with a normal or low reticulocyte count. Autoimmune hemolytic anemia may precede, accompany, or follow the development of CLL and be characterized by a secondary reticulocytosis, positive direct antiglobulin test, and an elevated indirect serum bilirubin level. A decreased platelet count is not uncommon in CLL and is related to bone marrow replacement by leukemic cells, hypersplenism, and/or platelet antibodies.

The lymphocytes of CLL may be morphologically indistinguishable from normal mature lymphocytes when examined with Wright's stain. Alternatively, the leukemic lymphocytes may have exaggerated nuclear chromatin clumping with numerous dark-staining chromatin aggregates separated by light-staining areas of parachromatin. The staining pattern that results from the contrast between the nuclear chromatin and parachromatin resembles the surface pattern of a soccer ball and may be a helpful image to recall in distinguishing the lymphocytes of CLL from those of other lymphoproliferative disorders. The morphology of peripheral blood lymphocytes in CLL is duplicated in the bone marrow aspiration and biopsy specimen (Fig. 20–6). The extent of marrow infiltration varies from patchy accumulations of lymphocytes to diffuse sheets that involve the entire marrow space.

Although the morphological characteristics of the lymphocytes involved in most cases of CLL are quite distinctive, the membrane phenotype of the proliferating neoplastic cells needs to be determined for a definitive diagnosis. Immunologic features and methods used to characterize lymphocytes as B cells or T cells were discussed earlier in the section entitled "Immunologic Features and Methods for Studying Lymphocytes."

Immune dysfunction within the proliferating B cells is indicated by the presence of hypogammaglobulinemia or hypergammaglobulinemia and monoclonal gammopathy. The frequent expression of autoantibodies in CLL contributes to a variety of autoimmune phenomenon, including those leading to anemia and thrombocytopenia.

Chromosomal Abnormalities

A number of chromosomal abnormalities have been associated with distinct forms of malignant lymphocytes. Genetic abnormalities, including the most common chromosomal abnormalities and gene rearrangements, are listed in Table 20–4.[33–44] The presence of additional chromosomes and multiple chromosomal abnormalities in B-CLL have been implicated as indicators of a poor prognosis.[38] Additionally, oncogenes,

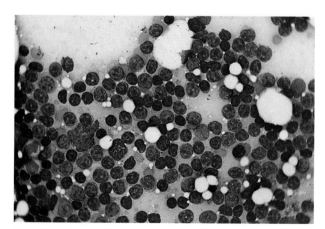

FIGURE 20–6 Photomicrograph of bone marrow aspirate smear from a patient with CLL. Note monotonous appearance of mature-appearing lymphocytes with condensed nuclear chromatin.

TABLE 20–4 Genetic Abnormalities

Disorders	Chromosomal Abnormalities
CLL	14q⁺, 6,11,12,13*
B-CLL	Trisomy 12†
B lymphoids neoplasms	14q32 translocations
Burkitt's lymphoma	t(8;14)(q24;q32)
T-CLL	Inv(14)(q11;32) an extra 8q, 7*

Disorder	Oncogene Abnormalities
CLL	Rearrangement of proto-oncogenes bcℓ-1 and bcℓ-2
T-CLL	Rearrangement patterns in the alpha and/or beta TCR genes

†May occur alone or with other abnormalities
*Structural abnormalities
Abbreviations:
t = Translocation; inv = Inversion; p = Short arm of a chromosome;
q = Long arm of the chromosome; numbers listed immediately after the "q" designations represent the regions and bands along the q arm of the chromosome.

the cellular genes that when genetically altered have the potential to cause or contribute to malignant expression, have been detected in certain chromosomal segments.[39]

Clinical Course, Prognostic Factors, and Staging

The overall median survival for CLL is currently 4 to 5 years. Half of patients are alive 5 years after diagnosis, and 30% of patients have a 10-year survival. CLL can be an indolent disease with an asymptomatic presentation and may not require any treatment until progressive lymphocytosis of the peripheral blood and marrow, lymphadenopathy, splenomegaly, anemia, neutropenia, thrombocytopenia, autoimmune phenomena, and infection develop. This may be as late as 10 to 15 years from initial diagnosis. In contrast to those with an indolent course, approximately 20% of patients with CLL have a very aggressive clinical course that progresses rapidly from initial diagnosis and results in death within 1 to 2 years. The wide variation seen among patients is not fully understood, but clinical and physical data have been used to try to predict the CLL patient's prognosis and identify various stages and risk groups.

The Rai system,[27] the Binet system,[28] and the International Workshop on CLL system[29] are the three major staging systems developed for CLL; however, only the Rai system is widely used in the United States. The Rai and Binet staging systems, along with median survival for each system by stage, are shown in Table 20–5. The Binet and Rai systems are combined according to the International Workshop on CLL recommendations in the following manner: A(O), A(I), A(II); B(I), B(II); C(III), C(IV). Staging systems for CLL cannot predict consistently whether a patient's clinical course is more likely to be indolent or progressive. The most reliable predicting factors for indolent CLL are blood lymphocyte doubling time (LDT) greater than 12 months[45] and a nondiffuse pattern of bone marrow lymphocyte infiltration,[46,47] along with a Rai stage of O, I, or II. A short LDT (less than 12 months), a diffuse lymphocyte infiltration of the bone marrow, a Rai staging of III or IV, and the presence of chromosomal abnormalities[48] are associated with a more progressive clinical course and shorter survival duration.

Three types of transformation in B-CLL have been described: prolymphocytoid transformation, which is relatively low grade and slowly progressive; Richter's syndrome (diffuse large-cell lymphoma); and immunoblastic transformation, which is rapidly progressive and accounts for about 5% of all deaths in CLL.[49]

TABLE 20–5 Staging Systems for Chronic Lymphocytic Leukemia

Stage		Clinical Features	Median Survival (years)
Original Rai System	**Modified Rai System**		
0	Low	Lymphocytosis in PB and BM ($\geq 5 \times 10^9$ lymphs/L in PB, $\geq$ 30% lymphs in BM)	>12.5
I	Intermediate	Lymphocytosis + enlarged lymph nodes	8.5
II	Intermediate	Lymphocytosis, lymphadenopathy, adenopathy, splenomegaly and ± enlarged spleen	6
III	High	Lymphocytosis + anemia (hgb < 11 g/dL)	1.5
IV	High	Lymphocytosis + thrombocytopenia (platelets $< 100 \times 10^9$/L)	1.5
Binet System			
A		2 or less node-bearing regions* + no anemia or thrombocytopenia (Hgb $\geq$ 10 g/dL, platelets $> 100 \times 10^9$/L)	>10
B		3 or more node-bearing regions + no anemia or thrombocytopenia	5
C		Anemia and/or thrombocytopenia independent of regions involved	2

Abbreviations: PB = Peripheral blood; BM = Bone marrow.
* = Cervical, axillary, inguinal, palpable spleen and liver

Transformation to acute leukemia is unusual in CLL, unlike the blast cell transformation that is responsible for almost all deaths in chronic myeloid leukemia. Most patients with CLL die without a major or recognizable morphological change of the leukemic cell population and usually succumb to infection or a cause totally unrelated to their CLL, such as cardiovascular disease. When there is a proliferation of a new population of lymphoid cells, namely larger cells with immature-appearing morphological features, finer nuclear chromatin pattern and a prominent nucleolus, the onset of the terminal transformation of CLL is suggested. This morphological transformation is often accompanied by the appearance of complex chromosomal changes not present earlier or in addition to the commonly present trisomy 12. The proliferation of a more malignant clone of cells is accompanied by an increasing resistance to therapy and an exceptionally poor prognosis. Because of the leukemogenic potential of agents used to treat CLL, it is likely that the exposure to therapeutic doses of radiation and chemotherapy plays a role in its transformation; however, the possibility of the transformation representing an end phase of the natural history of CLL cannot be ruled out. A variety of techniques are available to help determine whether the transformation represents a clonal evolution of the original CLL or an independent disease; these include cytogenetic analysis, immunoglobulin gene rearrangement by Southern blot analysis, and anti-idiotypic antibodies.[50] Recently molecular studies have shown that the development of Richter's syndrome in CLL may represent either the identical clone of cells present in the preceding CLL or may represent a different malignant clone.[51] Additionally, p53, a tumor-suppressor gene frequently mutated in a variety of human cancers, has been discovered in 15% of CLL patients and 40% of patients with Richter's syndrome.[52-54] The close association of p53 with transformation of CLL into a very aggressive lymphoma may also be a prognostic indicator for resistance to chemotherapy by interfering with normal programmed cell death and apopotic pathways in tumor cells.[55,56]

Treatment

Some patients diagnosed with CLL do not require immediate treatment; however, when the signs and symptoms of progressive disease appear, it is time to begin therapeutic intervention. Major physical and clinical signs and symptoms identify advancing disease and are indications for treatment. These include progressive marrow failure with resulting anemia; thrombocytopenia and neutropenia; progressive lymphocytosis; progressive lymphadenopathy; enlarging spleen; autoimmunity (autoimmune hemolytic anemia or idiopathic thrombocytopenic purpura); increased susceptibility to infection by bacteria, fungi, or viruses; and persistent constitutional symptoms such as night sweats, fever, and weight loss. There is currently no curative therapy for CLL; therefore, the goal of treatment is to reduce signs and symptoms of disease with minimal discomfort or risk to the patient.

Conventional treatment for CLL is chemotherapy. Combinations of chemotherapeutic agents are used for patients refractory to conventional therapy or those with advanced disease.[57-62] Table 20-6 summarizes the initial management of patients with CLL according to Rai staging groups.

Radiation therapy is an alternative or adjunctive therapeutic approach in treating CLL.[63-65] Leukemic lymphocytic masses in enlarged lymph nodes and in the spleen may respond to focused, local irradiation to relieve discomfort or eliminate obstruction. Like chemotherapy, irradiation also has its detrimental effects, especially in terms of causing life-threatening neutropenia.

In addition to chemotherapeutic intervention, the use of high-dose intravenous gamma globulin therapy prevents major bacterial infections,[66,67] and the immunosuppressant cyclosporin, a fungal metabolite, aids in the prevention or treatment of red cell aplasia, both of which can be management problems in the CLL patient. Experimental therapies are also being studied. They include not only new drugs but the use of various monoclonal antibodies and biological mediators.[68-82]

Bone marrow transplantation (autologous and allogeneic) is being explored as a possible curative therapy for patients with aggressive CLL, especially in patients under 50 years of age.[83]

Differential Diagnosis

As previously outlined in Table 20-1, CLL is a lymphoproliferative disorder that must be differentiated from other malignant or reactive lymphoid proliferations, namely acute lymphoblastic leukemia (ALL);

TABLE 20-6 **Management Recommendations for CLL**	
RAI System Risk Group	**Management Recommendation**
Low (Stage O)	Observation each 1-3 months
Intermediate (Stage I and II)	Chlorambucil, cytoxan, or radiation if symptomatic. Observation only if asymptomatic
High (Stage III and IV)	Combination chemotherapy: prednisone with chlorambucil or cyclophosphamide or Intensive regimens: CHOP (cyclophosphamide, hydroxydaunomycin, oncovin, prednisone), M-2 protocol (vincinstine, carmustine/BCNU, cyclophosphamide, melphalan, prednisone)

				Disorder				
Identifying Characteristic	ALL	CLL	PL	PDLL	HCL	Sézary Syndrome	T-Gamma Lymphocytosis	Infectious Mononucleosis
Predominating or significant cell type	Lymphoblast	"Mature" lymphocyte	Prolymphocyte	"Abnormal" lymphocyte	Hairy cell	Sézary cell	Large granular lymphocyte	Atypical lymphocyte
Nuclear chromatin pattern	Fine	Condensed; "soccerball"	Moderately condensed	Condensed	Fine to moderately condensed	Dark-staining	Condensed	Varies but generally less condensed than normal lymphocyte
Nuclear shape	Varies; round/oval	Regular	Regular	Irregular with clefts, notches, folds	Regular to slightly irregular; may have some folding	Irregular; many folds	Regular	
Nucleoli	Prominent	Not prominent	Prominent	Not prominent	Not prominent	Not prominent	Not prominent	May be prominent
Cytoplasm	Scanty	Scanty	Scanty to moderate	Scanty	Moderate with hairlike projections	Scanty	Moderately abundant with prominent vacuoles and/or azurophilic granules	Abundant; may have azurophilic granules and/or vacuoles
Cell size	Varies; generally homogeneous population with some variation in size and age	Varies; homogeneous population	Varies; heterogeneous population	Varies	Varies	Varies	Large	Large
Immunologic marker profile	Common ALL (early B) (70%) HLA-DR TdT CD19 CD10 (CALLA) CD20 Early T-cell ALL (15-20% of ALL is T-cell type)	B-cell CLL (98%) Weak sIg (IgM, IgD) HLA-DR CD5 CD19/20/24 T-cell CLL (2%) CD2 (E rosette) CD3 CD8	B-cell PL (80%) Strong sIg HLA-DR CD19/20/24 CD22 ±CD10 T-cell PLL (20%) CD2 (E rosette) CD3, CD4, CD5 CD7, ±CD8	B-cell Strong sIg HLA-DR CD19/20/24 ±CD10 (CALLA)	B-cell Subset Strong sIg HLA-DR CD19/20/24 CD22 CD25 (IL-2 Receptor, Tac)	T-cell Lymphoma E rosette CD2, CD3, CD4 CD5	T-cell CLL (LGL) Fc gamma receptor CD2 (E rosette) CD3 CD8 CD57 (HNK-1)	Reactive T Cells CD3 CD8 or CD4

Abbreviations: ALL = Acute lymphoblastic leukemia; CLL = Chronic lymphocytic leukemia; PL = Prolymphocytic leukemia; PDLL = poorly differentiated lymphocytic lymphoma; HCL = Hairy-cell leukemia; HNK = Human natural killer cell.

prolymphocytic leukemia (PL); non-Hodgkin's lymphomas, especially well-differentiated lymphocytic lymphoma (WDLL) and poorly differentiated lymphocytic lymphoma (PDLL); hairy cell leukemia (HCL), Sézary syndrome, T-gamma lymphocytosis, and reactive lymphocytosis associated with viral infection such as infectious mononucleosis or infection with cytomegalovirus. The morphological and immunologic characteristics of these lymphoproliferative disorders are

shown in Table 20–7. In addition to these disorders, other hematologic malignancies may be confused with CLL. These include adult T-cell leukemia/lymphoma (ATLL)[84,85] (Chap. 23) and Waldenstrom's macroglobulinemia[86] (Chap. 22).

The diagnosis of CLL is relatively straightforward and requires a sustained absolute lymphocytosis of mature-appearing lymphocytes in the absence of other causes. When the peripheral blood lymphocyte count

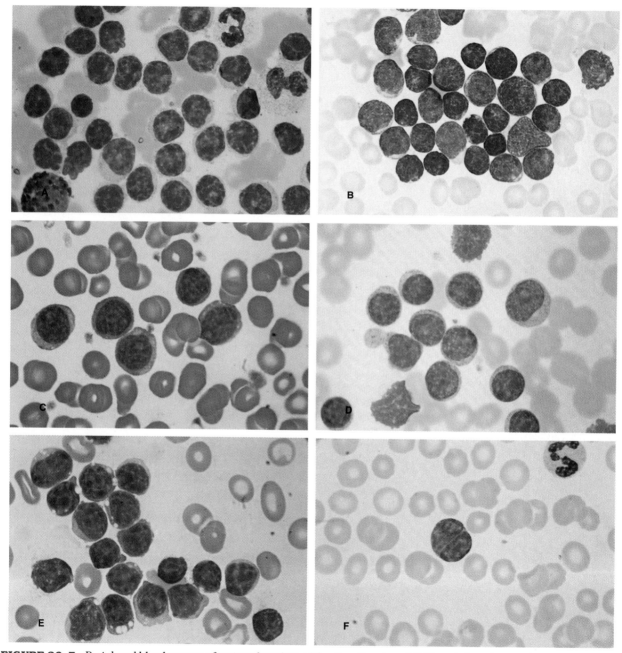

FIGURE 20–7 Peripheral blood smears of various lymphoproliferative disorders. (*A*) Chronic lymphocytic leukemia (CLL). (*B*) Acute lymphoblastic leukemia (ALL). (*C*) Prolymphocytic leukemia (PL). (*D*) CLL with occasional prolymphocyte. (*E*) Well-differentiated lymphocytic lymphoma (WDLL) in leukemic phase. (*F*) Poorly differentiated lymphocytic lymphoma (PDLL) in leukemic phase.

is $\geq 10 \times 10^9$/L (which is typically the case), the finding of either a lymphocyte infiltration of the bone marrow of >30% lymphocytes of all nucleated cells or a B-cell phenotype of the circulating lymphocytes is consistent with a diagnosis of CLL. When lymphocyte counts are between 5 and 10×10^9/L, both bone marrow infiltration of >30% lymphocytes and B-cell phenotype are necessary for the diagnosis of CLL.

The distinction between CLL and ALL is generally not a problem and is easily made in most instances based on morphological differences of the proliferating cell population (Fig. 20–7A–L). The smoother nuclear chromatin pattern of the lymphoblast in ALL as compared to the heavy condensation of nuclear chromatin in the CLL lymphocyte is readily appreciated when examining an appropriate monolayer area or feather edge of a well-stained blood smear. The age of the patient is also helpful when considering a diagnosis of lymphocytic leukemia. CLL is typically seen in patients over 50 years of age and only rarely reported in childhood,[87] whereas ALL is the most common form of childhood leukemia. The dramatic prognostic and therapeutic

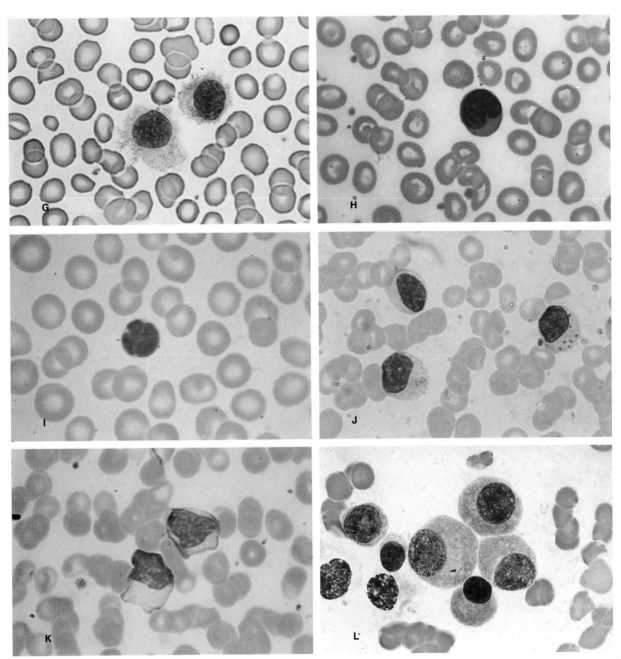

FIGURE 20–7 (Continued)   (G) Hairy cell leukemia (HCL). (From Hyun, BH et al: Practical Hematology. A Laboratory Guide with Accompanying Filmstrip. Saunders, Philadelphia, 1975, with permission.) (H) Sézary syndrome. (I) Adult T-cell leukemia/ lymphoma. (J) T-gamma lymphocytosis with large granular lymphocytes (LGL). (K) Infectious mononucleosis with atypical lymphocytes. (L) Plasma cell dyscrasia.

implications of misdiagnosing a chronic leukemia for an acute leukemia or vice versa cannot be overstated. All available laboratory diagnostic tools, that is, morphology, immunophenotyping, and molecular probes, should be used when necessary to make a final diagnosis.

Prolymphocytic leukemia (PL) is characterized by a predominance of circulating prolymphocytes (>55%, usually >70%). Prolymphocytes are larger, less-mature-appearing cells than the typical lymphocytes seen in CLL, with moderately condensed nuclear chromatin and a prominent vesicular nucleolus (Fig. 20–7C). The clinical and laboratory features that make PL a distinct lymphoproliferative disorder include extreme leukocytosis (often >100 × 10⁹/L) and prominent splenomegaly without substantial lymphadenopathy.[88–90] As in all disorders accompanied by leukocytosis, morphological detail of the predominating cell may not be appreciated unless appropriate areas of well-stained blood and bone marrow smears are examined. Prolymphocytes may be seen in patients with CLL, but are less than 10% of the circulating cells (Fig. 20–7D). When 11% to 55% prolymphocytes are present, a mixed-cell type of CLL, designated CLL/PL, is diagnosed.[91] This category includes patients with prolymphoid transformation.[92] Most cases of PL are B-cell in nature (B-PL) as demonstrated by strong sIg (as compared to weak sIg in CLL) and reactivity with the B-cell markers CD19, CD20, CD24, and CD22. T-PL does exist but is rare. If four positive criteria for B-CLL are set: weak sIg, > 30% mouse erythrocyte binding (M-rosettes), <50% CD5⁺ cells and <30% CD22⁺ cells, a combination of three or four of these markers is seen in 80% of typical CLL, in 65% of CLL/PL cases, and none in B-PL.[93] For cases of T-cell CLL or PL, two cytochemical techniques are helpful in distinguishing T cells from B cells, namely the alpha-naphthol acetate esterase (ANAE) stain and the acid phosphatase (AP) reaction.[94] The typical T-lymphocyte pattern with ANAE and AP is one large, localized dot of reaction product positivity (Fig. 20–8).

Well-differentiated lymphocytic lymphoma (WDLL) is a diffuse non-Hodgkin's lymphoma characterized by neoplastic transformation of B lymphocytes (Fig.

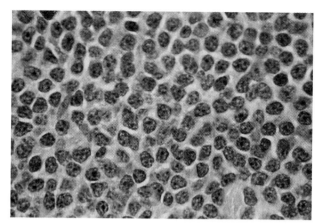

FIGURE 20–9 Well-differentiated lymphocytic lymphoma (WDLL), lymph node.

20–9). When WDLL progresses to a leukemic phase, the circulating cells cannot be morphologically differentiated from those of CLL (Fig. 20–7E);[95] however, the treatment and prognosis are often quite similar for both.

Poorly differentiated lymphocytic lymphoma (PDLL) is also a non-Hodgkin's lymphoma consisting of B lymphocytes that may be nodular (follicular) or diffuse in distribution[96] (Fig. 20–10) and can progress to a leukemic phase. The circulating cells of PDLL are morphologically characterized by nuclei that are irregular in shape and demonstrate irregular clefts, notches, or folds that may traverse the entire width of the nucleus (Fig. 20–7F). These "abnormal" lymphocytes typically have very scanty cytoplasm and were formally called *lymphosarcoma cells*,[97] a term that is no longer used as a result of more definitive means of classification. As compared to immunologic markers in B-CLL, PDLL shows strong sIg, low M-rosette positivity, CD22 positivity, CD5 negativity, and often CD10 positivity.

Another form of B-lymphocyte-derived chronic leukemia is hairy cell leukemia (HCL), so named because of the fine, hairlike, irregular cytoplasmic projections

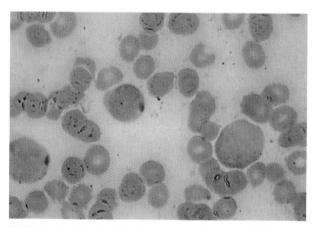

FIGURE 20–8 Naphthol acetate esterase (ANAE) stain showing localized "dotlike" positivity in two T lymphocytes.

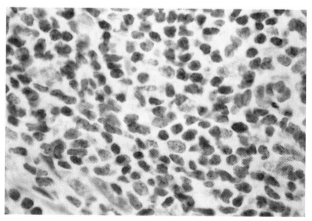

FIGURE 20–10 Poorly differentiated lymphocytic lymphoma (PDLL), lymph node.

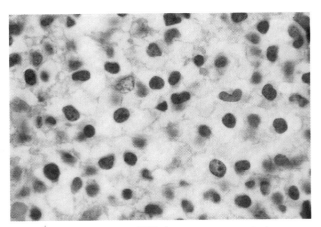

FIGURE 20-11   HCL, bone marrow aspirate.

that typify the disease (Fig. 20–7G). Pancytopenia is common in HCL, unlike the other lymphoid disorders discussed in this chapter, along with splenomegaly, marrow fibrosis, and responsiveness to interferon and pentostatin. Because a bone marrow aspirate is often difficult to obtain as a consequence of associated fibrosis (the so-called dry tap), a bone marrow biopsy section is essential for diagnosis and shows hairy cells surrounded by a clear zone that separates one cell from another, creating a fried-egg appearance (Fig. 20–11). The most characteristic cytochemical feature of hairy cells is a strong acid phosphatase reaction that is not inhibited by tartaric acid, known as the tartrate-resistant acid phosphatase stain (TRAP) (Fig. 20–12); this enzyme corresponds to the isoenzyme 5 demonstrable on polyacrylamide gel electrophoresis.[98] Immunologic markers that support the diagnosis of HCL are reactivity with B-cell-associated antigens (CD19, CD20, CD22, 79a), CD11c, and CD25 (the monoclonal antibody that recognizes the interleukin-2 receptor: Tac), FMC7, and CD103.[99] CD103 is the most useful marker for distinguishing HCL from other B-cell leukemias. A HCL variant with splenomegaly and a leukocytosis has been described,[100] as well as a splenic

form of non-Hodgkin's lymphoma that resembles HCL, called splenic lymphoma with villous lymphocytes (SLVL).[101] SLVL has a distinct immunologic profile, underscoring the importance of using immunophenotyping to differentiate SLVL from CLL, HCL, and other lymphoproliferative disorders.[102]

The leukemic phase of the most common cutaneous T-cell lymphoma, mycosis fungoides, is called Sézary syndrome, and is hallmarked by abnormal circulating lymphocytes, called Sézary cells.[103] A Sézary cell is typically the size of a small lymphocyte and has a dark-staining, hyperchromatic nuclear chromatin pattern with numerous folds and grooves referred to as *cerebriform* (see Fig. 20–7H). Nuclear folding is best appreciated at the ultrastructural level using electron microscopy. A less common large-cell variant of the Sézary cell is larger than a neutrophil and often larger than a monocyte, but has the same grooved nuclear chromatin pattern as the smaller Sézary cell. The bone marrow is infrequently involved. The diagnosis of Sézary syndrome is dependent on the primary diagnosis of the cutaneous T-cell lymphoma mycosis fungoides in which a skin biopsy shows the typical pattern of infiltration in the upper dermis with accumulation of lymphocytes, histiocytes, and Sézary cells within a vacuole, forming structures called *Pautrier microabcesses* (Fig. 20–13). The nuclear folding of a Sézary cell may at first glance suggest a monocytic cell line; however, a monocyte gives a diffuse pattern of cytoplasmic positivity with the nonspecific esterase stain ANAE mentioned earlier, as compared to a localized dotlike positivity pattern that identifies T cells. Immunologic marker studies of Sézary cells show a mature T-lymphocyte phenotype with reactivity for CD2, CD3, and CD4 (the monoclonal antibody that recognizes the helper-inducer subset of T lymphocytes). CD8, the monoclonal antibody that recognizes the cytotoxic-suppressor subset, does not show reactivity with Sézary cells. When conventional histomorphologic and immunophenotypic analysis is unable to distinguish neoplastic T cells from reactive T cells, newer molec-

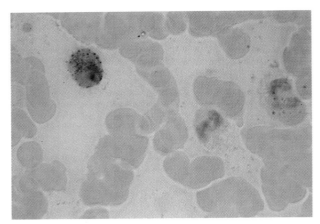

FIGURE 20-12 Tartrate-resistant acid phosphatase (TRAP) stain of peripheral blood showing positivity in hairy cell and no staining in neutrophils.

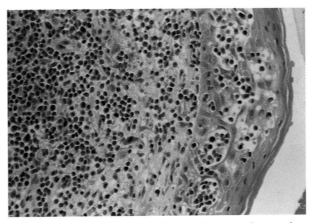

FIGURE 20-13 Infiltration of the epidermis and upper dermis by lymphocytes, many with convoluted (cerebriform) nuclei, histiocytes, and formation of Pautrier microabcesses, characteristic of the cutaneous T-cell lymphoma mycosis fungoides.

ular techniques may be used. The detection and amplification of markers of T-cell clonality at the T-cell receptor (TCR), β, and γ loci by PCR can significantly improve the sensitivity in detecting a clonal T-lymphoid population.[104]

Adult T-cell leukemia/lymphoma (ATLL), common in Japan and the Caribbean, is caused by of the human T-cell lymphotrophic virus type I (HTLV-1). Although there is a large heterogeneity in the clinical manifestations of the disease, characteristic clinical features include generalized lymphadenopathy, hypercalcemia, bone and skin lesions, and 10% to 80% abnormal lymphoid cells in the blood and bone marrow.[105,106] The most outstanding feature of these abnormal lymphocytes is the highly convoluted nuclear shape, which often is "cloverleafed" (see Fig. 20–7I). There is marked variation in size of the cells ranging from that of a small lymphocyte to a large monocyte. Nucleoli are typically inconspicuous, but when present may be prominent and cause confusion with prolymphocytes. The clinical course of ATLL can be acute, with a high white count and survival less than 1 year; chronic, with a lower white count and survival of more than 1 year, or "smoldering," in which the white count is normal with low numbers of abnormal T lymphocytes. Like T-PL and Sézary syndrome, ATLL cells show reactivity with T-cell-associated antigens (CD2, CD3, and CD5), most are CD4+, CD25+, but usually lack CD7. Rare CD8+ cases have been reported; 30% to 50% of patients have mutation in the tumor-suppressor gene p53.[107]

Chronic T-gamma lymphoproliferative disease, also called large granular lymphocytes (LGL), has the morphological distinction of persistent circulating lymphocytes that have abundant pale blue cytoplasm with azurophilic granules (see Fig. 20–7J). These granular lymphocytes usually constitute 50% to 95% of the circulating white cells. LGL was first described in patients with CLL of T-cell origin,[108] then subsequently in patients with chronic neutropenia.[109] Three distinct clinical syndromes are now described in patients with an increased number of circulating LGL.[110] When LGL carries a phenotype of T-LGL leukemia (a clonal proliferation of CD3+ LGL), chronic neutropenia and autoimmunity, especially rheumatoid arthritis, are characteristic.[111,112] Natural killer (NK-) LGL leukemia is characterized by a clonal CD3− LGL proliferation with an aggressive clinical course and multiorgan involvement. Most patients with increased numbers of CD3− LGL do not have features of NK-LGL leukemia, but rather demonstrate a more indolent clinical course.[113] Since quantitative abnormalities of LGL are fairly common and their presence in peripheral blood may represent a transient reactive phenonenom associated with viral infections, it is important to perform immunophenotyping and correlate these data with the clinical picture. Oral low-dose methotrexate has been shown to be an effective treatment for some patients with LGL leukemia.[114]

Reactive (atypical) lymphocytosis is self-limiting, rarely exceeds 5×10^9/L, and is most commonly caused by a viral infection such as infectious mononucleosis, viral hepatitis, cytomegalovirus in adults, and Bordetella pertussis in children.[115] The large reactive lymphocytes that characterize viremia are polyclonal and T-cell in origin. Abundant cytoplasm that may vary in degree of basophilia from very pale to deep blue is the most prominent feature of the reactive lymphocyte. These cells often have an irregular nuclear outline resembling a monocyte, and the nuclear chromatin is mostly coarse. Cytoplasmic vacuolization may be present (see Fig. 20–7K). Reactive B-cell lymphocytosis is rare. See Chapter 17 for discussion of infectious mononucleosis and other causes of reactive lymphocytosis.

The plasma cell dyscrasias, namely Waldenstrom's macroglobulinemia, multiple myeloma, and plasma cell leukemia, may be associated with the presence of abnormal circulating plasma cells (see Fig. 20–7L). Plasma cells and plasmacytoid lymphocytes are characterized by abundant basophilic cytoplasm, an eccentric nucleus with clumped nuclear chromatin, and a prominent perinuclear clear zone. Plasma cells are end-stage B lymphocytes with the aforementioned characteristic morphology and distinctive immunologic markers, namely the presence of monoclonal cy-

TABLE 20–8	**Typical Features of Chronic Lymphocytic Leukemia**
Feature	
Clinical	>50 years of age, lymphadenopathy, lymphocytosis
Morphology	Mature-appearing lymphocytes in blood and marrow often showing hyperclumped nuclear chromatin pattern; smudge cells
Immunophenotype	Positive sIg, CD19, CD20, CD5, CD23, CD43
Treatment	Varies from no treatment to use of single or combination chemotherapeutic agents with or without radiation therapy
Prognosis	50% 5-year survival; 30% ≥ 10-year survival
Differential diagnosis	ALL, PL, WDLL, PDLL, HCL, Sézary syndrome, LGL, ATLL, Waldenström's macroglobulinemia, viral infection

Abbreviations: ALL = Acute lymphoblastic leukemia; PL = Prolymphocytic leukemia; WDLL = Well-differentiated lymphocytic lymphoma; PDLL = Poorly differentiated lymphocytic lymphoma; HCL = Hairy cell leukemia; LGL = Large granular lymphocytosis; ATLL = Adult T-cell leukemia/lymphoma

toplasmic immunoglobulin and expression of CD38. Plasma cell disorders are covered extensively in Chapter 22.

The typical features summarizing CLL's significant clinical, morphological, and immunophenotypic features as well as treatment, prognosis, and differential diagnosis are shown in Table 20–8.

CASE STUDY

A 74-year-old African-American woman had a medical history of chronic obstructive pulmonary disease (COPD), hypertension, renal insufficiency, sickle trait, and CLL. CLL had been diagnosed 13 years ago and treated with chlorambucil and prednisone; an exacerbation of symptoms 11 years later required treatment with chlorambucil, vincristine, and bleomycin. A follow-up bone marrow study showed no lymphoid infiltrates. The patient had done well until approximately 2 weeks before admission, when she noted generalized fatigue. On the day before admission, she was noted by her nephew to be confused, minimally communicative, and quite weak. She had a diarrheal stool at the time. She was admitted to the hospital after being found unable to speak and rubbing her stomach. In the emergency room she became gradually more unresponsive and appeared to be guarding her abdomen. Blood was found rectally and in the nasogastric tube that was placed in the patient during the initial exam. She was also found to be markedly acidotic with a pH of 6.7. Her lactic acid level was 15.8 mg/dL with no acetone or ketones present and her glucose level was less than 10 mg/dL. She was also found to be in disseminated intravascular coagulation (DIC) with positive fibrinogen degradation products, a fibrinogen of 48 mg/dL with a prolonged prothrombin time (PT) and partial thromboplastin time (PTT). The patient was thought to be clinically septic and started on clindamycin, gentamycin, and ampicillin therapy. She was treated with sodium bicarbonate for her acidosis and the DIC was treated with platelets, fresh frozen plasma, and blood products. Blood pressure maintenance was difficult and the patient became oliguric. A Swan-Ganz catheter was placed and supportive care with fluid, blood products, sodium bicarbonate, and pressor agents was continued, but the patient became progressively less responsive. She became edematous, particularly around the facial area. Blood and urine cultures were negative. Tracheal sputum study showed gram-negative rods, and x-rays showed an abdominal ileus and increased congestion in the lungs with some left lower lobe atelectasis. The patient had an episode of bradycardia and expired.

Autopsy findings were remarkable for a monomorphic lymphocytic infiltrate of lymph nodes, liver, and the spleen, which also showed the presence of sickled red blood cells. The pyloric region of the stomach showed a large ulcer present that contained necrotic tissue, chronic inflammation, adenocarcinoma, and colonization with nonseptate fungus resembling *Candida*. Sections of the trachea showed multiple colonies of fungus with hyphae present along the tracheal epithelium and invading the tracheal mucosa, which upon staining with gamori silver (GMS) showed no septation and branching of the hyphae to be present consistent with *Candida* infection.

Note This case illustrates how susceptibility to opportunistic infections and immunologic deficiency can contribute to morbidity and mortality in a patient with CLL. Although patients with CLL frequently have a prolonged survival and succumb to an unrelated disorder, the course of CLL varies widely in different patients.

Questions

1. What would you expect the level of specific immunoglobulins to be in this case?
2. If marker studies were performed on the lymphocytic infiltration of lymph nodes would plasma cells be identified? Why or why not?
3. What chromosomal abnormalities coincide with this diagnosis?
4. Relate the finding of DIC with CLL in this case.
5. What percentage of lymphocytes found in the bone marrow is consistent with a diagnosis of CLL?

CHRONIC MYELOGENOUS LEUKEMIA

Chronic myelogenous leukemia (CML), also known as chronic granulocytic leukemia (CGL) or chronic myeloid leukemia, is a clonal myeloproliferative disorder of the hematopoietic pluripotent stem cell that has undergone neoplastic transformation and is characterized by excessive production of granulocytes and their precursors.[116-119] Although CML was first described in 1845,[120-122] it was not until 1960 that the association with a consistent chromosomal abnormality was made. This chromosome was called the Philadelphia chromosome (Ph) because it was first identified at the University of Pennsylvania School of Medicine in Philadelphia.[123] This was the first report of a chromosomal abnormality associated with a malignancy and was described as a small, deleted G-group chromosome in the metaphases recovered from the bone marrow of patients with CML. Approximately 90% to 95% of patients with the typical picture of CML carry the Ph chromosome in their leukemic cells[124] and consequently its presence is virtually diagnostic of the disease. Another hallmark of CML is that found at the molecular level. The Ph chromosome results from the aberrant conjoining of the proto-oncogene c-*abl* from chromosome 9 with the breakpoint cluster region gene (bcr) on chromosome 22. The new fusion protein bcr/*abl* produced is considered essential in the pathogenesis of CML.[125,126] In addition to the presence of the Ph chromosome, CML is characterized by marked leukocytosis with the presence of all stages of granulocytic maturation, organomegaly, especially splenomegaly and low levels of leukocyte alkaline phosphatase (LAP). The clinical course may be characterized by three separate phases: (1) the chronic phase, which is generally controllable with chemotherapeutic agents and lasts 2 to 5 years; (2) the chemotherapy-resistant phase called the *accelerated phase*, which lasts approximately 6 to 18 months; and (3) the blastic acute leukemialike phase, which averages 3 to 4 months and is generally unresponsive to treatment (including treatments used for de novo acute leukemia[116,127,128]) or has a biphasic course, in which case the chronic phase progresses directly to blast crisis.

CML is primarily considered an "adult leukemia" because it usually occurs in individuals between 30 and 50 years old. However, the disease can strike any age group, including elderly people, infants, and toddlers. Although rare, in infants and toddlers the disease is called *juvenile* CML and demonstrates marked hematopoietic, cytogenetic, and clinical differences from the adult form.[129,130] CML accounts for approximately 20% to 25% of all leukemia cases and in western countries is diagnosed in about 2 out of every 100,000 people annually, resulting in an estimated 5000 new cases each year.[131] There is a slight male sex predominance and the median survival is 3 to 4 years once the diagnosis of CML is made.

Etiology, Pathogenesis, and Pathophysiology

CML is a clonal stem cell disorder.[132] Although most patients with CML have no history of excessive exposure to ionizing radiation or chemical leukemogens, the implication of causation or presumed role in leukemogenesis of a variety of agents is well documented. These include exposure to ionizing radiation,[133] such as that seen in radiologists before the use of safety shielding techniques; in patients treated for ankylosing spondylitis; in survivors of nuclear explosions, as in the atomic bomb explosions in Hiroshima and Nagasaki; and following the administration of cytotoxic drugs, especially alkylating agents and biologically active chemicals such as benzene.[134] The cause is unknown in more than 95% of CML cases. A viral etiology continues to be explored using animal models.[135] CML is not an inherited disease, but it appears to be acquired as suggested by the rarity of familial aggregations of CML[136] and the failure of the second member of pairs of identical twins to have or develop the chronic leukemia.[137] The Ph chromosome is not present in nonhematopoietic tissues, nor is it found in the parents or offspring of patients.

The Ph chromosome has been found in neutrophil, monocyte, erythrocyte, platelet, and basophil precursors from CML patient's blood and bone marrow.[138] This unicellular stem cell origin helps to define the translocation that produces the Ph chromosome as a clonal abnormality and provides the subsequent progeny with a growth advantage over normal cells. Chromosomal banding analysis using Giemsa-trypsin (G-bands) or quinacrine fluorescent (Q-bands) techniques shows that the Ph chromosome is derived from the G-group chromosome 22 rather than chromosome 21 as originally thought.[139–141] The notation t(9;22) refers to the specific chromosomal translocation found in the majority of CML patients.[142] In CML, the main portion of the long arm of chromosome 22 is deleted and translocated most often to the distal end of the long arm of chromosome 9 (or to another chromosome in variant translocations), resulting in an elongated chromosome

9 (9q+). A small part of chromosome 9 is reciprocally translocated to the broken end of the deleted chromosome 22 (22q−). The unequal exchange of chromosomal material results in the tiny or "minute" chromosome 22, which is smaller than any normal chromosome and is easily recognized as the Ph chromosome under the microscope following appropriate cell culture, harvesting, chromosome preparation, and staining (Fig. 20–14). Thus, the notation for the most common translocation in CML is t(9;22) (q34.1;q11.1), frequently simply referred to as the 9/22 translocation.

Approximately 5% of CML patients have the deleted portion of chromosome 22 translocated to other chromosomes,[143] that is, t(4;22), t(12;22), and t(19;22)—called simple-variant Ph translocations, while other patients have complex-variant Ph translocations involving more than one chromosome in addition to chromosome 22[144] that is, t(9;11;22). Additionally, it has been found that on occasion the Ph chromosome may be "masked" by the presence of chromatin material translocated to the deleted chromosome 22 from one of the other chromosomes involved in the rearrangement.[145] Nonrandom chromosomal abnormalities such as duplication of the Ph chromosome, trisomy 8, and isochromosome 17 are detected in at least 50% of patients in accelerated phase of CML and in up to 80% of those who develop the blastic phase.[146]

Changes at the gene level in proliferating leukemic cells appear to endow clonal advantage on the cell because of gene deregulation or because qualitatively altered gene products are produced. Some of the genes involved in chromosomal alterations have been identified as cellular proto-oncogenes. Proto-oncogenes are normal cellular genes that, when activated by a molecular process such as mutations, deletions, and insertions of DNA sequences, can be converted to an oncogene, a gene that can cause malignant transformation. Human transforming DNA sequences have been found to be homologous to various viral oncogenes (v-*onc*) and are called cellular oncogenes (c-*ong*).[147] The proto-oncogene c-*abl* is the human counterpart to the Abelson murine leukemia virus (v-*abl*) and normally resides on chromosome 9 at band 9q34, the same location involved in the 9/22 translocation in CML. Since chromosome rearrangements have been shown to be associated with activated genes in appropriate

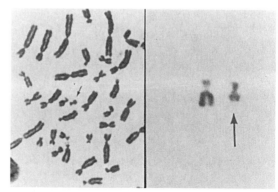

FIGURE 20–14 Philadelphia chromosome.

cells,[148] it is possible that regulation of cell growth and differentiation may be expressed inappropriately as a result of chromosomal changes. The term breakpoint cluster region (bcr) refers to the narrow 5.8-kilobase DNA fragment localized on chromosome 22 that defines the chromosomal break associated with the Ph chromosome abnormality and is based on restriction enzyme patterns of DNA probes from normal subjects and those with CML.[149] In CML, the balanced translocation between chromosomes 9 and 22 results in c-*abl* shifting from 9q34 to the bcr gene at 22q11. The subsequent formation of a bcr-*abl* hybrid gene product, a 210-kilodalton (kd) protein possessing increased tyrosine kinase activity, provides an important mediator of oncogenesis that may have potential in the pathophysiology of CML. It has been shown that the bcr-*abl* fusion protein expressed in CML acts as an antiapoptosis gene. *Apoptosis*, also known as programmed cell death, is the major form of cell death associated with the action of chemotherapeutic agents on tumor cells. The suseptibility of CML cells to treatment-induced cell death may be dependent on the expression of genes that interfere with apoptosis such as bcr-*abl*.[150,151] Most patients with CML have both the Ph chromosome and the bcr-*abl* gene, whereas some patients with clinically documented CML lack the Ph

chromosome but have the bcr-*abl* gene.[152] The gene rearrangement of the bcr region of chromosome 22 can be detected using DNA technology in Southern blots[153] or biotin-labeled gene probes.[154] The use of fluorescence in situ hybridization (FISH) to detect bcr-*abl* genes has also been shown to be an effective method of monitoring the effectiveness of therapy.[155] The molecular basis of the Ph chromosome is summarized in Fig. 20–15.

Another cellular oncogene, c-*sis*, the homologue of the transforming gene of simian sarcoma virus, has been mapped to chromosome 22. In CML, c-*sis* is translocated from chromosome 22 to a recipient chromosome, usually chromosome 9.[156] c-*sis* encodes sequences for the B chain of platelet-derived growth factor (PDGF),[157] which may play a role in the myelofibrosis that accompanies some cases of CML. The involvement of the cellular proto-oncogenes c-*abl* and c-*sis* in the pathogenesis of CML continues to be studied.[158]

The category of Ph-negative CML has led to much discussion in the past.[159-161] Patients at one time diagnosed as having Ph-negative CML may be rediagnosed as a result of the development of criteria for the myelodysplastic syndromes (Chap. 19) and other myeloproliferative disorders (Chap. 21). The conditions

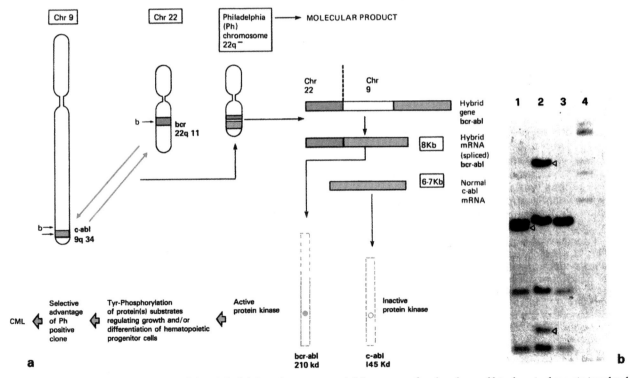

FIGURE 20–15 Molecular basis of the Philadelphia chromosome. (*a*) Sequence of molecular and biochemical events involved in generating the Ph chromosome and its phenotypic consequences. (*b*) Southern blot analysis of DNA from chronic myelogenous leukemia (CML) cells analyzed with a bcr probe to show clonal rearrangements in the bcr region. Lane 1: Ph positive CML DNA showing one rearranged band; lane 2; Ph positive CML as in lane 1 but with different break point in bcr region; lane 3: Ph negative leukemic cell DNA showing no rearranged bcr; lane 4: molecular weight markers. (From Greaves, MF: Cellular identification and markers. In Zucker-Franklin, D, Greaves, MF, et al (eds): Atlas of Blood Cells. Lea & Febiger, Philadelphia, 1988, p. 43, with permission.)

TABLE 20–9 **Clinical Signs and Symptoms of Chronic Myelocytic Leukemia (CML)/Chronic Granulocytic Leukemia (CGL)**

1. Symptoms related to hypermetabolism	Weight loss; anorexia; low-grade fever; warm, moist skin; night sweats; sternal tenderness (characteristic sign present in 2/3 of patients)
2. Splenomegaly	Present in >90% of patients and frequently massive: associated discomfort, pain, and indigestion
3. Symptoms related to anemia	Pallor, dyspnea, tachycardia
4. Other physical signs or symptoms	Bruising or ecchymoses over the extremities, epitaxis, retinal hemorrhages, menorrhagia in women or hemorrhage from other sites

that are characterized by the absence of the Ph chromosome and are readily distinguishable from CML on clinical and hematologic grounds include chronic neutrophilic leukemia,[162] the myelodysplastic syndrome chronic myelomonocytic leukemia (CMML),[163] and juvenile CML.[129] Rarely, true Ph-negative CML does exist and is diagnosed by the same clinical and hematologic parameters, other than the presence of Ph chromosome, as classical CML. However, in most of these patients the molecular defect, namely the juxtaposition of c-*abl* and bcr genes as seen in typical CML, can be demonstrated, even though there is no cytogenetic evidence of the Ph chromosome. Occasionally patients are encountered who lack the Ph translocation, bcr rearrangement, and a bcr-*abl* gene product, yet have a disease phenotype at diagnosis that is a morphological facsimile of classic chronic-phase CML and have a clinical course that is not marked by increases in blast cells.[164]

Clinical Features

Patients with CML may be asymptomatic or symptomatic. Detecting CML in its early stages may be difficult, and it is not uncommon for the disease to be discovered accidentally during a routine physical examination or hematologic evaluation, analogous to the incidental discovery of chronic lymphocytic leukemia. When symptoms do appear, the most common complaints of patients are general malaise; complaints attributable to anemia such as weakness, fatigue, diminished exercise tolerance, dizziness, headache, fever, and irritability; complaints resulting from a hypermetabolic state such as excessive perspiration, night sweats and weight loss, bone tenderness and aching due to marked marrow expansion, and fullness in the upper abdomen with accompanying easy satiation or loss of appetite resulting from hepatomegaly and splenomegaly. Excessive bleeding after a minor injury or surgical procedure, bleeding in the form of purpura, retinal hemorrhages, or hematuria caused by quantitative or qualitative platelet defects, or abnormal or unexplained bruising may also occur. Less commonly, patients may experience an increase in infections, attacks of gouty arthritis caused by the accumulating uric acid from myeloid cell breakdown, ankle edema, menorrhagia, peripheral vascular insuf-

ficiency, and priapism. On rare occasions, the presenting sign of a patient with CML is an infiltrating skin tumor or chloroma, so named because of the characteristic green color of the tumorous mass. Table 20–9 summarizes the clinical signs and symptoms of CML.

Laboratory Features

The laboratory features of CML, like the clinical features, are predominantly caused by the increased body load of myeloid cells that may be increased more than a hundredfold. The bone marrow produces and releases large numbers of cells, resulting in extreme leukocytosis often in excess of 100×10^9/L. A spectrum of myeloid forms is seen in the peripheral blood ranging from blast forms to mature neutrophils (Fig. 20–16); however, the segmented neutrophil and the myelocyte are the most numerous forms in the differential count. The immaturity seen in the granulocytic series is referred to as a *left shift*. Eosinophil, basophil, and platelet numbers may be increased and pelgeroid granulocytes may also be present at any phase of CML (Fig. 20–17). As in other myeloproliferative disorders, the blood smears of patients with CML may demonstrate giant platelets and/or megakaryocytic frag-

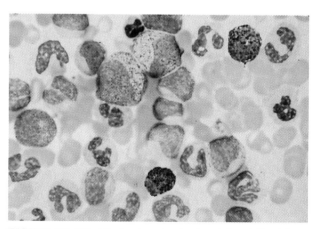

FIGURE 20–16 Photomicrograph of peripheral blood from a patient with CML.

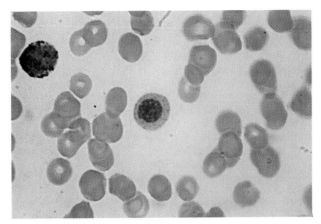

FIGURE 20–17 Pelgeroid granulocyte (pseudo-Pelger cell) in a patient with CML, peripheral blood. Note that the nucleus is round with condensed chromatin and should not be mistaken for a normal myelocyte or a nucleated red blood cell.

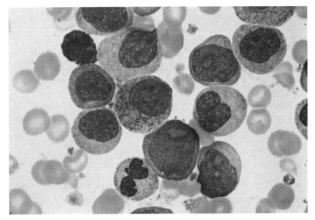

FIGURE 20–19 Photomicrograph of bone marrow aspirate from patient with CML. Note marked myeloid hyperplasia. (×54 magnification.)

ments (Fig. 20–18). A normocytic, normochromic anemia that varies in degree from patient to patient but is frequently associated with hemoglobin levels below 10 g/dL is typically present. Nucleated red blood cells may be present with varying degrees of anisocytosis, poikilocytosis, polychromasia, basophilic stippling, and reticulocytosis. As the disease progresses, the degree of anemia may worsen, thrombocytopenia develops, and there may be a shift toward the younger myeloid forms with increasing numbers of blasts.

The bone marrow is hypercellular with a marked myeloid hyperplasia. The myeloid:erythoid (M:E) ratio is generally at least 10:1 instead of the normal M:E ratio of 3:1 (Fig. 20–19). A secondary myelofibrosis may accompany the CML and is diagnosed by examining the bone marrow biopsy stained for reticulin or collagen fibers using a silver stain (see Fig. 20–20). Sea-blue histiocytosis, the appearance of storage cells with deep sea-blue pigmentation, may be seen scattered throughout the marrow of patients with CML. These contain accumulated glycolipids secondary to the expanded membrane turnover of the myeloid cell pool[165,166] (Fig. 20–21).

As mentioned earlier, in 90% to 95% of CML pa-

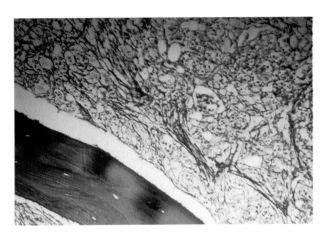

FIGURE 20–20 Silver stain for reticulin and collagen fibers on bone marrow biopsy in a patient with CML and secondary myelofibrosis.

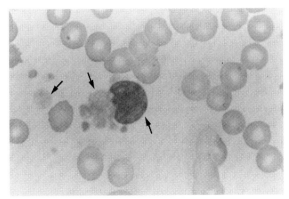

FIGURE 20–18 Photomicrograph of peripheral blood from demonstrating giant platelets and a megakaryocytic fragment (*arrow*).

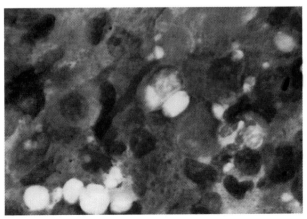

FIGURE 20–21 Sea-blue histiocytes (pseudo-Gaucher cells) in the bone marrow aspirate of a patient with CML.

tients, cytogenetic studies on the peripheral blood and bone marrow reveal the hallmark Ph chromosome t(9;22) (q34;q11) resulting from the translocation of the c-*abl* proto-oncogene from chromosome 9 to the *bcr* gene of chromosome 22, and the reciprocal translocation of the c-*sis* proto-oncogene from chromosome 22 to chromosome 9.

Another characteristic laboratory finding in CML is low to absent leukocyte alkaline phosphatase (LAP), also called, neutrophilic alkaline phosphatase (NAP) (see Figs. 13–3 and 20–22 to contrast absent LAP activity in CML with increased LAP activity in leukemoid reactions). During remission, LAP levels may increase as a reflection of enhanced maturation.[167] Although there is abnormal biochemical reactivity of LAP, not all bacteriocidal and phagocytic functions of the leukemic granulocytes are compromised; however, immunologic function such as adhesion to endothelial cells may be depressed.[168]

Other laboratory findings include elevated uric acid levels, elevated LDH level, and increased levels of serum vitamin B_{12}—findings resulting from the increased catabolism of large numbers of granulocytes common to the myeloproliferative disorders.

Clinical Course and Prognostic Factors

As mentioned earlier, CML can be divided into two or three phases: chronic, accelerated, and/or acute (blastic). The median survival from time of diagnosis is generally 3 to 4 years, and fewer than 30% of patients survive 5 years.[169] However, the chronic phase of CML is unstable and the transformation to the accelerated or blastic phase can occur at any time. In most patients, transformation is associated with development of chromosomal abnormalities in addition to Ph. The blood picture changes from the spectrum of myeloid cells with neutrophils and myelocytes predominating to an increase in the number of blasts and promyelocytes. Systemic symptoms of fever, night sweats, or weight loss reappear or worsen, as does hepatosplenomegaly and extramedullary disease in the lymph nodes, bone, skin, and soft tissue.[170] The median time from development of extramedullary disease to blastic

crisis is 4 months and median survival is 5 months. Acute blastic phase is the terminal event in CML and resembles acute leukemia in that the cells no longer differentiate to mature granulocytes and there are ≥30% blasts present in the bone marrow. The term *maturation arrest* refers to the absence of cellular differentiation beyond the blast or promyelocyte stage. The blasts of the blastic phase are usually myeloid, as demonstrated by myeloperoxidase activity. However, approximately 25% of patients develop a lymphoid blast crisis as demonstrated by the immunologic markers terminal deoxynucleotidyl transferase (Tdt) and common acute lymphoblastic leukemia antigen (CALLA). Less than 10% of patients develop megakaryocytic or erythroid blast crisis. Most patients die of complications arising during blast crisis, the most common of which are bleeding caused by thrombocytopenia, infection, therapy-related marrow aplasia, or aplasia exacerbated by progressive myelofibrosis.

The prognosis in CML can be predicted by several factors present at the time of diagnosis that are associated with early transformation to blast crisis. These "poor-risk" factors include absence of the Ph chromosome or presence of other karyotypic abnormalities in addition to the Ph chromosome, large spleen or liver size, thrombocytopenia ($<150 \times 10^9$/L) or thrombocytosis ($>500 \times 10^9$/L), extreme leukocytosis ($>100 \times 10^9$/L), peripheral blood blasts >1%, bone marrow blasts >5%, and peripheral blood basophils >15%.[171–174] CML in myeloid blast crisis is also considered a poor-risk discriminant as compared to lymphoid blast crisis, which traditionally is more responsive to chemotherapy. The morphological, cytochemical, and immunologic characteristics of blast cells in CML have been widely studied.[175,176] In addition to the aforementioned prognostic factors, analysis at the molecular level in one study correlated the sublocation of bcr breakpoint with differences in the duration of the chronic phase.[153] The number and morphological characteristics of megakaryocytes in bone marrow sections have also been used to identify histologic types of CML that may have prognostic significance.[177] The presence of p53, a tumor suppressor gene, is altered in 20% to 30% of CML patients in blast crisis. Mutations in the p53 gene may have prognostic significance, since these mutations could induce drug resistance by interfering with normal programmed cell death pathways in leukemic CML cells.

Treatment

The usual objective of therapy for the chronic phase of CML is to reduce the proliferating myeloid mass; relieve the symptoms of hyperleukocytosis, thrombocytosis, and splenomegaly; and maintain the patient in a symptom-free condition without causing therapy-related complications. This objective can be achieved by the conventional chemotherapeutic agents busulfan (Myleran) and hydroxyurea (Hydrea); however, neither cytotoxic drug postpones, prevents, or controls blast crisis. The only curative treatment for CML is bone marrow transplantation.[178] Cure is defined as a persistence of Ph-negative and bcr-*abl*-negative cells.

Bone marrow transplantation (BMT) can be syngeneic (the donor is the patient's identical twin), alloge-

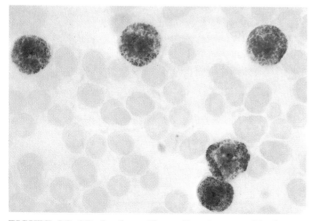

FIGURE 20–22 Leukemoid reaction: increased leukocyte alkaline phosphatase (LAP) activity.

neic (the donor is genetically compatible, most often HLA-identical siblings), or autologous (the patient's own "chronic-phase" marrow or peripheral blood is transplanted). Syngeneic or HLA-identical allogeneic bone marrow transplantation following high-dose chemotherapy is capable of eradicating the Ph-chromosome-containing leukemic clone and is recommended within 1 year of diagnosis for patients in the chronic phase under the age of 40 (under the age of 55 at some centers),[179] and for any child with juvenile chronic myelogenous leukemia as soon as possible after diagnosis and identification of a suitable donor.[180] For patients without a suitable family donor, donor registries are being established to tally the names of volunteer unrelated allogeneic bone marrow donors. The importance of transplantation in the chronic phase rather than in the accelerated or blast phase is emphasized when considering the survival data. Earlier studies show 49% to 64% of patients receiving allogeneic transplants while in chronic phase have long-term survival as compared with 15% to 30% for those transplanted in accelerated phase, and approximately 10% for patients transplanted in acute blastic phase.[181,182] A more recent progress report from the International Bone Marrow Registry reports that allogeneic BMT with a matched sibling donor can produce long-term disease-free survival in 45% of cases, but points out that this accounts for relatively few patients since mortality and morbidity are dependent on age.[183] Although transplantation gives CML patients a hope for a cure, transplant-related mortality is high (20% to 30%), with graft-versus-host disease (GVHD) a major cause of death. The use of autologous BMT avoids the debilitating effects of GVHD. In one study, 56% of patients lived 5 years after undergoing autograft;[184] however, earlier studies show less than a 10% long-term survival, with treatment most often failing because of leukemic relapse.[185] The incidence of acute GVHD can be reduced by depleting the donor marrow of the cells responsible for the GVHD reaction, namely T lymphocytes, by using various methods, including T-cell monoclonal antibodies, E-rosetting, and soybean lectin agglutination. Additionally, attempts to prevent GVHD utilizing methotrexate with or without cyclosporine,[186] glucocorticoids, or a combination are used by many transplant teams. Unfortunately, the use of T-cell depletion for GVHD prophylaxis significantly increases the incidence of leukemic relapse,[187–189] suggesting that the graft-versus-leukemia effect mediated by T lymphocytes is important in the successful cure of CML. Research is ongoing to retain the graft-versus-leukemia effect in spite of T-cell depletion.[190] Several approaches are under investigation for purging contaminating leukemic cells from nonleukemic hematopoietic cells collected for autographing.[191,192] The ability to determine the success of BMT in terms of detecting minimal residual disease has been dramatically enhanced by the DNA amplification technique called the *polymerase chain reaction* (PCR) described briefly in the CLL section of this chapter (under the heading, "Immunologic Features and Methods for Studying Lymphocytes").[193–195]

A popular chemotherapeutic agent used to treat CML palliatively is the oral alkylating agent busulfan (Myleran). Busulfan controls myelopoiesis and thrombopoiesis by acting on stem cells. This results in a slower but more prolonged control of disease than hydroxyurea, another commonly used cell-cycle-specific chemotherapeutic drug preferred by some clinicians. Both busulfan and hydroxyurea are administered until there is a 50% reduction in the white cell count. As with most therapies, busulfan has side effects that consist mainly of life-threatening pancytopenia if dosage is not carefully monitored and rare, but nonetheless severe, nonhematopoietic toxicity resulting in pulmonary fibrosis or a wasting syndrome resembling Addison's disease. Hydroxyurea is less toxic than busulfan[196] and, because of its rapid cytoreductive capabilities, is invaluable in treating patients with leukostasis resulting from hyperleukocytosis syndrome. High-dose hydroxyurea is also being analyzed as a potential treatment to induce partial or complete restoration of Ph chromosome negative hematopoiesis.[197] Other single chemotherapeutic agents used in CML include cyclophosphamide (Cytoxan), 6-mercaptopurine, chlorambucil, thioguanine, melphalan, and dibromomannitol. Adjunctive or alternative measures for treating CML include leukopheresis, splenic irradiation or splenectomy, intensive combination chemotherapy,[198] and immunotherapy; however, none of these approaches is guaranteed to prolong the duration of the chronic phase or improve overall survival. Cytogenetic response have been reported with some combination regimens.[199]

The response to standard chemotherapeutic regimens is poor once the patient progresses to the accelerated or blast phase of CML. Standard AML therapy (cytosine arabinoside and thioguanine), when used in patients with myeloid blast crisis, rarely results in survival beyond 5 months, whereas patients with lymphoid blast crisis have a median survival of approximately 8 months when treated with standard ALL therapy (vincristine and prednisone). Chemotherapeutic agents for myeloid blast crisis in CML do not kill leukemic blasts in preference to normal hematopoietic blasts. It is the similarity in response of these cell populations to chemotherapy that constitutes the major obstacle to chemotherapeutic treatment of CML in myeloid blast crisis.

Interferons (IFN), naturally occurring proteins that exist in alpha, beta, and gamma forms, have antitumor activity and have shown promise as single components or as part of a combined modality to achieve hematologic remission.[200–203] Although its exact mechanism of action is unclear, alpha-interferon (IFNα) has been shown to prolong overall median survival, especially when there is a cytogenetic response.[204] Currently, the median survival in CML is about 60 to 65 months, with survival rates of 75% to 85% percent at 3 years, and 50% to 60% at 5 years.[205]

Differential Diagnosis

CML is a myeloproliferative disorder that must be distinguished from the other hematologic disorders in this group, which include polycythemia vera, essential thrombocythemia, and agnogenic myeloid metaplasia (Chap. 21). The presence of the Ph chromosome and/or bcr rearrangement and low to absent LAP activity are virtually pathognomonic for CML and clearly dis-

TABLE 20–10   Differential Diagnosis between Leukemoid Reaction and CML

	Leukemoid Reaction	CML
Toxic vacuoles	2–4+	0–1+
Toxic granules	2–4+	0–1+
Döhle bodies	Frequent	Rare
Eosinophilia	0	1–3+
Basophilia	0	1–3+
Pseudo-Pelger-Huët	0–1+	Occasional
Karyorrhexis	0–1+	1–2+
Giant bizarre nuclei	1–1+	1–3+
Leukemic hiatus	0	Occasional
LAP score	High	Low (most cases) Normal or high (rare)
Ph chromosome	—	+ (85% of cases)

tinguish it from the other myeloproliferative disorders. Reactive granulocytic leukocytosis, such as the leukemoid reaction or leukoerythroblastic blood picture that may accompany bacterial infection or acute hemolysis, may be differentiated from CML mainly by their lack of the Ph chromosome and typical molecular aberrations of CML as well as their normal to high LAP levels. Table 20–10 summarizes the differential laboratory diagnosis between leukemoid reaction and CML. The typical features that summarize CML's significant clinical and diagnostic laboratory features, as well as treatment, prognosis, and differential diagnosis, are shown in Table 20–11.

CASE STUDY

A 60-year-old white man initially sought medical attention complaining of fatigue and fever. At that time, his white blood cell count was 45×10^9/L with a left shift; hemoglobin, 11.4 g/dL; hematocrit, 35% platelet count 500×10^9/L; LAP score 0; and his spleen was palpable 8 cm below the left costal margin. The patient's history is significant for multiple exposures to a variety of herbicides and insecticides as a result of his occupation as a farmer. A bone marrow examination and cytogenetic studies revealed hypercellularity with marked granulocytic hyperplasia, a M:E ratio greater than 10:1, and the Philadelphia chromosome t(9q+,22q−). Treatment with the alkylating agent busulfan (Myleran) was started and continued at various intervals for the next 2 years. His white blood cell count began to drop within 2 weeks and the symptoms of fatigue and fever subsided. The patient continued to do well for 2 more years, when he again complained of chronic fatigue and was again found to have marked leukocytosis. He received hydroxyurea for the next 6 months with minimal improvement of his white blood cell count. He was admitted to the hospital 1 month later for further evaluation, which included

TABLE 20–11   Typical Features of Chronic Myelogenous Leukemia

Clinical	Any age group, but usually 30–50 years of age; splenomegaly, constitutional symptoms, i.e., fatigue, weight loss, night sweats
Morphological	"Left shift" of the granulocytic series, thrombocytosis, basophilia and/or eosinophilia in blood and marrow
Cytogenetic	Philadelphia chromosome–positive t(9;22)(q34:q11)
Molecular marker	Breakpoint cluster region (bcr) gene
Other lab findings	Decreased/absent LAP activity; increased uric acid, LDH and serum B_{12}
Treatment	Chemotherapy/BMT
Prognosis	Median survival = about 5 years; 75%–85% 3-year survival; 50%–60% 5-year survival
Differential diagnosis	Leukemoid reaction; the other myeloproliferative disorders, namely polycythemia vera, essential thrombocythemia and myelofibrosis

another bone marrow examination and cytogenetic studies. This bone marrow study showed hypercellularity with granulocytic hyperplasia, and M:E ratio of 8:1 with foci of blasts was noted on scanning the bone marrow aspirate and biopsy specimen. In addition to the Ph chromosome, an isochromosome of the long arm of chromosome number 17 (i[17q]) was present. A CBC at this time revealed a white blood cell count of 62×10^9/L, hematocrit, 38%; hemoglobin, 12.8 g/dL; platelet count, 269×10^9/L, 36 segs, 5 bands, 1 metamyelocyte, 3 myelocytes, 13 promyelocytes, 21 blasts, 13 basophils, 3 lymphocytes, and 5 monocytes; pelgeroid granulocytes were also noted.

The patient was once again started on busulfan. More aggressive therapy was considered and discussed, but the patient refused further treatment and discharged himself from the hospital against the advice of his physicians.

Questions

1. What is meant by a "left shift" in this case?
2. The LAP score given in this case rules out what other leukocyte abnormality?
3. Given this patient's desire to refuse treatment, what are his chances for survival?
4. Describe the effect of Busulfan on leukocytosis.
5. What is the significance of pelgeroid granulocytes in this case?

REFERENCES

1. Bennett, JM, et al: The French American British (FAB) Cooperative Group: Proposals for the classification of chronic (mature) B and T lymphoid malignancies. J Clin Pathol 42(6):567, 1989.
2. Gallo, RC, et al: Association of type C retrovirus with a subset of adult T-cell cancers. Cancer Res 43:3892, 1983.
3. Popovic, RC, et al: Isolation and transmission of human retrovirus. Science 219:856, 1983.
4. Poisez, BJ, et al: Detection and isolation of type c-retrovirus particles from fresh and cultured lymphocytes with cutaneous T-cell lymphoma. Proc Nat Acad Sci USA 77:7415, 1980.
5. Garver, FA, et al: Characterization of a human retrovirus from cultured chronic lymphocytic leukemia B-cells (abstr). Blood 64:202, 1984.
6. Mann, DL, et al: HTLV-I associated B-cell CLL: indirect role for retrovirus in leukemogenesis. Science 236:1103, 1987.
7. Gale, PR and Foon, KA: Chronic lymphocytic leukemia—Recent advances in biology and treatment. Ann Intern Med 103:101, 1985.
8. Chikkappa, G, et al: Pure red cell aplasia in patients with chronic lymphocytic leukemia. Medicine 65:339, 1986.
9. Kipps, TJ and Carson, DA: Autoantibodies in CLL and related systemic autoimmune diseases. Blood 81:2475, 1993.
10. Patrick, CW: Chronic lymphocytic leukemia—A biologically diverse disease. Lymphocyte workshop, University of Wisconsin, 1985.
11. Knapp, W, et al: CD antigens 1989. Blood 4:1448, 1989.
12. Conley, CL, et al: Genetic factors predisposing to chronic lymphocytic leukemia and to autoimmune disease. Medicine 5:323, 1980.
13. Caligaris-Cappio, F, et al: Lineage relationship of chronic lymphocytic leukemia and hairy cell leukemia with TPA. Leuk Res 8:567, 1984.
14. Ikematsu, W, et al: Surface phenotype and Ig heavy-chain gene usage in chronic B-cell leukemias and expression of myelomonocytic markers in CD5⁻ chronic B-cell leukemia. Blood 83:2602, 1994.
15. Newman, R, et al: Phenotypic markers and bcl-1 gene rearrangement in B-cell chronic lymphocytic leukemia: a cancer and leukemia group B study. Blood 82:1239, 1993.
16. Rouby, SE, et al: p53 gene mutation in B-cell chronic lymphocytic leukemia is associated with drug resistance and is independent of MDR1/MDR3 gene expression. Blood 82:3452, 1993.
17. Molica, S, et al: CD11$_C$ expression in B-cell CLL. Blood 81:2466, 1993.
18. Knowles, DM: Lymphoid cell markers. Am JCP 9:85, 1985.
19. Korsmeyer, SJ: Antigen receptor genes as molecular markers of lymphoid neoplasms. J Clin Invest 79:1291, 1987.
20. Foroni, L, et al: Rearrangement of the T-cell receptor delta genes in human T-cell leukemias. Blood 73:559, 1989.
21. Dimond, P: About PCR. Diagnostics and clinical testing. Lab Med 27:12, 1989.
22. Stevenson, MS, et al: Detection of occult follicular lymphoma by specific DNA amplification. Blood 72:1822, 1988.
23. Crescenzi, M, et al: Thermostable DNA polymerase chain amplification of t(14;18) chromosome breakpoints and detection of minimal residual disease. Proc Nat Acad Sci USA 85:4869, 1988.
24. Spier, CM, et al: Chronic lymphocytic leukemia in young adults. Am J Clin Pathol 84:675, 1985.
25. Johnson, LE: Chronic lymphocytic leukemia. Am Fam Physician 38:167, 1988.
26. Conlan, MG and Mosher, DF: Concomitant chronic lymphocytic leukemia, acute myeloid leukemia, and thrombosis with protein C deficiency. Cancer 63:1398, 1989.
27. Rai, KR, et al: Clinical staging of chronic lymphocytic leukemia. Blood 46:216, 1975.
28. Binet, JL, et al: A clinical staging system for chronic lymphocytic leukemia. Cancer 48:198, 1981.
29. Binet, JL, et al: Chronic lymphocytic leukemia: proposals for a revised prognostic staging system. Br J Haematol 48:365, 1981.
30. Binet, JL, et al: Chronic lymphocytic leukemia: recommendations for diagnosis, staging and response criteria, International workshop on CLL. Ann Intern Med 110:236, 1989.
31. Chenson, BD, et al: Guidelines for clinical protocols for CLL: recommendations of the NCI-sponsored working group. Am J Hematol 29:152, 1988.
32. Harris, N, et al: A revised European-American classification of lymphoid neoplasms: a proposal from the International Lymphoma Study Group. Blood 84:1361, 1994.
33. Rowley, JD and Testa, JR: Chromosomal abnormalities in malignant hematologic diseases. Adv Cancer Res 36:103, 1982.
34. Knuutila, S, et al: Trisomy 12 in B cells of patients with B-cell chronic lymphocytic leukemia. N Engl J Med 314:865, 1986.
35. Que, TH, et al: Trisomy 12 in chronic lymphocytic leukemia detected by fluorescence in situ hybridization: Analysis by stage, immunophenotype and morphology. Blood 82:571, 1993.
36. Yunis, JJ: Chromosomal basis of human neoplasia. Science 221:227, 1983.
37. Gahrton, G, et al: Role of chromosomal abnormalities in chronic lymphocytic leukemia. Blood Rev 1:183, 1987.

38. Croce, CM and Kloin G: Chromosome translocations and human cancer. Science 3:54, 1985.

39. Whang-Peng, J and Knutsen, T: Cytogenetics: Methods and findings in hematologic disease. Lab Manag 4:19, 1986.

40. Athan, E, et al: Bcl-1 rearrangement: Frequency and clinical significance among B cell chronic lymphocytic leukemia and non-Hodgkin's lymphoma. Am J Pathol 138:591, 1991.

41. Dyer, MJS, et al: BC1-2 translocations in leukemias of mature B cells. Blood 83:3682, 1994.

42. Miyashita, T and Reed, JC: bcl-2 oncoprotein blocks chemotherapy-induced apoptosis in a human leukemia cell line. Blood 81:151, 1993.

43. Campos, L, et al: Effects of bc1-2 antisense oligode-oxynucleotides on in vitro proliferation and survival of normal marrow progenitors and leukemic cells. Blood 84:595, 1994.

44. Korsmeyer, SJ: Immunoglobulin and T-cell receptor genes reveal the clonality, lineage and translocations of lymphoid neoplasms. Important Adv Oncol 3, 1987.

45. Montserrat, E, et al: Lymphocyte doubling time in chronic lymphocytic leukaemia: analysis of its prognostic significance. Br J Haematol 62:567, 1986.

46. Rozman, C and Montserrat, E: Bone marrow histologic pattern—the single best prognostic parameter in chronic lymphocytic leukemia: a multivariate survival analysis of 329 cases. Blood 64:642, 1984.

47. Rozman, C, and Montserrat, E: Bone marrow biopsy in chronic lymphocytic leukemia. Nouv Rev Fr Hematol 30:369, 1988.

48. Han, T, et al: Prognostic significance of karyotypic abnormalities in B-cell chronic lymphocytic leukemia: an update. Semin Hematol 24:257, 1987.

49. Galton, DA: Terminal transformation in B-cell chronic lymphocytic leukemia. Bone Marrow Transplant 4:156, 1989.

50. Foon, KA and Gale, RP: Clinical transformation of chronic lymphocytic leukemia. Nouv Rev Fr Hematol 30:385, 1988.

51. Matolcsky, A, et al: Molecular genetic demonstration of the diverse evolution of Richter's syndrome (chronic lymphocytic leukemia and subsequent large cell lymphoma). Blood 83:1363, 1994.

52. Imamura, J, et al: p53 in hematologic malignancies. Blood 84:2412, 1994.

53. Gaidano, G, et al: p53 mutation in human lymphoid malignancies associated with Burkit lymphoma and chronic lymphocytic leukemia. Proc Nat Acad Sci USA 88:5413, 1991.

54. Fenaux, P, et al: Mutations of the p53 gene in B-cell CLL. A report of 39 cases with cytogenetic analysis. Leukemia 6:246, 1993.

55. El Ronby, S, et al: p53 gene mutation in B-cell chronic lymphocytic leukemia is associated with drug resistance and is independent of MDR1/MDR3 gene expression. Blood 82:3452, 1993.

56. Wattel, E, et al: p53 mutations are associated with resistance to chemotherapy and short survival in hematological malignancies. Blood 84:3148, 1994.

57. Liepman, M and Votaw, ML: The treatment of chronic lymphocytic leukemia with COP chemotherapy. Cancer 41:1664, 1978.

58. Oken, MM and Kaplan, ME: Combination chemotherapy with cyclophosphamide, vincristine and prednisone in the treatment of refractory chronic lymphocytic leukemia. Cancer Treat Rep 63:441, 1979.

59. Hansen, MM, et al: CHOP versus prednisolone + chlorambucil in chronic lymphocytic leukemia (CLL): preliminary results of a randomized multicenter study. Nouv Rev Fr Hematol 3:433, 1988.

60. Kempin, S, et al: Combination chemotherapy of advanced chronic lymphocytic leukemia; the M − 2 protocols (vincristine, BCNU, cyclophosphamide, melphalan, and prednisone). Blood 60:1110, 1982.

61. Cheson, BD: Current approaches to the chemotherapy of B-cell chronic lymphocytic leukemia: a review. Am J Hematol 32:72, 1989.

62. O'Brien, S, et al: Results of fludarabine and prednisone therapy in 264 patients with CLL with multivariate analysis-derived prognostic model for response to treatment. Blood 82:1695, 1993.

63. Richards, F, et al: The control of chronic lymphocytic leukemia with mediastinal irradiation. Am J Med 64:947, 1978.

64. Yam, LT and Crosby, WH: Early splenectomy in lymphoproliferative disorders. Arch Intern Med 133:270, 1974.

65. Spiers, ASD: Chronic Lymphocytic Leukemia. In Gunz, FW and Henderson, ES (eds): Leukemia, ed 4. Grune and Stratton, New York, 1983, p 709.

66. Cooperative Group for the Study of Immunoglobulin in CLL: Intravenous immunoglobulin for the prevention of infection in CLL. New Engl J Med 319:902, 1988.

67. Bunch, C: Immunoglobulin replacement in chronic lymphocytic leukemia. Nouv Rev Fr Hamatol 30:419, 1988.

68. Grever, MR, et al: Low dose deoxycoformycin in lymphoid malignancies. J Clin Oncol 9:1196, 1985.

69. O'Dwyer, PJ, et al: 2'-deoxycoformycin (pentostatin) for lymphoid malignancies. Ann Intern Med 108:733, 1988.

70. Grever, MR, et al: Fludarabine monophosphate: A potentially useful agent in chronic lymphocytic leukemia, Nouv Rev Fr Hematol, 30:457, 1988.

71. Keating, MJ, et al: Fludarabine (FLU), prednisone (PRED): A safe effective combination in refractory chronic lymphocytic leukemia (CLL). Proc Am Soc Clin Oncol 780:201, 1989.

72. O'Brien, S, et al: Results of fludarabine and prednisone in 264 patients with chronic lymphocytic leukemia with multivariate analysis-derived prognostic model for response to treatment. Blood 82:1695, 1993.

73. Johnson, SA, et al: Complete remission after fludarabine for chronic lymphocytic leukemia. Blood 81:560, 1993.

74. Piro, LD, et al: 2-chlorodeoxyadenosine: An effective new agent for the treatment of chronic lymphocytic leukemia. Blood 72:1069, 1988.

75. Foon, KA, et al: Effects of monoclonal antibody therapy in patients with chronic lymphocytic leukemia. Blood 64:1085, 1984.

76. Grossbord, ML, et al: Serotherapy of B-cell neoplasms with anti-B4 blocked recin: a phase I trial of daily bolus infusion. Blood 79:576, 1992.

77. Foon, KA, et al: Phase II trial of recombinant leukocyte A interferon in patients with advanced chronic lymphocytic leukemia. Am J Med 78:216, 1985.

78. O'Connell, MJ, et al: Clinical trial of recombinant leukocyte A interferon as initial therapy for favorable histology non-Hodgkin's lymphomas and chronic lymphocytic leukemia. J Clin Oncol 4:128, 1986.

79. Pangalis, GA, and Griva, E: Recombinant alpha-2b-interferon therapy in untreated, stages A and B chronic lymphocytic leukemia. Cancer 61:869, 1988.

80. Rozman, C, et al: Recombinant a₂-interferon in the treatment of B chronic lymphocytic leukemia in early stages. Blood 71:1295, 1988.

81. Kay, NE, et al: Evidence for tumor reduction in refractory or relapsed B-CLL patients with infusional interleukin-2. Nouv Rev Fr Hematol 30:475, 1988.

82. Nierodzik, ML, et al: Treatment of CD4 chronic lymphocytic leukemia (CLL) with etoposide (abstr). Blood 74:1039, 1989.

83. O'Brian, S, et al: Advances in the biology and treatment

of B-cell chronic lymphocytic leukemia. Blood 85:307, 1995.

84. Rai, KR, et al: Chronic lymphocytic leukemia. Med Clin North Am 68:697, 1984.

85. Uchiyama, T, et al: Adult T-cell leukemia: clinical and hematologic features of 16 cases. Blood 50:481, 1977.

86. Krajny, M and Pruzanski, W: Waldenstrom's macroglobulinemia: Review of 45 cases. Can Med Assoc J 114:899, 1976.

87. Sonnier, JA, et al: Chromosomal translocation involving the immunoglobulin kappa-chain and heavy-chain loci in a child with chronic lymphocytic leukemia. N Engl J Med 309:590, 1983.

88. Galton, DAG, et al: Prolymphocytic leukemia. Br J Haematol 27:7, 1974.

89. Katayama, I, et al: B-lineage prolymphocytic leukemia as a distinct clinical pathological entity. Am J Pathol 99:399, 1980.

90. Lampert, I, et al: Histopathology of prolymphocytic leukemia with particular reference to the spleen: A comparison with chronic lymphocytic leukemia. Histopathology 4:3, 1980.

91. Melo, JV, et al: The relationship between chronic lymphocytic leukemia and prolymphocytic leukemia. I. Clinical and laboratory features of 300 patients and characterization of an intermediate group. Br J Haematol 63:377, 1986.

92. Enno, A, et al: "Prolymphocytoid" transformation of chronic lymphocytic leukaemia. Br J Haematol 41:9, 1979.

93. Melo, JV, et al: The relationship between chronic lymphocytic leukaemia and prolymphocytic leukemia. In Gale, RP and Rai, K (eds): Chronic lymphocytic leukemia: Recent progress and future direction. Alan Liss, New York, 1987, p 205.

94. Catovsky, D, and Costello, C: Cytochemistry of normal and leukaemic lymphocytes: a review. Basic Appl Histochem 23:255, 1979.

95. Mann, RB, et al: Malignant lymphomas, conceptual understanding of morphologic diversity. Am J Pathol 94:105, 1979.

96. Aisenberg, AC: Cell lineage in lymphoproliferative disease. Am J Med 75:110, 1983.

97. Mintzer, DM and Hauptman, SP: Lymphosarcoma cell leukemia and other non-Hodgkin's lymphoma in leukemic phase. Am J Med 75:110, 1983.

98. Yam, LT, et al: Tartrate-resistant acid phosphatase isoenzyme in the reticulum cells of leukemic reticuloendotheliosis. N Engl J Med 284:357, 1971.

99. Visser, L, et al: Monoclonal antibodies reactive with hairy cell leukemia. Blood 74:320, 1989.

100. Catovsky, D, et al: Hairy cell leukemia (HCL) variant: An intermediate between HCL and B-prolymphocytic leukemia. Semin Oncol 11:362, 1984.

101. Melo, JV, et al: Splenic B cell lymphoma with circulating villous lymphocytes: Differential diagnosis of B cell leukemias with large spleens. J Clin Pathol 40:642, 1987.

102. Matutes, E, et al: The immunophenotype of splenic lymphoma with villous lymphocytes and its relevance to the differential diagnosis with other B-cell disorders. Blood 83:1558, 1994.

103. Flandrin, G and Brouet, JC: The Sezary cell: cytologic cytochemical and immunologic studies. Mayo Clin Proc 49:575, 1974.

104. Bottaro, M, et al: Heteroduplex analysis of T-cell receptor γ gene arrangements for diagnosis and monitoring of cutaneous T-cell lymphomas. Blood 83:3271, 1994.

105. Poiesz, BJ, et al: Detection and isolation of type C retrovirus particles from fresh and cultured lymphocytes of a patient with cutaneous T cell lymphoma. Proc Nat Acad Sci USA 77:7415, 1980.

106. Shimoyama, M and members of the Lymphoma Study Group (1984-87): Diagnostic criteria and classification of clinical subtypes of adult T-cell leukemia-lymphoma. Br J Haematol 79:428, 1991.

107. Sakashita, A, et al: Mutations of the p53 gene in adult T-cell leukemia. Blood 70:477, 1992.

108. Brouet, JC, et al: Chronic lymphocytic leukemia of T-cell origin: Immunological and clinical evaluation in eleven patients. Lancet 2:890, 1975.

109. McKenna, RE, et al: Chronic lymphoproliferative disorder with unusual clinical morphological, ultrastructural and membrane surface characteristics. Am J Med 62:588, 1977.

110. Loughran, TP: Clonal diseases of large granular lymphocytes. Blood 82:1, 1993.

111. Scott, CS, et al: Disorders of the large granular lymphocytes and natural killer-associated cells. Blood 83:301, 1994.

112. Kaushik, AS and Logue, GI: Autoimmune neutropenia. Blood 8:1984, 1993.

113. Tefferi, A, et al: Chronic natural killer cell lymphocytosis: A descriptive clinical study. Blood 84:2721, 1994.

114. Loughran, TP, et al: Treatment of LGL leukemia with oral low dose methotrexate. Blood 84:2164, 1994.

115. Bennett, JM, et al: Proposals for the classification of chronic (mature) B and T lymphoid leukemias. J Clin Pathol 42:567, 1989.

116. Kantarjian, HM, et al: Chronic myelogenous leukemia—past, present, and future. Hematol Pathol 2:91, 1988.

117. Champlin, RE: Chronic myelogenous leukemia. In Gale, R (ed): Leukemia Therapy. Blackwell, Boston, 1986, p 147.

118. Champlin, RE and Golde, DW: Chronic myelogenous leukemia: Recent advances. Blood 65:1039, 1985.

119. Koeffler, HP and Golde, DW: Chronic myelogenous leukemia—New concepts. N Engl J Med 304:1201, 1269, 1981.

120. Bennett, JH: Case of hypertrophy of the spleen and liver, in which death took place from suppuration of the blood. Edinburgh Med Surg J 64:413, 1845.

121. Craigie, D: Case of disease of the spleen in which death took place in consequence of the presence of purulent matter in the blood. Edinburgh Med Surg J 64:400, 1854.

122. Virchow, R: Weisses blut. Froiep Notizen 36:151, 1845.

123. Nowell, PC and Hungerford, DA: A minute chromosome in human chronic granulocytic leukemia. Science 132:1497, 1960.

124. Rowley, JD: Ph-positive leukemia, including chronic myelogenous leukemia. Clin Haematol 9:55, 1980.

125. Litz, CE, et al: Duplication of small segments with the major breakpoint cluster region in chronic myelogenous leukemia. Blood 81:1567, 1993.

126. Melo, JV, et al: The abl-bcr fusion gene is expressed in chronic myeloid leukemia. Blood 81:158, 1993.

127. Goldman, JM and Lu, DP: New approaches in chronic granulocytic leukemia-origin, prognosis and treatment. Semin Hematol 19:241, 1982.

128. Spiers, ASD: Chronic granulocytic leukemia. Med Clin North Am 68:713, 1984.

129. Glassy, EF and Sun, NCJ: Juvenile variant of chronic myelogenous leukemia. ASCP check sample H85-11, 1985.

130. Chi-Sing, NG, et al: Juvenile chronic myeloid leukemia. Am J Pathol 90:575, 1988.

131. Bertino, JR, et al: Chronic myelogenous leukemia. Leukemia Society of America: Public education and information department booklet, January 1988.

132. Fialkow, PJ, et al: Chronic myelocytic leukemia: Clonal origin in a stem cell common to the granuocytic, erythrocytic, platelet and monocyte/macrophage. Am J Med 63:125, 1977.

133. Gunz, FW: Ionizing radiation and human leukemia. In

Gunz, FW and Henderson, ES (eds): Leukemia, ed 4. Grune and Stratton, New York, 1983, p 359.

134. Askoy, M, et al: Leukemia in shoeworkers exposed chronically to benzene. Blood 44:837, 1974.

135. Van Etten, RA, et al: A mouse model for chronic myelogenous leukemia (abstr). Blood 74:185, 1989.

136. Baikie, AG, et al: Cytogenetic studies in familial leukemias. Austral Ann Med 18:7, 1969.

137. Jacobs, EM, et al: Chromosome abnormalities in human cancer: report of a patient with chronic myelocytic leukemia and his nonleukemic monocygotic twin. Cancer 19:869, 1966.

138. Sandberg, AA: The chromosomes in human cancer and leukemia. Elsevier, New York, 1980.

139. Whang-Peng, J and Knutsen, T: Cytogenetics: methods and findings in hematologic disease. Lab Manag 4:19, 1986.

140. Caspersson, T, et al: Identification of the Philadelphia chromosome on a number 22 by quinacrine mustard fluorescence analysis. Exp Cell Res 63:238, 1970.

141. Prieto, F, et al: Identification of the Philadelphia (Ph) chromosome. Blood 35:23, 1970.

142. Paris conference: Standardization in human cytogenetics. Birth Defects, Orig Article Ser 8, No. 7, 1971.

143. Oshimura, M, et al: Variant Ph translocations in CML and their incidence, including two cases with sequential lymphoid and myeloid crises. Cancer Genet Cytogenet 5:187, 1982.

144. Cork, A: Chromosomal abnormalities in leukemia. Am J Med Tech 49:703, 1983.

145. London, B, et al: A new translocation in chronic myeloid leukemia—t(4;9;22)—resulting in a masked Philadelphia chromosome. Cancer Genet Cytogenet 20:5, 1986.

146. Kantarjian, HM, et al: Characteristics of accelerated disease in chronic myelogenous leukemia. Cancer 61:1441, 1988.

147. Bishop, MJ: Cellular oncogenes and retroviruses. Annu Rev Biochem 52:301, 1984.

148. Hunter, T: Oncogenes and protooncogenes: How do they differ? J Nat Cancer Inst 73:773, 1984.

149. Groffen, J, et al: Philadelphia chromosomal breakpoints are clustered within a limited region, bcr, on chromosome 22. Cell 36:93, 1984.

150. Sandberg, AA, et al: The Philadelphia chromosome: A model of cancer and molecular cytogenetics. Cancer Genet Cytogenet 21:129, 1986.

151. McGahon, A, et al: Bcr-abl maintains resistance of chronic myelogenous leukemia cells to apoptotic cell death. Blood 83:1179, 1994.

152. Ganesan, TS, et al: Rearrangement of the bcr gene in Philadelphia chromosome-negative chronic myeloid leukemia. Blood 68:957, 1986.

153. Shtalrid, M, et al: Analysis of breakpoints within the bcr gene and their correlation with the clinical course of Philadelphia-positive chronic myelogenous leukemia. Blood 72:485, 1988.

154. Telzer, LL and Concepcion, EG: Detection of the gene rearrangement in chronic myelogenous leukemia with biotinylated gene probes. Am J CP 91:464, 1989.

155. Bemtz, M, et al: Detection of chimeric bcr-abl genes on bone marrow samples and blood smears in chronic myeloid and acute lymphoblastic leukemia by in situ hybridization. Blood 83:1922, 1994.

156. Groffen, J, et al: C-sis is translocated from chromosome 22 to chromosome 9 in chronic myelocytic leukemia. J Exp Med 158:9, 1983.

157. Doolittle, RF, et al: Simiam sarcoma virus gene, v-sis is derived from the gene (or genes) encoding a platelet derived growth factor. Science 221:275, 1983.

158. Champlin, R, et al: Chronic leukemia: oncogenes, chromosomes and advances in therapy. Ann Intern Med 104:671, 1986.

159. Travis, LB, et al: Ph-negative chronic granulocytic leukemia: a nonentity. Am J CP 85:186, 1986.

160. Fitzgerald, PH, and Beard, MEJ: Ph-negative chronic myeloid leukemia. Br J Haematol 66:311, 1987.

161. Pugh, WC, et al: Philadelphia-negative chronic myelogenous leukemia: A morphological reassessment. Br J Haematol 60:457, 1985.

162. Krause, JR: Chronic neutrophilic leukemia. ASCP tech sample H-2, 1989.

163. Bennet, JM, et al: The French-American-British (FAB) cooperative group. Proposals for the classification of the myelodysplastic syndromes. Br J Haematol 51:189, 1982.

164. Kurzrock, R, et al: Philadelphia-negative CML without bcr rearrangement: a chronic myeloid leukemia with a distinct clinical course (abstr). Blood 74:102, 1989.

165. Brigden, ML and Preece, EV: An electrolyte abnormality in a case of chronic granulocytic leukemia. Lab Med 15:761, 1984.

166. Ulirsch, R: Sea-blue histiocytosis in chronic myelocytic leukemia. ASCP Tech Sample H-4, 1985.

167. Rosner, F, et al: Leukocyte alkaline phosphatase: fluctuations with disease status in chronic granulocytic leukemia. Arch Intern Med 130:892, 1972.

168. Gordon, MY, et al: Adhesive defects in chronic myeloid leukemia. Curr Top Microbiol Immunol 149:151, 1989.

169. Sokal, JE: Evaluation of survival data for chronic myelocytic leukemia. Am J Hematol 1:493, 1976.

170. Terjanian, T, et al: Clinical and prognostic features of patients with Philadelphia chromosome positive chronic myelogenous leukemia and extramedullary disease. Cancer 59:297, 1987.

171. Gomez, GA, et al: Prognostic features at diagnosis of chronic myelocytic leukemia. Cancer 47:2470, 1981.

172. Tura, S, et al: Staging of chronic myeloid leukemia. Br J Haematol 47:105, 1981.

173. Sokal, JE, et al: Prognostic discrimination in "good-risk" chronic granulocytic leukemia. Blood 63:789, 1984.

174. Cervantes, F and Rozman, C: A multivariate analysis of prognostic factors in chronic myeloid leukemia. Blood 60:1298, 1982.

175. Polli, N, et al: Characterization of blast cells in chronic granulocytic leukaemia in transformation, acute myelofibrosis and undifferentiated leukaemia. I. Ultrastructural morphology and cytochemistry. Br J Haematol 59:277, 1985.

176. San Miguel, JF, et al: Characterization of blast cells in chronic granulocytic leukaemia in transformation, acute myelofibrosis and undifferentiated leukaemia. II. Studies with monoclonal antibodies and terminal transferase. Br J Haematol 59:297, 1985.

177. Lorand-Metze, IJ et al: Histological and cytological heterogeneity of bone marrow in Philadelphia-positive chronic myelogenous leukaemia at diagnosis. Br J Haematol 67:45, 1987.

178. Alfan, NC: Therapeutic options in chronic myeloid leukemia. Blood Rev 3:45, 1989.

179. Thomas, ED and Clift, RA: Indications for marrow transplantation in chronic myelogenous leukemia. Blood 73:861, 1989.

180. Sanders, JE, et al: Allogeneic marrow transplantation for children with juvenile chronic myelogenous leukemia. Blood 71:1144, 1988.

181. Goldman, JM, et al: Bone marrow transplantation for chronic myelogenous leukemia in chronic phase. Ann Intern Med 108:806, 1988.

182. McGlave, PB, et al: Therapy of chronic myelogenous leu-

kemia with allogeneic bone marrow transplantation. J Clin Oncol 5:1033, 1987.

183. Borten, MM, et al: 1993 progress report from the International bone marrow registry. Bone Marrow Transplant 12:97, 1993.

184. Hoyle, C, et al: Autografting for patients with chronic myelocytic leukemia in chronic phase: an update. Br J Haematol 85:76, 1994.

185. Butturini, MM, et al: Autotransplants in chronic myelogenous leukemia: Strategies and results. Lancet 335:1244, 1990.

186. Clift, RA, et al: Treatment of chronic myeloid leukemia by marrow transplantation. Blood 82:1954, 1993.

187. Santos, GW: Problems and strategies for bone marrow transplantation in acute leukemia and chronic myelogenous leukemia. Cancer Detect Prev 12:589, 1988.

188. Apperley, JF, et al: Bone marrow transplantation for chronic myeloid leukemia in first chronic phase: Importance of a graft-versus-leukaemia effect. Br J Haematol 69:239, 1988.

189. Goldman, JM: Allogeneic bone marrow transplantation: state of the art and future directions. Bone Marrow Transplant 4:131, 1989.

190. Champlin, R, et al: Selective CD8 depletion of donor marrow: retention of graft-versus-leukemia effect following bone marrow transplantation for chronic myelogenous leukemia (abstr). Blood 74:95, 1989.

191. Leemhuis, T, et al: Identification of bcr-abl negative primitive hematopoietic progenitor cells within chronic myeloid leukemia marrow. Blood 81:801, 1993.

192. Dekter, TM and Chang, J: New strategies for the treatment of chronic myeloid leukemia. Blood 84:673, 1994.

193. Kohler, S, et al: Application of the polymerase chain reaction to the detection of minimal residual disease after bone marrow transplantation for patients with chronic myelogenous leukemia (abstr). Blood 74:96, 1989.

194. Synder, DS, et al: Definition of remission based on the expression of bcr-abl RNA following bone marrow transplant for chronic myelogenous leukemia in chronic phase (abstr). Blood 74:97, 1989.

195. Lee, M, et al: Clinical usage of polymerase chain reaction to analyze the bcr/abl splicing patterns and minimal residual disease in Philadelphia chromosome-positive chronic myelogenous leukemia (abstr). Blood 74:745, 1989.

196. Hehlmann, R, et al: The German CML study group: Randomized comparison of busulfan and hydroxyurea. Blood 82:398, 1993.

197. Kolitz, JE, et al: Phase II trial of high-dose hydroxyurea in chronic myelogenous leukemia (abstr). Blood 74:577, 1989.

198. Clift, RA, et al: Marrow transplantation for chronic myeloid leukemia: A randomized study comparing cyclophosphamide and total body irradiation with busulfan and cyclophosphamide. Blood 84:2036, 1994.

199. Kantarjian, H, et al: High doses of cyclophosphamide, BCNU and etoposide induce cytogenetic responses in most patients with advanced stages of Philadelphia chromosome-positive chronic myelogenous leukemia (abstr). Blood 74:1032, 1989.

200. Talpaz, M, et al: Chronic myelogenous leukemia: hematologic remissions and cytogenetic improvements induced by recombinant alpha A interferon. N Engl J Med 314:1065, 1986.

201. Niederle, N, et al: Interferon alpha-2B in the treatment of chronic myelogenous leukemia. Semin Oncol 16:29, 1987.

202. Higno, CS, et al: Alpha interferon induced cytogenetic remissions in patients who relapse with chronic myelogenous leukemia after allogeneic bone marrow transplantation (abstr). Blood 74:307, 1989.

203. Talpaz, M, et al: Sustained complete cytogenetic responses among Philadelphia positive chronic myelogenous leukemia patients treated with alpha interferon (abstr). Blood 74:289, 1989.

204. Kloke, O, et al: Impact of interferon alpha-induced cytogenetic improvement on survival in chronic myelogenous leukemia. Br J Haematol 83:399, 1993.

205. Kantarjian, HM, et al: Chronic myelogenous leukemia: A concise update. Blood 82:691, 1993.

QUESTIONS

1. The cells of CLL are morphologically identical to those of:
   a. ALL
   b. WDLL
   c. Infectious mononucleosis
   d. Sézary syndrome

2. Surface immunoglobulin is the most reliable surface marker for:
   a. T lymphocytes
   b. Plasma cells
   c. B lymphocytes
   d. Histiocytes

3. Cells that demonstrate a positive reaction with the tartrate-resistant acid phosphatase (TRAP) stain are most likely:
   a. T lymphoblasts of ALL
   b. Atypical lymphocytes of a viral infection
   c. Large granular lymphocytes of T-gamma lymphoproliferative disorder
   d. Hairy cells of hairy cell leukemia

4. A mutated tumor suppressor gene found in a variety of human cancers including CLL and CML is:
   a. p53
   b. MDM2
   c. HLA-DR
   d. CD4

5. The typical immunophenotypic profile for B-CLL cells is:
   a. Positivity for polyclonal T cell antigens
   b. CD5, CD20, and CD19 positivity
   c. Intense surface IgG/kappa and lambda positivity
   d. CD25/CD22 positivity

6. The translocation that results in formation of the Philadelphia chromosome (Ph) involves chromosomes:
   a. 21 and 22
   b. 22 and 9
   c. 8 and 14
   d. 21 and 9

7. Blast crisis in CML is:
   a. Followed by the chronic phase and the accelerated phase
   b. Only seen in the juvenile form of CML
   c. The terminal phase of CML characterized by increased number of blasts in the bone marrow and peripheral blood
   d. The first phase of a typical case of CML

8. Each of the following favors a diagnosis of CML rather than a leukemoid reaction except:
   a. Absence of eosinophils and basophils in the peripheral blood
   b. Low LAP score with myeloblasts through segs in the peripheral blood
   c. Ph chromosome
   d. Enlarged spleen

9. The only curative treatment for CML is:
   a. Combination chemotherapy
   b. Total body radiation
   c. Bone marrow transplantation
   d. None

10. At the molecular level, the aberrant conjoining of genetic material from chromosome 9 and chromosome 22 in patients with CML results in the formation of a new gene product called the:
   a. bcr-*abl* gene
   b. bcl-2 gene
   c. Multidrug resistance gene
   d. Blast crisis gene

ANSWERS

1. **b** (p 358)
2. **c** (pp 348, 349)
3. **d** (p 359)
4. **a** (p 360 and 366)
5. **b** (p 348)
6. **b** (p 362)
7. **c** (p 366)
8. **a** (pp 364–365) (incl. Table 20–9)
9. **c** (p 366)
10. **a** (p 363)

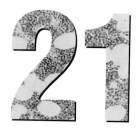

Chronic Myeloproliferative Disorders

Barbara S. Caldwell, BS, MT(ASCP)SH

Objectives

At the end of this chapter, the learner should be able to:

1. Describe the origin of myeloproliferative disorders.
2. List characteristics of chronic myeloproliferative disorders.
3. Identify the predominant abnormal erythrocyte morphology associated with idiopathic myelofibrosis.
4. Select features of myelofibrosis that distinguish it from chronic myelogenous leukemia.
5. Name conditions that may cause an absolute erythrocytosis.
6. List laboratory findings for polycythemia vera.
7. Describe the therapeutic control of polycythemia vera.
8. Select features of secondary polycythemia and relative erythrocytosis that distinguish them from polycythemia vera.
9. State the diagnostic criteria for essential thrombocythemia.
10. List the most common cause of reactive thrombocytosis.

INTRODUCTION TO MYELOPROLIFERATIVE DISORDERS

Historic Perspective

The term *myeloproliferative disorder* (MPD) was proposed in 1951 by Dr. William Damashek[1] to describe a closely related group of acquired malignant disorders that share several common clinical and hematologic features. He speculated on the presence of a common myelostimulatory factor that, under certain conditions, would cause excessive proliferation of both hematopoietic cells and fibroblasts in the bone marrow. According to Damashek, this factor also appeared to activate dormant embryonal hematopoietic tissue in the spleen and liver (extramedullary hematopoiesis).[1] Although recent discoveries regarding hematopoiesis have necessitated certain modifications to the original hypothesis, the Damashek concept of myeloproliferative syndrome has been widely accepted.

Definition and Classification

MPDs are characterized by a hypercellular bone marrow with increased quantities of one or more cellular lineages (i.e., erythrocytes, leukocytes, and platelets in the peripheral blood). The physical hallmark feature in 60% to 100% of patients is splenomegaly.[2]

TABLE 21–1 Myeloproliferative Disorders (MPDs)

Acute MPDs
Acute nonlymphocytic leukemia
    Acute myeloblastic leukemia
    Acute promyelocytic leukemia
    Acute myelomonocytic leukemia
    Acute monocytic leukemia
    Erythroleukemia
Unusual Variants
    Megakaryocytic leukemia
    Eosinophilic leukemia
    Basophilic leukemia

Chronic MPDs
Chronic myelogenous leukemia
Idiopathic myelofibrosis
Polycythemia vera
Essential or idiopathic thrombocythemia

The MPDs may be subdivided into two groups, acute and chronic. The former include all the variants of acute nonlymphocytic leukemia (ANLL) that are morphologically designated according to the predominant cell type. The ANLLs have been classified according to the French-American-British (FAB) system as M0 to M7 and all are characterized by excessive proliferation of immature cells (see Chap. 18 for complete discussion of these diseases). The chronic MPDs include chronic myelocytic leukemia (CML), polycythemia vera (PV), idiopathic myelofibrosis (IMF), and essential thrombocythemia (ET) (Table 21–1).

These specific myeloproliferative disorders are distinguished by the predominant cell type involved. The most prominent feature of CML is excessive production of granulocytes; of PV, overproduction of erythrocytes; and of ET, overproduction of platelets. Idiopathic myelofibrosis (IMF) is recognized by a prominence of marrow fibrosis and extramedullary hematopoiesis in the liver and spleen. The finding of a variable amount of fibrosis may complicate any of the chronic MPDs (Fig. 21–1).

The evidence for the clonal and therefore neoplastic nature of the MPDs is derived from cytogenetic analysis isoenzyme studies of glucose-6-phosphate dehydrogenase (G6PD) and clonogenic assays.[3,4] These studies demonstrate that the hemopoietic abnormalities arise from a neoplastic transformation of a single multipotential stem cell, a progenitor cell that is committed to differentiation of myeloid cell lines (that is, granulocytes, monocytes, platelets, and erythrocytes).[5] Adams and coworkers[6] postulate that the increased sensitivity of the precursor granulocyte-macrophage, megakaryocytic, and erythroid progenitor cells to small amounts of growth factor accounts for the variably programmed predisposition of the affected stem cells to undergo transformation into abnormal blast-forming cells, as well as the subsequent deranged production of a spectrum of mature cells.

Marrow fibroblasts, however, do not share a common ancestry with the pluripotent hemopoietic precursor cell responsible for the hyperplasia and dysplasia that characterize each of the MPDs. Cell karyotypes and G6PD expression have both revealed the bone marrow fibroblasts to be polyclonally derived.[4,7] Therefore, fibrosis is thought to reflect a reactive rather than an intrinsic neoplastic process. (As mentioned earlier, the acute MPDs are discussed in Chap. 18 and the reader is referred to Chap. 20 for a discussion of chronic myelocytic leukemia.)

There is a close qualitative and quantitative identity at the committed precursor cell level for IMF, PV, and

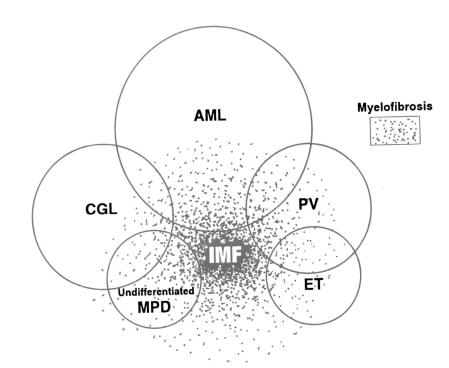

FIGURE 21–1 Myelofibrosis in the myeloproliferative variants. Myelofibrosis occurs in a wide spectrum of myeloproliferative diseases but is a predominant feature of idiopathic myelofibrosis (IMF). AML = acute myeloblastic leukemia, PV = polycythemia vera, ET = essential thrombocythemia, CGL = chronic granulocytic leukemia (Adapted from Lewis,[29] p. 17.)

ET, and these diseases will be discussed at length in this chapter. Cell culture studies by Adams and associates[6] suggest a progression of increasing abnormality in the stem cells, from the least abnormal in PV to the intermediate abnormality in ET to the most abnormal state in IMF. The pathophysiology, clinical and laboratory findings, and therapy for each of these chronic MPD variants are reviewed in detail.

COMMON CLINICAL AND HEMATOLOGIC FEATURES OF CHRONIC MYELOPROLIFERATIVE DISORDERS

All of the clinical variants of the chronic myeloproliferative diseases (CMPDs) may share, to varying extents, the following characteristics:

1. Predominantly affects middle-aged and older groups
2. Insidious, sometimes silent, asymptomatic onset[8]
3. Panhyperplasia of bone marrow (granulocytic with or without monocytic, erythrocytic, and megakaryocytic elements)
4. Extramedullary hematopoiesis; myeloid metaplasia manifesting primarily in the spleen and less frequently in the liver, causing portal hypertension
5. Bone marrow fibroblastic proliferation and reticulin-collagen formation (see Fig. 21–1)
6. Transitions often occur between these disorders, with overlapping manifestations causing difficulty in classification (Fig. 21–2)
7. Increased propensity for terminating in acute leukemia

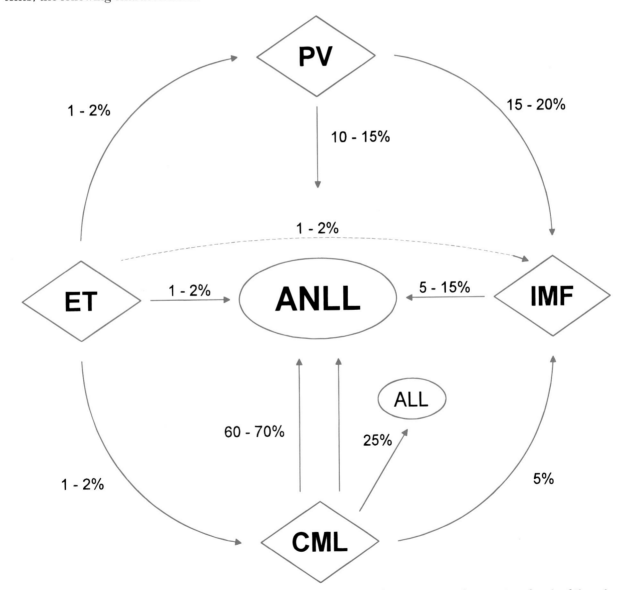

FIGURE 21–2 Relationship among the various myeloproliferative disorders. Transition frequencies of each of these bone marrow stem cell disorders are shown. ANLL = acute nonlymphocytic leukemia; ALL = acute lymphoblastic leukemia; PV = polycythemia vera; IMF = idiopathic myelofibrosis; ET = essential thrombocythemia. (A solid line indicates a strong relationship between disorders; a dashed line indicates a weak relationship.)

TABLE 21–2 Differential Characteristics of the Chronic MPDs

	CML	Idiopathic Myelofibrosis	Polycythemia Vera	Essential Thrombocythemia
Erythrocytes	N or ↓	N or ↓	4+	0–1+
Granulocytes	4+	1–2+	1–2+	0–1+
Platelets	0–3+	0–3+	1–3+	4+
Fibroblasts	0–2+	2–4+	0–2+	0–2+
NRBCs	Rare	Common	Rare	Rare
LAP	↓↓	N–↑↑	Usually ↑	N
Bone marrow	Marked myeloid hyperplasia	Fibrosis, dry tap	Hypercellular, ↓ iron stores	Hypercellular, ↑↑↑ megakaryocytes
Splenomegaly (% patients)	60–80%	80–99%	70%	40–50%
Blastic transformation	90%	5–20%	10–15%	5%
Special studies	Ph¹ chromosome	Marrow imaging	RBC mass ↑	Abnormal platelet function tests ↓↓ IL 6

N = normal

8. Bone marrow may demonstrate large numbers of megakaryocytes, sometimes atypical in appearance
9. Elevation of platelet count, giant and/or bizarre platelets
10. Hemorrhagic and thrombotic complications as a result of platelet dysfunction
11. Cytogenetic abnormalities; the most common, in decreasing order of frequency, are 20q−, +8, +9, 13q−, +6;9, +23p, +34q[16] and partial trisomy 1q7 (the Philadelphia chromosome +9;22 is present in about 90% of patients with CML)

Although the CMPDs share clinical manifestations, each disorder is well defined in regard to important differences between the subtypes, pathophysiology, laboratory findings, clinical course, therapeutic options and prognosis. A comparison of the type and amount of cellular proliferations and other specific findings in the CMPDs is provided in Table 21–2.

IDIOPATHIC MYELOFIBROSIS

Definition and History

Within the family of myeloproliferative disorders, idiopathic myelofibrosis (IMF) is an important entity. The syndrome is characterized by the classic triad of findings of: (1) fibrosis of the marrow, at first patchy and later widespread, that may or may not be accompanied by sclerosis; (2) extramedullary hematopoiesis or myeloid metaplasia of the spleen and liver giving rise to moderate to marked splenomegaly and hepatomegaly; and (3) leukoerythroblastosis and teardrop poikilocytosis of the peripheral blood.

IMF was first reported in 1879 by Heuck,[11] who described the case of a 24-year-old butcher who had been afflicted with severe fatigue for 1 year. On examination, severe anemia, leukocytosis with myeloid immaturity, and marked hepatosplenomegaly were noted. The patient survived for only 2 years, and on autopsy was demonstrated to have severe osteosclerosis and extra-medullary hematopoiesis. Heuck[11] thus concluded, based on the unique features of the case, that myelofibrosis with myeloid metaplasia was distinct from leukemia.

At least 20 synonyms have been assigned to this disease. Some of the most frequently employed are agnogenic myeloid metaplasia, myelosclerosis, osteosclerosis, chronic erythroblastosis, aleukemic myelosis, and chronic or primary myelofibrosis. Recently the term idiopathic myelofibrosis with myeloid metaplasia (IMF/MM), or just idiopathic myelofibrosis (IMF) for brevity, has been applied to this disorder, highlighting the essential features of fibrosis and extramedullary hematopoiesis.

Incidence, Epidemiology, and Etiology

There have been a limited number of epidemiologic studies in IMF. An overall annual incidence of 0.6 per 100,000 was found by Woodliffe and Douigan;[12] the disease was stated to be one quarter as common as chronic myelocytic leukemia by Ward and Block.[13] The male-to-female ratio is approximately 2:1. The age distribution is generally between 50 and 70; therefore, as with other MPDs, most IMF cases occur in middle-aged and elderly people. In the below-30 age group, fewer than 30 cases of this disorder have been reported.[14] Certain racial factors of interest have been studied. IMF is said to be rare in African Americans and Spanish Americans[13] and is still occurring in Japanese as a sequela of the atomic bomb. It is generally more prevalent in white persons born in Europe who have subsequently moved to Australia than in other ethnic groups in that country.[9]

Familial CMPDs have been reported in several generations within the same family in which no environmental causative agent was found.[15] This finding suggests a possible genetically inherited etiology.

As the name implies, the cause is unknown in most patients with IMF. Exposure to ionizing radiation is most likely a factor in the development of some cases;

an increased incidence of IMF has been reported in survivors of the Hiroshima atomic bomb blast.[16] Myelofibrosis secondary to exposure to toxins such as benzene, toluene, arsenic, lead, and fluorine has been documented.[17,18] Conditions associated with abnormal immunologic mechanisms have been implicated in the genesis of IMF, as evidenced by its development in patients with lupus erythematosus[19] and the existence in most IMF patients of a high proportion of peripheral leukocytes containing immune complexes.[20] Myelofibrosis has also occurred secondary to chronic infections, especially tuberculosis; to histoplasmosis; and after myocardial infarction. However, the fibrosis seen in these disorders represents a secondary or reactive process.

In the setting of myeloproliferative disorders, a virtually identical syndrome develops in up to 20% of patients with polycythemia vera, as well as a small number of patients with essential thrombocythemia, and can be related to previous radioactive phosphorus (^{32}P) therapy.[21]

Pathogenesis

Stem Cell Defect

The hemopoietic abnormalities in idiopathic myelofibrosis arise from the mutation of a single multipotential stem cell, with bone marrow fibrosis occurring as a secondary, non-neoplastic process. The pathogenesis of the progenitor cell defect must be considered separately from that of the fibrosis.

The clonal proliferation of abnormal progenitor cells colony-forming unit–granulocyte-monocyte (CFU-GM) and colony-forming unit–megakaryocyte (CFU-MK) has been well documented by isoenzyme and cytogenetic studies. Khan and associates[22] and Jacobson and colleagues[4] showed that in women heterozygous for G6PD isoenzymes A and B, the bone marrow fibroblasts express both isoenzymes but the blood cells express only one type. This finding, therefore, suggests that the blood cells are clonally derived, whereas the fibroblasts do not proliferate as a result of the malignant clone. Furthermore, Van Slych and associates[23] showed that the blood cells from an IMF patient had a consistent chromosomal abnormality, in comparison to bone marrow fibroblasts, which had normal karyotypes.

Marrow Fibrosis

The pathogenesis of fibro-osteosclerotic changes characterizing IMF is controversial. However, there is general agreement that the myelofibrosis is related to an increase in marrow collagen accumulation and that the source of collagen synthesis is in the fibroblasts. Hematopoietic cells, their products, or both, provide the provoking stimulus to activate the marrow collagen-producing cells, thus establishing the reactive nature of fibrosis.

A number of factors have been described that are capable of stimulating fibroblastic proliferation. There is current evidence that megakaryocytes are intimately involved in the pathway whereby increased collagen deposition takes place and are a prerequisite for osteo-sclerotic changes. One of the most fully characterized changes in terms of its biologic properties is platelet-derived growth factor (PDGF), which is released from abnormal megakaryocytes and platelets and is found in elevated levels in patients with IMF.[24] An essential feature causally promoting the release of PDGF is ineffective megakaryopoiesis with intramedullary death of megakaryocytes.[17,25] Several reports postulate that immune complexes also interact with platelets to cause release of PDGF with subsequent activation of fibroblastic proliferation and collagen deposition.

A new study by Gersuk[26] has shown consistently impaired natural killer (NK) cells in patients with myelofibrosis. The CD16+ NK cells had detectable PDGF on their surface, and this finding was correlated to significantly inhibited NK cytotoxicity.

Furthermore, platelet factor 4, a cationic polypeptide synthesized by megakaryocytes and contained in platelet alpha granules, inhibits collagenase activity, thereby offsetting the natural balance between marrow collagen production and degradation. This action conversely leads to enhancement of myelofibrosis.[27]

Vitamin D appears to play a role in the regulation of collagen deposition in the marrow. Calcitriol (1,25-dihydroxyvitamin D_3), the active metabolite of vitamin D_3, inhibits collagen synthesis by suppressing megakaryocyte proliferation.[28] A deficiency of this factor would allow abnormal accumulation of marrow collagen, hence leading to development of myelofibrosis (Fig. 21–3).

The histologic course of IMF encompasses several phases. In the so-called cellular phase of IMF, the bone marrow displays panhyperplasia with a predominance of megakaryocytes. As the disease progresses, there is deranged marrow architecture with an increase in reticulin (or a neutral-soluble collagen type III) and a progressive change to and deposition of the type I collagen that are insoluble and cross-linked. It is this type that occurs in osteosclerosis.[29]

The disturbance to the normal hemopoietic microenvironment is responsible for the hematologic abnormalities characteristic of IMF: increase in circulating stem cells, trilineage proliferation and dysplasia (particularly dysmegakaryocytopoiesis), and extravascular hemopoiesis.[29]

Clinical Features

Myelofibrosis is a chronic progressive disorder with such an insidious onset that the patient may be symptom-free for many years. Athens and associates[30] reported a case in which a patient with a palpable spleen was known to have had the enlarged spleen for 15 years before diagnosis. In about one third of the cases, diagnosis is made following a routine physical examination and the incidental finding of unexplained splenomegaly and/or abnormal peripheral blood results. As the myeloid metaplasia gradually increases, with eventual enlargement of the spleen and sometimes the liver, the patient presents with the customary sensation of splenomegaly, namely left or midabdominal fullness and distension and early satiety for food intake, resulting from decreased abdominal capacity caused by splenic encroachment. With massive splenomegaly, urinary frequency and incontinence

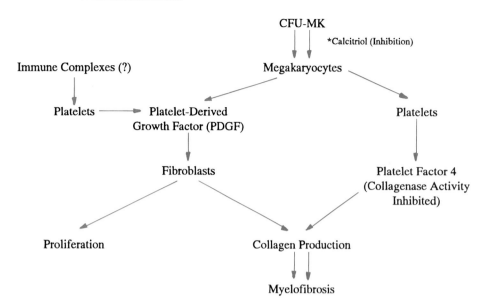

FIGURE 21-3 Schematic representation of possible relationships involved in collagen deposition in myelofibrosis. CFU–MK = colony-forming unit—megakaryocyte. *Calcitriol, 1, 25 (OH)$_2$ D$_3$ is the active metabolite of vitamin D$_3$.

may be a problem. Splenomegaly is more pronounced in IMF than in almost any other disease (Fig. 21–4).

Patients also present with the signs and symptoms of anemia such as weakness, pallor, lethargy, and dyspnea on exertion. Fifteen percent of patients present with a serious bleeding diathesis[2] secondary to thrombocytopenia or thrombocytosis; qualitative platelet defects; and coagulation abnormalities that may cause petechiae, ecchymoses, and gastrointestinal or urogenital bleeding. Bone pain is an occasional feature, usually occurring later in the disease process.

The metabolic consequences of myelofibrosis often result in the symptoms of night sweats, fever, itching, anorexia, and weight loss. Gout may be a complication stemming from hyperuricemia. Ward and Block[13] found gout in 16% of the patients with massive splenomegaly. Although hepatomegaly is found in about 50% of patients,[30] it is not generally excessive but may be accompanied by mild to moderate jaundice and/or ascites.

Extramedullary Hematopoiesis

Splenomegaly and hepatomegaly are present to a varied degree in all patients. The spleen is mildly enlarged in one third of patients, palpable 5 cm below the left costal margin in another third, and massively enlarged in the remaining third.[31] The extraordinary splenic hyperplasia present in IMF is multifactorial in origin. The enlargement is the result of a combination of extramedullary hematopoiesis and fibrosis, as well as congestion from increased blood flow through the celiac axis. Extramedullary hematopoiesis may be present in liver and/or spleen (Fig. 21–5). The exaggeration of red cell pooling is so pronounced that up to two thirds of the red cell mass may be detained in transit through the splenic cords. Hematopoietic precursors evicted from the bone marrow find a hospitable surrogate microenvironment in the spleen and, to some extent, in the liver and lymph nodes. Stem cells capable of self-renewal give rise to neoplastic islands

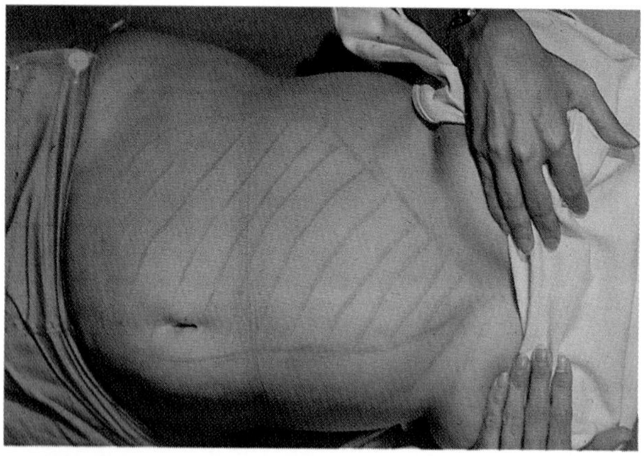

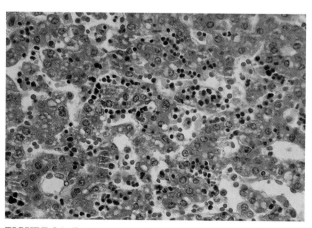

FIGURE 21-4 Hepatosplenomegaly, a characteristic finding in patients with idiopathic myelofibrosis with myeloid metaplasia (IMF-MM).

FIGURE 21-5 Extramedullary hematopoiesis in the liver of a patient with IMF.

that may circulate via the splenic vein to other reticuloendothelial system organs. Extramedullary tumors may occasionally arise in the central nervous system, accounting for symptoms of speech impairment, semiblindness, partial paralysis, coma, and possibly death if the intracranial space has been invaded.[27]

Radiologic Features

Myelofibrosis is defined as an increase in fine fibers (reticular) in the marrow; *myelosclerosis* means an increase in coarse fibers (collagen); and *osteomyelosclerosis* refers to an additional new bone formation.[29] Approximately 40% to 50% of patients demonstrate radiologic osteosclerosis. The most readily recognizable pattern is diffuse increase in bone density in the long bones. In most cases this finding is readily visible on chest x-ray examinations.

Hematologic Features

A normocytic, normochromic anemia is found in most patients at presentation and becomes more severe as the myelofibrosis progresses. The anemia results from a complex reaction of factors representing the additive effects of bone marrow failure, ineffective or dyserythropoiesis, pooling of over 35% of the erythrocyte mass in the enlarged spleen (dilutional anemia), and an underlying hemolysis caused by hypersplenism. In half of the anemic patients, there is shortened red cell survival, again the result of the ineffective erythropoiesis combined with hyperplasia. When severe hemolytic anemia occurs as evidenced by marked reticulocytosis, it is generally antiglobulin (Coombs') test negative. However, in some cases of IMF, the erythrocytes are mildly Coombs-positive as a result of deposition of IgG and IgM immune complexes and complement on the erythrocyte surfaces.[27]

Occasionally patients develop a hypochromic, microcytic anemia secondary to gastrointestinal bleeding or peptic ulcer, and sometimes the hyperproliferative state induces folate deficiency and a concomitant megaloblastic macrocytosis.

As the myelofibrosis progresses, the morphological changes become increasingly abnormal and the classic leukoerythroblastic blood picture unfolds (see Fig. 15-8). The characteristic findings are the appearance of abundant nucleated red cells, immature granulocytes, and teardrop poikilocytosis (Fig. 21-6). Improvement or even normalization of red cell morphology after splenectomy supports the concept of a causative relationship between splenic fibrosis and red cell changes.[32] Marrow fibrosis in conjunction with splenic fibrosis presumably accounts for teardrop formation, as the erythrocytes assume the teardrop shape on passage through narrow, fibrotic sinusoids of the bone marrow and spleen (Fig. 21-7).

The leukocyte count is variable in IMF. In about 50% of cases the white blood cell (WBC) count exceeds 10.0 $\times$ 10^9/L; in approximately 35%, the WBC count is normal; and in nearly 15%, the WBC count is below normal.[13,33] As the disease evolves, the leukocyte count declines with an increase of immature myeloid cells dominating the peripheral blood picture, but not to the

degree seen in acute myelocytic leukemia. In rare cases in which the WBC count exceeds 100 $\times$ 10^9/L, the diagnosis of chronic myelocytic leukemia (CML) may be erroneously applied. The leukocyte alkaline phosphatase (LAP) score is typically normal or moderately increased. Serum levels of vitamin B$_{12}$ are increased, but not to the degree found in untreated CML. Eosinophils and basophils may also be increased in number in many patients.

The platelet count may be normal, elevated, or decreased. In approximately 50% of IMF patients, platelet counts are increased at time of diagnosis, and the concentration may occasionally be more than 1000 $\times$ 10^9/L. As the disease progresses, thrombocytopenia becomes increasingly prevalent. Giant dysplastic platelets are often conspicuous, and megakaryocytic fragments or even dwarf megakaryocytes may be present in the peripheral blood (see Fig. 21-6). These findings attest to malignant platelet physiology and support the correlation of platelet dysfunction found in up to 50% of patients.[34] Platelet adhesiveness is often reduced and, conversely, spontaneous aggregation may occur, clinically resulting in increased risk of hemorrhage or thrombosis. According to one study by Silverstein,[31] the bleeding time (a measure of platelet number and function) was prolonged in 20% of the patients, which is particularly important in relation to gastrointestinal or cerebral hemorrhage.

Bone Marrow Findings

Attempts at bone marrow aspirations are unsuccessful in nearly 90% of patients, resulting in the so-called dry tap of myelofibrosis. The reticulin and collagen fibrosis locks in the marrow contents, making a needle biopsy essential for a reliable diagnosis (Fig. 21-8). Trilineage hyperplasia is found early in the disease, along with nonuniform fibrosis. At later stages, there is a decreasing number of hematopoietic islands with residual foci consisting mainly of clumps of dysplastic megakaryocytes. Finally, marked hypocellularity is observed, and fibrotic features begin to predominate. In less than 10% of patients, osteosclerosis (new bone deposition) occurs (Table 21-3). The bone marrow hypocellularity and peripheral blood pancytopenia prevail because the myeloid metaplasia does not compensate for the loss of bone marrow function resulting from the marrow fibrosis.

Coagulation Abnormalities

Platelet dysfunction (mentioned earlier) can cause troublesome hemostatic complications in IMF patients. Both hypoplatelet and hyperplatelet function have been reported, with hypofunction seen more often.[35] In addition, patients in approximately half of the cases demonstrate prolonged prothrombin and thrombin times, as well as elevated levels of fibrin degradation products and reduced levels of factors V and VIII. These features suggest occult disseminated intravascular coagulation (DIC).[5]

Hepatic dysfunction is found in many patients in the later stages of the disease, setting the scene for coagulation factor deficiencies, chronic DIC, and fibrinolytic activation.

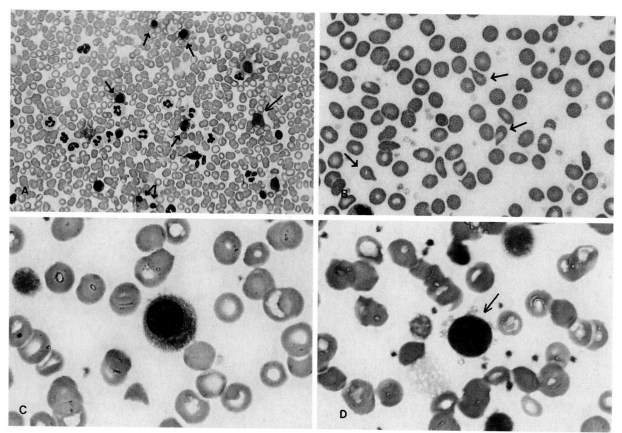

FIGURE 21-6 Leukoerythroblastosis, teardrop poikilocytosis, and abnormal platelet morphology associated with idiopathic myelofibrosis. (*A*) Leukoerythroblastosis. Note the myeloblast at the large arrow and the numerous nucleated red blood cells at the small arrows. (*B*) Teardrop poikilocytosis. (*C*) Dwarf megakaryocyte (or micromegakaryocyte). This pathologic alteration of a megakaryocyte may be found in any of the myeloproliferative disorders. Although this cell is often difficult to distinguish from cells of other lineages, observation of the marked cytoplasmic granularity and further comparision of this cytoplasm to that of other platelets present on the peripheral smear will aid in identification. (*D*) Dwarf megakaryocyte. The cell at the pointer displays cytoplasmic blebs or budding of platelets, which is another characteristic of a micromegakaryocyte. Also note the giant platelets present on this peripheral blood smear.

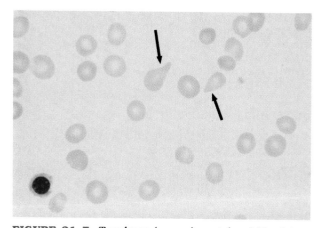

FIGURE 21-7 Teardrops (*arrows*): peripheral blood in a patient with myelofibrosis.

Miscellaneous Findings

Most patients have some type of chromosome abnormality; particularly common are deletions of the long arm of chromosome 13 (13q−) and t(1;13) translocations.[36]

Hyperuricemia and elevated liver enzyme levels are found in one third of IMF patients. Circulating anti-Gal antibodies directed against a terminal galactosyl α(1,3) galactose molecules have been shown to increase in correlation with disease activity and may provide a future sensitive tool to detect IMF.[37]

Differential Diagnosis

Idiopathic myelofibrosis must be distinguished from other diseases within the spectrum of the CMPDs and differentiated from fibrosis secondary to infiltrative disorders (Tables 21-2 and 21-4).

The American Polycythemia Vera Study Group (PVSG) has defined myelofibrosis as encompassing the following features:

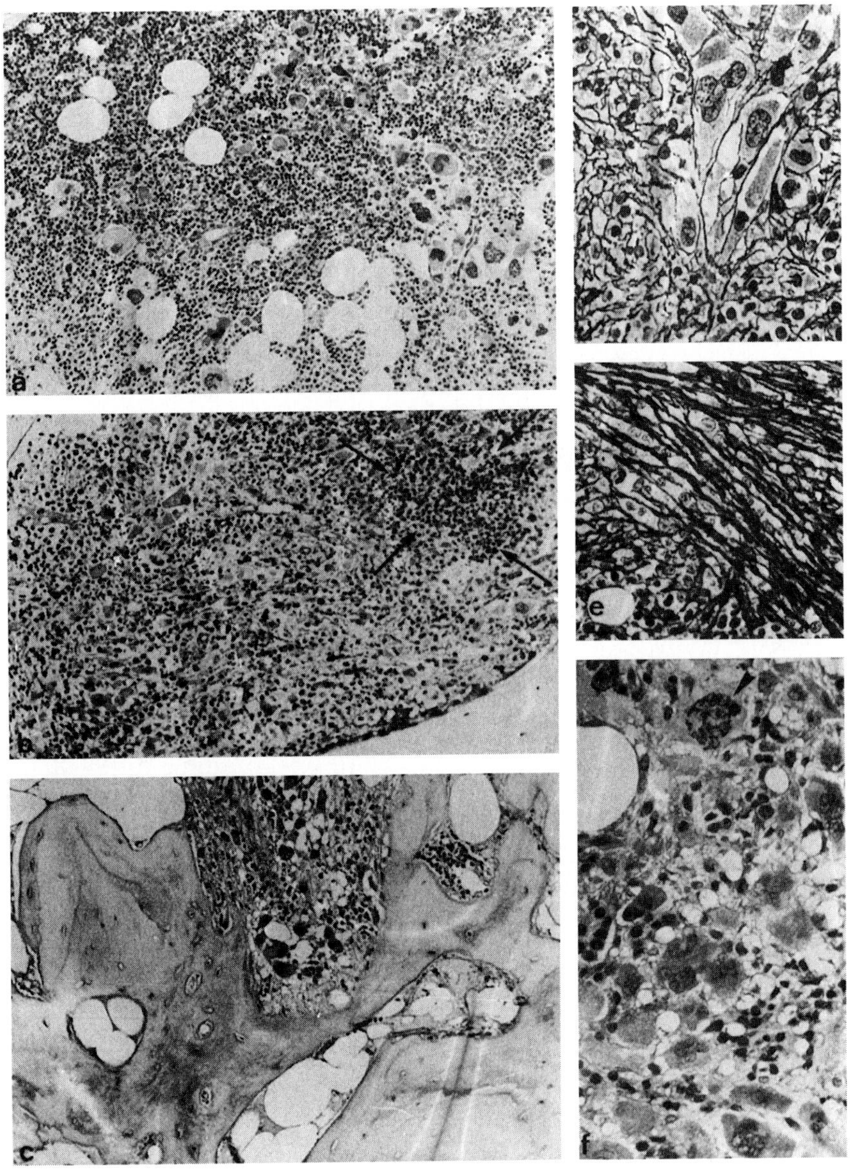

FIGURE 21-8 Histopathology of the bone marrow in idiopathic myelofibrosis. (*A*) Early hyperplastic state without fibrosis. (*B*) Advanced stage with a conspicuous increase in reticulin fibers and a still hypercellular marrow and a lymphoid infiltrate (*arrows*). (*C*) Late osteosclerotic state with endophytic bone formation, a residual cluster of hematopoiesis, and large areas of fatty tissue. (*D*) Moderate degree of reticulin fibers surrounding atypical megakaryocytes in early IMF. (*E*) Coarse bundles of obvious collagen fibers encompassing a few hematopoietic elements in terminal stages of IMF. (*F*) Clusters of pleomorphic megakaryocytes displaying abnormal maturation and mitosis (*arrowhead*). a–c, ×140; d–f, ×350. a–c, f PAS stain; d,e Gomori's silver impregnation. (From Thiele, J et al: Primary myelofibrosis–osteosclerosis. Agnogenic mecloid metaplasia. AntiCa Res 9:430, 1989, with permission.)

1. Splenomegaly
2. Fibrosis involving more than one third of the sectional area of an adequate bone marrow biopsy specimen
3. A leukoerythroblastic blood picture
4. Absence of increased red cell mass
5. Absence of Philadelphia (Ph[1]) chromosome
6. Exclusion of systemic disorders
7. A diagnosis of osteomyelosclerosis requiring the presence of sclerotic changes detected radiologically in axial skeleton long bones[17]

CML is the diagnosis considered most frequently in the differential diagnosis of IMF. In chronic cases of CML, there is marked leukocytosis, whereas in IMF the WBC count is usually less than 30×10^9/L. Red cell morphology in CML is generally normal or may show a slight amount of anisocytosis and poikilocytosis, compared with the significant teardrop poikilocytosis in IMF. The presence of the Ph[1] and LAP score are the strongest differentiating features that distinguish CML from IMF. Ordinarily, differentiation from CML is not difficult. However, in atypical cases such as Ph[1]-negative CML, it may be virtually impossible to characterize CML as a separate entity from IMF with leukocytosis and minimal fibrosis (the cellular phase of IMF).

Approximately 15% to 20% of patients with known PV undergo a transition to terminal myelofibrosis with marked anemia, bone marrow fibrosis and hypofunction, and progressive splenomegaly. An intermediate or transitional myeloproliferative disease has been described as occurring in a group of patients with polycythemic peripheral blood counts and concomitant

TABLE 21–3 Histological Course of Idiopathic Myelofibrosis as Seen in Bone Marrow

Cellular Phase
Diffusely hyperplastic; normal maturation of erythropoiesis and granulopoiesis
Megakaryocytes may predominate; some immature forms
Reticulin ± increase
Fibrotic Phase
Megakaryocytes still predominant; decreasing numbers of other hemopoietic cells
Altered sinus architecture
Reticulin ++
Collagen +
Sclerotic Phase
Grossly disturbed architecture
Markedly reduced hematopoiesis
Megakaryocyte and megakaryoblast clusters
Fibroblasts +++
Reticulin +++
Collagen +++
Osteosclerotic Phase
Fibroblasts +++
Collagen +++
Osteocyte proliferation with bone formation

Source: Lewis,[2] p. 4, with permission.

features of myelofibrosis, including myeloid metaplasia, leukoerythroblastic blood picture, and extensive reticulin-collagen fibrosis of the marrow. This subset of transitional patients seems to remain in a steady state for several years, whereas patients in the terminal post-PV spent phase of myelofibrosis undergo a more aggressive course.

Idiopathic myelofibrosis must be differentiated from secondary causes of myelofibrosis. Metastatic carci-

TABLE 21–4 Differential Diagnosis of Myelofibrosis

Idiopathic Myelofibrosis
Other chronic myeloproliferative disorders
  Chronic myelogeneous leukemia
  Polycythemia vera
  Essential thrombocythemia
  Transitional myeloproliferative disorders
Secondary to infiltrative disorders
  Metastatic carcinoma
  Hematologic malignancies involving bone marrow
    Acute leukemia
    Myelodysplastic syndromes (preleukemia)
    Hairy-cell leukemia
    Non-Hodgkin's lymphoma
    Myeloma
Secondary to nonmalignant conditions

Granulomatous disorders	Osteoporosis
Sarcoidosis	Vitamin D deficiency
Tuberculosis	Systemic lupus
Histoplasmosis	erythematosus
Toxic exposure to	Systemic sclerosis
chemicals	
Hypoparathyroidism and	
hyperparathyroidism	

noma and lymphoma are frequent causes of fibrosis.[38] Granulomatous disorders such as tuberculosis, histoplasmosis, or sarcoidosis of the marrow can cause myelofibrosis. Other hematologic diseases including acute leukemia, hairy cell leukemia, and myelodysplastic syndromes may induce secondary fibrosis (see Table 21–4). The cause of the infiltrative disorders can usually be established by careful scrutiny of the blood and bone marrow for evidence of abnormal cells that characterize the disease, by use of microbiologic cultures, and other diagnostic tests such as chest x-rays or skin tests. In certain situations (such as when a patient has acute leukemia) techniques of cytochemistry, immunologic surface markers, and electron microscopy studies may help to define the nature of the malignancy.

Treatment

The primary aim of treatment in IMF is to improve the quality of life, since few patients with IMF have been cured. Approximately 30% of patients are asymptomatic at diagnosis, and because there is no evidence that treatment increases survival time, these patients are best left untreated. Eventually most patients manifest symptoms caused by anemia, splenic enlargement, bleeding, bone pain, or hypermetabolism. Treatment of these complications is palliative and invasive procedures should be limited.

One of the major problems requiring therapy is anemia. It has been estimated that 60% of patients with IMF sooner or later manifest signs of anemia during their clinical course.[31] Transfusion dependence develops as the anemia becomes more severe. In most cases, the anemia is normochromic, normocytic, whereas 5% of patients develop iron-deficiency anemia, and rare patients demonstrate folate or vitamin B_{12} deficiency. When nutritional deficiencies are suspected, patients are treated with iron, folate, or pyridoxine as appropriate. If inefficient erythropoiesis is the predominant mechanism, androgen therapy is indicated. Approximately 40% of anemic individuals respond to androgen therapy and should be given a trial of either oxymetholone (50 to 200 mg orally daily) or testosterone enamthate (400 mg intramuscularly every 3 to 4 weeks). Patients receiving oxymethalone require careful monitoring of liver function tests.[29]

Patients with thrombocytopenia may be treated with adrenal steroids.[2] About 50% of patients respond to the combination of androgen and glucocorticoid therapy (prednisone, 30 mg daily). The benefit of androgen therapy in IMF is still debatable[35] and long-term treatment may have annoying side effects, particularly fluid retention and hirsutism (excessive unusual growth of hair, especially in women).[25]

The main aim of treatment in patients with progressive splenomegaly is to remove the spleen or reduce its size, thereby relieving the severe pain caused by pressure and ameliorating the constitutional symptoms of serious digestive disturbances, weight loss, and diarrhea.

Although there is no general agreement on the indications and value of this invasive modality, splenectomy is important in the management of patients with IMF who have profoundly enlarged spleens. The main problem is that patients with symptoms that can be relieved by splenectomy are poor surgical risks and "good risk patients seldom need palliative surgery."[39] Timing for a splenectomy operation is difficult and the postoperative complication rate is above average.[40]

Four major life-threatening conditions have been espoused as situations warranting consideration of splenectomy:[41]

1. Painful splenic enlargement that is unresponsive to irradiation
2. Severe refractory hemolytic or dilutional anemia sufficient to cause cardiopulmonary symptoms
3. Severe life-threatening thrombocytopenia
4. Portal hypertension with bleeding varices

Whenever splenectomy is contemplated, an extensive coagulation workup is necessary because bleeding is a major hazard.

Because the spleen may become the major hematopoietic organ in patients whose marrow has been replaced by fibrosis, it is vital to ensure that splenectomy is considered only when splenic hematopoiesis constitutes a minor (less than 15% to 20%) proportion of total hematopoiesis. This can be quantified by bone imaging and measurement of transferrin-bound ^{52}Fe uptake. Mean survival following splenectomy is approximately 25 months. This procedure does not seem to alter the overall clinical course, and the mortality and morbidity, estimated at 10% to 25%, are mainly the result of bleeding, thromboembolism, and infection (the same causes as in patients who have not had splenectomy). After splenectomy, approximately 16% of patients will develop a compensatory myeloid metaplasia of the liver, further increasing the amount of hepatomegaly.[2]

Chemotherapy is an alternative to splenectomy to reduce spleen size and control thrombocytosis, but it has little or no beneficial effect on the anemia. The alkylating agents busulfan (2 to 4 mg daily), chlorambucil (4 to 6 mg daily), and more recently hydroxyurea[42] have been used. Other additional agents such as radiophosphate and 6-thioguanine have also been advocated. If antitumor therapy is used, the treatment must be strictly monitored by regular blood counts in order to avoid inducing dangerous cytopenias in the patient.

Radiation therapy is also considered in patients with massive mechanical splenomegaly, although, as with the use of chemotherapy, the duration of the reduction in splenic size is usually measured in months. In patients having acute splenic infarction, ascites demonstrating prominent megakaryocytosis, or focal but severe bone pain, the use of radiation may produce gratifying effects.[31]

Allogeneic marrow transplantation following ablative chemotherapy or radiotherapy has been attempted in a few patients and offers a rational means of curing myelofibrosis. However, it is controversial whether or not the application of this rigorous therapy to a chronic disease, generally limited to the elderly, is judicious. Disappearance of fibrosis and regeneration of normal medullary hematopoiesis have been achieved in responsive patients, yet it is still to be ascertained whether the fibrosis found in IMF and the reactive fibrosis of other disorders is reversible and therefore curable.

Allopurinol therapy is warranted in almost all patients to prevent the hyperuricemia from progressing to gout or urate nephropathy.[43]

A new, significant approach to the treatment of myelofibrosis is the utilization of antifibrosing agents such as penicillamine or colchicine. Biochemically, as myelofibrosis progresses, there is increasing conversion of soluble to insoluble collagen. Penicillamine interferes with the cross-linkage of collagen and, therefore, with its use, a decrease in fibrous tissue occurs. It is still unclear whether penicillamine has a significant effect on the natural course of this disease.

Another agent, colchicine, appears to produce its antifibrosing effect through two mechanisms: (1) it produces a decreased rate of procollagen and (2) it increases the secretion of collagenases.[29,44]

Prognosis

Patients with IMF make up extremely heterogeneous populations and survival varies considerably. Median survival is approximately 5 years from the time of diagnosis; however, at least two major subpopulations have been identified. The first (low-risk) group is characterized by a benign or slowly progressive disease with a median survival of 10 years or longer and a young age (under 45). The second, less fortunate (high-risk) group is distinguished by a short survival of 2 years and older age group (over 45). Many patients in this subgroup die after acute blastic transformation.[45]

Besides age, a number of prognostic indicators have been identified; the most important in regard to long survival include the following:

1. Lack of symptoms
2. Effective erythropoiesis evidenced by hemoglobin level greater than 10 g/dL, reticulocyte count greater than 2%, bone marrow showing normal erythropoiesis
3. Platelet counts above 100×10^9/L
4. Absence of significant hepatosplenomegaly

Conversely, patients with severe ineffective hematopoiesis and marrow failure, marked splenomegaly with plasma volume expansion and portal hypertension, red cell mass reduction, or excessive hemolysis fare poorly, having an average survival of only 1 to 2 years. The major causes of death are acute myocardial infarction, congestive heart failure, gastrointestinal and cerebral hemorrhage, and infection.

Between 5% and 15% of patients have a terminal transformation to leukemia, acute myelogenous leukemia in most instances, with a rapidly progressive, fatal outcome. Rarely, patients die of liver or renal failure, and development of acute lymphocytic leukemia[46] and erythroleukemia[47] has been reported.

Major scientific advances and application of new knowledge have taken place in recent years. Relevant discoveries in the areas of collagen biochemistry and histochemistry, bone marrow ultrastructure, cell culture studies, and cell growth regulation have allowed a more in-depth understanding of the pathologic processes involved in the disease of myelofibrosis. As new, innovative strategies are applied to the treatment of this complex disease, it is hoped that there will be a significant improvement in both the survival and quality of life of patients with IMF.

THE POLYCYTHEMIAS

A number of diverse conditions may cause an elevation in the hematocrit (Hct). Initially these disorders can be separated into two groups based on the determination of the red cell (RC) mass (Table 21–5). In the absolute polycythemias, the RC mass (or RC volume) is elevated, implying a true increase in the number of circulating erythrocytes. By contrast, in relative polycythemia, there is an increased Hct in the absence of an elevation in RC volume. This state is the result of an increase in the ratio of RC mass to the plasma volume, as would occur with dehydration (in which the plasma volume is contracted or decreased).

The absolute polycythemias may be further divided into three distinct groups: (1) the chronic myeloproliferative disorder, polycythemia vera, arising as a clonal hematologic malignancy of the bone marrow; (2) secondary polycythemias representing a physiologic response to abnormal stimulus (e.g., tissue hypoxia, increased erythropoietic activity); or (3) an idiopathic group for which neither a myeloproliferative nor secondary cause of sustained erythrocytosis can be implicated. An overall comparison of these three groups of polycythemia can be found in Table 21–6. Primary polycythemia vera is discussed in length first.

Polycythemia Vera: Description, History, and Pathogenesis

Polycythemia vera (PV) is a hematopoietic stem cell disorder predominantly characterized by accelerated erythropoiesis and, to varying degrees, excessive proliferation of myeloid and megakaryocytic elements of the bone marrow (Figs. 21–9 and 21–10). As mentioned earlier, the absolute increase in RC mass is the sine qua non for establishing the diagnosis of PV. In keeping with other myeloproliferative disorders, the manifestations of splenomegaly, myeloid metaplasia, and myelofibrosis are variably expressed at diagnosis and throughout the course of the disease. Most commonly, at the time of initial presentation the degree of extramedullary hematopoiesis is usually mild and marrow fibrosis is most often minimal. However, 15% to 20% of patients transform to a spent phase with progressive anemia and increasing splenomegaly, this development being virtually indistinguishable from idiopathic myelofibrosis.

The nature of this disease has been controversial over the years. Hippocrates recognized "plethora vera,"[48] and Von Haller in 1730[49] associated throm-

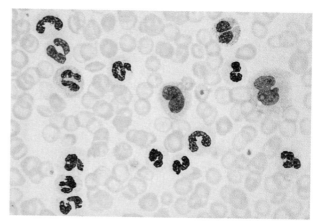

FIGURE 21–9 Polycythemia vera (PV) (peripheral blood). Note hypochromia and increased cellularity. (Magnification ×400)

bosis with the frequent occurrence of gangrene. Vasques, Cabot, and, in 1903, Olsen first characterized the disease as autonomous erythrocytosis, additionally noting the concurrent feature of splenomegaly.[50] Turk[51] in 1904 described the leukoerythroblastic blood picture as well as documenting the finding of increased granulocytic and megakaryocytic activity. The replacement of normal marrow by fibrotic and sclerotic tissue was reported by Hirsch[52] in 1935,

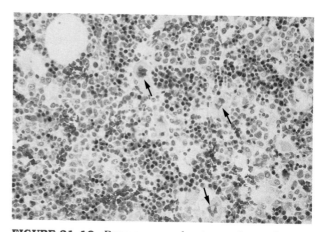

FIGURE 21–10 Bone marrow showing panhyperplasia in PV. Note increased number of megakaryocytes (*arrow*). Hematoxylin and eosin stain (low power).

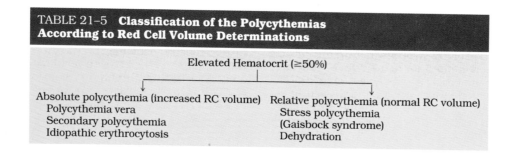

TABLE 21–5 Classification of the Polycythemias According to Red Cell Volume Determinations

Elevated Hematocrit (≥50%)

Absolute polycythemia (increased RC volume)	Relative polycythemia (normal RC volume)
Polycythemia vera	Stress polycythemia
Secondary polycythemia	(Gaisbock syndrome)
Idiopathic erythrocytosis	Dehydration

and by 1938, Rosenthal and Bassen[53] had delineated the natural history and cause of the disease. The concept of the myeloproliferative diseases was originally proposed in the 1950s by Damshek,[1] and since that time the body of knowledge encompassing polycythemia has greatly expanded.

It has now been clearly established that the cell of origin in PV is an abnormal pluripotent stem cell. This has been demonstrated by studies of black women with PV who were heterozygous for the two different G6PD isoenzymes. In these women, only one of the isoenzymes was present in the progenitors and progeny of erythroid, granulocytic, monocytic, and megakaryocytic cell lines, whereas nonhematopoietic tissue displayed both isoenzymes A and B.[2] In normal, healthy women, equal amounts of isoenzyme types would be found in blood cells. These findings strongly suggest that the abnormal hematopoietic cells arise from a single malignant clone. Furthermore, some patients eventually develop marrow fibrosis, and this occurrence appears to be a reactive process. Just as in myelofibrosis, the excessive fibroblastic proliferation is a result of the release of certain growth factors from abnormal megakaryocytes.[54]

When blood and bone marrow cells from patients with PV are cultured on semisolid media, erythroid colonies (colony-forming unit—erythroid [CFU-E] and burst-forming unit—erythroid [BFU-E]) will be formed without the addition of exogenous erythropoietin. This led to the original presumption that erythroid colonies grew spontaneously, because in normal individuals, formation of erythroid colonies is dependent on erythropoietin, which acts in the committed erythroid cell line causing increased proliferation. It has now been suggested that the erythroid progenitors are extremely sensitive to low levels of erythropoietin supplied by the serum that is inherently present in the basic culture medium. Cultures of erythroid precursor cells are one of the tests currently advocated in the differential diagnosis of PV versus secondary polycythemia.[55]

Epidemiology

PV is a relatively rare disease with an annual incidence of approximately 2 cases per 100,000 population. The median age at diagnosis is 60 years, but onset may occur from adolescence to old age. According to Danish,[56] nine cases of childhood PV have been documented. The disease has a slightly higher incidence in men than in women. Familial occurrences, although rare, have been reported. A cluster of MPDs, including PV cases, has been reported in Ashkenazi Jews in northern Israel, where the incidence of MPDs in Jews was 10 times higher than in the Arab population.[57] The etiology of PV remains unknown, as it is in other MPDs.

Clinical Features

PV has an insidious onset and is often discovered quite incidentally when an elevated hemoglobin (Hgb) or Hct level is discovered following a routine examination. In other cases, development of characteristic symptoms related to increased RC volume or hyperviscosity may herald the recognition of the disease (Fig. 21–11). Common complaints caused by cerebral circulatory disturbances and transient ischemic attacks include headaches, dizziness, vertigo, visual phenomena (blurred vision, diplopia, scotomas), tinnitus, and rarely mild dementia. Vascular complications are manifested equally in arteries and veins. Thrombotic episodes, such as phlebitis, myocardial infarction, erythromelalgia (painful red extremities), paraesthesia, and burning sensations, particularly in the feet, reflect impairment of blood flow to the peripheral circulation. Dawson and coworkers[58] proposed that the coexistent thrombocytosis acts in conjunction with the hyperviscosity and high blood volume to increase the incidence of thrombosis, thromboembolism, and hemorrhage in these patients. Incidence of morbidity and mortality from vessel wall disease is already high in this age group, and concomitant high Hct level adversely influences the outcome of occlusive events.

Hemorrhagic diathesis is often seen in patients with PV. Life-threatening hemorrhage may occur in association with trauma, surgery, or peptic ulcer. Spontaneous minor hemorrhages in the form of epistaxis, gingival bleeding, and ecchymoses are common events almost certainly caused by qualitative platelet abnormalities.

The presence of splenomegaly in about 75% of patients is a finding of significant differential importance. The splenic enlargement is usually mild to moderate and is the result of extramedullary hematopoiesis and not of the expanded blood volume per se (the spleen size does not diminish as blood volume is reduced by phlebotomy). Patients having moderate splenomegaly appear more likely to evolve to IMF at an early stage. Modest hepatomegaly is observed in one third of patients at the time of initial presentation (Table 21–6).

Portal hypertension and esophageal variceal hemorrhage are sometimes reported. These occur because of the excessive flow of blood from the spleen into the portal system.[2]

A common physical finding is ruddy cyanosis of the face, nose, ears, and lips. This facial plethora results from conjunctival and mucosal blood vessel congestion. Patients have stated that the appearance of their ruddy complexion has prompted friends to comment that they "look wonderful."[59]

Pruritus, occurring in about 30% of patients, is especially troublesome after a hot shower. The pathogenesis of the persistent itching and urticaria, occurring in 10% of patients, is related to elevated levels of histamine produced by basophils and other granulocytes.

Fever, night (and day) sweats, and weight loss may occur as a result of the hypermetabolic state. Gout ascribed to increased nucleoprotein turnover occurs in 5% to 10% of patients. Uric acid calculi or urate nephropathy may arise from the increased uric acid excretion.

Laboratory Features (see Table 21–6)

Elevation of the Hgb and Hct levels is the most important finding in PV; however, polycythemia may be masked if accompanying iron deficiency is present. The diagnosis of PV requires the demonstration of an increase in red cell mass as part of the initial evaluation of erythrocytosis. The ^{51}Cr dilution technique is a simple, well established method for direct measure-

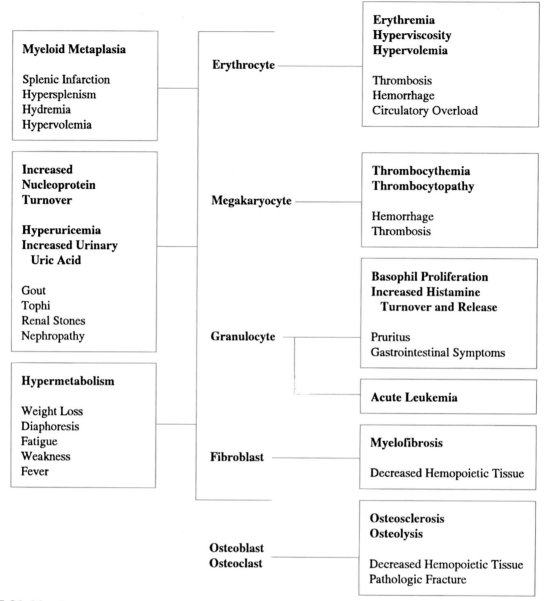

FIGURE 21-11 Physiological complications of polycythemia vera. The clinical features of this disorder are attributable to the excessive proliferation of the three main hematopoietic cell lines and reactive proliferation in bone marrow fibroblasts. (From Gilbert,[103] p. 359, with permission.)

ment of total red cell mass. Absolute erythrocytosis is present in men with values at least 36 mL/kg and in women with at least 32 mL/kg. The plasma volume can be measured with human serum albumin labeled with I^{125} or I^{131}, and is normal or slightly reduced. A calculation of RC mass from plasma volume gives unreliable results, because a disproportionate increase in plasma volume occurs in pronounced splenomegaly as a result of red cell pooling.

Characteristically, at presentation there is increased red cell production at intramedullary sites. The erythrocytes are normochromic, normocytic, and have a normal life span. As the disease progresses, extramedullary ineffective hematopoiesis leads to an increasing anisocytosis and poikilocytosis, as well as shortened red cell life span secondary to splenic sequestration.[60] Some patients demonstrate the microcytosis and hypochromia associated with iron deficiency as low serum iron occurs in about one half of patients[2] (see Fig. 21-9). This iron deficiency has been attributed to consumption of iron because of the tremendous increase in erythropoiesis as well as possible occult gastrointestinal blood loss and defective platelet function.[61] The reticulocyte count is usually normal, and only

TABLE 21–6 Features of PV, Secondary (Hypoxic) Polycythemia, and Relative Erythrocytosis			
Manifestations	Polycythemia Vera	Secondary Polycythemia	Relative Erythrocytosis
Clinical features			
Cyanosis (warm)	Absent	Present	May be present
Heart or lung disease	Absent	Present	Absent
Splenomegaly	Present in 75%	Absent	Absent
Hepatomegaly	Present in 35%	Absent	Absent
Laboratory features			
Arterial oxygen saturation	Normal	Decreased (rarely normal)	Normal
Red cell mass	Increased	Increased	Normal
Leukocyte	Increased in 80%	Normal	Normal
Platelet count	Increased in 50%	Normal	Normal
Nucleated red cells, poikilocytes	Often present	Absent	Absent
Leukocyte alkaline phosphatase (LAP)	Elevated	Normal	Normal
Bone marrow	Hypercellular; increased erythropoiesis and myelopoiesis; increased megakaryocytes; fibrosis	Increased erythropoiesis	Normal
Erythropoietin (Epo)	Decreased (rarely normal)	Increased (rarely normal)	Normal
Serum vitamin B_{12}	Elevated in 75%	Normal	Normal
Culture studies	Autonomous, erythroid proliferation	Epo-dependent colony formation	Not applicable

rarely are immature erythrocytes found in the peripheral blood.

Relative and absolute granulocytosis occurs in two thirds of the patients. The elevation in total WBC count is usually moderate, with counts in the range of 12 to 25×10^9/L. Occasionally basophilia and eosinophilia are apparent and few metamyelocytes, myelocytes, and even more immature cells may be seen on examination of the peripheral smear.

Thrombocytosis is present at the time of diagnosis in about 50% of the patients with PV. The platelet count is most often moderately elevated, with counts between 450 and 800×10^9/L, but in about 5% the platelet count exceeds 1000×10^9/L. Morphological alterations of platelets include the presence of giant platelets and deficient granulation. Studies show that most patients with PV form spontaneous megakaryocytic colonies analogous to spontaneous erythroid colony formation seen in all MPDs.[62] Platelets from most patients demonstrate some abnormality in aggregation studies, but the results of these laboratory tests correlate poorly with clinical thrombotic and hemorrhagic episodes. Also of interest is the fact that in most patients, even those with bleeding diathesis, the bleeding time, which is the best measurement of in vivo platelet function, is nearly always normal.[63]

When performing coagulation tests on PV patients, such as prothrombin time (PT), activated partial thromboplastin time (APTT), and thrombin time (TT), the anticoagulant-blood ratio must be maintained at 1:9. Sodium citrate functions as an anticoagulant by binding calcium in plasma. In the case of erythrocytosis, in which plasma volume is decreased, citrate is left in excess in the vacutainer tube. This residual citrate is then available to bind calcium in the test system, thus causing falsely prolonged clotting times.

When the Hct is greater than 55%, the following adjustment for the volume of anticoagulant should be applied:

$$(0.00185) \ (V) \ (100 - Hct) = C$$

where V = volume of whole blood
C = volume of anticoagulant, in milliliters

The PT, APTT, TT and fibrinogen levels are generally normal in patients with PV. The bone marrow is hypercellular with decreased fat content in nearly all cases. Panhyperplasia is evident to a varying extent, in contrast to the exclusive erythroid hyperplasia seen in secondary polycythemia (see Fig. 21–10). Besides the striking increase in the number of megakaryocytes, they are often increased in size. Marrow iron stores, demonstrated by Prussian blue staining, are reduced or absent. As previously mentioned, this apparently relates to the increased utilization of iron in the process of excessive erythropoiesis and the subsequent expansion of red cell mass, in addition to the chronic occult blood loss. Early in the course of PV, fibrosis is a rare finding. If serial biopsies are performed, a progressive increase in reticulin deposits can often be demonstrated during the active phase of the disease and before the spent phase develops.[64] As the disease runs its course, cellularity usually decreases, although megakaryocytosis may persist. The transition to frank myelofibrosis occurs in 15% to 20% of patients.

The arterial oxygen saturation is normal in most patients with PV; however, infrequently the oxygen saturation may be slightly lowered (88% to 92%). This feature is helpful in excluding erythrocytosis secondary to pulmonary and cardiac abnormalities, wherein the oxygen saturation is routinely decreased.

Patients with PV have absent or reduced plasma and urine erythropoietin, which can now be measured by a very sensitive radioimmunoassay procedure. There is no significant rise in the levels of erythropoietin following phlebotomy and normalization of the Hgb and Hct. As mentioned previously, autonomous or spontaneous erythroid colonies can be grown in culture medium without the addition of exogenous erythropoietin, which demonstrates that endogenous erythroid colony (EEC) formation can occur from culture of peripheral blood of patients with PV. This finding is considered by many investigators to be of diagnostic value. The addition of both interleukin-3 (IL-3) or alpha-interferon (alpha-IFN) and subsequent increase in EEC has given an even better diagnostic discrimination between PV and secondary polycythemia patients.[65]

The LAP activity is increased in 75% of PV cases[17] (Fig. 21–12). The determination of the LAP may be inconsequential in differential diagnosis of erythrocytosis because some patients with PV have a normal LAP score, as do most patients with secondary erythrocytosis (in the absence of inflammation, infection, or hormonal therapy).

Two of the three vitamin B_{12}–binding proteins, transcobalamin I and III, are frequently elevated in PV, as in other MPDs. Transcobalamin III is the binding protein most commonly elevated in PV, whereas transcobalmin I is predominantly increased in chronic myelogeneous leukemia.[66] These increased serum values are attributed to the excessive granulocyte turnover. Furthermore, the unsaturated B_{12} binding capacity ($UB_{12}BC$) is increased in approximately 75% of patients.[67]

Hyperuricemia and uricosuria are present in 40% of patients with PV at the time of presentation. This is a frequent finding in many hypoproliferative disorders where there is increased synthesis and degradation of cellular nucleotides. Most patients remain asymptomatic, but uncommonly clinical gout may develop.

Two new criteria have been described by Westwood and colleagues.[65] The mean platelet distribution width (MPV as measured by a Coulter Counter analyzer) is significantly increased in PV as compared to secondary polycythemia. The platelet nucleotide ratio (ATP:ADP

as determined by a lumiaggregometer) was also increased compared to values seen in secondary polycythemia.

A low-normal erythrocyte sedimentation rate (ESR) is commonly present in patients with PV. The increased Hct as well as the elevated ratio of red cell membrane to plasma fibrinogen and globulins may account for this finding.[2] Nonrandom chromosome abnormalities are seen in about 15% of patients, increasing to 50% with disease progression. Trisomies and deletions are especially common, particularly 20q.[68]

Differential Diagnosis

The diagnostic criteria for evaluating a patient with erythrocytosis should encompass procedures that systematically exclude the various causes of secondary and relative polycythemia (Table 21–7). In 1968 the Polycythemia Vera Study Group (PVSG) developed a set of criteria that indicated with a high degree of probability the establishment of the diagnosis of PV (Table 21–8). Because of the sensitivity and specificity of these criteria, they have become the standard approach to this diagnostic problem worldwide.

TABLE 21–7 Classification of the Disorders Associated with Polycythemia

Primary Polycythemia
  Polycythemia vera
Secondary Polycythemia
  Physiologically appropriate increase in erythropoietin
    (hypoxic activation)
    High altitude
    Chronic pulmonary disease
    Cyanotic congenital heart disease
    Cirrhosis
    Alevolar hypoventilation (obesity/sleep apnea,
      pickwickian syndrome, intrinsic lung disease)
  Defective oxygen transport
    Smoking (carboxyhemoglobinemia)
    Methemoglobinemia
    High oxygen affinity hemoglobinopathies
    Defective oxidative metabolism (cobalt therapy)
  Physiologically inappropriate increase in erythropoietin
    Renal ischemia
      Renal tumors
      Renal cysts
      Renal transplant rejection
      Renal artery stenosis
      Hydronephrosis
    Neoplasms
      Uterine fibroids
      Hepatoma
      Cerebellar hemangioblastoma
    Endocrine disorders
      Pheochromocytoma
      Conn's syndrome
      Ovarian tumors (androgen secreting)
      Cushing's syndrome
    Miscellaneous causes
      Neonatal polycythemia
      Androgen therapy
Hypertransfusion
Relative Polycythemia
  Stress polycythemia (Gaisböck's syndrome)
  Dehydration

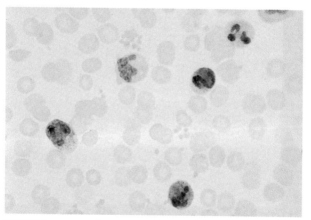

FIGURE 21–12 LAP stain of peripheral blood showing increased activity in PV (red staining).

TABLE 21–8 PVSG Criteria for Diagnosis of PV*

Category A (Major Criteria)
1. Elevated red cell mass
2. Normal arterial oxygen saturation
3. Splenomegaly

Category B (Minor Criteria)
1. Leukocytosis
2. Thrombocytosis
3. Elevated leukocyte alkaline phosphatase score
4. Increased serum vitamin B_{12} or vitamin B_{12}-binding proteins

*To establish a diagnosis of polycythemia vera, either all three diagnostic criteria from category A or an elevated red cell mass and normal arterial oxygen saturation *in addition to* two criteria from category B must be present.

Source: From Beck, WS: Hematology, ed 3. MIT Press, Cambridge, 1982, p 297, with permission.

As always, a careful history and physical should preclude more extensive (and costly) diagnostic procedures. Of particular importance are such items as smoking, cardiopulmonary status, alcohol intake, family history, and examination for evidence of hepatosplenomegaly. It is imperative that the initial laboratory investigation include documentation of absolute increase in total red cell mass; this finding is associated with a variety of conditions causing absolute polycythemia.

Once it has been established that an increased red cell mass is present, other specific diagnostic studies are warranted to assist in the differential diagnosis of secondary polycythemia versus (primary) PV (Fig. 21–13). Normal arterial O_2 and oxygen saturation (at least 92%), along with a normal chest x-ray, can help to rule out chronic pulmonary or cardiac disease. Additionally, patients have symptoms and other complications as a consequence of their primary underlying disorder.

If evidence of tissue hypoxia is lacking, investigation for the presence of an occult erythropoietin-secreting tumor or other cause of inappropriate erythropoietin production should be undertaken. Common procedures at this level of evaluation include an intravenous pyelogram (IVP), renal ultrasound, abdominal and/or head computed tomography (CT) scan, and a liver scan. Carboxyhemoglobin levels should be measured in patients who smoke, since Hct levels above normal have been demonstrated in some of these patients.

Erythrocytosis in the absence of characteristic features of either PV or cardiopulmonary secondary polycythemia should prompt consideration of the possibility of inherited hemoglobin abnormality (high oxygen affinity hemoglobin). Hemoglobin electrophoresis is abnormal in most of these cases; however, the measurement of the oxygen affinity ($P_{50}O_2$) can help reveal those few cases in which the hemoglobin mutation is electrophoretically silent. Furthermore, family history can be very useful, since the inheritance mode of these disorders is autosomal dominant.

A serum erythropoietin assay is helpful in distinguishing between primary and secondary polycythemia. Most values in PV are decreased, indicating autonomous production of red cells by the bone marrow;

however, sometimes the result may be in the normal range. In difficult cases, culture studies of peripheral blood and/or bone marrow may identify autonomous producing erythroid colonies and hence verification of a MPD.

In summary, the most significant characteristic findings in PV are increased red cell mass, splenomegaly, pancytosis, and elevated LAP score. Occasionally a patient may present with a normal or near-normal Hgb reading, iron deficiency, splenomegaly, leukocytosis, and thrombocytosis; and the disease may therefore be difficult to distinguish from essential thrombocythemia. In this case, the presumed blood loss and iron deficiency are masking the erythrocytosis of the underlying PV, and a trial of iron administration is warranted to establish a definitive diagnosis. In PV, the Hgb and Hct can be expected to rise to polycythemic levels, thus clarifying the diagnosis. Conversely, the combination of heavy smoking and excessive alcohol consumption has led to false-positive diagnoses of PV. In this setting, the smoker's polycythemia and alcoholic liver disease, manifested by splenomegaly, elevated serum vitamin B_{12} levels, leukocytosis, and in some cases elevated LAP, has erroneously prompted diagnosis of PV.[69] Again, measurement of carboxyhemoglobin levels, bone marrow examination for presence of panhyperplasia, and erythropoietin assay (expected decrease) can help to rule in PV.

Treatment

Early descriptions indicated that the life expectancy of untreated patients with PV averaged 6 to 36 months.[70,71] Over the years, therapeutic modalities have been complex and controversial. Today, however, these patients can enjoy a relatively normal life span if their disease is adequately controlled and monitored by their physician. No present treatment can completely eradicate this disease.

The major complications of PV are those of thrombotic events arising from hyperviscosity and complications caused by transition to a MPD (myelofibrosis or leukemia or both). The primary objective of therapy is the reduction of the total red cell mass. The use of cytotoxic myelosuppressive agents to control the malignant proliferative process is currently a controversial issue because this traditional therapeutic approach is now being questioned by some investigators.[72] The treatment of the erythrocytic phase may be divided into induction and maintenance therapy.

Induction Rapid reduction of the blood volume to normal can be accomplished by phlebotomy, thereby relieving the patient of the characteristic painful symptoms of hyperviscosity. This is a safe and relatively inexpensive method of controlling the erythrocytosis and is the cornerstone of treatment in PV.[2] Removal of 350 to 500 mL may be done every 2 to 3 days until the Hct is reduced to 40% to 45%. Recent studies have demonstrated the cerebral blood flow is significantly improved and mental alertness heightened if the Hct can be maintained within this range.[73] Phlebotomies can then be performed on a bimonthly basis. In elderly patients or those with a history of cardiovascular disease, it is undesirable to remove more than 200 to 300 mL at a time. Surgery in an untreated patient is hazardous

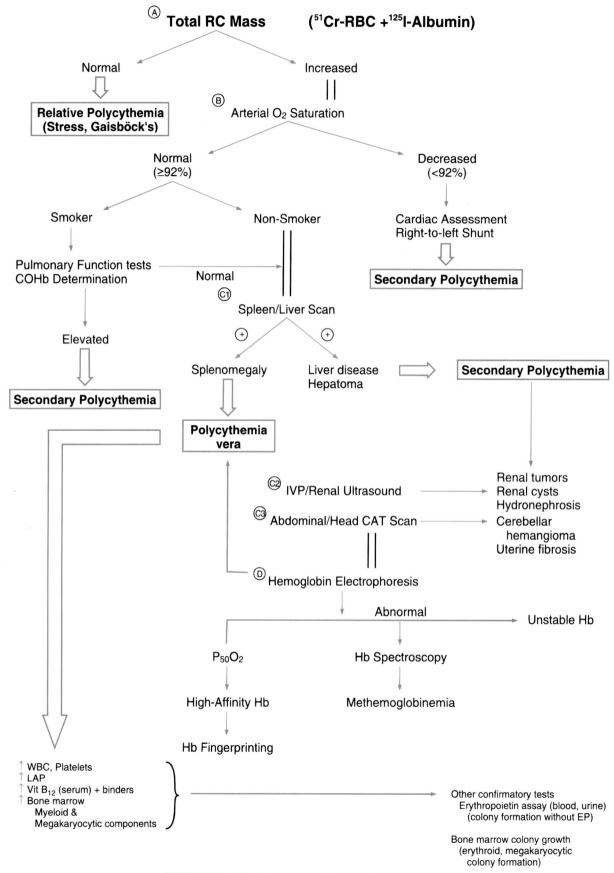

FIGURE 21–13 Diagnostic evaluation of polycythemia.

owing to the increased risk of thrombohemorrhagic complications. In such emergency situations, intensive phlebotomy accompanied by plasma infusion is advisable to maintain intravascular volume.

Because removal of every unit of blood causes a loss of approximately 250 mg of elemental iron, nearly all patients regularly treated by phlebotomy develop iron deficiency with microcytic, hypochromic red cell changes. Development of this iron deficiency and concomitant disruption of normal erythropoiesis allow maintenance of the Hct at acceptable level with the decreased frequency of phlebotomies required. Most patients do not show the classic symptoms of glossitis, dysphagia, cheilosis, weight loss, and so on generally associated with iron deficiency; however, some patients do have unexplained fatigue. Iron therapy is not usually required, but if iron is administered, the Hct must be carefully monitored because it may rise quickly, necessitating more frequent phlebotomies. The microhematocrit method is preferable over the automated cell counter method, because the Hct may be overestimated by up to 10% at low mean corpuscular hemoglobin (MCH) and mean corpuscular hemoglobin concentration (MCHC) values.[17]

Management by phlebotomy alone is recommended for patients under age 40, particularly women in the childbearing years, unless specific thrombosis-associated risk factors are present (that is, high platelet counts, pre-existing vascular disease). The major limitation of phlebotomy is that it has no suppressive effect on the abnormal bone marrow proliferation, particularly that of thrombocytosis. It does not alleviate pruritus or control any symptoms related to splenomegaly. Myelosuppression is often advocated to repress these manifestations.

Maintenance Long-term control of the peripheral blood counts is essential to minimize the risk of thrombotic complications. Although phlebotomy relieves the burden of erythrocytosis, the reduction is short-term, and all patients require close supervision by a physician to cope with the increased risk of thrombosis during the first years of treatment, especially those patients with elevated platelet counts. Apparently no single therapy is optimal for patients of all ages and stages of this disease, and therefore decisions as to the most effective approach must be based primarily on individual patient characteristics.

Extensive data on the management of PV by use of phlebotomy alone and/or in combination with the various myelosuppressive modalities are now available, thanks to the past 20 years of investigation by the PVSG. In this long-term study, 431 patients were randomized into three modes of treatment: phlebotomy alone, chlorambucil with phlebotomy as needed, and radioactive phosphorus ^{32}P and phlebotomy as needed. An additional study examined the results of long-term control of PV with a nonalkalating agent, hydroxyurea (HU). Patients treated with phlebotomy only exhibited an increased incidence of thrombotic complications, whereas significantly greater percentages of patients who were regulated by either radioactive phosphorus or an alkalating agent subsequently developed acute leukemia and other neoplasms. The comparison studies also show that HU, supplemented by phlebotomy, is *not* accompanied by excessive thrombotic complications.[74] Recent studies by Weinfeld and colleagues[72] have demonstrated that patients treated with HU, an agent originally not considered leukemogenic, have indeed shown an increased rate of development of acute leukemia. Additionally, since myelosuppressive treatment has not been shown to prolong survival in PV patients, the indications for the use of cytotoxic chemotherapy must outweigh the risk of inducing leukemia.

As a result of the PVSG's systematic study of prognostic indicators, complications, and effective therapeutic modalities, and because no form of treatment for PV is risk-free, the PVSG suggests the following guidelines to provide the best control of the disease:

1. Because of the increased risk of vascular occlusion associated with age, patients over age 70 are most simply and effectively treated with phlebotomy and radioactive phosphorus (^{32}P) as needed.
2. In patients under age 40, the disease should be controlled with phlebotomy alone unless thrombosis-associated risk factors are demonstrated. If the requirement for phlebotomy is excessive or there is a history of a previous thrombotic episode, myelosuppression with HU may be cautiously used even in this young age group.
3. Because the role of myelosuppression is controversial in patients aged 40 to 70, phlebotomy alone can be used if no thrombosis-associated risks are present. If the aforementioned risk is identified, HU may be used judiciously.
4. Symptomatic hypersplenomegaly, resistant pruritus, bone pain, or poor veins may be other indications for the additive use of myelosuppression.[69,75]

Either chemotherapy or irradiation may be used to effect myelosuppression. Radioactive phosphorus, ^{32}P, is still probably the most convenient form of delivering myelosuppressive radiation. [32]P should be administered intravenously at a dosage of 2.3 to 5 mCi/m². In many cases, a single dose is sufficient to reduce spleen size and normalize the peripheral blood count. However, the response takes 2 to 3 months for maximal effect of chemotherapy. Sometimes a second small dose of 2 to 3 mCi/m² of ^{32}P is required after 3 to 4 months to completely arrest the disease. Satisfactory control of PV occurs in 75% to 85% of patients, and the duration of remission is typically 6 to 36 months. Since there are very few side effects, this agent is of particular advantage to patients who live lengthy distances from their physicians.[76] Although a low incidence of acute leukemia is a characteristic of the natural history of this disease, there is no doubt that there is a greatly increased risk for leukemic transformation in ^{32}P-treated patients. Approximately 10% to 15% of patients convert to an acute, usually nonlymphocytic leukemia, and, according to Williams,[41] this incidence is 20 to 40 times greater than that expected for a human population exposed to similar radiation doses and times at risk.

The average dose of 1 g/day of HU is sufficient to maintain a normal hematocrit and platelet count. Supplemental phlebotomies may be necessary. The initial respone to HU treatment is positive, with between 80% and 90% achieving good control of the disease and more than 60% retaining long-term control after 5 years. Weinfeld and coworkers[72] report that most of the acute leukemia transformations will take place during the first 4 years of treatment. In a high percentage of patients, HU also seems to have a beneficial effect on pruritus and splenomegaly.[77] Possible side effects include rashes, drug fever, and megaloblastoid changes.

Adjuvant therapy is often necessary to control hyperuricemia and hyperuricosuria. In addition to standard colchicine therapy, allopurinol (300 mg/day), an agent that blocks the formation of uric acid from its precursors, is used to prevent and/or control acute attacks of gout. In patients receiving myelosuppressive therapy, the need for allopurinol is diminished because of the decreased nucleic acid turnover effected by suppression of cellular proliferation.[41] Allopurinol may be continued indefinitely in patients treated by phlebotomy alone.

Severe pruritus is a distressing symptom in many cases. It is best managed by controlling the erythrocytosis; however, it may persist in some patients despite a normal Hct and physical exam. The antihistamine cyproheptadine and cimetidine may be of benefit. Cholestyramine, an anion-exchange resin that functions by binding bile acids, has been reported to provide some relief of pruritus.

Course and Prognosis

The course of patients with PV is determined by the natural history of the disease and the development of complications that may or may not be related to the mode of therapy employed.

As previously mentioned, this disease progresses through several stages, each of variable duration. In the active erythrocytic phase, the red cell mass can be maintained at satisfactory levels with administration of treatment that is dictated by age and the presence of certain risk factors. Many patients eventually enter a period characterized by increasing anemia, and this spent phase is associated with transformation to frank myelofibrosis in 15% to 20% of cases. The progressive splenomegaly appears to be a manifestation of the natural course of the disease, but splenectomy carries a high incidence of morbidity and mortality in this group of patients. The treatment of this phase is predominantly supportive and may be very difficult. The cause of the anemia may be multifactorial, being the result of one or more of the following factors: (1) iron, folic acid, or vitamin B_{12} deficiency; (2) inefficient hematopoiesis; or (3) splenic sequestration and destruction of erythrocytes, leukocytes, and platelets. Treatment of the anemia may involve appropriate nutritional replacement and/or administration of steroids to help control the ineffective erythropoiesis. Ongoing transfusion of packed red cells is often required. Despite possible splenic sequestration, thrombocytosis and leukocytosis may persist. Myelosuppressive therapy may be indicated to control the myelofibrotic proliferation. Prognosis is poor for this phase of the disease and median survival is about 2 years.

Malignant transformation to acute leukemia, usually acute myeloblastic leukemia (AML), occurs in 10% to 15% of cases. This complication is almost universally fatal. As discussed earlier, the therapeutic modality affects the rate of leukemic transformation. In patients treated by phlebotomy alone, the incidence of transition to leukemia is only 1% to 2%, whereas those treated by chemotherapy have a risk approaching 15%. A few cases each have been documented of PV transforming into a myelodysplastic syndrome, myeloma, and also chronic lymphocytic leukemia.[17]

Reported survival rates in PV range from 8 to 15 years. Thrombohemorrhagic incidents account for 40% of deaths and acute leukemia and myeloid metaplasia each account for 15%.[41] As the mean age of diagnosis is 60 years, many other patients die of additional unrelated reasons.

Continued research of the pathophysiologic abnormalities associated with this disease as well as the effects of various treatment modalities will undoubtedly lengthen the future life expectancy of patients with PV.

The Secondary Polycythemias

Absolute erythrocytosis may have a wide variety of causes (see Table 21–7). The secondary polycythemias differ from PV in that autonomous bone marrow proliferation occurs in PV. Increased secretion of erythropoietin has been implicated as the responsible stimulus for all cases of secondary erythrocytosis. These causes can be separated into three groups: those in which there is an appropriate, compensatory increase in erythropoietin; those resulting from an inappropriate or pathologic secretion of erythropoietin; and a miscellaneous category.

Relative Polycythemia

Relative polycythemia may be seen in patients with an elevated Hct reading, normal red cell mass, and decreased plasma volume. Two groups can be clearly distinguished among patients with relative erythrocytosis (see Table 21–5). First, it is most often clinically seen in the group of patients having a depletion in circulating plasma volume caused by acute or subacute dehydration resulting from a number of conditions (such as burns). The second group of patients is characterized predominantly by asymptomatic middle-aged white men who are hypertensive and obese and have a long history of heavy smoking. In 1905, Gaisbock[78] first described a condition of "polycythemia hypertonica" in several hypertensive patients who had increased red cell counts, plethora, but no accompanying splenomegaly. Today, this condition is variously termed Gaisbock's syndrome, stress or benign polycythemia, or pseudopolycythemia. It is well documented that excessive smoking causes mild to moderate erythrocytosis and a decreased plasma volume, hence the term *smokers' polycythemia*. Undoubtedly some patients with erythrocytosis merely represent the extreme physiologic range of Hct. The combined effect of a high-normal red cell mass and a low-normal plasma volume resulting in a so-called spurious erythrocytosis is not considered pathologic. Physical stress, extreme alcohol consumption, and diuretic therapy have also been documented as possible causes of plasma volume reduction.

This condition usually follows a benign course; however, a few patients may progress to an absolute polycythemia with an obvious underlying cause becoming apparent. A few nonspecific symptoms such as headache, nausea, and dyspepsia may be reported in these patients. Hypertension, with possible increased risk of thromboembolic complications, is seen in approximately one third of the patients. The Hct value is generally between 50% and 60%. Therapy indicated is in the form of encouragement of the cessation of smoking and/or alcohol intake, reduction of obesity, treatment of hypertension, stress counseling, and discontinuance of diuretic therapy when appropriate. Ongoing studies are investigating the efficacy of maintaining the Hct below 50% by phlebotomies. The risk of vascular occlusive episodes is presumably greatly decreased in this manner.

ESSENTIAL THROMBOCYTHEMIA

Essential thrombocythemia (ET) is a rare chronic MPD characterized by marked thrombocytosis associated with abnormal platelet function. ET was the last of the MPDs to be identified as a distinct entity, owing to the fact that extreme thrombocytosis is also frequently observed in CML, IMF, and PV. Sex-linked G6PD cell-marker studies established ET as a clonal disorder involving the multipotential stem cell, which supported the placement of ET within the MPD classification.[79]

Diagnostic criteria that define ET were proposed by the PVSG in the mid 1970s. These guidelines include: (1) platelet count in excess of 600×10^9/L (and generally >$1,000 \times 10^9$/L, (2) megakaryocytic hyperplasia in the marrow, (3) absence of identifiable causes of reactive thrombocytosis, (4) the absence of the Ph[1], (5) hemoglobin no higher than 13 g/dL or normal red cell mass, (6) absence of significant marrow fibrosis, and (7) presence of stainable iron in marrow or failure of iron trial.[79–81]

Synonyms for this condition include idiopathic thrombocythemia, primary thrombocythemia and primary hemorrhagic thrombocythemia.

Epidemiology

The mean age at time of diagnosis is approximately 60 years, most patients being over 50. This disease has occasionally been described in the 20- to 40-year age group, and very rarely in patients under age 20. Most studies do not demonstrate a statistical difference between frequency of males and females affected. The incidence of the disease has been estimated at 7 per million population per year. The etiology of thrombocythemia remains unknown.

Clinical Features

Many patients are asymptomatic at diagnosis. With the introduction of automated instruments that routinely perform whole blood platelet counts, asymptomatic patients with coincidental high platelet counts are being discovered more frequently. Two thirds of patients in a recent study by Bellucci and colleagues[82] were found to be asymptomatic. Patients who are symptomatic present with hemorrhagic vaso-occlusive

symptoms, or both. In a more recent study of patients under 45, Mitus[83] found a 39% incidence of hemorrhage, thrombosis, or both. In most instances bleeding is mild and manifestations are primarily mucocutaneous (epistaxis and ecchymoses); however, life-threatening hemorrhage may occur following accidental trauma or, rarely, following surgery. Bleeding of gastrointestinal as well as esophageal varices has also been reported. Hemorrhage has been attributed to several mechanisms: (1) platelet functional abnormalities; (2) thrombosis with infarction, ulceration of the infarction, and subsequent bleeding; (3) consumption of coagulation factors; and (4) increased numbers of circulating platelets causing excessive production of prostacyclin (PGI_2) by endothelial cells (increased level of PGI_2 suppresses platelet granule release and aggregation[61]).

Thrombosis is the other major manifestation of ET and is caused by intravascular clumping of sludged, hyperaggregable platelets. Vascular occlusive symptoms are usually related to small-vessel obstruction (microvascular occlusion), although larger-vessel occlusive events such as myocardial infarction and stroke may occur. Erythromelalgia of the toes, feet, and occasionally fingers (localized painful redness, burning, and "pins-and-needles" tingling sensation) is a characteristic vaso-occlusive symptom and may progress to cyanosis and/or necrosis of the extremities. The involvement of the hands and feet may simulate a diabetic neuropathy.[84] The toxic effect of the metabolites of platelet arachidonic acid appears to be responsible for the erythromelalgia, and this may be relieved by decreasing the platelet count or by use of anti-inflammatory agents such as aspirin.[85,86] Singh and Wetherly-Mein[87] suggest that thrombotic complications may be more common when the platelet count is greater than 2000×10^9/L.

Neurologic manifestations are usually of a transient ischemic nature and include visual disturbances, headaches, paresthesia, dizziness, transient ischemic attacks, and, rarely, seizures. Complete stroke is an uncommon occurrence. In older patients, underlying degenerative vascular disease in combination with thrombocytosis and platelet functional defects all contribute to the thrombohemorrhagic complications.

Other signs and symptoms that have been observed in this disease are recurrent abortions and fetal growth retardation,[88,89] pruritus, gout, and priapism. Modest splenomegaly is present in approximately 50% of patients with ET. Splenic atrophy resulting from splenic vascular thrombosis and silent infarctions occurs in up to 20% of patients. According to Silverstein,[30] patients with splenomegaly have a more favorable prognosis than do patients without splenomegaly. This is thought to be attributable to the beneficial effect of splenic sequestration of platelets.

Laboratory Features

The platelet count is always elevated, in the range 600 to 2500×10^9/L. Platelets are usually morphologically normal, although some degree of platelet anisocytosis may be apparent. When present, this correlates with an elevation of the platelet distribution width (PDW) as determined by automated instruments. Abnormal morphological findings may include giant platelets (megathrombocytes) as well as microthrombocytes, platelet aggregates, abnormally granulated platelets, and megakaryocytic cytoplasmic fragments (Fig. 21–14).

A mild normocytic, normochromic anemia may be present in 15% to 20% of patients, although the hemoglobin value is not usually less than 10 g/dL. When associated bleeding leads to iron deficiency anemia, the mean corpuscular volume (MCV) and mean corpuscular hemoglobin concentration (MCHC) will be decreased and a microcytic, hypochromic blood picture will be apparent on examination of the peripheral smear. Erythrocyte morphological findings reflective of hyposplenism that occurs in the occasional patient with splenic infarction and atrophy include the presence of Howell-Jolly bodies, Pappenheimer bodies (siderotic granules), target cells, and acanthocytes.

Leukocytosis is present in about one third of patients, with WBC counts rarely exceeding 50×10^9/L. Neutrophilia is observed in most patients with elevated WBC, but a mild eosinophilia and/or basophilia may occasionally be seen. Rarely, nucleated red cells and immature granulocytes may also be evident. The LAP score is variable but most commonly is normal.

The bone marrow in patients with ET demonstrates trilineage hyperplasia with a marked increase in the megakaryocytic component.[90] The megakaryocytes are typically larger than normal and may be dysplastic in appearance (Fig. 21–15). Stainable iron is normal to slightly decreased in most cases, and increased reticulin content is often seen. Marrow karyotype is generally normal; however, the deletion of the long arm of chromosome number 21 (21q−) has been reported in some patients.[91]

Plasma levels of interleukin-6 (IL-6), which is primarily produced by monocytes, are increased during acute phase response, such as the reactive thrombocytosis that may accompany acute and chronic inflammatory states. Tefferi[89] and associates reported an increased IL-6 level in 60% of patients with reactive thrombocytosis, whereas IL-6 levels were not detected

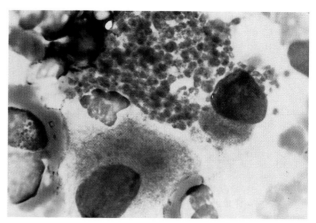

FIGURE 21–15 Essential thrombocythemia, bone marrow. Note increased megakaryocytes. (From Hyun, BH: Morphology of Blood and Bone Marrow. American Society of Clinical Pathologists, Workshop 5121, Philadelphia, September 7, 1983, with permission.)

in all patients with ET. Plasma fibrinogen and C-reactive protein (CRP) levels also are both increased with reactive thrombocytosis but are normal with ET.[92]

Platelet function studies reveal a variety of abnormalities in some patients. Abnormal platelet aggregation to epinephrine, collagen, and adenosine diphosphate (ADP) are quite frequent. Studies have demonstrated both normal bleeding times (even in the case of patients with hemorrhagic tendencies[93]) and prolonged bleeding times. Reduced level of platelet factor 3 (PF3), reduced platelet adhesion, low protein S levels,[94] and nucleotide storage pool defects have all been reported in association with ET. Despite all of these identified abnormalities, there is poor correlation with any of these findings and the incidence of clinical thrombohemorrhagic manifestations.

Differential Diagnosis

ET must be differentiated from the various causes of reactive thrombocytosis (Table 21–9), from other chronic MPDs with associated thrombocytosis (Fig. 21–16), and from the myelodysplastic syndromes (MDSs) in which the platelet count is markedly ele-

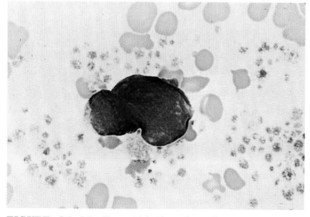

FIGURE 21–14 Essential thrombocythemia; peripheral blood megakaryocyte and numerous platelets. (From Hyun, BH: Morphology of Blood and Bone Marrow. American Society of Clinical Pathologists, Workshop 5121, Philadelphia, September 7, 1983, with permission.)

TABLE 21–9 **Causes of Reactive Thrombocytosis**
Acute hemorrhage
Postsplenectomy and hyposplenism
Postoperative
Malignancy
Chronic inflammatory disorders
Chronic infection
Myelophthisic diseases
Hemolytic anemia
Iron-deficiency anemia
Drug-induced
Rebound recovery from thrombocytopenia
Exercise

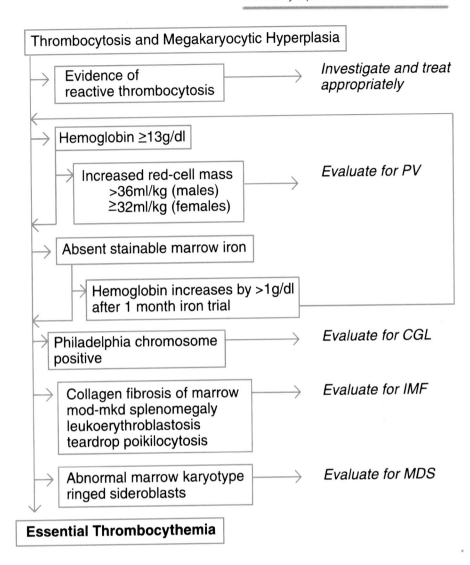

Thrombocytosis and Megakaryocytic Hyperplasia

Evidence of reactive thrombocytosis → *Investigate and treat appropriately*

Hemoglobin ≥13g/dl

Increased red-cell mass >36ml/kg (males) ≥32ml/kg (females) → *Evaluate for PV*

Absent stainable marrow iron

Hemoglobin increases by >1g/dl after 1 month iron trial

Philadelphia chromosome positive → *Evaluate for CGL*

Collagen fibrosis of marrow mod-mkd splenomegaly leukoerythroblastosis teardrop poikilocytosis → *Evaluate for IMF*

Abnormal marrow karyotype ringed sideroblasts → *Evaluate for MDS*

Essential Thrombocythemia

FIGURE 21-16 Differential criteria for diagnosis of essential thrombocythemia. PV = polycythemia vera, CGL = chronic granulocytic leukemia, IMF = idiopathic myelofibrosis, MDS = myelodysplastic syndrome. (Adapted from Iland et al,[102] with permission.)

vated. This distinction is important because hemorrhagic complications are more common in ET than reactive thrombocytosis and there is a considerable variation in prognosis and therapy in ET versus chronic MPDs.

Most cases of extreme thrombocytosis represent incidental findings in patients with a wide variety of inflammatory and trauma-associated conditions. Reactive thrombocytosis, even when persistently present for weeks or months, is usually well tolerated in these patients, and is not generally associated with thrombosis or hemorrhage. Bone marrow examination, virtually always performed in patients suspected of having MPD, is rarely done in instance of reactive thrombocytosis. The platelet count in secondary thrombocytosis seldom exceeds 1000×10^9/L, and commonly falls in the range of 500 to 750×10^9/L. Platelet morphology and function is generally normal in chronic reactive states compared to the variety of abnormalities seen in MPDs.

When the platelet count is persistently greater than 600×10^9/L and the bone marrow demonstrates predominant megakaryocytic hyperplasia, the diagnosis

of ET should be investigated (see Fig. 21–16). As there are no unique clinical, hematologic, or histopathologic findings in this disease, it is by nature a diagnosis of exclusion. At presentation, the hemoglobin should be less than 13 g/dL and the red cell mass should be normal in order to shift the diagnosis from PV with thrombocytosis (one third of PV cases) to ET. To ensure that masked PV has not been overlooked in those patients having a normal or decreased red cell mass caused by iron deficiency, the establishment of the absence of marrow iron stores helps to exclude the diagnosis of ET. Additionally, if the clinical situation permits, a 1-month trial of iron therapy should be administered. The response to iron therapy should be carefully monitored, and if a rise in the Hct and red cell volume is observed, the patient should be evaluated for evidence of PV, evidence of blood loss, or both.

Chromosome analysis of the bone marrow should be performed to ensure that the Ph[1] chromosome is not present, thereby excluding CML. In those approximately 15% of patients with CML and thrombocytosis that are Ph[1]-chromosome-negative, the findings of profound myeloid metaplasia, low LAP score, and moderate to marked splenomegaly are important for supporting the diagnosis of CML.

Early IMF is often associated with extreme thrombocytosis. However, there is usually marked splenomegaly, a leukoerythroblastic blood picture, teardrop poikilocytosis, and the characteristic myelofibrotic involvement of the bone marrow (increased reticulin and collagen fibrosis). Additionally, the platelet morphology in ET has been described as nondysplastic, in comparison to the abundance of bizarre and atypical platelets seen in IMF.[95]

MDSs associated with thrombocytosis usually present with a more severe degree of anemia that is often macrocytic in appearance as compared with that seen in patients with ET. Additionally, the presence of either the 5q− syndrome or of ringed sideroblasts in the bone marrow denotes a MDS as the cause of associated thrombocytosis rather than essential thrombocythemia.

Treatment

The therapeutic approach to ET depends upon a number of factors, including the patient's age and childbearing potential, the elevation of the platelet count, and, most important, the presence and duration of symptoms. Careful monitoring, without therapy specifically aimed at lowering the platelet count, is generally advocated for asymptomatic patients with extreme thrombocytosis. Young patients with few or no symptoms do not require treatment unless surgery is indicated or childbirth is imminent. In these cases, plateletpheresis is useful in controlling the elevated platelet count. Additionally, a young patient with vaso-occlusive manifestations may respond to aspirin therapy alone.

Treatment in patients over age 50 who are symptomatic is divided into control of hemorrhage and manifestation of vascular occlusion, and the control of the progressive megakaryocyte proliferation. Thrombotic events have been reported to occur more often than hemorrhagic events. It is interesting to note that the degree of thrombocytosis does not correlate with the risk of thrombosis.[89] There may be an even greater incidence of occlusive ischemic complications in the presence of cardiovascular risk factors, particularly smoking.[96] Acute hemorrhage and occlusive events, which occur in approximately 30% of patients, indicate the necessity for immediate therapy. Plateletpheresis achieves a dramatic reduction in the platelet count in the matter of hours; however, this reduction is transient. Chemotherapy should be initiated in addition to plateletpheresis[97] whenever thrombohemorrhagic complications develop. A number of effective myelosuppressive agents have been used, but their use has been associated with a increased potential for induction of acute leukemia. The antimetabolite hydroxyurea is generally considered to be the drug of choice because of its efficacy. Hydroxyurea administration should be continued daily at a dosage of 15 mg per kilogram of body weight with adjustment according to response. In 90% of patients the platelet count will be decreased to less than 600×10^9/L in 2 to 6 weeks.[85] A lower continuous dosage is required to maintain disease control because, once this treatment is halted, the platelet count rises again. The only common side effects are dose-related, reversible leukopenia and macrocytic red cell changes.

Platelet antiaggregating agents, aspirin (300 mg daily), and dipyridamole (50 mg three times a day) have been shown to reverse incipient gangrene in patients with limb ischemia and provide long-lasting relief of symptoms of erythromelalgia.[84,98] There is also some evidence that neurologic manifestations in ET are also improved through this therapy.[99] An important role for aspirin may be found in patients with recurrent miscarriages, since this treatment does not carry the risk of teratogenicity of the other treatment options.[100] However, continuous use of aspirin once symptoms have abated or myelosuppression has controlled the platelet count, or both, is not advisable because of the significant risk of hemorrhage, particularly from the gastrointestinal tract.

Investigation of the drug anagrelide for treatment of thrombocytosis has shown great promise.[90] Alpha-interferon has also been advocated for treatment in ET.[96,101] This agent exerts an inhibitory effect on the growth of megakaryocyte progenitors that correlates clinically with a marked decrease in platelet count following treatment with interferon.

If surgery is indicated, the platelet count should be controlled preoperatively by use of plateletpheresis or myelosuppression or both. Platelet concentrates may be needed to provide normal functional platelets.

Course and Prognosis

Recent follow-up studies by the PVSG and others suggest that survival time in ET is lengthy. Eighty percent will survive 5 years, with the prognosis particularly good for younger patients. Leukemic transformation can occur but seems to be an extremely rare event compared to the incidence of transitions that occurs in other MPDs.[102,103]

CASE STUDY 1

A 74-year-old man presented with complaints of increasing weakness, night sweats, shortness of breath, easy bruising, and a fever of 10 days' duration. The patient had lost about 10 lb over a 6-month period and noted early satiety. On physical examination he was pale and underweight, and had a fever of 103°F. Massive splenomegaly, moderate hepatomegaly, and pulmonary congestion were noted. Purpuric lesions were present on the upper extremities.

Initial laboratory studies disclosed the following values: WBC, 30.5×10^9/L; RBC, 2.9×10^{12}/L; Hb, 8.3 g/dL; Hct, 25.8%; MCV, 89 fL; MCH, 28.6 pg; MCHC, 32.2%; platelets, 650×10^9/L. The differential count revealed 45% segmented neutrophils, 6% band neutrophils, 20% lymphocytes, 9% monocytes, 3% eosinophils, 3% basophils, 4% metamyelocytes, 3% myelocytes, 2% promyelocytes, 5% "dwarf" megakaryocytes, and 15 nucleated red blood cells (NRBC) per 100 WBCs. Erythrocyte morphology demonstrated anisocytosis and poikilocytosis with prominent teardrop red cells, polychromasia, and basophilic stippling. Platelet number was increased and platelet morphology was abnormal, as evidenced by the presence of giant platelets and hypergranulated and hypogranulated platelets and megakaryocytic fragments. Other laboratory tests included reticulocyte count, 3.6%; LAP score, 132 (normal 22 to 124); LDH, 3054 μ/L; uric acid, 13.2 mg/dL; stool occult blood, negative; Ph[1] chromosome, negative; and direct antiglobulin test (DAT), negative. A bone marrow aspirate was attempted several times but was unsuccessful because of a dry tap. The bone marrow biopsy revealed trilineage hyperplasia with many clumps of dysplastic atypical megakaryocytes. Extensive fibrosis was also noted. Bacterial and fungal bone marrow cell cultures were performed and all results were negative.

Comment The diagnosis of idiopathic myelofibrosis with myeloid metaplasia was made based on the classic findings of leukoerythroblastic anemia, marked splenomegaly, thrombocytosis with circulating megakaryocyte precursors, teardrop erythrocytes, and increased fibrosis of the bone marrow. Chronic myelogeneous leukemia was excluded, as most of these patients have the Philadelphia chromosome, a low LAP, a higher proportion of myelocytes and myeloblasts, and a bone marrow showing predominantly granulocytic hyperplasia. Additionally, the red cell morphological changes—in particular teardrop red cells—are more prominent in myelofibrosis.

Of patients with known PV, 15% to 20% undergo a transition to IMF; however, since there is no prior history of PV, this disease can be ruled out. Granulomatous disorders and acute leukemia can be excluded by careful scrutiny of the bone marrow and the negative microbiologic cultures. An increased platelet count and marked proliferation of bizarre megakaryocytes would be highly unusual in acute leukemia.

Another disorder involved in differential diagnosis is essential thrombocythemia. Again, these patients rarely show the red cell abnormalities associated with fibrosis in the marrow and splenic hematopoiesis, and the bone marrow is easily aspirated. The platelet count in ET is almost always greatly elevated, generally greater than 1000×10^9/L, and immature granulocytes are rarely prominent.

Busulfan therapy was administered to this patient and continued over the course of 1 year. Blood transfusions were required every 3 to 4 weeks to counteract the impending anemia. Androgen therapy (danazol) was also initiated. The patient's condition gradually worsened and it was evident that the chemotherapy was only mildly effective in decreasing splenic size. Splenectomy was performed in an attempt to ameliorate his anemia and relieve the constitutional symptoms of splenomegaly.

Four years after initial presentation, this patient developed acute myelogenous leukemia and underwent a rapidly progressive fatal course. This case illustrates a typical course of myelofibrosis. The me-dian survival is approximately 5 years and treatment has little effect in prolonging the survival.

Questions

1. Referring to the WBC differential, is a "left shift" evident in this case? Why or why not?
2. What is the corrected WBC count, given the number of NRBCs?
3. Give reasons why the bone marrow aspirate resulted in a "dry tap" in this case?

CASE STUDY 2

A 58-year-old white man was admitted to the hospital with pain and swelling of the left arm suggestive of thrombophlebitis. He had presented to his physician 2 days earlier with complaints of pounding headaches, blurred vision, tinnitus, and generalized pruritus, especially after bathing. The patient had been treated for gout for the past 2 months. Family history is unremarkable for any hematologic disorders. The patient is a nonsmoker.

On physical examination, the patient's face appeared flushed and the retinal veins were engorged. Several ecchymoses were apparent on the legs. The spleen tip was palpable three fingerbreaths below the costal margin. No hepatomegaly or lymphadenopathy were observed.

Complete blood count revealed the following: WBC, 20.3×10^9/L; RBC, 7.53×10^{12}/L; Hb, 18.2 g/dL; Hct, 58.0%; MCV, 77 fL; MCH, 24.2 pg; MCHC, 31.4%; platelets, 710×10^9/L. The differential count demonstrated 80% segmented neutrophils, 8% band neutrophils, 9% lymphocytes, and 3% monocytes. Red cell morphology was consistent with a microcytic, hypochromic classification.

Subsequent investigations were undertaken as part of the diagnostic workup of the erythrocytosis. Determination of the red cell mass (utilizing the ^{51}Cr dilution method) was performed and found to be 41 mL/kg (normal, male, less than or equal to 36 mL/kg). The plasma volume was 40 mL/kg. Arterial oxygen saturation was 94%. The serum iron level was 30 μg/dL (normal, 50 to 150) and total iron-binding capacity (TIBC), 460 μg/dL (normal 250 to 450). Serum vitamin B_{12} level was 925 pg/mL (normal, 205 to 876) and vitamin B_{12}-binding capacity was 2600 pg/mL (normal 1000 to 1022). The LAP score was 198, and the uric acid determination was 10.3 mg/dL. A bone marrow examination revealed 95% cellularity with panhyperplasia, and many large megakaryocytes. Iron stores were absent and the reticulin content was slightly increased.

Comment Several findings in the history and physical examination suggest a presumptive diagnosis of PV. The nonspecific symptoms of headache and blurred vision are a result of cerebral circulatory disturbances because of hyperviscosity. Thrombotic episodes, such as the phlebitis recorded in this patient, are vascular manifestations resulting from the thrombocytosis in conjunction with the hyperviscosity and increased blood volume. The facial plethora and engorged retinal veins are findings associated with conjunctival and mucosal blood vessel congestion. Generalized pruritus occurs in 30% of patients with polycythemia and is related to hyperhistaminemia. The lack of cardiac or respiratory abnormalities and the presence of normal arterial saturation are helpful in ruling out secondary polycythemia. The splenomegaly noted is a frequent finding in myeloproliferative disorders.

The most important clinical findings supportive of polycythemia are the elevation of the Hgb and Hct, increased red cell mass, and normal plasma volume. Furthermore, evidence of trilineage involvement, leukocytosis, and thrombocytosis in addition to erythrocytosis and bone marrow panhyperplasia strongly suggests a diagnosis of PV. Abnormal elevation of the vitamin B_{12} and B_{12}-binding proteins, uric acid, and LAP are all consistent with a myeloproliferative process and are helpful in establishing a diagnosis of PV. The low serum iron level and absence of iron store indicates concomitant iron deficiency. In most patients this is attributed to occult gastrointestinal blood loss and defective platelet function.

This patient fulfills all the diagnostic criteria for PV set forth by the PVSG. Since this 58-year-old patient has an elevated Hct and platelet count and is symptomatic (thrombophlebitis), both phlebotomy and myelosuppressive therapy were initiated. Colchicine and allopurinol were used to control the gout. Pruritus was a persistent complaint despite the management of erythrocytosis by phlebotomy and hydroxyurea. Cyproheptadine was prescribed and found to be successful in controlling the pruritus.

Questions

1. What laboratory parameters listed in this case indicate a microcytic, hypochromic anemia?
2. How do the iron studies present in this case differ from a patient diagnosed with iron-deficiency anemia?
3. Are the white cells demonstrating a "shift to the left" in this case? Explain your answer
4. What is the reason for splenomegaly in this patient?

CASE STUDY 3

A 35-year-old woman initially presented with the thrombocytosis (platelet count 1200×10^9/L) discovered on routine physical examination. Her WBC and Hgb levels were normal. The history was unremarkable except for occasional epistaxis and minor bruising. She was advised to have a routine follow-up examination and complete blood count (CBC) every 3 months and, despite a continually elevated platelet count, remained asymptomatic for 3 years. At that time she was seen by her physician with complaints of dizziness, visual disturbances, and erythromelalgia. She has also had recent dental surgery and experienced a major perioperative bleeding episode. Mild splenomegaly was noted. Her platelet count was 2500×10^9/L and platelet distribution width (PDW) was increased. Other laboratory values were as follows: WBC, 18.5×10^9/L;

Hct, 28.5%; prolonged bleeding time; reduced platelet adhesion; and defective platelet aggregation with epinephrine. Bone marrow biopsy demonstrated megakaryocytic hyperplasia with massive platelet clumping. Erythroid and myeloid hyperplasia and a mild increase in reticulin content were also observed.

Plateletpheresis was performed to rapidly reduce the marked thrombocytosis. The patient was treated with the myelosuppressive agent hydroxyurea in dosages varying from 1 g/day to 500 mg five times per week, depending on the platelet counts. The bleeding and vaso-occlusive symptoms were resolved and coagulation abnormalities were corrected. Close follow-up is necessary for this patient to ensure continued beneficial clinical and laboratory response to all.

Comment   This case highlights the common findings in essential thrombocythemia: namely, marked increased platelet counts, thrombohemorrhagic events, splenomegaly, and bone marrow megakaryocytic hyperplasia. Although this is primarily a disease of upper middle age (50 to 70), a second population of younger, predominantly female patients exists. Two thirds of patients are asymptomatic, as was this patient initially. With the advent of automated cell counters that routinely generate platelet count, asymptomatic patients are being discovered more frequently.

The erythromelalgia noted in this patient represents one of the most characteristic vaso-occlusive manifestations. Prolonged bleeding after trauma or surgery is a common finding related to platelet dysfunction.

In an asymptomatic young patient it is advisable to withhold myelosuppressive therapy, as these patients do well for many years untreated. When a patient requiring surgery presents with markedly increased platelet count and hemorrhagic complications, plateletpheresis will lower the platelet count dramatically. Additionally, myelosuppression is necessary to control the hyperproliferative process.

Causes of reactive thrombocytosis, such as iron-deficiency anemia, malignancy, inflammatory disorders, splenectomy, and so on, are generally easy to exclude based upon the clinical and hematologic features of the individual patient. In order to reliably exclude the other chronic MPDs, the PVSG guidelines should be followed. To distinguish a patient with ET from an iron-deficient PV patient, a 1-month trial of oral iron should be instituted. The Hgb should not rise by more than 1 g/dL to support a diagnosis of ET. In patients with anemia, splenomegaly, and thrombocytosis, the presence of the Ph^1 chromosome conclusively rules out the diagnosis of ET.

The outlook for long-term survival in ET is encouraging as long as appropriate measures are taken to minimize thrombohemorrhagic complications. Many patients can tolerate markedly increased platelet counts for years without any complications. The introduction of plateletpheresis has allowed dramatic response in life-threatening or urgent surgical situations. Furthermore, hydroxyurea has proven to be an effective chemotherapeutic agent.

Questions

1. What is the meaning of the PDW result in this case?
2. Erythromelalgia can progress into what clinical manifestation?
3. Give reasons for megakaryocytic hyperplasia seen in the bone marrow biopsy.

REFERENCES

1. Damashek, W: Some speculations on the myeloproliferative syndrome. Blood 6:372, 1951.
2. Bick, RL, et al: Hematology, Clinical and Laboratory Practice, vol 2. Mosby-Year Book, Chicago, 1993, pp 533–542, 1239–1257.
3. Fialkow, PJ: The origin and development of human tumors studies with cell markers. N Engl J Med 291:26, 1974.
4. Jacobson, RJ, Solo, A, and Fialkow, PJ: Agnogenic myeloid metaplasia: A clonal proliferation of hemopoietic cells and secondary myelofibrosis. Blood 51:189, 1978.
5. Hoogstraten, B and Duiant, JR: Hematologic Malignancies. International Union Against Cancer, Current Treatment of Cancer. Springer-Verlag, Berlin Heidelberg, 1986.
6. Adams, JA, Berrett, AJ, and Beard, J: Primary polycythemia, essential thrombocythemia and myelofibrosis—three facets of a single disease process? Acta Haematol (Basel) 79:33–37, 1988.
7. Greenberg, BR and Wilson, FD: Cytogenetics of fibroblastic colonies in Ph¹–positive chronic myelogenous leukemia. Blood 51:1039, 1978.
8. Vadher, BD, et al: Life-threatening thrombotic and haemorrhagic problems associated with silent myeloproliferative disorders. Br J Haematol 85:213, 1993.
9. Muller, EW, De Wolf, JT, and Haagsma, EB: Portal hypertension as presenting feature of a myeloproliferative disorder. Diagnosis and therapeutic dilemmas. Scand J Gastroenterol Suppl 200:74, 1993.
10. Soekarman, D, et al: The translocation (6;9) (p23;q34) shows consistent rearrangement of two genes and defines a myeloproliferative disorder with specific clinical features. Blood 79:2990, 1992.
11. Hueck, G: Zwei Falle von Leukamia mit eigenthum Lichem Blut-resp Knoch en Markesbefund. Virchow Arch, Pathol Anat 78:475, 1879.
12. Woodliffe, HJ and Douigan, L: Myelofibrosis: Incidence and prevalaence in Western Australia. In Dahlem Workshop on Myelofibrosis-Osteosclerosis Syndrome, Oxford, Pergramon Press, 1974.
13. Ward, HP and Block, MH: The natural history of agnogenic myeloid metaplasia and a critical evaluation of its relationship with the myeloproliferative syndrome. Medicine 50:357–420, 1971.
14. Boxer, LA, et al: Myelofibrosis-myeloid metaplasia in childhood. Pediatrics 55:861, 1975.
15. Perez-Encinas, M, et al: Familial myeloproliferative syndrome. Am J Hematol 46:225, 1994.
16. Anderson, RE, Hoshino, T, and Yamamoto, T: Myelofibrosis with myeloid metaplasia in survivors of the atomic bomb in Hiroshima. Ann Intern Med 60:1, 1964.
17. Hoffbrand, AV and Lewis, SM: Postgraduate Hematology, ed 3. Heineman Professional Publishing, Oxford, 1989.
18. Bosch, W, et al: Toluene-associated myelofibrosis. Blut 58:219, 1989.
19. Rosen, PS, et al: Systemic lupus erythematosus (SLE) and myelofibrosis: A possible pathogenic relationship. Clin Res 21:565, 1973.
20. Lewis, CM and Pegrum, GD: Immune complexes in myelofibrosis: A possible guide to management. Br J Haematol 39:233, 1978.
21. Silverstein, MN: The evolution into and the treatment of late-stage polycythemia vera. Semin Hematol 3:79, 1976.
22. Khan, A, et al: A deficient G6PD variant with hemizygous expression in blood cells of a woman with primary myelofibrosis. Humangenetik 30:41, 1975.
23. Van Slyck, EJ, Weiss, L, and Dully, M: Chromosomal evidence for the secondary role of bone marrow fibroblast proliferation in acute myelofibrosis. Blood 36:729, 1970.
24. Takimoto, Y and Kimura, A: Basic and clinical study of platelet-derived growth factor gene expression. Rinsho Ketsueki 35:364, 1994.
23. Assoian, RK, et al: Cellular transformation by coordinated action of three peptide growth factors from human platelets. Nature 309:804, 1984.
26. Gersuk, GM, et al: Quantitative and functional studies of impaired natural killer (NK) cells in patients with myelofibrosis, essential thrombocythemia, and polycythemia vera. I. A potential role for platelet-derived growth factor in defective NK cytotoxicity. Nat Immun 12:136, 1993.
27. Jandl, JH: Blood, Textbook of Hematology. Little Brown, Boston, 1987.
28. McCarthy, DM: Fibrosis of the bone marrow: Content and causes. Br J Haematol 59:1, 1985.
29. Lewis, SM: Myelofibrosis, Pathology and Clinical Management, Hematology, vol 4. Marcel Dekker, New York, 1985.
30. Lee, GR, et al: Wintrobe's Clinical Hematology, ed 9. Lea & Febiger, Philadelphia, 1993.
31. Silverstein, MN: Agnogenic Myeloid Metaplasia. Publishing Science, Boston, 1975.
32. Manoharan, A, Hargrave, M, and Gordon, S: Effect of chemotherapy on tear drop poikilocytes and other peripheral blood findings in myelofibrosis. Pathology 20:7, 1988.
33. Njoku, OS, et al: Anemia in myelofibrosis: Its value in prognosis. Br J Haematol 54:79, 1983.
34. Weinfield, A, Branehog, I, and Kutti, J: Platelets in the myeloproliferative syndromes. Clin Haematol 4:373, 1975.
35. Baker, RI and Manoharan, A: Platelet function in myeloproliferative disorders: Characterization and sequential studies show multiple platelet abnormalities, and change with time. Eur J Haematol 40:267, 1988.
36. Babior, BM and Stossed, TP, Hematology A Pathophysiological Approach, ed 3. Churchill Livingstone, 1994.
37. Leoni, P, et al: Antibodies against terminal galactosyl alpha (1-3) galactose epitopes in patients with idiopathic myelofibrosis. Br J Haematol 85:313, 1993.
38. Dickstein, JI and Vardiman JW: Issues in the pathology and diagnosis of the chronic myeloproliferative disorders and the myelodysplastic syndromes. (Review). Am J Clin Pathol 99:515, 519, 1993.
39. Benbasset, J, et al: Splenectomy in patients with agnogenic myeloid metaplasia: An analysis of 321 published cases. Br J Haemotol 42:207, 1979.
40. Ketley, NJ, et al: Haematological splenectomy. Changing indications and complications. Clin Lab Haematol 14:179, 1992.
41. Williams, JW: Hematology, ed 3. McGraw-Hill, New York, 1983.
42. Laszlo, J, et al: The use of hydroxyurea in myelofibrosis. Minutes of Polycythemia Vera Study Group, November 1983.

43. Hoffbrand, AV, and Pettit, JW, Essential Haematology, ed 3. Blackwell Scientific, Oxford, 1993.

44. Rojkind, M: Anti-inflammatory and antifibrotic actions of colchicine. Myelofibrosis and the Biology of the Connective Tissue Symposium, New York, November 1982.

45. Barosi, G, et al: A prognostic classification of myeloid metaplasia. Br J Haematol 70:400, 1988.

46. Polliock, A, Prokocimer, and M, Matzner, Y: Lymphoblastic leukemia transformation (lymphoblastic crisis) in myelofibrosis and myeloid metaplasia. Am J Hematol 9:211, 1980.

47. Garcia, S, et al: Idiopathic myelofibrosis terminating in erythroleukemia. Am J Hematol 32:70, 1989.

48. Hippocrates: Dehumoribus. Chapter 1.

49. Von Haller: Elementa physiologiae corporis humani. (Lausanne) 2:34, 1757.

50. Wasserman, LR: Polycythemia Vera Study Group: A Historical Perspective. Semin Hematol 23:183, 1986.

51. Turk, W: Beitrage zur Kenntnis des Symptomenbildes Polycythamie mit Milztumor und Zyanose. Wein Klin Wochenschr 17:153, 1904.

52. Hirsch, R: Generalized osteosclerosis with chronic polycythemia vera. Arch Pathol 19:91, 1935.

53. Rosenthal, N and Sessen, FA: Course of polycythemia. Arch Intern Med 62:903, 1938.

54. Castro-Malaspina, H, et al: Human megakaryocyte stimulation of proliferation of bone marrow fibroblasts. Blood 57:781, 1981.

55. Kung, C, et al: Polycythemia: primary or secondary: The differential diagnostic value of stem cell cultures. Schweiz Med Wochenschr 123:53, 1993.

56. Danish, EH, Rasch, CA, and Harris, JW: Polycythemia vera in childhood: Case report and review of the literature. Am J Hematol 9:421, 1980.

57. Chaiter, Y, Brenner, B, et al: High incidence of myeloproliferative disorders in Askenazi Jews in northern Israel. Leukemia Lymphoma 6:252, 1992.

58. Dawson, AA and Ogston, D: The influence of platelet counts on the incidence of thrombotic and hemorrhagic complications in polycythemia vera. Postgrad Med J 46:76, 1970.

59. Rogers, BA: Want to live with polycythemia vera for a few hours? Lab World, 12:33, 1981.

60. Pollycove, M, Winchell, HS, and Lawrence, JH: Classification and evolution of patterns of erythropoiesis in polycythemia vera as studied by iron kinetics. Blood 28:807, 1966.

61. Reich, PR: Hematology, Physiopathologic Basis for Clinical Practice, ed 2. Little, Brown, 1984.

62. Juvonen, E: Megakaryocytic colony formation in polycythemia vera and secondary erythrocytosis. Br J Hematol 69:441, 1988.

63. Murphy, S, et al: Template bleeding time and clinical hemorrhage in myeloproliferative disease. Arch Intern Med 138:1251, 1978.

64. Ellis, JT, et al: Studies of bone marrow in polycythemia vera and the evolution of myelofibrosis and second hematologic malignancies. Semin Hematol 23:154, 1986.

65. Westwood, N, et al: Primary polycythaemia: Diagnosis by nonconventional positive criteria. Eur J Haematol 51:228, 1993.

66. Zittoun, G, et al: The three transcobalamins in myeloproliferative disorders and acute leukemia. Br J Haemotol 31:287, 1975.

67. Gilbert, HS, et al: Serum vitamin B_{12} content and unsaturated vitamin B_{12}-binding capacity in myeloproliferative disease. Ann Intern Med 71:719, 1969.

68. Dutcher, TF: Hematologic morphology for teachers and learners. ASCP National Meeting, ASCP Press, Chicago, 1994.

69. Berk, PD, et al: Therapeutic recommendations in polycythemia vera based on Polycythemia Vera Study Group Protocols. Semin Hematol 23:132, 1986.

70. Videbalk, A: Polycythemia vera, course and prognosis. Act Med Scand 138:179, 1950.

71. Chievitz, E and Thiede, T: Complications and causes of death in polycythemia vera. Acta Med Scand 172:513, 1962.

72. Weinfeld, A, Swolin, B, and Westin, J: Acute leukaemia after hydroxyurea therapy in polycythemia vera and allied disorders: Prospective study of efficacy and leukaemogenicity with therapeutic implications. Eur J Haematol 52(3):134, 1994.

73. Thomas, DJ, et al: Cerebral blood flow in polycythemia. Lancet 2:161, 1977.

74. Kaplan, M, et al: Long-term management of polycythemia vera with hydroxyurea: A progress report. Semin Hematol 23:167, 1986.

75. Wasserman, LR: Polycythemia Vera Study Group: A historical perspective. Semin Hematol 23:183, 1986.

76. Donovan, PB: Progress in diagnosis and treatment of polycythemia vera. Lab World 12:25, 1981.

77. Sharon, R, Tatarsky, I, Ben-arieh, Y: Treatment of polycythemia vera with hydroxyurea. Cancer 57:718, 1986.

78. Gaisbock, F: Die Bedeutung des Blutdruckmessung fur die arztlichen Praxis. Dtsch Arch Klin Med 83:363, 1905.

79. Fialkow, PJ, et al: Evidence that essential thrombocythemia is a clonal disorder with origin in a multipotent stem cell. Blood 58:916, 1981.

80. Murphy, S, et al: Essential thrombocythemia: An interim report from the Polycythemia Vera Study Group. Semin Hematol 23:177, 1986.

81. Iland, HJ, et al: Differentiation between essential thrombocythemia and polycythemia vera with marked thrombocytosis, Am J Hematol 25:191, 1987.

82. Belluce, S, et al: Essential thrombocythemia, clinical evolutionary and biological data. Cancer 58:2440, 1986.

83. Mitus, AJ, et al: Hemostatic complications in young patients with essential thrombocythemia. Am J Med 88:371, 1990.

84. Rosenthal, DS: Clinical aspects of chronic myeloproliferative diseases (Review). Am J Med Sci 304:109, 1992.

85. Williams, WJ, et al: Hematology, ed 4. McGraw-Hill Publishing, 1990.

86. Michiels, JJ, and Ten Kate, FJ: Erythromelalgia in thrombocythemia of various myeloproliferative disorders. Am J Hematol 39:131, 1992.

87. Singh, AK, and Wetherling-Mein, G: Microvascular occlusive lesions in primary thrombocythemia. Br J Haematol 36:553, 1977.

88. Falconer, J, et al: Essential thrombocythemia associated with recurrent abortions and fetal growth retardation. Am J Hematol 25:345, 1987.

89. Tefferi, A, and Hoagland, HC: Issues in the diagnosis and management of essential thrombocythemia. Mayo Clin Proc 69:651, 1994.

90. Silverstein, MN, et al: Anagrelide: A new drug for treating thrombocytosis. N Engl J Med 318:20, 1988.

91. Fuscaldo, KE, et al: Correlation of a specific chromosomal marker, 21q−, and retroviral indicators in patients with thrombocythemia. Cancer Lett. 6:51, 1979.

92. Randi, ML, et al: Which tests are most useful in distinguishing between reactive thrombocytosis and the thrombocytosis of myeloproliferative disease? Clin Lab Haematol 14:267, 1992.

93. Murphy, S, Douis, JJ, Walsh, PN, et al: Template bleeding time and clinical hemorrhage in myeloproliferative disease. Arch Intern Med 138:1251, 1978.

94. Conlon, M and Haire, W: Low protein S in essential thrombocythemia with thrombosis. Am J Hematol 32:553, 1989.

95. Thiele, J, et al: Primary (essential) thrombocythemia versus initial (hyperplastic) stages of agnogenic myeloid metaplasia with thrombocytosis—a critical evaluation of clinical and histomorphological data. Acta Haematol 81:200, 1989.
96. Van Genderen, PJ and Michiels, JJ: Primary thrombocythemia: diagnosis, clinical manifestations and management. Ann Hematol 67:57, 1993.
97. Baron, BW, Mick, R, and Baron, JM: Combined plateletpheresis and cytotoxic chemotherapy for symptomatic thrombocytosis in myeloproliferative disorders. Cancer 72:1209, 1993.
98. Michiels, JJ, et al: Erythromelagia caused by platelet mediated arteriolar inflammation and thrombosis in thrombocythemia. Ann Intern Med 102:466, 1985.
99. Jabaily, J, et al: Neurologic manifestations of essential thrombocythemia. Ann Intern Med 99:513, 1983.
100. Beard, J, et al: Primary thrombocythemia in pregnancy. Br J Haematol 77:371, 1991.
101. Gugliotta, L, et al: In vivo and in vitro inhibiting effect of alpha-interferon on megakaryocytic colony growth in essential thrombocythemia. Br J Haematol 71:177–181, 1989.
102. Iland, HJ, et al: Essential thrombocythemia: Clinical and laboratory characteristics at presentation. Trans Assoc Am Physicians 96:165, 1983.
103. Gilbert, HS: The spectrum of myeloproliferative disorders. Med Clin North Am 57:355, 1973.

QUESTIONS

1. What is the origin of MPDs?
   a. Fibroid infiltration of major organs
   b. Neoplastic transformation of multipotential stem cells
   c. Widespread deterioration of cellular function
   d. Splenic sequestration of normal blood cells

2. Which of the following is not a characteristic of a chronic MPD?
   a. Extramedullary hematopoiesis
   b. Possible termination in acute leukemia
   c. Cytogenetic abnormalities
   d. Hypoplasia of bone marrow

3. What is the predominant abnormal erythrocyte morphology associated with idiopathic myelofibrosis?
   a. Schistocytes
   b. Ovalocytes
   c. Teardrop cells
   d. Target cells

4. Which features are the most important characteristics of chronic myelogenous leukemia that distinguish it from myelofibrosis?
   a. Presence of increased platelets and fibroblasts
   b. Decreased erythrocytes with abnormal morphology
   c. Increased leukocytes with hypercellular bone marrow
   d. Low LAP score and presence of Ph[1] chromosome

5. What are the laboratory findings in polycythemia vera?
   a. Decreased hemoglobin and/or hematocrit, increased RBCs and granulocytes, decreased platelets
   b. Increased hemoglobin and/or hematocrit; increased RBCs, granulocytes, and platelets
   c. Normal hemoglobin and hematocrit, normal RBCs, increased granulocytes and platelets
   d. Increased hemoglobin and/or hematocrit, increased RBCs, decreased granulocytes and platelets

6. Which features help to distinguish secondary polycythemia and relative erythrocytosis from polycythemia vera?
   a. Absence of splenomegaly; normal leukocyte, platelet, and LAP levels
   b. Presence of splenomegaly; increased leukocyte, platelet, and LAP levels
   c. Presence of hepatomegaly; decreased leukocyte, platelet, and LAP levels
   d. Presence of both splenomegaly and hepatomegaly; increased leukocytes and platelets; decreased LAP score

7. What is the safest and least expensive treatment for patients with polycythemia vera?
   a. High altitude
   b. Decrease of iron levels
   c. Therapeutic phlebotomy
   d. Decrease of erythropoietin levels

8. Which condition will not cause an absolute erythrocytosis?
   a. High altitude
   b. Chronic pulmonary disease
   c. Polycythemia vera
   d. Dehydration

9. What condition is defined by a platelet count >600 × 10^9/L, megakaryocytic hyperplasia, absence of Ph[1] chromosome, and hemoglobin ≤13 g/dL (or normal red cell mass)?
   a. Essential thrombocythemia
   b. May-Hegglin anomaly
   c. Acute myelogenous leukemia
   d. Polycythemia vera

10. What condition is not characteristically associated with reactive thrombocytosis?
    a. Acute hemorrhage
    b. Aplastic anemia
    c. Chronic inflammatory disorders
    d. Iron-deficiency anemia

ANSWERS

1. **b** (p 376)
2. **d** (pp 377–378)
3. **c** (p 378)
4. **d** (p 383)
5. **b** (pp 387–389)
6. **a** (pp 390–391)
7. **c** (p 393)
8. **d** (p 390) (Table 21–7)
9. **a** (p 395)
10. **b** (p 396) (Table 21–9)

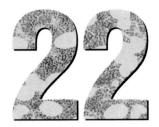

Multiple Myeloma and Related Plasma Cell Disorders*

James M. Long, MD, LtCol (sel), USAF

Multiple Myeloma
    Laboratory and Radiologic Evaluation of
      Plasma Cell Disorders
    Diagnosis and Differential Diagnosis of
      Multiple Myeloma
Monoclonal Gammopathy of Undetermined
Significance

Waldenström's Macroglobulinemia
Heavy-Chain Disease
Case Study 1
Cast Study 2
Case Study 3

Objectives

At the end of this chapter, the learner should be able to:
1. List laboratory tests that are useful for the evaluation of immunoglobulin disorders.
2. Describe the significance of an M-spike and its evaluation by immunoelectrophoresis.
3. State what Bence-Jones proteins are, how they are detected, and why they are important.
4. List the diagnostic criteria for multiple myeloma.
5. List tests useful for staging and prognosis of patients with multiple myeloma.
6. List diagnostic criteria for monoclonal gammopathy of undetermined significance.
7. List diagnostic criteria for Waldenström's macroglobulinemia.
8. Describe heavy-chain disease.

MULTIPLE MYELOMA

Overview

Multiple myeloma is a disorder characterized by the overproduction of abnormal plasma cells. This single cellular excess has far-reaching effects, as listed in Table 22–1. Patients with multiple myeloma may have markedly different symptoms at the time of diagnosis because of the variety of body functions affected by the disease. Multiple myeloma may cause bone destruction, high serum calcium levels, kidney failure, infections, nerve compression with paralysis, and changes in mental status ranging from mild confusion to coma. This disease is diagnosed in some patients with no symptoms after a screening blood test reveals abnormally high serum protein levels or x-rays reveal excess calcium loss from the bones. In some rare cases, patients are diagnosed only after they have developed marked changes in their mental status with extensive bone destruction, high calcium levels, and kidney failure. Most patients found to have multiple myeloma fall somewhere between these two extremes.

The causes of multiple myeloma and the population it affects will be discussed. The wide-ranging effects of myeloma on the body will follow in a "cause-and-effect" format. The use of the clinical laboratory in evaluating plasma cell disorders is then discussed, followed by an introduction to the various radiologic procedures used in the evaluation of these diseases. The evolving field of molecular biology and its relevance to the study of multiple myeloma will be briefly introduced.

Following this technical information, the clinical usefulness of this testing will be presented. Specifically, it will be shown how physicians are able to use this information to determine whether a patient has multiple myeloma or one of the other related plasma

---

*The views expressed in this material are those of the author and do not reflect the official policy or position of the U.S. Government, the Department of Defense, or the Department of the Air Force.

TABLE 22-1 **Signs and Symptoms of Plasma Cell Disorders**

Signs	Symptoms
Anemia	Tiredness
	Fatigue
	Shortness of breath
Hypercalcemia	Mental status changes
	Bone pain
	Kidney stones
	Constipation and abdominal pain
Renal failure	None (until late)
Bone lesions on radiograph	Bone pain
	Mass
	Pathologic fractures
Elevated serum globulins	Possible hyperviscosity syndrome
Serum hyperviscosity	Confusion
	Increased bleeding tendency
	Raynaud's phenomenon
	Visual complaints

cell disorders listed in Table 22–2. These other disorders are briefly introduced. Since the prognosis of the patient and treatment decisions depend on the extent and aggressiveness of the disease, various "staging" systems have been developed. These systems attempt to group together patients with similar disease conditions and expected outcome and will be briefly presented.

Principles of the treatment of multiple myeloma will be summarized, but extensive discussion of the details of treatment is beyond the scope of this text. References are supplied for those seeking further information.

Plasma Cell Development and Abnormal Clones

The plasma cell is the final stage in the development of B lymphocytes (refer to Chapter 1 and Fig. 22–1). It is characterized by the production and release of specific immunoglobulin molecules (see Fig. 22–1).

During cellular replication and differentiation, a genetic mistake may occur. Evolving evidence supports

TABLE 22-2 **Plasma Cell Disorders**

Solitary plasmacytoma
Multiple myeloma
  Smoldering myeloma
  Classic multiple myeloma
  Advanced myeloma
  Nonsecretory myeloma
Monoclonal gammopathy of undetermined significance (MGUS)
Waldenström's macroglobulinemia
Heavy-chain disease (HCD)
  Gamma HCD
  Mu HCD
  Alpha HCD

the theory that mutations in multiple myeloma occur during the period when mature B lymphocytes are becoming plasmablasts. A mutated plasmablast is then relocated via the blood to the bone marrow, where it produces a colony of identical mutated plasma cells referred to as a *clone*. A single tumor mass composed of a clone of abnormal plasma cells is called a *plasmacytoma*. Some of these abnormal cells travel by the blood to other locations in the bone marrow where new colonies are established.[1] These multiple plasmacytomas lead to the name multiple myeloma.

There is clear evidence that one of the primary changes that occur as a result of these mutated plasma cells is the production of interleukin-6 (IL-6). IL-6 is one of a broad class of molecules referred to as *cytokines*. Cytokines provide "communication" among cells leading to stimulation or suppression of cellular reproduction, production of cell products, or secretion of other cytokines (see Chap. 1). Abnormal plasma cells in multiple myeloma proliferate when exposed to IL-6 and other growth factors. Blocking IL-6 stops the growth of myeloma cells in the laboratory. Although it is not the only cytokine involved, it appears to be one of the most important.[2] As these mutated plasma cells induce the production of the IL-6 and other cytokines that cause further replication, the malignancy known as multiple myeloma develops.

Etiology and Epidemiology

The overall incidence of myeloma is 5 cases per 100,000 persons each year. Men have approximately 50% greater risk than women. The rates of occurrence in black individuals (8 per 100,000) are double the rates in white individuals (4 per 100,000). Hawaiians, Alaskans, female Hispanics, and female Native Americans also have higher rates than whites, whereas those of Japanese and Chinese descent experience less. There is a steady increase in incidence of multiple myeloma with age, the disease being distinctly rare under the age of 40 and the highest risk (70 cases per 100,000 population) being in black men over the age of 80 (Fig. 22–2).[3]

Environmental factors play a clear role in causing multiple myeloma. Atomic bomb survivors and individuals exposed to radiation in the workplace (such as radium watch dial painters and radiologists) have an increased risk of multiple myeloma. Studies of workers at nuclear power plants also suggest that chronic exposure to low levels of radiation may lead to increased risk of myeloma. Chronic stimulation of the immune system has been a suspected cause of myeloma. Increased risk of myeloma in the agricultural industry has implicated grain dust, molds, engine exhaust, viruses, insecticides, fertilizers, herbicides, and other agricultural chemicals. Workers in the metal, rubber, wood, leather, and textile industries may be at increased risk, as are those who work with benzene and other organic solvents. The debate still rages about the significant evidence linking use of hair dyes to increased risk of myeloma in women and men. No relationship to tobacco or alcohol use has been shown. Certain medical conditions such as rheumatoid arthritis, chronic allergic conditions, and chronic infections may also increase the risk for myeloma.[4]

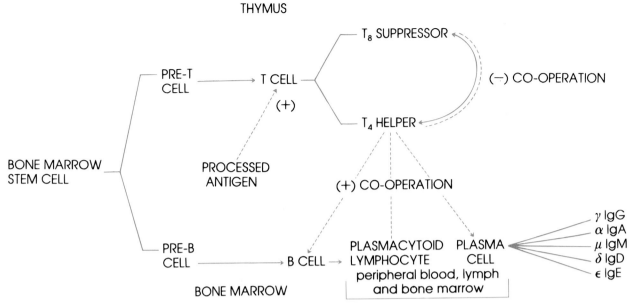

FIGURE 22–1 Development of T and B lymphocytes showing interaction. T_4 and T_8 are equivalent to CD4 and CD8, respectively.

Pathophysiology of Multiple Myeloma

Overview

There are three primary disease processes that lead to the complex disruption of various organ systems. The understanding of multiple myeloma can be simplified by examining these processes. Each has multiple effects and will be discussed in turn. First, the effects of the expanding plasma cell mass will be presented, followed in turn by discussions of the overproduction of monoclonal immunoglobulins, and the production of osteoclast activating factor and other cytokines.

Expanding Plasma Cell Mass

Mutated plasmablasts in the bone marrow undergo continued clonal replication under the influence of IL-

Myeloma incidence per 100,000

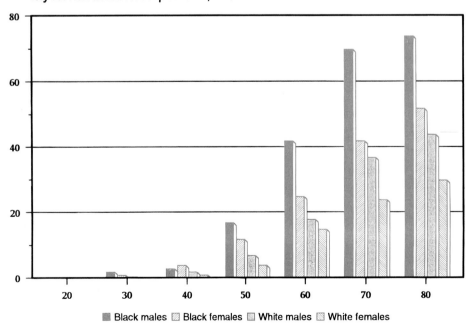

Decade of age (years)

FIGURE 22–2 Average annual age-specific incidence of multiple myeloma in the United States, 1973–1988. Age is plotted as the average of two 5-year age groups. Rates are per 100,000 persons per decade of age in years. (From Ries LAG, Hankey BF, Miller BA, et al: Cancer Statistics Review 1973–1988 Washington, DC, US Government Printing Office, 1991 [DHHS publication (NIH) No. 9 2789.]

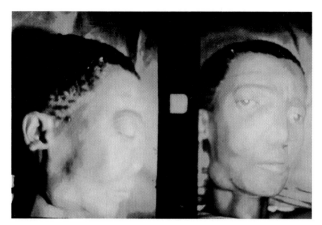

FIGURE 22–3 Plasmacytomas of the face and jaw in a patient with multiple myeloma.

6 and other growth factor cytokines.[2] As this relentless growth proceeds, individual actively dividing cells again circulate in the blood to find rest at other locations in the bone marrow. Each new colony establishes an independent local production of growth factor, and the process continues.

Normal bone marrow is gradually replaced by the steadily growing individual malignant plasma cell colonies. As the replacement progresses, normal circulating blood cells decrease in number, a condition referred to as *pancytopenia*. These cellular deficiencies commonly appear in sequence. First, a decrease in the number of red blood cells (anemia) is observed. Later, decreases in the numbers of platelets occur (throm-

bocytopenia), and in advanced myeloma, neutrophils also decrease (neutropenia). Anemia results in fatigue, shortness of breath, and rapid heart rate. Thrombocytopenia results in delayed hemostasis with resultant prolonged bleeding with injuries. Neutropenia causes a dramatically increased susceptibility to bacterial infections.

The expanding cell masses originating in the bone marrow frequently cause destruction of the surface "cortex" of the bone. Stretching of the overlying nerve-rich periosteum leads to pain. Pain is present at diagnosis in more than two-thirds of patients.[5] The expanding plasmacytoma may extend beyond the boundaries of the bone to compress adjacent neurologic structures. This occurs most frequently in the vertebrae, where the nerve roots exiting from the spine and even the spinal cord itself may be compressed. This causes pain and may lead to paralysis and loss of sensation. Less commonly plasmacytomas may occur in areas other than the bone and bone marrow (Fig. 22–3). These "extramedullary plasmacytomas" may occur in the nasopharynx, paranasal sinuses, liver, spleen, skin, kidneys, and gastrointestinal tract. Symptoms result from the growing tumor and vary according to the site involved.

Production of Immunoglobulin: "Monoclonal Gammopathy"

Normal Immunoglobulin Structure Most malignant plasma cells actively produce immunoglobulin. Immunoglobulin units are composed of two identical heavy chains (50,000 daltons) and two identical light chains (25,000 daltons) (Fig. 22–4). These chains are

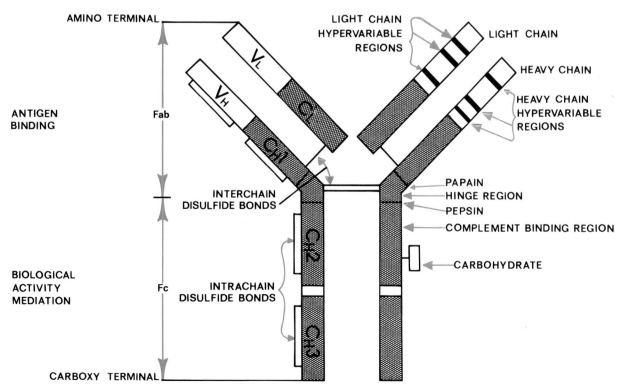

FIGURE 22–4 Structure of the basic immunoglobulin unit.

held together by varying numbers of disulfide bonds. The antibody produced by each plasma cell has only one type of light chain and one type of heavy chain. There are two types of light chains named kappa and lambda. There are five types of heavy chains named gamma, alpha, mu, delta, and epsilon. They correspond to the five classes of antibodies named IgG, IgA, IgM, IgD, and IgE. The heavy-chain subunit identifies the immunoglobulin class. Each immunoglobulin class has a specific function. IgG is the primary antibody class involved in fighting infection and is produced in measurable amounts long after the antigen stimulus is removed. IgA is characteristically a secretory antibody providing protection of body surfaces in the gastrointestinal tract and the airways. IgM is produced as the earliest, but temporary, response to infections and becomes unmeasurable within weeks after it first appears. The IgE class is involved in allergic or hypersensitivity reactions. The role of IgD remains unclear. IgA and IgG have varying numbers and location of the disulfide bonds linking the heavy chains together and the heavy chains to the light chains. These differing "isotypes" are named IgG1, IgG2, IgG3, IgG4, IgA1, and IgA2. The functions and properties vary slightly as a result of these differences.

Most antibodies are composed of two identical heavy chains and two identical light chains making a single immunoglobulin unit. IgM, however, exists primarily as a "pentamer" molecule composed of five such units. IgA and IgG2 tend to exist in pairs of units as "dimers" or may polymerize to larger molecules. An antibody is named by its heavy-chain class as well as the type of light chain (e.g., IgG kappa or IgA lambda, etc.)

Monoclonal and Incomplete Immunoglobulins In multiple myeloma the normally controlled and purposeful production of antibodies is replaced by the inappropriate production of even larger amounts of use-

less immunoglobulin molecules. The normally equal production of light chains and heavy chains may be imbalanced. The result is the release of excess free light chains or free heavy chains. The immunoglobulins produced by a clone of myeloma cells are identical. Any abnormal production of identical antibodies is referred to by the general name of monoclonal gammopathy. Rarely (<1%), myelomas may produce no antibodies; 6% produce only light chains. Two antibody classes are produced in 3.5% of cases and probably represent the coexistence of two different malignant clones (Fig. 22–5). The overproduction of immunoglobulin is one of the hallmarks of multiple myeloma. IgG is the most common (52%), but IgA also accounts for 25% of cases. IgD, IgE, and IgM together account for less than 1% of cases.

Hyperviscosity Syndrome The presence of excess immunoglobulin can lead to alteration in the physical characteristic of blood known as viscosity. Overly viscous blood has higher resistance to flow. The result is decreased flow through the smallest blood vessels of the brain, heart, and other organs as well as an increased workload on the heart. Patients suffering from hyperviscosity syndrome may complain of confusion, blurred vision, headache, chest tightness or angina, or numbness or tingling of the fingertips. The increased oncotic pressure caused by these proteins leads to expansion of blood volume. The heart may be unable to tolerate these changes, leading to congestive heart failure. Such patients experience fluid weight gain, swelling of the ankles, and difficulty breathing.

Any class of immunoglobulins can cause hyperviscosity syndrome if the blood levels are sufficiently high. IgM, a large molecule composed of five immunoglobulin units, causes a much higher increase in viscosity than would five individual units (of IgG, for example). For this reason, most cases of clinical hyperviscosity

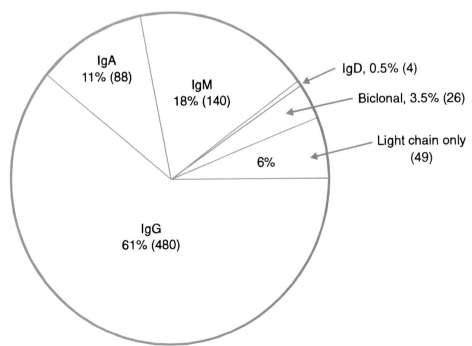

FIGURE 22–5 Monoclonal serum protein in 787 Mayo Clinic patients.

syndrome are seen due to excess IgM. IgA and IgG3 may exist as dimers or polymers and are somewhat more likely to cause hyperviscosity syndrome than IgG monomers.[6]

Decreased Production of Normal Immunoglobulins Patients with multiple myeloma often have decreased levels of the normal circulating antibody classes. The low levels are probably caused by suppressed function of normal B lymphocytes and plasma cells as a response to the presence of the abnormal immunoglobulins. The lower level of immunoglobulins leads to increased susceptibility to infections such as sinusitis, bronchitis, and pneumonia. Infection remains the leading cause of death of patients with multiple myeloma.

Bence-Jones Protein and Kidney Damage Imbalanced immunoglobulin production most frequently yields an excess of light chains. These light chains are rapidly metabolized in the blood and are small enough to be filtered into the urine. The excess is thus most frequently detected by finding light chains in the urine and are often not detected in the blood. Light chains have the unique property of precipitating out of solution when urine is heated to approximately 56°C, and then dissolving again as the temperature rises. As the urine is allowed to cool to 56°C, a precipitate will again form, followed by dissolution on further cooling. These urinary light chains are named Bence-Jones proteins after the physicians who first noted this unusual property. Light chains are toxic to the kidneys and can lead to leakage of protein into the urine (proteinuria) and kidney failure.

Amyloidosis Immunoglobulin kappa or lambda light chains may settle or deposit in many organs such as the heart, kidneys, nerves, liver, spleen, gastrointestinal tract, and skin. Accumulation of this nonstructural protein is called *amyloid* (Fig. 22–6). Amyloidosis causes progressive loss of function of the involved organs and may lead to death caused by heart or kidney failure.

Autoimmune Phenomena Rarely, the antibodies produced by myeloma plasma cells are specifically targeted on the patient's own cells. If the targeted cells are red cells, this may lead to the red cell destruction known as *autoimmune hemolytic anemia*. If the anti-

bodies are directed against one of the clotting factor proteins, the patient may develop a bleeding disorder. Although rare, many different manifestations of this type of autoimmune phenomena have been reported.

Bleeding Disorders and Cryoglobulins Increased levels of immunoglobulins in the blood may interfere with the function of the clotting factor proteins of the coagulation cascade. This is usually not clinically significant, but may result in prolongation of tests of blood coagulation such as the prothrombin time (PT) and activated partial thromboplastin time (APTT). In advanced stages, bruising and abnormal gum or nose bleeding may occur.

Cryoglobulins are immunoglobulins that precipitate on exposure to cold. Cryoglobulinemia may rarely occur in patients with multiple myeloma. Patients with this syndrome often complain of pain in the extremities on exposure to cold. This usually affects the fingers, nose, and ears. Cryoglobulins can cause more serious complications such as vasculitis and kidney damage after cold exposure.

Production of Osteoclast-Activating Factor and Cytokines

Osteoclasts and Bone Destruction Normal bone is a dynamic structure with ongoing remodeling as a result of a balance between bone resorption and new bone formation. Osteoclasts are bone cells active in locally reabsorbing bone and releasing calcium into the blood. Nearby osteoblasts are equally active in utilizing calcium in the blood to form new bone.

Multiple myeloma interrupts this balance by the secretion of at least two substances. These are IL-6, mentioned above, and osteoclast-activating factor (OAF). OAF, as its name implies, stimulates osteoclasts to increase bone resorption and release of calcium. Since osteoblasts are not stimulated, the net result is progressive destruction of the bone, with corresponding loss of calcium and weakening of the bone structure. In x-rays, bone appears dense because of the calcium in the cortex. Since the individual plasmacytomas growing in the marrow each stimulate local destruction of the cortical bone and loss of calcium, radiographs demonstrate clear or lucent areas referred to as lytic lesions (Fig. 22–7). These weakened areas may break under everyday stresses such as standing up, lifting objects, or even bending over (see Fig. 22–8). Such breaks caused by weakening of the bone from malignancy are called *pathologic fractures*.

Interleukin-6 (IL-6) as well as other factors have been found to have a critical role in stimulating osteoclast activity as well as inhibiting osteoblasts and new bone formation. It is likely that the inhibition of osteoblastic activity is as important as the stimulation of osteoclasts in the formation of lytic bone lesions. IL-6 has both a local effect on bone destruction, as does OAF, but also is found in measurable levels in the blood. Occasionally myeloma patients have a generalized loss of calcium from the bones known as osteoporosis that may appear earlier than the lytic lesions. It is possible that circulating IL-6 or other cytokines may be partly responsible for this finding.[7]

Hypercalcemia Balance of calcium in the body is critical because of its role in many cellular processes.

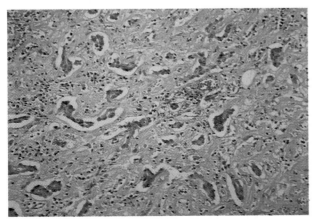

FIGURE 22–6 Amorphous amyloid deposits replacing normal liver architecture.

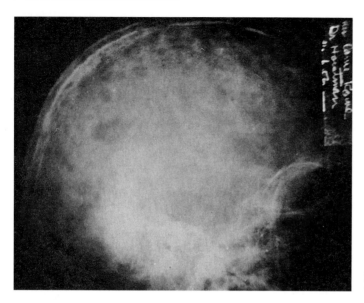

FIGURE 22–7 Extensive lytic skull lesions in a patient with multiple myeloma.

As calcium is released from the bones, the result is excess free calcium in the blood. This may cause several symptoms. One of the earliest is constipation and cramping from altered motility of the intestine. Muscle weakness may occur. Varying degrees of change in mental status may develop, such as confusion, psychosis, and even coma. The extent of mental status change is dependent on both the level of calcium and the rate of rise. Bone pain is common with high calcium levels. Increased calcium in the urine can lead to formation of kidney stones and kidney failure. Figure 22–9 outlines the disorders associated with multiple myeloma.

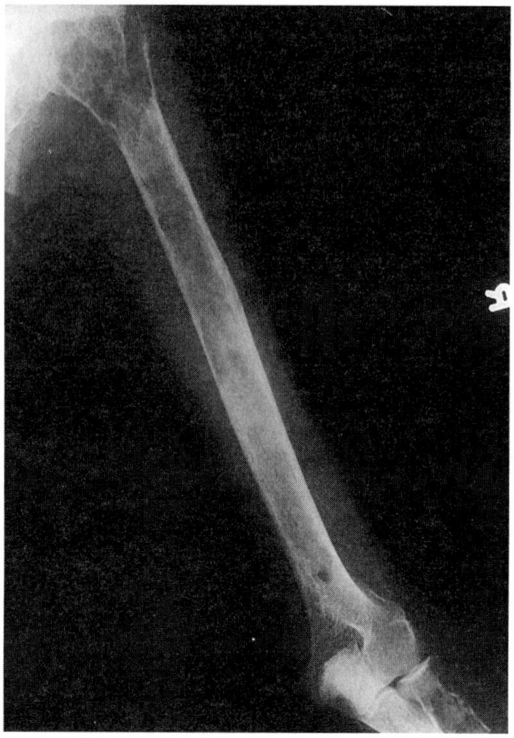

Laboratory and Radiologic Evaluation of Plasma Cell Disorders

Laboratory Studies

Protein Electrophoresis Protein in the serum consists primarily of albumin, immunoglobulins, and smaller amounts of other proteins. Serum proteins are measured as total protein on routine automated chemistry panels. Measurement of albumin allows approximate quantitation of the immunoglobulin-containing fraction by subtraction (i.e., Total protein − Albumin = Immunoglobulin fraction). Thus, one can detect a substantial increase in immunoglobulins by an automated chemistry panel alone. It is important to differentiate between increased immunoglobulins formed as a result of normal processes and the monoclonal antibodies seen in disorders of plasma cell function such as multiple myeloma. This can best be performed by protein electrophoresis. Figure 22–10 illustrates and compares different patterns of protein electrophoresis for the various plasma cell disorders.

The spike on protein electrophoresis caused by monoclonal immunoglobulins is called a monoclonal spike or M-spike (see Fig. 22–10). Thus, a primary reason for performing a protein electrophoresis is to determine whether an M-spike is present or not. The same procedure is used for analyzing urine samples for M-spikes. It is performed on an aliquot of a 24-hour urine collection. Further identification of the proteins causing the M-spike is carried out by a technique called *immunoelectrophoresis*, which is critical in the diagnostic evaluation of multiple myeloma.

Immunoelectrophoresis In immunoelectrophoresis, the proteins are separated by electrical charge and

FIGURE 22–8 Radiographic film of the left humerus of a patient with multiple myeloma. Areas with severe cortical bone destruction may be fractured by everyday activities such as lifting or walking (pathological fractures).

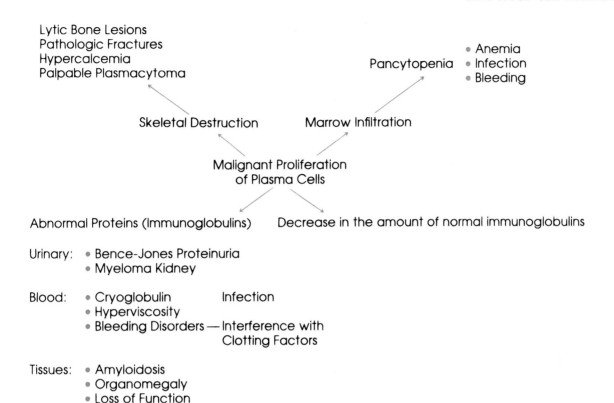

Lytic Bone Lesions
Pathologic Fractures
Hypercalcemia
Palpable Plasmacytoma

Pancytopenia
• Anemia
• Infection
• Bleeding

Skeletal Destruction   Marrow Infiltration

Malignant Proliferation
of Plasma Cells

Abnormal Proteins (Immunoglobulins)   Decrease in the amount of normal immunoglobulins

Urinary: • Bence-Jones Proteinuria
           • Myeloma Kidney

Blood: • Cryoglobulin   Infection
           • Hyperviscosity
           • Bleeding Disorders — Interference with
                                   Clotting Factors

Tissues: • Amyloidosis
           • Organomegaly
           • Loss of Function

FIGURE 22-9 Mechanisms of disease in multiple myeloma. Skeletal destruction, abnormal immunoglobulin production, marrow failure, and decreased production of normal immunoglobulins all play a role.

antibodies to IgG, IgM, IgA, kappa light chains, and lambda light chains are then diffused into the gel. Precipitation occurs when the antibody from the reagent meets the corresponding light-chain or heavy-chain molecule. An M-spike may be identified because it will form a line of precipitation only with the antibody targeted to its specific heavy-chain class and with the antibody targeted toward its specific light chain.

Quantitative Immunoglobulins Immunoglobulin classes IgG, IgA, and IgM and both kappa and lambda light chains are quantitated by either radial immunodiffusion or rate nephelometry. The latter is the most accurate technique (less than 5% variation in results) and is based on light scatter caused by antigen-antibody complexes formed by mixing a serum sample with an appropriate specific antibody reagent.[8] Decreased levels of normal immunoglobulins are characteristic of multiple myeloma.

Complete Blood Count and Peripheral Blood Smear The automated complete blood count (CBC) is the most readily available assessment of bone marrow function. The most common finding in multiple myeloma is a decrease in the number of red blood cells with no change in size (normocytic anemia). In more advanced disease, the platelet count and even the white blood count may also decrease.

The peripheral smear allows microscopic examination of the blood cells. The most characteristic finding

in multiple myeloma is rouleaux formation of the red cells. Rouleaux is the stacking of red cells together like coins (Fig. 22-11). It is caused by increased amounts of immunoglobulins in the blood causing red blood cells to adhere to each other. The same phenomenon results in the increased erythrocyte sedimentation rate described below. With progressive replacement of bone marrow by myeloma, plasma cells may be identified in the peripheral blood (Fig. 22-12). Replacement of bone marrow may also cause teardrop-shaped red cells and earlier forms of white blood cells such as metamyelocytes and myelocytes to appear in the blood. Gross examination of the stained glass slide may reveal a bluish background tint because of the staining of immunoglobulin in the plasma.

Erythrocyte Sedimentation Rate The erythrocyte sedimentation rate (ESR) is often performed, but adds little to the evaluation of or treatment decisions in myeloma. An increased ratio of serum protein to number of red cells results in adherence of the red cells together. Stacked red cells have an increased weight compared to their surface area, resulting in a faster rate of settling out of solution because of gravity. The ESR is measured in millimeters settled per hour and is often elevated in myeloma.

Bone Marrow Biopsy In evaluations for possible multiple myeloma, the bone marrow biopsy is performed to evaluate the numbers of plasma cells present and to examine the appearance of the cells. Be-

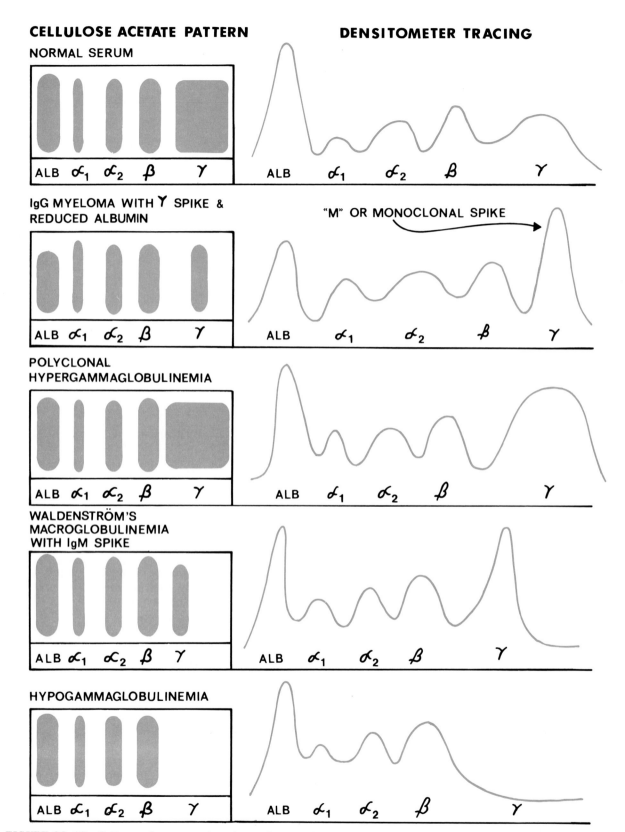

FIGURE 22–10 Patterns of serum protein electrophoresis showing characteristic patterns of normal serum, monoclonal M spike, polyclonal antibody production, IgM M spike, and the absence of antibody production seen in hypogammaglobulinemia.

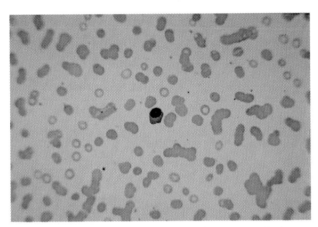

FIGURE 22-11 Peripheral blood showing marked rouleaux formation. Note the "stacked-coin" appearance of the red cells.

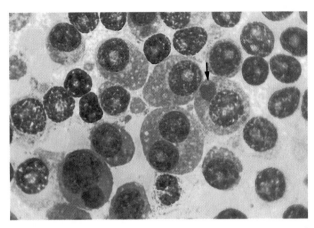

FIGURE 22-13 Bone marrow aspirate showing atypical and binucleated plasma cells and Russell bodies (*arrow*).

cause myeloma may be a patchy process, biopsies are usually taken at two different sites. Characteristic findings on marrow biopsy in patients with myeloma include increased numbers of plasma cells, often forming "sheets," with immature, binucleate, and large forms commonly seen (Fig. 22–13). A differential count of marrow cells, usually from 300 to 1000 cells counted, is performed to establish percentages of various cell types present. Patients with myeloma have more than 10% plasma cells, often more than 30%, and in some cases much higher percentages (Fig. 22–14). Flame cells (Fig. 22–15) are large, intensely staining plasma cells sometimes found in the bone marrow of patients with IgA myeloma.

Chemistry Studies Routine chemistry panels yield useful information in myeloma. Serum BUN and creatinine are measures of kidney function that directly correlate with survival of myeloma patients. Serum LDH is another nonspecific marker of disease activity with shorter survival correlating with high levels of LDH. Calcium levels are elevated in the great majority of patients at some time in the course of the disease.

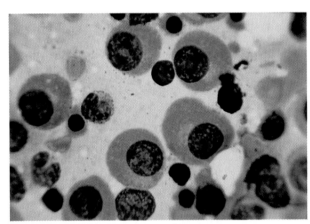

FIGURE 22-14 Bone marrow biopsy showing replacement of marrow by plasma cells.

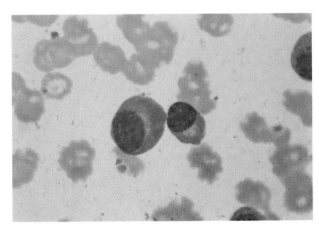

FIGURE 22-12 Plasma cells in a patient with multiple myeloma, peripheral blood.

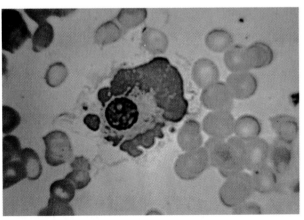

FIGURE 22-15 Flame cell, sometimes associated with IgA myeloma.

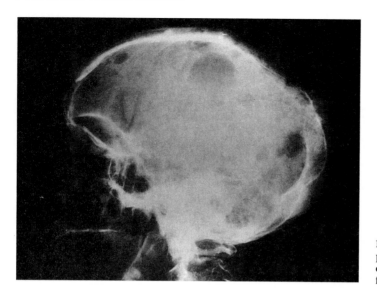

FIGURE 22-16 Skull radiograph showing discrete punched-out lesions characteristic of multiple myeloma, caused by production of osteoclast-activating factor by clusters of malignant plasma cells.

Calcium is primarily bound to albumin. It is the unbound or free calcium that is of concern and calcium levels must always be interpreted with the albumin level in mind. For each 1 g/dL of albumin below normal, the serum calcium should be considered increased by 0.8 mg/dL. High serum uric acid levels may be seen and can cause kidney damage. This should be evaluated initially and when increased disease activity is suspected.

Beta$_2$ Microglobulin and C-Reactive Protein
Beta$_2$ microglobulin (β2M) is the light chain of the histocompatability locus antigen (HLA). It is a nonspecific but useful predictor of disease activity and prognosis in multiple myeloma. A level of 6 μg/mL or greater is associated with decreased survival. It takes on even more significance when considered along with serum albumin, as will be discussed later.

C-reactive protein (CRP) is another marker of disease activity, reflecting activity of IL-6, the importance of which has been previously discussed. It also has prognostic value and will probably play an increasingly prominent role in the future.

Radiologic Studies

Plain Film Radiography Plain film radiography is what is usually known as x-rays. Definition of soft tissues is poor because of small differences in density to x-rays. Bones are visualized quite well in most areas of the body because of the calcium in the cortex of the bones. Multiple myeloma decreases the calcium in bones, producing both discrete lytic or "punched-out" lesions (Fig. 22–16) and the general decrease in bone density known as *osteoporosis* (Fig. 22–17). A full skeletal survey is usually performed to evaluate patients with possible myeloma. Special attention is given to the weight-bearing bones such as the femurs, spine, and humeri. Extensive destruction in these areas may lead to pathologic fractures. Multiple lytic lesions are very suggestive of multiple myeloma and are present in 76% of patients at diagnosis.

Nuclear Medicine Studies In multiple myeloma, the usefulness of nuclear medicine studies is very limited. This is because technetium radioisotope used in bone scans is actively taken up by osteoblasts. Since

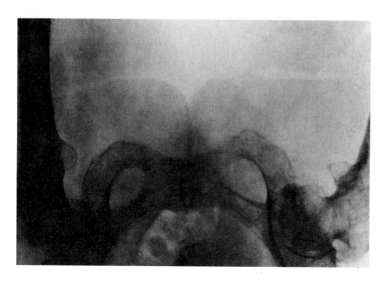

FIGURE 22-17 Pelvis radiograph of a patient with multiple myeloma showing the diffuse loss of bone seen in this disease.

there is little osteoblastic activity in myeloma, most myeloma lesions are not detected.

Magnetic Resonance Imaging Magnetic resonance imaging (MRI) produces computer-generated images based on tissue absorption of radiofrequency energy while in a powerful magnetic field. It excels at imaging neurologic tissues and the spine because of its ability to detect differences between normal and abnormal soft tissues and its ability to image the spine longitudinally. MRI can clearly demonstrate the presence of plasmacytomas in the spine and evaluate for nerve compression. Myeloma involving the bone marrow in vertebrae can be seen even with no destruction of the cortical bone visible on spinal radiographs.

Diagnosis and Differential Diagnosis of Multiple Myeloma

Diagnostic Criteria for Multiple Myeloma

The currently agreed-upon diagnostic criteria are listed in Table 22–3. Multiple myeloma is considered present if (1) two major criteria, (2) one major criterion and one unrelated minor criterion, or (3) three minor criteria are present. Thus, an M-spike of 5 g/dL of IgG kappa light chains with multiple lytic lesions would fulfill the criteria for diagnosis. Forty percent plasma cells in the bone marrow with a IgG kappa M-spike of 1.8 g/dL without bone lesions would fulfill the criteria. Plasma cells comprising 15% of the bone marrow with an M-spike measuring 1.2 g/dL with an IgA level of 20 mg/dL and an IgM level of 30 mg/dL would also fulfill the criteria.

TABLE 22–3 Diagnostic Criteria for Multiple Myeloma

I. Biopsy proven plasmacytoma
II. >30% plasma cells in bone marrow
III. Monoclonal protein (M spike)
>3.5 g/dL of serum IgG or
>2.0 g/dL of serum IgA or
>1.0 g/24 hr of lambda or kappa urinary light chains (in absence of amyloidosis)
Minor Criteria
a. 10–30% plasma cells in bone marrow
b. M spike present but less than levels above
c. Multiple lytic bone lesions
d. Low normal immunoglobulins
IgM <50 mg/dL
IgA <100 mg/dL
IgG <600 mg/dL
Rules of Combination
A. One major and one minor criterion
1. I + b; I + c; I + d (not I + a)
2. II + b; II + c; II + d (not II + a)
3. III + a; III + c; III + d (not III + b)
B. Three minor criterion (must include a + b)
1. a + b + c
2. a + b + d

Source: Adapted from Durle, BGM and Salmon, SE: Staging kinetics and flow cytometry of multiple myeloma. In Wiernik, P, et al (eds): Neoplastic Diseases of the Blood. New York, Churchill Livingstone, 1985.

Only six tests are required to make or exclude the diagnosis of multiple myeloma. These include bone marrow biopsy, serum protein electrophoresis, urine protein electrophoresis, immunoelectrophoresis, serum quantitative immunoglobulins, and a radiologic bone survey. If a mass is present, it should also be biopsied to evaluate for plasmacytoma. Other tests are important in the staging and prognosis of myeloma.

Differential Diagnosis

Frequently a patient has a monoclonal gammopathy and fails to meet the criteria for diagnosis of multiple myeloma. A list of other disorders that may be responsible must then be considered. Such a list of alternative diagnoses is called a *differential diagnosis*. A review of 856 patients at Mayo Clinic who underwent evaluation for monoclonal gammopathy is shown in Fig. 22–18.[9] Table 22–4 lists the standard battery of tests used for evaluating monoclonal gammopathies and plasma cell disorders. A complete physical examination (always done), CT scans of the chest and abdomen, with biopsies of suspicious enlarged lymph nodes, may also be required. "Monoclonal gammopathy of undetermined significance" is often diagnosed after multiple myeloma, B-cell lymphoma, and chronic lymphocytic leukemia are excluded. Much less commonly, Waldenström's macroglobulinemia, heavy-chain disease, or amyloidosis may be diagnosed. The spectrum of plasma cell disorders is listed in Table 22–2.

Staging

Once a diagnosis of multiple myeloma has been established, an estimate is made of the extent of disease to help determine the appropriate treatment plan and the patient's prognosis. This procedure, called *staging*, is also useful for reporting treatment outcomes and providing a common means of communication between physicians.

Various staging systems have been proposed and are currently in use. The older and probably most used staging system, described by Durie and Salmon in 1975,[10] is outlined in Table 22–5. This system uses hemoglobin, M-spike magnitude, serum calcium level, bone radiographs, and serum creatinine level (kidney function) to estimate the mass of myeloma cells in the body. It associates low myeloma mass (stage I) with a median survival of greater than 5 years. An intermediate myeloma mass (stage II) is associated with a survival of approximately 3½ years, although a patient with a high myeloma mass (stage III) may survive less than 2 years.

Other systems have been proposed that make use of serum beta$_2$ microglobulin and albumin, or beta$_2$ microglobulin (β2M) and C-reactive protein (CRP). The use of serum albumin and β2M is illustrated in Table 22–6 and demonstrates identification of groups surviving 55 months, 29 months, and 4 months. A similar staging system may be used for β2M and CRP levels to establish survival groups of 54, 27, and 6 months.[11] In practice, it is common to collect all this information to use in formulating a composite prognosis.

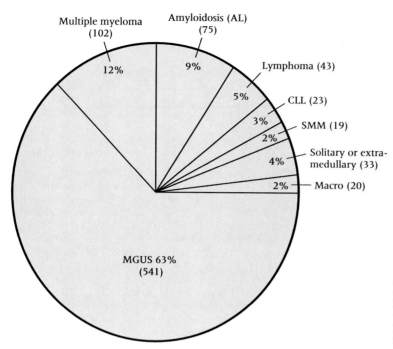

Multiple myeloma (102)
Amyloidosis (AL) (75)
Lymphoma (43)
12%
9%
5%
CLL (23)
3%
SMM (19)
2%
Solitary or extra-medullary (33)
4%
2%
Macro (20)
MGUS 63% (541)

FIGURE 22–18 Monoclonal gammopathies in 856 Mayo Clinic patients (1990). CLL = chronic lymphocytic leukemia; SMM = smoldering multiple myeloma; Macro = macroglobulinemia; MGUS = monoclonal gammopathy of undetermined significance.

TABLE 22–4 Standard Evaluation of Plasma Cell Disorders

Determine whether monoclonal protein is present
    Serum protein electrophoresis (SPEP)
    24-hour urine protein and protein electrophoresis (UPEP)
Characterize monoclonal protein
    Immunoelectrophoresis (IEP) of urine and serum
    Immunofixation electrophoresis if results are questionable
Evaluate bones with skeletal survey
Evaluate renal function
    Serum BUN
    Serum creatinine
    24-hour urine for creatinine clearance
Screening serum chemistry panel
    Calcium
    Total protein
    Albumin
    Uric acid
Evaluate bone marrow function
    CBC with reticulocyte count and WBC differential
    Bone marrow aspirate and biopsy
Evaluate for suppression of normal immunoglobulins
    Quantitative immunoglobulins
Serum viscosity
Miscellaneous
    Erythrocyte sedimentation rate (ESR)
    C-reactive protein
    Biopsy of mass or bone lesion if bone marrow is normal
    Beta$_2$ microglobulin if multiple myeloma diagnosed

TABLE 22–5 Myeloma Staging System

Criteria	Median Survival

Stage I (low myeloma mass) (*all* criteria *must* be met)
1. Hemoglobin >10 g/dL
2. Corrected serum calcium <12 mg/dL
3. Less than 2 lytic bone lesions
4. Small M spike
    IgG <5 g/dL
    IgA <3 g/dL
    Urine light chains <4 g/24 hr
	> 60 months

Stage II (intermediate myeloma mass) 1. Does not meet *all* stage I criteria 2. Does not meet *any* stage III criteria	41 months

Stage III (high myeloma mass) (any of the following criteria)
1. Hemoglobin <8.5 g/dL
2. Corrected serum calcium >12 mg/dL
3. ≥2 lytic bone lesions
4. Large M spike
    IgG >7 g/dL
    IgA >5 g/dL
    Urine light chains >12 g/24 hr
	23 months

Substaging A. Serum creatinine <2.0 mg/dL B. Serum creatinine >2.0 mg/dL	

Source: Adapted from Durie, BGM and Salmon, SE: Staging kinetics and flow cytometry of multiple myelomas. In Wiernik, P, et al (eds): Neoplastic Diseases of the Blood. New York, Churchill Livingstone, 1985.

TABLE 22–6 **Myeloma Staging Based on β_2 Microglobulin and Serum Albumin**			
Stage	**β_2 Microglobulin**	**Serum Albumin**	**Median Survival**
I. Low risk	<6 μg/mL	>3.0 g/dL	55 months
II. Intermediate risk	>6 μg/mL	>3.0 g/dL	29 months
III. High risk	>6 μg/mL	<3.0 g/dL	4 months

Source: Adapted from Bataille, R, et al.[11]

Treatment of Multiple Myeloma and Its Variants

General Principles of Treatment

Chemotherapy is the primary treatment of multiple myeloma. Radiation therapy may be used for treating localized painful areas, lytic lesions endangering the strength of a bone, or masses compressing nerve structures. It is highly effective for localized processes, but has limited usefulness for treating the full extent of the disease.

Although various combinations of chemotherapy have been used, the standard treatment remains the use of alkylators and glucocorticoids.

Standard chemotherapy does not cure myeloma. Of all patients, 50% to 60% have at least a 50% reduction in the size of the M-spike. There is a clear prolongation of survival in patients receiving chemotherapy compared to those not so treated.

Patients under the age of 65 who are otherwise in good health may consider high-dose chemotherapy with autologous marrow or peripheral stem cell support. This treatment first removes bone marrow or peripheral blood stem cells (or both) and preserves them by freezing in liquid nitrogen. High doses of chemotherapy are given (often high-dose melphalan with or without other agents) followed by reinfusion of the thawed stem cells or bone marrow. This technique is relatively safe (<10% mortality), and can induce remissions in up to 30% of patients who are resistant to the more standard chemotherapy agents.

Younger patients (under the age of 55) may be treated experimentally with allogeneic bone marrow transplants using a treatment regimen similar to that just mentioned, but infusing donor marrow, usually from an HLA-matched brother or sister. This has the benefits of not reintroducing myeloma cells with the bone marrow and possibly allowing the new bone marrow to reject the myeloma (graft-versus-disease effect). The procedure is associated with a 30% to 50% chance of death from infections or complications from the donor-recipient mismatch known as graft-versus-host disease. Although prolonged complete responses are reported with both procedures, it remains doubtful that cures are yet possible.[12]

Smoldering Myeloma

If a patient meets the criteria for the diagnosis of stage I, low-mass multiple myeloma, and has normal kidney function, normal serum calcium, and no lytic bone lesions, then he or she falls into the category of smoldering myeloma. Since there is no curative treatment, and since these patients are not suffering ill effects from the myeloma, treatment may often be delayed with close monitoring for signs of disease progression. Treatment is usually required within 1 to 3 years when progression to stage II or III occurs.

Multiple Myeloma

When a patient has stage II or III (intermediate or high-mass) multiple myeloma, treatment is initiated with chemotherapy at the time the diagnosis is made. Supportive care is given to resolve high calcium levels with intravenous saline and medications that inhibit osteoclasts such as glucocorticoids, bisphosponates, and calcitonin. If needed, radiation treatments for plasmacytomas or large lytic bone lesions may be given. Vaccines for the encapsulated bacteria (*Streptococcus pneumoniae*, *Hemophilus influenzae*, and *Neisseria meningitidis*) should be given early. In patients with recurrent bronchitis or sinusitis, intravenous pooled immunoglobulins given at monthly intervals may be of significant benefit. Chemotherapy continues until maximum reduction in M-spike is achieved. Interferon injections have been shown to prolong the remission achieved by chemotherapy. When the disease progresses, chemotherapy is reinstituted.

Nonsecretory Myeloma

Less than 1% of multiple myelomas may be found to have no abnormal immunoglobulins in the blood or urine. The numbers of plasma cells in the bone marrow, elevation of serum calcium, and formation of plasmacytomas with bone pain all still occur. The immunoglobulin levels are usually normal. Treatment is the same as for multiple myeloma. Because of a normal immune response, infectious complications are fewer. Absence of light-chain excretion via the kidneys preserves renal function and survival is often improved. Evaluation of response to therapy is impaired because of the lack of M-spike. Treatment decisions are commonly based on changes in β2M or CRP levels.

Solitary Plasmacytoma

Of patients with plasmacytomas, 5% are found to have a single tumor. The usual presentation is pain at the site of the growing tumor. The tumor may secrete immunoglobulin resulting in a small serum M-spike, but no other signs of myeloma are present, including lytic bone lesions. The bone marrow has less than 10% plasma cells. Solitary plasmacytomas occur more often in men and with an average age 7 years younger than the average age of multiple myeloma patients. The standard treatment for solitary plasmacytomas is radiation therapy given over 4 to 6 weeks. It is estimated that only 15% of patients treated for solitary plasmacytoma remain disease-free. On relapse, the myeloma tends to have a comparatively mild course with an average survival of 10 years or more. Treatment decisions on relapse are the same as for multiple myeloma.[13]

Solitary plasmacytomas of nonbone structures also occur. These extramedullary plasmacytomas can be found in the sinuses, gastrointestinal tract, skin, and other locations (see Fig. 22–3). Principles of treatment are the same as for skeletal plasmacytomas, but the risk of conversion to multiple myeloma is less.[14]

Plasma Cell Leukemia

The presence of significant numbers of plasma cells in the peripheral blood constitutes plasma cell leukemia (Fig. 22–19). Half of these rare cases are found in advanced multiple myeloma, late in the course of the illness, in the final weeks of the disease. Near complete replacement of the bone marrow by malignant plasma cells results in increased numbers of circulating cells.

Half of cases are caused by a variation of multiple myeloma referred to as primary plasma cell leukemia. This variant has circulating plasma cells at the time of diagnosis. It is complicated by more frequent high-calcium levels, more kidney failure, and much more anemia and thrombocytopenia. Liver, spleen, and lymph node enlargement are common. Treatment is the same as for multiple myeloma, often using one of the more aggressive regimens. Prognosis is poor with expected survival of only several months.[15]

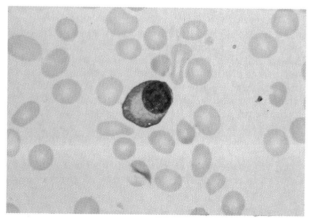

FIGURE 22–19 Peripheral blood in plasma cell leukemia showing presence of circulating plasma cells. (From Dutcher, T: Hematology. In Listen, Look and Learn. Health and Education Resources, Inc., Bethesda, MD, with permission.)

TABLE 22–7 **Diagnostic Criteria for Monoclonal Gammopathy of Undetermined Significance**
I. M spike present IgG <3.5 g/dL IgA <2.0 g/dL Urinary light chains <1.0 g/24 hr II. <10% plasma cells in bone marrow III. No bone lesions IV. No symptoms (*all* criteria must be met)

Source: Adapted from Durie, BGM and Salmon, SE: Staging kinetics and flow cytometry of multiple myeloma. In Wiernik, P, et al (eds): Neoplastic Diseases of the Blood. New York, Churchill Livingstone, 1985.

MONOCLONAL GAMMOPATHY OF UNDETERMINED SIGNIFICANCE

Monoclonal gammopathy of undetermined significance (MGUS) was previously named benign monoclonal gammopathy. The only clinical finding is a small M-spike on serum protein electrophoresis and no other findings of multiple myeloma. This is found in approximately 1% of individuals over the age of 50 and up to 3% of those over the age of 70. Considering that the incidence of multiple myeloma in the same age group is 70 per 100,000 or less, most patients with a small M-spike will not have multiple myeloma. By definition, MGUS is diagnosed when a patient has a small M-spike, urine light chains less than 1 g per 24 hours, no lytic bone lesions, and less than 10% plasma cells in the bone marrow as listed in Table 22–7. No treatment is indicated.

It is no longer referred to as benign monoclonal gammopathy because it is well recognized that as many as 11% of such patients eventually develop an overt malignant process such as lymphoma, chronic lymphocytic leukemia, or multiple myeloma over a 5-year period (Table 22–8). After completing the initial screening tests for multiple myeloma, a second M-spike measurement is made approximately 3 months later. If it remains stable, the patients are followed at 6-month intervals for life. If significant changes occur, appropriate testing is repeated.

TABLE 22–8 **Monoclonal Gammopathy of Undetermined Significance: 5-Year Follow-up**	
Course of Illness	**Fraction of Patients**
No significant progression of M-spike	57%
>50% increase in M-spike	9%
Progression to malignant monoclonal gammopathy	11%
Death from unrelated cause	23%

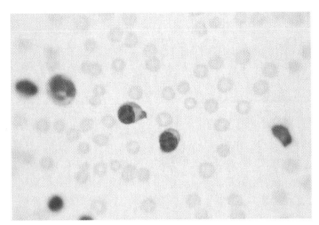

FIGURE 22-20 Plasmacytoid lymphocytes; note the red staining accumulation of immunoglobulin in the cytoplasm.

WALDENSTRÖM'S MACROGLOBULINEMIA

Waldenström's macroglobulinemia (WM) is the overproduction of monoclonal IgM antibodies by cells called *plasmacytoid lymphocytes* or prolymphs (Fig. 22-20). Prolymphs appear to be an intermediate stage of maturation between mature B lymphocytes and early plasma cells. It is diagnosed by finding a monoclonal IgM M-spike and the presence of plasmacytoid lymphocytes infiltrating the bone marrow (Fig. 22-21).

WM is most commonly diagnosed in individuals in the seventh decade of life and is found equally in both men and women. Patients with this disease come to a physician with early complaints of fatigue, weight loss, and generalized weakness. As the levels of IgM rise, the liver, spleen, and lymph nodes may become enlarged because of infiltration with abnormal lymphocytes. Prolymphocytes may also infiltrate nerves, the meninges, and even the brain, resulting in a variety of neurologic manifestations.

When levels of IgM rise sufficiently, symptoms of "hyperviscosity syndrome" may arise. Clinical features

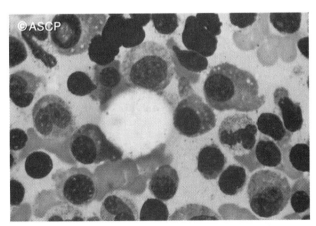

FIGURE 22-21 Plasmacytoid lymphocytes in marrow aspirate from a patient with Waldenström's macroglobulinemia. (From Hyun, BH: Morphology of Blood and Bone Marrow, American Society of Clinical Pathologists, Workshop 5121, Philadelphia, September 7, 1983, with permission.)

TABLE 22-9 Clinical Features of Hyperviscosity Syndrome

Sign or Symptom	Fraction of Patients
Neurologic changes	20%
Retinopathy	35%
Hypervolemia/congestive heart failure	20%
Abnormal bleeding	20%
Enlarged liver and spleen	35%
Enlarged lymph nodes	45%

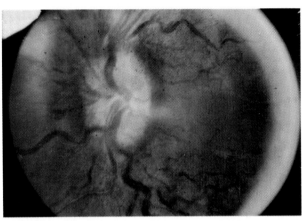

FIGURE 22-22 Tortuous veins with sausage-link appearance present in the fundus of the eye.

of hyperviscosity syndrome are listed in Table 22-9. Blurred vision, headache, and confusion are common neurologic changes. Worsening can lead to somnolence and even coma. Examination of the eyes may reveal characteristic "sausage-link" veins in 50% of patients with WM caused by hyperviscosity (Fig. 22-22). Congestive heart failure may occur because of the high protein levels resulting in an expansion of fluid volume within the blood vessels.

Patients with WM often have extensive bruising called *cryoglobulinemic purpura* (Fig. 22-23) and may have bleeding from the gums and nose. More severe bleeding may be seen. This is caused by interference with platelets and blood clotting factor proteins by the abnormal IgM. Bleeding time is often prolonged, as are the clotting factor assays, PT and APTT (see Chap. 34).

Cryoglobulins are proteins (often IgM) that precipitate on exposure to cold. Some patients with WM de-

TABLE 22-10 Comparison of Multiple Myeloma and Waldenström's Macroglobulinemia

	Macroglobulinemia	Myeloma
Organomegaly	+++	+
Hyperviscosity	+++	+
Lytic bone lesions	+	+++
Renal failure	+	+++
Length of survival	++	+

TABLE 22–11	**Heavy Chain Diseases (HCD)**			
Disease	**Antibody Heavy Chain (M-spike)**	**Organ Involvement**	**Other Characteristics**	**Survival Rate**
Gamma HCD	Gamma chains (IgG)	Liver and spleen may be enlarged Enlarged lymph nodes	Disease of elderly people	Few weeks to a few years
Alpha HCD	Alpha chain (IgA)	GI tract (abdominal mass)	Commonly called Mediterranean lymphoma because it is frequently reported in younger individuals in the Mediterranean area	Few months
Mu HCD	Mu chains (IgM)	Enlargement of liver and spleen	May be a variation of CLL because of high number of lymphs in blood BM: vacuolated plasma cells	Not available

Abbreviations: BM = bone marrow findings; CLL = chronic lymphocytic leukemia

velop symptoms of cryoglobulinemia. Patients with cryoglobulinemia may develop pain and color changes in cold exposed areas (Raynaud's phenomenon), clotting or thrombosis of small blood vessels, and kidney damage.

WM is not curable at this time. Chemotherapy is the primary treatment, using alkylators such as chlorambucil, cyclophosphamide, and L-phenylalanine mustard. If severe symptoms are present at diagnosis, IgM may be quickly removed by plasmapheresis, resulting in rapid improvement in symptoms. Table 22–10 compares WM with multiple myeloma.

Survival is estimated based on the percentage of prolymphs in the bone marrow. Less than 20% replacement of bone marrow by prolymphs results in survival approaching 5 years, whereas 50% replacement or more results in survival of less than 1 year.

HEAVY-CHAIN DISEASE

Heavy-chain disease (HCD) is the excessive production of the heavy-chain portion of the antibody unit. It appears to be a disorder in which the plasma cells have

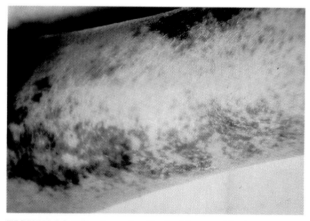

FIGURE 22–23 Arm of patient with cryoglobulinemic purpura. Note the skin manifestations.

lost the ability to synthesize the light-chain component. An HCD has been identified for each of the major immunoglobulin classes: IgG, IgA, and IgM. These diseases are very rare. Table 22–11 summarizes the characteristics of heavy-chain diseases.

CASE STUDY 1: MULTIPLE MYELOMA

A 71-year-old man went to his doctor with complaints of a constant aching in his back that had progressively worsened over a 6-month period. His wife noted that he was frequently confused, slept much of the day, and made occasional nonsensical statements.

On examination, the patient appeared normal. However, he was unable to state the correct date and could not name the current president of the United States. His spine was tender to examination. There were no enlarged lymph nodes, liver, or spleen. His examination was otherwise normal.

Radiographs of the spine were ordered and revealed osteoporosis with compression fractures of the third and fourth lumbar vertebrae. Blood tests revealed a mild normocytic anemia with an Hgb level of 10 g/dL and an MCV of 91 fL. Platelets and white cells were normal. The laboratory reported that rouleaux were noted on his blood smear. His chemistry panel revealed a calcium level of 10.6 mg/dL (normal range, 8.8 to 10.5) with a low albumin level of 2.6 g/dL. Total protein was 8.2 g/dL. The physician subtracted the albumin from the total protein and realized that the antibody-containing protein level was elevated at 5.6 g/dL. He corrected the serum calcium because of the low albumin and found that the equivalent calcium level was 11.7 g/dL. The patient's kidney function was normal.

The patient was hospitalized. Hydration with normal saline rapidly lowered the calcium levels and the patient's mental status quickly improved over the following 3 days. Because of continued back pain, an MRI of his spine was obtained that revealed destruction of the bone structure at several levels, with bone marrow signal alteration consistent with malignancy, but no compression of the spinal cord. Serum protein electrophoresis revealed an M-spike measuring 4.7 g/dL. Immunoelectrophoresis revealed that the M-spike was composed of an IgG kappa antibody. His serum IgM level was 63 mg/dL and IgA was 120 mg/dL. A 24-hour urine collection demonstrated no protein. Bone marrow biopsies were obtained and revealed 32% plasma cells, forming sheets, with binucleated forms present. A radiologic skeletal survey revealed classic lytic lesions in the skull, pelvis, both arms, and both femurs with diffuse osteoporosis.

Questions

1. What major and minor criteria for multiple myeloma are met in this patient?
2. What stage myeloma does he have?
3. What other tests could be ordered to help estimate his survival prognosis?
4. Should he be considered for a bone marrow transplant? Why?

Answers

1. Major criteria met were: a. Greater than 30% plasma cells in the bone marrow, b. IgG kappa M-spike greater than 3.5 g/dL. Minor criteria met: a. lytic bone lesions, low-normal immunoglobulins (see Table 22–3).
2. He has stage III disease based on the presence of multiple lytic bone lesions. Any single stage III criterion is sufficient (see Table 22–5).
3. Low albumin is an adverse prognostic factor. Beta$_2$ microglobulin and C-reactive protein are also useful in determining prognosis (see Table 22–6).
4. He is not a candidate for bone marrow transplant. His age makes it likely that the danger to him would outweigh the potential benefit.

CASE STUDY 2: MGUS

A 55-year-old man was seen by a primary care clinic for prolonged back pain after lifting some heavy boxes several months before. Examination of his back revealed some tenderness in the muscles with no bone tenderness. X-rays of the back were read as normal. As part of his evaluation, a serum protein electrophoresis was ordered and revealed an M-spike measured at 1.1 g/dL. Immunoelectrophoresis identified the M-spike as IgG lambda. He was referred to a hematologist to rule out multiple myeloma.

The hematologist performed a thorough physical examination and found no significant abnormalities, including normal lymph nodes, liver, and spleen. He ordered a full skeletal survey, 24-hour urine collection for protein evaluation, serum calcium, serum quantitative immunoglobulins and performed bilateral iliac crest bone marrow biopsies. The x-rays were normal. No protein was detected in the urine. Calcium, IgM, and IgA levels were normal. The bone marrow revealed 6.4% normal-appearing plasma cells. To be thorough, he also ordered CT scans of the chest and abdomen, which revealed no enlarged lymph nodes suspicious

for lymphoma, and confirmed a normal size spleen. He felt satisfied that this patient had MGUS.

Questions

1. Which explanation should be given to the patient?
   a. You have an incurable disease, probably a cancer that has not yet been found. I want to see you back every 3 months for tests.
   b. Nothing of concern was found. There is nothing to worry about. Have a nice life.
   c. Your body is producing some abnormal antibodies. It is a common disorder that will probably never cause you any problems. A small percentage of patients may develop a more serious problem later, so I need to see you back in 3 months, then periodically to see if there has been any change.
2. Besides multiple myeloma, what other malignancies can be associated with monoclonal gammopathies?
   1. Lung cancer
   2. Chronic lymphocytic leukemia
   3. Acute myeloid leukemia
   4. Non-Hodgkin's lymphoma
      a. 1, 2, and 3
      b. 1 and 3
      c. 2 and 4
      d. All of the above
3. What follow-up schedule would be appropriate?
   a. Monthly serum protein electrophoresis.
   b. Bone marrow biopsy repeated every 6 months for 2 years. If there is no evidence of myeloma at that time, the patient does not have to return any more.
   c. Repeat the complete evaluation every 6 months.
   d. Repeat the serum protein electrophoresis in 3 months, then every 6 months thereafter if there has been no change.

Answers

1. c. Although a few patients develop multiple myeloma, non-Hodgkin's lymphoma, or chronic lymphocytic leukemia, most patients with MGUS are not adversely affected by this disorder. (Table 22–8)
2. c. Choices 2 and 4 are correct. Lymphoid malignancies may produce measurable amounts of immunoglobulin. Nonlymphoid malignancies such as lung cancer and acute myeloid leukemia do not (see Fig. 22–18).
3. d. Once the initial evaluation is complete, no further testing needs to be done unless there is a change in the production of the M-spike immunoglobulin. Three months is considered a reasonable interval because of the known growth rate of these disorders. If it is stable after that time interval, the period of time may safely be increased to 6-month follow-ups for life.

CASE 3: WALDENSTRÖM'S MACROGLOBULINEMIA

A 59-year-old woman was seen by her physician for a 35-lb unintentional weight loss from her usual

165 lb over the last 18 months. She had been having trouble concentrating at work, had decreased energy, and had two frightening episodes during which she could not make sense of the words she was reading in a novel. She was otherwise in excellent health.

On physical examination, she was noted to be a tall, thin woman with no enlarged lymph nodes. Her spleen was enlarged, easily felt approximately 7 cm below her left ribs. Her neurologic exam was normal. Blood tests revealed an Hgb of 9.7 g/dL; Hct, 29.2%; MCV was 89 fL. Platelets, white cells, and white cell differential were normal. Chemistry panel was normal with the exception of a total protein level of 8.7 g/dL with a low albumin at 2.7 g/dL. Calcium level was 8.3 mg/dL. A serum protein electrophoresis was ordered and revealed a 5.7 g/dL M-spike.

Immunoelectrophoresis identified the protein as an IgM kappa. A bone marrow biopsy revealed that 23% of the marrow consisted of abnormal plasmacytoid lymphocytes consistent with Waldenström's macroglobulinemia. Blood viscosity was measured and found to be moderately increased.

Questions

1. Which of the following is a possible cause of the patient's problems in concentrating and reading?
   a. The calcium level is actually high when the low albumin level is considered. High calcium is well known to cause mental status changes.
   b. The increased viscosity of the blood is causing poor circulation through the blood vessels in the brain, resulting in these symptoms.
   c. On exposure to cold, cryoglobulins in the patient's head precipitate and block blood vessels.
   d. Osteolytic lesions in the spine.
2. Which statement is most correct about the patient's diagnosis?
   a. This is a terminal disease that may end her life within the next year.
   b. This is a chronic disorder that often requires treatment, but she will probably live a relatively normal life.
   c. This disease is rapidly fatal and does not respond to treatment.
   d. This is a terminal disease, but the numbers of abnormal cells in the bone marrow suggest that, with treatment, she may live another 4 or 5 years.
3. If the patient developed more severe neurologic problems, what could be done to rapidly lower the IgM in the blood?

   The following questions do not pertain to the cases above.

Answers

1. b. Hyperviscosity syndrome is common with Waldenström's macroglobulinemia, and these are classic symptoms. The plasmacytoid lymphocytes may infiltrate nerves, meninges, and the brain and may be a less common cause of mental status changes and neurologic changes. Hypercalcemia is uncommon with WM, and cor-

recting the albumin to 4 g/dL (1.3 g/dL increase) would result in a correction of serum calcium of $0.8 \times 1.3 = 1.04$ mg/dL, totaling 9.34 mg/dL. This is within the normal range. Chilling of the scalp would not result in precipitation of cryoglobulins in the brain, but might affect the tips of the ears and nose. (p 420)
2. d. The prognosis for patients with WM is associated with extent of plasmacytoid lymphocytes in the bone marrow. This patient may live for 3 to 4 years after diagnosis. (p 420)
3. Plasmapheresis is useful in removing IgM-rich plasma from the patient within 1 to 2 hours and may result in dramatic resolution of symptoms. (p 420)

REFERENCES

1. Potter, M: Perspectives on the origins of multiple myeloma and plasmacytomas in mice. Hematol Oncol Clin North Am 6:211, 1992.
2. Klein, B and Bataille, R: Cytokine network in human multiple myeloma. Hematol Oncol Clin North Am 6:273, 1992.
3. Ries, LAG, et al: Cancer Statistics Review 1973–1988. Washington, DC, US Govt Printing Office, 1991.
4. Riedel, DA and Pottern, LM: The epidemiology of multiple myeloma. Hematol Oncol Clin North Am 6:225, 1992.
5. Kyle, RA: Multiple myeloma, an update on diagnosis and management. Acta Oncol 29:1, 1990.
6. Patterson, WP, Caldwell CW, and Doll, DC: Hyperviscosity syndromes and coagulopathies. Semin Oncol 17:210, 1990.
7. Bataille, R, Chappard, D, and Klein, B: Mechanisms of bone lesions in multiple myeloma. Hematol Oncol Clin North Am 6:285, 1992.
8. Steele, PE, Penn, GM, and Hurtubise, PE: Laboratory evaluation of malignant immunoproliferative diseases. In Bick, RL (ed.): Hematology, Clinical and Laboratory Practice, Mosby-Year Book, St Louis, 1993, p 741.
9. Kyle, RA: Diagnostic criteria of multiple myeloma. Hematol Oncol Clin North Am 6:347, 1992.
10. Durie, BGM and Salmon, SE: A clinical staging system for multiple myleoma: correlation of measured myeloma cell mass with presenting clinical features, response to treatment, and survival. Cancer 36:842, 1975.
11. Bataille, R, et al: C-reactive protein and beta 2-microglobulin produce a simple and powerful myeloma staging system. Blood 80:733, 1992.
12. Boccadoro, M and Pileri, A: Standard chemotherapy for myelomatosis: an area of great controversy. Hematol/Oncol Clin North Am 6:371, 1992.
13. Dimopoulos, MA, et al: Solitary plasmacytomas of bone and asymptomatic multiple myeloma. Hematol/Oncol Clin North Am 6:359, 1992.
14. Holland, J, et al: Plasmacytoma: Treatment results and conversion of myeloma. Cancer 69:1513, 1992.
15. Noel, P and Kyle, RA: Plasma cell leukemia: An evaluation of response to therapy. Am J Med 83:1062, 1987.

QUESTIONS

1. Which laboratory test(s) for whole blood is/are used in the evaluation of plasma cell disorders?
   a. CBC
   b. Peripheral blood smear
   c. ESR
   d. All of the above

2. What laboratory serum tests are used for evaluation of plasma cell disorders, and how are they used?

   a. First SPEP; if M spike is seen, then IEP or immunofixation to determine the specific antibody class

   b. Immunoelectrophoresis used to determine the antibody group and immunofixation or SPEP used to determine if light or heavy chain is increased

   c. First SPEP; if no abnormalities, then IEP or immunofixation used, as more sensitive indicators of increased antibody class(es)

   d. Either SPEP or IEP first; if M spike is seen, then immunofixation to determine the specific antibody class

3. Which of the following tests can directly detect urinary light chains and is used to distinguish between kappa and lambda light chains?

   a. Heat precipitation test

   b. Urine immunoelectrophoresis

   c. Sulfosalicylic acid test

   d. Both urine immunoelectrophoresis and sulfosalicyclic acid test

4. Which list would contain diagnostic criteria for multiple myeloma?

   a. Biopsy proven plasmacytoma and 10 to 30% plasma cells

   b. >30% plasma cells in bone marrow

   c. Biopsy-proven plasmacytoma and M spike present

   d. Monoclonal protein and M spike present

5. Which of the following would be diagnostic criteria for Waldenström's macroglobinemia?

   a. IgM M spike and hyperviscosity

   b. Lytic bone lesions and rouleaux

   c. Renal failure and >30% plasma cells

   d. M spike of IgM, IgG, or IgA; low-normal other immunoglobulins; inability to make light chains

6. What are the characteristics of heavy chain disease? (Use answer choices for question 5.)

ANSWERS

1. **d** (p 411)
2. **a** (p 410)
3. **b** (pp 410–411)
4. **c** (p 415)
5. **a** (p 420)
6. **d** (p 420) (Table 22–11)

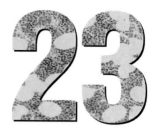

The Lymphomas

Dan M. Hyder, MD

Objectives

At the end of this chapter, the learner should be able to:

1   Name and describe the cell characteristics of Hodgkin's disease.
2   List distinguishing features for lymphocyte predominance, mixed cellularity, lymphocyte depletion, and nodular sclerosing Hodgkin's disease.
3   List the distinguishing features of the four stages of Hodgkin's disease.
4   Describe the classification criteria for non-Hodgkin's lymphomas.
5   List some distinguishing features for various lymphomas.
6   Name tests that may be needed to provide a differential diagnosis for lymphomas.

The malignant lymphomas are a heterogeneous group of diseases that arise from cells of the lymphoid tissue (lymphocytes, histiocytes, and reticulum cells). They are broadly divided into the two major categories of Hodgkin's disease and the non-Hodgkin's lymphomas (NHL). Although the vast majority of lymphomas within the second category are of lymphocytic origin, occasional cases do appear to arise from nonlymphoid cells. This subdivision of the malignant lymphomas into two general categories has both biologic and therapeutic implications.

HODGKIN'S DISEASE

Hodgkin's disease was the first of the lymphomas to be recognized. In 1832 Thomas Hodgkin described what he believed to be a primary yet benign disease of the lymphoid tissue.[1] Samuel Wilks in 1865 suggested that the disorder described by Hodgkin was a malignant process and was the first to apply the term *Hodgkin's disease* in honor of Hodgkin's original description of the process.[2] In 1898 Sternberg[3] and in 1902 Reed[4] described the distinct histologic features of Hodgkin's disease, including the peculiar cell that is the morphologic hallmark of Hodgkin's disease and that now bears their names, that is, the Sternberg-Reed (or Reed-Sternberg) cell (Fig. 23–1).

Etiology and Pathogenesis

The continued use of the term Hodgkin's disease rather than Hodgkin's lymphoma attests to the fact that the etiology and even the very nature, that is, inflammatory/reactive versus malignant, of Hodgkin's disease remains uncertain.

An infectious cofactor appears to be operational in the pathogenesis of Hodgkin's disease. The probable infectious agent is Epstein-Barr virus (EBV), although cytomegalovirus and herpesvirus 6 have also been implicated. EBV nucleic acids can be demonstrated in the lesions of approximately 80% of patients with Hodgkin's disease and EBV antigens such as latent membrane protein (LMP) can be detected in approximately 50% of patients.

The current view of Hodgkin's disease is that it is truly a malignant proliferation and that the malignant cells are the morphologically characteristic Reed-Sternberg cell and its variants (Fig. 23–2A–E). The weight of the data strongly favors a lymphocyte origin of the Reed-Sternberg cell.[5] Depending on the specific histologic subtype of Hodgkin's disease, the Reed-Sternberg cell appears to be derived from either a B lymphocyte (nodular lymphocyte predominance subtype) or a T lymphocyte (all other subtypes).

Pathology

A major success of twentieth-century medicine has been the development of a single, clinically useful classification scheme for Hodgkin's disease, namely the Rye classification[6] (Table 23–1). To those confronted with the challenge of making a histologic diagnosis of Hodgkin's disease, utilization of the more complicated schemes such as the Lukes and Butler classification[7] (Table 23–2) is common practice.

The cytologic hallmark of Hodgkin's disease is the presence of an unusual giant cell, the Reed-Sternberg cell. The features of this cell include large size (up to 45 μm in diameter), abundant acidophilic cytoplasm, multinucleated or polylobated nucleus, and gigantic (>5 μm in diameter), inclusionlike nucleoli (see Fig. 23–1). There is often clearing of the chromatin around the macronucleoli resulting in a distinct halo effect. It is necessary to identify at least one of these "diagnostic" Reed-Sternberg cells before a primary diagnosis of Hodgkin's disease is made. The identification of Reed-Sternberg (or Reed-Sternberg-like) cells, however, is not a sufficient condition for the diagnosis of Hodgkin's disease. Reed-Sternberg-like cells are commonly seen in a variety of benign and malignant conditions other than Hodgkin's disease (Table 23–3). The diagnosis of Hodgkin's disease should be based on finding Reed-Sternberg cells in the proper cellular, stromal, and clinical setting. Many nondiagnostic variants of Reed-Sternberg cells have been described (see Fig. 23–2). Observation of these cells is helpful in suggesting the possibility of Hodgkin's disease and in the subclassification of Hodgkin's disease.

Lymphocyte-Predominance Hodgkin's Disease

Lymphocyte-predominance (LP) Hodgkin's disease is a relatively uncommon variety of Hodgkin's disease. The descriptive name is somewhat of a misnomer since lymphocytes do not always predominate. Benign histiocytes, which are always a component of this disorder, may in fact predominate. The histologic importance of both lymphocytes and histiocytes in this subcategory of Hodgkin's disease is acknowledged in the Lukes and Butler designation for this disorder, namely lymphocytic and histiocytic (L&H) Hodgkin's disease. Although not distinguished by the Rye classification, both nodular and diffuse forms of LP Hodgkin's disease are recognized in the Lukes and Butler classification.

The nodular variant is generally characterized by a vague nodularity, although in some cases it may be well developed. The cellular milieu in both the diffuse and nodular varieties is composed of a mixture of small, normal-appearing lymphocytes, benign histiocytes, rare Reed-Sternberg cells, and variable numbers of a characteristic but nondiagnostic Reed-Sternberg variant referred to as an *L&H cell* (see Fig. 23–2C). This cell has a variable amount of pale-staining cytoplasm, a convoluted nucleus commonly referred to as popcorn-shaped, and an indistinct nucleolus. Plasma cells, eosinophils, fibrosis, and necrosis are usually absent. The paucity of Reed-Sternberg cells often makes definitive diagnosis difficult. The histologic features of LP Hodgkin's disease must be distinguished from various reactive conditions such as infectious mononucleosis as well as certain low-grade non-Hodgkin's lymphomas. Such differentiation may require special phenotypic and genotypic studies.

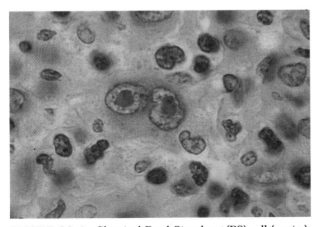

FIGURE 23–1 Classical Reed-Sternberg (RS) cell (*center*), characterized by large size, multilobed nucleus, and inclusionlike nucleoli.

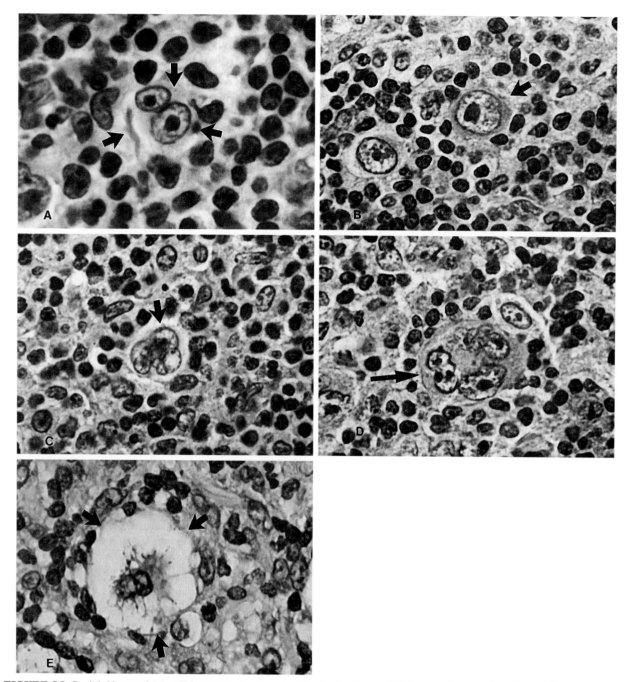

FIGURE 23–2 (*A*) Classical RS cell (*arrows*), characterized by large size, multilobed nucleus, and inclusionlike nucleoli. (*B*) Mononuclear variant (*arrow*) with single monolobed nucleus and inclusionlike nucleolus. (*C*) L and H cell (*arrow*), a variant RS cell characteristic of Hodgkin's disease with lymphocyte predominance. (*D*) Pleomorphic RS variant (*arrow*) commonly seen in mixed-cellularity and lymphocyte-depletion subtypes of Hodgkin's disease. (*E*) Lacunar cell (*arrow*), a variant RS cell characteristic of nodular sclerosing Hodgkin's disease.

Mixed-Cellularity Hodgkin's Disease

As its name implies, mixed-cellularity (MC) Hodgkin's disease is characterized by a heterogeneous mixture of cells including lymphocytes, histiocytes, plasma cells, eosinophils, Reed-Sternberg cells, and Reed-Sternberg variants (Fig. 23–3). Specifically, the number of Reed-Sternberg cells and mononuclear

Hodgkin's cells in MC Hodgkin's disease has been defined as between 5 and 15 per high-power microscopic field.[8]

In addition to the cellular milieu there is usually an increase in the background stroma in the form of a disorderly, noncollagenous fibrosis distinct from that seen in nodular sclerosing (NS) Hodgkin's disease. Small areas of necrosis are commonly present. In some

TABLE 23–1 Rye Classification of Hodgkin's Disease

Nodular sclerosis
Lymphocyte predominance
Mixed cellularity
Lymphocyte depletion
Unclassified

Source: From Lukes et al,[6] with permission.

TABLE 23–2 Lukes and Butler Classification of Hodgkin's Disease

Nodular sclerosis
Lymphocytic and histiocytic
  Nodular
  Diffuse
Mixed cellularity
Reticular
  Sarcomatous
  Nonsarcomatous
Diffuse fibrosis
Unclassified

Source: From Lukes and Butler,[7] with permission.

TABLE 23–3 Diseases or Disorders in which Reed-Sternberg-Like Cells Have Been Reported

Viral infection, e.g., infectious mononucleosis
Anticonvulsant-induced lymphadenopathy
Epithelial and stromal malignancies
Melanoma
Various lymphomas and leukemias
Myeloproliferative disorders

cases, clusters of epithelioid histiocytes may be numerous, making distinction from Lennert's lymphoma (a T-cell lymphoma with high content of epithelioid histiocytes) difficult. The lymphocytes of Lennert's lymphoma are cytologically atypical as opposed to the small, uniform features of the lymphocytes in all forms of Hodgkin's disease, including MC Hodgkin's disease. There is often only partial involvement of nodes involved by MC Hodgkin's disease.

Lymphocyte-Depletion Hodgkin's Disease

Lymphocyte-depletion (LD) Hodgkin's disease is at the opposite end of the cellular spectrum from LP Hodgkin's disease. Lymphocytes are sparse in this disorder, whereas Reed-Sternberg cells and Reed-Sternberg variants predominate. Other types of cells such as plasma cells, histiocytes, and eosinophils are infrequently found. In addition, irregular sclerosis is a major histologic component of LD Hodgkin's disease. This sclerosis ranges from a hypocellular reticular pattern of connective tissue to hypercellular proliferative fibrosis.

In the Lukes and Butler classification, two subtypes of LD Hodgkin's disease are recognized, namely the reticular and diffuse fibrosis types. The reticular subtype has been further divided into sarcomatous and nonsarcomatous variants. In the sarcomatous form of reticular LD Hodgkin's disease, numerous bizarre, pleomorphic Reed-Sternberg variants (see Fig. 23–2D) are present. The pattern of fibrosis and presence of bizarre Reed-Sternberg variants creates a pattern quite akin to that seen in pleomorphic sarcomas such as malignant fibrous histiocytoma. The nonsarcomatous form, on the other hand, is characterized by large numbers of classic Reed-Sternberg cells.

The diffuse fibrosis variant of LD Hodgkin's disease is truly cell-poor because of the presence of abundant acellular, amorphous fibrillar connective tissue. Reed-Sternberg cells are less frequently found than in the reticular form of LD Hodgkin's disease.

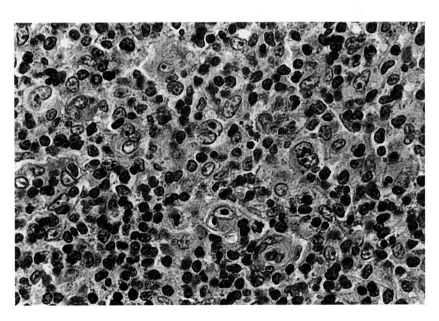

FIGURE 23–3 Hodgkin's disease of mixed cellularity, characterized by a polymorphous cellular milieu including small lymphocytes, eosinophils, plasma cells, and frequent RS cells and RS variants.

There has been a marked decrease in the diagnosis of LD Hodgkin's disease during the past decade. This is not a result of a decreased incidence of this form of Hodgkin's disease but of the recognition that many cases previously diagnosed as LD Hodgkin's disease are actually misdiagnosed cases of non-Hodgkin's lymphoma, particularly polymorphous T-cell lymphomas.[9] In fact, it may be impossible in some cases, even after detailed study including phenotypic and genotypic studies, to resolve the differential diagnosis between a pleomorphic NHL and LD Hodgkin's disease.

Nodular Sclerosing Hodgkin's Disease

The cardinal histologic features of nodular sclerosing (NS) Hodgkin's disease are the presence of birefringent collagenous sclerosis, classic Reed-Sternberg cells, and a distinctive Reed-Sternberg variant called a *lacunar cell*. The sclerosis observed in NS Hodgkin's disease is different from that seen in the other subtypes of Hodgkin's disease. It is found in the form of well-organized bands of collagen that subdivide the tissue into distinct nodules (Fig. 23–4). Within the nodules is a variable mixture of lymphocytes, classic Reed-Sternberg cells, lacunar cells, plasma cells, eosinophils, and neutrophils. The lacunar cells often form distinct collections within the central region of the nodule ("grouped lacunars"), and these collections may be associated with focal necrosis. The lacunar cell is best identified in formalin-fixed tissue sections where the artifact of formalin fixation produces a distinctive appearance of this Reed-Sternberg variant. The lacunar cell is separated from the surrounding cells by a large clear or pale-staining space (lacuna) (see Fig. 23–2E). Wisps of cytoplasm may be seen in this space. The nucleus is large, often polylobated, and the nucleoli are small to intermediate in size.

In some cases of Hodgkin's disease the characteristic cellular milieu of NS Hodgkin's disease may be seen, including the presence of large numbers of lacunar cells; however, the sclerotic bands are absent. These cases have been assigned by some authorities to a subcategory of NS Hodgkin's disease referred to as the cellular phase of NS Hodgkin's disease.[10] Others have as-

signed cases with this pattern to MC Hodgkin's disease.[11]

Sclerosis alone, even when present as orderly bands of collagen, is not sufficient for a diagnosis of NS Hodgkin's disease.

Unclassified Hodgkin's Disease

A small percentage of cases of Hodgkin's disease exhibit sufficient histologic features for a diagnosis of Hodgkin's disease but insufficient features to be assigned to one of the above subcategories. These cases are assigned to the unclassified subcategory.

Histologic Progression

The concurrent evaluation of multiple sites of involvement with Hodgkin's disease usually demonstrates similar histology at each site. On the other hand, with the passage of time, re-evaluation often reveals histologic progression in the sequence: LP Hodgkin's disease to MC Hodgkin's disease to LD Hodgkin's disease.

Clinical Features

In the United States, Hodgkin's disease accounts for approximately one third of newly diagnosed cases of lymphoma. The incidence of Hodgkin's disease exhibits a bimodal distribution with peaks between the ages of 15 and 35 and in the over-50 age group.

Most patients with Hodgkin's disease present with a complaint of nonpainful lymph node swelling. Each subtype of Hodgkin's disease is associated with rather characteristic, but not totally specific, clinical features. LP Hodgkin's disease demonstrates a male predominance and is generally a disease of younger patients. The disease is usually localized at presentation to one peripheral node or node group. NS Hodgkin's disease, on the other hand, shows a female predominance and is usually associated with cervical, scalene, and/or supraclavicular adenopathy. An anterior mediastinal mass is often detected by chest radiograph. Most patients with NS Hodgkin's disease are asymptomatic on presentation. MC and LD Hodgkin's disease are most often seen in symptomatic patients with widely disseminated disease. Extranodal involvement is common in these two subcategories of Hodgkin's disease.

Diagnostic Evaluation and Staging

The diagnosis of Hodgkin's disease requires tissue biopsy and microscopic evaluation. Because of the complexities involved in accurate diagnosis and subclassification, adequate tissue should be obtained at the time of initial biopsy for routine light microscopic studies as well as for ancillary studies such as immunophenotypic and genotypic analysis if these are found to be necessary.

Following a tissue diagnosis of Hodgkin's disease, the patient should be appropriately staged to determine the extent of disease and permit selection of appropriate therapy. The staging evaluation of Hodgkin's disease has become standardized and can be divided into clinical and pathologic staging. Clinical staging

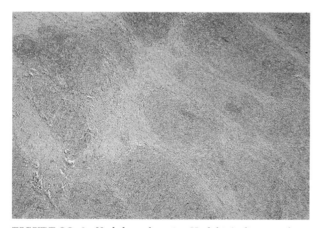

FIGURE 23–4 Nodular sclerosing Hodgkin's disease, characterized by orderly bands of collagen that subdivide the tissue into cellular nodules containing a mixture of cell types including large numbers of lacunar cells.

TABLE 23–4 Staging Workup for Hodgkin's Disease

1. Initial tissue biopsy demonstrating Hodgkin's disease
2. Careful history
3. Detailed physical exam
4. Laboratory studies (CBC; sedimentation rate; chemistry panel to include liver, kidney, and bone profiles)
5. Chest x-ray (anterior and lateral)
6. Bipedal lymphangiography

TABLE 23–6 "B" Symptoms

1. Unexplained loss of more than 10% of body weight in the 6 months before admission
2. Unexplained fever with temperature above 38°C
3. Drenching night sweats

should be performed on all newly diagnosed patients with Hodgkin's disease. The elements of clinical staging are listed in Table 23–4. The most widely used staging scheme is the Ann Arbor Classification (Table 23–5).[12] This scheme may be used with the data obtained from either clinical and/or pathologic staging. In addition to the anatomic extent of the disease implicit in the staging categories, the disease is further classified based on the presence or absence of specific symptoms (Table 23–6). The letter "A" (asymptomatic) or "B" (symptomatic) is then appended to the appropriate stage number.

The clinical utility of the Ann Arbor staging scheme stems from the predictable behavior of Hodgkin's disease. Hodgkin's disease is a lymph-node-based disease and rarely, if ever, starts in extranodal sites. It spreads by the lymphatic route in an orderly and predictable pattern to contiguous lymph nodes. Only late in the disease course, when hematogenous spread may occur, does a more disorderly pattern appear.

Treatment and Prognosis

Current modalities for the therapy of Hodgkin's disease are radiation, chemotherapy, or a combination of the two. The selection of therapy is directed by the results of the staging evaluation rather than the specific histologic subtype.

Long-term disease-free survival can be accomplished in approximately 75% of patients with early-stage Hodgkin's disease and recurrences after radiotherapy are generally responsive to chemotherapy. With appropriate therapy, the 10-year survival for stage I and II Hodgkin's disease now exceeds 80%. Ten-year survival for stage III and IV Hodgkin's disease has been improved with aggressive chemotherapy and now approaches 70%.[13]

NON-HODGKIN'S LYMPHOMA

Virchow (1858)[14] and Billroth (1871)[15] were the first to employ the terms *lymphoma* and *malignant lymphoma*. The distinction between the two major categories of malignant lymphoma, that is, the lymphocytic lymphomas and Hodgkin's disease, was suggested in 1893 by Dreschfield[16] and Kundrat.[17]

Etiology and Pathogenesis

It seems certain that a prerequisite for the development of lymphoma is damage to those regions of the genetic code that regulate the growth and reproduction of cells of the immune system. The inciting agents for this damage remain unknown; however, it is felt that mutagenic factors such as chemicals, ionizing radiation, and certain viruses may play a role in initiating and promoting the damage. Although viruses such as the Epstein-Barr virus (EBV) do not appear to be directly mutagenic, they may function via persistent antigenic stimulation as polyclonal mitogens that somehow favor the eventual selection of a single clone of non-growth-regulated (malignant) cells. Support for this hypothesis comes from the increased incidence of lymphomas in individuals with conditions associated with primary or acquired immunodeficiency (Table 23–7).

TABLE 23–5 Ann Arbor Staging

Stage I	Involvement of single lymph node region or localized involvement of a single extralymphatic organ or site (I_E).
Stage II	Involvement of two or more lymph node regions on the same side of the diaphragm or localized involvement of a single associated extralymphatic organ or site and its regional lymph node(s) with or without involvement of other lymph node regions on the same side of the diaphragm (II_E)
Stage III	Involvement of lymph node regions on both sides of the diaphragm, which may also be accompanied by localized involvement of an associated extralymphatic organ site (III_E)
Stage IV	Disseminated (multifocal) involvement of 1 or more extralymphatic organs, with or without associated lymph node involvement, or isolated extralymphatic organ involvement with distant (nonregional) nodal involvement.

Source: From Carbone et al,[12] with permission.

TABLE 23–7 Conditions Associated with Increased Risk of Developing Lymphoma (NHL)

Sjögren's syndrome
Sarcoidosis
Systemic lupus erythematosus
Rheumatoid arthritis
Celiac disease
Dermatitis herpetiformis
AIDS
Organ transplant recipients
Congenital immunodeficiency disorders

TABLE 23–8   **Common Chromosomal Abnormalities Associated with Malignant Lymphomas**

Abnormality	Genetic Loci Involved	Associated Lymphoma
Trisomy 12		B-CLL/PLL
t(11;14)	bcl-1/IgH (Prad 1)	Mantle cell lymphoma
t(14;18)	IgH/bcl-2	Follicle center lymphoma
t(11;18)		Marginal zone lymphoma (extranodal)
Trisomy 3		Marginal zone lymphoma (extranodal)
t(8;14)	c-*myc*/IgH	Burkitt's lymphoma
t(2;8)	kappa/c-*myc*	Burkitt's lymphoma
t(8;22)	c-*myc*/lambda	Burkitt's lymphoma
t(3;14)	*bcl*-6/IgH	Diffuse large B-cell lymphoma
inv 14 (q11;q32)		T-CLL/PLL
t(2;5)	ALK-NPM	CD30+ Anaplastic large cell

Abbreviation: ALK = kinase gene; NPM = nucleolar protein gene.

The genetic damage associated with the development of a lymphoma is often associated with numeric and/or structural alterations of chromosomes.[18] With high-resolution karyotyping techniques, nonrandom chromosomal abnormalities can be demonstrated in approximately 60% of cases of lymphoma. Certain types of lymphoma are highly correlated with specific chromosomal abnormalities, particularly translocations involving chromosomes 2, 8, 14, and 22 (Table 23–8). For many T-cell lymphomas, a common breakpoint is in the region of one of the T-cell receptor genes. The other breakpoint is in the vicinity of a gene important in the regulation of cell growth and division. This growth-regulating gene, referred to as a *proto-oncogene* when it is normally located in the genome, is translocated to the region of one of the immunoglobulin genes (B-cell lymphomas) or T-cell receptor genes (T-cell lymphomas). In this new location the growth-regulating gene functions abnormally and is now referred to as an *oncogene*. One of the best-studied examples of this process occurs in Burkitt's lymphoma, a B-cell lymphoma, in which the c-*myc* proto-oncogene located at region q24 on chromosome 8, is translocated to the immunoglobulin heavy-chain locus at 14q32 (Fig. 23–5). This occurs in about 90% of Burkitt's lymphoma cases. It also is found in about 40% of high-grade large-cell lymphomas and therefore is not specific for Burkitt's lymphoma.

Chromosomal translocations are only one mechanism for oncogene activation. Other mechanisms include deletions, base pair mutations, and gene amplification. Oncogene activation and deregulation is believed to play a role in the development of most, if not all, lymphomas.

Pathology

Since the original suggestion by Dreschfield[16] that the lymphocytic lymphomas represent distinct histologic entities, a number of lymphoma classification schemes have been proposed. At least seven major classification schemes have been extensively used since the mid-1960s. Most of the classification schemes are based on the growth pattern, for example, nodular or diffuse (Fig. 23–6A and B), and the cytologic features of the malignant cells. Later modifications of some of the original classification schemes have added immunophenotypic-genotypic characteristics to the subclassification of the non-Hodgkin's lymphomas. At present, the scheme most widely used by pathologists and clinicians in the United States is the modified Rappaport classification[19] (Table 23–9) and in Europe it is the modified Kiel (Lennert's) classification[20] (Table 23–10).

A critical analysis of the existing schemes conducted by the National Cancer Institute in the late 1970s

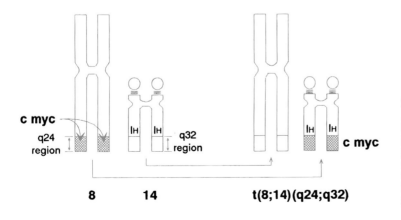

FIGURE 23–5 Reciprocal translocation t(8;14)(q24;q32) is seen in most cases of Burkitt's lymphoma as well as some non-Burkitt's high-grade lymphomas. A reciprocal translocation of genetic material occurs between chromosomes 8 and 14. A distal portion of the long arm of chromosome 8, containing the c-myc oncogene, is translocated to a site adjacent to the immunoglobulin heavy-chain locus on chromosome 14.

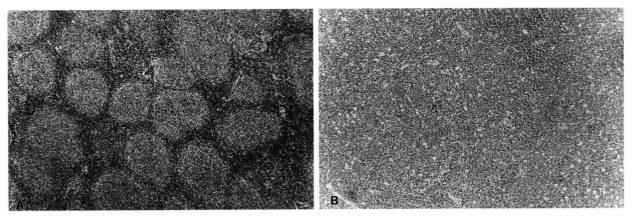

FIGURE 23-6   Growth patterns of the non-Hodgkin's lymphomas. (*A*) Nodular (follicular) pattern resulting from closely packed neoplastic follicles without mantle zones. (*B*) Diffuse pattern in which neoplastic cells are distributed as sheets of cells without follicular organization.

revealed no significant differences in the various schemes with regard to their clinical utility. In acknowledgment of this fact and recognizing the clinical confusion created by the lack of a standard classification scheme, the investigators in this multi-institutional study group proposed the Working Formulation for Clinical Usage[21] (Table 23-11). Although not proposed as a lymphoma classification, it is nevertheless commonly used as such.

More recently, the pathologists of the International Lymphoma Study Group have proposed a Revised European-American Classification of Lymphoid Neoplasms[22] that includes accepted lymphoma entities not recognized by the earlier classification schemes or the Working Formulation. The utility of this more "biologically correct" classification scheme remains to be tested by both the pathologist and clinician communities.

A conceptual understanding of the common classification schemes requires knowledge of the morphological ontogeny of normal lymphocytes. The lymphocytic lymphomas may be conceptualized as a malignant population of lymphocytes arrested at a particular stage (morphological, genotypic, phenotypic, or functional) of lymphocyte maturation (see Chap. 18). Thus, we would expect to see lymphomas that express the attributes of normal lymphoid cells found in each of the various normal lymphoid com-

partments, that is, the precursor (bone marrow), intrafollicular, mantle zone, marginal zone, and interfollicular compartments. As illustrated in Fig. 23-7 and Fig. 23-8A,B each of the lymph node compartments is occupied by morphologically characteristic cells. These cells are also immunophenotypically and genotypically distinct.

Lymphomas Related to Intrafollicular (Follicular Center) Lymphocytes

Two principal morphologically distinct lymphocyte cell types are found in the normal follicle (see Fig. 23-7), namely the small cleaved (centrocyte) and large noncleaved (centroblast) lymphocytes. The follicular-center lymphomas are composed of various mixtures of these two cell types.

Follicular-center lymphomas composed predominantly of small cleaved lymphocytes (centrocytes) are referred to as poorly differentiated lymphocytic (Rappaport); centroblastic-centrocytic, small cell type (Kiel); or small cleaved cell (Working Formulation) lymphomas. The predominant malignant cell in this lymphoma is the counterpart of the small cleaved follicular-center cell (centrocyte), although a few large lymphocytes (centroblasts) are always present. The small cleaved cell is relatively small (6 to 12 μm di-

TABLE 23-9 **Modified Rappaport Classification**	
Nodular	**Diffuse**
Lymphocytic, poorly differentiated	Lymphocytic, well differentiated
Mixed lymphocytic-histiocytic	Lymphocytic, intermediate differentiated
Histiocytic	Lymphocytic, poorly differentiated
	Mixed, lymphocytic-histiocytic
	Undifferentiated, Burkitt's type
	Undifferentiated, non-Burkitt's type
	Histiocytic
	Lymphoblastic

Source: From Berard and Dorfman,[19] with permission.

TABLE 23–10	**Updated Kiel (Lennert) Classification (1991)**
Low-Grade Malignant B-Cell Lymphomas	**Low-Grade Malignant T-Cell Lymphomas**

Lymphocytic
   CLL
   PLL
   HCL
Immunocytoma
Plasmacytic
Centroblastic-centrocytic
Centrocytic
Monocytoid
	Lymphocytic
	   CLL
	   PLL
	Small cell, cerebriform (Mycosis fungoides,
	   Sézary's syndrome)
	Lymphoepithelioid
	AILD (LgX) type
	T-zone lymphoma
	Pleomorphic, small cell

High-Grade Malignant B-Cell Lymphomas	**High-Grade Malignant T-Cell Lymphomas**

Centroblastic
   Monomorphic
   Polymorphic
   Multilobated
   Centrocytoid
Immunoblastic
Burkitt's lymphoma
Large cell anaplastic
Lymphoblastic
	Pleomorphic, medium-sized and large cell
	Immunoblastic
	Large cell anaplastic
	Lymphoblastic

Source: From Lennert et al,[20] with permission.

ameter) with scant cytoplasm, slightly to distinctly irregular nucleus (angulated, clefted), and indistinct nucleoli (Fig. 23–9). A predominantly follicular or mixed follicular and diffuse pattern is most commonly found. Pure diffuse lymphomas of this type are rare and most cases classified as such are usually some other type of lymphoma, most commonly mantle cell lymphoma. This lymphoma is classified as low grade (indolent) if follicular (with or without diffuse areas), and intermediate grade if purely diffuse (Working Formulation).

Follicular-center lymphomas composed predominantly of large lymphocytes are referred to as histiocytic (Rappaport); centroblastic-centrocytic, large cell (Kiel); and large cell (Working Formulation) lymphomas. These lymphomas are composed predominantly (>75%) of large cleaved (large centrocytes) and large noncleaved cells. Large cleaved (Fig. 23–10) cells are from 15 to 20 μm in diameter and have modest amounts of cytoplasm, irregular vesicular nuclei, and indistinct nucleoli. Large noncleaved cells (centroblasts) (Fig. 23–10) are 20 to 40 μm in diameter, have a modest amount of pyranophilic (RNA-rich) cytoplasm, round to oval vesicular nuclei, and small but distinct nucleoli. All three growth patterns (follicular, diffuse, or mixed follicular and diffuse) may be observed, and this group falls into the intermediate-grade category of the Working Formulation regardless of growth pattern. For biologic and possibly prognostic reasons, purely diffuse large cell lymphomas of follicular origin should be distinguished from diffuse large cell lymphomas of nonfollicular origin.

All follicular-center lymphomas are a mixture of small cleaved and large cells (Table 23–12). When neither cell type dominates, a mixed pattern is recognized by some classification schemes (e.g., Working Formulation and Rappaport classification). The specific criteria for the diagnosis of mixed small cleaved and large cell vary with the different classification schemes and are largely subjective. Berard[23] has developed specific criteria for the follicular (nodular) variety of the follicular-center cell lymphomas: between 5 and 15 *large noncleaved cells* (centroblasts) per high-power field qualifies as mixed small and large cell, <5 per high-power field is small cleaved, and >15 per high-power field is large cell. Mixed small cleaved and large cell lymphoma is classified as low grade if follicular and intermediate if diffuse.

Lymphomas derived from follicular-center cells are by definition B-cell lymphomas. The expected immunophenotype of a follicular-center lymphoma can be found in Table 23–13. Follicular lymphomas are distinguished at the genetic level by a unique chromosomal translocation t(14;18), which is present in 70% to 95% of cases (see Table 23–8).

Follicular-center lymphomas account for approximately 40% of adult non-Hodgkin's lymphomas in the United States. The disease most commonly affects adults and is usually widespread at diagnosis (Table 23–14). Although the disease course is usually indolent, it is not often curable with current therapy. Prognosis is dependent on the number of large cells (centroblasts) and the degree of follicularity. Progression with time from a follicular pattern to a more aggressive diffuse large cell pattern occurs in approximately 40% of cases (Table 23–15), however, spontaneous remissions have also been described.

TABLE 23–11 **Working Formulation for Clinical Usage**

Low Grade
Malignant lymphoma, small lymphocytic
   Consistent with CLL
   Plasmacytoid
Malignant lymphoma, follicular, predominantly small cleaved cell
   Diffuse areas
   Sclerosis
Malignant lymphoma, follicular, mixed small cleaved and large cell
   Diffuse areas
   Sclerosis

Intermediate Grade
Malignant lymphoma, follicular, predominantly large cell
   Diffuse areas
   Sclerosis
Malignant lymphoma, diffuse, small cleaved cell
   Sclerosis
Malignant lymphoma, diffuse, mixed, small and large cell
   Sclerosis
   Epithelioid cell component
Malignant lymphoma, diffuse, large cell
   Cleaved cell
   Noncleaved cell
   Sclerosis

High Grade
Malignant lymphoma, large cell, immunoblastic
   Plasmacytoid
   Clear cell
   Polymorphous
   Epithelioid cell component
Malignant lymphoma, lymphoblastic
   Convoluted cell
   Nonconvoluted cell
Malignant lymphoma, small noncleaved cell
   Burkitt's
   Follicular areas

Source: From Rosenberg et al,[21] with permission.

Lymphomas Related to Mantle Zone Lymphocytes (Mantle Cell Lymphoma)

Lymphomas composed of lymphocytes with the morphological and immunophenotypic features of mantle cells have only recently been accepted as a distinctive subcategory of non-Hodgkin's lymphoma.[24] Of the commonly used classification schemes, only the modified Kiel classification recognizes an entity, centrocytic lymphoma, that corresponds to mantle cell lymphoma. The cytologic features of mantle cell lymphoma are somewhat variable; however, the cells are most commonly small to medium-sized lymphocytes with scant pale cytoplasm, irregular nuclei, and inconspicuous nuclei (Fig. 23–11). Occasionally the cells are very similar to small lymphocytes creating an appearance similar to small lymphocytic lymphoma. Growth centers as described in the section on small lymphocytic lymphoma, however, are absent. Centroblasts and immunoblasts are rarely found. Most often, mantle cell lymphoma has a diffuse or faintly nodular pat-

tern; however, occasionally a distinct mantle zone pattern is observed. In this form the malignant cells are distributed as an expanded mantle zone surrounding benign (polyclonal) germinal centers. This pattern of mantle cell lymphoma must be distinguished from mantle zone hyperplasia.

The immunophenotype of mantle cell lymphomas aids in differentiating this subcategory of lymphoma from other morphologically similar lymphomas (see Table 23–13). This immunophenotype corresponds to the normal CD5+, CD23– B cell of the inner follicle mantle.[25] Most cases of mantle cell lymphoma demonstrate a unique chromosomal translocation t(11;14) that results in the overexpression of the cell cycle protein cyclin D1 (see Table 23–8).

Mantle cell lymphoma is a disease of older adults with high male:female ratio (Table 23–14). The disease is usually widespread at diagnosis and, despite its moderately aggressive course, behaves like other low-grade lymphomas in that it is generally not curable with current therapies. A peculiar presentation of the disease in the intestine is referred to as *lymphomatous polyposis* (Fig. 23–12). A more aggressive form of mantle cell lymphoma with median survival of 3 years is termed *blastoid* variant because of the lymphoblast-like appearance of the cells. Transformation to a typical large-cell lymphoma, however, does not appear to occur.

Lymphomas Related to Marginal Zone Lymphocytes

The marginal zone of lymph nodes is a poorly defined anatomic compartment.[26] However, in other lymphoid tissues, that is, spleen and Peyer's patches, the marginal zone is better defined.[27] The typical marginal zone cell is a centrocytelike cell (small cleaved cell) with more abundant pale-staining cytoplasm than a true centrocyte. Under antigenic stimulation these marginal zone B cells are believed by some investigators to be capable of differentiation into monocytoid (parafollicular) B cells and plasma cells (see Fig. 23–8A). Monocytoid B cells are medium-sized lymphocytes morphologically resembling monocytes that are found predominantly in the lymphoid sinuses and paracortex of some reactive lymph nodes but not in normal lymph nodes. They are particularly common in the reactive lymphadenopathies associated with HIV infection and toxoplasmosis.

Lymphomas related to marginal zone cells are a group of recently described and controversially related entities.[28] A common form of presentation of marginal cell lymphoma is at extranodal sites, particularly stomach, salivary gland, lung, thyroid, and orbit, where they have been referred to as lymphomas of mucosal-associated lymphoid tissue (MALT lymphomas).[29] Collections of lymphoid tissue normally occur in extranodal mucosal sites such as the small bowel (Peyer's patches). MALT, however, does not normally occur in the most common sites for MALT lymphomas. Under conditions of chronic antigenic stimulation, for example, infection or autoimmune disease, such lymphoid tissue may develop in these sites. Examples of

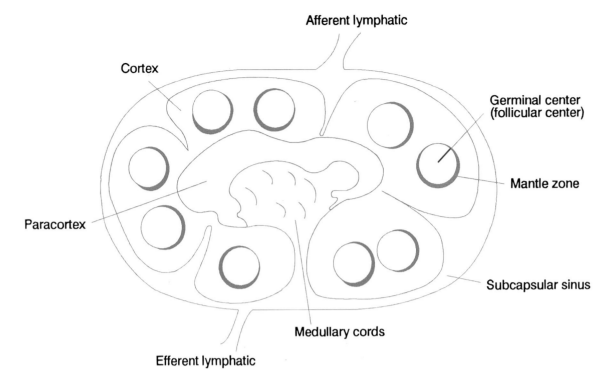

FIGURE 23-7 Anatomic compartments of the lymph nodes.

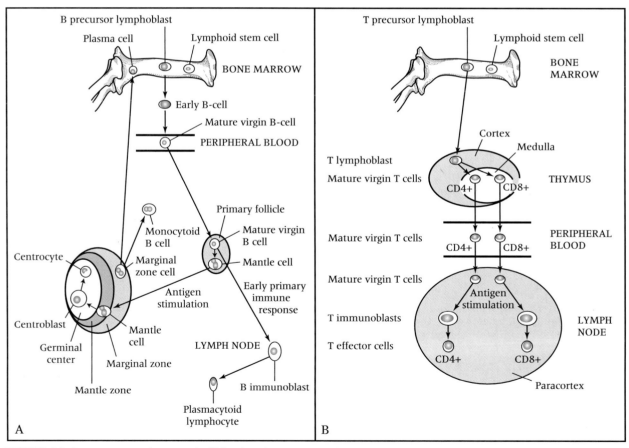

FIGURE 23-8 Maturation (ontogeny) of (*A*) B-lymphocytes and (*B*) T-lymphocytes in relation to the pertinent anatomic compartments.

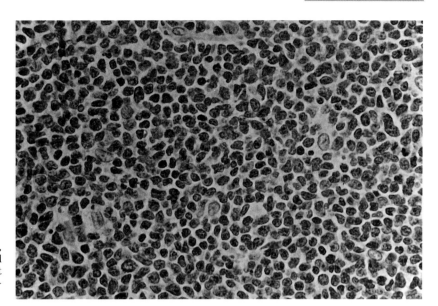

FIGURE 23-9 Malignant lymphoma, small cleaved cell composed of small cells (6–12 μm in diameter) with scant cytoplasm and angulated or clefted nuclei with indistinct nucleoli.

such conditions are *Helicobacter pylori* gastritis, Sjögren's syndrome, and Hashimoto's thyroiditis. Lymphomas that develop in the setting of chronic antigenic stimulation may remain dependent on the presence of benign antigen-driven T cells, a fact that has important therapeutic and prognostic implications. For example, in the case of the MALT-type marginal cell lymphoma of the stomach, eradication of the offending antigen (*H. pylori*) with antimicrobial therapy has been demonstrated to be effective in treating this specific lymphoma.[30]

The histologic features of extranodal marginal cell lymphoma (MALT) are highly characteristic. Reactive follicles or their remnants are uniformly present (Fig. 23–13). Subjacent to the mucosal lining or glandular epithelium of involved organs and surrounding the reactive follicles are collections of small to medium-sized lymphocytes with a moderate amount of pale-staining cytoplasm and irregular nuclei (centrocyte-like cells) (Figs. 23–14, 23–15). In addition to centrocyte-like cells, neoplastic cells with features similar to small lymphocytes and/or monocytoid B cells are present. Plasma differentiation in a portion of the cells is also a common finding. A constant feature of these lymphomas is infiltration of the associated epithelium by neoplastic lymphocytes resulting in the formation of lymphoepithelial lesions (Fig. 23–16). The neoplastic cells may also infiltrate the reactive follicles, giving the impression of a follicular-center cell lymphoma, a process referred to as follicular colonization.

A second pattern of marginal cell lymphoma is lymph-node-based and is often referred to as *monocytoid B-cell lymphoma* by hematopathologists in the United States.[31]

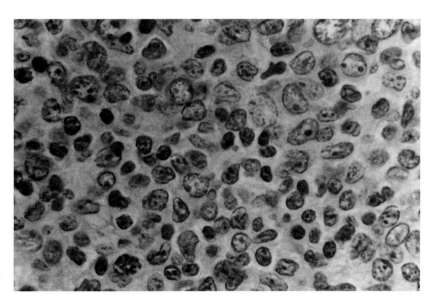

FIGURE 23-10 Malignant lymphoma, large diffuse cell composed of a mixture of large cleaved and large noncleaved cells.

TABLE 23–12 Low-Grade B-Cell Lymphomas: Morphological Features

Lymphoma Subtype	Small Cells	Large Cells
B-cell CLL/SLL	Round (rarely cleaved)	Paraimmunoblasts/prolymphocytes
Mantle cell	Cleaved (rarely round)	Usually absent
Follicular-center cell (CB/CC)	Cleaved (centrocytes)	Centroblasts
Immunocytoma	Round	Immunoblasts
Marginal cell	Round, cleaved, and/or monocytoid	Centroblasts/immunoblasts

Abbreviations: CLL = Chronic lymphocytic leukemia; SLL = Small lymphocytic lymphoma; CB/CC = Centroblastic/centrocytic.

TABLE 23–13 Low-Grade B-Cell Lymphomas: Immunophenotypic Profile

Lymphoma Subtype	CD5	CD10	CD23	CD43	Leu 8
B-cell CLL/SLL	+	−	+	+	+
Mantle cell	+	−/+	−	+	+
Follicular-center cell (CB/CC)	−	+/−	−	−	−
Immunocytoma	−/+	−	−	−/+	+/−
Marginal cell					
Extranodal	−	−	−	−/+	+/−
Nodal	−	−	−	+/−	+

Abbreviations: −/+ = less than 50% of cases positive; +/− = greater than 50% of cases positive; CLL = Chronic lymphocytic leukemia; SLL = Small lymphocytic lymphoma; CB/CC = Centroblastic/centrocytic.

TABLE 23–14 Low-Grade B-Cell Lymphomas: Clinical Features

Lymphoma Subtype	Male:Female	Stage 1 (%)	Extranodal (%)	BM (%)	PB (%)	NED @5 yrs (%)	Survival Rate @5 yrs (%)
B cell CLL/SLL	2:1	0	Rare	100	>90	<10	90
Mantle cell	3:1	<10	>50	>50	25	0	<40
Follicular-center cell (CB/CC)	1:1	<10	<50	>50	<15	<25	>60
Immunocytoma	1.3:1	Rare	Rare	100	<30	0	>70
Marginal cell							
Extranodal	1:2	>80	100	<15	Rare	>80	100
Nodal	1.2	50?	?*	50?	Rare	50?	50

*Pure nodal marginal cell lymphomas are uncommon.
Abbreviations: BM = Bone marrow involvement; PB = Peripheral blood involvement; NED = No evidence of disease.

TABLE 23–15 Low-Grade B-Cell Lymphomas: Large Cell Transformation

Lymphoma	Secondary Large Cell Type	Incidence of Transformation
Chronic lymphocytic leukemia	Richter's transformation (diffuse large cell)	5%
Small lymphocytic leukemia	Paraimmunoblastic/prolymphocytoid transformation	15%
Mantle cell lymphoma	Blastic variant (lymphoblastoid)	7%
	Centrocytoid/centroblastic (centroblastoid variant)	?%
Follicular center cell lymphoma	Secondary centroblastic (diffuse large cell)	40%
Immunocytoma	Secondary immunoblastic	5%
Marginal zone cell lymphoma	Secondary high grade lymphoma	?%

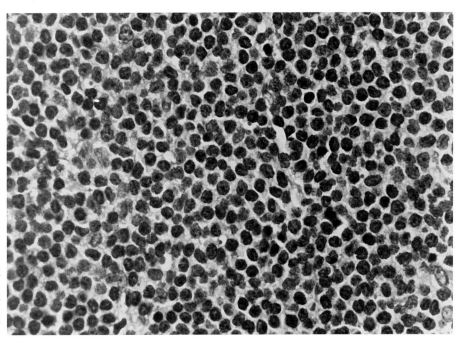

FIGURE 23-11 Mantle-cell lymphoma. The cytologic features are "intermediate" between those of small lymphocyte lymphoma and small cleaved cell lymphoma.

Histologically, node-based marginal zone lymphoma is characterized by infiltration of the paracortex and sinuses with a monoclonal population of monocytoid B cells. These cells have oval, reniform, or sometimes quite irregular nuclei, bland chromatin pattern, and relatively abundant pale-staining cytoplasms with distinct cytoplasmic borders. Benign secondary follicles with hyperplastic germinal centers are present. These serve to accent the pale-staining infiltrate of monocytoid B cells.

The characteristic immunophenotype of the marginal zone lymphomas is found in Table 23–13. The extranodal form (MALT lymphoma) is associated with the chromosomal abnormalities trisomy 3 and t(11;18) (see Table 23–8).

The clinical features of marginal zone lymphoma correspond to the two modes of presentation discussed above (see Table 23–14). The extranodal (MALT) form is a disease of adults with a slight female predominance and is highly associated with autoimmune dis-

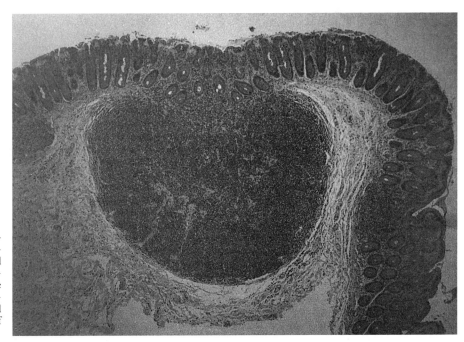

FIGURE 23-12 Lymphomatous polyposis, a form of mantle-cell lymphoma, is characterized by the presence of multiple malignant lymphoid polyps of the gastrointestinal tract. The malignant cells have the cytological and phenotypical features of mantle cells.

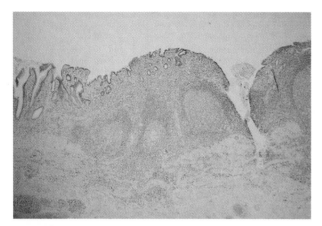

FIGURE 23-13 Mucosal associated lymphoid tissue (MALT) lymphoma of the stomach. The gastric mucosa is replaced and expanded by a lymphoid infiltrate including benign secondary follicles with germinal centers and a diffuse population of malignant cells.

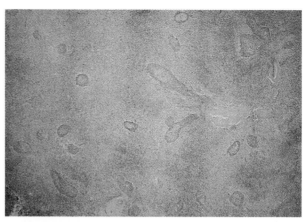

FIGURE 23-14 MALT lymphoma of the parotid gland. Pale zones of malignant cells surround and infiltrate remnants of parotid gland epithelium. Collections of dark-staining cells are benign (reactive) lymphocytes.

ease or infection (*Helicobacter* gastritis). Transformation to a large cell lymphoma occasionally occurs (see Table 23–15).

Adding to the complexity and controversy of the category of marginal cell lymphomas is the entity splenic marginal zone lymphoma with or without villous lymphocytes.[32] Its relationship to nodal and extranodal marginal zone lymphoma is not well understood, although to some investigators splenic marginal zone lymphoma is more closely related to the rare chronic lymphoid leukemia referred to as splenic lymphoma with circulating villous lymphocytes.[33]

Lymphomas Related to Interfollicular Lymphocytes

These lymphomas may express either a B- or T-cell phenotype. Morphological features alone are unreliable in assessing the B- or T-cell nature of these lymphomas.

Small Lymphocytic Lymphoma This low-grade lymphoma is also commonly referred to as *well-differentiated lymphocytic lymphoma* (Rappaport classification). The growth pattern is diffuse, although a pseudofollicular pattern may be observed (Fig. 23–17A).

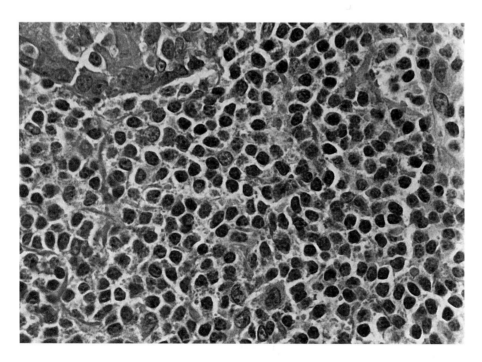

FIGURE 23-15 MALT lymphoma of the parotid gland, a type of lymphoma thought to be related to marginal zone lymphocytes, is composed of a mixture of cells with features of lymphoplasmacytoid cells, centrocytelike cells, and monocytoid B cells. One of the morphologic types often predominates.

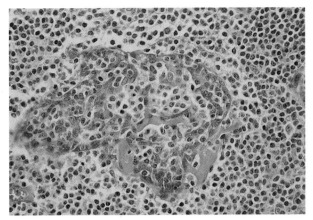

FIGURE 23–16 Detailed view of a lymphoepithelial lesion MALT lymphoma of the parotid gland, composed of metaplastic parotid gland epithelium infiltrated by the atypical lymphoid cells of MALT lymphoma.

These pseudofollicles, also called growth centers, do not have the cytologic or histologic features of true neoplastic follicles.[34] Most of the neoplastic cells are small, uniform lymphocytes with scant cytoplasm, round nucleus, clumped chromatin, and absent to small nucleoli, that is, they appear cytologically similar to normal small lymphocytes (Fig. 23–17B). Admixed with these small lymphocytes are variable numbers of intermediate to large lymphocytes referred to as prolymphocytes and paraimmunoblasts. These cells are most commonly found in increased numbers within the pseudofollicles (growth centers). In approximately 40% of the cases of small lymphocytic lymphoma, a leukemic phase identical to chronic lymphocytic leukemia will develop. Small lymphocytic lymphoma and chronic lymphocytic leukemia are now considered to represent different clinical expression of the same basic disease process.

Small lymphocytic lymphomas may show evidence of plasmacytoid differentiation, including the presence of cytoplasmic immunoglobulin and a small amount of circulating monoclonal immunoglobulin in the peripheral blood. These cases are phenotypically and clinically similar to small lymphocytic lymphoma and as such should be distinguished from true immunocytoma (see section below). Transformation to a large cell lymphoma (Richter's transformation) can occur and portends a more aggressive clinical course (see Table 23–15).

The normal counterpart cell to the malignant cell of small lymphocytic lymphoma is believed to be a recirculating B or T lymphocyte. The vast majority of small lymphocytic lymphomas express a B-cell phenotype (98% in western countries). In addition to the expression of B-cell-associated antigens (CD19, 22, 24), with sensitive techniques, low-density monoclonal surface immunoglobulin is detectable. The B-cell small lymphocytic lymphomas are also positive for CD5, CD23, and CD43, but lack CD10. A small number of patients are weakly positive for CD11c. The remaining 2% usually express a mature T-cell phenotype usually of the "helper" type [CD2(+)/CD3(+)/CD4(+)/CD5(+)/CD7(+)/CD8(−)]. Approximately 20% of T-cell cases coexpress CD4 and CD8 and only very rare cases show CD8+, CD4−.

Trisomy 12 has been reported in one third of patients with B-cell small lymphocytic lymphoma, whereas T-cell small lymphocytic lymphoma is characterized genotypically in 75% of the cases by inv 14 (q11;q32) (see Table 23–8).

Small lymphocytic lymphoma or chronic lymphocytic leukemia is a disease of older adults and is usually widespread at diagnosis. The disease, although indolent in behavior, is considered incurable with standard therapy. Aggressive treatment, including bone marrow transplantation in the hope of achieving durable remission or even cure, is under investigation.

Lymphoplasmacytoid Cell Lymphoma/Immunocytoma A phenotypically and clinically distinct form of lymphoma of small lymphoid cells exists in which the cells exhibit maturation to plasma cells and a phenotype distinct from typical small lymphocytic lymphoma. Specifically, they express surface and cytoplasmic immunoglobulin, usually of the IgM class; are

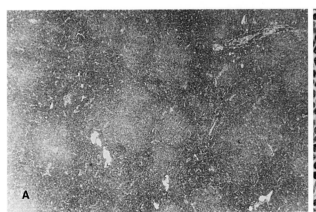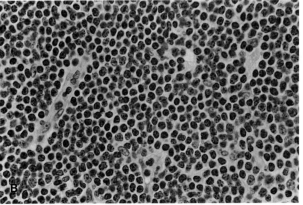

FIGURE 23–17 Small lymphocytic malignant lymphoma. (A) Pseudofollicular pattern is evident because of presence of numerous growth centers. (B) Outside the growth centers, this subtype of lymphoma is composed predominantly of sheets of small, mature-appearing lymphocytes.

positive for B-cell-associated antigens (CD19, 20, 22, 79a); but lack CD10. Less than 50% of cases are positive for CD43 and CD5. The normal counterpart of this lymphoma is believed to be a recirculating CD5 negative cell that has been stimulated to differentiate to plasma cells. Clinically, these lymphomas usually correspond to the syndrome of Waldenström's macroglobulinemia. A monoclonal gammopathy of the IgM type is often present and is associated with hyperviscosity symptoms.

Immunoblastic Lymphomas Lymphomas corresponding to the immunoblast stage of differentiation and morphologically resembling immunoblasts are referred to as *immunoblastic lymphomas*. This category of lymphoma falls within the broad category of diffuse large cell lymphoma. Diffuse large cell lymphomas are conceptualized in the Working Formulation as made up of two subcategories, namely diffuse large cell lymphomas of follicular origin and diffuse large cell lymphomas of nonfollicular origin (immunoblastic). Controversy exists as to whether these two subcategories can be reliably distinguished on morphological grounds alone and whether there is any clinical justification for separating these two subcategories of large cell lymphoma.

Morphologically four cellular patterns of immunoblastic lymphoma have been described and are distinguished within the Working Formulation. Specifically, these are the plasmacytoid, clear cell, polymorphous, and epithelioid subcategories. Normal immunoblasts are large cells with intensely basophilic cytoplasm, large round nuclei, and large central, often solitary nucleoli. The cytologic features of the plasmacytoid variant of immunoblastic lymphoma best correspond to features of the normal immunoblast (Fig. 23–18). The clear cell variant is distinguished by relatively abundant clear cytoplasm but otherwise typical immunoblast nuclear features. Marked variation in nuclear

size and contour characterizes the polymorphous subtype. The malignant cells of the epithelioid variant may be plasmacytoid, clear, and/or polymorphous; however, there is a large admixture of benign epithelioid histiocytes. Mitotic activity is high in all subtypes of immunoblastic lymphoma.

Immunoblastic lymphomas may be of either T- or B-cell immunophenotype. The histologic features are helpful but not infallible in predicting the immunophenotype, namely, plasmacytoid immunoblastic lymphomas most often express a B-cell phenotype, whereas the clear cell, polymorphous, and epithelioid patterns are usually associated with a T-cell phenotype, commonly of the CD4+ type. In keeping with their nonfollicular origin, the B-cell immunoblastic lymphomas are CD5− and CD10− and at the molecular level do not show rearrangement of the *bcl*-2 gene or the t(14;18) translocation characteristic of follicular lymphomas. Those few large cell lymphomas with immunoblastic morphology that express follicular-center cell antigens or *bcl*-2 rearrangement probably represent transformation of a pre-existing follicular lymphoma. Such cases serve to illustrate the difficulty in distinguishing follicular from nonfollicular (immunoblastic) types of diffuse large cell lymphoma.

The clinical behavior of immunoblastic lymphoma is similar to that of diffuse large cell lymphomas in general. The disease is aggressive but potentially curable with multiagent chemotherapy. Relapse is more common with the T-cell type than with B-cell immunoblastic lymphoma.

Lymphomas Related to Precursor Lymphocytes (Lymphoblastic Lymphomas)

The cells of lymphoblastic lymphoma are cytologically identical to the lymphoblasts of acute lymphoblastic leukemia (Fig. 23–19). They have scant cyto-

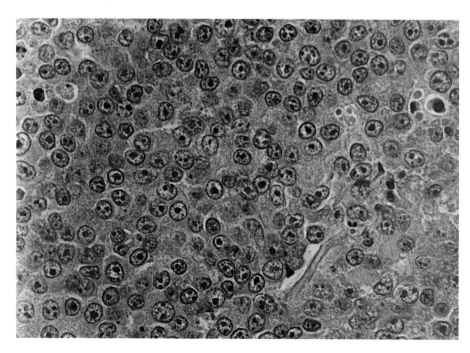

FIGURE 23–18 Immunoblastic lymphoma, plasmacytoid type. The malignant cells are large, with eccentrically placed nuclei and prominent central nucleoli.

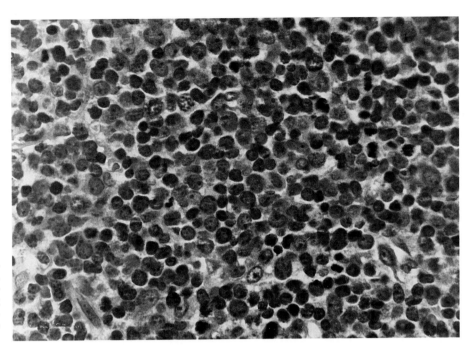

FIGURE 23–19 Lymphoblastic lymphoma, a form of high-grade lymphoma, is cytologically characterized by cells with scant cytoplasm, finely dispersed chromatin ("blastic"), and brisk mitotic rate.

plasm and nuclei with finely dispersed chromatin and absent or indistinct nucleoli. The nuclear contour may be either convoluted or nonconvoluted and mitotic activity is high. The cells are slightly larger than normal lymphocytes and the cytologic and histologic features of this lymphoma may be confused with those of small, noncleaved lymphoma. Attention to nuclear features as well as immunophenotypic and cytogenetic data can resolve the distinction between these two lymphoma types.

Approximately 70% of lymphoblastic lymphomas are of the T-cell type. Their phenotype is complex; however, most are terminal deoxynucleotidal transferase positive (see Chap. 18), which serves to distinguish them from other categories of lymphoma. In addition to TdT, most T-cell lymphoblastic lymphomas are CD7+ and CD3+, whereas cases of T-cell acute lymphoblastic leukemia usually express a more immature phenotype (CD7+, CD3−). The B-cell type of lymphoblastic lymphoma also shows a high frequency of expression of TdT. It is usually CD19+, CD79a+, CD22+, CD20−/+, CD10+/−, HLA-DR+, and CD34+/−. Surface immunoglobulin is rarely present. Both the B- and T-cell types of lymphoblastic lymphomas are believed to be derived from committed precursor B and T cells, respectively.

Lymphoblastic lymphoma most commonly affects adolescent and young adult males. The disease is very aggressive, with rapidly enlarging mediastinal mass and/or peripheral lymph nodes. Central nervous system involvement is frequent and a leukemic phase is a common terminal event. Despite the aggressive course, which is rapidly fatal if untreated, lymphoblastic lymphoma is potentially curable with multi-agent chemotherapy.

Common Lymphomas Whose Normal Counterpart Cell is Poorly Defined

The normal counterpart cell of many of the rare lymphomas has not been defined; however, this is also true for some relatively common lymphomas, such as Burkitt's lymphoma and the related Burkitt-like lymphoma.

Burkitt's lymphoma, first described in 1958 by Dennis Burkitt,[35] is endemic to Africa but also accounts for approximately one-third of non-African pediatric lymphomas and a high percentage of lymphomas in immunocompromised patients, particularly patients with acquired immunodeficiency syndrome (AIDS).

The monotonously uniform cells of Burkitt's lymphoma are described as small noncleaved cells in the Working Formulation as well as the Lukes and Collins classification. They are medium-sized cells with uniformly round nuclei, multiple small nucleoli, and a modest amount of intensely basophilic cytoplasm (Fig. 23–20). Lipid vacuoles are readily evident in the cytoplasm on smears or imprints of the tissue. The mitotic rate of Burkitt's lymphoma is very high and the estimated volume doubling time of this lymphoma is the highest of any tumor (approximately one day). Programmed tumor cell death (apoptosis) is also very high and a starry-sky pattern of tingible-body macrophages is usually evident because of phagocytosis of the apoptotic debris (Fig. 23–21). The normal counterpart to the Burkitt lymphoma cell is controversial with different lines of evidence pointing to either an early B cell or a follicular center cell.

As previously discussed, Burkitt's lymphoma is cytogenetically characterized by a t(8;14) translocation

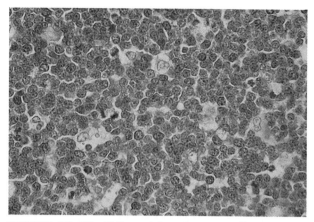

FIGURE 23–20 Malignant lymphoma, small noncleaved cell (Burkitt's lymphoma). This subtype of lymphoma is characterized by relatively uniform cells (15–20 μm in diameter) having a moderate amount of pyranophilic cytoplasm and round nuclei with multiple small distinct nucleoli.

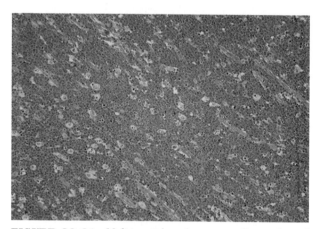

FIGURE 23–21 Malignant lymphoma, small noncleaved cell type. "Starry sky" pattern is produced by the clear cytoplasm of numerous tingible body macrophages admixed with the neoplastic small noncleaved cells.

in the majority of cases or less often by t(2;8) or t(8;22). In the endemic (African) form of this disease, the breakpoint on chromosome 14 involves the heavy-chain joining region, suggesting an early B-cell origin of the Burkitt cell. However, in the nonendemic form, the breakpoint is in the heavy-chain switch region consistent with origin at a latter stage (follicular center cell?) of B-cell development. The endemic and immunodeficiency-related cases are also associated with a high frequency of tumor-cell-incorporated Epstein-Barr virus genomes. The immunophenotype of Burkitt's lymphoma is surface IgM+, B-cell-antigen positive, CD10+, CD5−, CD23−, TdT−.

The male-to-female ratio for Burkitt's lymphoma is approximately 2.5 to 1. The facial bones, particularly the jaw, are the most common sites of involvement for the African (endemic) variety (Fig. 23–22). In the nonendemic variety, an abdominal mass is the most common presenting pattern. Involvement of the distal ileum, cecum, and mesentery are the most frequent sites of involvement. Other less common sites of involvement include the kidneys, ovaries, and breasts. Burkitt's lymphoma is a highly aggressive and rapidly fatal disease if untreated; however, this disease is potentially curable and prognosis correlates with tumor bulk (see staging).

Another lymphoma with histologic features very similar to Burkitt's lymphoma is the high-grade B-cell lymphoma, Burkitt-like, also referred to as undifferentiated, non-Burkitt (Rappaport classification) and small noncleaved cell, non-Burkitt (Working Formulation). This lymphoma is distinguished from true Burkitt's lymphoma by the lack of uniformity of the nuclei, lack of c-*myc* rearrangement (chromosome 8) and frequent presence of *bcl*-2 rearrangement. Immunophenotypically this lymphoma is sIg+/−, cytoplasmic Ig−/+, B-cell-antigen-positive, CD5−, CD10−/+. The normal counterpart cell is uncertain. The disease most commonly affects adults and is highly aggressive and usually fatal.

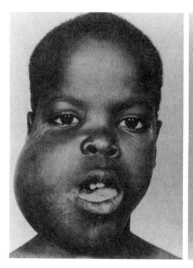
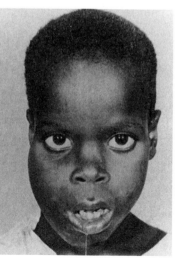

FIGURE 23–22 Burkitt's lymphoma (*left*) before and (*right*) after treatment.

Miscellaneous Lymphomas

A plethora of uncommon, unusual, and sometimes difficult to classify lymphomas have been described (Table 23–16). Most fall within the general cateogry of peripheral T-cell lymphomas, also referred to as post-thymic T-cell lymphomas. Peripheral T-cell lymphomas are defined immunologically as TdT/CD1-negative, CD3-positive T-cell lymphomas, that is, they correspond to normal T cells at the post-thymic stage of T-cell ontogeny. Although many peripheral T-cell lymphomas can be assigned to specific categories within the common classification schemes, their unique clinical presentation warrants further distinction of these disorders.

Primary Cutaneous T-Cell Lymphoma

The category of cutaneous T-cell lymphoma includes a broad group of dysplastic and frankly malignant T-cell proliferations with a predilection for infiltration of the skin.[36] Disorders within this category include mycosis fungoides, Sézary's syndrome, lymphomatoid papulosis, and primary cutaneous anaplastic large cell lymphoma.

Mycosis fungoides and Sézary's syndrome, two related disorders, are characterized by infiltration of the dermis and epidermis by malignant T cells with a peculiar cerebriform nucleus. In many cases, mycosis fungoides progresses through three clinical phases. In the premycotic (erythroderma) phase, lasting from 6 months to 50 years, the T-cell infiltrate produces a nonspecific eczematous dermatosis that is difficult to differentiate from a benign inflammatory infiltrate. As the disease progresses, the infiltrate thickens to form distinct plaques (plaque stage) and finally tumor nodules (tumor stage) (Fig. 23–23). Systemic dissemination with lymph node, peripheral blood, and visceral organ involvement are more likely to develop in the later stages. Transformation to a large cell lymphoma

TABLE 23–16 **Miscellaneous Lymphomas**	
Types of Lymphoma	**Characteristics**
Cutaneous T-cell lymphomas Mycosis fungoides	• T cell infiltrate of skin • Plaques and tumor nodules • Systemic, extracutaneous dissemination • Transformation to large cell lymphoma
Sézary syndrome	• Sézary cells circulate • T-cell leukemia
Subcutaneous panniculitic T-cell lymphoma	• Rare T-cell lymphoma confined to subcutaneous tissue • Associated with fatal hemophagocytic syndrome
Angioimmunoblastic lymphadenopathy with dysproteinemia (AILD)-like T-cell lymphoma	• Atypical lymphoid cells • Hyperimmunity following exposure to certain drugs and infectious agents
Angiocentric T-cell lymphomas	• Atypical lymphoreticular cells causing a variety of angiodestructive disorders • Lung is most common site of involvement
HTLV-I associated T-cell lymphoma/leukemia	• Associated with type C retrovirus, HTLV-I infection • Widely disseminated at presentation • Rapidly fatal disorder
Intestinal T-cell lymphoma with or without enteropathy	• Rare, peripheral T-cell lymphoma with intestinal involvement
Anaplastic large cell lymphoma	• Large, atypical malignant cells with peculiar sinus pattern infiltration of lymph node • Often occurs in children
Hepatosplenic gamma/delta T-cell lymphoma	• Rare T-cell lymphoma primarily affecting spleen and liver • Often occurs in young adults
Angiotropic large cell lymphoma	• Rare T- or B-cell lymphoma of blood vessels of skin and central nervous system • Normally occurs in adults
True histiocytic lymphoma	• Lymphomas with enzyme and immunophenotypic profiles similar to that of histiocytes/monocytes

Source: Compiled from Edelson,[36] Willemze et al,[37] Gonzalez et al,[38] Shimoyama et al,[39] Jaffe,[40] Gallo,[41] Chott et al,[42] Lennert et al,[43] Farcet et al,[44] Drobacheff et al,[45] Ferry et al,[46] and Sangueza et al.[47]

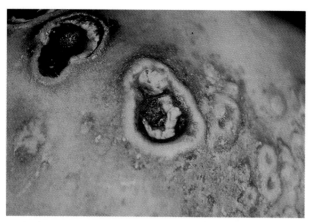

FIGURE 23-23 Mycosis fungoides, tumor stage. Tumor nodules are produced by massive local infiltrates of the skin by the characteristic cerebriform cells of mycosis fungoides.

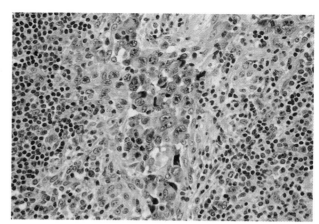

FIGURE 23-25 Anaplastic large cell lymphoma. Large pleomorphic cells of anaplastic large cell lymphoma infiltrate in a sinus pattern that may be easily misinterpreted as metastic carcinoma or melanoma.

similar to anaplastic large cell lymphoma may occur and is most frequently seen as a terminal event. The prognosis for mycosis fungoides confined to the skin is relatively good with median survival of greater than 10 years. Extracutaneous spread, however, is associated with a median survival of less than 1 year.

In the related Sézary syndrome, the early erythroderma stage is associated with a leukemia of the characteristic cerebriform T cells (Sézary cells) (Fig. 23–24). Progression to the tumor stage is unusual in Sézary's syndrome.

HTLV-I–Associated T-Cell Lymphoma/Leukemia

This aggressive lymphoma is associated with infection by the type C retrovirus, human T-cell lymphotropic virus I (HTLV-I) and is most common in the endemic areas of southwestern Japan, the Caribbean basin, and the tropical islands of the Pacific and Indian oceans.[41] A low frequency of infection is observed in the United States, mainly among blacks of the southeastern region. This type of lymphoma is, therefore, rare in the United States. It is often widely disseminated at presentation and clinically is characterized by lymphadenopathy, hepatosplenomegaly, and involvement of the peripheral blood, skin, and cerebrospinal fluid. Hypercalcemia is usually present. Skin involvement is common and mimics mycosis fungoides.

Table 23–16 lists and summarizes the characteristics of the following miscellaneous lymphomas: subcutaneous T-cell lymphoma, angioimmunoblastic lymphadenopathy with dysproteinemia (AILD)-like T-cell lymphoma, angiocentric T-cell lymphomas, intestinal T-cell lymphomas, anaplastic large cell lymphoma (Fig. 23–25), hepatosplenic gamma/delta T-cell lymphoma, angiotropic large cell lymphoma (Figs. 23–26 through 23–28), and true histiocytic lymphoma.

Diagnostic Evaluation

Tissue biopsy is required for the diagnosis and subcategorization of non-Hodgkin's lymphoma. Ancillary

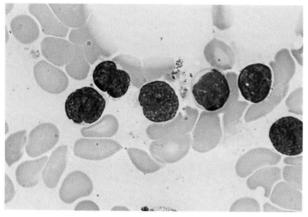

FIGURE 23-24 Sézary cells observed in the peripheral blood from a patient with Sézary's syndrome. (From Hyun, BH: Morphology of Blood and Bone Marrow. American Society of Clinical Pathologists, Workshop 5121. Philadelphia, September 1983, with permission.)

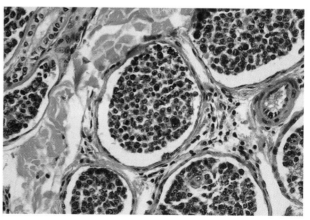

FIGURE 23-26 Angiotropic large-cell lymphoma. Malignant cells are confined to vascular spaces.

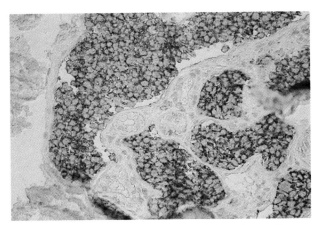

FIGURE 23–27 Angiotropic large cell lymphoma. Immunoperoxidase stain demonstrates positive staining (*red*) of the malignant cells for leukocyte common antigen.

TABLE 23–17 **Routine and Ancillary Tests Useful in the Evaluation of Lymph Node Biopsies**

I. Fresh Tissue
  A. Bacterial and viral studies
  B. Cell suspension for surface marker, cytogenetic studies, and genotypic studies
  C. Frozen material for rapid diagnosis, histochemical and immunohistochemical stains
II. Fixed Tissue
  A. Paraffin-embedded for light microscopy and limited histochemical, immunohistochemical, and genotypic studies
  B. Resin (plastic) embedded for electron microscopy and thin-section light microscopy

studies, however, are often required and these include immunophenotypic studies, nucleic acid (DNA and RNA) content analysis, cytogenetics, gene rearrangement, and functional studies (Table 23–17).

The diagnostic difficulties fall into a relatively small number of categories, namely, differentiating (1) benign versus malignant lymphoproliferations, (2) lymphoma versus nonlymphoma, (3) T-cell versus B-cell lymphoma, and (4) non-Hodgkin's lymphoma versus Hodgkin's disease. One or more of the ancillary tests may be required to resolve the differential diagnostic dilemma, and rarely the dilemma may be unresolvable.

Benign versus Malignant

If light microscopic evaluation fails to distinguish a benign from a malignant lymphoproliferation, the demonstration of immunophenotypic or genotypic monoclonality would favor a malignant diagnosis. For B cells, immunophenotypic monoclonality is defined as restriction of immunoglobulin light-chain produc-

tion by a population of cells to a single light-chain class, either kappa or lambda.[48–51] Operationally, light-chain monoclonality is present if the percentage of kappa-positive cells to lambda-positive cells (kappa-lambda ratio) falls outside of the expected ("normal") range or if "clonal excess" can be demonstrated by statistical comparison (Kolmogorov-Smirnov test)[52] of the kappa and lambda fluorescence intensity distributions. An example of monoclonality demonstrated by two-color flow cytometry is illustrated in Figure 23–29A and B.

Unfortunately, at present no practical method exists to define immunophenotypic T-cell clonality. Evidence for T-cell malignancy, however, may be suggested by immunophenotypically demonstrating an aberrant T-cell phenotype. Benign T-cell proliferations generally express a "normal" T-cell phenotype in which all pan-T-cell antigens (CD2, CD3, CD5, CD7) are expressed by the individual T cells. On the other hand, T-cell malignancies that might be confused with a benign T-cell proliferation often express an aberrant T-cell phenotype in which one or more of the pan-T-cell antigens are not expressed. Approximately 60% of peripheral T-cell lymphomas express such an aberrant phenotype, with CD5 and CD7 being the most frequently absent antigens.[53]

A genotypic definition of both B- and T-cell clonality is possible. Clonal rearrangements of the T-cell receptor or immunoglobulin genes are detectable by several methods including Southern analysis and the polymerase chain reaction (PCR) (Chap. 35). Figure 23–30 illustrates the results of Southern analysis, in which a clonal population of T cells is indicated by the presence of nongermline bands in the Southern blot. The identification of a clonal rearrangement is presumptive evidence of a malignant proliferation.[54–56]

The development of DNA probes for specific chromosomal alterations may obviate the necessity of performing karyograms in the cytogenetic evaluation of lymphoproliferations. Southern analysis, PCR, and fluorescence in situ hybridization (FISH) are commonly used techniques for demonstrating diagnostically important chromosomal translocation (see Table 23–8) without the need for complete karyotype analysis.

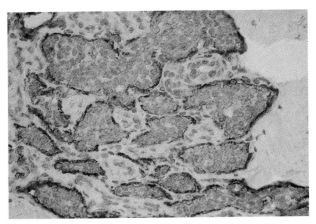

FIGURE 23–28 Angiotropic large cell lymphoma. Staining for factor VIII antigen is confined to the endothelial cells lining the vascular spaces.

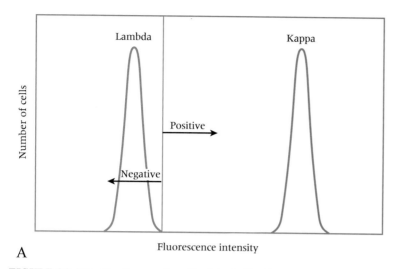
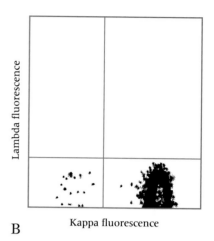

A

B

FIGURE 23–29   B-cell monoclonality detected by flow cytometry. (A) Dual parameter (two-color) histogram of simultaneous staining for kappa and lambda light chains. (B) The presence of a dense cluster of fluorescence in the lower right quadrant indicates a monoclonal kappa population of a B cell (for details, see Chap. 24).

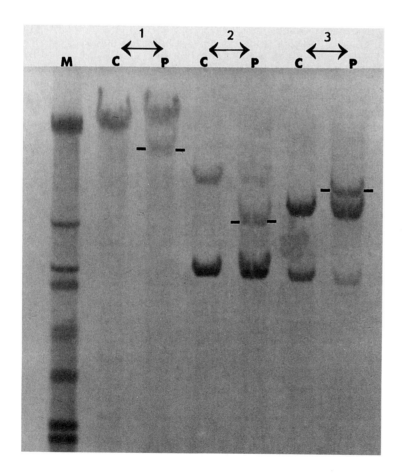

FIGURE 23–30   T-cell monoclonality demonstrated by Southern analysis. Abnormal bands designated by small bars indicate clonal rearrangement of the T-cell receptor gene. M = molecular weight markers; C = control DNA to locate position of germ-line (nonrearranged) bands; P = patient DNA; 1 = Bam HI digest; 2 = Eco RI digest; 3 = Hind III digest (for details, see Chap. 35).

TABLE 23–18 Antibody Panel for Distinguishing Among the Four Major Categories of Cancer

Cancer Type	Antibody			
	Cytokeratin*	Vimentin[†]	LCA[‡] (CD45)	S100[§]
Carcinoma	+	−	−	−
Sarcoma	−	+	−	−
Lymphoma	−	±	+	−
Melanoma	−	±	−	+

*Antibody directed against the cytokeratin group of intermediate filament proteins found in epithelial cells.
[†]Antibody directed against the 58-kilodalton intermediate filament protein found in mesenchymal cells.
[‡]Antibody directed against the 200-kilodalton leukocyte common antigen found in various hematopoietic and lymphoreticular cells.
[§]Antibody directed against the 25-kilodalton protein found in selected cells of the nervous system, melanocytes, interdigitating reticulum cells, etc. The antibody HMB-45 is more specifically restricted to melanocytes than anti-S100.

Lymphoma versus Nonlymphoma

The differential diagnoses of large cell lymphoma and nonlymphoid malignancies such as amelanotic melanoma, poorly differentiated carcinoma, germ cell neoplasms, and round cell sarcomas is a frequent problem in surgical pathology. A differential diagnosis is facilitated by determining the antigenic phenotype of the tumor cells. This is most commonly done by staining the cells with an immunoenzyme technique using a panel of antibodies directed against normal cellular differentiation antigens (Table 23–18).[57]

Hodgkin's Disease versus Non-Hodgkin's Lymphoma

The literature is replete with contradictory studies concerning the significance of various tests in distinguishing Hodgkin's disease from non-Hodgkin's lymphoma.[58] At present the only specific immunophenotypic distinction between these disorders is the presence of light-chain monoclonality in B-cell non-Hodgkin's lymphomas and its absence in Hodgkin's disease. Clonal rearrangement of the immunoglobulin heavy-chain and T-cell receptor genes has been described in some cases of Hodgkin's disease and therefore limits the utility of such tests in the differential diagnosis of Hodgkin's disease from non-Hodgkin's lymphomas.[59]

The differential diagnosis of Hodgkin's disease, excluding lymphocyte-predominance Hodgkin's disease, generally includes peripheral T-cell lymphoma and anaplastic large cell lymphoma. The Reed-Sternberg cells and Hodgkin's cells of Hodgkin's disease are characteristically CD45−, CD15+, CD30+ (Table 23–19), whereas peripheral T-cell lymphomas are usually CD45+, CD15−, CD30−. Unfortunately, the Reed-Sternberg-like cells of peripheral T-cell lymphoma are occasionally CD15+ and/or CD30+[60] and careful attention to histologic features and the presence of CD45 positivity on the Reed-Sternberg-like cells is required to prevent misdiagnosis in these cases. Similarly, anaplastic large cell lymphomas are by definition CD30+, yet the usual absence of CD15 and presence of CD45 on the large atypical cells usually aids in distinguishing anaplastic large cell lymphoma from Hodgkin's disease. Nodular lymphocyte-predominant Hodgkin's disease must be distinguished from low-grade non-Hodgkin's lymphomas, particularly follicular-center lymphomas and reactive conditions such as progressive transformation of follicle centers. The expression of monoclonal surface immunoglobulin by the low-grade lymphomas definitively distinguishes them from nodular lymphocyte predominance Hodgkin's disease. The presence of epithelial membrane antigen (EMA) polylobated L&H cells (see Table 23–19) and rare classic Reed-Sternberg cells differentiates this form of Hodgkin's disease from various reactive conditions.

Staging

The staging evaluation of the non-Hodgkin's lymphomas is similar to that for Hodgkin's disease. The same staging scheme, the Ann Arbor classification (see

TABLE 23–19 Immunophenotype of Hodgkin's Disease

Antibody	RS Cells and Variants*	L & H Cells
CD45	−	+/−
CD15	+	−/+
CD30	+	−/+
CD20	−/+	+/−
CD74	+	+
CD75	−/+	+
EMA[†]	−	+/−

*Excludes L&H cells.
[†]Epithelial membrane antigen.
Abbreviations: +/− = Usually positive; −/+ = Usually negative.

TABLE 23–20 **Staging Classification of Burkitt's Lymphoma**	
Stage A	Single extra-abdominal site
Stage B	Multiple extra-abdominal sites
Stage C	Intra-abdominal tumor
Stage D	Intra-abdominal tumor with multiple extra-abdominal sites
Stage AR	Stage C disease with >90% of tumor surgically removed

Table 23–5), which was designed for Hodgkin's disease, is also used for the staging of non-Hodgkin's lymphomas. Since the natural history of Hodgkin's disease is different from that of non-Hodgkin's lymphoma, there are certain problems with using the Ann Arbor classification in staging the non-Hodgkin's lymphomas. Despite these drawbacks, the Ann Arbor scheme remains the staging scheme of choice. One major exception to this statement is Burkitt's lymphoma. In this lymphoma the bulk of tumor, rather than sites of involvement, is a primary determinant of prognosis. Consequently, a different staging scheme is in use for Burkitt's lymphoma (Table 23–20).

Treatment and Prognosis

For the purposes of prognostic assessment and therapeutic selection, the non-Hodgkin's lymphomas can be grouped into two broad categories: the indolent lymphomas and the diffuse aggressive lymphomas. Figure 23–31 illustrates metastatic lymphoma involving the kidney. The indolent lymphomas are composed of the low-grade lymphomas of the Working Formulation (Table 23–11) and the more recently described group of mantle cell and marginal zone lymphomas. They are so designated because the median survival without therapy for this group of lymphomas is relatively long (7 to 9 years). The diffuse aggressive lymphomas encompass the intermediate and high-grade lymphomas of the Working Formulation. Without treatment, these

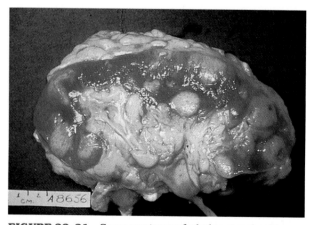

FIGURE 23–31 Gross anatomy of a kidney involved in metastatic lymphoma. Note the white nodular lymphocytic infiltration. (Courtesy of Dr. John Sutherland.)

lymphomas are rapidly fatal (median survival is 6 to 12 months).

Therapy for the indolent lymphomas is controversial. The disease is essentially incurable with standard or aggressive multiagent chemotherapy. Furthermore, because existing therapies were ineffective in prolonging survival in the low-grade lymphomas, a "watch and wait" approach was adopted by many oncologists during the 1970s and 1980s.[61] When symptoms warranted, or the lymphoma progressed to a higher grade, therapy was instituted. More recently, aggressive multiagent chemotherapy has been shown to be effective at prolonging survival; however, this does not equate to cure. The diffuse aggressive lymphomas are rapidly fatal if untreated but are potentially curable with aggressive chemotherapeutic strategies.

CASE STUDY

A 68-year-old male auto mechanic presented to his primary care physician with a chief complaint of bilateral, painless masses in the neck region of at least 6 months' duration. He had a 120-pack-year smoking history and his family history included a father and brother with thyroid cancer. His past medical history was positive for rheumatoid arthritis. On physical examination, the patient was found to have bilateral supraclavicular and cervical lymphadenopathy consisting of matted groups of lymph nodes that were painless to palpation. The patient was afebrile and had experienced an unintentional decrease in weight from 195 to 180 lb over a 6-month interval.

Questions

1. What pathologic processes must be considered in the evaluation of lymphadenopathy?
2. What are some of the important *diagnostic* tests that should be performed?

All parameters of the initial CBC were normal and the peripheral smear was without morphological abnormality. A chest x-ray demonstrated hilar adenopathy without any recognizable parenchymal lung lesions. Excisional biopsy of a group of nodes was performed. On microscopic examination there was diffuse effacement of lymph node architecture by a population of relatively uniform cells, averaging 20 to 40 μm in diameter with round to slightly irregular nuclei and occasional prominent nucleoli. Immunophenotypically, the cells were characterized by the expression of CD45, CD10, CD19, CD20 and kappa light chains. No T-cell antigens were detected on the abnormal cells.

3. What is the most likely diagnosis based on the available data?
4. What additional studies should be performed before therapy is instituted?

Bilateral bone marrow biopsies demonstrate several aggregates of abnormal cells, similar to those observed in the lymph nodes, randomly distributed within the marrow. A computed tomography (CT) scan of the abdomen and pelvis reveals para-aortic adenopathy and modest enlargement of the spleen.

5. What stage is this lymphoma?

6. What therapy would be appropriate?
7. What is the probability of cure?

Answers

1. The causes of lymphadenopathy are myriad and include various benign and malignant causes. Benign disorders producing localized or generalized adenopathy are most commonly infectious or inflammatory in nature, for example, viral illness or cat-scratch fever, but may be secondary to autoimmune disorders such as lupus or rheumatoid arthritis. Metastatic malignancies (carcinoma, melanoma, or sarcoma) produce lymphadenopathy, but on physical examination they are usually more localized. Lymphoma must always be considered in the differential diagnosis of lymphadenopathy, regardless of age.

2. The formed elements (white cells, red cells, and platelets) of the peripheral blood often exhibit changes helpful in determining the cause of lymphadenopathy. Therefore, a CBC with peripheral smear evaluation is indicated. A chest x-ray should be performed in a search for intrathoracic disease, particularly lung lesions. The definitive test to distinguish benign from malignant processes is microscopic examination of an enlarged lymph node. This may be achieved by fine needle aspiration or excisional biopsy. Excisional biopsy is preferred if lymphoma is high on the differential diagnostic list.

3. Malignant lymphoma, diffuse large cell, B-cell type of probable follicular center cell origin.

4. For staging purposes bilateral bone marrow biopsies and CT scanning of the abdomen and pelvis should be performed.

5. Stage IV.

6. Multiagent chemotherapy.

7. The probability of 2-year relapse-free survival is 40% to 70% for advanced aggressive grade non-Hodgkin's lymphomas. If relapse does not occur within 2 years after achieving complete remission, the patient is considered cured. Therefore, the probability of cure in this case is 40% to 70%.

REFERENCES

1. Hodgkin, T: On some morbid appearances of the absorbent glands and spleen. Med Chir Trans 17:68, 1832.
2. Wilks, Sir S: Cases of enlargement of the lymphatic glands and spleen (or, Hodgkin's disease), with remarks. Guy's Hosp Rep 11:56, 1865.
3. Sternberg, C: Uber eine eigenartige unter dem Bilde der Pseudoleukamie verlaufende Tuberculose des lymphatischen Apparates. Ztschr Heilk 19:21, 1898.
4. Reed, DM: On the pathological changes in Hodgkin's disease, with special reference to its relation to tuberculosis. Johns Hopkins Hosp Rep 10:133, 1902.
5. Banks, PM, et al: Mantle Cell Lymphoma. A proposal for unification of morphologic, immunologic and molecular data. Blood 84:1005, 1994.
6. Lukes, RJ, et al: Report of the Nomenclature Committee. Cancer Res 26:1311, 1966.
7. Lukes, RJ and Butler, JJ: The pathology and nomenclature of Hodgkin's disease. Cancer Res 26:1063, 1966.
8. Correa, P, et al: International comparability and reproducibility in histologic subclassification of Hodgkin's disease. J Nat Cancer Inst 50:1429, 1973.
9. Kant, JA, et al: A critical reappraisal of the pathologic and clinical heterogeneity of "lymphocyte depleted Hodgkin's disease." J Clin Oncol 4:284, 1986.
10. Kadin, ME, Glatstein, E, and Dorfman, RF: Clinicopathologic studies of 117 untreated patients subjected to laparotomy for the staging of Hodgkin's disease. Cancer 27:1277, 1971.
11. Lukes, RJ: Criteria for involvement of lymph node, bone marrow, spleen, and liver in Hodgkin's disease. Cancer Res 31:1755, 1971.
12. Carbone, PP, et al: Report of the Committee on Hodgkin's Staging Classification. Cancer Res 31:1860, 1971.
13. DeVita, VT, et al: Curability of advanced Hodgkin's disease with chemotherapy. Ann Intern Med 92:587, 1980.
14. Virchow, RLK: Die cellulare Pathologie in ihrer Begruendung auf physiologische und pathologische Gewebelehre. Berlin, Hirschwald, 1858.
15. Billroth, T: Multiple Lymphome: Erfolgreiche Behandlung mit Arsenik. Wien Med Wochenschr 21:1066, 1871.
16. Dreschfield, J: Ein Beitrag Zur Lehre von den Lymphosarkomen. Dtsch Med Wochenschr 17:1175, 1893.
17. Kundrat, H: Uber Lympho-sarkomatosis. Wien Klin Wochnschr 6:211, 234, 1893.
18. Heim, S and Mitelman, F: Cancer Cytogenetics. Alan R Liss, New York, 1989.
19. Berard, CW and Dorfman, RF: Histopathology of malignant lymphomas. Clin Hematol 3:39, 1974.
20. Lennert, K, et al: Histopathology of Non-Hodgkin's Lymphoma, ed 2. Springer-Verlag, New York, 1992.
21. Rosenberg, SA, et al: National Cancer Institute sponsored study of classification on non-Hodgkin's lymphomas: Summary and description of a working formulation for clinical usage. Cancer 49:2112, 1982.
22. Harris, NL, et al: A Revised European-American Classification of Lymphoid Neoplasms: A Proposal from the International Lymphoma Study Group. Blood 84:1361, 1994.
23. Mann, RB and Berard, CW: Criteria for the cytologic subclassification of follicular lymphomas: A proposed alternative method. Hematol Oncol 1:187, 1983.
24. Banks, PM, et al: Mantle Cell Lymphoma. A proposal for unification of morphologic, immunologic, and molecular data. Am J Surg Pathol 16:637, 1992.
25. Inghirami, G, et al: Autoantibody-associated cross-reactive idiotype-bearing human B lymphocytes: Distribution and characterization, including IgVH gene and CD5 antigen expression. Blood 78:1503, 1991.
26. Van den Oord, J, et al: The marginal zone in the human reactive lymph node. Am J Clin Pathol 86:475, 1986.
27. VanKrieken, JHJM, et al: Splenic marginal zone lymphocytes and related cells in the lymph: a morphologic and immunohistochemical study. Human Pathol 20:320, 1989.
28. Harris, NL: Low-Grade B-Cell Lymphoma of Mucosa-Associated Lymphoid Tissue and Monocytoid B-Cell Lymphoma: Related entities that are distinct from other low-grade B-cell lymphomas. Arch Pathol Lab Med, 117:771, 1993.
29. Isaacson, P: Malignant Lymphoma of Mucosa-Associated Lymphoid Tissue. Histopathology 445, 1987.
30. Wotherspoon, A, et al: Regression of primary low-grade B-cell gastric lymphoma of mucosa-associated lymphoid tissue after eradication of Helicobacter pylori. Lancet 342:575, 1993.
31. Ngan, B-Y, et al: Monocytoid B-cell lymphoma: A study of 36 cases. Human Pathol 22:409, 1991.
32. Schmid, C, et al: Splenic marginal zone cell lymphoma. Am J Surg Pathol 16:455, 1992.

33. Milo, J, et al: Splenic B cell lymphoma with circulating villous lymphocytes: Differential diagnosis of B cell leukaemias with large spleens. J Clin Pathol 40:642, 1987.

34. Nathwani, BN: Classifying Non-Hodgkin's Lymphomas. In Berard, CW, et al (eds): Malignant Lymphoma (IAP Monographs in Pathology, no. 29). Williams & Wilkins, Baltimore, 1987.

35. Burkitt, D: A sarcoma involving the jaws in African children. Br J Surg 46:218, 1958.

36. Edelson, RL: Cutaneous T cell lymphoma. J Dermatol Surg Oncol 6:358, 1980.

37. Willemze, R, et al: Spectrum of primary cutaneous CD30 (Ki-1)-positive lymphoproliferative disorders. J Am Acad Dermatol 28:973, 1993.

38. Gonzalez, CL, et al: T-cell lymphoma involving subcutaneous tissue. A clinicopathologic entity commonly associated with hemophagocytic syndrome. Am J Surg Pathol 15:17, 1991.

39. Shimoyama, J, et al: Immunoblastic lymphadenopathy (IBL)-like T cell lymphoma. Jpn J Clin Oncol 9(Suppl):347, 1979.

40. Jaffe, ES: Post Thymic Lymphoid Neoplasia. In Jaffe, ES, and Bennington, JL (ed): Surgical Pathology of the Lymph Nodes and Related Organs. WB Sanders, Philadelphia, 1985.

41. Gallo, RC: Human T cell leukemia/lymphoma virus and T cell malignancies in adults. Cancer Surv 3:113, 1984.

42. Chott, A, et al: Peripheral T-cell lymphomas of the intestine. Am J Pathol 141:1361, 1992.

43. Lennert, K, et al: Large Cell Anaplastic Lymphoma of T-cell type (Ki-1+) in Histopathology of Non-Hodgkin's Lymphomas, ed 2, Springer-Verlag, New York, 1992.

44. Farcet, J, et al: Hepatosplenic T-cell lymphoma. Sinusal/sinusoidal localization of malignant cells expressing the T-cell receptor gamma/delta. Blood 75:2213, 1990.

45. Drobacheff, C, et al: Malignant Angioendotheliomatosis: Reclassification as an angiotropic lymphoma. Int J Dermatol 28:454, 1989.

46. Ferry, JA, et al: Intravascular lymphomatosis (Malignant angiotheliomatosis): A B cell neoplasm expressing surface homing receptors. Mod Pathol 1:444, 1988.

47. Sangueza, O, et al: Intravascular lymphomatosis: Report of an unusual case with T cell phenotype occurring in an adolescent male. J Cutan Pathol 19:226, 1992.

48. Picker, LJ, et al: Immunophenotypic criteria for the diagnosis of non Hodgkin's lymphoma. Am J Pathol 128:181, 1987.

49. Tubbs, R, et al: Tissue immunomicroscopic evaluation of monoclonality of B cell lymphomas. Am J Clin Pathol 76:24, 1986.

50. Hsu, SM: The use of monoclonal antibodies and immunohistochemical techniques in lymphoma: Review and Overlook. Hematol Pathol, 2:183, 1988.

51. Little, JV, et al: Flow cytometric analysis of lymphomas and lymphoma-like disorders. Semin Diagn Pathol 6:37, 1989.

52. Ault, KA: Detection of small numbers of monoclonal B lymphocytes in blood of patients with lymphoma. N Engl J Med 300:1401, 1979.

53. Weiss, LM, et al: Morphologic and immunologic characterization of 50 peripheral T cell lymphoma. Am J Pathol 118:316, 1985.

54. Korsmeyer, SJ and Walkman, TA: Immunoglobulin Genes: rearrangement and translocation in human lymphoid malignancy. J Clin Immunol 4:1, 1984.

55. Bertness, VO, et al: T cell receptor gene rearrangements as clinical markers of human T cell lymphomas. J Engl J Med 313:534, 1985.

56. Cossman, J, et al: Molecular genetics and the diagnosis of lymphoma. Arch Pathol Lab Med 112:117, 1988.

57. Battifora, H: Recent progress in the immunohistochemistry of solid tumors. Semin Diagn Pathol 1:251, 1984.

58. Grogan, T: Hodgkin's Disease in Surgical Pathology of the Lymph Nodes and Related Organs, ed 2. WB Saunders, Philadelphia, 1995.

59. Griessler, H, et al: Clonal rearrangements of T-cell receptor and immunoglobulin genes and immunophenotypic antigen expression in different subclasses of Hodgkin's disease. Int J Cancer 40:157, 1987.

60. Chittal, SM, et al: Monoclonal antibodies in the diagnosis of Hodgkin's disease. Am J Surg Pathol 12:9, 1988.

61. Horning, SJ and Rosenberg, SA: The natural history of untreated low grade non Hodgkin's lymphomas. N Engl J Med 311:1471, 1984.

QUESTIONS

1. What infectious agent is most commonly associated with the pathogenesis of Hodgkin's disease?
   a. Echovirus
   b. Herpesvirus
   c. *Helicobacter pylori*
   d. Epstein-Barr virus

2. The cell characteristic of all types of Hodgkin's disease is the:
   a. Lacunar cell
   b. L&H cell
   c. Reed-Sternberg cell
   d. Sézary cell

3. Burkitt's lymphoma is histologically characterized by which of the following:
   a. Uniform nuclei
   b. High mitotic rate
   c. "Starry-sky" pattern
   d. All of the above

4. Lymphoblastic lymphomas are associated with all the following except:
   a. High frequency of developing acute lymphoblastic leukemia
   b. Mediastinal mass
   c. Usually express B-cell phenotype
   d. Potentially curable in young patients

5. All of the following are T-cell disorders except:
   a. Mycosis fungoides
   b. Sézary's syndrome
   c. Hepatosplenic gamma/delta lymphoma
   d. Burkitt's lymphoma

6. A lymphoma associated with infection by a type C retrovirus is:
   a. Endemic to Japan
   b. Associated with hypercalcemia
   c. Usually rapidly fatal
   d. All of the above

7. The immunophenotypic definition of B cell monoclonality is:
   a. Clonal rearrangement of the IgH gene
   b. Loss of B cell antigens by the malignant cells
   c. Expression of a single light-chain class
   d. Expression of a single heavy-chain class

8. All of the following are true regarding the low-grade non-Hodgkin's lymphomas except:
   a. Survival without treatment averages greater than 5 years.
   b. Disease is usually advanced at diagnosis.
   c. Multiagent chemotherapy can prolong survival.
   d. Cure is possible in more than 50% of cases.

9. The diffuse aggressive lymphomas are:
   a. Seldom curable
   b. Rapidly fatal if untreated
   c. Best treated with a combination of surgery and radiotherapy
   d. Preferably treated with single-agent chemotherapy.

10. The staging system for Hodgkin's disease and the non-Hodgkin's lymphomas is:
   a. The Working Formulation
   b. The Duke's staging system
   c. The Rye staging system
   d. The Ann Arbor staging system

ANSWERS

1. **d** (p 425)
2. **c** (p 425)
3. **d** (p 441)
4. **c** (pp 440–441)
5. **d** (pp 443–444)
6. **d** (p 444)
7. **c** (p 445)
8. **d** (p 448)
9. **b** (p 448)
10. **d** (pp 447–448; Table 23–5, p 429)

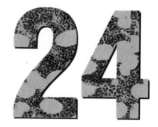

Introduction to Flow Cytometry

Bette Jamieson, MEd, SH(ASCP)

Definition and History
Flow Design
Monoclonal Antibodies
Immunophenotyping

Leukemias and Lymphomas
DNA Analysis
Other Applications of Flow Cytometry

Objectives

At the end of this chapter, the learner should be able to:
1   Define flow cytometry.
2   List the technological improvements that contributed to the implementation of the flow cytometer in the clinical laboratory.
3   Name the four main components of the flow cytometer.
4   Describe the importance of monoclonal antibodies in the use of the flow cytometer.
5   Name two of the most important fluorochromes used in flow cytometry.
6   Define CD (cluster designation).
7   Describe the mechanism by which HIV infects lymphocytes.
8   Describe the importance of immunophenotyping in the classification of lymphomas and leukemias.
9   Define mixed-lineage leukemia.
10 Define biphenotypic leukemia.
11 Explain DNA analysis by flow cytometry.
12 List newer applications of the flow cytometer in the hematology laboratory.

DEFINITION AND HISTORY

Flow cytometry (FCM) is the measurement of cellular properties as they move in a fluid past a stationary set of detectors. The microscope, invented by Robert Hooke in 1665, has been and still is the "gold standard" for the morphological observation of cells. Improved optics and better staining techniques have improved the laboratory worker's ability to define and distinguish cells. However, the interpretation of a microscopic image is based on training and experience and is limited by the resolution of the human eye and the decision-making process of the individual. In contrast to the labor-intensive review of cells under a microscope, the flow cytometer is rapid and objective. The flow cytometer permits the analysis of 10^5 to 10^6 cells per minute, simultaneously measuring physical and biological properties.

The essence of FCM, as defined by Mendelssohn, is the "bringing of suspended cells one by one to a detector by means of a flow channel" (Mendelssohn, 1979.) FCM is an automated method used to measure cells or particles as they flow single-file through a sensing area. Sensing can be accomplished electronically, as done by the Coulter principle, or optically. The term *flow cytometry* is commonly used to denote the optical type of sensing. Optical sensing is done with an intense light source, usually a laser or mercury arc lamp. These instruments measure light scatter and fluorescent signals generated as cells pass through a light beam. Table 24–1 compares the features of light microscopy and flow cytometry.

FCM had its origin in the early 1970s. The instruments were the result of several decades of scientific research. The first generation of flow instruments, available in the early 1980s, were expensive, cumber-

TABLE 24–1 Comparative Features of Light Microscopy and Flow Cytometry

Parameter	Light Microscopy	Flow Cytometry
Cells analyzed	10^2–10^3 cells/assay	10^5–10^6 cells/assay
Speed of analysis	5 minutes/specimen	1 minute/specimen
Final results	Subjective	Objective
Complexity of analysis	Positive/negative	Multiparametric
Reproducibility	Low	High
Labor	Labor intensive	Semiautomated

Source: From Riley, R: "Flow Cytometry for the Nineties and Beyond," ASCP Workshop presented Orlando, Florida, 1993, p 2, with permission.

some, and labor-intensive. The new generation of commercial flow instruments is less expensive, easy to operate, and stable for everyday use in the clinical laboratory.

Table 24–2 follows the historical developments in flow cytometry. Flow instruments used during the seventies were primarily used for research; however, the eighties were the decade for the clinical adaptation of the flow cytometer. Simultaneously, research instruments were designed with multiparametric analysis as well as cell-sorting capabilities. Two or three lasers are common in the research flow cytometer, with greatly improved software capability for storage and analysis.

Parallel developments in monoclonal antibodies, computers, electronics, and fluorochrome chemistry collectively hastened the implementation of the flow cytometer from the research laboratory to the clinical laboratory.

The AIDS epidemic and a better understanding of leukemias and lymphomas were also significant factors in the rapid introduction of the flow cytometer.

FLOW DESIGN

Components

The four main components of FCM include the fluidics (or cell transportation system), a laser for cell illumination, photodetectors for signal detection, and a computer-based management system. The fluidics are regulated by pressurized gas, usually nitrogen. Cells suspended in fluid are transported to a flow tip, where the sample is surrounded by a sheath fluid. The sheath and sample stream both exit the flow chamber through a small orifice (usually 75 μm). This laminar flow design confines cells to the center of the sheath and can be adjusted to obtain single-file alignment of cells (Fig. 24–1).

Light Scatter

The flow cytometer is a system in which a very narrow beam of light must intersect with a very narrow sample stream to obtain maximum efficiency. The point at which the laser beam and the cell stream meet is called the *interrogation point.*

As a cell enters the laser beam, light is scattered through 360 degrees. Forward-angle light scatter (FS, 2 to 10 degrees) provides information regarding particle size. Light scattered at 90 degrees or right-angle light scatter (side scatter, SS) studies the particle's internal features or granularity (Fig. 24–2).

Laser light differs from conventional sources in two fundamental ways: (1) the light is coherent, that is, all of the waves of light are parallel; (2) the light is monochromatic; that is of a single wavelength or frequency. Flow cytometers now in clinical use have more efficient optical systems and operate with lower-power, air-cooled lasers.

TABLE 24–2 Historical Developments in Flow Cytometry

Year	Development	Investigator
1934	Photoelectric counting of white cells in a stream	Moldaven
1949	Invention of cell counter and volume analyzer	Coulter
1953	Application of laminar sheath principle to cell counting	Crosland-Taylor
1956	"Model A" Coulter Counter	Coulter
1965	Multiparametric analysis, 2-D histograms, computerization	Kamentsky et al.
1965	Electrostatic cell sorter	Fulwyler
1968	Development of cytophotometer	Dittrich and Gohde
1969	Orthogonal axes, argon-ion laser	Van Dilla et al.
1970s	Research applications	
1980s	Research and clinical applications	

Source: From Riley, R: "Flow Cytometry for the Nineties and Beyond," ASCP Workshop presented Orlando, Florida, 1993, p 4, with permission.

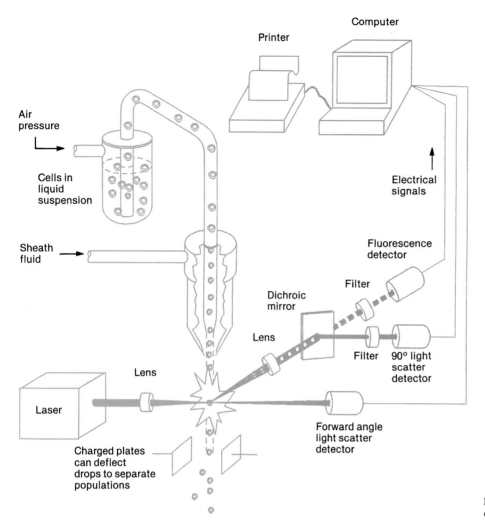

FIGURE 24–1 Components of a laser-based flow cytometer.

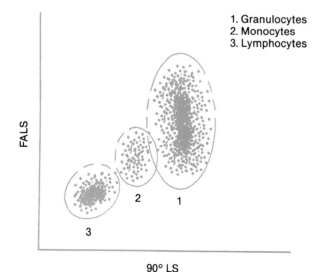

1. Granulocytes
2. Monocytes
3. Lymphocytes

FIGURE 24–2 Peripheral blood leukocyte analysis by simultaneous evaluation of forward-angle light scatter (FALS) and 90° light scatter (LS).

Detectors in most clinical cytometers, designated FL1, FL2, and FL3, are sensitive to green, orange, and red fluorescence, respectively. On excitation by the laser beam, these colors are emitted by fluorochrome-tagged antibodies or other fluorescent markers, such as propidium iodide, which is used as a DNA stain.

Gating

Gating is in essence an electronic window that sets upper and lower limits on the type and amount of material that passes through. Gates may be rectilinear or amorphous and are used to separate a subpopulation from a heterogeneous population. Gates are typically used to separate lymphocytes from other white cells for analysis. In other cases, the malignant population is gated for analysis. Gating permits very specific questions to be asked about a particular population.

Sorting

Some flow cytometers also have the capability of "sorting" subpopulations of cells. These cells can be separated by single or multiple characteristics and remain unaltered during the process. The sorting process can be accomplished under sterile conditions enabling the cell preparations to be cultured. These purified or sorted cells can be studied for additional morphological, functional, biochemical, or cytogenetic properties. Flow cytometers with cell-sorting capabilities are used extensively in research laboratories, but at present have limited used in the clinical laboratory.

MONOCLONAL ANTIBODIES

Description

Monoclonal antibodies are antibodies developed from one clone; therefore, the concentration of a particular antibody should remain unchanged from batch to batch. In addition, the ability to stain discrete epitopes (antigenic sites on the cell surface) with minimal cross-reactivity has made monoclonal antibodies the reagent of choice in flow cytometry.

Kohler and Milstein in 1975 developed highly specific monoclonal antibodies. Commensurate with the importance of this discovery, they received the Nobel Prize in physiology and medicine. Production of monoclonal antibodies is based on the fusion of immune B cells with a myeloma partner to produce an immortal hybridoma cell that will secrete a unique antibody (Fig. 24–3).

Cluster Designations

Because of the profusion of lineage-specific monoclonal antibodies by different laboratories, it was realized that a universal mechanism for adequately categorizing the antigens being defined by monoclonal antibodies would be a worthwhile goal. The first International Workshop on Human Leukocyte Differentiation Antigens was held in 1982 in Paris, France. As originally defined, a cluster designation (CD) groups antibodies that all recognize the same antigen. The CD nomenclature is synonymous with a given protein antigen, or in the case of some carbohydrate antigens, a given epitope.

The CDs now number more than 130, with activation antigens and cytokines included in the increasing number of cell "markers" recognized by new monoclonal antibodies. For the clinical laboratory technologist, the most important CDs are the ones that were first discovered, not only because they have been studied longer but also because there is more clinical data to support their usefulness.

The following CD designations are mentioned both as an example and because of their common usage.

CD2: Pan T-cell marker
CD4: Helper-inducer T cell
CD8: Cytotoxic/suppressor T cell
CD20: Mature B cell
CD19: Immature B cell

Fluorescence and Fluorochromes

The coupling of monoclonal antibodies with fluorescent dyes is necessary for recognition and enumera-

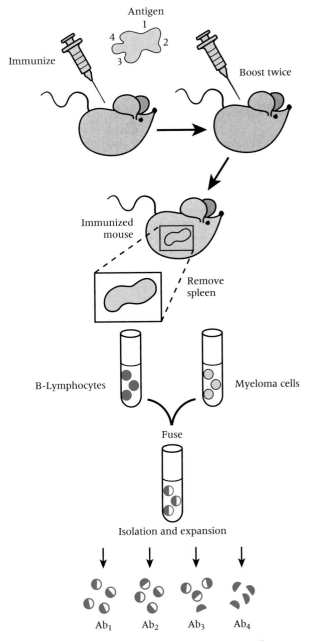

FIGURE 24–3 Monoclonal antibody (MAB) production requires immunization of animals, fusion of a myeloma cell line with B lymphocytes from the immunized animal, and in vitro selection and growth of the antibody-secreting hybrids. (From Keren, D, Hansen, C, and Hurtubise, P: Flow Cytometry and Clinical Diagnostics. ASCP Press, Chicago, 1989, with permission).

tion by the flow cytometer. Each fluorochrome possesses a distinctive spectral pattern of absorption (excitation) and emission. Lasers emit monochromatic light, or light of a single wavelength. To be of value in FCM, a fluorochrome or chromophore must absorb light at the wavelength or at one of the wavelengths the

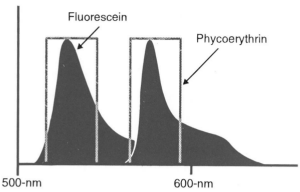

FIGURE 24–4 Selection of optical filters matched to emission spectra. (From Flow Cytometric Immunophenotyping—Procedure and Lecture Manual, U.S. Department of Health and Human Services, Atlanta, GA.)

laser emits. Consequently, not all fluorochromes can be used with all lasers. The fluorochromes present on or in the cell absorb the laser light and re-emit the light at a lower energy and longer wavelength. This is the property known as fluorescence. It occurs very rapidly, in about 10 seconds. With multiple fluorochromes, their emission spectra must have minimal overlap so as to be separately quantitated.

The most popular fluorochrome used in immunofluorescence is fluorescein isothiocyanate (FITC), which has an absorption maximum between 450 and 540 nm. If multiple fluorochromes are used, their emission spectra must have minimal overlap to be quantitated separately. An example of an excellent combination would be to use phycoerythrin (PE) as a second fluorochrome since it can absorb light from the same laser beam but emits most of its light at higher wavelengths than FITC. FITC emits light detectable in FL1 on the flow cytometer and PE emits light detectable in FL2 with third-color reagents having emission detectable in FL3. Any of these fluorochromes can be coupled to specific monoclonal antibodies, which can be used to identify individual cells by attaching to cell surface or cytoplasmic antigens (Fig. 24–4).

Compensation

Compensation is a tool that is used in multicolor assays to correct for fluorochromes with spectral overlap. This bleeding over of emissions is corrected by *compensation*, an electronic method that subtracts a percentage of the fluorescence signal empirically determined to be caused by this overlap. The amount of compensation varies with the brightness of the individual fluorochromes and the instrument being used, so caution must be exercised to avoid both overcompensation and undercompensation.

IMMUNOPHENOTYPING

Definition

Immunophenotyping is the term used in the identification of cells by labeling with monoclonal antibod-

ies, identified as CD markers. It is performed by labeling the cells with red, green, and/or orange-labeled monoclonal antibodies. The cells are then interrogated in the flow cytometer and the number and percentage of positive cells are recorded.

Lymphocytes

Immunophenotyping or labeling of the various epitopes or antigens on lymphocytes has been and continues to be the most important clinical application of the flow cytometer in hematology.

In the late 1960s, lymphocytes were broadly divided into T (thymus-derived) lymphocytes and B (bursal equivalent) lymphocytes. T lymphocytes are responsible for cell-mediated immunity and B lymphocytes are responsible for humoral or antibody-mediated immunity. These cell populations were originally distinguished because it was discovered that sheep red cells formed rosettes around the T lymphocyte. It was a convenient, albeit unreliable, marker of T cells. After the introduction of monoclonal antibodies, the CD2 marker (known as the E-rosette equivalent because of the sheep cell phenomena) began to be exclusively used for marking this T-lymphocyte subset. Originally, the cells were labeled with monoclonal antibody conjugated with a fluorochrome and these cells were read under a fluorescent microscope, evaluating individual cells for positivity. The introduction of the flow cytometer gave the laboratorian a new tool for enumerating large numbers of cells rapidly (10,000 cells per second) and also making multivariate analysis of these cells at the same time.

Human Immunodeficiency Virus Disease

Lymphocyte immunophenotyping laid the groundwork for the evaluation of normal lymphocytes in the study of immunosuppressed patients, such as those infected with the human immunodeficiency virus (HIV) and other immune deficiency diseases. One such disease is DiGeorge syndrome, in which T cells are present but in decreased numbers; another is severe combined immunodeficiency (SCID), in which there are no T cells. Lymphocytes that mature in the thymus carry with them differentiation antigens that are unique and distinguish them from lymphocytes maturing in the bone marrow.

After the CD2 monoclonal antibody was discovered, identifying the T lymphocyte that had been previously demonstrated by E-rosetting with sheep red cells, several new antibodies quickly followed. They were given CDs corresponding to the order in which they were discovered. For example, CD1 was the thymocyte marker, CD4, the T helper cell, and CD8, the T suppressor cell.

Panel for Human Immunodeficiency Virus Disease

Coincidentally and significantly, the full understanding of HIV disease emerged at approximately the same time. The human immunodeficiency viral particle first binds to a receptive cell surface via specific CD4 glycoproteins, then fuses to the membrane, and finally enters the cell. Viral single-stranded (ss)-RNA is converted to double-stranded (ds)-DNA by a specific reverse transcriptase and then integrates into the nuclear DNA via specific enzymes. This incorporation into the cellular DNA causes a lifelong persistent infection. HIV infection and replication causes the progressive loss of CD4+ lymphocytes.

The quantitation of CD4+ (helper) lymphocytes and CD8+ (suppressor) lymphocytes is important in the staging and monitoring of patients with HIV disease. The T-lymphocyte subsets change dramatically during the evolution of HIV disease. Clinical staging closely follows the changes in the CD4+ T lymphocytes, and their progressive loss correlates with the immunosuppression of the individual. Interestingly, there is a corresponding increase in CD8+ lymphocytes as the CD4+ lymphocytes decrease.

Normal values for CD4 lymphocytes are 32% to 66% of the lymphocyte population with an absolute count of 389 to 1868×10^9/L. The normal values for CD8 are 14% to 42% of the lymphocyte population with the absolute count 185 to 1045×10^9/L. The normal CD4/CD8 ratio is 1.0 to 3.3. The CD4/CD8 ratio is frequently used by clinicians to evaluate disease stage and response to therapy (Fig. 24–5). These numbers are based on an adult population of a large Veterans' Administration medical center. Normal values for CD4 and CD8 are age-dependent and should be determined at each institution performing these procedures. Table 24–3 lists the Centers for Disease Control (CDC)-recommended panel for lymphocyte immunophenotyping.

Peripheral Blood Stem Cell Transplantation

Peripheral blood stem cell harvest has become an acceptable alternative for the transplantation of hematopoietic progenitor cells. The strategy in high-dose chemotherapy as a treatment for cancer patients is to intensify the drug level to a concentration at which all hematopoietic cells are killed. This is followed by "rescue," and either bone marrow or peripheral blood stem cell transplantation is an effective means of reconstituting the patient's hematopoietic cells.

Progenitor cell mobilization is accomplished by the use of G–CSF (granulocyte colony-stimulating factor) or GM–CSF (granulocyte-macrophage colony-stimulating factor). The maximum number of circulating progenitor stem cells is reached 5 to 10 days after the induction procedure and the peripheral stem cell harvest is initiated at that time.

The use of the CD34 monoclonal antibody enables the detection of stem cells present in the harvest, enabling the clinician to determine how many harvests will be required and the effectiveness of the procedure. Because the percentage of stem cells present in a peripheral stem cell harvest may be lower than 1%, it is necessary to use as many different characteristics as possible to distinguish the true progentior cells. The CD34 antibody is combined with other antibodies to help accurately define this small population of cells.

LEUKEMIAS AND LYMPHOMAS

Immunophenotyping has become an essential component in the study of hematologic malignancies. Complementing traditional morphological examination, it has increased both our ability to classify these cells and provided new insight into their lineage and differentiation.

Acute Leukemias

The choice of monoclonal antibodies chosen for a new leukemia/lymphoma workup is directed by: (1) clinical features, (2) morphology of the peripheral smear and bone marrow, and (3) cytochemical stains. The panel is selected for maximum results with minimum number of reagents. As a general rule, reactivity with one antibody is not enough to determine the lineage of acute leukemia.

Careful attention must be paid to the cell preparation used for FCM analysis. Density-gradient separation of the mononuclear cells or whole blood lysis may be used to separate or lyse out the red blood cells. It is essential to review the smear or cytospin preparation for assurance that the cellular preparation is representative of the tissue in question.

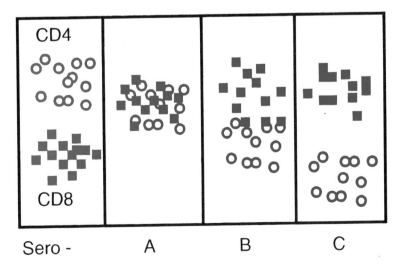

FIGURE 24–5 Changes in T-lymphocyte subsets during HIV disease progression. (Normal, A = asymptomatic, B = symptomatic, C = AIDS.) (From Flow Cytometric Immunophenotyping—Procedure and Lecture Manual, U.S. Department of Health and Human Services, Atlanta, GA.)

TABLE 24–3 **CDC Recommended Panel for Lymphocyte Immunophenotyping**

Fluorescein Isothiocyanate (FITC)	Phycoerythrin (PE)	Reason for Using
CD45	CD14	To draw gates; lymphocytes are brightly positive for CD45 and negative for CD14
Isotype	Isotype	To set cursors, or discriminators for positivity in the samples to follow
CD3	CD4	To measure CD4+ T cells; only cells + for both CD4 and CD3 should be considered CD4+ T cells
CD3	CD8	To measure CD8+ T cells; only cells that are positive for both CD8 and CD3 should be considered CD8+ T cells. The remainder of the CD8 cells (CD3–) are natural killer (NK) cells
CD3	CD19	To measure B-cells for quality assurance and to account for all lymphocytes
CD3	CD16 and/or CD56	To measure NK cells (negative for CD3, positive for CD16 and/or CD56) for quality assurance and to help account for all lymphocytes

Target Cells	Monoclonal Antibodies
CD14	Monocytes
CD45	Leukocyte common antigen
CD3	T-cell receptor complex
CD4	T subset, helper/inducer
CD8	T subset, cytotoxic, suppressor, NK
CD19	B cells
CD16	T subset, NK
CD56	T subset, NK cell

Isotype: Patient cells with fluorochrome and no antibodies

There are now hundreds of lineage-specific antigens associated with hematopoietic cells, as well as differentiation-specific antigens that are expressed at various developmental stages within a series. The selection of monoclonal antibodies can be done case by case, or a standardized panel can be used. Table 24–4 lists the monoclonal antibodies useful in the study of leukemia and lymphoma.

An example of a base panel used in a large hospital for immunophenotyping acute leukemias is the following: B lineage—CD19, kappa, lambda, T lineage—CD5, CD7; T & B lineage—CD10, TdT (terminal deoxynucleotidyl transferase); myelomonocytic lineage—CD13, CD33; "blasts"—CD34, HLA-DR.

Immunophenotyping is useful in defining B-cell versus T-cell lineage in the acute lymphocytic leukemias (ALLs) and lymphomas. B-lineage ALL can be divided into subgroups based on expression of HLA-DR, CD19, CD10, CD20, cytoplasmic immunoglobulin, and the TdT.

T-lineage ALLs are reasonably screened by one or two antibodies to pan T-associated antigens (e.g., CD3 and CD7). When these are positive, T-subset markers may be added for appropriate lineage identification. These markers may include CD2, CD4, CD5, CD8, CD16, or CD56.

The myeloid or monocytoid monoclonal antibodies are of most value in the poorly differentiated AML when diagnosis by standard morphologic examination and the use of cytochemical stains is unclear. The monoclonal antibodies most often used are CD13 and CD33, which characterize most of the myeloid leukemias. Other monoclonal antibodies are available and may be useful in determining specific lineage, such as CD14 and HLA-DR.

Glycophorin A antibody has been useful in the diagnosis of M6 erythroleukemia and CD61 in the diagnosis of M7 megakaryoblastic leukemia. The elucidation of more specific markers for M6, M7, and the few leukemias that remain undifferentiated continues to be investigated.

Chronic Leukemias

More than 95% of chronic lymphocytic leukemia (CLL) cases are of B-cell origin. They characteristically coexpress the CD5 antigen and a low-density surface membrane immunoglobulin (sIg) with monoclonal light chain. Pan-B monoclonal antibody markers such as CD19, CD20, and CD22 are present in virtually all cases of CLL.

It is important to separate PLL (prolymphocytic leu-

TABLE 24–4 Monoclonal Antibodies Useful in the Study of Leukemia and Lymphoma*

CD Group	Antibodies	Reactivity
Lymphoid-B		
CD19	B4, Leu 12	B lymphocytes
CD20	B1, Leu16	B lymphocytes
CD22	Leu 14, SHC11	B lymphocytes
CD21	B2, CR2	B lymphocytes
CD10	CALLA, J5	Immature B cells; granulocytes
CD23	B6, Leu20	B lymphocytes
Lymphoid-T		
CD1	T6, Leu6	Thymocytes
CD2	T11, Leu5b	T lymphocytes; subset of NK cells
CD3	T3, Leu4	T lymphocytes; subset of NK cells
CD4	T4, Leu3a	T helper/inducer cells
CD5	Leu1, T1	T lymphocytes; small subset of B cells
CD7	Leu9, 3A1, WT1	T lymphocytes; subset of NK cells
CD8	T8, Leu2a	T cytotoxic/suppressor cells; subset of NK cells
Myelomonocytic		
CD33	MY9, LeuM9, L4F3	CFU–GEMM to promyelocytes and mature monocytes
CD13	MY7, LeuM7	CFU–GM to mature granulocytes and monocytes
CD14	MY4, LeuM3, MO2	Monocytes
CD15	LeuM1, MY1	Promyelocytes to granulocytes; monocytes
—	17F11, 95C3, YB5.B8	Early myeloid precursors; mast cells
Platelets and red blood cells		
CD41	GPIIbIIIa, PL-273	Platelets and megakaryocytes
CD42	GPIb, FMC-25	Platelets and megakaryocytes
—	Glycophorin A, 10F7	Mature erythrocytes and erythroid precursor cells
NK cells		
CD16	Leu11, OKNK	NK cells
CD56	Leu19, NKH1	NK cells
Others		
CD34	MY10, HPCA-1	Progenitor cells
—	HLA-DR, Ia	B lymphocytes; monocytes; activated T cells

*CD indicates cluster designation; NK, natural killer; CFU–GEMM, granulocyte-erythrocyte-macrophage-megakaryocyte colony-forming unit; and CFU–GM, granulocyte-macrophage colony-forming unit.

Source: From Huh, YO: Surface markers in acute and chronic leukemia and non-Hodgkins lymphoma. Reprinted with permission from The Cancer Bulletin. Copyright 1993. The University of Texas M.D. Anderson Cancer Center, Houston, Texas.

kemia) and HCL (hairy cell leukemia) from CLL. Prolymphocytic leukemia usually demonstrates a high white count, predominance of prolymphocytes, and is usually CD5-negative with strong expression of SIg. HCL expresses CD19, CD20, CD22, and SIg.

Mixed-Lineage and Biphenotypic Leukemias

Mixed-lineage leukemias (expression of two or more markers of different lineage on the same malignant cell) have received no consensus regarding definition, terminology, or diagnostic criteria. The reported incidence in adults is much higher than in children. Biphenotypic leukemia is another classification of leukemia in which two leukemias exist simultaneously. In this case, the selection of monoclonal antibodies is predicated by the morphology of the two leukemias present.

Immunophenotyping for both acute and chronic leukemias is not an exact science. It requires careful assessment of the patient population served, clinical and morphologic correlation, continued research as to the availability and utility of monoclonal antibodies, and finally synthesis and interpretation of this information.

DNA ANALYSIS

Description

DNA analysis is performed by staining cells with one of several fluorescent dyes that intercalate between DNA base pairs. Fluorescent dyes such as propidium iodide (PI), acridine orange (AO), ethidium bromide mithramycin, and diamidine phenylindole (DAPI) stoichiometrically bind to DNA. The fluorescent intensity of the dye in each cell is a direct measure of the amount of nuclear DNA.

Aneuploidy

Populations of aneuploid (any chromosome number other than the normal diploid number of 46 chromosomes) can be detected and quantified by analysis of the data. In addition, the precise number of cells in each phase of the cell cycle (G0/G1, S, and G2/M) can be determined (Fig. 24–6).

Aneuploidy is believed to reflect the high incidence of numerical or structural chromosomal aberrations present in neoplastic cells. Clones of cells that differ in DNA content by 4% (one or two chromosomes) can be differentiated by the flow cytometer. The expression of DNA content abnormalities are regarded as reliable (but not absolute) diagnostic features of malignancy. Aneuploidy has been associated with worsened survival in ovarian cancer, early-stage breast cancer, colorectal cancer, non–small cell lung cancer, and bladder carcinoma. Conversely, it is considered a positive prognostic indicator in childhood acute lymphoblastic leukemia (ALL), neuroblastoma, and rhabdomyosarcoma. Current cancer therapy selectively destroys aneuploid cell lines; consequently, some of these malignancies with extra chromosomes respond well to chemotherapy.

Proliferative activity, determined by the flow cytometer has been difficult to evaluate because of technical variables in the measurement of this activity. Newer software packages with statistically significant mathematical models have helped standardize this evaluation.

One of the advantages of DNA analysis is that it can be performed on fixed, embedded tissue without any

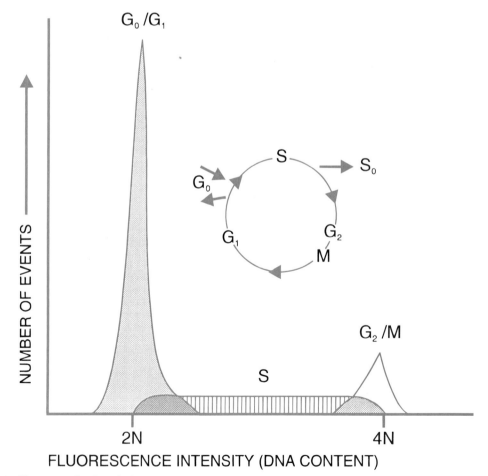

FIGURE 24–6 Histogram display of relative DNA-bound dye fluorescence contains areas separable into corresponding phases of the cell cycle. (From Keren, D, Hansen, C, and Hurtubise, P: Flow Cytometry and Clinical Diagnostics. ASCP Press, Chicago, 1989, with permission.)

loss of data. This has allowed for retrospective studies of DNA content in a variety of malignant conditions in which the outcome in terms of survival has been determined.

Quality Assurance

For accurate DNA analysis of tissue, there must be a monodispersed suspension of cells devoid of cellular aggregates. Preparation for FCM may require mechanical or enzymatic cell disaggregation. Nuclei can be stripped from their cytoplasm with detergent-containing media and then stained with a fluorescent dye, or they may be minced and filtered through nylon mesh before enzymatic digestion.

The resolution of DNA analysis is determined by measuring the coefficient of variation (CV) of the G0/G1 peak of a normal, nonmalignant cell population. CVs of less than 2% are desirable with a human blood lymphocyte population. Precise CVs are necessary so that an aneuploid peak located close to the normal diploid peak is not obscured by a broad diploid peak.

DNA analysis by flow has proven an independent prognostic indicator in certain malignancies. Improvements in FCM instruments, reagents, procedures, and software packages has decreased the subjectivity present in the interpretation of DNA by flow cytometry, permitting better clinical correlation and prognostication.

OTHER APPLICATIONS OF FLOW CYTOMETRY

Reticulocytes

The concept of flow cytometric determination of reticulocytes depends on the binding of a suitable fluorescent dye to RNA. Pyronine Y, DiOC (cyanine dye), propidium iodide, thioflavin T, acridine orange, and thiazole orange are all dyes that have been used in flow cytometric analysis of reticulocytes.

The cost efficiency of performing reticulocyte counts by FCM depends on individual factors in each laboratory. Software packages for many of the commonly used hematology instruments now feature programs for automated reticulocyte analysis.

Antiplatelet Antibodies

Immunofluorescent assays have been developed for the recognition of antiplatelet antibodies, including complement fixation or lysis, immunologically mediated platelet alteration, cell-mediated assays, and immunoglobulin binding assays. These assays have been adapted to the flow cytometer with considerable success.

Flow Cytometry Cross Match

Cross matching donor and recipient products by the use of flow cytometry and fluorescent anti-immunoglobulin reagents provide a level of sensitivity beyond that obtainable by traditional blood banking methodology. This type of cross match has shown to have in-

creased sensitivity in detecting anti-HLA antibodies adsorbed to cells.

Nucleic Acid Probe Technology

Nucleic acid probe assays are now being used for the diagnosis of infectious disease and FISH (fluorescence in situ hybridization). Both of these techniques can be adapted to the flow cytometer.

Other Assays

Assays of neutrophil function including those for the diagnosis of chronic granulomatous disease, antineutrophil antibodies, antinuclear antigens, detection of minimal residual disease, and cytogenetic analysis are all procedures that have been implemented or in the formative stages for use on the flow cytometer.

BIBLIOGRAPHY

Carey, J: Teleconference, "Flow Cytometric Immunophenotyping of Leukemias and Lymphomas," presented November 4 and 11, 1992.

Centers for Disease Control: Flow Cytometric Immunophenotyping Quality Assurance & Quality Control Procedures for CD4+ T-Lymphocyte Determinations, procedure manual and lecture manual, U.S. Department of Health & Human Services, April, 1993.

Hubbard, RA: "Future Clinical Applications of Flow," Advance for Administrators of the Laboratory, Vol. 4, No. 4, April, 1995.

Huh, YO: The Cancer Bulletin, University of Texas MD Anderson Cancer Center, Volume 45, Number 1, January-February, 1993, "Surface Markers in Acute and Chronic Leukemia and Non-Hodgkin's Lymphoma," pp 78–85.

Keren, D: Flow Cytometry in Clinical Diagnosis. ASCP Press, Chicago, 1989.

Keren, D, Hansen, C, and Hurtubise, P: Flow Cytometry and Clinical Diagnosis. ASCP Press, Chicago, 1994.

Kohler G, and Milstein, C.: Nature, 256:495, 1975.

Kotylo, P, and Moriarty, A: Teleconference, "Flow Cytometric Analysis of Acute Leukemias," presented ASCP National Meeting, Spring, 1994.

McCarthy, R: Teleconference, "Basic Immunology for Laboratorians: Advantages and Limitations of Monoclonal Antibodies as Immunological Reagents," presented Chicago, Illinois, May 16, 1989.

Melamed, MR, Lindmo, T, and Mendelsohn, ML (eds): Flow Cytometry and Sorting. Wiley-Liss, New York, 1990, pp 415–444.

Owens, M and Loken, M: Flow Cytometry Principles for Clinical Laboratory Practice, Wiley-Liss, New York, 1995.

Riley, R, Mahin, E, and McCoy, JP: "Flow Cytometry for the Nineties and Beyond." ASCP workshop presented Orlando, Florida, October, 1993.

QUESTIONS

1. What is the definition of flow cytometry?
   a. The measurement of cellular (or particle) properties as they move in a fluid (flow) past a stationary set of detectors
   b. The measurement of ionic particles as they move in a fluid (flow) past a stationary set of detectors

c. An instrument that measures light intensity; composed of a source of radiant energy, filter for wavelength selection, cuvette holder, detector, and a readout device
d. A device used to isolate a certain wavelength or range of wavelengths

2. What other area of science contributed to the development of flow cytometry?
   a. Monoclonal antibody production
   b. Electronics
   c. Fluorochrome chemistries
   d. All of the above

3. What is (are) the main component(s) of the flow cytometer?
   a. Laser light source
   b. Fluidics
   c. Photodetectors
   d. All of the above

4. What is meant by "gating"?
   a. The chromatic arrangement of cellular populations
   b. Process by which one cell population adheres to another population
   c. An electronic window separating one subpopulation of cells
   d. An electronic device measuring all populations of cells

5. How is a monoclonal antibody produced?
   a. The fusion of immune B cells with a myeloma partner to produce an immortalized hybridoma cell producing a unique antibody
   b. The fusion of immune T cells with a myeloma partner to produce an immortalized hybridoma cell producing a unique antibody
   c. The fusion of immune B cells with a myeloma partner to produce an immortalized hybridoma cell producing a unique antigen
   d. The fusion of immune T cells with a myeloma partner to produce an immortalized hybridoma cell producing a unique antigen

6. What does CD mean when used to describe monoclonal antibodies?
   a. It refers to cellular designation and is used in numbering the monoclonal antibodies as they were and are discovered.
   b. It refers to cluster designation and is used to describe the blood group antigens.
   c. It refers to cluster designation and is used in numbering the monoclonal antibodies as they were and are discovered.
   d. It refers to cluster designation and is used to describe the white cell antigens.

7. Why was the development of fluorochrome chemistry such an important event in the implementation of the flow cytometer?
   a. Fluorochrome chemistry is the basis for plasma cell and monoclonal antibody production.
   b. The coupling of fluorochrome dyes to monoclonal antibodies is necessary for recognition and enumeration.
   c. The coupling of fluorochrome dyes to polyclonal antibodies is necessary for recognition and enumeration.
   d. All of the above.

8. What is the importance of flow cytometry in the evaluation of HIV disease?

a. Enumeration of CD4 helper cells
b. Enumeration of CD34 stem cells
c. Enumeration of CD10 B cells
d. Enumeration of plasma cells

9. What procedure is necessary in preparation for a peripheral blood stem cell transplantation in a cancer patient?
   a. Induction therapy using erythropoietin
   b. Induction therapy using G–CSF and GM–CSF
   c. Cytokine suppression
   d. LAP score

10. What is the "gold standard" for classifying lymphomas and leukemias?
    a. Immunophenotyping
    b. Morphological classification
    c. Crossmatching
    d. Immunoelectrophoresis

11. All of the following are considered pan T cell markers except:
    a. CD2
    b. CD7
    c. CD33
    d. CD3

12. How is DNA measured in flow cytometry?
    a. A fluorescent dye is used that stoichiometrically binds to the cell nucleus and is a direct measurement of nuclear DNA.
    b. A fluorescent dye is used that stoichiometrically binds to the cell cytoplasm and is a direct measurement of nuclear DNA.
    c. A fluorescent dye is used that stoichiometrically binds to the cell nucleus and is an indirect measurement of nuclear DNA.
    d. A fluorescent dye is used that stoichiometrically binds to the cell cytoplasm and is an indirect measurement of nuclear DNA.

13. All of the following are applications of flow cytometry except:
    a. Antiplatelet antibodies
    b. Reticulocyte analysis
    c. Platelet aggregation
    d. Cross-matching

ANSWERS

1. **a** (p 452)
2. **d** (p 453)
3. **d** (p 453)
4. **c** (p 454)
5. **a** (p 455)
6. **c** (p 455)
7. **b** (p 455)
8. **a** (p 457)
9. **b** (p 457)
10. **b** (p 457)
11. **c** (p 458)
12. **a** (p 461)
13. **c** (p 461)

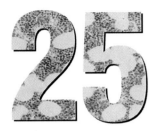

Lipid (Lysosomal) Storage Diseases and Histiocytosis

Denise M. Harmening, PhD, MT(ASCP), CLS(NCA)
Catherine M. Spier, MD

Lipid (Lysosomal) Storage Diseases
  Gaucher's Disease
  Niemann-Pick Disease
  Tay-Sachs Disease
  Mucopolysaccharidoses

Histiocytoses
  Sea-Blue Histiocyte Syndrome
  Other Histiocytic Disorders (Eosinophilic
    Granuloma, Hand-Schüller-Christian
    Disease, Letterer-Siwe Disease)

Case Study

Objectives

At the end of this chapter, the learner should be able to:
1. Name the enzyme deficiency seen in Gaucher's disease.
2. List characteristics for type I, type II, and type III Gaucher's disease.
3. Describe the appearance of Gaucher's cells.
4. Name the enzyme deficiency seen in Niemann-Pick disease.
5. List clinical features of Niemann-Pick disease.
6. Name the enzyme deficiency seen in Tay-Sachs disease.
7. List clinical features of Tay-Sachs disease.
8. Describe clinical features of Hurler's syndrome, Hunter's syndrome, and other mucopolysaccharidoses.
9. List laboratory findings in mucopolysaccharidosis disorders.
10. Describe the characteristic cell of sea-blue histiocyte syndrome.

LIPID (LYSOSOMAL) STORAGE DISEASES

The lipid storage diseases are rare, autosomally inherited disorders. They are known as lysosomal storage diseases because there is subcellular accumulation of unmetabolized material in the lysosomes of various cells. Lipid or lysosomal storage diseases are caused by various enzyme defects (inborn errors) in lipid metabolism linked to an enzyme deficiency (Fig. 25–1). Although many different types of lipid storage disorders have been documented, the most widely known and well-established include Gaucher's, Niemann-Pick, and Tay-Sachs diseases and mucopolysaccharidoses (Table 25–1). Although all ethnic groups are known to be affected by lipid storage diseases, there is an increased incidence of some selected disorders such as Gaucher's and Tay-Sachs diseases in

certain ethnic groups, most notably Ashkenazi Jews (Jews who trace their origin to the Baltic Sea region). Lipid storage diseases have a wide clinical expression, ranging from essentially asymptomatic to severe and incapacitating with early death. The aim of control in these disorders has been directed at prenatal detection. The only currently effective practical therapy is enzyme replacement, which has initiated a new age of treatment for genetic disorders and has improved the lives of many patients. The greatest controversy, however, regarding enzyme replacement therapy is the optimum amount and frequency of treatment.[1] In addition, allogeneic bone marrow transplantation (BMT) has been used to treat some patients and can be considered curative.[2] However, bone marrow transplantation is an extremely aggressive, expensive, and high-risk therapy considering that these conditions now

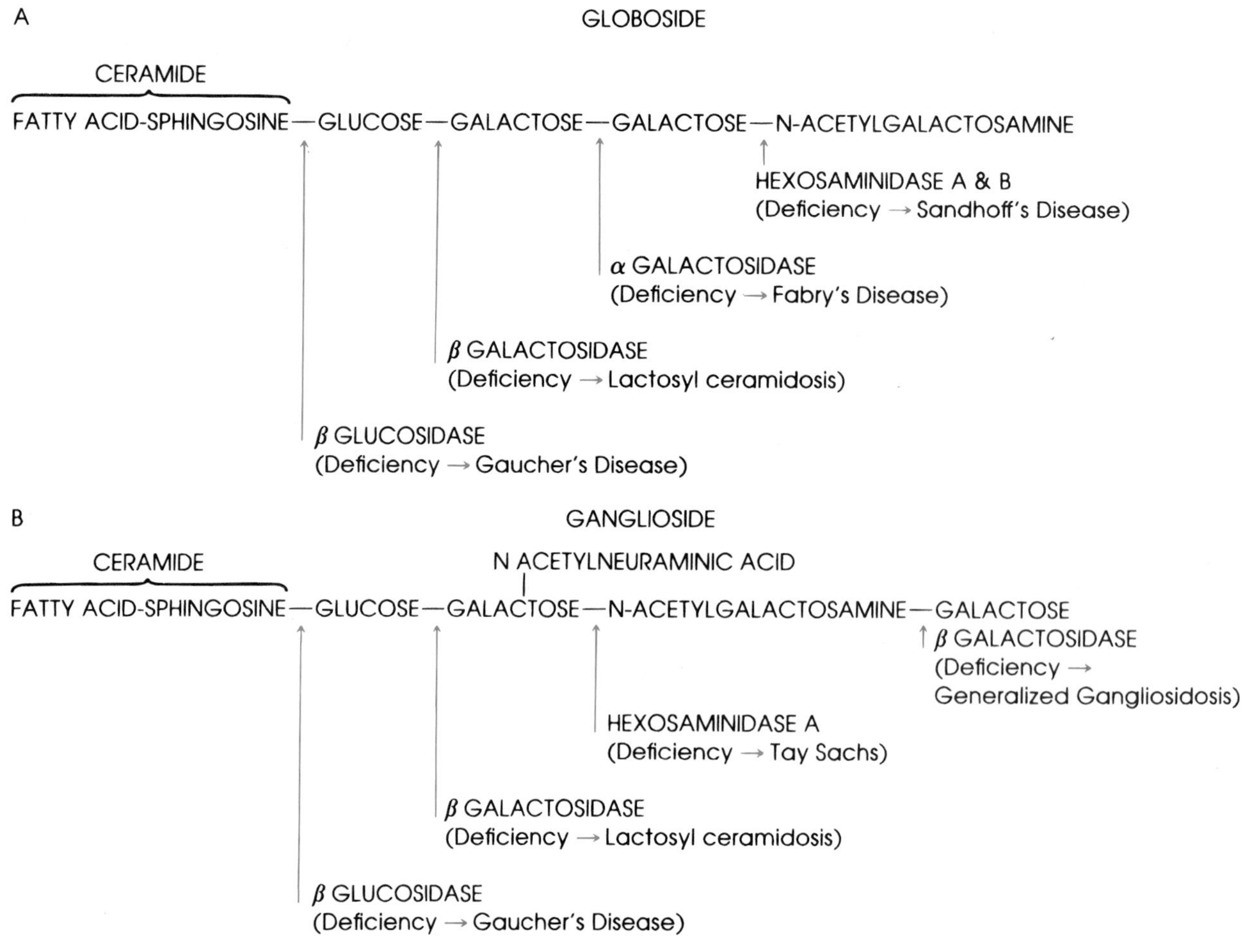

A
GLOBOSIDE

CERAMIDE

FATTY ACID-SPHINGOSINE — GLUCOSE — GALACTOSE — GALACTOSE — N-ACETYLGALACTOSAMINE

HEXOSAMINIDASE A & B
(Deficiency → Sandhoff's Disease)

α GALACTOSIDASE
(Deficiency → Fabry's Disease)

β GALACTOSIDASE
(Deficiency → Lactosyl ceramidosis)

β GLUCOSIDASE
(Deficiency → Gaucher's Disease)

B
GANGLIOSIDE

CERAMIDE

N ACETYLNEURAMINIC ACID

FATTY ACID-SPHINGOSINE — GLUCOSE — GALACTOSE — N-ACETYLGALACTOSAMINE — GALACTOSE

β GALACTOSIDASE
(Deficiency →
Generalized Gangliosidosis)

HEXOSAMINIDASE A
(Deficiency → Tay Sachs)

β GALACTOSIDASE
(Deficiency → Lactosyl ceramidosis)

β GLUCOSIDASE
(Deficiency → Gaucher's Disease)

FIGURE 25–1 Schematic structure of globoside and ganglioside to show site of action of the several catabolic enzymes, which, when defective, result in one of the storage diseases. (From Wintrobe, MM, et al: Clinical Hematology, ed 8. Lea & Febiger, Philadelphia, 1981, p. 1341, with permission.)

have an effective and practical treatment in enzyme replacement therapy. Table 25–2 summarizes the general characteristics of lipid storage diseases.

Gaucher's Disease

Historical Perspectives

This disorder was first described in 1882 by Philippe C. Gaucher in a 32-year-old woman with an enlarged spleen. Gaucher believed that the abnormal cells found in her spleen at autopsy were part of a primary splenic tumor. This abnormal cell, later named Gaucher's cell, is the result of the deficiency of the enzyme β-glucocerebrosidase, which leads to an accumulation

of unmetabolized substrate glucocerebroside in cells, predominantly the monocyte-macrophage system (the reticuloendothelial system, Fig. 25–2). Gaucher's observations were studied further and the entity known as Gaucher's disease was defined and characterized as a familial disorder at the turn of the century.[3] In 1920,

---

TABLE 25–1 Lipid Storage Diseases

* Gaucher's disease
* Niemann-Pick disease
* Tay-Sachs disease
* Mucopolysaccharidoses

TABLE 25–2 General Characteristics of Lipid Storage Disease

* Rare, inherited autosomal-recessive disorders
* Also known as lysosomal storage diseases because of accumulation of unmetabolized material in lysosomes
* Caused by enzyme deficiencies in lipid metabolism
* Increased incidence of some lipid storage diseases in certain ethnic groups (i.e., Gaucher's disease in Ashkenazi Jews)
* Great variation in clinical expression (i.e., asymptomatic to severe with early death)
* Effective therapy: enzyme replacement
* Most well-known and characterized: Gaucher's disease, Niemann-Pick disease, Tay-Sachs disease, and mucopolysaccharidoses

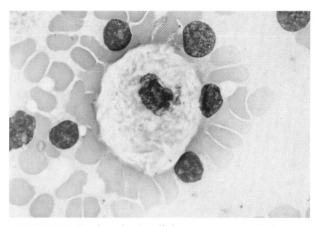

FIGURE 25–2   Gaucher's cell, bone marrow aspirate.

another variation or type of Gaucher's disease that is characterized by neurologic involvement was first described. It was after this date that Gaucher's disease was classified as a lysosomal storage disorder resulting from an enzyme deficiency with an autosomal recessive inheritance pattern. Although Gaucher's disease is the most frequent lysosomal storage disease, it was not until 1965 that the actual enzyme deficiency was identified as glucocerebrosidase. In 1984 the gene for glucocerebrosidase was cloned and in 1991 an important breakthrough occurred with the initiation of clinical trials for enzyme replacement therapy at the National Institutes of Health (NIH).[2] Gaucher's disease became the first enzyme-deficiency disorder to be successfully treated with infusion of replacement enzyme.[4–7] Table 25–3 summarizes the chronology of Gaucher's disease.

Classification and Clinical Features

Gaucher's disease has three clinically recognizable types: the adult or non-neuronopathic form (type I); the infantile, acute, or malignant neuronopathic form (type II); and the juvenile or subacute neuronopathic form (type III). Gaucher's types I, II, and III all have in common the triad of hepatosplenomegaly, Gaucher's cells in the bone marrow, and an increase in serum acid phosphatase (Table 25–4).[8] The severity of the disease and the patient's age when the disease is first

TABLE 25–3   **Gaucher's Disease: Chronology**
• 1882: first described by Philippe Gaucher
• Abnormal cell named Gaucher's cell
• 1900: Gaucher's disease defined as a familial disorder
• 1920: Another type of Gaucher's disease described characterized by neurologic involvement
• Gaucher's disease classified as a lysosomal storage disorder inherited as autosomal recessive
• 1965: Enzyme deficiency identified as glucocerebrosidase
• 1984: Gene for glucocerebrosidase cloned
• 1991: Enzyme replacement therapy in clinical trials

TABLE 25–4   **The Common Clinical Triad of Gaucher's Disease**
Hepatosplenomegaly
Gaucher's cells in the bone marrow
Increase in serum acid phosphatase

manifested are related to the magnitude of the enzyme deficiency. Table 25–5 briefly summarizes the characteristics of each type of Gaucher's disease.

The accumulation of glucocerebrosides, the result of the enzyme deficiency of β-glucocerebrosidase, produces the distinctive Gaucher's cells (see Fig. 25–2). These cells are histiocytes that are 20 to 100 μm in diameter with a displaced nucleus. One or more round to oval nuclei are present in each cell. The cytoplasm is faintly blue with white stain and has a "crumpled tissue paper" or finely folded appearance, possibly a result of glycolipid deposition. The presence of Gaucher's cells alone is not pathognomonic for Gaucher's disease, since these cells are also found in other lymphoproliferative disorders. Gaucher's cells can be deposited in any bone in the body, which leads to a predisposition for fractures, loss of bone, and avascular necrosis (particularly in the femoral head).[2] Bone involvement in Gaucher's disease may be presented as chronic bone pain or severe crises similar to those described in patients with sickle cell anemia. The accuracy and severity of such episodes of bone involvement are unpredictable. Skeletal involvement in Gaucher's disease includes a spectrum of findings radiographically ranging from minimal bone loss and osteopenia to severe evidence of bone destruction, including osteolytic and sclerotic lesions.[2] Table 25–6 summarizes the radiologic classification of bone pathology.[9] Figure 25–3 demonstrates the osteolytic lesions seen in the x-ray of the knee of a patient with Gaucher's disease. The underlying mechanisms of the bone complications of Gaucher's disease are not well defined. It is assumed that Gaucher's cells infiltrate the medullary space and eventually replace trabecular bone and initiate a series of events that lead to osteopenia, osteolytic lesions, and osteonecrosis. Gaucher's disease is clearly a multisystemic disorder characterized not only by skeletal disease but also by organomegaly, hematologic complications, and occasionally pulmonary involvement.[8]

Type I: Adult Gaucher's Disease (Chronic Non-neuronopathic)   Type I non-neuronopathic Gaucher's disease is the most common type of this disorder and the most common of the lipidoses. It is the most frequently inherited disorder in the Ashkenazi Jewish population. There is a remarkable degree of variability in the clinical signs and symptoms. Some patients with type I Gaucher's disease may display anemia, thrombocytopenia, massively enlarged livers and spleens, and extensive skeletal disease. In contrast, other type I Gaucher's disease patients have no symptoms at all and the disorder is identified in their adult years only during the screening or evaluation for other diseases. The average age of onset is between 30 and 40 years old. In most cases of a severe disorder, the diagnosis is made in childhood or early adulthood. Approximately two thirds of the patients with type I Gaucher's

TABLE 25–5	Gaucher's Disease—Clinical Subtypes		
Clinical Features	**Type I: Non-Neuronopathic (Adult Form)**	**Type II: Acute Neuronopathic (Infant Form)**	**Type III: Subacute Neuronopathic (Juvenile Form)**
Clinical onset	Childhood/Adult	Infancy	Childhood/juvenile
Estimated frequency	1/450–1/1,000	1/100,000	1/100,000
Hepatosplenomegaly	+	+	+
Hematologic complications secondary to hypersplenism	+	+	+
Skeletal deterioration (Bone crises/fractures)	+	−	+
Neurodegenerative course	−	+++	++
Life expectancy	6–80+ years	<2 years	20–40 years
Ethnic predilection	Ashkenazi Jew	Panethnic	Swedish (Norrbottnian)

disease are of Ashkenazi Jewish descent.[2] The remaining one third of patients with type I have a panethnic distribution. Three clinical presentations occur in the type I nonneuronopathic form of Gaucher's disease: (1) the mild presentation, which represents from 10% to 25% of patients who are essentially asymptomatic and live without the need for any treatment or intervention; (2) the moderate clinical presentation, in which the patient has hepatosplenomegaly, near normal blood counts, and a normal physical appearance; and (3) the most severe form, in which patients present with massive hepatosplenomegaly, significant thrombocytopenia, anemia, and skeletal complications.[10] A few patients with the severe forms of the disease may develop central nervous system damage, delayed sexual maturation, severe wasting, and eventually death. It should be noted that clinical presentations can be misleading since some of these patients may still develop underlying skeletal complications (Table 25–7). It is important, therefore, to perform a baseline skeletal evaluation even in patients with a mild case of the disease. The femoral heads are the most common initial bone site to be affected by the disease, and this area should be evaluated by magnetic resonance imaging (MRI) to assess for avascular necrosis.[2] The definitive diagnosis of Gaucher's disease is made with an assay for the enzyme acid β-glucocerebrosidase activity of the leukocytes. Bone marrow examination alone is insufficient for confirming the diagnosis since Gaucher's cells may be present in other disorders.

The gene for the enzyme glucocerebrosidase is located on chromosome 1q21-31. Since the characterization, cloning, and sequencing of the glucocerebrosidase gene in 1984, more than 40 genetic mutations have been described.[1] The mutations include both single insertional and point mutations as well as crossover mutations. All of the mutations that cause Gaucher's disease have complex effects on the properties of this enzyme.[11] The normal enzyme, glucocerebrosidase (acid β-glucosidase), is a lysosomal enzyme responsible for the degradation of the glucosylceramide molecule, preventing its buildup in tissue cells.[12] Protein synthesis of the normal enzyme occurs in the endoplasmic reticulum with transport to the Golgi apparatus for glycosylation and delivery to the lysosomes of the cell. Mutations at the genetic level that code for the production of this enzyme have direct effects on the catalytic activity with decreases from 5- to 100-fold.[13] In addition, enzyme stability and half-life activity (normal = 60 hours) is also decreased for acid β-glucosidase as a result of these mutations.[14]

Type II: Infantile Gaucher's Disease (Acute or Malignant Neuronopathic) Type II Gaucher's disease is a much rarer form that occurs in infancy and patients rarely survive past the age of 2 years old. Type II acute neuronopathic Gaucher's disease is seen in all ethnic groups, although it is uncommon in the Jewish population.[2] The frequency of type II disease is estimated at approximately 1 in 100,000.[2] The hallmark of type II Gaucher's disease is neurologic involvement that in-

TABLE 25–6	Radiologic Classification of Gaucher Bone Pathology[9]
Stage	**Description**
1 Osteopenia	Coarse trabecular pattern of decreased bone density, which may be localized or diffuse
2 Medullary expansion	Loss of normal concavity above femoral condyles
3 Localized destruction (osteolysis)	Small erosions, well-defined or moth-eaten, cortex rarefied and endosteally notched, ground-glass veiling
4 Ischemic necrosis of long bone, sclerosis, osteitis	Patchy densities and erosions, serpiginous sclerotic streaks, layered periostitis, sequestra
5 Diffuse destruction, epiphyseal collapse, osteoarthrosis	Flattening or irregular destruction of fermoral heads with mixed lytic and sclerotic foci, larger "soap bubble" pattern

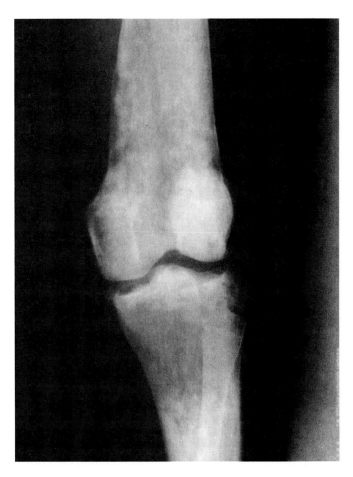

FIGURE 25-3 Anteroposterior radiograph of the knee shows diffuse mottled increased density of the distal femur and proximal tibia characteristic of widespread bone infarction in Gaucher's disease. The metaphyseal regions are broader than normal, resembling an Erlenmeyer flask deformity. (Courtesy of Charles S. Resnik, M.D., Department of Diagnostic Radiology, University of Maryland Medical Center, Baltimore, Maryland.)

cludes multiple signs such as difficulty swallowing, opisthotonos (extreme arching of the spine), and other manifestations of brainstem involvement that are noted early in infancy.[15] The infant has difficulty in feeding and fails to grow. Death usually occurs before the age of 2 years. Familial intermarriage is frequently found in the infant's family history. The clinical presentation of this type II disease is much more uniform than that observed with type I Gaucher's disease and is very severe. The disease exhibits a progressive pattern of clinical symptoms with hepatosplenomegaly evident within the first 6 months of life and is often discovered by 3 months of age. The principle cause of death in these infants with type II Gaucher's disease is brainstem damage.

Type III: Juvenile Gaucher's Disease (Subacute Neuronopathic) Type III Gaucher's disease may be present from early childhood to the teenage years and is characterized by clinical and physical findings and survivals ranging between those of type I and type II.[2] Type III has been noted, especially in a group of children from northern Sweden, the offspring of several related intermarriages. The frequency of type III Gaucher's disease among some Swedes is approximately 1 in 100,000.[2] Neurologic involvement is also characteristic of type III Gaucher's disease; however, the clinical manifestations are much more heterogenous than those observed in type II. Two distinct subtypes of type III Gaucher's disease have been described.[16] The classic form, type IIIa, usually presents itself clinically between early childhood and midadult life. It is characterized by mild to moderately severe systemic disease. Neurologic involvement is recognized at the onset of the disease with multifocal, rapid jerky movements observed in several muscle groups of the patient, either at rest or with movement.[16] Gener-

TABLE 25-7 **Clinical Presentations of Type I Gaucher's Disease**		
Mild	**Moderate**	**Severe**
10%–25% of patients	Hepatosplenomegaly	Massive hepatosplenomegaly
Asymptomatic	Near-normal blood counts	Significant thrombocytopenia
No need for treatment	Normal physical appearance	Anemia
		Skeletal complications

TABLE 25–8   Comparison of Type IIIa and IIIb Gaucher's Disease

	Type IIIa	Type IIIb
Clinical onset	Early childhood to mid-adult	Infancy to early childhood
Clinical course	Mild to moderately severe	Aggressive systemic disease
Neurologic involvement	At onset; multifocal rapid jerky movements, ataxia, spasticity, dementia, and seizures	Ocular motor disorder, horizontal supranuclear gaze palsy; mild cognitive impairment

alized seizures occur as the neurologic illness progresses. The seizure episodes are frequently refractory to any conventional treatments. In addition, ataxia, spasticity, and dementia frequently occur. Type IIIb Gaucher's disease is characterized by a clinically aggressive systemic disease with neurologic involvement of isolated horizontal supranuclear gaze palsy as the major sign.[17] Ocular motor disorder is the distinctive neurologic feature of type IIIb Gaucher's disease. This neurologic disorder usually appears during infancy or early childhood. The clinical presentation of type IIIb Gaucher's disease is very severe with aggressive systemic disease and death typically occurring in childhood or adolescence, primarily from hepatic or pulmonary complications.[16] Generally, in type III Gaucher's disease regardless of the subtype, the more severe the neurologic disease, the shorter the survival. Table 25–8 compares the clinical characteristics of type IIIa and type IIIb Gaucher's disease.

Laboratory Diagnosis

Peripheral blood, bone marrow, and spleen are the sites most frequently examined in patients with Gaucher's disease. The peripheral blood nearly always demonstrates a moderate normocytic, normochromic anemia with thrombocytopenia because of the replacement of normal hematopoietic cells with Gaucher's cells in the bone marrow. There is pooling of blood in the enlarged spleen and some degree of ineffective erythropoiesis, with decreased incorporation of iron in erythroid precursors in the bone marrow. As a result, active signs of a compensated anemia such as polychromasia and nucleated red blood cells are usually *absent* on the peripheral smear.[18] Leukocytes are commonly decreased in number. Platelets are also usually decreased in number as a result of splenic sequestration. These patients may have a bleeding tendency, with nosebleeds especially common. Gaucher's cells are noted only rarely in the peripheral blood.

Bone marrow aspirates are often the first tissue in which Gaucher's cells are detected; these cells are required for diagnosis (see Fig. 25–2). They are histiocytes, 20 to 100 μm in diameter, found in moderate numbers and as clumps of cells in the thickest areas of the smear. One or more round to oval nuclei are present in each cell. The cytoplasm is faintly blue with Wright's stain and has a "crumbled tissue paper" or finely folded appearance possibly as a result of glycolipid deposition. Electron microscopy has demonstrated that this appearance is the result of lamellar bodies stacked inside secondary phagolysosomes.

These cells stain positive with periodic acid-Schiff (PAS), acid phosphatase, Giemsa, iron, Sudan black B, and oil red O stains because of the accumulation of the unmetabolized glucocerebroside. It is important to note that the presence of Gaucher's cells is not pathognomonic for Gaucher's disease, since these cells are also found in other lymphoproliferative disorders.

The spleen is variably enlarged, owing to the accumulation of masses of Gaucher's cells. The enlargement is commonly up to 10 times normal splenic weight and can cause considerable discomfort to the patient. Other organs and systems commonly affected include the liver and, in type II, the nervous system, pituitary gland, kidneys, lung, and ovaries. These organs contain massive deposits of Gaucher's cells.

The serum acid phosphatase level is increased, and isozyme measurement of this enzyme has shown that the tartrate-resistant fraction is what is increased in patients with Gaucher's disease.

With the advance of molecular techniques in the diagnosis of disease, new knowledge has been gained regarding Gaucher's disease.[19] Recently it has been shown through the use of polymerase chain reaction (PCR) that the severity of disease in type I Gaucher's disease could be predicted based on the type of genetic mutation within the glucocerebrosidase gene that was detected using this type of deoxyribonucleic acid (DNA) analysis.[20] In this study, the single nucleotide substitution of adenine for guanine was the most common finding in patients with type I Gaucher's disease.[20] These types of advances are rapidly expanding the ability to diagnose Gaucher's disease, predict its severity, and perhaps even aid in its treatment. Table 25–9 summarizes the laboratory findings in Gaucher's disease.

Although the Gaucher's cell is associated with the disease, so-called pseudo-Gaucher's cells have also

TABLE 25–9   Gaucher's Disease: Laboratory Findings

Normocytic, normochromic or normocytic, hypochromic anemia
Leukopenia
Thrombocytopenia
Gaucher's cells in bone marrow (BM) aspirate
Increased serum acid phosphatase
Positive staining of Gaucher's cells in BM with PAS, acid phosphatase, Giemsa, iron, Sudan black B, and oil red O stains

TABLE 25-10 Disorders in Which "Pseudo-Gaucher's" Cells Have Been Described
AML
CLL
Plasma cell myeloma
Aplastic anemia
ITP
Thalassemia major
Rheumatoid arthritis

TABLE 25-12 Immunologic Abnormalities Described in Gaucher's Disease
Increased helper-to-suppressor (T_4:T_8) cell ratio
Decreased natural killer (null) cells
Polyclonal B-cell lymphocytosis
Plasmacytosis

been described. They are seen in disease states with increased cellular turnover, especially chronic myelogenous leukemia, in which the phenomenon was first described. In theory, the increased cell turnover presents so much glycosyl ceramide to the reticuloendothelial system (RES) that its enzyme system is overwhelmed and cannot adequately metabolize all of the material. The excess is therefore stored in histiocytes, with their end morphological expression identical to that of true Gaucher's cells. This phenomenon is also seen in a variety of other disorders, including acute myelocytic leukemia, chronic lymphocytic leukemia, plasma cell myeloma, aplastic anemia, idiopathic thrombocytopenic purpura (ITP), thalassemia major, and rheumatoid arthritis (Table 25-10).[21] The presence of Gaucherlike cells in patients with these diseases has no known prognostic significance. It should be emphasized that in each of these diseases there is no deficiency of the β-glucocerebrosidase, as there is in Gaucher's disease, but rather an overtaxation of a normal system.

Prognosis

As previously stated, the length of survival in patients with Gaucher's disease is variable and depends on the type. The adult form (type I) has the longest survival, with patients surviving commonly into adulthood. In the infantile form (type II), survival beyond 2 years of age is rare. Like the clinical features, survival in the juvenile form (type III) is intermediate between the first two, and patients usually live into adolescence. A relatively increased risk of cancer in patients with Gaucher's disease has been reported,[22] primarily because of an increased incidence of hematologic malignancy (14.7:1). Table 25-11 lists the most frequently reported hematologic malignancies. This increased risk of malignancy may be associated with immunologic abnormalities found in patients with Gaucher's disease. These abnormalities include increased helper to suppressor (T_4:T_8) cell ratio, de-

TABLE 25-11 Most Frequently Reported Hematologic Malignancies in Gaucher's Disease
Multiple myeloma
CLL (chronic lymphocytic leukemia)
Hodgkin's disease and non-Hodgkin's lymphoma
Acute leukemia

creased natural killer (null) cells, polyclonal B cell lymphocytosis, and plasmacytosis.[22] Table 25-12 lists the immunologic abnormalities described in Gaucher's disease.

Treatment

Before the advent of the newer treatment modality of enzyme replacement therapy, Gaucher's disease was traditionally managed by supportive therapy. Total or partial splenectomy was frequently performed. In addition, transfusions, orthopedic procedures, and occasionally bone marrow transplantation were used in some patients. Although potentially curative, allogeneic bone marrow transplantation (BMT) is an extremely aggressive and high-risk therapy. In 1991, a major advancement occurred in the treatment of Gaucher's disease type I. The United States Food and Drug Administration approved the use of enzyme replacement therapy for this disorder. Gaucher's disease is the first lysosomal storage disorder for which enzyme replacement therapy is available. Enzyme replacement therapy has successfully reversed many of the clinical complications of this disorder, including correcting blood counts and reducing the organomegaly that occurs in these patients.[23-27]

The first enzyme replacement therapy utilized was a purified enzyme from human placenta. This enzyme, which is an alglucerase injection, is manufactured by Genzyme Corporation as Ceredase and has demonstrated effectiveness by the reversal of signs and symptoms of Gaucher type I, nonneuronopathic disease.[28] Another form of the enzyme, the recombinant form, which is also produced by Genzyme Corporation as Cerezyme, is genetically engineered and has the advantage of being unlimited in supply. In addition, the recombinant Cerezyme has the advantage of a very low risk of transmitting any infectious agent and also has a lower rate of patients developing IgG antibodies to the glucocerebrosidase enzyme.[28]

Niemann-Pick Disease

This inherited form of lipid storage disease was first described in 1914 by Niemann and subsequently by Pick in 1933.[29]

Niemann-Pick disease is caused by a deficiency of the enzyme sphingomyelinase with a secondary accumulation of the unmetabolized lipid sphingomyelin as well as cholesterol. Sphingomyelin is a sphingophospholipid that is a common constituent of cell membranes as well as cellular organelles. As a result, a deficiency of sphingomyelinase is a serious disorder. Table 25-13 summarizes the general characteristics of

TABLE 25–13 General Characteristics of Niemann-Pick Disease

Inherited lipid storage disease
Caused by a deficiency of the enzyme sphingomyelinase
Niemann-Pick cells (lipid-laden giant foam cells) found in
    BM aspirate, tissues, and organs
Increased incidence in the Jewish population
Five types A to E have been described
Wide variety of clinical manifestations

Niemann-Pick disease. A wide variety of clinical manifestations of variable severity have been reported in patients with Niemann-Pick disease. These include growth retardation, hepatosplenomegaly, lymphadenopathy, pigmentation, and impaired neurologic functions (Table 25–14).[30] A large number of lipid-laden giant foam cells known as Niemann-Pick cells can be found in affected tissues and organs (Fig. 25–4). The detection of Niemann-Pick cells in patients with this disorder is essential for the diagnosis of this disease. There is an increased incidence of Niemann-Pick disease in the Jewish population, especially in consanguinous groups. Because of the very different clinical manifestations of the disease, five types, A through E have been described.[31] Only types A, B, and C will be discussed. Type E, which is very rare, has been found only in adults and is characterized by a mild chronic course and a lack of neurologic manifestations. Table 25–15 compares types A, B, and C of Niemann-Pick disease.

Classification and Clinical Features

Type A This form is also known as infantile or classic Niemann-Pick disease. It is the most common form, accounting for up to 85% of all cases of Niemann-Pick disease. The onset is early in infancy and is associated with failure to thrive, difficulty feeding, and retarded physical and mental development. The skin has a waxy consistency. There is often jaundice at birth and usually hepatosplenomegaly with a distended abdomen. The lymph nodes are enlarged as well. A cherry-red spot in the macula of the eye is found in approximately 50% of the affected infants. The neurologic symptoms are more pronounced in this type of Niemann-Pick disease than in any of the other types. Deterioration is rapid, and survival past the age of 1 or 2 years is rare.

Type B Also called the chronic or adult form, this type of Niemann-Pick disease is much more rare than type A, with approximately 20 reported cases in the literature. Clinical onset consisting of hepatospleno-

TABLE 25–14 Clinical Manifestations of Niemann-Pick Disease

Growth retardation
Hepatosplenomegaly
Lymphadenopathy
Pigmentation
Neurologic impairment

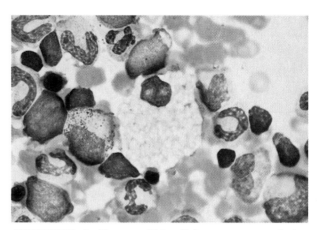

FIGURE 25–4 Niemann-Pick cell, bone marrow aspirate.

megaly is usually found in infancy, but the central nervous system is not involved. Individuals with this type of disease may live longer than those with type A, but they do not survive beyond childhood or early adolescence.

Type C Type C Niemann-Pick disease has been described in two forms, an infantile or juvenile form with a prolonged life span, and an adolescent or adulthood form, which is generally slower in evolution and progression.[32] The primary defect in type C Niemann-Pick disease still remains unknown. However, it is characterized by a milder defect in sphingomyelinase activity and an abnormality in cholesterol transport reflected in an alteration in cholesterol esterification from exogenous cholesterol. Type C Niemann-Pick disease is an autosomal-recessive disease characterized by a gradual and ill-defined onset of neurologic abnormalities, which include unsteady gait, poor motor coordination, slurred speech, dysphagia, and ophthalmoplegia.[31] When neurologic symptoms appear, psychotic manifestations may also be predominant. Neuro-ophthalmologic findings in which the oculomotor system is often affected are also characteristic. In addition, seizures often appear with neurologic involvement, with grand mal seizures most frequently observed. Frequent seizures may contribute to the mental deterioration observed in patients with type C Niemann-Pick disease. Hepatosplenomegaly is a constant finding in the infantile or juvenile form, whereas hepatomegaly is often absent in the adult form. Splenomegaly, however, is present in the adult form, with thrombocytopenia being a sign of hypersplenism. The characteristic foam cell, Niemann-Pick cell, and/or sea-blue histiocytes are a consistent finding in the bone marrow of patients with type C Niemann-Pick disease. Diagnosis of type C Niemann-Pick disease is made with the finding of the characteristic abnormality in cholesterol transport and esterification from exogenous cholesterol.

Laboratory Diagnosis

There is a distinct pattern to the histiocytes in Niemann-Pick disease. These cells are most commonly seen in bone marrow and spleen, although they ac-

TABLE 25-15	Comparison of Types A, B, and C Niemann-Pick Disease		
Classification	**Type A, Infantile or Classic**	**Type B, Chronic or Adult**	**Type C, Two Forms: Infantile or Juvenile Form and Adolescent or Adult Form**
Incidence	Accounts for 85% of all cases	Rare	Rare
Clinical manifestations	Jaundice at birth, hepatosplenomegaly, enlarged lymph nodes, cherry-red spot in macula of the eye, neurologic symptoms, retarded physical and mental development	Hepatosplenomegaly	Hepatosplenomegaly in infantile form, splenomegaly in the adult form, neurologic abnormalities, neuro-ophthalmologic findings, seizures
Survival	1–2 yrs	Childhood or early adolescence	Juvenile or adulthood

cumulate throughout the body and in the nervous system in patients with type A disease. They are large cells, 20 to 90 μm in diameter, with an inconspicuous nucleus. The cytoplasm is filled with and distended by round, uniformly sized droplets of accumulated lipid, turning the cell a very pale or light blue when Wright-stained (see Fig. 25–4). Stains producing a positive reaction with Niemann-Pick cells are the lipid stains oil red O, Sudan black, and luxol fast blue; and acid phosphatase and nonspecific esterase. The PAS staining is weak, and the myeloperoxidase stain is negative.

The bone marrow of some adult patients with certain varieties of Niemann-Pick disease contains a mixture of Niemann-Pick cells and sea-blue histiocytes (histiocytes distended with blue-staining ceroid on Wright's stain). It is believed that the sphingomyelin is gradually metabolized to ceroid, thus generating the sea-blue histiocytes. A marrow specimen with these findings would then need to be distinguished from the entity of sea-blue histiocytosis (see section at the end of this chapter).

Other disorders that may cause Niemann-Pick-like cells in the bone marrow are GM_1 gangliosidosis, lactosyl ceramidosis, and Fabry's disease.

The peripheral blood is most remarkable for the vacuoles that may be found in lymphocytes and monocytes of a routine peripheral blood smear (Fig. 25–5). These vacuoles are round, and from 2 to 20 may be found within one cell. Anemia and leukopenia may be present but do not usually present any threat to the patient. Serum lipids are not usually increased. An assay of the enzyme sphingomyelinase activity in leukocytes and fibroblasts can also be performed.

Prognosis and Treatment

There may be a slightly longer survival in patients with the other types of Niemann-Pick disease, but those with type A have a very short life expectancy. Survival past the age of 2 years is uncommon. Currently there is no treatment for Niemann-Pick disease. However, successful allogeneic bone marrow transplants have been reported for type B.[18] In addition, research studies have focused on finding a source of enzyme replacement for sphingomyelinase[33] and gene therapy using retroviruses.[34]

Tay-Sachs Disease

Also known as GM_2 gangliosidosis, Tay-Sachs disease was first described in 1881 by the British ophthalmologist Warren Tay. In 1886, the New York neurologist Bernard Sachs used the term *familial amaurotic infantile idiocy* to describe this disorder. Its incidence in the Ashkenazi Jewish population is 100 times greater than that in the non-Jewish population.[35] It is estimated that this high-risk group has a 1 in 30 carrier rate. This autosomal-recessive sphingolipidosis is the result of a deficiency of the enzyme hexosaminidase A, with an increase of the other isoenzyme, hexosaminidase B. The gene for hexosaminidase A is located on chromosome 15.[35] Inheritance of two abnormal alleles (one from each parent) accounts for almost all infantile Tay-Sachs cases in the Ashkenazi Jewish population. The severity of the disease correlates with the level of residual enzyme activity. The unmetabolized GM_2 ganglioside accumulates in almost all tissues and has its most devastating effects within the central nervous system and eye.[36] Table 25–16 summarizes the general characteristics of Tay-Sachs disease.[37]

Clinical Features

Although affected infants appear normal at birth, by 6 months of age both physical and mental deteriora-

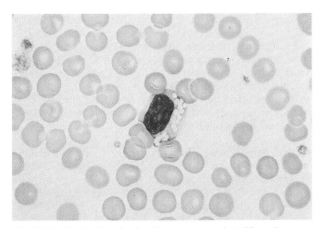

FIGURE 25-5 Tay-Sachs disease, vacuolated lymphocytes (also characteristic of Niemann-Pick disease).

TABLE 25–16 General Characteristics of Tay-Sachs Disease

Known as GM$_2$ gangliosidosis
Inherited autosomal recessively
Caused by a deficiency of hexosaminidase A
Higher incidence in Ashkenazi Jewish population
CNS degeneration
Physical and mental deterioration
Cherry-red spot in the macula of each eye
Macrocephaly (enlargement of head)
Seizures and paralysis
Death by 4 years old

tion are notable. They have an exaggerated physical response to noise (the startle reflex) beginning at age 3 to 5 months. There is a progressive loss of motor function with weakness, decreased attentiveness to surroundings, hypotonia (diminished tone of skeletal muscles), and poor head control between the ages of 6 and 10 months.[37] In addition, a cherry-red spot in the macula of each eye is found; this is the most characteristic feature of Tay-Sachs disease. The central nervous system steadily degenerates after 1 year of age. Along with the continual deterioration, there is enlargement of the head (macrocephaly), seizures, and paralysis. Spasticity with hyperactive reflexes, deafness, and blindness follow. The neurons are greatly enlarged by accumulation of the unmetabolized ganglioside in vacuoles in the cytoplasm. In contrast to many other lipid storage diseases, the spleen, liver, and lymph nodes are *not* enlarged. Feeding is poor, and death occurs by 4 years of age. It should be noted that cherry-red spots are not pathognomonic for Tay-Sachs disease; however, this clinical finding in a Jewish infant with the absence of organomegaly is strongly suggestive of Tay-Sachs disease.[36]

Variant forms of GM$_2$ gangliosidoses are known. Although these variant forms are less common than infantile Tay-Sachs, they still occur most frequently among the Ashkenazi Jews. These forms are commonly referred to as juvenile and adult (chronic) onset. These patients have physical disabilities related to the cerebellum and neurons controlling motor functions. Functions of intelligence vary considerably, but may be less severely affected in the adult form. Survival is quite variable.

Laboratory Diagnosis

A deficiency of hexosaminidase A is the basic cause of this disease. Hexosaminidase A is the enzyme responsible for hydrolyzing GM$_2$ ganglioside, the glycolipid that accumulates in neurons. This deficiency can be demonstrated in the serum, plasma, leukocytes, and cultured fibroblasts of infants with Tay-Sachs disease.

The major site of pathology is in the central nervous system, and examination of other tissues is less informative. The peripheral blood contains vacuolated lymphocytes (see Fig. 25–5). The number and size of the vacuoles are related to the duration of the disease. It is postulated, but not definitely proven, that they con-

tain the unmetabolized lipid GM$_2$ ganglioside. Vacuolated lymphocytes, however, are not pathognomonic for Tay-Sachs disease, as they are also seen in Niemann-Pick disease and in certain types of leukemias. Foam cells, or vacuolated histiocytes, are found in the bone marrow. The presence of these cells is helpful but not diagnostic for the disease.

Because of the high frequency of this disease in certain populations, prenatal detection has taken on greater importance. Culture of fetal fibroblasts from the amniotic fluid can be undertaken to detect hexosaminidase A levels in the fetus. Mass screening programs of adults at possible risk for transmitting the disease have been undertaken, with variable success.

The ability to examine the messenger ribonucleic acid (mRNA) and DNA in patients with noninfantile forms of Tay-Sachs, using the molecular techniques of RNAase detection assays and PCR, has pinpointed the defect to an amino acid substitution in the α-subunit of the β-hexosaminidase enzyme.[38] These results will undoubtedly be incorporated into genetic counseling for families.

Prognosis and Treatment

The infantile form of Tay-Sachs disease is uniformly fatal before age 4. Enzyme replacement is now being attempted, and the final results of the potential therapy are not yet known. Patients with the juvenile and adult forms of Tay-Sachs disease have longer survival than those with the infantile form, although it is quite variable. Supportive treatment remains the mainstay of this disorder, which includes management of hydration, recurrent infections, and seizures with conventional fluids, antibiotics, and drugs, respectively. Prenatal diagnosis can be performed by measuring hexosaminidase A in amniotic fluid, cultured amniocytes, or chorionic villus samples.

Mucopolysaccharidoses

The mucopolysaccharidoses (MPSs) are rare disorders that constitute a group of lysosomal storage diseases caused by a deficiency in one of the enzymes involved in the breakdown of mucopolysaccharides.[39]

Like the previously described disorders, the MPSs show accumulations of unmetabolized material within lysosomes (Fig. 25–6); however, it is mucopolysaccharides, not sphingolipids, that accumulate. Products are found in the reticuloendothelial system (spleen, bone marrow, liver), lymph nodes, blood vessels, brain, heart, connective tissue, and urine. The clinical severity of these disorders varies widely, with mild, intermediate, and severe forms. Multiple clinical presentations exist, including skeletal abnormalities, organomegaly, facial dysmorphism, and corneal opacities.

The original description of children affected with different forms of the MPSs was published within a relatively short time span at the turn of the century. In London in 1900, Dr. John Thompson first described three young brothers with the characteristics of MPS. Gertrud Hurler elaborated on his description, describing two unrelated boys in Munich in 1919 with very similar characteristics, now known as Hurler's syn-

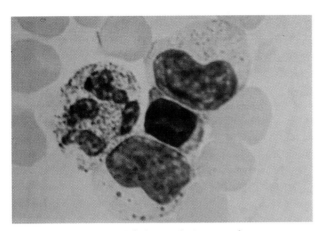

FIGURE 25-6 Hurler's anomaly.

drome. In 1917, Hunter described two brothers with a constellation of abnormalities now recognized as Hunter's syndrome. Table 25–17 summarizes the general characteristics of MPSs.

Classification

The MPSs have been arranged into seven categories, but there are only four possible unmetabolized products that build up in tissues: keratan sulfate, dermatan sulfate, heparan sulfate, and chondroitin sulfate. Table 25–18 gives an abbreviated classification scheme for MPSs.[39] With the exception of Hunter's syndrome, which is X-linked recessive, these disorders have an autosomal-recessive mode of inheritance. There does not appear to be a significant increase of affected individuals within any one ethnic group.

In terms of the biochemical classification of MPS, very different clinical phenotypes can result from different mutations at the same locus. Characterization of these mutations showed deletions for MPS I, II, and III and point mutation for MPS IV.[40]

For example, in MPS I H (Hurler's disease) and in MPS I S (Scheie's syndrome), mutations at the same locus of the enzyme α-iduronidase occur for both disorders, producing quite different clinical phenotypes.[41] In Hurler's disease, there is a progressive mental and physical deterioration, with death occurring usually in the first decade of life. This is in contrast to the course in Scheie's disease, in which the condition is milder, intellect is normal into adult life, and life expectancy is normal. The presence of many different mutations at the α-iduronidase enzyme locus that may be inherited in either the homozygous or het-

erozygous state accounts for the wide variation in clinical phenotypes. The use of molecular probes to characterize these mutations will eventually allow correlations to be made between mutations and phenotypes.

Clinical Features

Many clinical abnormalities are found within each type of MPS, and there are seven categories of MPS; therefore a detailed description of each is not possible in this chapter. Profound mental retardation is found in MPS I H (Hurler's syndrome), MPS II (the severe form of Hunter's syndrome), and MPS III (all four subtypes of Sanfilippo syndrome). Normal intelligence is maintained in MPS I S (Scheie's syndrome), MPS IV (Morquiois syndrome), and MPS VI (Maroteaux-Lamy syndrome).[39] The findings in Hurler's syndrome will be given in the most detail, because it is considered the prototype of the MPSs.

In patients with Hurler's syndrome (MPS I), there may be a short period of apparently normal development, but this is only temporary. These individuals are abnormally short and have coarse facial features, with a broad, flat nose, widely spaced eyes, and thickened tongue and lips.[42] Some authors have described their appearance as similar to that of a gargoyle (the carved heads sometimes found on older European churches). The amount of body hair is increased, dark, and especially prominent on the forehead. The skin is thickened. Patients are mentally retarded. Clouding of the corneas of the eyes is present. These individuals may have hearing loss or be completely deaf. The heart is damaged, owing to the accumulation of mucopolysaccharides in the valves and blood vessels. There is a hump on the back and a prominent abdomen, with enlarged liver and spleen. The arms and legs are abnormal, with contractures of many joints. In addition, the hands are very wide and the fingers shortened.

In Hunter's syndrome (MPS II), the changes are similar, although not as severe. Corneal clouding is much less common. Patients affected with Sanfilippo's syndrome (MPS III) have a more normal stature but unfortunately many more severe neurologic problems and decreased survival. Compared with patients with Hurler's syndrome, those with Scheie's syndrome (MPS I S) have more prominent corneal clouding but less abnormality in stature, facial appearance, and mental development. Patients with Maroteaux-Lamy syndrome (MPS VI) have growth and skeletal abnormalities but no mental retardation. In Morquio's syndrome (MPS IV), patients have numerous skeletal changes, giving a markedly abnormal physical appearance; however, there is no mental retardation.[39]

Laboratory Diagnosis

An accurate enzymatic diagnosis should be established for all suspected cases of MPS, since clinical diagnosis alone is often impossible because of overlapping phenotypes. The diagnosis of MPS can be made by performing simple enzyme assays using leukocytes, serum, or fibroblasts.[43] The identification of heterozygotes, however, is still a difficult process because of the overlays of normal and heterozygous levels of en-

---

TABLE 25-17 **General Characteristics of Mucopolysaccharidoses**
Rare lyosomal storage disease
Autosomal recessive inheritance
Deficiency of one of the enzymes involved in the breakdown of mucopolysaccharides
Panethnicity
Different clinical phenotypes resulting from different mutations at the same locus

TABLE 25–18	**Mucopolysaccharidoses (MPSs)**				
Category	Mode of Inheritance	Accumulated Product	Enzyme Deficiency	Clinical Features	Life Expectancy
MPS I H (Hurler's)	Autosomal recessive	Heparan sulfate Dermatan sulfate	α-L-iduronidase	Onset 6-8 months, severe mental retardation, dwarfism, large long head, flat broad nose with upturned nostrils (coarse facies), corneal clouding, hepatosplenomegaly, valvular lesions, coronary artery lesions, skeletal deformities, joint stiffness	6–10 yr
MPS I S (Scheie's)	Autosomal recessive	Heparan sulfate Dermatan sulfate	α-L-iduronidase	Onset after 5 yr, normal intelligence, stiff joints (especially of the hands), near normal height, corneal clouding, valvular lesion, coronary artery lesions	Normal
MPS I H-S (Hurler-Scheie)	Autosomal recessive	Heparan sulfate Dermatan sulfate	α-L-iduronidase	Onset infancy, mild retardation (may be normal), dwarfism, facial and bony lesions of Hurler's syndrome, cardiac lesions	3rd decade
MPS II (Hunter) (wide range of severity)	X-linked recessive	Heparan sulfate Dermatan sulfate	Iduronate α-sulfatase	Mild retardation to normal intelligence, similar to Hurler's syndrome, but no corneal clouding, retinal degeneration, deafness, nodular skin infiltrates	2nd decade to normal
MPS III (Sanfilippo's A) (Sanfilippo's B) (Sanfilippo's C) (wide range of severity)	Autosomal recessive	Heparan sulfate	Heparan N-sulphatase α-N-Acetylglucosaminidase Acetyl-CoA: α-glucosaminide N-acetyltransferase	Onset after 3 yr, mild to severe mental retardation, normal growth, Hurler facies, no corneal clouding, no heart disease, no hepatosplenomegaly, mild skeletal changes	2nd-3rd decade
MPS IV A (Morquio's) (wide range of severity)	Autosomal recessive	Keratan sulfate Chondroitin sulfate	N-Acetylgalactosamine 6-sulphate sulphatase	Normal intelligence, severe skeletal deformities, dwarfism, thoracolumbar gibbus, kyphoscoliosis, facies similar to Hurler's syndrome, corneal clouding, valvular and coronary artery lesions, joint hypermobility, genu valgum	3rd-6th decade
MPS IVB (Morquio's)			β-Galactosidase		
MPS VI (Maroteaux-Lamy)	Autosomal recessive	Dermatan sulfate	N-Acetylgalactosamine 4-sulphate sulphatase (arylsulphatase B)	Similar to Hurler's syndrome, but normal intelligence, longer survival	2nd decade

TABLE 25-18 **Mucopolysaccharidoses (MPSs)** (*Continued*)					
Category	Mode of Inheritance	Accumulated Product	Enzyme Deficiency	Clinical Features	Life Expectancy
MPS VII (Glucuronidase deficiency disease)	Autosomal recessive	Dermatan sulfate Heparan sulfate Chondroitin sulfate	β-Glucuronidase	Variable from severe mental retardation with dysostosis multiplex and hepatosplenomegaly to a milder form; also severe neonatal form with hydrops fetalis	Variable, 1–40 Yr

Source: Modified from Fensom and Benson,[42] pp 2–3.

zyme activity. Molecular studies such as the cloning of complementary DNAs (cDNAs) can complement accurate enzyme assays.[43]

Several specialized substrates used for the diagnosis of MPS are now available commercially. In addition, several new assays have been described for the diagnosis of MPS. These include a photometric test for MPS III D,[44] a fluorometric test for MPS III B[45] and MPS IV A,[46] a sensitive test for MPS VI using radiolabeled oligosaccharides,[47] and the use of a monoclonal antibody for the diagnosis of MPS VI.[48]

In contrast to findings in the other lysosomal storage diseases, nonmetabolized products may be detected in the urine of patients with MPS.[42] Using the toluidine blue spot test or the turbidity test to detect acid mucopolysaccharides is the initial screening test. The spot test may be unreliable, however, with up to 32% false-negative test results in patients with Hurler's syndrome reported. Also of note is that the urine of normal healthy newborn infants may give false-positive results, a phenomenon that disappears by 2 weeks of age. Any positive screening test result should be confirmed by lysosomal enzyme assays.

An interesting but somewhat inconsistent finding in the MPS in the peripheral blood is the presence of large granules in leukocytes, especially lymphocytes. These are known as Alder-Reilly bodies (see Fig. 16–11). In polymorphonuclear leukocytes this needs to be distinguished from toxic granulation, but the large size of the granules in MPS usually leaves little doubt. A metachromatic stain, such as toluidine blue, will aid in confirmation. These granules are found with much greater regularity, however, in histiocytes and lymphocytes in the bone marrow.

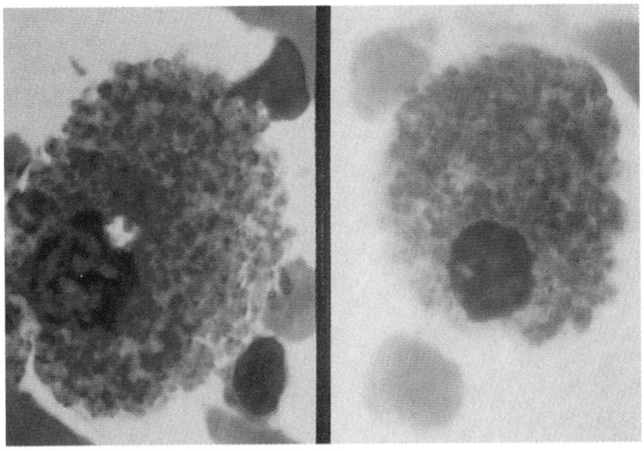

Prognosis

The prognosis of the MPS varies somewhat with the type. Patients with Hurler's syndrome may live only one decade, whereas those affected with Hunter's syndrome may live into their 20s.[42] The theoretical aid of enzyme replacement therapy has yet to be translated into practical results.

Treatment

Bone marrow transplantation (BMT) has been used successfully in treating some patients with MPS.[49] More studies are needed, however, to prove that BMT can be a practical treatment leading to a complete cure. Prenatal diagnosis is still important, including first-trimester diagnosis by chorionic villus sampling, early amniocentesis for more sensitive lysosomal enzyme assays, the use of DNA analysis for detecting mutations, and the possibility of preimplantation diagnosis of early embryos after in vitro fertilization.

HISTIOCYTOSES

Sea-Blue Histiocyte Syndrome

Although initially described in isolated case reports of young adults with an enlarged spleen, the syndrome

FIGURE 25–7 Sea-blue histiocytes. Note the abnormally coarse azurophilic granules present in neutrophils, lymphocytes, and monocytes. (From Hyun, BH, Ashton, JK, and Dolan, K: Bone marrow. In Practical Hematology. A Laboratory Guide with Accompanying Filmstrip. WB Saunders, Philadelphia, 1975, with permission.)

TABLE 25-19 **General Characteristics of Sea-Blue Histiocytosis**
Autosomal-recessive benign genetic disorder Striking blue histiocytes with Wright's stain Splenomegaly and hepatomegaly Thrombocytopenia

TABLE 25–20 Characteristics of Histiocytic Disorder

Disease	Age at Onset	Main Site(s) of Involvement	Disease
Eosinophilic granuloma	Children and young adults, especially males, often no symptoms until bone fracture	Unifocal—skull, rib, femur most common	Rare spontaneous healing; most require surgical removal; occasional patients develop recurrence later
Hand-Schüller-Christian disease	Usually <5 yr old	Multifocal—bones, skin, lymphoid tissue; triad of pituitary, eye, and skull involvement is characteristic but uncommon	50%: spontaneous recovery 50%: recovery with chemotherapy
Letterer-Siwe disease	Usually <3 yr old	Generalized—skin, lymphoid tissue, bones, +/− bone marrow; more severe and extensive than Hand-Schüller-Christian disease	Chemotherapy has improved prognosis, which was previously considered poor

of the sea-blue histiocyte is a genetic disorder with a benign course. The striking blue color of the histiocytes after staining with Wright's or May-Grünwald-Giemsa stain gives the syndrome its name.

The mode of transmission has not been clearly established, but autosomal-recessive inheritance, with a variable degree of expression, appears most likely. Most patients receive the diagnosis before they reach 40 years of age. The earlier in life the disease is found, the more severe it is likely to be. Major findings on physical examination are splenomegaly and usually hepatomegaly. Also described, but occurring less consistently, are abnormalities of the eyes, skin, and nervous system. Involvement of the lung may be noted on radiographic examination. Involvement of the lymph nodes is not seen.

Significant laboratory findings are usually confined to the blood. In the peripheral blood, thrombocytopenia is found with great frequency. Consequently, clinical manifestations such as epistaxis, gastrointestinal tract bleeding, and purpura may be expected. However, there is no correlation of the degree of thrombocytopenia with the size of the spleen. Blood lipid levels are normal. Abnormal liver function study results are only rarely seen.

The bone marrow aspirate is usually the site of diagnosis. Histiocytes of variable size (20 to 60 μm) are present in greatly increased numbers. They contain the blue-to-green staining granules that vary in size, shape, and ability to take up the stain (Fig. 25–7). Thus, not all cells will have the same staining intensity. It is not currently known why the granules stain blue with these stains. The cells will also react with the PAS, Sudan black B, and acid-fast stains, but not with toluidine blue or iron stains.[50]

The great majority of patients with this syndrome do well and have normal life spans. Splenectomy is not always required; many patients never have the spleen removed. As previously mentioned, manifestations of the disease at an early age may imply more severe symptoms. Table 25–19 summarizes the general characteristics of sea-blue histiocytosis.

Other Histiocytic Disorders (Eosinophilic Granuloma, Hand-Schüller-Christian Disease, Letterer-Siwe Disease)

This group of "histiocytic" disorders represents an abnormal proliferation and accumulation of mature histiocytes, or Langerhans' cells. Langerhans' cells are large but inconspicuous cells in the skin whose function is to process and present antigen to other cells in the area, including lymphocytes.[31] These cells, as well as histiocytes, are normally found in small numbers in the skin and reticuloendothelial system (RES). Most patients with these disorders are either children or young adults. A favorable outcome may be expected in most cases, with the exception of Letterer-Siwe disease, which may be fatal. These disorders may actually represent a continuum, from the unifocal and benign eosinophilic granuloma to the generalized and sometimes fatal Letterer-Siwe disease.[31] The term *histiocytosis X* is generally used to describe these disorders. Table 25–20 summarizes the major characteristics of histiocytic disorders.

CASE STUDY

A 32-year-old man visited his doctor complaining of pain in his forearms and fatigue. Physical examination revealed an enlarged spleen (2 cm) and multiple bruises down the patient's forearms. His physician ordered the following laboratory workup:

RBC count	3.1×10^{12}/L
WBC count	4.9×10^{9}/L
Hemoglobin	11.0 g/dL
Hematocrit	32%
MCV	92 fL
MCHC	31%
Reticulocytes	0.4%

Differential:

Segmented neutrophils	52%
Lymphocytes	41%
Monocytes	4%
Bands	3%

A bone marrow aspiration was performed at the left posterior iliac crest and revealed a histiocytic-appearing cell (see Fig. 25–2). These cells stained positive with PAS, Sudan black B, and Prussian blue.

Questions

1. This case history is representative of what lipid storage disease?
2. What further testing must be done to confirm diagnosis?
3. Is "effective erythropoiesis" apparent in this case? Why or why not?
4. Classify the anemia according to the RBC indices.
5. What treatment is available to this patient?

REFERENCES

1. Barranger, JA (ed): Gaucher Clinical Perspectives 4(1):1, 1996.
2. Gaines, BA and Idstad, ST: Mixed chimerism and Gaucher disease. Gaucher Clinical Perspectives 3(3):5, 1995
3. Desnick, RJ: Gaucher disease (1882–1982): Centennial perspectives on the most prevalent Jewish genetic disease. Mt Sinai J Med 49:443, 1982.
4. Barton, NW, Brady, RO, Dambrosia, JM, et al: Replacement therapy for inherited enzyme deficiency: macrophage-targeted glucocerebrosidase for Gaucher's disease. N Engl J Med 324:1464, 1991.
5. Pastores, GM, Sibille, AR, and Grabowski, GA: Enzyme therapy for Gaucher disease type 1: Dosage efficacy and adverse effects in 33 patients treated for 6 to 24 months. Blood 82:408, 1993.
6. Erikson, A, Johannson, K, Mansson, JE, et al: Enzyme replacement therapy of infantile Gaucher disease. Neuropediatrics 24:237, 1993.
7. Bembi, B, Zanatta, M, Carrozzi, M, et al: Enzyme replacement treatment in type 1 and type 3 Gaucher's disease. Lancet 344:1679, 1994.
8. Brady, RO, O'Neill, RR, and Barton, NW: Glucosylceramide lipidosis: Gaucher disease. In Rosenberg, RN, Prusiner, SB, DiMauro, S, et al (eds): The Molecular and Genetics Basis of Neurological Disease. Stoneham, MA, Butterworths, 1993, pp 467–484.
9. Hermann, G, Goldblatt, J, Levy, RN, et al: Gaucher's disease type 1: Assessment of bone involvement by CT and scintigraphy. Am J Roentgenol 147:943, 1986.
10. Grewal, RP, Doppelt, SH, Thompson, MA, et al: Neurologic complications of nonneuronopathic Gaucher disease. Arch Neurol 48:1271, 1991.
11. Grace, ME, et al: Analysis of human acid beta-glucosidase by site-directed mutagenesis and heterologous expression. J Biol Chem, 269:2283.
12. Berg-Fusman A, Grace, ME, Ioannou, Y, et al: Human acid beta-glucosidase. N-glycosylation site occupancy and the effect of glycosylation on enzymatic activity. J Biol Chem 268:14861, 1993.
13. Miao, S, McCarter, JD, Grace, ME, et al: Identification of Glu340 as the active-site nucleophile in human glucocerebrosidase by use of electrospray tandem mass spectrometry. J Biol Chem 269:10975, 1991.
14. Sibille, A, Eng, CM, Kim, SJ, et al: Phenotype/genotype correlations in Gaucher disease type I: clinical and therapeutic implications. Am J Hum Genet 52:1094, 1993.
15. Brady, RO, Barton, NW and Grabowski, GA: The role of neurogenetics in Gaucher disease. Arch Neurol 50:1212, 1993.
16. Pastores, GM and Lenz, P: Growth and development in children with Type I Gaucher disease. Gaucher Clinical Perspectives 3(1):1, 1995.
17. Patterson, MC, Horowitz, M, Abel, RB, et al: Isolated horizontal supranuclear gaze palsy as a marker of severe systemic involvement in Gaucher's disease. Neurology 43:1993, 1993.
18. Athens, JW: Disorders involving the monocyte-macrophage system. The storage disease, In Lee, GR (ed): Wintrobe's Clinical Hematology. Lea & Febiger, Philadelphia, 1993, p 1631.
19. Weiler, S, Carson, W, Lee, Y, et al: Synthesis and characterization of a bioactive 82-residue sphingolipid activator protein, saposin C. J Molec Neurosci 4:161, 1993.
20. Beutler, E: Gaucher disease: New molecular approaches to diagnosis and treatment. Science 256:794, 1992.
21. Savage, RA: Specific and not-so-specific histiocytes in bone marrow. Lab Med 15:467, 1984.
22. Shiran, A, Brenner, B, Laor, A, et al: Increased risk of cancer in patients with Gaucher disease. Cancer 72:219, 1993.
23. Grabowski, GA and Pastores, GM: Enzyme replacement therapy in type 1 Gaucher disease. Gaucher Clin Persp 1:8, 1993.
24. Pastores, GM, Sibille, AR, and Grabowski, GA: Enzyme therapy in Gaucher disease type 1: Dosage efficacy and adverse effects in 33 patients treated for 6 to 24 months. Blood 82:408, 1993.
25. Bembi, B, Zanatta, M, Carrozzi, M, et al: Enzyme replacement treatment in type 1 and type 3 Gaucher's disease. Lancet 344:1679, 1994.
26. Richards, SM, Olson, TA, and McPherson, JM: Antibody response in patients with Gaucher disease after repeated infusion with macrophage-targeted glucocerebrosidase. Blood 82:1402, 1993.
27. Gaucher Disease Conference, NIH, Bethesda MD, Feb 27–Mar 1, 1995.
28. Grabowski, GA, Barton, NW, Pastores, G, et al: Enzyme therapy in Gaucher disease type 1: Comparative efficacy of mannose-terminated glucocerebrosidase from natural and recombinant sources. ASH Gaucher Disease, Beyond the Hematologic Parameters. Workshop presented at ASH, Nashville, TN, Dec 2, 1994.
29. Pick, L: Niemann-Pick's disease and other forms of so called xanthomatosis. Am J Med Sci 185:601, 1933.
30. Das, S, Begum, B, and Sen, NN: J Indian Med Assoc 92:1994.
31. Robbins, SL and Cotran, RS: Pathologic Basis of Disease. WB Saunders, Philadelphia, 1994.
32. Turpin, JC, Masson, M, and Baumann, N: Clinical Aspects of Niemann-Pick, Type C Disease in the Adult. Dev Neurosci 13:304, 1991.
33. Bembi, B, Comelli, M, Scaggiante, B, et al: Treatment of sphingomyelinase deficiency by repeated implantations of amniotic epithelial cells. Am J Med Genet 44:427, 1992.
34. Dinur, T, Schuchman, EH, Fibach, E, et al: Toward gene therapy for Niemann-Pick disease (NPD): Separation of retrovirally corrected and noncorrected NPD fibroblasts using a novel fluorescent sphingomyelin. Hum Gene Ther 3:633, 1992.
35. Triggs-Raine, BL, Geigenbaum, ASJ, Natowicz, M, et al: Screening for carriers of Tay-Sachs disease among Ashkenazi Jews. N Engl J Med 323:6, 1990.
36. Robb, RM: Ocular abnormalities in childhood metabolic disease and leukemia. In Nelson, LB, Calhoun, JH and Harley, RD (ed): Pediatric Ophthalmology ed 3. WB Saunders, Philadelphia, 1991, p 468.
37. Sandhoff, K, Conzelmann, E, Neufeld, EF, et al: The GM$_2$ gangliosidoses. In Scriver, CR, Beaudet, AL, Sly, WS, Valle, D (eds): The Metabolic Basis of Inherited Disease, ed 6, McGraw-Hill, New York, 1989, pp 1807–1839.
38. Paw, BH, Kaback, MM, and Neufeld, EF: Molecular basis

of adult-onset and chronic GM_2 gangliosidoses in patients of Ashkenazi Jewish origin: Substitution of serine for glycine at position 269 of the α-subunit of β-hexosaminidase. Proc Nat Acad Sci USA 86:2413, 1989.

39. Di Natale, P, Annella, T, Daniele, A, et al: Biochemical diagnosis of mucopolysaccharidoses: Experience of 297 diagnoses in a 15-year period (1977–1991). J Inher Metab Dis 16:473, 1993.
40. Wicker, G, Prill, V, Brooks, D, et al: Mucopolysaccharidosis VI (Maroteaux-Lamy syndrome). An intermediate clinical phenotype caused by substitution of valine for glycine at position 137 of arylsulfatase B. J Biol Chem 266:21386, 1991.
41. Roubicek, M, Geller, J, and Spranger, J: The clinical spectrum of α-L-iduronidase deficiency. Am J Hum Genet 20:471, 1985.
42. Hopwood, JJ and Morris, C: The mucopolysaccharidoses. Diagnosis, molecular genetics and treatment. Mol Biol Med 7:381, 1990.
43. Fensom, AH and Benson, PF: Recent advances in the prenatal diagnosis of the mucopolysaccharidoses. Prenatal Diagn 14:1, 1994.
44. Nowakowski, RW, Thompson, JN and Taylor, KB: Sanfilippo syndrome, type D. A spectrophotometric assay with prenatal diagnostic potential. Pediatr Res 26:462, 1991.
45. Marsh, J and Fensom, AH: 4-Methylumbelliferyl alpha-N-acetylglucosaminidase activity for diagnosis of Sanfilippo B disease. Clin Genet 27:258, 1985.
46. van Diggelen, OP, Zhao, H, Kleijer, WJ, et al: A fluorimetric enzyme assay for the diagnosis of Morquio disease type A (MPS IV A). Clin Chem Acta 187:131, 1990.
47. Hopwood, JJ, Elliott, H, Muller, VJ, et al: Diagnosis of Maroteauz-Lamy syndrome by the use of radiolabelled oligosaccharides as substrates for the determination of arylsulphatase B activity. Biochem J 234:507, 1986.
48. Brooks, DA, Gibson, GH, McCourt, PAG, et al: A specific fluorogenic assay for N-acetylgalactosamine-4-sulphatase activity using immunoabsorption. J Inher Metab Dis 14:5, 1991.
49. Hoogerbrugge, PM, and Vossen, JMJJ: Bone marrow transplantation in the treatment of lysosomal storage disease. In Fernandes, J, Saudubray, JM, and Tada, K (eds): Inborn Metabolic Diseases. Diagnosis and Treatment. Berlin, Springer-Verlag, 1990, pp 659–670.
50. Henry, JB: Clinical Diagnosis and Management by Laboratory Methods. WB Saunders, Philadelphia, 1990, p 454.

QUESTIONS

1. What defect is found in lipid storage diseases?
   a. Subcellular accumulation of unmetabolized material in lysosomes
   b. Cellular accumulation of metabolites in cytoplasm
   c. Protein accumulation in cellular mitochondria
   d. Abnormal sequestration of minerals and trace elements in cellular nuclear organelles

2. What is the enzyme deficiency seen in Gaucher's disease?
   a. Sphingomyelinase
   b. Hexosaminidase A
   c. β-Glucocerebrosidase
   d. α-Galactosidase

3. Which description best characterizes type I Gaucher's disease?
   a. Found in any ethnic group, multiple neurologic signs including difficulty in swallowing and manifestations involving brain stem, enlargement of liver and spleen
   b. Found primarily in Ashkenazi Jews, enlargement of liver and spleen, anemia, thrombocytopenia
   c. Found in northern Sweden, neurologic disorders, bone disorders, skin pigment changes
   d. Found in Mediterranean; hypermetabolic manifestations; fever, lethargy, poor musculature, bone deformities

4. What are the characteristics of Gaucher's cells?
   a. Atypical lymphocytes with foamy cytoplasm
   b. Hypersegmented neutrophils with Auer's rods
   c. Large, multilobed monocytes with prominent red granules
   d. Histiocytes with blue, folded cytoplasm

5. What is the enzyme deficiency seen in Niemann-Pick disease?
   a. Sphingomyelinase
   b. Hexosaminidase A
   c. β-Glucocerebrosidase
   d. α-Galactosidase

6. What are the characteristics of Niemann-Pick cells?
   a. Atypical lymphocytes with large vacuoles
   b. Cytoplasm filled with lipid droplets, inconspicuous nucleus
   c. Vacuolated histiocytes or foam cells
   d. Lymphocytes with Alder-Reilly bodies

7. What is the enzyme deficiency seen in Tay-Sachs disease?
   a. Sphingomyelinase
   b. Hexosaminidase A
   c. β-Glucocerebrosidase
   d. α-Galactosidase

8. What are the clinical features of Tay-Sachs disease?
   a. Waxy, jaundiced skin; retarded physical and mental development; cherry-red spot in macula of eye
   b. Startle reflex; blindness; macrocephaly; no enlargement of liver, spleen, or lymph nodes
   c. Abnormal facial features; deafness; increased body hair, mental retardation; heart damage; structural deformities
   d. Splenomegaly; hepatomegaly; eye, skin, nervous system, and lung abnormalities

9. Which cell is found in Tay-Sachs disease, but is not considered diagnostic?
   a. Atypical lymphocytes with large vacuoles
   b. Cytoplasm filled with lipid droplets; inconspicuous nucleus
   c. Vacuolated histiocytes or foam cells
   d. Lymphocytes with Alder-Reilly bodies

10. Which cell may be found in MPS disorders?
    a. Large, foamy histiocytes with blue or green granules
    b. Neutrophils with toxic granulation
    c. Neutrophils with Döhle bodies
    d. Lymphocytes with Alder-Reilly bodies

ANSWERS

1. **a** (p 463)
2. **c** (p 464)
3. **b** (p 465)
4. **d** (p 465)
5. **a** (p 469)
6. **b** (p 471)
7. **b** (p 471)
8. **b** (p 472)
9. **c** (p 472)
10. **d** (p 475)

Part IV

HEMOSTASIS AND INTRODUCTION TO THROMBOSIS

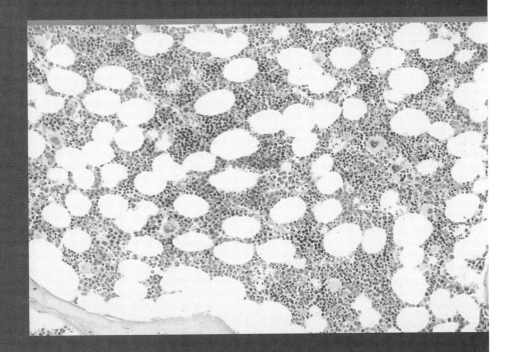

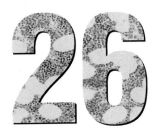

Introduction to Hemostasis

AN OVERVIEW OF HEMOSTATIC MECHANISM, PLATELET STRUCTURE AND FUNCTION, AND EXTRINSIC AND INTRINSIC SYSTEMS

Denise M. Harmening, PhD, MT(ASCP), CLS(NCA)
Linda D. Lemery, MBA, MT(ASCP)DLM

Objectives

At the end of this chapter, the learner should be able to:

1   Define the terms *homeostasis, hemostasis, coagulation, fibrinolysis, petechiae, ecchymosis,* and *hemorrhage.*
2   List the major and minor systems involved in maintaining hemostasis.
3   Describe the events that take place in primary hemostasis.
4   Name the three structural zones of platelets.
5   Describe the composition and functions of the peripheral zone, sol-gel zone, and organelle zone.
6   List steps in platelet plug formation and describe the process of platelet adhesion and aggregation.
7   Describe the events that take place in secondary hemostasis.
8   Name the product responsible for stabilization of the hemostatic plug.
9   List characteristics for the contact coagulation proteins, prothrombin proteins, and fibrinogen group.
10   Define the extrinsic system, intrinsic system, and common pathway.
11   Describe the events that take place in fibrinolysis.
12   Describe the use of the prothrombin time test in monitoring hemostasis.
13   Describe the use of the activated partial thromboplastin time test in monitoring hemostasis.

PLATELETS AND HEMOSTATIC MECHANISMS

Hemostasis is the process by which the body spontaneously stops bleeding and maintains blood in the fluid state within the vascular compartment. Hemostasis contributes to homeostasis by holding the body's tendency toward clotting and bleeding in balance (Fig. 26–1).

Four major systems and three minor systems are involved in maintaining hemostasis (Table 26–1).

The hemostatic mechanisms are designed rapidly to repair any vascular breaks and maintain blood flow within the vessels. However, potential risks are associated with this rapid localized hemostasis: imbalance leads to excessive bleeding or thrombosis. Since the process of hemostasis involves consumption of platelets and coagulation factors, there are also limits to the degree of vascular injury that may be controlled. If the requirements of the vessel breach exceed the capacity of the platelets and coagulation factors for sealing and reinforcement, complications ensue, and a hemostatic balance is not achieved without some form of treatment.

Table 26–2 outlines the structure of the vessel wall, which includes: the outermost layer, or adventitia, the middle layer, or media, and the inner layer, the intima.[1]

In general, the relative importance of the hemostatic mechanisms varies with vessel size (Table 26–3). Generally, the larger the area of bleeding, the larger the vessel involved. Some sources and types of bleeding are listed in Table 26–4. Vessel vasoconstriction is controlled by local, humoral, and neural factors.[2]

Vascular System

The vascular system acts to prevent bleeding by: (1) contraction of vessels (vasoconstriction) and reflex stimulation of adjacent vessels, (2) diversion of blood flow around damaged vasculature, (3) initiation of contact-activation of platelets with subsequent aggregation, and (4) contact-activation of the coagulation sys-

TABLE 26–1 **Systems Involved in Maintaining Hemostasis**	
Major Systems	**Minor Systems**
Vascular system	Kinin system
Platelets	Serine protease inhibitors
Coagulation system	Complement system
Fibrinolytic system	

tem (both extrinsic and intrinsic) leading to fibrin formation (Table 26–5). Vascular integrity, which is influenced by vitamin C intake, is important in maintaining the fluidity of the blood. The blood vessel, with its smooth and continuous endothelial lining and fibrous coat, is designed to facilitate blood flow as well as participate in the process of hemostasis. The endothelial surface of the blood vessel is usually inert to coagulation factors and platelets. It is termed a nonwettable surface in that the physical and chemical characteristics of the endothelium allow a minimum of interaction between blood and the endothelial surface. However, when the endothelial lining is disrupted, underlying collagen and basement membrane are exposed, activating platelets and the plasma coagulation factors. This break in endothelium leads to platelet adhesion (Fig. 26–2) and thrombus formation because the endothelial cells contain adenosine diphosphate (ADP), which is important in inducing aggregation of platelets. In addition, released tissue thromboplastin initiates fibrin formation through the extrinsic pathway of the coagulation system. In response to substances such as ADP, platelet aggregation and degranulation follow, and eventually a thrombus forms. In addition, released tissue thromboplastin initiates fibrin formation through the extrinsic pathway of the coagulation system. Some other substances that bind to endothelial cells and thus play a role in coagulation are listed in Table 26–6.[3] The vascular response involved in the hemostatic mechanisms usually lasts less than 1 minute. Underneath the endothelial layer lies the subendothelium, an extracellular matrix secreted by the endothelial cells.[3] Together the endothelium and/or subendothelium contain some hemostasis-related substances such as collagen and others listed in Table 26–7.

PLATELET STRUCTURE AND FUNCTION

Platelets are intimately involved in primary hemostasis, which is the interaction of platelets and the vascular endothelium in halting bleeding after vascular injury.

As discussed in Chapter 1, platelets are anucleate cellular fragments containing several kinds of granules. Platelets, also called thrombocytes, are derived from the cytoplasm of megakaryocytes present in the bone marrow. Platelets are released and circulate approximately 9 to 12 days as small, disc-shaped cells with an average diameter of 2 to 4 μm. On a Wright-stained peripheral blood smear, platelets appear as

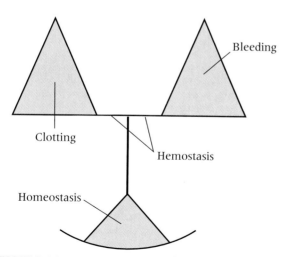

FIGURE 26–1 Hemostasis: a system in balance.

TABLE 26–2   Vessel Layer Composition and Function

Vessel Layer	Composition and Function
Tunica adventitia	Connective tissue cell support
Tunica media	Elastic tissue and smooth muscle, controlling vasoconstriction and sometimes vasodilation
Tunica intima	Broad flat endothelial cells with an underlying basement membrane supported by a few connective tissue cells, providing a smooth nonwettable surface but facilitating migration of cells through the spaces as needed

TABLE 26–3   Vessels and General Breach-Sealing Requirements

Vessel	Relative Sizes	General Breach-Sealing Requirements*
Capillary	Smallest	Generally direct-sealing
Venule		Mostly fused platelets
Arteriole		Mostly fused platelets
Vein		Vascular contraction, fused platelets, perivascular and intravascular hemostatic factor activation
Artery	Largest	Greater vascular contraction, more fused platelets, greater perivascular and intravascular hemostatic factor activation

*In general, the larger the vessel, the more hemostatic system involvement required to seal the breach

TABLE 26–4   Some Sources and Types of Bleeding

Source	Type
Arteriole, venule	Pinpoint petechial hemorrhage (diapedesis or leakage of blood out of small vessels)
Veins	Ecchymosis (large, ill-defined soft tissue bleeding)
Artery	Rapidly expanding "blowout" hemorrhage

TABLE 26–6   Some Substances That Bind to Endothelial Cells

Factor V
Factor IXa
Factor X and Xa
HMWK (high-molecular-weight kininogen)

Source: Reproduced from Jaffe,[3] with permission.

TABLE 26–5   Actions of the Vascular System to Prevent Bleeding

1. Contraction of vessels (vasoconstriction) and reflex stimulation of adjacent vessels
2. Diversion of blood flow around damaged vasculature
3. Initiation of contact activation of platelets with subsequent adhesion, release reaction, and aggregation
4. Contact activation of the coagulation system (both extrinsic and intrinsic) leading to fibrin formation

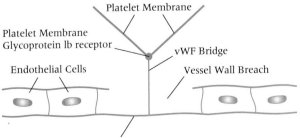

FIGURE 26–2 Platelet adhesion to subendothelium through vWF bridge.

TABLE 26–7 **Some Hemostasis-Related Substances Present in the Endothelium and/or Subendothelium and Some of Their Functions**

Substance(s)	Some Function(s) in Hemostasis
Collagen	Binds to platelet membrane receptor GP Ia/IIa, activates plasma coagulation factors
Mucopolysaccharide	Contains substances such as heparan sulfate that have anticoagulant activity and contribute to activation of antithrombin III
von Willebrand factor	Primarily binds to platelet membrane receptor GP Ib to promote adhesion, may bind to fibronectin, and sometimes binds to GP IIb/IIIa in some conditions such as high shear stress to anchor the platelet to the vessel breach
Fibrinogen and fibrin	Present in healing blood vessel subendothelium (fibrinogen), binds to endothelial cells (fibrinogen/fibrin), eventually reinforces platelet plug
Vitronectin	Present in and binds to endothelial cells, released by activated platelets, probably binds to platelet GP IIb/IIIa, helps endothelial cells bind to the substratum
Tissue thromboplastin	Activates factor VII with ionized calcium (extrinsic pathway)
Factor V	Plays a role in prothrombin activation; synthesized both by endothelial cells and hepatocytes
Thrombomodulin	Binds thrombin, facilitating the activation of protein C in the presence of free protein S
Fibronectin	May function as an adhesive protein for platelets, promoting spreading
Laminin	May function as an adhesive protein for platelet, but does not promote spreading

Source: Adapted from Jaffe[3] and Bennett and Shattil.[7]

round or oval granular purple dots. The platelet's typical stained morphology consists of a clear zone of cytoplasm, termed *hyalomere*, that surrounds a highly stained granulomere (Fig. 26–3).

The normal platelet count ranges from 130,000 to 400,000 per microliter (µL) depending on the methodology employed. Normal platelet function in vivo and in vitro requires more than 100,000 platelets per microliter.[2] It is unusual for a patient with a platelet count greater than 20,000 per microliter to have major hemorrhages. Assuming normal platelet function, a platelet count greater than 50,000/µL will minimize the chance of hemorrhage during surgery.

In the peripheral blood, approximately 30% of the platelets are sequestered in the microvasculature or spleen as functional reserves after their release from the bone marrow. It is possible that newer and larger platelets travel more slowly through the spleen, adhering to splenic cord reticular cells and endothelial cells present in the sinuses, resulting in splenic pooling. Aged or nonviable platelets are removed by both spleen and liver.

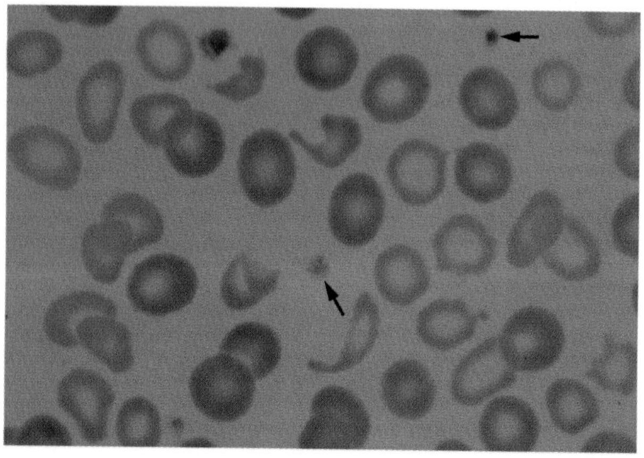

Though platelets are anuclear cytoplasmic fragments, they contain a number of interesting organelles, which are listed in Figure 26–4.

Platelet Structure

The platelet structure is quite distinct, leading to subdivision into three defined zones that possess unique functional capabilities. Table 26–8 summarizes the three described zones and their contents. These zones are prominently delineated by the circumferential band of microtubules found in the platelet (Fig. 26–5).

Peripheral Zone

The peripheral zone is a complex region of the platelet consisting of the glycocalyx (an amorphous exterior coat), platelet membrane, numerous deeply penetrating surface-connecting channels known as the *open canalicular system* (OCS), and a submembranous area of specialized microfilaments.

The glycocalyx intimately surrounds the platelet and is considered an important component of the platelet membrane. A number of glycoproteins present in this area are responsible for blood group specificity (ABO), tissue compatibility (human leukocyte antigen [HLA]), and platelet antigenicity. Platelet membrane glycopro-

FIGURE 26–3 Normal platelets; Wright-stained blood smear (peripheral blood).

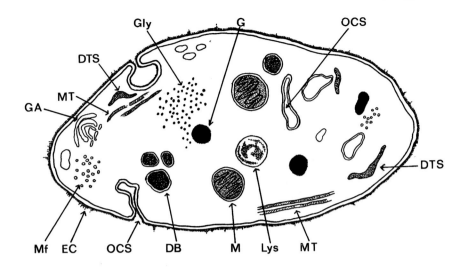

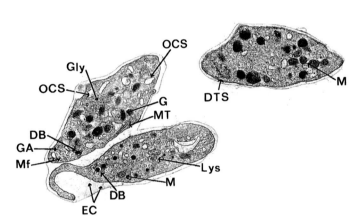

MT —— Microtubules

G —— Other Granules

DB —— Dense Bodies

DTS —— Dense Tubular System

M —— Mitochondria

Gly —— Glycogen Lakes (particles)

Lys —— Lysosomes

OCS —— Open Canalicular System

Mf —— Microfilaments

EC —— Exterior Coat (Glycocalyx)

GA —— Golgi Apparatus

FIGURE 26–4   Discoid platelets; (*Top*) summary diagram of the platelet organelles; (*Bottom*) transmission electron micrograph (TEM) of cross-sectioned platelets illustrating basic ultrastructure.

TABLE 26–8   **Platelet Ultrastructural Zones**

I. Peripheral zone (stimulus receptor/transmitter region)
   A. Glycocalyx
   B. Platelet membrane
   C. Open canalicular system
   D. Submembraneous region
II. Sol-Gel zone (cytoskeletal/contractile region)
   A. Circumferential microtubules
   B. Microfilaments
III. Organelle zone (Metabolic/organellar region)
   A. Granules
      1. Alpha granules
      2. Dense granules
      3. Lysosomes
      4. Glycogen granules
   B. Mitochondria
   C. Dense tubular system
   D. Peroxisomes

teins serve as receptors and facilitate transmission of stimuli across the platelet membrane. Platelet membrane glycoprotein Ib appears to be a primary receptor for von Willebrand factor (vWF), which serves to mediate the initial adhesion of platelets to subendothelium (see Fig. 26–2).

Platelet membrane GP IIb/IIIa functions as a receptor for substances such as fibrinogen (a necessary precursor for fibrin strand formation, which will eventually reinforce the platelet plug), fibronectin (an adhesive protein), and vWF (binding may help expose the site for binding to fibrinogen), thereby mediating platelet aggregation. Although the primary receptor for vWF seems to be GP Ib, vWF is more likely to bind to GP IIb/IIIa under high shear stress (rapid flow within a small blood vessel with the accompanying increased chances of cellular shearing) because the vWF molecules distort to form extended filaments,[4] thus strengthening the chances for platelet attachment,[5] or to enhance platelet-to-platelet interaction.[6] Calcium

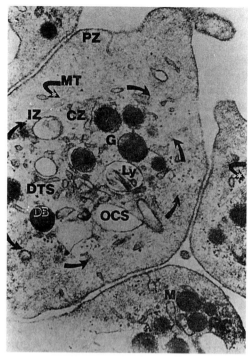

FIGURE 26-5 Internal anatomy of a stimulated platelet. Circumferential band of microtubules (MT) leads to reorganization of the internal structure of the platelet into three zones. The peripheral zone (PZ) is the region external to a circumferential band of microtubules (MT with * on curved arrows). The intermediate zone (IZ) (*encircling arrows*) includes the microtubules and the closely adjacent cytoplasmic material. The central zone (CZ) is internal to the microtubule band and contains many organelles such as granules (G), dense bodies (DB), dense tubular system (DTS), lysosomes (Ly), mitochondria (M), and many profiles of the open canalicular system (OCS). Magnification ×49,700. (From Barnhart, MI: Platelet responses in health and disease. Mol Cell Biochem 22:115, 1978, with permission.)

TABLE 26-9	**Platelet Factors (PF) 1 to 7**
PF 1	Coagulation factor V
PF 2	Thromboplastin-like material
PF 3	Platelet thromboplastin*
PF 4	Antiheparin factor*
PF 5	Fibrinogen coagulant factor
PF 6	Antifibrinolytic factor
PF 7	Platelet cothromboplastin

*Most important
Source: Adapted from Bick and Murano.[2]

PF4 seem to be the most important PFs. In addition to containing receptors for various stimuli, the peripheral zone of the platelet also contains the mechanism for the development of stickiness, which is essential for adhesion and aggregation.

The membranous surface-connecting system referred to as the OCS consists of tubular invaginations of the plasma membrane that articulate throughout the platelet even though it is part of the peripheral zone. Platelet-stored products are released to the exterior through the OCS, just as squeezing a sponge might express the contained fluid. The OCS also facilitates collection of plasma procoagulants that aid in fibrin formation by providing increased surface absorptive area.

Sol-Gel Zone

The term *cytoskeleton* is often used to describe this zone. Within the matrix of the platelet are microtubules, microfilaments, and submembranous filaments. Submembranous filaments are found within the peripheral zone and have been previously discussed. Microtubules and microfilaments are found within the sol-gel zone. The most numerous of the three fibers is the circumferential band of microtubules.

Microtubules encase the entire platelet, maintaining its discoid shape.[8] In the stimulated platelet (see Fig. 26-5), contraction of the circumferential band of microtubules toward the center of the platelet appears to be responsible for both the movement of organelles toward the interior and their reorganization, which facilitates the secretory process.[8] After secretion, the microtubules disappear from the center of the platelet and reappear in other peripheral areas such as pseudopods.[8] Microtubules appear to monitor the internal contraction of platelets, preventing secretion in response to only minimal stimulation and thereby regulating the degree of platelet response.

Microfilaments are interwoven throughout the cytoplasm of the platelet and are composed of actin and myosinlike contractile proteins. Actin is the major contractile protein in the platelet cytosol, accounting for 20% to 30% of the total platelet protein, whereas myosin composes 2% to 5% of the total platelet protein (a sizable percentage for a nonmuscle cell). Also present is thrombosthenin, a contractile protein similar to actomyosin.[2] Actomyosin is complexed actin and myosin.[8] In the platelet, actin and myosin complex in a ratio of about 100:1.[8] Microfilaments can convert from

and/or magnesium in the form of divalent cations are also required for fibrinogen binding.[7] It appears that, in a high-shear field, vWF is the required GP IIb/IIIa ligand, rather than fibrinogen,[4] but that in a low-shear field, vWF is less relevant.[4] The relationship among and binding time sequence of GP IIb/IIIa, vWF, and fibrinogen are not completely understood.

The platelet membrane also includes receptors for substances such as ADP, thrombin, epinephrine, and serotonin, which play a role in platelet aggregation.[2] Various enzymes have also been isolated in the platelet plasma membrane.

The platelet membrane, similar to other plasma membranes, represents a fluid lipid bilayer composed of glycoproteins, glycolipids, and lipoproteins. The membrane phospholipid portion of the activated platelet serves as a surface for the interaction of the plasma proteins involved in blood coagulation, which assemble in complexes on the platelet's surface. Coagulation factors V and VIII also are present on the surface of the platelet membrane, as are various platelet factors (PFs) that participate in the formation of fibrin. At least seven PFs have been identified (Table 26-9). PF3 and

an unorganized gelatinous state to organized parallel filaments capable of contraction within seconds as the platelet's shape changes.

Organelle Zone

The organelle region is responsible for the metabolic activities of the platelet. Generally, the most numerous organelles are the platelet granules, which are heterogeneous in size, electron density, and chemical contents. Platelets contain three morphologically distinct types of storage granules: dense granules, alpha granules, and lysosomes containing acid hydrolases. The alpha granules are more numerous (20 to 200 per platelet) and contain a number of different proteins, summarized in Table 26–10.[8] The physiologic role of these proteins present in the alpha granules of platelets has not been clearly defined.

Dense bodies are fewer in number (2 to 10 per platelet) and represent densely opaque granules in transmission electron microscope (TEM) preparations. Table 26–11 lists the contents of the dense body granules in the platelet.

The contents of both the alpha granules and dense bodies are released during the energy-dependent release reaction. Subsequent to ADP liberation from the dense bodies during the release reaction, additional platelets are drawn to the site of the vascular injury, resulting in the formation of platelet aggregates.

Other granules such as lysosomes, peroxisomes, and glycogen granules can be found in the platelet as well as in other cells.

The dense tubular system (DTS) is another important structure present in the cytoplasm of the organelle zone of platelets. Like the sarcotubules in skeletal muscle, the DTS is derived from the smooth endoplasmic reticulum (ER) of immature megakaryocytes. The

TABLE 26–11 **Contents of Platelet Dense Body Granules**
Adenosine diphosphate (ADP)
Adenosine triphosphate (ATP)
Calcium
Catecholamines (epinephrine, norepinephrine)
Serotonin
Pyrophosphate
Magnesium

DTS is the site of prostaglandin and thromboxane synthesis and sequestration of calcium. It is primarily the release of calcium from the DTS that triggers platelet contraction and subsequent internal activation of platelets.

Platelet activation is an energy-dependent process that relies on the metabolic function of mitochondria. The approximately 10 to 60 mitochondria present per platelet require glycogen as their source of energy for metabolism. Resting platelet ATP (energy) production is generated by glycolysis and the oxidative Krebs cycle. In the activated state, about half the ATP production in platelets occurs through the glycolytic pathway.

Platelet Function

Platelets must be adequate in number and function to participate optimally in hemostasis. The functions of platelets in hemostasis are listed in Table 26–12.

Numerous stimuli can trigger platelet activation, which may be transient, reversible, or irreversible. Activation refers to several separate responses of platelet function that include stickiness, adhesion, shape change, secretion release, and aggregation. Platelets respond in a graded fashion depending on the strength and duration of the stimuli as well as the physiologic or pathologic state of the platelet.

In the initial stage of activation, platelets form pseudopods as they begin to contract.[2] As activation progresses, contraction and pseudopod formation progress, organelles including the alpha granules and dense bodies are reorganized to the center of the platelet, and further contraction causes the granules to spill their contents into the OCS, which shunts the contents to the outside of the platelet.[2] Adjacent platelets are activated through receptor contact with the granule contents, amplifying the activation process.[2] Hence, it may be said that platelet activation spans platelet adhesion, platelet secretion, and platelet aggregation.

Before proceeding further, the reader should review the structure of the platelet in order to visualize and

TABLE 26–10 **Some Proteins Present in Platelet Alpha Granules**
Platelet-Specific Proteins
1. Platelet factor (PF) 1–7
2. Beta-thromboglobulin
3. Platelet-derived growth factor*
4. Basic protein
5. Chemotactic factor*
6. Permeability factor
7. Bactericidal factor
Plasma Proteins
1. Fibrinogen
2. von Willebrand factor (vWF)
3. Factor V
4. Albumin
5. Fibronectin
6. Plasminogen
7. High-molecular-weight kininogen (HMWK)
8. Protein S
9. Immunoglobulin G
Other Proteins
1. Osteonectin
2. Thrombospondin

*Possibly identical
Source: From Holmson,[8] with permission.

TABLE 26–12 **Platelet Function in Hemostasis**
Maintenance of vascular integrity
Initial arrest of bleeding by platelet plug formation
Stabilization of hemostatic plug by contributing to fibrin formation

understand subsequent events that occur in the platelet at the ultrastructural level during hemostasis (see Fig. 26–4).

Maintenance of Vascular Integrity

Platelets are involved in the nurturing of endothelial cells lining the vascular system. The platelets are incorporated into the vessel wall, releasing a substance called platelet-derived growth factor that nurtures the endothelial cells, maintaining normal vascular integrity.

When a platelet adheres to the endothelial cell, the amount of cytoplasm between platelet and cell is reduced and the platelet may eventually become incorporated into the endothelial cell. This process has the effect of nurturing or feeding the tissue cells by releasing endothelial growth factor. Through the release of this mitogen (platelet-derived growth factor or PDGF), vascular healing is also promoted by stimulating endothelial cell migration and medial smooth muscle cell migration in the vessel wall. Figure 26–6 shows a scanning electron micrograph (SEM) demonstrating platelet adherence at the site of endothelial loss compared with the normal smooth contour of the endothelial cell.

In the absence of platelets, a large number of red cells migrate through the vessel wall, enter the lymphatic drainage, and appear as petechiae or purpura in the skin or mucous membranes. The process of maintenance of normal vascular integrity, involving nourishment of the endothelium by the platelet or actual incorporation of platelets into the vessel wall, utilizes a small minority of the platelets in the circulation but is nevertheless an important function.

Platelet Plug Formation

Various processes that are involved in the initial formation of a platelet plug can be grouped as follows: platelet adhesion (in which activation and shape change are also discussed), platelet release reaction (secretion), and platelet aggregation.

Adhesion Exposure to subendothelial connective tissue, such as collagen fibers, initiates platelet adhesion. Adhesion is a reversible process whereby platelets stick to foreign surfaces. This process of platelet adhesion involves the interaction of platelet surface glycoproteins with the connective tissue elements of the subendothelium.

Adhesion of platelets to subendothelial fibers is dependent on a plasma protein called von Willebrand factor (vWF), discussed earlier in this chapter. vWF is a component of the factor VIII complex and varies in size of multimer (the structural unit of the molecule with inheritance).

Evidence indicates that vWF is synthesized by endothelial cells and megakaryocytes (precursors of platelets). Absorption of vWF occurs both on exposed subendothelial fibers and on the surface of the platelet as the vWF attaches to the appropriate platelet membrane surface glycoprotein Ib (see Fig. 26–2).

Platelets thus adhere (stick to a nonplatelet surface) to the area of injury at the endothelial lining, acting to arrest the initial episode of bleeding. In Figure 26–7, a

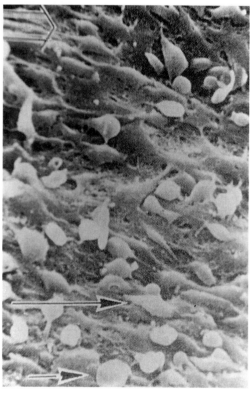

FIGURE 26–6 SEM of platelet adherence at the site of endothelial loss. Short arrow points to a discoid intact platelet with a single pseudopod, long arrow points to an elongated adherent platelet, double arrow marks densely adherent platelets appearing as elongated humps fused to the subendothelial layer. (From Cotran, E: Robbins Pathologic Basis of Disease, ed 1, WB Saunders, Philadelphia, 1979, p 120, with permission.)

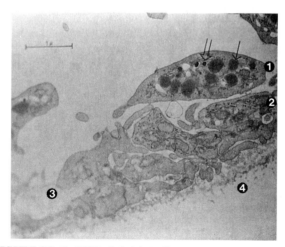

FIGURE 26–7 TEM of platelet adherence to subendothelial connective tissue at the focus of endothelial loss. (1) Intact platelet with pseudopod (thin arrow indicates alpha granule; thick arrow indicates dense body), (2) partially degranulated platelet, (3) degranulated platelet "ghost," (4) internal elastic lamina. (From Cotran, E: Robbins Pathologic Basis of Disease, ed 1, WB Saunders, Philadelphia, 1979, p 116, with permission.)

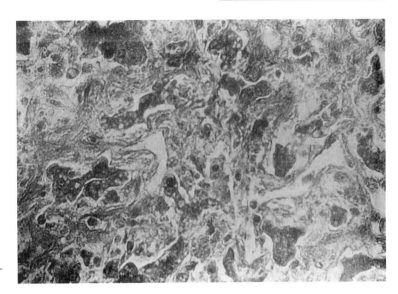

FIGURE 26-8 TEM of viscous metamorphosis.

TEM demonstrates platelet adherence to subendothelial connective tissue at the focus of endothelial loss. A decrease in platelet number, therefore, leads to failure to block the site of injury, resulting in increased bleeding. Facilitated by chemical messengers, other platelets may cohere (stick to each other) to the original contact platelets (adhering to the site of injury), producing the phenomenon of aggregation and resulting in thrombus formation to stop bleeding. Platelet adhesion consumes little energy as measured by ATP use.

Release Reaction (Secretion) The platelet release reaction and platelet aggregation are intimately related and may sometimes occur almost simultaneously; therefore, the discussion of the two topics is very difficult to separate. A sufficiently strong stimulus is necessary for the release reaction to occur. The release reaction from dense granules involves the secretion of ADP, serotonin (a vasoactive amine), and calcium. Responsible for both initial and further aggregation of platelets (depending on the amount secreted), ADP

serves to amplify the process. Elevation of intracellular Ca^{2+} further amplifies the process by activating more calcium-sensitive phospholipases, leading to further formation of thromboxane A_2 (TXA_2), a potent platelet aggregator. Amplification of the initial aggregation of platelets (a reversible phenomenon) results in secondary aggregation of many other platelets into an irreversible aggregation of a mass of degenerative platelet material without membranes. This transformation of the mass is termed *viscous metamorphosis* (Fig. 26–8).

Different substances are released at different rates, suggesting a heterogenicity of granules. The release of substances such as fibrinogen and beta-thromboglobulin confirms the degranulation of alpha granules. Secretion is an energy-dependent process that occurs only after internal reorganization and transformation have occurred, given a sufficiently strong platelet stimulus that results in an irreversible process (Fig. 26–9).

Aggregation Aggregation follows adhesion in the presence of sufficient activation or stimulation. During

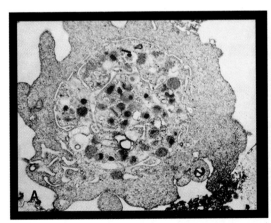
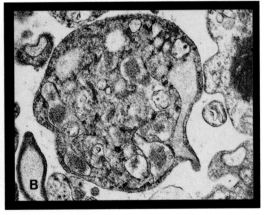

FIGURE 26-9 TEM of an activated and a degranulated platelet. (*A*) Early aggregation of activated platelet (the primary wave of aggregation, a reversible process). (*B*) Degranulated platelet (the secondary wave of aggregation, an irreversible process). (From Barnhart, MI: Platelet responses in health and disease. Mol Cell Biochem 22:117, 1978, with permission.)

early platelet aggregation, the platelet shape is spherical with pseudopods (Fig. 26–10). Initial aggregation of platelets is caused by release of ADP from adherent platelets in an initial release wave.[2] This initial aggregatory wave is called *primary* or *reversible aggregation* because aggregation is still reversible at this point.[2]

ADP is a weak platelet agonist (unable to signal secretion without primary aggregation)[7] and gives the signal for ambient discoid platelets to change their shape and transform themselves into reactive spiny spheres. These spheres react with one another to form a mass of aggregated platelets.

Both ionized calcium and the plasma protein fibrinogen (coagulation factor I) are necessary for platelet aggregation. Other platelet agonists can play a role in platelet stimulation and the ensuing fibrinogen-binding site exposure.[7]

The platelet-to-platelet interaction (initial aggregation) is a process of Ca^{2+}-dependent ligand formation between membrane-bound fibrinogen molecules (fibrinogen is present inside platelets, on the platelet surface, and in the circulation). Fibrinogen binds to the divalent cation (calcium or magnesium) complex of platelet membrane glycoproteins IIb/IIIa (GPIIb/IIIa).[7] Once fibrinogen binds to this complex, extracellular ionized calcium-dependent fibrinogen bridges form between adjacent platelets, thereby promoting platelet aggregation.

Platelets will not aggregate in the absence of membrane glycoprotein, fibrinogen-binding sites, fibrinogen, or divalent cations (usually thought of as ionized calcium).

Binding of ADP to the platelet membrane activates phospholipase, an enzyme that cleaves the phospholipids present in the platelet membrane, freeing fatty acids such as arachidonic acid.[5] Released arachidonic acid is converted in the cytoplasm of the platelet into the (prostaglandin) endoperoxides by prostaglandin synthetase, commonly known as cyclooxygenase. These endoperoxides are converted to TXA_2, which is a potent aggregator of platelets, a mediator of platelet release reaction, and a promoter of vasoconstriction (Fig. 26–11). With its in vivo half-life of 30 seconds, TXA_2 activity is limited in time because it hydrolyzes spontaneously within the platelet to an inactive form thromboxane B_2 (TXB_2). As TXA_2 is generated with subsequent aggregating effects on platelets, calcium, sequestered in the dense-tubular system of the platelet, is extruded in the sol-gel zone. Thrombin, also a potent platelet aggregator, can induce secretion of all types of granules (dense, alpha, and lysosomes).

In vitro platelet aggregation can be initiated by a variety of agents (listed in Table 26–13). In vitro aggregation can be visualized as a two-phase process that may be reversible or irreversible, depending on the

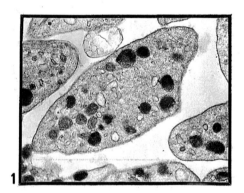

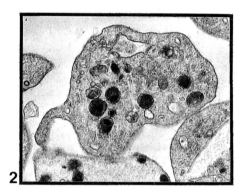

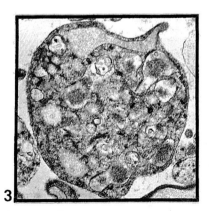

FIGURE 26–10   TEM showing disk-to-sphere transformation of an activated platelet. Note progression from (*1*) disk shape to (*2*) pseudopod formation to (*3*) degranulated ballooned sphere.

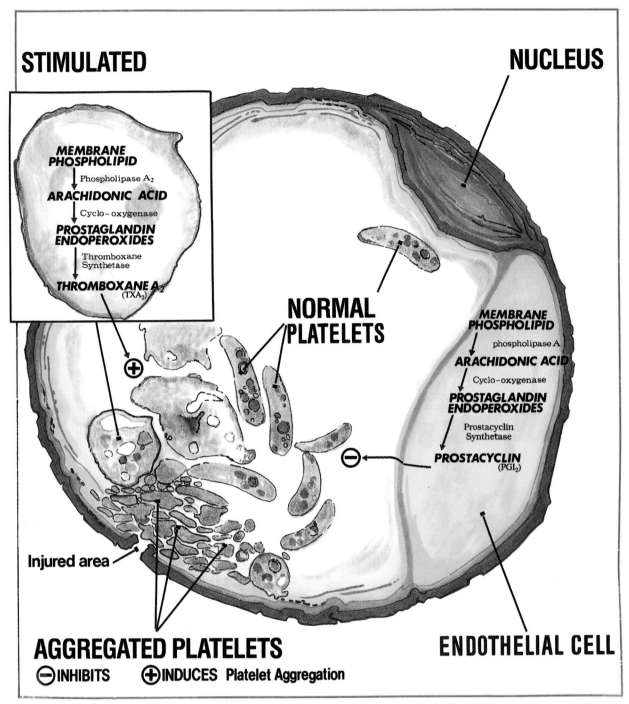

STIMULATED

NUCLEUS

MEMBRANE
PHOSPHOLIPID

Phospholipase A₂

ARACHIDONIC ACID

Cyclo-oxygenase

PROSTAGLANDIN
ENDOPEROXIDES

Thromboxane
Synthetase

THROMBOXANE A₂
(TXA₂)

⊕

**NORMAL
PLATELETS**

MEMBRANE
PHOSPHOLIPID

phospholipase A

ARACHIDONIC ACID

Cyclo-oxygenase

PROSTAGLANDIN
ENDOPEROXIDES

Prostacyclin
Synthetase

PROSTACYCLIN
(PGI₂)

⊖

Injured area

AGGREGATED PLATELETS

ENDOTHELIAL CELL

⊖INHIBITS   ⊕INDUCES Platelet Aggregation

FIGURE 26–11   Synthesis of prostaglandins in platelets and endothelial cell during platelet plug formation.

strength of the activation stimulus. Early aggregation, the primary (initial or first) wave of aggregation, involves contraction of the circumferential microtubules and reorganization and centralization of platelet organelles. When using a platelet aggregometer, platelet aggregation results in decreased absorbance or optical density (because of optical clearing as the aggregates fall out of solution). Decreased optical density results in increased light transmitted through the cuvette (or increased percent transmission) as measured by the platelet aggregometer.

An intriguing new test[9] presents a method for performing functional platelet aggregation screening by slide kit called the slide platelet aggregation test (SPAT). For a review of the laboratory procedure for platelet aggregation and some helpful sample aggregation curves using common laboratory aggregating agents, see Chapter 34.

TABLE 26–13 **Some in Vitro Platelet Aggregators**
Adenosine diphosphate (ADP)* (low, optimal, and high concentrations)
Collagen*
Epinephrine*
Thrombin*
Ristocetin*
Serotonin
Arachidonic acid
Immune products
Snake venoms

*More commonly used.

The secondary wave of aggregation is dependent on the activation stimulus being strong enough to evoke the secretion of platelet granules (described previously) as a consequence of stronger more complete contraction. Ultrastructurally, the internal reorganization of organelles is more severe, and degranulation is evident by the lack of density of the granules with TEM (see Fig. 26–10). Biochemical studies have confirmed the release of substances such as ADP, serotonin, and epinephrine; these are responsible for the secondary wave of aggregation, which is usually irreversible.

Figure 26–12 depicts a typical biphasic response of in vitro platelet aggregation to ADP, as recorded by an aggregometer. It should be noted that aggregation is an energy-dependent process that greatly exhausts the platelet energy resources.

Effect of Aspirin on Platelet Plug Formation

Aspirin interferes with platelet plug formation by blocking platelet aggregation through inhibiting production of prostaglandin endoperoxide and TXA_2.

Aspirin induces irreversible acetylation and inactivation of platelet cyclo-oxygenase, leading to the inhibition of endoperoxide and TXA_2 synthesis, thus pre-venting aggregation.[10] Because platelets cannot synthesize cyclo-oxygenase, TXA_2 synthesis is inhibited for the entire life span of the platelet. Megakaryocytes are capable of synthesizing cyclo-oxygenase, and therefore newly released platelets show enzyme activity.

Prostaglandins (PGs) are present in many different tissues, including endothelium. In endothelium, there is a pathway similar to the one described in platelets (see Fig. 26–11). Arachidonic acid in endothelium is converted to PGG_2 by cyclo-oxygenase, but thromboxane is not formed. Instead prostacyclin PGI_2 is formed from the cyclic endoperoxides by the enzyme prostacyclin synthetase. PGI_2, produced in the endothelium, has an effect opposite to that of thromboxane on the platelet. Prostacyclin (PGI_2) is a potent inhibitor of platelet aggregation and a vasodilator. Therefore, as long as the endothelium is intact and PGI_2 is made and secreted, platelet aggregation is limited in time.

Aspirin also inhibits cyclo-oxygenase produced by the endothelial cells. Endothelial cells, however, possess the organelles necessary to synthesize cyclo-oxygenase, thereby regenerating enzyme activity as the level of circulating aspirin decreases. However, if very high doses of aspirin are ingested, both the endothelial

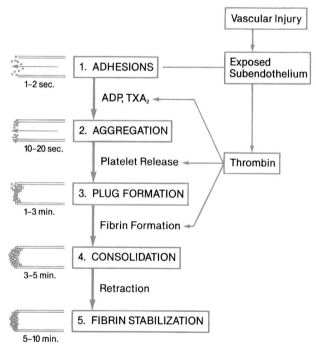

FIGURE 26–13 Sequence of events in hemostatic plug formation. (*1*) Platelet adhesion to exposed subendothelial connective tissue structures. (*2*) Platelet aggregation by ADP, thromboxane A_2, and thrombin recruitment through transformation of discoid platelets into reactive spiny spheres that interact with one another through calcium-dependent fibrinogen bridges. (*3*) Contribution of platelet coagulant activity to the coagulation process, which stabilizes the plug with a fibrin mesh. (*4*) Consolidation of the platelet mass to provide a dense thrombus. (*5*) Fibrin polymerization and fibrin stabilization by factor XIII. (From Thompson, AR and Harker, LA: Manual of Hemostasis and Thrombosis, ed 3. FA Davis, Philadelphia, 1983, with permission.)

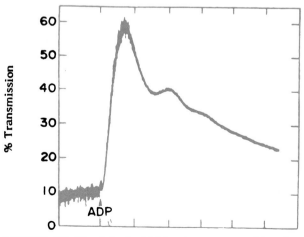

FIGURE 26–12 A typical biphasic response of in vitro platelet aggregation to ADP, as recorded by an aggregometer.

and platelet cyclo-oxygenase will be affected and the effect will cancel out. Thus, a potential for thrombosis may occur.

Stabilization of Hemostatic Plug

The last stage involved in arresting bleeding after vessel damage is the formation of a stable platelet plug. This stabilization is achieved through the formation and deposition of fibrin, the end product of coagulation, which interweaves through and over the platelet plug, compressing the plug into place in the vessel breach. Fibrin is formed as a result of a series of reactions that involve not only platelets but also various blood proteins, lipids, and ions (see the following section on the fibrin-forming system).

As mentioned previously, platelets provide an optimal environment for fibrin formation by exposing certain phospholipids (PF3) on the platelet membrane surface during aggregation. These membrane phospholipids provide a catalytic surface for the activation of various clotting enzymes or factors, such as factor X. In addition, certain coagulation factors (V and VIII) are present on the platelet membrane. Figure 26–13 provides a reivew of the sequence of events involved in platelet plug formation and the approximate time involved in each stage.

FIBRIN-FORMING (COAGULATION) SYSTEM

The fibrin-forming (coagulation) system is that system through which coagulation factors interact to eventually form a fibrin clot. The purpose of fibrin clot formation (secondary hemostasis) is to reinforce the platelet plug (primary hemostasis).

This system is mediated by many coagulation proteins normally present in the blood in an inactive state (coagulation factors). Table 26–14 lists the coagulation factors and their most commonly used designations. The factor VI designation was dropped because a substance originally thought to be factor VI was found to be a precursor to factor V, and to avoid confusion, fac-

tor VI has not been reassigned.[11] Secondary hemostasis is the phrase used to encompass the coagulation factors' role in the hemostatic mechanism (see Table 26–14 for a review of the appropriate nomenclature).

Most of the coagulation factors are designated by Roman numerals. The numerical system adopted assigns the number to the factors according to the sequence of discovery and not to the point of interaction in the cascade. Some factors are routinely referred to by their common names, such as fibrinogen and prothrombin, whereas others are more commonly referred to by Roman numeral (such as factor XI, plasma thromboplastin antecedent factor).

Activation of a factor is designated by addition of a small "a" next to the Roman numeral in the coagulation cascade (e.g., XII → XIIa) unless convention dictates otherwise (e.g., most references incorporate "thrombin" into the coagulation cascade rather than using its alternate designation, IIa). Some of the common names are derived from the original patients who exhibited symptoms leading to elucidation of that factor deficiency and an understanding of the role of that factor in the cascade (e.g., Christmas factor, Hageman factor). Other common names describe the action of the factor in the coagulation system (e.g., fibrin-stabilizing factor).

All the coagulation proteins are produced in the liver. The von Willebrand's portion of factor VIII is produced in other body sites as well, namely endothelial cells and megakaryocytes.

Hemostatic Function

In terms of general hemostatic function, the coagulation factors can be divided into three categories: substrate, cofactors, and enzymes.

Factor I, fibrinogen, is regarded as the main substrate of the blood coagulation system because the formation of a fibrin clot from fibrinogen is the ultimate goal. Cofactors are proteins that accelerate the enzymatic reactions involved in the coagulation process. Some examples of blood coagulation cofactors include factors III (tissue factor or tissue thromboplastin), V

TABLE 26–14	**Nomenclature of Coagulation Factors**
Factor I	Fibrinogen
Factor II	Prothrombin
Factor III	Tissue thromboplastin (tissue factor)
Factor IV	Ionized calcium (Ca^{2+})
Factor V	Labile factor (proaccelerin)
Factor VI	Not assigned
Factor VII	Stable factor (serum prothrombin conversion accelerator or SPCA)
Factor VIII	Antihemophilic factor (AHF), factor VIII:C (coagulant portion)
Factor IX	Christmas factor (plasma thromboplastin component or PTC)
Factor X	Stuart-Prower factor
Factor XI	Plasma thromboplastin antecedent (PTA)
Factor XII	Hageman factor (contact factor)
Factor XIII	Fibrin-stabilizing factor (FSF)
Fitzgerald factor	High-molecular-weight kininogen (HMWK)
Fletcher factor	Prekallikrein

(labile factor), VIII:C (antihemophilic factor, or AHF), and Fitzgerald factor (high-molecular-weight kininogen, or HMWK).

The last general category of blood coagulation factors is the enzyme category. Enzymes involved in coagulation can be subdivided into two groups: serine proteases or transaminases. Except for factor XIII (fibrin-stabilizing factor), all the enzyme examples listed above are serine proteases when they are in their activated form. These proteases have serine as a portion of their active enzymatic site and function to cleave peptide bonds.

Factor XIII (fibrin-stabilizing factor) is the only member of the transamidase subgroup. It functions to create cross-linkages between the fibrin monomers formed during the coagulation process to produce a stable fibrin clot.

Physical Properties

On the basis of their physical properties, the coagulation proteins may also be conveniently divided into three other groups: (1) the contact proteins, (2) the prothrombin proteins, and (3) the fibrinogen or thrombin-sensitive proteins. Refer to Table 26–15 for details on each group.

The contact group (see Table 26–15) includes factor XII (Hageman factor), factor XI (plasma thromboplastin antecedent), prekallikrein (Fletcher factor), and HMWK (Fitzgerald factor). These proteins are involved in the initial phase of intrinsic system activation. Although deficiencies of these coagulation proteins are associated with markedly abnormal laboratory tests, an isolated factor XI deficiency is associated with a mild bleeding disorder. Interestingly, problems with thrombosis have been reported in patients with factor XII (Hageman factor) and prekallikrein (Fletcher factor) deficiencies.

The prothrombin proteins (see Table 26–15) are generally low molecular weight proteins that include factors II (prothrombin), VII (stable factor), IX (Christmas factor), and X (Stuart-Prower factor). This group is also known as the vitamin K–dependent coagulation proteins. Each member of this group contains a unique amino acid—gamma carboxyglutamic acid—that is necessary for both calcium binding and attraction of

these coagulation factors to the surface of activated platelets, where the formation of a fibrin clot occurs.

If the patient is deficient in vitamin K, vitamin K–dependent coagulation factors are produced, but they function abnormally because of a lack of calcium-binding sites.[2] These dysfunctional factors are called *proteins induced by vitamin K absence or antagonists* (PIVKAs).[2]

Drugs that act as antagonists to vitamin K (such as coumadin, which is commonly used for oral anticoagulant therapy, and indanedione, which is used in therapy for individuals who exhibit coumadin sensitivity)[12] inhibit this vitamin K–dependent reaction, which is required for functionally active coagulation factors of the prothrombin group.

Factors II (prothrombin), VII (stable factor), IX (Christmas factor), and X (Stuart-Prower factor) and proteins C and S are still synthesized by the liver but are not complete because they lack specific binding receptors for calcium.[12] These proteins may be present physically but are impaired functionally as they cannot enter into the formation of an enzyme-substrate complex.[12] Therefore, patients who are vitamin K–deficient exhibit decreased production of functional prothrombin proteins (normal amounts of the proteins may be present, but the proteins themselves are dysfunctional). Thus, PIVKAs are produced.

Acquired deficiencies of the vitamin K–dependent coagulation factors are relatively common because the body does not contain appreciable stores of vitamin K. Characteristic prototypes for developing a vitamin K deficiency include patients who have just had surgery and are receiving parenteral feeding, patients who are receiving high doses of intravenous antibiotics, and patients suffering from liver disease. Protein C status is important too because some patients who are protein C–deficient may develop coumadin-induced skin necrosis,[13] although this occurrence is rare.

The fibrinogen group (see Table 26–15) consists generally of high-molecular-weight proteins that include factors I (fibrinogen), V (labile factor), VIII:C (antihemophilic factor), and XIII (fibrin-stabilizing factor). During coagulation, generated thrombin acts on all the factors in the fibrinogen group. Thrombin enhances the activity of factors V (labile factor) and VIII:C (antihemophilic factor) by converting these proteins to ac-

TABLE 26–15	**Categorization of Coagulation Proteins by Physical Properties**		
	Protein Groups		
	Contact	**Prothrombin**	**Fibrinogen**
Factors	XII, XI, PK, HMWK	II, VII, IX, X	I, V, VIII, XIII
Consumed during coagulation	No	No (except II)	Yes
Present in serum	Yes	Yes (except II)	No
Present in stored plasma	Yes	Yes	No*
Absorbed by BaSO$_4$	No	Yes	No
Present in adsorbed plasma	Yes	No	Yes
Vitamin K–dependent	No	Yes	No

*Factors V and VIII are not present in stored plasma because of their labile nature, but factors I and XIII are present.
Abbreviations: PK = prekallikrein; HMWK = high-molecular-weight kininogen

tive cofactors, which are involved in the assembly of macromolecular complexes on the surface of activated platelets. Thrombin also activates factor XIII (fibrin-stabilizing factor) and converts fibrinogen to fibrin.

Factors V (labile factor) and VIII:C (antihemophilic factor) are the least stable factors, since their activity is relatively labile to degradation and denaturation. Therefore, testing for factor V (labile factor) and VIII:C (antihemophilic factor) should be rapid, or else appropriate storage measures should be taken.

In addition to the presence of the fibrinogen group in plasma, these factors are also found within plate-lets. The fibrinogen group of coagulation factors has been reported to increase with inflammation in pregnancy and with the use of oral contraceptives.

Blood Coagulation: The "Cascade" Theory

The process of blood coagulation involves a series of biochemical reactions that transforms circulating substances into an insoluble gel through conversion of soluble fibrinogen to fibrin. This process requires plasma proteins (coagulation factors) as well as phospholipids and calcium.

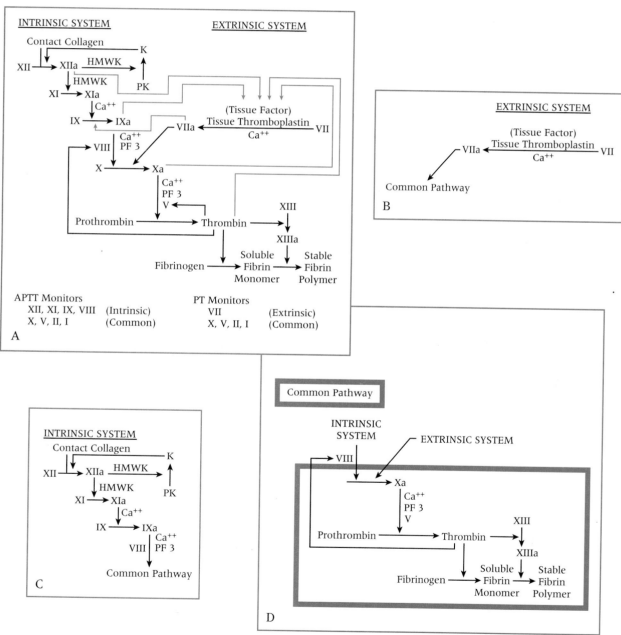

FIGURE 26–14   The "cascade" theory of coagulation. (*A*) Overview. (*B*) The extrinsic system. (*C*) The intrinsic system. (*D*) The common pathway.

Blood coagulation leading to fibrin formation can be separated into two pathways, extrinsic and intrinsic, both of which share specific coagulation factors with the common pathway (Fig. 26–14). Both pathways require initiation, which leads to subsequent activation of various coagulation factors in a cascading, waterfall, or domino effect. Useful demonstrations can be derived from the waterfall or domino concept. According to the cascade theory, each coagulation factor is converted to its active form by the preceding factor in a series of biochemical chain reactions. Ionized calcium (Ca^{2+}) participates in some of the reactions as a cofactor. Each reaction is promoted by the preceding reaction, and if there is a deficiency of any one of the factors, the consequences listed in Table 26–16 result.

Eventually, both the extrinsic and intrinsic systems lead to generation of the enzyme thrombin, which converts fibrinogen to fibrin (see Fig. 26–14A, D).

The term *extrinsic* is used because this pathway is initiated when factor III (tissue thromboplastin or tissue factor), a substance not found in blood, enters the vascular system (see Fig. 26–14A, B). The tissue factor includes a phospholipid component that is the source of required phospholipid in the extrinsic system. Phospholipid provides a surface for interaction of various factors. The phospholipids required in the intrinsic pathway are provided by the platelet membrane. In the intrinsic pathway, all the factors necessary for clot formation are intrinsic to the vascular compartment because they are all found within the circulating blood (see Fig. 26–14A, C).

Extrinsic Pathway

In the extrinsic pathway, factor VII is activated to factor VIIa in the presence of ionized calcium (factor IV) and the tissue factor (factor III), which is released from the injured vessel wall. In the extrinsic coagulation system, it is important to realize that this pathway bypasses the activation of factors XII, XI, IX, and VIII:C, requiring only factor VIIa, factor IV (Ca^{2+}), and factor III (tissue thromboplastin) to activate factor X to Xa, although there may be some additional interaction (see section on current concepts).

Figure 26–14 (A and B) shows that the extrinsic pathway provides a means for very quickly producing small amounts of thrombin leading to fibrin formation. In addition, the thrombin generated by this pathway can accelerate the intrinsic pathway by enhancing the activity of factors V and VIII. In the laboratory, the prothrombin time (PT) test is used to monitor the extrinsic pathway (for a review of the procedure, see Chap. 34).

Intrinsic Pathway

Following exposure to foreign substances ("contact") such as collagen, subendothelial collagen, phospholipids, or kallikrein (activated prekallikrein or Fletcher factor),[2] activation of factor XII to XIIa initiates clotting through the intrinsic pathway. Factor XII is only partially activated by this contact with a foreign substance. Prekallikrein (Fletcher factor) and HMWK (Fitzgerald factor) are additionally needed to enhance or amplify the contact factors involved in the intrinsic system (see Fig. 26–14A, C). Specifically, factor XIIa in the presence of HMWK converts prekallikrein to kallikrein. Kallikrein feeds back to accelerate the conversion of factor XII to XIIa, speeding up intrinsic system processes.

The activation of factor XII acts as the common link between many aspects of the hemostatic mechanism, including the fibrinolytic system, the kinin system, and the complement system (Fig. 26–15 and section on fibrin-lysing system). Contact activation occurs in the absence of ionized calcium and also refers to the activation of factor XI to factor XIa by factor XIIa in the presence of HMWK.

Once generated, factor XIIa in the presence of HMWK converts factor XI to XIa. Factor XIIa is capable of activating factor XI without HMWK, but the activation takes place much more slowly.[2]

The next reaction in the intrinsic pathway is the activation of factor IX to factor IXa by factor XIa, in the presence of ionized calcium. Activated factor IX (IXa) participates, along with the essential cofactor VIII:C, in the presence of ionized calcium and PF3, a source of phospholipid, to activate factor X, which leads to the generation of thrombin and formation of fibrin. The complex consisting of factor IXa-factor VIII:C-phospholipid-Ca^{2+} has been called *tenase complex* because it activates factor X[14] (Fig. 26–16).

The macromolecular complex of factors IXa, VIII:C, X, PF3, and Ca^{2+} assembles on the surface of the activated platelet (providing the phospholipid) during the intrinsic pathway of blood coagulation. This surface provides a protective environment that facilitates the enzymatic reactions of the coagulation cascade without interference from the physiologic anticoagulants normally present in plasma.

In regard to the intrinsic pathway, it is also important to be familiar with the properties of the factor VIII complex (Table 26–17). Factor VIII complex consists of two main portions, factor VIII:C (the procoagulant portion) and vWF (the carrier protein).

It should be noted that factor VIII requires enhancement by the generated enzyme thrombin to amplify its activity. In the laboratory, the activated partial thromboplastin time (APTT) test is used to evaluate the intrinsic pathway (for a review of this procedure see Chap. 34).

Factor VIII complex, which consists of several components, comprises the largest protein involved in the coagulation cascade. The major portion of this protein complex is considered to be the carrier protein called von Willebrand factor (vWF), although this is not the portion active in the coagulation cascade. There seems to be a movement to use the designation "vWF" rather than factor VIII:vWF when referring to the vWF portion of the factor VIII complex.[14]

TABLE 26–16 Consequences of Factor Deficiency

- Coagulation cannot proceed at a normal rate
- Initiation of the next subsequent reaction is delayed
- The time required for the clot to form is prolonged
- Bleeding from the injured vessel continues for a longer time (or there may be a physiologic tendency toward thrombosis present if the patient is deficient in factor XII or prekallikrein)

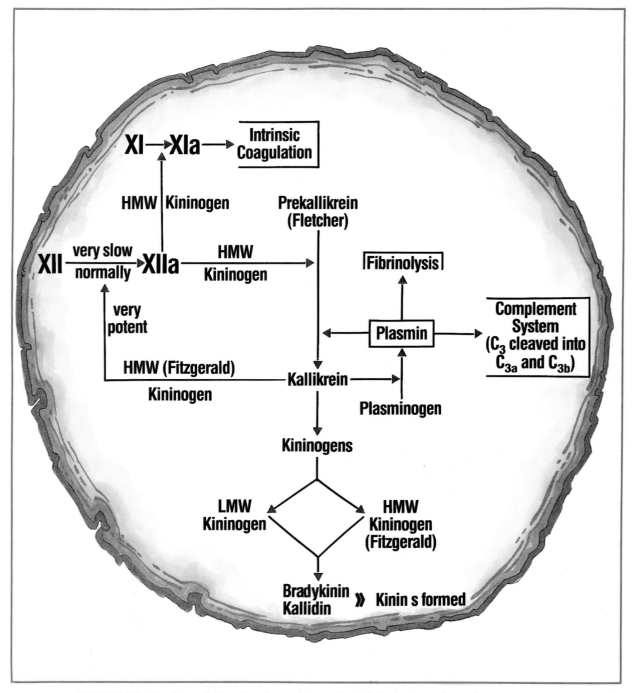

FIGURE 26–15 Interrelationship of coagulation, fibrinolytic, kinin, and complement systems.

A smaller subunit or protein that is associated with factor VIII is responsible for the clotting or procoagulant activity of factor VIII (VIII:C). The C in the expression VIII:C stands for "coagulant." It is factor VIII:C that is functionally active in the coagulation cascade.

The vWF portion of the complex carries the VIII:C procoagulant portion. The vWF portion may exhibit a stabilizing effect over factor VIII:C by protecting it from proteolytic activity.[6] Because of vWF's extremely large size and its ability to bind to the platelet membrane GPIb and IIb/IIIa receptors, it appears to have a role in anchoring the platelet plug to the vessel breach.

Common Pathway

The common pathway begins with the activation of factor X by the intrinsic system, the extrinsic system, or both (see Fig. 26–14A–D). Factor Xa, in the presence of factor V, Ca^{2+}, and phospholipid (PF3), converts prothrombin to its active form, thrombin. Thrombin then

Factor X

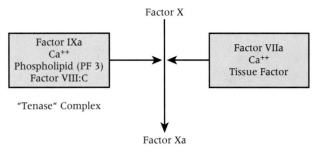

"Tenase" Complex

Factor Xa

FIGURE 26–16 Activation of factor X at the beginning of the common pathway and the "tenase" complex.

takes the following actions: it feeds back to activate factors VIII and V, converts fibrinogen to soluble fibrin monomer, and helps to stabilize the fibrin monomer by converting factor XIII to XIIIa, which crosslinks the fibrin monomers to form stable fibrin polymer. Thrombin also takes other actions not listed in this section (see Chap. 30). Since the common pathway contains the factors X, V, II, and I, these factors may be monitored by both the prothrombin time and the activated partial thromboplastin time.

TABLE 26–17 **Factor VIII Complex**

I. Smaller Protein Subunit
   1. Nomenclature
      VIII (referring to the procoagulant portion)
      VIII:C (for coagulant)
      VIII:AHF (the antihemophilic factor)
   2. Components
      a. VIII:CAg—antigen determinant of VIII, measured by immunoassays with human antibodies to VIII
      b. VIII:C—procoagulant property of normal plasma measured in the APTT test as procoagulant activity
   3. Characteristics
      a. Inherited as sex-linked recessive
      b. Acts as a cofactor in a complex with factor IXa, Ca^{2+}, and PF3 to activate factor X to Xa
II. Major Protein Portion
   1. Nomenclature
      a. vWF (von Willebrand factor)
      b. VIII:vWF
      c. VIII:R (factor VIII-related protein)
   2. Components
      a. vWF:Ag—antigen determinant on vWF that is detected by using the heterologous antibodies to von Willebrand's factor
      b. Ristocetin cofactor (VIIIR:RCₒ)—the property of normal plasma VIIIR that supports ristocetin-induced agglutination of washed normal platelets
   3. Characteristics
      a. Usually inherited as autosomal dominant
      b. Responsible for platelet adhesion
      c. Responsible for ristocetin-induced aggregation of platelets
      d. Stabilizes VIII:C when bound to vWF during circulation, and functions in prevention or protection of VIII:C from proteolytic inactivation or removal from the circulation

---

From the extrinsic system, factor VIIa in the presence of cofactor tissue thromboplastin (factor III) and ionized calcium convert factor X to Xa. From the intrinsic system, the tenase complex (factor IXa in the presence of factor VIII:C, phospholipid (PF 3), and Ca^{2+}) converts factor X to Xa (see Fig. 26–16).

After the formation of factor Xa, this activated factor, along with cofactor V, in the presence of Ca^{2+} and phospholipid (PF3), converts factor II, prothrombin, to the active enzyme thrombin (Fig. 26–17). The phospholipid is present to provide surfaces so that prothrombin and factor X can be bound by bridges of ionized calcium.[14] The association of factor Xa, factor V, phospholipid, and Ca^{2+} is called the *prothrombinase complex* (or the prothrombin activator) because it enzymatically converts the substrate prothrombin to the enzymatically active thrombin (see Fig. 26–17). This additional macromolecular complex of factors Xa, V, IV (Ca^{2+}), PF3 (the platelet membrane phospholipid), and prothrombin also assembles on the surface of activated platelets.

An interesting corollary to this discussion is that, as prothrombin is converted to thrombin, a prothrombin F1.2 fragment splits off. F1.2 may be useful as adjunct testing in assessing thrombosis.[15]

Activation of thrombin is slow, but once generated, it further amplifies coagulation. Thrombin does the following and more (see Chap. 30):
   1. Converts fibrinogen to fibrin
   2. Activates factor XIII
   3. Enhances factor V and VIII activity
   4. Induces platelet aggregation

Thrombin acts on fibrinogen to form fibrin monomers. Fibrinogen is composed of three pairs of polypeptide chains (two alpha chains, two beta chains, and two gamma chains) (Fig. 26–18). Thrombin cleaves a portion of each of the alpha and beta polypeptides to form fibrinopeptides A and B. Most of the alpha and beta chains are still left on the fibrinogen molecule.[2] After this cleavage, resulting in removal of fibrinopeptides A and B, the remainder of the fibrinogen molecule is called fibrin monomer (see Fig. 26–18).

By using the PT and APTT test results in the laboratory, one can identify defects or deficiencies as occurring in the intrinsic, extrinsic, or common pathways of blood coagulation with the exception of factor XIII functional deficiency. Using Table 26–18, the reader can practice interpretation of these tests in identifying possible factor deficiencies. It may be helpful to refer to Table 26–15 for a review of physical prop-

Prothrombin

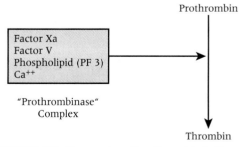

"Prothrombinase" Complex

Thrombin

FIGURE 26–17 Conversion of prothrombin to thrombin by prothrombinase complex.

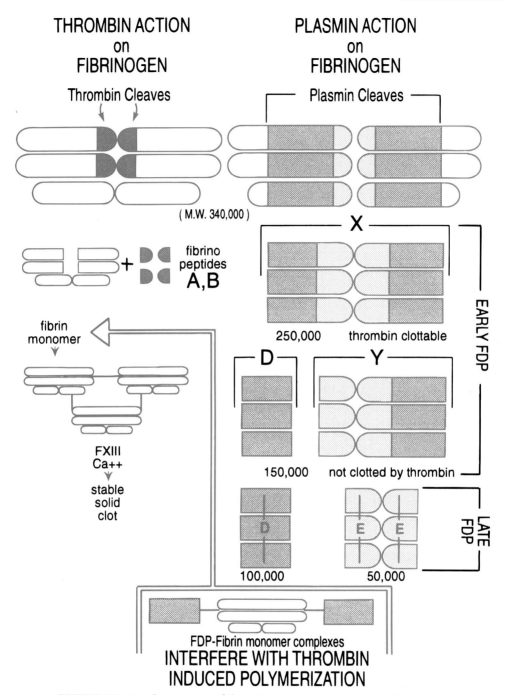

FIGURE 26–18 Comparison of thrombin and plasmin activity of fibrinogen.

erties of the coagulation factors. Table 26–19 summarizes the properties of the coagulation factors.

Current Concepts of the Coagulation System

There is more interaction between the extrinsic, intrinsic, and common pathways of coagulation than first believed. Newer concepts are denoted by the dashed lines in Figure 26–14. These newer concepts are probably beyond the scope of the beginning student of hemostasis.

Division of the coagulation process into strictly defined extrinsic and intrinsic pathways has been abandoned because the cascade theory has been extensively modified. It has been reported that factor VIIa of the extrinsic pathway can directly activate factor IX of the intrinsic pathway (see dashed lines on Fig. 26–14). Additionally, it is reported that factor VII can be activated by factors XIIa, IXa, Xa, and thrombin (see dashed lines on Fig. 26–14). It has therefore been hypothesized that factor VII may be the key regulatory protein that initiates blood coagulation. In addition,

TABLE 26–18 Use of PT and APTT for Identification of Factor Deficiency in Coagulation Studies

Patient PT	Results PTT	PT Adsorbed Plasma Reagent	PT Serum Reagent	PTT Adsorbed Plasma Reagent	PTT Serum Reagent	Deficiency
N	Ab	—	—	C	NC	VIII
N	Ab	—	—	C	C	XI, XII*
N	Ab	—	—	NC	C	IX
Ab	Ab	C	NC	C	NC	V
Ab	Ab	NC	C	NC	C	X
Ab	Ab	NC	NC	NC	NC	II
Ab	N	NC	C	—	—	VII

N = normal time; Ab = abnormal time; C = time corrected to normal; — = not applicable; NC = time not corrected to normal.
*No associated bleeding occurs in this deficiency.

TABLE 26–19 Coagulation Factor Nomenclature at a Glance

Factor	Synonym	Clotting Pathway	Molecular Weight (daltons)	Site of Production
I	Fibrinogen	Intrinsic, extrinsic, common pathway	340,000	Liver
II	Prothrombin	Intrinsic, extrinsic, common pathway	71,600	Liver—Vitamin K-dependent
III	Tissue thromboplastin	Extrinsic system only	45,000	Thromboplastic activity present in most tissues
V	Labile factor proaccelerin	Intrinsic, extrinsic, common pathway	350,000	Liver
VII	Stable factor proconvertin	Extrinsic system only	50,000	Liver—Vitamin K-dependent
VIII	Antihemophilic factor (AHF)/ coagulant (VIII:C)	Intrinsic system only	330,000	Liver
IX	Christmas factor, plasma thromboplastin component (PTC)	Intrinsic only	60,000	Liver—Vitamin K-dependent
X	Stuart-Prower factor	Intrinsic, extrinsic, common pathway	58,800	Liver—Vitamin K-dependent
XI	Plasma thromboplastin antecedent (PTA)	Intrinsic only	143,000	Liver
XII	Hageman factor/ contact factor	Intrinsic only	76,000	Liver
XIII	Fibrin-stabilizing factor (FSF)	Intrinsic, extrinsic, common pathway	320,000	Liver or platelets
Prekallikrein	Fletcher factor	Intrinsic only	100,000	Liver
High-molecular-weight kininogen	Fitzgerald factor	Intrinsic only	200,000	Liver

Note: Although not a coagulation protein or factor, calcium is sometimes denoted as factor IV.

tissue factor pathway inhibitor (TFPI) is the most recently characterized protein involved in the regulation of hemostasis.[5] Until more information is generated, and for simplicity of presentation, the reader should still be able to assimilate the classic cascade presentation of fibrin formation, with an awareness of the underlying complexity of the protein and activation relationships.

FIBRIN-LYSING (FIBRINOLYTIC) SYSTEM

The fibrin-forming and fibrin-lysing systems are intimately related. Activation of coagulation also activates fibrin lysis. Fibrinolysis, the physiologic process of removing unwanted fibrin deposits, represents a gradual progressive enzymatic cleavage of fibrin to soluble fragments. These fragments are then removed from the circulation by the fixed macrophages of the reticuloendothelial system (RES). This action of the fibrinolytic system re-establishes blood flow in vessels occluded by a thrombus and facilitates the healing process following injury.

The fibrinolytic system is mediated mainly by the enzyme plasmin, which acts primarily on fibrin to produce lysis of the clot. Plasmin is generated from the inactive zymogen called *plasminogen.* Plasminogen is activated to plasmin by tissue plasminogen activator (TPA) and other substances listed in Table 26–20.

A number of plasmin inhibitors exist to keep fibrinolysis from getting out of control.

In addition to plasmin, plasminogen, and plasminogen activators, inhibitors of plasmin are a part of the fibrinolytic system. They include alpha-2 antiplasmin (a rapid inhibitor of plasmin), alpha-2 macroglobulin (a slower inhibitor of plasmin), and others (see section on protease inhibitors and Chap. 29).

It is important to realize that some of the same substances that initiate or enhance clot formation also initiate clot degradation. For example, in tissue, both tissue thromboplastin (initiator of extrinsic pathway of fibrin formation) and TPA (which activates plasmino-

TABLE 26–19	**Coagulation Factor Nomenclature at a Glance (*Continued*)**				
Plasma Concentration (μg/ml)	Half-life Disappearance (hr)	Minimum Hemostatic Level	Storage Stability	Active Form	Other Characteristics (all factors are present in normal fresh plasma)
2000–4000	120	50–100 mg%	Stable	Protein substrate	Activity destroyed during coagulation process/ present in absorbed plasma
100	100	40 concentration	Stable	Serine protease	Consumed during coagulation process
0	N/A	N/A	Stable	Cofactor	Found in tissues
5–12	25	10% concentration	Labile	Cofactor	Activity destroyed during coagulation process/ present in absorbed plasma
10–20	5	10% concentration	Stable	Serine protease	Present in serum
10–20	8–12	30% concentration	Labile	Cofactor	Activity destroyed during coagulation process/ present in absorbed plasma
3–4	20	30% concentration	Stable	Serine protease	Present in serum
6–8	65	10% concentration	Stable	Serine protease	Present in serum
2–7	65	20–30% concentration	Stable	Serine protease	Present in serum and absorbed plasma
30–40	60	0%	Stable	Serine protease	Present in serum and absorbed plasma
25	150	1% concentration	Stable	Transglutaminase	Actively destroyed during coagulation process/present in absorbed plasma
35–50	35	?	? Stable	Serine protease	Present in serum and absorbed plasma
70–90	156	?	? Stable	Cofactor	Present in serum and absorbed plasma

Note: Although not a coagulation protein or factor, calcium is sometimes denoted as factor IV.

TABLE 26–20 **Some Plasminogen Activators**
TPA (tissue kinase released from injured tissue and endothelium)
Kallikrein
Urokinase, streptokinase, staphylokinase
Factor XIIa (indirect activator through conversion of prekallikrein)
APSAC (the thrombolytic agent acyl-plasminogen-streptokinase activator complex)
Endotoxin
Antigen-antibody complex
Thrombin (indirectly through inducing release of TPA from endothelial cells)

Abbreviation: TPA = tissue plasminogen activator
Source: Information taken from Bick and Murano[2] and Canton.[19]

TABLE 26–21 **Plasmin Actions**
Destroys fibrinogen and fibrin
Produces FDPs, which increase vascular permeability and interfere with thrombin-induced fibrin formation (see Fig. 26–18)
Produces D-Dimer, a degradation product specifically derived from cross-linked stabilized fibrin polymer
Destroys factors V, VIII, IX, XI, and other plasma proteins
Indirectly enhances or amplifies conversion of factor XII to XIIa (see Fig. 26–15)
Enhances or amplifies conversion of prekallikrein to kallikrein, liberating kinins from kininogen
Cleaves C3 into fragments (see section on complement system)

Abbreviation: FDP = fibrin(ogen) degradation products
Source: Reproduced from Bick and Murano,[2] with permission.

gen) are released with endothelial damage. TPA is produced by vascular endothelial cells and selectively binds to fibrin as it activates fibrin-bound plasminogen. Because circulating plasminogen is not activated by TPA, this biologic substance is efficient in dissolving a clot without causing systemic fibrinolysis and serves as an ideal therapeutic fibrinolytic agent.

Biologic TPA has been successfully produced by recombinant deoxyribonucleic acid (DNA) technology and is currently available. TPA-I-1 and TPA-I-2, inhibitors of TPA, also exist and contribute to controlling its actions.[2]

It is also important to note that thrombin generates both fibrin and plasmin formation. In addition, prekallikrein (Fletcher factor) and HMWK (Fitzgerald factor) indirectly initiate clotting (via factor XIIa) as well as plasmin formation (see Fig. 26–15).

Action of Plasmin

Plasmin is a broad-spectrum endopeptidase (proteolytic enzyme) that acts nonspecifically, with a strong affinity for fibrin. Plasmin, however, cannot distinguish between the protein fibrin and fibrinogen. The action of plasmin begins by splitting off pieces of each of the alpha and beta polypeptides (a larger portion than that cleaved by thrombin) and a smaller piece of each of the two gamma polypeptides from fibrinogen. The remaining molecule is called the X monomer (which is still thrombin-clottable).

As plasmin continues its action, it further splits the X monomer into a Y fragment (not clottable by thrombin) and a smaller D fragment. Further action of plasmin cleaves the Y fragment into D and E fragments. Therefore, the final fibrin-split products are two D fragments and one E fragment generated from one molecule of fibrinogen (see Fig. 26–18). These products are collectively known as either fibrin(ogen) degradation products (FDPs) or fibrin(ogen)-split products (FSPs).

The term *fibrin(ogen)* means that the FDPs can come from either fibrinogen or fibrin. Early FDPs include X monomer and Y fragments; late FDPs include D and E fragments. These fragments are important clinically because they can increase vascular permeability and interfere with thrombin-induced fibrin formation. In patients with certain disease conditions, when plas-

min is activated, FDPs are measured (see Chap. 29 for further information).

In addition to its action on fibrin and fibrinogen, plasmin also destroys factors V, VIII, and other coagulation factors. Plasmin actions are summarized in Table 26–21.

KININ SYSTEM

The kinin system, important in inflammation, vascular permeability, and chemotaxis, is activated by both the coagulation and fibrinolytic systems.

In this system, prekallikrein (Fletcher factor) is activated to kallikrein by factor XIIa (Hageman factor) and plasmin. The kinin system is also involved in the contact activation phase of the intrinsic pathway of coagulation. Activation of factor XII to XIIa does not occur without kallikrein or HMWK. Kallikrein amplifies the generation of factor XII, and HMWK is an essential factor in the activation of factor XI to XIa. HMWK (Fitzgerald factor) is necessary in both the fibrin-forming and fibrin-lysing systems (see Fig. 26–15).

Kallikrein is an enzyme that can act on kininogens—low molecular weight (LMW) and high molecular weight (HMW, or Fitzgerald factor)—and convert them to kinins. The kinins generated may include substances such as kallidin and bradykinin. Bradykinin functions to:
1. Increase vascular permeability
2. Contract smooth muscle
3. Dilate small blood vessels
4. Induce inflammation and pain
5. Release prostaglandins from tissues

PROTEASE INHIBITORS

Because the fibrinolytic system is activated when coagulation is activated, extra fibrin is degraded and eliminated along with some of the coagulation factors. However, enzymes such as plasmin and kallikrein still circulate until they are eliminated by: (1) liver hepatocytes (which have an affinity for activated enzymes), (2) reticuloendothelial system (RES) cells (which picks

TABLE 26–22 **Some Important Serine Protease Inhibitors**
Antithrombin III
Alpha-2 macroglobulin
Alpha-2 antiplasmin
Alpha-1 antitrypsin
C1 esterase inhibitor
Protein C inhibitor
Protein S inhibitor

up particulate matter), or (3) serine protease inhibitors present in plasma.

Serine protease inhibitors attach to various enzymes and inactivate them. Some important serine protease inhibitors are listed in Table 26–22.

Antithrombin III, also termed heparin cofactor or factor Xa inhibitor, is the major inactivator of thrombin and Xa. It is considered the most important physiologic anticoagulant because possibly more than 90% of the antithrombin activity of normal human plasma is derived from AT-III.[16] In addition, AT-III inhibits factors XIIa, XIa, IXa, protein S, protein C, plasmin, and kallikrein.[16] AT-III may also be said to indirectly inactivate factor VIIIa and other factors through inhibition of thrombin, although the inactivation of factors VIIIa and Va is usually ascribed to activated protein C.

In its natural state, AT-III is a slow progressive inhibitor. However, in the presence of heparin it becomes a very potent inhibitor of coagulation. Therefore the efficacy of heparin therapy depends on the level of AT-III.

Alpha-2 macroglobulin is a nonspecific inhibitor that works on many coagulation factors as well as a plasmin inhibitor secondary to alpha-2 antiplasmin binding site saturation.[17] The major blood inhibitor of plasmin is alpha-2 antiplasmin. Alpha-1 antitrypsin inhibits coagulation factors such as Xa, XIa and thrombin[13] and some fibrinolytic factors such as plasmin.[18] C1 esterase inhibitor inhibits factor XIa, XIIa, XIIa fragments, kallikrein,[13] and plasmin.[19]

All of these protease inhibitors have broad spectrums of inhibition, even though specificity for one factor or more may be exhibited. Both kallikrein and plasmin are inhibited by all of these serine proteSe inhibitors.

Also included in this group is a vitamin K–dependent protein inhibitor known as protein C (autoprothrombin II-A). Protein C is a serine protease inhibitor that acts as an anticoagulant by proteolytically cleaving factors Va and VIIIa, resulting in their inactivation. For protein C to be activated, thrombin must first bind to thrombomodulin, which is present on the endothelial cell surface. Once the thrombin-thrombomodulin complex forms, thrombin loses its ability to convert fibrinogen to fibrin or to activate platelets,[16] but now can convert protein C to its activated form (protein CA). Activated protein C (APC), then, in the presence of its cofactor, free protein S (another vitamin K–dependent protein), can inactivate factors V and VIII:C. Deficiencies of proteins C and S are associated with a predisposition for thrombosis.[16]

Finally, it should be mentioned that the generation of activated protein C may be regulated by its own specific inhibitor. APC inhibitor, along with AT-III and

heparin cofactor II (which inhibits thrombin and chymotrypsin),[16] is the third heparin-sensitive protease inhibitor. Recent studies indicate that it appears to be a plasma-endothelial inhibitor.[16] Alpha-1 antitrypsin[19] and plasminogen activator inhibitor 3 (PAI-3) (former name protein C inhibitor I)[19,20] also inhibit APC. PAI-1 and PAI-2 also inhibit TPA.[20]

COMPLEMENT SYSTEM

The complement system is composed of approximately 22 serum proteins that, working together with antibodies and clotting factors, play an important role as mediators of both immune and allergic reactions. The reactions in which complement participates take place in the blood or in other body fluids. The most important biologic role of complement is the production of cell membrane lysis of antibody-coated target cells. Two independent pathways of activation of the complement cascade may occur along with a common cytolytic pathway. These are designated the classic and alternate pathways of complement activation (see Chap. 13 for a review of the complement system).

Plasmin activates complement by cleaving C3 into C3a and C3b. C1 esterase inhibitor inactivates complement and also has a role in hemostasis as described above.

Both the coagulation system and the fibrinolytic system are interrelated with complement. Plasmin is an important activator of complement, possessing the ability to cleave directly C3 into C3a and C3b.[21] C3a is an anaphylotoxin that causes increased vascular permeability via degranulation of mast cells releasing histamine. C3b is an opsonin causing immune adherence. C5a is a chemotactic agent and an anaphylatoxin. The hemostatic value of the C1 esterase inhibitor has already been stated above, and it is also an inactivator of the complement sequence.

The interrelationship of the coagulation, complement, and fibrinolytic systems is clinically demonstrated in the condition known as hereditary angioneurotic edema. In this disease, there is no inhibition of C1 enzyme activity. The allergic-type symptoms are increased in stressful conditions. Stress results in increased blood levels of plasmin and therefore complement activation. In the absence of adequate C1 inactivation, the body cannot rid itself of the complement products.

LABORATORY EVALUATION OF HEMOSTASIS

The diagnosis of any hemostatic disorder is made by the systematic evaluation of information obtained in the history and physical examination, along with the appropriate laboratory testing. Diagnostically, the most valuable data from a patient's history include:

1. Documentation of the physical appearance, site, severity, and frequency of bleeding episodes
2. A reliable family history of bleeding disorders
3. An accurate drug history
4. Other contributing or underlying illnesses

Bleeding disorders present themselves differently depending on the causative problem. Two general rules are operative. First, patients with platelet disor-

TABLE 26-23 Some Common Laboratory Screening Tests for Hemostatic Disorders

Platelet count
Peripheral blood smear examination
Prothrombin time (PT)
Activated partial thromboplastin time (APTT)
Template bleeding time (TBT)
Thrombin time (TT)*

*Included less often

ders usually exhibit petechiae and mucous membrane bleeding. In general, this is because a defect of primary hemostasis is present, resulting in the formation of a defective platelet plug. Second, patients with coagulation defects usually develop deep spreading hematomas and bleeding into the joints with evident hematuria. In general, this is because a defect of secondary hemostasis is present, resulting in the inadequate fibrin reinforcement of a functionally normal platelet plug.

Alteration of any aspect of the hemostatic mechanism may cause abnormal bleeding in a wide variety of familial and acquired clinical disorders. These defects may be classified into three broad categories that can be diagnostically approached by a systematic laboratory evaluation. These include vascular and platelet disorders, coagulation factor deficiencies, and fibrinolytic disorders.

Although many laboratories differ in their approach to a bleeding disorder, a general profile of laboratory tests is usually established. This profile can often be used as a means of differentiating various hemostatic problems. Laboratory screening tests routinely ordered to assess hemostatic dysfunction are listed in Table 26-23.

The PT and APTT are both variations of plasma recalcification times accelerated by the addition of a thromboplastic substance. The PT reagent contains thromboplastin and calcium that, when added to patient plasma, initiates rapid formation of a fibrin clot. The APTT reagent contains phospholipid substitute (cephalin), and, after incubation with plasma, calcium is added to the system to initiate fibrin clot formation.

As mentioned previously, the PT test measures the factors of the extrinsic pathway of coagulation (factors VII, X, V, II, and I). Factor VII is the only factor listed that is restricted to the extrinsic system, as factors X, V, II, and I are part of the common pathway (see Fig. 26-14). The PT test is ideally used to detect early vitamin K deficiencies, as factor VII has the shortest half-life of the coagulation factors and is vitamin K–dependent. The PT test is also used to monitor oral anticoagulant therapy. Any abnormalities of these factors, a vitamin K defect, liver disease, or the presence of inhibitors will result in an abnormally prolonged PT.

The APTT test measures factors of the intrinsic pathway of blood coagulation (XII, Fletcher, Fitzgerald, XI, IX, VIII, X, V, II, and I). It should be noted that factors XII, XI, IX, VIII, Fletcher, and Fitzgerald are limited to the intrinsic system. Deficiencies or inhibitors of any of these factors will result in an abnormally prolonged APTT. Both the PT and APTT tests will show prolonged results with an abnormality of the shared factors of the common pathway (X, V, II, and I). A factor abnormality refers to a deficiency of that factor in plasma for any one of the following reasons:

1. Decreased synthesis
2. Synthesis of a dysfunctional factor molecule
3. Excessive destruction of factors through acquired disorders
4. Inactivation of factors through circulating inhibitors

TABLE 26-24 Interpretation of Coagulation Test Results

Test Battery	Results	Possible Cause
APTT PT TT	Abnormal Abnormal Normal	1. Vitamin K defect 2. Liver disease 3. Inhibitor present 4. Factor deficiency in common pathway (X, V, II)
APTT PT	Abnormal Normal	1. Factor deficiency in the intrinsic pathway (XII, XI, IX, VIII, Fletcher, Fitzgerald) 2. Lupus anticoagulant 3. Specific factor inhibitor
APTT PT	Normal Abnormal	1. Factor deficiency in the extrinsic pathway (VII) 2. Specific factor inhibitor
APTT PT TT	Abnormal Abnormal Abnormal	1. Factor deficiency (I) 2. Severe liver disease 3. DIC 4. Potent inhibitor 5. Hypofibrinogenemia or dysfibrinogenemia
APTT PT TT	Normal Normal Normal	1. Factor deficiency (XIII) 2. Specific factor inhibitor 3. Normal patient or laboratory error

Abbreviations: PT = prothrombin time; APTT = activated partial thromboplastin time; TT = thrombin time; DIC = disseminated intravascular coagulation

Test	Vascular Disorder	Quantitative Platelet Disorder	Qualitative Platelet Disorder	Factor Deficiency	Fibrinolytic Disorder (Acquired)
Platelet count	N	AbN	N	N	AbN
PT	N	N	N	AbN*	AbN
APTT	N	N	N	AbN*	AbN
TBT	AbN	AbN	AbN	N	AbN

TABLE 26–25 Classification of Bleeding Disorders by Screening Tests

Abbreviations: N = normal; AbN = abnormal; PT = prothrombin time; APTT = activated partial thromboplastin time; TBT = template bleeding time
*Dependent on the factor deficiency; see Table 26–24 for specific information.

Table 26–24 summarizes the interpretation of the PT and APTT test results.

As the reader will note, neither the PT nor the APTT screens adequately for factor XIII activity. The PT and APTT test for the initial conversion of fibrinogen to fibrin.[12] Cross-linked stabilized fibrin, which develops later through mediation of factor XIIIa, does not impact on the PT or APTT.[12] Special testing to assess factor XIII activity must be done (see Chap. 34).

PT and APTT can be reported in a variety of ways, such as patient seconds and control seconds, percent activity, and ratio. Recent changes have occurred in PT reporting that bear mention. The international normalized ratio (INR) now seems to be the mode of choice for PT reporting[22–24] because it adjusts for source-related thromboplastin sensitivity differences through use of a mathematical exponent, the ISI. The ISI is unique to each batch of thromboplastin and is furnished by the manufacturer.

Numerous articles state the method for reporting INR values. INR standardizes PT reporting worldwide by adjusting all reported values to a World Health Organization international reference thromboplastin standard (so that all PT results reported by INR methodology are theoretically comparable), and facilitates optimal oral anticoagulant therapy in patients at risk for thrombosis, especially those on coumadin who travel extensively and require frequent monitoring. According to one source[25] thromboplastins with a low ISI (less than 1.2) may be preferable as they seem to correlate better to human brain thromboplastin.

The thrombin time is a measure of the ability of thrombin to convert fibrinogen to fibrin and is particularly useful in the evaluation of circulating anticoagulants (pathologic inhibitors). The thrombin time is prolonged in the following conditions:
1. Hypofibrinogenemia and dysfibrinogenemia
2. Treatment with heparin
3. Circulating FDPs
4. Pathologic circulating inhibitors

Table 26–25 can be used as a general guide toward categorizing bleeding disorders into the groups previously listed, using the suggested screening tests. Additional laboratory testing is designed to narrow down the abnormality to one of these specific areas. As a result, laboratory testing can be divided into the following categories:
1. Screening tests for vascular and/or platelet dysfunction (such as bleeding time, platelet adhesion, platelet aggregation, PF3 assay, and clot retraction)
2. Tests for coagulation (such as factor assays)
3. Special tests (e.g., for fibrinolytic disorders such as tests for determination of FDPs and protamine sulfate and ethanol gel tests for detection of fibrin monomers)

SUMMARY

It should be clear from the preceding pages that the human body with its accompanying physiology geared toward maintaining homeostasis is elegant, intricate, and intriguing. Hemostasis is a logical, fascinating contributor to the overall homeostatic mechanism and is well worth further study. The reader may refer to subsequent chapters for detailed discussion of vascular and platelet-related disorders, plasma clotting factor defects, hemostatic system interaction, thrombosis and anticoagulant therapy, and laboratory methods.

CASE STUDY

A 3-year-old boy was brought to the emergency room by his mother. The child had fallen off his tricycle, knocked out his two front teeth, and had been bleeding copiously since the accident. Patient history revealed that he bruised very easily, and family history revealed that several male relatives were "free bleeders," but that no female relatives seemed to have any bleeding problems. Coagulation studies demonstrated a prolonged activated partial thromboplastin time (APTT), a normal prothrombin time (PT), and a normal platelet count. The attending physician also post-ordered a bleeding time test, the result of which was normal.

Since the PT was normal and the APTT was prolonged, an intrinsic factor deficiency/defect was suspected (possibly factors XII, XI, IX, or VIII). Deficiencies involving common pathway factors (X, V, II, and I) and extrinsic pathway factor (VII) were ruled out because of the normal PT result. Factor XII deficiency was considered unlikely since a deficiency in this factor seems to predispose a patient to thrombosis rather than to bleeding (see Chap. 28), leaving factors XI, IX, and VIII as possibilities for the deficiency (inherited deficiencies usually occur singly, and this patient is young enough to have an inherited factor deficiency).

This laboratory routinely performs an APTT mixing study as a screen for circulating anticoagulants prior to performing correction studies (see Chap. 28). The mixing study was performed using a 1:1 ratio of the boy's plasma to normal plasma. The APTT corrected to high normal, ruling out the possibility of an anticoagulant disorder.

Correction studies using serum reagent and adsorbed plasma reagent were performed (see Table 26–18). The patient's APTT corrected downward to high normal using the adsorbed plasma reagent, but did not correct using the serum reagent. Using the chart in Table 26–18, the cause of the prolonged APTT was identified as factor VIII deficiency.

This was a true factor VIII deficiency, meaning that factor VIII:C was deficient (the procoagulant portion of the factor VIII complex). This is not to be confused with a deficiency of factor VIII:vWF (von Willebrand's factor), the transport portion of the factor VIII complex, deficiency of which causes von Willebrand's disease. Inheritance of a sex-linked, recessive deficiency of factor VIII:C causes hemophilia A. Hemophilia A patients are almost exclusively male (the female is the carrier, and only under very special conditions can a female inherit the disease). More information on hemophilia A and other factor deficiencies can be obtained in Chapter 28.

This case study illustrates the use of the correction studies in identification of a factor deficiency.

Questions

1. What active role does this factor play in the coagulation cascade?
2. Where is the factor produced?

REFERENCES

1. Kent, TH and Hart, MN: Introduction to Human Disease, ed 3. Appleton & Lange, Norwalk, 1993, p 144.
2. Bick, RL and Murano, G: Physiology of hemostasis. In Bick, RL (ed): Hematology: Clinical and Laboratory Practice. CV Mosby, St Louis, 1992, pp 1285–1309.
3. Jaffe, EA: The role of blood vessels in hemostasis. In Williams, WJ, Beutler, E, Erslev, AJ, et al (eds): Hematology, ed 4. McGraw-Hill, New York, 1990, pp 1322–1328.
4. Ruggeri, ZM: New Insights into the Mechanisms of Platelet Adhesion and Aggregation. Semin Hematol 31:229, 1994.
5. Brandt, JT: Overview of hemostasis. In McClatchey, KD (ed): Clinical Laboratory Medicine. Williams & Wilkins, Baltimore, 1994, pp 1045–1062.
6. Zimmerman, TS and Ruggeri, ZM: Laboratory diagnosis of von Willebrand disease. In Bick, RL (ed): Hematology: Clinical and Laboratory Practice. CV Mosby, St Louis, 1992, pp 1441–1445.
7. Bennett, JS and Shattil, SJ: Platelet function. In Williams, WJ, Beutler, E, Erslev, AJ, et al (eds): Hematology, ed 4. McGraw-Hill, New York, 1990, pp 1233–1243.
8. Holmson, H: Composition of platelets. In Williams, WJ, Beutler, E, Erslev, AJ, et al (eds): Hematology, ed 4. McGraw-Hill, New York, 1990, pp 1182–1191.
9. Speck, RE and Melvin, JR: A comparison of a slide platelet aggregation procedure with the bleeding time test. American Clinical Laboratory 12, 1994.
10. Harker, LA: Antithrombotic therapy. In Williams, WJ, Beutler, E, Erslev, AJ, et al (eds): Hematology, ed 4. McGraw-Hill, New York, 1990, pp 1569–1579.
11. Slide 18, 35: Functional aspects of hemostasis. In Slide Presentation, Cat. No. 5184. Helena Laboratories Hemostasis Systems, September 1993.
12. Bick, RL: Antithrombotic therapy. In Bick, RL (ed): Hematology: Clinical and Laboratory Practice. CV Mosby, St Louis, 1992, pp 1603–1617.
13. Comp, PC: Control of coagulation reactions. In Williams, WJ, Beutler, E, Erslev, AJ, et al (eds): Hematology, ed 4. McGraw-Hill, New York, 1990, pp 1304–1308.
14. Mammen, EF: Congenital coagulation protein disorders. In Bick, RL (ed): Hematology: Clinical and Laboratory Practice. CV Mosby, St Louis, 1992, pp 1391–1414.
15. Hursting, MJ: An enzyme-linked immunosorbent assay for prothrombin fragment 1.2 (F1.2). American Clinical Laboratory 32, 1992.
16. Bick, RL: Hypercoagulability and thrombosis. In Bick, RL (ed): Hematology: Clinical and Laboratory Practice. CV Mosby, St Louis, 1992, pp 1463–1493.
17. Lazarchick, J and Kizer, J: Interaction of the fibrinolytic, coagulation, and kinin systems and related pathology. In Harmening, DM (ed): Clinical Hematology and Fundamentals of Hemostasis, ed 2. FA Davis, Philadelphia, 1992, pp 486–497.
18. Alper, CA: The plasma proteins. In Williams, WJ, Beutler, E, Erslev, AJ, et al (eds): Hematology, ed 4. McGraw-Hill, New York, 1990, pp 1616–1626.
19. Canton, MM: Introduction to thrombosis and anticoagulant therapy. In Harmening, DM (ed): Clinical Hematology and Fundamentals of Hemostasis, ed 2. FA Davis, Philadelphia, 1992, pp 498–513.
20. Colorado Coagulation Consultants: The Fibrinolytic Mechanism. Coagulation Update, October 1993.
21. Warren, JS, Ward, PA, and Johnson, KJ: The Inflammatory Response. In Williams, WJ, Beutler, E, Erslev, AJ, et al (eds): Hematology, ed 4. McGraw-Hill, New York, 1990, pp 63–69.
22. Bick, RL: Oral anticoagulants and the INR: Confusion, controversy, fiction, and fact. American Clinical Laboratory 36, 1994.
23. Maldonado, WE and Melvin, JR: A Physician's Guide to the International Normalized Ratio. Ortho Diagnostic Systems, Raritan, NJ, August, 1989.
24. Brigden, ML and Preece, E: INR: A Better Way to Report Prothrombin Times. Medical Laboratory Observer 25:1991.
25. Hawkins, P and Vondergeest, J: An ultrasensitive PT reagent using recombinant human tissue factor. American Clinical Laboratory November 1993.

BIBLIOGRAPHY

Abrams, C: Case studies put consumptive coagulopathies in perspective. Advance for Medical Technologists 2(37):16, September 10, 1990.

Abrams, C: Consumptive coagulopathies: Many types and many cases. Advance for Medical Technologists 2(30):8, July 23, 1990.

Abrams, C: Logical approach simplifies APTT evaluation. Advance for Medical Laboratory Professionals 3(34):18, August 26, 1991.

Abrams, C: More lupus inhibitors being seen in coagulation labs. Advance for Medical Technologists 2(5):18, January 29, 1990.

Abrams, C: Quest continues for perfect thrombolytic therapy. Advance for Medical Laboratory Professionals 5(7):10, February 15, 1993.

Abrams, C: Treatment of thrombosis improves as causes are better understood. Advance for Medical Laboratory Professionals 3(9):16, March 4, 1991.

Barnhart, MI: Platelet responses in health and disease. Mol Cell Biochem 22:113, 1978.

Baruch, D, et al: Von Willebrand factor and platelet function. Clin Haematol 2:627, 1989.

Berndt, MC, Fournier, DJ, and Castaldi, PA: Bernard-Soulier syndrome. Clin Haematol 2:585, 1989.

Caen, JP: Glanzmann's thrombasthenia. Clin Haematol 2:609, 1989.

Cochran, D: Case study in hemostasis: Protein C deficiency. Advance for Medical Laboratory Professionals 7, November 22, 1993.

Daniel, L and Tuszynski, P: Platelet contractile proteins. In Coleman, R-V, et al (eds): Hemostasis and Thrombosis. JB Lippincott, Philadelphia, 1987, pp 641, 649.

Decary, F and Rock, G: Platelet membrane in transfusion medicine. S Karger AG, Basel, Switzerland, 1988.

Deykin, D and Miale, JB: Clinical Importance of the Bleeding Time Test. Reprint, General Diagnostics, October 1982.

Dolan, G, Ball, J, and Preston, FE: Protein C and protein S. Clin Haematol 2:999, 1989.

Evans, VJ: Looking at platelets. J Med Tech 1:9, 1984.

Evans, VJ: Platelet morphology and the blood smear. J Med Tech 1:9, 1984.

Giannelli, F: Factor IX. Clin Haematol 2:821, 1989.

Glassman, B: Platelet abnormalities in hepatobiliary diseases. Ann Clin Lab Sci 20:119, 1990.

Hill, JE and Ens, GE: Malignancy and Hemostasis. Clin Hemostasis Rev January 1988.

Hardisty, RM: Disorders of platelet secretion. Clin Haematol 2:673, 1989.

Hovig, T: Megakaryocyte and platelet morphology. Clin Haematol 2:503, 1989.

Jenny, RJ and Mann, KG: Factor V: A prototype pro-cofactor for vitamin K-dependent enzyme complexes in blood clotting. Clin Haematol 2:919, 1989.

Jensen, R and Ens, G: Hemostasis: A precarious balance assisted by naturally occurring anticoagulants. Advance for Medical Laboratory Professionals 10, September 13, 1993.

Kaplan-Gouet, C and Salmon, C: Platelet Immunology. S Karger AG, Basel, Switzerland, 1988.

Kaczor, D and Horner, AO: Protein C/Protein S Anticoagulant Pathway. American Clinical Laboratory 9, July 1993.

Koepke, JA: Duplicate PTs and PTTs. In Tips On Technology, Medical Laboratory Observer, September 1991.

Kuast, TVD, et al: Localization of VIII CAg using different monoclonal antibodies against VIII C. Thromb Haemost 50:17, 1983.

Kwan, HC and Samana, MM (eds): Clinical Thrombosis. CRC Press, Boca Raton, FL, 1989.

La Croix, KA and Davis, GL: A review of protein C and its role in hemostasis. J Med Tech 2:2, 1985.

Lane, DA and Caso, R: Antithrombin: Structure, genomic organization, function and inherited deficiency. Clin Haematol 2:961, 1989.

Lemery, LD: Hemostasis doesn't stop with the fibrin clot: A brief review of fibrinolysis. Advance for Medical Laboratory Professionals:10, November 29, 1993.

Lemery, LD: The other factor VIII: A brief review of von Willebrand's disease. Advance for Medical Laboratory Professionals 5, March 28, 1994.

Lemery, LD: The platelets can't do it alone: A brief review of secondary hemostasis. Advance for Medical Laboratory Professionals 5, November 22, 1993.

Lemery, LD: Spring a leak? Here come the platelets: A brief review of primary hemostasis. Advance for Medical Laboratory Professionals 5, November 15, 1993.

Longberry, J: Hemostasis: Part I. Screening tests to evaluate abnormal hemostasis. Am J Med Technol 48:100, 1982.

MacGillivray, RTA and Fung, MR: Molecular biology of factor X. Clin Haematol 2:897, 1989.

Mason, RG, et al: The endothelium: Roles in thrombosis and hemostasis. Arch Pathol Lab Med 101:61, 1977.

McGann, MA and Triplett, DA: Laboratory evaluation of the fibrinolytic system. Lab Med 14:18, 1983.

Menitove, JE and McCarthy, LJ: Hemostatic Disorders and the Blood Bank. American Association of Blood Banks, Arlington, VA, 1984.

O'Brien, DP: The molecular biology and biochemistry of tissue factor Clin Haematol 2:801, 1989.

Pati, HP, Gupta, MK, and Saraya, AK: Screening tests for platelet function defect: Evaluation and recommendation. Hem Rev Comm 4:1, 1990.

Peck, SD: Prolonged bleeding time: A differential diagnosis. Clin Hemost Rev 1(2):4, 1987.

Pennica, D, et al: Cloning and expression of human tissue-type plasminogen activator with DNA in E. coli. Nature 301:214, 1983.

Roberts, HR and Hussey, CU: Coagulation. In Listen, Look, and Learn Audiovisual Series, National Committee for Careers in the Medical Laboratory, Bethesda, MD.

Smith, C: Surgicutt: A device for modified template bleeding times (reprint). J Med Technol 3(4), 1986.

Speck, RE: An Accurate Assay for Platelet Factor 3. American Clinical Laboratory 16, September 1993.

Triplett, DA: Hemostasis: A Case-Oriented Approach. Igaku-Shoin, New York, 1985.

Triplett, DA, Brandt, JT: Lupus Anticoagulant: Clinical Implications and Laboratory Diagnosis. Bio/Data Corporation, Hatboro, PA, September 1944.

Tuddenham, EGD: Factor VIII and Haemophilia A. Clin Haematol 2:849, 1989.

Vermylen, J and Blockmans, D: Acquired disorders of platelet function. Clin Haematol 2:729, 1989.

Von Dem Borne, AEGK and Ouwehand, WH: Immunology of platelet disorders. Clin Haematol 2:749, 1989.

Walker, FJ: Protein C deficiency in liver disease. Ann Clin Lab Sci 20:106, 1990.

Questions

1. Which of the following is true concerning the organelle zone?
   a. Responsible for metabolic activities of the platelet
   b. Contains dense granules, alpha granules, and glycocalyx
   c. Contains the dense tubular system which is the site of prostaglandin synthesis, calcium release, and platelet relaxation
   d. Contains the OCS to deliver stored products to the platelet surface

2. What events are involved in the normal formation of a platelet plug?
   a. Adhesion, activation, fibrinolysis, secondary hemostasis
   b. Aggregation, coagulation, release reaction, lupus anticoagulant
   c. Release action, adhesion, lupus anticoagulant, secondary hemostasis
   d. Activation, adhesion, aggregation, release reaction

3. What product is resposible for stabilization of the hemostatic plug?
   a. Thromboxane A_2
   b. PF3
   c. Fibrin
   d. GPIIb

4. Which of the following are classified as contact group proteins?
   a. Factors II, VII, IX, X
   b. Factors XII, XI, PK, HMWK

c. Factors I, V, VIII, XIII
d. Factors I, II, V, X

5. Which of the following are classified as prothrombin group proteins?
   a. Factors II, VII, IX, X
   b. Factors XII, XI, PK, HMWK
   c. Factors I, V, VIII, XIII
   d. Factors I, II, V, X

6. Which of the following are classified as fibrinogen group proteins?
   a. Factors II, VII, IX, X
   b. Factors XII, XI, PK, HMWK
   c. Factors I, V, VIII, XIII
   d. Factors I, II, V, X

7. Which of the following factors are dependent on vitamin K for synthesis?
   a. Factors II, VII, IX, X
   b. Factors XII, XI, PK, HMWK
   c. Factors I, V, VIII, XIII
   d. Factors I, II, V, X

8. Which of the following factors are unique to the extrinsic system?
   a. XII, XI, X, IV, VIII, V, II, I
   b. III, VII
   c. VII, X, V, II, I
   d. XII, XI, IV, PF 3, VIII

9. What events take place in the extrinsic system?
   a. Activation of factor X to Va
   b. Acceleration of intrinsic pathway by enhancement of the activity of factors XII and XI
   c. Activation of factor XII to XIIa to initiate clotting
   d. Activation of factor VII to VIIa in the presence of Ca^{2+} and factor III

10. Which of the following factors are unique to the intrinsic system?
   a. Factors XII, XI, IX, VIII, X, V, II, I, Fletcher, Fitzgerald
   b. Factors XII, XI, IX, VIII, Fletcher, Fitzgerald
   c. Factors VII, X, V, II, I
   d. Factors III, VII, X, V, II, I

11. What factor is *not* found in the common pathway?
   a. Factor X
   b. Factor V
   c. PF3
   d. Factor XII

12. Which of the following is a function of thrombin?
   a. Conversion of fibrinogen to fibrin
   b. Activation of factor XIII to stabilize fibrinolysis
   c. Conversion of factor VII to XIIa
   d. Enhancement of factor V, VIII, and XI activity

13. Which of the following is a function of plasmin?
   a. Cleavage of TPA
   b. Destruction of fibrin
   c. Conversion of XII to XIa
   d. Inhibition of XIa

14. What is the purpose of the PT test in monitoring hemostasis?
   a. Measures factors of the extrinsic pathway
   b. Detects platelet decrease or dysfunction
   c. Detects presence of aspirin
   d. Monitors heparin therapy

15. What is the purpose of the APTT test in monitoring hemostasis?
   a. Measures factors of the intrinsic pathway
   b. Detects deficiency of factors for both intrinsic and extrinsic pathways
   c. Measures circulating FDPs
   d. Detects platelet dysfunction

Answers

1. **a** (p 487)
2. **d** (pp 488–492)
3. **c** (p 493)
4. **b** (p 494)
5. **a** (p 494)
6. **c** (p 494)
7. **a** (p 500, Table 26–19)
8. **b** (p 496)
9. **d** (p 496)
10. **b** (p 496)
11. **d** (p 498–499)
12. **a** (p 498)
13. **b** (p 502)
14. **a** (p 504)
15. **a** (p 504)

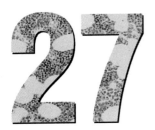

27 Quantitative and Qualitative Vascular and Platelet Disorders, Both Congenital and Acquired

Janis Wyrick-Glatzel, MS, MT(ASCP)

Objectives

At the end of this chapter, the learner should be able to:

1. Characterize von Willebrand's disease based on pathophysiology, clinical symptoms, and associated laboratory findings.
2. Characterize Bernard-Soulier syndrome based on pathophysiology, clinical symptoms, and associated laboratory findings.
3. Characterize Glanzmann's thrombasthenia based on pathophysiology, clinical symptoms, and associated laboratory findings.
4. Compare and contrast von Willebrand's disease with Bernard-Soulier syndrome.
5. Differentiate between congenital and acquired qualitative platelet disorders.
6. Describe disorders of platelet secretion based on abnormal laboratory findings.
7. Compare and contrast acute and chronic idiopathic thrombocytopenic purpura.
8. Characterize isoimmune neonatal thrombocytopenia by associated laboratory findings and clinical symptoms.
9. Differentiate between congenital and acquired vascular disorders.
10. Define thrombocytopenia, thrombocytosis, and thrombocythemia. State the expected platelet counts in each.

Numerous clinical manifestations are associated with platelet dysfunction (Table 27–1). Hemorrhagic manifestations of the skin and mucous membranes are commonly seen in platelet defects. Thromboembolic episodes occur less frequently. The most common symptoms associated with platelet defects include easy bruising, epistaxis, petechiae, prolonged bleeding from minor cuts, spontaneous gingival bleeding, menorrhagia, and gastrointestinal hemorrhage. Hemarthroses and the formation of deep hematomas after trauma generally do *not* occur.

Table 27–2 lists new and traditional screening tests used to assess the platelets' role in hemostasis. An automated platelet count and careful evaluation of the peripheral smear for estimation of platelet numbers are important initial screening tests. Evaluation of the peripheral smear for platelet morphology may yield clues in the diagnosis of inherited platelet defects or conditions associated with increased platelet destruction and decreased platelet survival. The bleeding time (BT) is the primary screening test of platelet and vascular function.

Platelet aggregation or lumiaggregation and antiplatelet antibody tests, as well as those listed in Table

TABLE 27–1 Clinical Manifestations Associated with Platelet Dysfunction

Petechiae*
Purpura*
Mild to moderate mucosal bleeding (bilateral epistaxis, gastrointestinal, genitourinary, pulmonary)
Gingival bleeding
Spontaneous bruising

*Petechiae and purpura associated with thrombocytopenia or platelet dysfunction are characteristically symmetric and found in both extremities as well as the trunk.

27–2, can be used to aid in the diagnosis of platelet dysfunction. Currently, some of these tests have limited clinical application.

New methods are available to assess platelet activity associated with hypercoagulable states (see Chaps. 30 and 34).

This chapter discusses the etiology, pathophysiology, clinical manifestation, and laboratory tests used to diagnose the various qualitative and quantitative platelet abnormalities (Table 27–3).

QUALITATIVE PLATELET DISORDERS

Congenital Disorders of Platelet Function

Congenital disorders of platelet function are considered rare and are often referred to as *thrombocytopathies*. The inherited platelet defects can be classified based on the platelet function or response that is abnormal. This classification currently includes defects of mechanisms involving: (1) platelet adhesion, (2) platelet aggregation, (3) platelet storage or secretion, (4) platelet–coagulant protein interaction, and (5) platelet–agonist interaction. Table 27–4 lists the various congenital disorders as they relate to abnormal platelet function.

Disorders of Adhesion

von Willebrand's Disease In 1926, Dr. von Willebrand documented investigation of a 5-year-old girl

TABLE 27–3 General Overview of Platelet Disorders

Platelet Defects
  Congenital
  Acquired
  Drug-induced
Thrombocytopenia
  Congenital
  Decreased production
  Increased destruction
Thrombocytosis
  Acquired
  Reactive
Thrombocythemia
Hyperactive platelets

with a history of severe bleeding. After studying the family members, of whom approximately one third had a positive history for bleeding, he noted three clinical manifestations that separated this bleeding disorder from hemophilia: mucocutaneous bleeding, an autosomal dominant inheritance, and a prolonged bleeding time.

Von Willebrand's disease (vWD) is a relatively common heterogeneous disorder characterized by quantitative or qualitative abnormalities of the large multimeric glycoprotein von Willebrand's factor (vWf).[1–4] vWD is the most common inherited bleeding disorder; affected individuals generally manifest with mild clinical bleeding (see Chap 28).

The relationship between vWF and VIII:C activity of the factor VIII complex has been intensively studied (Figs. 27–1 and 27–2). Certain functions of the molecules are known. VWF and VIII:C are individual molecules of different molecular weights capable of separation by gel filtration. vWF is an important adhesive protein following vascular injury. It serves as a ligand between platelets, vascular endothelium, and other adhesive proteins such as fibronectin. vWf has distinct domains for binding to platelet glycoprotein Ib/IX, glycoprotein IIb/IIIa[1,5] and subendothelial components heparin and collagen.[1] Platelet glycoprotein Ib serves

TABLE 27–2 Laboratory Test to Assess Platelet Functions

Peripheral blood smear (estimate of platelet numbers and morphology)
Platelet count
Bleeding time
Aggregation
Lumiaggregation (platelet release)
Platelet membrane glycoproteins (flow cytometry)
Platelet antibodies
Adhesion/retention*
Platelet factor 3 availability*
Molecular markers for platelet reactivity
Mean platelet volume (MPV)*
Platelet distribution width (PDW)*

*Limited clinical usefulness

TABLE 27–4 Congenital Disorders of Platelet Function

Disorders of Adhesion
von Willebrand's disease
Bernard-Soulier syndrome

Disorders of Aggregation
Glanzmann's thrombasthenia
Congenital afibrinogenemia

Disorders of Secretion
Storage pool deficiencies
Aspirinlike defects

Miscellaneous Congenital Disorders
May-Hegglin anomaly
Hermansky-Pudlak syndrome
Wiskott-Aldrich syndrome
Chediak-Higashi syndrome

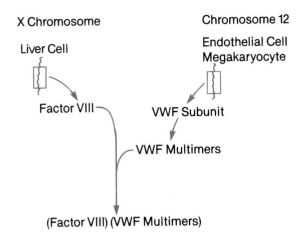

The Factor VIII/VWF Complex in Plasma

FIGURE 27-1   Factor VIII/vWF complex in plasma.

as the major receptor for vWf. Platelet adhesion is dependent upon subendothelium, GPIb, and vWf. In vWD, the platelets are intrinsically normal. A deficiency of vWf results in abnormal adhesion and coagulation. It is the interaction of platelet receptors with adhesive proteins that promote adhesion and aggregation. Congenital defects of adhesive proteins such as vWf and platelet glycoproteins are associated with impaired hemostasis and clinical hemorrhage.

The routine laboratory evaluation of patients suspected of having vWD includes a thorough clinical history, bleeding time, platelet count, factor VIII procoagulant activity measured by the activated partial thromboplastin time (APTT), quantitative measurements of plasma vWf by crossed immunoelectrophoresis or agarose gel electrophoresis, and functional assays of plasma vWf by ristocetin-induced platelet aggregation (see Chap. 28).

Bernard-Soulier Syndrome   Bernard-Soulier syndrome was first described in 1948 as a familial bleeding disorder characterized by a prolonged bleeding time and unusually large platelets. Today, it is known that Bernard-Soulier syndrome is a rare autosomal trait associated with a defect of platelet glycoprotein Ib/IX. Glycoprotein V (GP V), a thrombin substrate, has also been documented to be deficient in Bernard-Soulier platelets.[6] GPIb/IX plays a major role in various hemostatic events. GPIb/IX is the platelet receptor involved in the vWf-dependent contact adhesion of unactivated platelets to exposed subendothelium at high shear rates[7,8] and for the binding of platelets to fibrin.[9] It also serves as the high-affinity thrombin binding site important for thrombin activation of platelets.[10,11] Regulation of platelet shape and reactivity is also mediated by the GPIb/IX complex.[12] Data suggest that the platelet membrane is attached to the cytoskeleton via GPIb. The loss of normal membrane-cytoskeletal function may account for the abnormal morphology seen in Bernard-Soulier platelets.

Clinically, patients with Bernard-Soulier syndrome present with the typical symptoms of a platelet-mediated defect such as mucocutaneous bleeds of varying severity. Symptoms occur early in life and have a tendency to decrease with age. Gingival bleeds, epistaxis, purpura, and menorrhagia are frequent findings. Gastrointestinal bleeding has also been reported.

Patients with Bernard-Soulier syndrome are characterized by prolonged bleeding and mild or moderately reduced platelet counts with large irregularly shaped platelets noted on the peripheral smear (Table

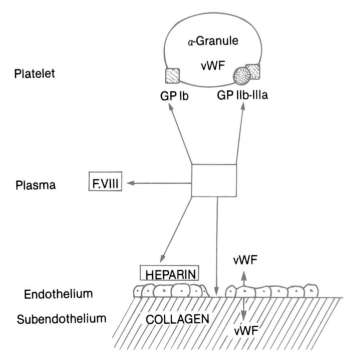

FIGURE 27-2   Schematic representation of the interactions among vWF, platelets, and collagen of the subendothelium. vWF synthesized by endothelial cells is released in plasma and in the subendothelium, is stored in the alpha granules of platelets, and can be released after stimulation. vWF mediates platelet adhesion through binding to collagen and to platelet GPIB in the presence of ristocetin, as well as the platelet GPIIB-IIIa in the presence physiologic agonists (thrombin, collagen, ADP). vWF also binds to F.VIII and to heparin.

27–5). Normal numbers of megakaryocytes are found on bone marrow examination. The observation of abnormally large platelets in patients with Bernard-Soulier syndrome is thought to be related to the role of GPIb/IX as a major connection between platelet membrane and cytoskeleton.[12] Platelet aggregation is normal with ADP, epinephrine, and collagen. Ristocetin-induced platelet aggregation is absent, whereas aggregation with thrombin is reduced. Defective ristocetin-induced platelet aggregation is also observed in vWD. This aggregation defect is corrected by the addition of normal plasma in patients with vWD, unlike Bernard-Soulier syndrome, in which normal plasma fails to correct ristocetin aggregation. The inability of normal plasma to correct the adhesion defect in Bernard-Soulier platelets highlights the fact that these platelets lack the vWf receptor, GPIb/IX, thereby reflecting an abnormal interaction of platelets with the vessel wall. Crossed immunoelectrophoresis or flow cytometry of platelet membrane glycoproteins should demonstrate a decrease in GPIb, GPIX, and GPV to confirm a diagnosis of Bernard-Soulier syndrome.

Heterogeneity among the glycoprotein abnormalities in Bernard-Soulier syndrome indicates that there are multiple genetic defects. Heterozygotes present with recognizable abnormalities such as occasional large platelets on the peripheral smear with a history of bleeding yet few clinical problems. Homozygotes present with abnormal platelet function and morphology,[13] thrombocytopenia, and hemorrhagic disease.

Rather specific criteria for the diagnosis of this bleeding syndrome have been established. These criteria are as follows:

1. An autosomal trait with clinical manifestations expressed in homozygotes (or double heterozygotes with two combined genetic abnormalities of GPIb, GPV, and GPIX)

2. Mild or moderate thrombocytopenia (despite a normal number of marrow megakaryocytes)

3. A significant number of giant or large platelets present on the peripheral blood smear and bleeding time, too prolonged for the degree of thrombocytopenia

4. Absent platelet aggregation in response to bovine vWF or to human vWF plus ristocetin

5. Normal platelet aggregation in response to ADP, collagen, and epinephrine; reduced aggregation in response to thrombin

6. Normal fVIII:C and vWf:Ag

Bernard-Soulier syndrome must be differentially diagnosed from other congenital disorders of thrombocytopenia associated with giant platelets such as May-Hegglin anomaly or Gray platelet syndrome. Patients with May-Hegglin anomaly, a rare disorder, present with bleeding episodes that correlate with the degree of thrombocytopenia; their platelet membrane glycoprotein and platelet function are normal. Gray platelet syndrome, a very rare disorder, presents with mild bleeding episodes, thrombocytopenia, large platelets, and decreased content of the alpha granules; however, membrane glycoproteins are normal. It is important to recognize that some patients with vWD may present with a normal APTT; therefore fVIII:C and vWF:Ag assays should be performed in patients suspected of having Bernard-Soulier syndrome. In the evaluation of this disorder, as with all other congenital platelet defects, it is necessary to exclude a drug-induced platelet defect. Hereditary platelet defects are considered rare; however, acquired platelet defects associated with underlying conditions are quite common and have a high incidence of clinically significant bleeding.

The nature of the bleeding episodes in patients with Bernard-Soulier syndrome is similar to that described for Glanzmann's thrombasthenia. Treatment for pa-

Laboratory Findings	Glanzmann's Thrombasthenia	Bernard-Soulier Syndrome
Platelet count	Normal	Decreased
Platelet morphology	Normal	Giant platelets
Bleeding time	Prolonged	Prolonged
Platelet adhesion	Normal	Abnormal
Platelet aggregation		
ADP	Abnormal	Normal
Thrombin	Abnormal	Abnormal
Collagen	Abnormal	Normal
Epinephrine	Abnormal	Normal
Ristocetin	Normal	Abnormal
vWF	Normal	Abnormal
Clot retraction	Abnormal	Normal
Platelet membrane		
Glycoprotein abnormality	GPIIb-IIIa	GPIb/IX
Inheritance	Autosomal recessive	Autosomal
Bleeding manifestations	Menorrhagia, purpura, easy bruising, mild severe mucocutaneous bleeds	Severe hemorrhage in homozygotes

TABLE 27–5 **Comparison of Clinical and Laboratory Findings in Glanzmann's Thrombasthenia and Bernard-Soulier Syndrome**

tients with Bernard-Soulier syndrome generally consists of supportive care. Iron replacement therapy is indicated in patients with persistent bleeding; red cell transfusions are utilized in uncontrollable hemorrhage. Platelet transfusion, often an unsatisfactory therapy, should be used judiciously to avoid alloimmunization to GPIb.

Disorders of Aggregation

Glanzmann's Thrombasthenia   Glanzmann's thrombasthenia was first described in 1918 by Glanzmann as "hereditary hemorrhagic thrombasthenia." Early observations in patients with this disorder showed heterogeneity of the disease.

Glanzmann's thrombasthenia is a rare autosomal recessive disorder of platelet function associated with an absence or deficiency of membrane glycoprotein IIb/IIIa (GPIIb/IIIa) complex. GPIIb/IIIa mediates aggregation of activated platelets by binding fibrinogen, vWf, and fibronectin.[8] The role of GPIIb/IIIa as the receptor for fibrinogen in platelet aggregation has been confirmed by the use of monoclonal antibodies, chemical cross-linking of fibrinogen to the glycoprotein complex, and purified complexes that are capable of binding fibrinogen. GPIIb/IIIa also serves to connect adhesive proteins with contractile proteins of the platelet following activation, thereby facilitating clot retraction, an abnormality seen in Glanzmann's thrombasthenia. Both megakaryocytes and platelets express the GPIIb/GPIIIa complex.

Clinical manifestations of Glanzmann's thrombasthenia are quite variable, ranging from minor bruising to severe and potentially fatal hemorrhages with the severity of bleeding consistent within single families. Glanzmann's thrombasthenia is an uncommon inherited platelet defect; however, it occurs with greater frequency than Bernard-Soulier syndrome. Glanzmann's appears to cluster in ethnic populations in which consanguity is prevalent. The most common bleeding symptoms include easy bruisability, epistaxis, spontaneous gingival bleeding, prolonged bleeding from minor cuts, and menorrhagia. Gastrointestinal hemorrhages are less common. The formation of deep hematomas and recurrent hemarthrosis after trauma do not occur in Glanzmann's thrombasthenia, which is a classic feature in patients with hemophilia. Certain criteria for diagnosing Glanzmann's thrombasthenia have been proposed:

1. A wide variation in hemorrhagic symptoms from minor bruising to severe mucocutaneous bleeding beginning during infancy
2. An autosomal recessive trait with clinical manifestations expressed in homozygotes only
3. Prolonged bleeding time
4. Normal platelet count; normal platelet morphology
5. Absent platelet aggregation to ADP, thrombin, collagen and epinephrine; normal platelet agglutination to ristocetin and bovine vWF

Laboratory findings that are hallmarks of this disorder include a normal platelet count; prolonged bleeding time; absent aggregation to ADP collagen, thrombin, and epinephrine; and absent clot retraction (see Table 27–5).

Patients with Glanzmann's thrombasthenia who present with severe bleeding episodes require platelet transfusions. Supportive therapy should be used judiciously, since patients may develop alloantibodies to normal platelet GPIIb and GPIIIa as well as anti-HLA antibodies and thus become refractory to supportive therapy.[14] The use of drugs that may interfere with platelet function is contraindicated.

Disorders of Platelet Secretion

Storage Pool Deficiencies   Platelet secretion is a process that involves the release of contents from alpha granules and dense granules into the surrounding environment. Release, initiated by an increase in cytoplasmic calcium, takes place when the membrane of the granule fuses with the membrane of the open canalicular system.

In platelets, ADP and ATP are stored in two pools, the metabolically active pool within the cytoplasm and the nonmetabolic storage pool in the electron-dense granules. On platelet stimulation, the electron-dense granules are released. Platelet aggregation is initiated by the release of ADP from the electron-dense granules. The glycoprotein IIb/IIIa complex binds one platelet to another by way of fibrinogen, thereby facilitating the aggregation response.

Inherited storage pool deficiencies are associated with abnormal platelet function and bleeding manifestations. This heterogeneous group of inherited platelet disorders is characterized by defects in platelet secretion. They may be classified based on impaired ADP secretion because of decreased stores of ADP and ATP in electron-dense granules (storage pool deficiencies) or defects in the metabolic pathways of the release mechanism (aspirinlike defects) leading to secretion and aggregation. Current knowledge of the mechanisms by which signal transduction in the platelet occurs will most assuredly redefine the classification of storage pool defects.

Clinically, bleeding manifestations are generally mild to moderate. Common features include easy bruising, postoperative bleeding, menorrhagia, and epistaxis.

Abnormal laboratory findings associated with these disorders include prolonged bleeding time, absent or diminished secondary aggregation in response to ADP and epinephrine, decreased aggregation to collagen, decreased platelet retention to glass beads, and impaired platelet factor 3 (PF 3) availability. The platelet count and platelet morphology are most often normal. Normal aggregation patterns have been observed in patients with storage pool defects and therefore a diagnosis of storage pool deficiency cannot be excluded based on normal aggregation studies. The use of electron microscopy is helpful in classifying the disorder as to storage pool deficiency or impaired release mechanism. Lumiaggregation is a useful and sensitive test that aids in the diagnosis of storage pool deficiencies. In the differential diagnosis of congenital storage pool defects, acquired defects such as those seen in hypercoagulable states and myeloproliferative disorders must be excluded.

Decreases in substances within the electron-dense granules are characteristic of storage pool deficiencies;

however, rare documented cases of alpha granules have been reported.[15] The gray platelet syndrome is a rare inherited disorder in which platelets lack alpha granules. Patients generally present with mild hemorrhagic symptoms, including easy bruising, epistaxis, and menorrhagia. Gray platelets are seen on Wright-stained blood smears. Thrombocytopenia, prolonged bleeding time, nonspecific abnormal platelet aggregation studies, and defective release of platelet factor 4 (PF 4) characterize this disorder. Electron microscopy shows absence of alpha granules. Weiss and associates[16] has suggested a system for classification based on morphological evaluation of platelet granules by electron microscopy and analysis of granule substances.[16]

Storage pool deficiencies also include rare, inherited disorders of arachidonic acid and prostaglandin synthesis. Deficiencies of cyclo-oxygenase and thromboxane synthetase have been observed. This group of storage pool deficiencies presents with abnormal aggregation in response to ADP, epinephrine, collagen, and arachidonic acid. Because aspirin and many aspirin-containing drugs inhibit cyclo-oxygenase, it is critical to exclude a drug-induced platelet dysfunction in the diagnosis of storage pool deficiencies.

Other Congenital Disorders of Platelet Secretion
In many patients, reference has been made to storage pool deficiencies associated with other congenital conditions. Table 27–6 lists and summarizes the other congenital disorders of platelet secretion.

Patients with storage pool defects present with mild or moderate clinical bleeding and therefore ordinarily do not require supportive treatment. When bleeding as a result of trauma or surgery is excessive, the treatment of choice is platelet concentrates. Patients who have a very mild bleeding syndrome may not be detected.

Acquired Qualitative Platelet Disorders

Renal Disease—Uremia

Bleeding has long been recognized as a common yet sometimes severe complication of uremia. Patients with acute and chronic renal failure hemorrhage predominantly from mucous membranes. Petechiae, purpura, epistaxis, ecchymoses, and gastrointestinal bleeds are common.[17] Severe hemorrhages within serous cavities and muscles may also occur. Paradoxically, other patients with uremia manifest with thrombosis. Although both may occur, bleeding is more often the common clinical manifestation.

A number of different laboratory findings and clinical symptoms suggest that platelet dysfunction with abnormal platelet–vessel wall interaction is the major cause of hemorrhage. Studies have shown an abnormality in the interaction of vWf and platelet glycoprotein IIb/IIIa complex in uremic patients; however, platelet membrane glycoproteins Ib, IIb, and IIIa are quantitatively normal.[18] Other platelet abnormalities seen in uremia include abnormal prostaglandin synthesis, decreased membrane procoagulant activity, decreased platelet serotonin, abnormal beta thromboglobulin (β-TG), elevated intracellular calcium, and decreased thromboxane synthesis. Increased levels of "uremic toxins" such as guanidosuccinic acid and phenols are rather consistent findings in patients with uremia. The acquired platelet defects associated with uremia are thought to be primarily mediated by these products. A correlation of the metabolic changes with the exact mechanisms of the functional defect has not yet been firmly established.

Thrombocytopenia wherein platelet counts are within the range of 100×10^9/L, decreased adhesion, abnormal aggregation, and increased bleeding times

TABLE 27–6 **Other Congenital Disorders of Platelet Secretion**	
Hermansky-Pudlak	Platelet deficiency of nonmetabolic ADP Oculocutaneous albinism Increased ceroid of reticuloendothelium
Chediak-Higashi	Partial oculocutaneous albinism Increased susceptibility to pyogenic infections Storage pool defect of dense granules
TAR baby syndrome	Multiple skeletal and cardiac abnormalities Storage pool defect
Wiskott-Aldrich	Disorders of dense granules Recurrent pyogenic infections Eczema Thrombocytopenia
May-Hegglin anomaly	Thrombocytopenia Giant platelets Dohle bodies
Alport's disorder	Giant platelets Thrombocytopenia Deafness Nephritis Epistaxis

are abnormal laboratory findings often seen in patients with uremia. As with other acquired platelet defects, aggregation studies in uremic patients show no characteristic patterns.

The anemia of renal failure may contribute to the hemostatic defects observed in uremic patients. Hematocrit values of less than 25% may prolong bleeding times.[19] Red cells may play a role in hemostasis by improving factor VIII function and by providing adenosine diphosphate (ADP), a platelet-aggregating agent.[20] Erythropoietin (Epo) therapy has proven effective in improving hemostasis and decreasing the bleeding tendencies in uremic patients on dialysis. It is thought that Epo may increase platelet numbers and help in aggregation.[21]

Hemodialysis or peritoneal dialysis, or both, is the treatment of choice to correct the hemostatic defect in uremia; however, platelet function abnormalities may remain. Administration of cryoprecipitate to patients unresponsive to dialysis has also been used as a means of therapy.[22] The use of the vasoactive peptide, 1-deamino-8-D-arginine-vasopressin (DDAVP) in uremic patients has prevented clinical bleeding in patients following surgical procedures and has shortened the bleeding time temporarily.[23]

Dysproteinemias

Patients with malignancies may exhibit both hemorrhagic diathesis and hypercoagulability. These hemostatic alterations are complex and multifactorial. Clinically significant bleeding is a manifestation associated with multiple myeloma, Waldenström's macroglobulinemia, and other related malignant paraprotein disorders (Figs. 27–3 and 27–4). The pathogenesis of hemorrhage and other recognized hemostatic abnormalities has been proposed to be caused by the interaction of the paraprotein with platelets and coagulation factors. Clinical bleeding and platelet dysfunction are seen in approximately 60% of the patients with IgM myeloma or Waldenström's macroglobulinemia as compared to approximately 40% of the patients with IgA myeloma and 15% of patients with IgG myeloma.[24]

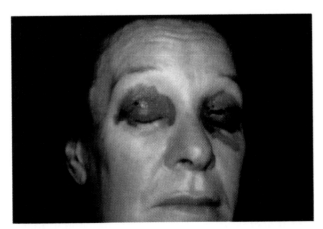

FIGURE 27–3 Amyloid purpura. Note characteristic periorbital distribution.

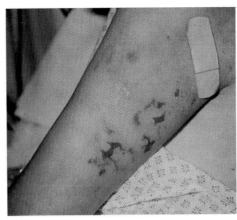

FIGURE 27–4 Cryoglobulinemic purpura (skin manifestations).

The hemorrhagic diathesis is characterized by a prolonged bleeding time and platelet dysfunction.[25] The occurrence of bleeding correlates with the impairment of platelet function. Patients may present clinically with spontaneous epistaxis and ecchymoses, or unexplained postoperative bleeding in the face of a normal platelet count and coagulation profile. Patients with malignant paraprotein disorders should not ingest aspirin or aspirin-containing drugs because this may exacerbate the platelet defect. Uremic platelet dysfunction associated with renal failure often seen in the malignant paraproteinemias may also contribute to the hemorrhagic episodes.

Platelet abnormalities are demonstrated and often confirmed by decreased aggregation in response to various aggregating agents, altered shape change, abnormal release reactions, and a prolonged bleeding time. Acquired von Willebrand's syndrome owing to reduced levels of vWf–factor VIII complexes, amyloid-associated coagulopathies, impaired fibrin formation and polymerization, acquired lupus anticoagulants, hyperviscosity syndrome, nephrosis, and DIC represent additional abnormalities that predispose patients to bleeding.

Thrombocytopenia, unrelated to the paraprotein effect, may result from marrow replacement, chemotherapy, or hypersplenism and is a common finding contributing to the incidence of significant bleeding.

Therapy for patients with qualitative defects resulting from multiple myeloma and related disorders include plasmapheresis, the administration of platelet concentrates, and the use of vasopressin. Various other therapies may be required when additional hemostatic abnormalities are present.

Myeloproliferative Disorders

Concomitant hemorrhage and thromboembolic episodes are frequent in patients with myeloproliferative disorders (MPDs). The hemorrhagic manifestations include ecchymoses, epistaxis, and mucocutaneous bleeding of the gastrointestinal and genitourinary tracts. Thrombosis occurs in both the arterial and venous circulation and includes deep vein thrombosis; stroke; pulmonary emboli; and thrombosis of the hepatic, portal, splenic, and mesenteric veins. The exact mechanism of platelet dysfunction and hemostatic defect is uncertain. In many cases, the degree of thrombocytosis is a contributing factor to the complications seen in the MPDs.[26-28] Patients may present with bleeding and thrombosis simultaneously, or alternate with bleeding and thrombotic episodes as the disease progresses (refer to Chap. 21).

Acute Leukemia and Malignancy

Altered hemostasis is seen in malignancy and the acute leukemias. Both bleeding and thrombosis are observed in these disease states owing to the activation of platelets, coagulation factors, endothelial cell injury, and the intiation of fibrinolysis.

In acute leukemia, hemorrhage is a common clinical manifestation seen in 35% to 80% of the patients. Hemorrhage is attributed to thrombocytopenia (less than 10,000/μL), DIC, vascular abnormalities, primary fibrinolysis, and defective protein synthesis. Severe, often fatal hemorrhages are attributed to gastrointestinal, intracranial, and disseminated bleeding (see Chap. 18).

Acquired von Willebrand's Disease

Acquired von Willebrand's disease (vWD) is a bleeding disorder that has been found in patients with MPDs, lymphoproliferative diseases, monoclonal gammopathies, and collagen vascular diseases. Most patients are 40 years or older, with no previous history of bleeding. Bleeding presents with an insidious onset and manifests as mucocutaneous or post-traumatic hemorrhage.

Laboratory findings seen in acquired vWD include a prolonged bleeding time (variable); decreases in plasma levels of factor VIII:C, vWF:Ag, ristocetin cofactor, and variable decreases in vWF multimers. Platelet vWF is generally normal. Following infusion of plasma or cryoprecipitate, there is an absence in the rise in plasma factor VIII:C levels observed in most patients with classic vWD.

Spontaneous remission and remission after therapy for the underlying disease is often seen. Therapeutic use of DDAVP has been observed to correct the bleeding time and increase the level of vWF. A response to the use of corticosteroid therapy has been documented.

Cardiopulmonary Bypass

In the United States, more than 200,000 patients per year undergo cardiopulmonary bypass (CPB) surgery. Alterations in hemostasis and the potential for life-threatening hemorrhage have been well documented. Various hemostatic abnormalities have been implicated in the development of the hemorrhagic manifestations of CPB surgery. They include decreases in platelet numbers and function, factor deficiencies owing to consumption and hemodilution, increased fibrinolytic activity for a short period following bypass,

DIC, and inadequate or excess neutralization of heparin with protamine.[29] Postbypass diffuse microvascular bleeding occurs with greater frequency in patients undergoing repeat surgery or complicated cardiac procedures than in patients undergoing first-time surgery.[29] During CPB, a prolonged bleeding time in the face of a platelet count of 100,000/μL is often seen. Bleeding as a result of platelet activation and platelet dysfunction accounts for most hemostatic alterations seen during this procedure.[29] Proposed mechanisms include platelet activation with alpha granule release during exposure to the extracorporeal unit and plasmin degradation of platelet membrane receptors.[30]

Platelet concentrates are administered to stop the bleeding. Fresh frozen plasma and cryoprecipitate should be given only to treat bleeding associated with coagulation factor deficiencies. Recently, aprotinin has been licensed for use in the United States to decrease postoperative bleeding in bypass patients, particularly those undergoing repeat or complicated procedures. It is thought that aprotinin maintains platelet function by inhibiting plasmin degradation of platelet membrane receptors.[31]

Liver Disease

The liver is the site of synthesis of nearly all coagulation factors, naturally occurring protease inhibitors, and fibrinolytic factors (with the exception of vWf, tissue plasminogen activator [tPA] and plasminogen activator inhibitor [PAI-1]). It also serves to clear fibrin(ogen) degradation products (FDPs) and activated factors from circulation. The severity of liver pathology often determines the complexity of hemostatic disorders. Chronic liver disease is often associated with a significant hemorrhagic diathesis as a result of multiple alterations in hemostasis. A patient with liver disease may have a single factor deficiency, multiple factor deficiencies, and structural or functional abnormalities of coagulation factors. Increased fibrinolytic activity, platelet dysfunction, thrombocytopenia, and DIC are also observed in patients with liver disease.

Mild to moderate thrombocytopenia is seen in approximately one third of patients with chronic liver disease as a result of splenic sequestration secondary to congestive splenomegaly associated with portal hypertension.[32] Abnormal platelet function tests found in patients with chronic liver disease include reduced platelet adhesion; abnormal platelet aggregation to ADP, epinephrine, and thrombin; and abnormal PF 3 availability.

Acquired Storage Pool Deficiencies

Acquired storage pool deficiencies have been reported in patients with systemic lupus erythematosus (SLE), idiopathic thrombocytopenic purpura (ITP), thrombotic thrombocytopenic purpura (TTP), DIC, hemolytic uremic syndrome (HUS), MPDs, hairy cell leukemia, acute nonlymphocytic leukemia, and in those who have had cardiopulmonary bypass. The acquired platelet defect is probably secondary to the underlying disease process.

Disseminated Intravascular Coagulation

Disseminated intravascular coagulation (DIC) represents altered hemostasis seen in association with well-defined clinical disorders. Clinical manifestations include the spectrum of both hemorrhage and microvascular thrombosis. Thrombosis accounts for the high morbidity and mortality seen in DIC owing to ischemia and organ damage. Historically, DIC was known as a "consumptive coagulopathy." The pathophysiology of DIC is defined by simultaneous activation of coagulation and fibrinolysis by a triggering event with both thrombin and plasmin generated and circulating systemically. Thrombocytopenia is usually present and results from decreased platelet survival and increased platelet destruction relating to the pathophysiology of DIC (see Chap. 29).

Drug Therapy

A large variety of pharmacologic drugs have quite a pronounced effect on platelets. Many drugs induce thrombocytopenia. In general, most drugs inhibit platelet response. Drug-induced alterations of hemostasis that cause activation of platelet function clinically manifest as thrombosis (see Chap. 30); drugs that inhibit platelet function clinically manifest as hemorrhage. Most often, the acquired drug-induced hemostatic abnormalities observed are transitory and disappear when the drug is discontinued; however, other effects may be irreversible and disappear only after time. Table 27–7 lists the drugs that inhibit platelet function.

Platelet Antibodies

Disorders such as ITP, SLE, and Graves' disease have been reported in association with increased platelet-associated antibodies.[33] Platelet antibodies have been demonstrated to cause platelet lysis, platelet aggregation, increased PF 3 availability, and serotonin release. These events can lead to platelet destruction resulting in thrombocytopenia or acquired platelet defects.

Other conditions may be associated with an acquired qualitative platelet defect. Massive transfusion, defined as replacement of the majority of a patient's blood volume, is quite often associated with severe trauma and results in many hemostatic defects. A large percentage of patients who have been massively transfused may acquire hemostatic defects as a result of the use of stored blood and blood components and dilutional effects. Platelets lose their viability when stored at 4°C to 6°C and are considered nonfunctional. Massive transfusion of packed red cells or plasma dilutes the remaining platelets. This dilutional effect is somewhat proportional to the number of transfusions. Trauma and tissue injuries are believed to cause qualitative defects in platelet function.

QUANTITATIVE PLATELET DISORDERS

Platelets must be present in adequate numbers to maintain normal hemostasis. The average platelet count ranges from 150 to 400×10^9/L of whole blood. The platelet count is a routine screening test used to detect quantitative changes such as thrombocytosis (platelet counts greater than 400×10^9/L) and thrombocytopenia (platelet counts less than 50×10^9/L). Quantitative changes in platelet counts may result from a primary disorder of the bone marrow or secondary to a variety of underlying conditions. Often the presence of qualitative defects may coexist with quantitative changes.

Thrombocytopenia

Decreased Platelet Production

Decreased platelet production resulting in thrombocytopenia may be associated with congenital or acquired disorders. These disorders generally affect the bone marrow, resulting in megakaryocytic hypoplasia. Concomitant anemia and leukopenia are also found in many patients with these disorders. A list of disorders associated with quantitative platelet changes is found in Table 27–8.

TABLE 27–7 **Drugs That Inhibit Platelet Function**	
Drug	**Effect**
Heparin	Thrombocytopenia
Aspirin	Inhibits platelet aggregation and secretion
Nonsteroidal anti-inflammatory agents (NSAIDs) (indomethacin, ibuprofen, phenylbutazone, sulfinpyrazone)	Inhibit prostaglandin synthesis
Antimicrobial drugs (penicillin, ampicillin, carbenicillin)	Interfere with platelet membrane and membrane receptors
Dextran	Interferes with platelet's surface membrane
Cardiovascular drugs	Alters prostaglandin synthesis and interferes with platelet membrane and membrane receptors

TABLE 27–8 Classification of Thrombocytopenia

Decreased Production of Platelets
Leukemias
Lymphomas
Myelodysplastic syndrome
Aplastic anemia
Fanconi's anemia
Metastatic carcinoma
Myelofibrosis
Chemotherapeutic and immunosuppressive agents
Thrombocytopenia with absent radii (TAR baby syndrome)
Osteoporosis
Viral infections
Drugs
May-Hegglin anomaly
Bernard-Soulier syndrome

Ineffective Thrombopoiesis
Vitamin B_{12} deficiency
Folic acid deficiency
Alcohol ingestion
Myelodysplastic syndrome
Paroxysmal nocturnal hemoglobinuria (PNH)
Di Guglielmo's syndrome
Drug ingestion

Abnormal Distribution of Platelets
Hypersplenism

Increased Destruction
Immune mediated thrombocytopenia
  Idiopathic thrombocytopenic purpura (ITP)
    Acute
    Chronic
    Recurrent
  Isoimmune neonatal
  Drug-induced thrombocytopenia
  Post transfusion purpura
Secondary immune-mediated
  Viral, bacterial, parasitic infections
  Lymphoproliferative disorders
  Collagen vascular diseases (eg, SLE)
  HIV-1
  Drugs (eg, heparin)
  Transfusions
Non-immune-mediated thrombocytopenia
  Disseminated intravascular coagulation
  Thrombotic thrombocytopenic purpura
  Hemolytic uremic syndrome
  Heparin
  Complications of pregnancy
  Viral, bacterial, mycotic infections

Ineffective Thrombopoiesis

Ineffective thrombopoiesis is a state in which the number of megakaryocytes in the bone marrow is normal to increased, but maturation and release of platelets to the circulation is abnormal. Conditions that prevent normal maturation or platelet release result in ineffective thrombopoiesis (that is, megaloblastic anemia, myelodysplastic syndromes, and paroxysmal nocturnal hemoglobinuria).

Abnormal Distribution of Platelets

Normally, the spleen pools approximately one third of all circulating platelets. Splenomegaly is associated with many conditions, causing increased pooling of circulating platelets, thereby producing thrombocytopenia. Increased platelet destruction has been observed in splenomegaly.

Increased Destruction of Platelets

A sudden decrease in the platelet count without evidence of a hemorrhage suggests a condition of increased platelet sequestration by the spleen and liver or increased destruction of platelets in these organs, thereby reducing platelet life span. Increased sequestration or destruction of platelets is either immune- or non-immune-mediated. This section will discuss the various disorders of non-immune-mediated thrombocytopenia.

Nonimmunologic Thrombocytopenias

Thrombotic Thrombocytopenic Purpura The hallmarks of this syndrome, first described in 1924 by Moschowitz,[34] are thrombocytopenia, microangiopathic hemolytic anemia, fluctuating neurologic abnormalities, fever, and renal disease. The pathologic feature characteristic of thrombotic thrombocytopenic purpura (TTP) is the hyaline microthrombi composed of platelets and fibrin that occlude arterioles and capillaries in multiple organs (Fig. 27–5). Localized fibrinolytic activity is absent in the vessels occluded by these microthrombi. The microthrombi are not solely diagnostic for TTP; they occur in DIC as well. The composition of the thrombotic lesion, being predominantly platelets rather than fibrin, and the normal coagulation studies help to differentiate TTP from DIC.

The exact pathogenic mechanisms responsible for this disorder remain uncertain. Evidence suggests that a genetic predisposition or an underlying disorder is necessary for expression of the disease. Endothelial damage caused by drugs, virus, or bacteria appears to be critical in the development of vascular injury. A few concepts help explain the pathogenesis of TTP. These are: (1) that predisposing factors such as genetics, pregnancy, underlying disease, and circulating immune complexes may initiate TTP; (2) that large

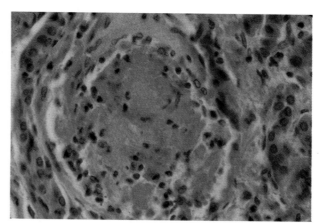

FIGURE 27–5 Renal biopsy from a case of thrombotic thrombocytopenic purpura (TTP) showing glomerular deposits of platelet-fibrin microvascular occlusion.

vWF–factor VIII multimers secreted by endothelial cells persist in circulation, promoting microvascular thrombosis; (3) that endothelial cell damage from various causes inhibits fibrinolysis and promotes thrombosis by platelets and coagulation factors interacting with damaged endothelium; and (4) that, as a consequence of endothelial cell damage, there is a deficiency of PGI_2 synthesis and release leading to platelet aggregation and thrombosis.[35]

The incidence of TTP is thought to be approximately one per million.[36] However, increased awareness and diagnosis may change these statistics. Women appear to be affected more often than men, with a female-to-male ratio of 3:2. The peak incidence occurs between the third and fourth decades of life. Patients who are pregnant, have viral infection, ingest drugs, and have autoimmune disorders appear to be predisposed to TTP.

Patients with TTP initially present with nonspecific symptoms of malaise, weakness, fatigue, and often fever or abdominal pain associated with the hallmark neurologic complication and bleeding manifestations of thrombocytopenia. Clinical features of TTP are those of a severe microangiopathic hemolytic anemia with associated poikilocytosis (see Fig. 14–11), reticulocytosis, and nucleated red blood cells indicating a compensatory marrow response. Signs of hemolysis are reflected by increases in serum lactate dehydrogenase (LDH), indirect bilirubin, and decreased haptoglobin levels. There is a severe thrombocytopenia and evidence of decreased platelet survival despite megakaryocytic hyperplasia in the bone marrow.

Prothrombin time (PT), activated partial thromboplastin time (APTT), and fibrinogen levels are generally normal in patients with TTP, with slight elevations in the FDP levels. Renal involvement is characterized by signs of hematuria, proteinuria, and acute renal failure. Neurologic abnormalities manifest as dysphasia or aphasia, headache, pareses, seizures, obtundation, and paresthesias. Abdominal pain, pancreatitis, and gastrointestinal bleeding may also be associated findings. Any organ system may show involvement; cardiac damage with arrhythmias is not unusual. Table 27–9 lists the common characteristics of TTP.

Over the last 20 years there has been a significant improvement in the survival of patients with TTP. Although recovery from TTP has been reported as a result of numerous therapeutic modalities, the rarity of this disorder and its variable nature make evaluation of these therapies difficult. In early case histories it was often fatal, with a term survival rate of less than 10%.[37] Corticosteroid therapy, when used as the sole therapeutic agent, is ineffective; however, corticosteroids in combination with other agents appear to have a greater efficacy. Splenectomy is considered in patients who fail to respond to other therapies. Most patients undergoing splenectomy have also received corticosteroids and blood products with an increase in the response rate. Antiplatelet drugs such as aspirin, dipyridamole, dextran, and sulfinpyrazone have been used. Often these antiplatelet drugs are used in variable combinations, making their efficacy difficult to evaluate. Therapy involving dextran may be somewhat beneficial. Plasma exchange and the infusion of large amounts of plasma have met with a variable degree of success and are currently being used as the "treatment of choice." Heparin therapy is discouraged because of its associated toxicity. Immunosuppressive drugs such as vincristine[38] have been used, as well as intravenous synthetic prostacyclin.[37] Both have been reported to induce remission. Most often, patients with TTP are treated by a combination of therapeutic modalities.

Hemolytic Uremic Syndrome   Hemolytic uremic syndrome (HUS) is characterized clinically by microangiopathic hemolytic anemia, thrombocytopenia, and renal failure (see Fig. 14–17). Renal vascular damage may initiate intravascular hemolysis with subsequent red cell ADP and membrane phospholipid platelet release. Renal damage may also promote coagulant activity resulting in fibrin deposition and endothelial damage but no consumption of clotting factors.

HUS may clinically resemble TTP, but there is a difference in the age of the patients affected (see Table 27–9).

Respiratory Distress Syndrome

This syndrome is characterized by excessive fibrin deposition localized in the lungs of infants considered to be at high risk for this disorder. The fibrinolytic response is absent in these infants.

Severe cases of multiple trauma are also associated with pulmonary dysfunction or adult respiratory distress syndrome subsequent to pulmonary vascular obstruction and numerous thrombi.

TABLE 27–9 **Comparison of TTP and HUS**		
Characteristics	**TTP**	**HUS**
Epidemiology		
Age	Peak incidence at 40 years	Childhood
Sex Prediliction	Female	Equal
Organ Involvement	Multiple	Limited to kidney
Hematologic		
Microangiopathic hemolytic anemia	Severe	Severe
Thrombocytopenia	Severe	Moderate
Neurologic	Common, severe	Uncommon, less severe
Renal Failure	Uncommon, mild	Common, severe

Heparin Therapy

Thrombocytopenia is frequently associated with heparin therapy, occurring more often in patients given bovine heparin than in patients given porcine heparin. The incidence of heparin-induced thrombocytopenia in patients is estimated at approximately 8% to 15%. At therapeutic levels, heparin induces platelet aggregation, whereas large doses inhibit aggregation. In relatively few patients, spontaneous platelet aggregation has been noted on platelet exposure to heparin. More often, previous exposure of platelets to heparin for a period of 6 to 10 days, enough to develop antibody titers, is required for antibody-mediated thrombocytopenia.

Heparin-induced thrombocytopenia may be classified into two types. Type I is characterized by a mild idiopathic thrombocytopenia occurring early in the course of heparin therapy. Patients generally do not bleed despite the fact that they are receiving anticoagulant therapy and are thrombocytopenic. Type II heparin-induced thrombocytopenia is characterized by a severe thrombocytopenia occurring late in the course of heparin therapy. Venous or arterial thrombosis is often an associated complication accounting for a high incidence of morbidity and mortality in 20% of the patients who present with this type.[40,41] In these patients, heparin must be discontinued to return the platelet count to normal, generally within 4 to 6 days. Warfarin and low-molecular-weight heparin—associated with a lower incidence of thrombocytopenia—may be substituted should therapy be required (see Chap 30).

Disseminated Intravascular Coagulation A syndrome that results in the pathologic generation of thrombin and plasmin, DIC presents with clinical manifestations of hemorrhage (Fig. 27–6) and thrombosis. A significant thrombocytopenia is seen in DIC as a result of increased platelet destruction and decreased platelet life span (Fig. 27–7). The hemorrhagic diathesis is attributed to the activation of platelets, coagulation factors, and increased fibrinolytic activity. In Chapter 29, DIC is discussed in greater detail.

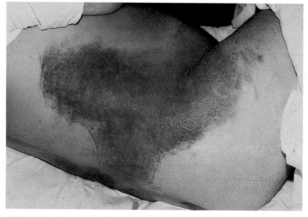

FIGURE 27–6 Diffuse hemorrhage, a clinical manifestation in a patient with disseminated intravascular coagulation (DIC). Note the multiple cutaneous ecchymoses.

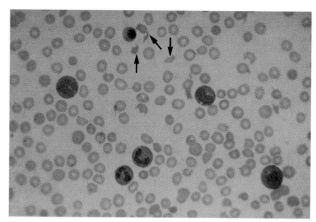

FIGURE 27–7 DIC (peripheral blood). Note presence of schistocytes (*arrows*) and nucleated red cell (*top border*).

Thrombocytopenia in Pregnancy Various alterations in hemostasis have been seen in the obstetric population during pregnancy, the birthing process, and the postpartum period. Abruptio placentae and amniotic fluid embolism are generally associated with forms of acute intravascular coagulation leading to the consumption of plasma clotting factors. In pre-eclampsia and eclampsia, thrombocytopenia occurs as a result of platelet consumption. The nature of the mechanism for the associated thrombocytopenia is not clearly understood; however, abnormal platelet to endothelial tissue interaction has been reported.

Immunologic Thrombocytopenias

Thrombocytopenias of this group all have an immune-mediated mechanism by which there is increased platelet sequestration and destruction.

Idiopathic Thrombocytopenic Purpura This is one of the most common causes of thrombocytopenia as a result of immune-mediated platelet destruction. A clinical syndrome characterized by thrombocytopenia, ITP may arise by several different mechanisms or may have no known etiologic factor. The diagnosis of ITP is made by exclusion; the disease may occur in acute, chronic, or recurrent form.

Acute ITP occurs predominantly in young children in the 2- to 5-year age group, with no predilection for either sex. In as many as 84% of the cases, thrombocytopenia develops within 1 to 3 weeks following an acute viral illness.[42] The onset of bleeding is usually abrupt, with initial platelet counts of less than 20,000/μL. This disorder is usually self-limiting, and spontaneous remissions, with or without therapy, occur in a large majority of these patients (Table 27–10). Spontaneous remission rarely occurs after a year from onset. Patients who do not have remissions within 6 months are generally considered to have chronic ITP.

The bone marrow is characterized by megakaryocytic hyperplasia (Fig. 27–8), and young, abnormally large platelets with variation in shape are seen on the peripheral smear. Platelet life span is decreased.

Cases of acute ITP may range from mild to severe, with manifestations of scattered petechiae (Figs. 27–9 and 27–10) in more mild cases and gastrointestinal

TABLE 27–10	**Comparison of Acute and Chronic ITP**	
Characteristics	**Acute**	**Chronic**
Age of onset	Childhood	20–50 years; females over males (2:1 to 3:1)
Previous infection	Common	Usually not associated
Platelet count	<20,000/µL	Variable, 30,000 to 80,000/µL
Bleeding	Abrupt	Insidious
Duration of thrombocytopenia	Few weeks	Months to years
Spontaneous remissions	Occurs in majority of patients	Relatively rare

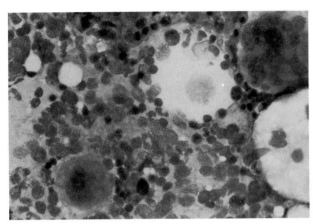

FIGURE 27–8   Idiopathic thrombocytopenic purpura (ITP), bone marrow aspirate. Note increased number of megakaryocytes with normal cellularity (M/E 3:1).

bleeding, hematuria, retinal hemorrhage, and generalized purpura in more severe cases. Of all cases of ITP, 3% to 4% are severe, with about one fourth to one half of these cases at risk for life-threatening intracranial hemorrhage. This complication accounts for the 1% to 2% morbidity rate for patients with acute ITP.[43]

Levels of platelet-associated IgG (PAIgG)[44] and other platelet-associated proteins are increased in cases of acute ITP. In general, elevations of amounts of these platelet-associated proteins are a nonspecific consequence of platelet destruction. Platelets in acute ITP are thought to be destroyed by immune complexes or foreign antigens adsorbed by platelets following an infection. Serologic studies in cases of acute ITP are generally not considered diagnostic.

Most patients with acute ITP do not require treatment. Their clinical manifestations are mild, and spontaneous remissions are the general rule. Therapy is used in serious cases of ITP and may include intravenous gamma globulin, splenectomy, platelet transfusion, corticosteroids, plasma exchange, and immunosuppressive drugs. Intravenous gamma globulin (IVIgG) appears to be effective in most cases of childhood acute ITP when the bleeding is rather severe. Splenectomy is considered for life-threatening intracranial hemorrhages. Splenectomy removes the primary site of platelet destruction and antibody production. Complications of sepsis in children with acute ITP have been reported following splenectomy. Corticosteroid therapy is considered ineffective in most cases

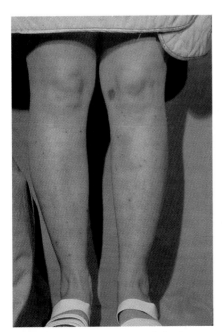

FIGURE 27–9   Petechial bleeding of the lower extremities in a patient with ITP.

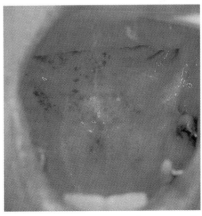

FIGURE 27–10   Oral cavity of patient with ITP.

of acute ITP. The shortened life span of transfused platelets makes their use effective only as a means of treating severe hemorrhage. Plasma exchange appears to be more effective in treating acute ITP than chronic ITP.

Chronic ITP is most common in adults 20 to 50 years of age, with a greater predilection for women between the ages of 20 to 50. The onset of bleeding is generally insidious, with variable platelet counts. Chronic ITP is characterized by a variable clinical course. Bleeding manifestations such as menorrhagia, recurrent epistaxis, or easy bruisability may persist for a few days or weeks, with intermittent asymptomatic periods. Spontaneous remissions, as seen in acute ITP, are uncommon and no known associated findings can be attributed to the thrombocytopenia.

In chronic ITP, the bone marrow is characterized by megakaryocytic hyperplasia, as in the acute form of ITP. Circulating platelets are young, since platelet life span is shortened and appears more effective at maintaining hemostasis.

The differential diagnosis between acute and chronic ITP is not always possible at the onset, but platelet counts are generally lower in acute than in chronic ITP. Acute ITP and chronic ITP also differ in age of onset, prior infection, duration of thrombocytopenia, and method and response to therapy (see Table 27–10). Chronic ITP must also be differentiated from ITP-like syndromes. The diagnosis of ITP is always one of exclusion.

In some patients with chronic ITP, antiplatelet antibodies have been shown to react with specific platelet membrane glycoproteins, thus favoring the possibility of an immune mechanism involved in platelet sensitization.[45,46] Various methods have shown that PAIgG is elevated in thrombocytopenic patients with chronic ITP and that there is somewhat of an inverse relationship between PAIgG levels and platelet counts.[47] In patients with chronic ITP, increased platelet destruction mediated by autoantibodies to platelet membrane glycoproteins occurs primarily through splenic sequestration. Splenectomy and corticosteroids are the conventional therapies used to treat patients with chronic ITP. Patients with chronic ITP are initially treated with corticosteroids. Corticosteroids are thought to suppress splenic sequestration of moderately sensitized platelets, thereby increasing the platelet life span and ameliorating the thrombocytopenia. The aim of therapy is to give an initial dose of prednisone sufficient to obtain a satisfactory increase in the platelet count and to reduce the dosage to a level that maintains the platelet count at hemostatic levels. Approximately 70% to 90% of patients treated respond favorably to steroids.[48] This therapy has been effective in increasing platelet counts in some patients with ITP.

Splenectomy is the treatment of choice for chronic ITP refractory to steroid therapy. Significant improvement following splenectomy is obtained in 70% to 90% of patients.[49] The benefit from splenectomy results from the removal of the organ responsible for the sequestration of moderately sensitized platelets. Splenectomy may be contraindicated in ITP in certain circmstances. Other, less frequently employed therapies to treat chronic ITP include such drugs as vincristine, Danazol, colchicine, immunosuppressive agents, plasma exchange, intravenous gamma globulin (IVIgG), and epsilon aminocaproic acid (EACA). Extracorpuscular immunoadsorption of plasma by staphylococcal protein A has been shown to be effective in reducing circulating immune complexes and platelet-associated IgG antibodies.[46]

A recurrent form of ITP also occurs, characterized by alternating intervals of thrombocytopenia and periods in which the platelet count is normal. This recurrent form is seen in children and adults.

Secondary Immune Thrombocytopenia Lymphoproliferative disorders such as Hodgkin's disease and non-Hodgkin's lymphoma have been reported with an ITP-like thrombocytopenia associated with decreased platelet survival and increased PAIgG levels.[50] Chronic lymphocytic leukemia (CLL) is also associated with an ITP-like thrombocytopenia. In SLE, roughly 14% of the patients develop thrombocytopenia resembling ITP during the course of the disease. Thrombocytopenic purpura is often the presenting sign, preceding the other clinical manifestations of the disease. Bleeding in SLE as a result of thrombocytopenia responds well to corticosteroid therapy. Qualitative tests for antiplatelet antibodies and tests for PAIgG frequently are positive in disorders associated with immune-mediated thrombocytopenia.

Thrombocytopenia as a result of viral, bacterial, or parasitic infections has been well documented. An immunologic mechanism appears likely in the development of thrombocytopenia as a result of infection. Viral infections such as mumps and rubeola may be complicated by severe thrombocytopenia. In bacterial sepsis, thrombocytopenia is generally present with or without DIC. Malaria is frequently associated with thrombocytopenia as a result of increased destruction and splenic sequestration.

HIV-Related Immune Thrombocytopenic Purpura An array of hemostatic complications have been described in association with the human immunodeficiency virus (HIV). The most common hemostatic abnormality in these patients is ITP. The incidence of ITP appears to vary according to the stage of the disease. Significant hemorrhagic complications may occur but are difficult to predict based solely on the platelet count.

The pathogenesis of HIV-related ITP appears to be heterogeneous and at present is still speculative. Autoantibody probably plays a role in the mechanism of ITP in mucosally infected patients, whereas immune complex formation mediates platelet destruction in parenterally acquired HIV. The pattern of IgG subclasses found in HIV-infected patients,[51] as well as the level of anti-IgG immune complexes on platelet surfaces[51] in HIV disease, are significantly different from patients with "classic ITP." Immunohistochemical markers show increased CD8+ T cells in the spleen of patients with HIV-related ITP.[52] Viral infection of hematopoietic cells, altered platelet production, and dysfunction of the reticuloendothelial system may all play a prominent role in HIV-mediated thrombocytopenia.

To date, the optimal treatment modality for HIV-related ITP appears to be intravenous gamma globulin (IVIgG).

ITP has also been reported in patients with HIV infection. Circulating anticoagulants, most notably the lupus anticoagulant and the anticardiolipin antibodies, are found in 44% to 94% of HIV-infected patients. Rarely do these patients manifest with clinical evidence of bleeding. The hemostatic problems seen in this disease are thought to be part of the autoimmune process triggered by HIV.

Drug-Induced Thrombocytopenia   Quinine-induced thrombocytopenia was observed as early as 1928. It was noted that, after discontinuing quinine therapy and after an initial recovery, thrombocytopenia could again be induced on readministering the drug.[51] The drug appears to act as a hapten, eliciting an antibody response when complexed with a larger carrier molecule. The antibody-drug-platelet complex leads to thrombocytopenia. Antibody combining with drug appears to be the initial step in the formation of the complex. Cellular binding or adsorption of the antibody-drug complex to the platelet membrane results in platelet injury and splenic sequestration.

The list of drugs that can cause immune drug purpura is rather extensive. A few of the drugs most frequently implicated are quinine, quinidine, digitoxin, gold, thiazides, salicylates, and the various sulfa drugs.

Drug-immune purpura appears to occur more frequently in the elderly population as a result of the increased usage of medication; however, cases have been reported in children and young adults. Purpura occurs approximately 7 days after first-time use of the drug but may occur within 3 to 5 days as in an anamnestic response on re-exposure to the drug. It is estimated that 1 in 100,000 drug users per year will require hospitalization as a result of a drug-induced blood disorder.[54] The frequency for users of quinine and quinidine is roughly 1 in 1000.[54] The disorder is generally self-limiting since the platelet count returns to normal once the drug has been removed from circulation. Readministration of a drug known to cause purpura should be avoided.

Several serologic techniques are used to detect drug-induced platelet antibodies such as platelet agglutination, complement fixation, platelet aggregation, inhibition of clot retraction, and platelet release of granular contents.

Post-Transfusion Purpura   In this disorder, sudden onset of thrombocytopenia occurs one week after transfusion of blood or blood products containing platelets (Fig. 27–11). It is believed that post-transfusion purpura (PTP) results from an anamnestic response. In the cases that have been studied thus far, the antibody present in the patients sera has been directed against the platelet antigen Pl^{A1}, also referred to as HPA-1a.[55] This antigen is found in approximately 97% of the normal population; the 3% of people who lack the Pl^{A1} (HPA-1a) antigen on their platelets are considered at risk for developing post-transfusion purpura. Most reported cases have been in middle-aged women who have had children. It is believed that primary immunization occurs in pregnancy; Pl^{A1}-positive fetal platelets sensitize a Pl^{A1}-negative mother (see section on isoimmune neonatal thrombocytopenia). Other mechanisms for the development of PTP have been suggested.[56]

Complement fixation, release of ^{51}Cr-labeled or ^{14}C-labeled serotonin have been some of the reliable

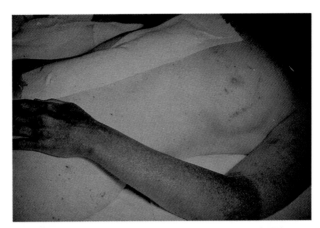

FIGURE 27–11   Post-transfusion purpura (PTP).

laboratory tests used to detect and measure anti-Pl^{A1} (HPA-1a) antibodies in PTP. Currently, direct and indirect laboratory tests have been developed to increase specificity and sensitivity in the detection of platelet antibodies. These tests employ some of the following techniques: enzyme-linked immunoabsorbent assay (ELISA), Western blot followed by ELISA or radioimmunoassay (RIA), platelet suspension immunofluorescence, and immunoprecipitation of radiolabeled GPIIa. To confirm the presence of a platelet-specific antibody, a panel with Pl^{A1}-positive cells should be run. The patient's platelets should also be phenotyped. In some cases of PTP, isosensitization to HLA antigens found on platelets occurs as well as the appearance of platelet-specific antigens other than Pl^{A1},[57] making serologic typing difficult.

Plasmapheresis, exchange transfusion, and the use of IVIgG have been effective means in treating the hemorrhagic complications associated with PTP. There have been a number of cases in which patients have had repeated episodes of PTP following re-exposure to Pl^{A1}-positive blood.[58] Pl^{A1}-negative blood is indicated for all subsequent transfusions when possible, since all patients are considered at risk for recurrence of PTP.

Isoimmune Neonatal Thrombocytopenia   Similar to the pathogenesis of erythroblastosis fetalis, isoimmune neonatal thrombocytopenia results from immunization of the mother by fetal platelet antigens and placental transfer of maternal antibody. The Pl^{A1} (HPA-1a) antigen is most often associated with isoimmune neonatal thrombocytopenia and is considered to be strongly immunogenic. It is an uncommon disorder, generally affecting the firstborn child. Based on gene frequency of the Pl^{A1} (HPA-1a) antigen in fathers, there is a high probability that a Pl^{A1}-negative mother will have a Pl^{A1}-positive child. Once isoimmune neonatal thrombocytopenia has developed, there appears to be an increased risk of the next child being affected, since most fathers are Pl^{A1}-homozygous.

A large percentage of Pl^{A1}-negative mothers who give birth to an affected child are phenotype-positive for the HLA-B8 antigen. It has been suggested that the HLA-B8 antigen serves to protect from immunization, which accounts for the relatively low incidence of isoimmune neonatal thrombocytopenia, despite the frequency of the Pl[A1] antigen and the chance for maternal sensitization. ABO incompatibility and its relation to symptomatic isoimmune neonatal thrombocytopenia are unclear.

Infants who develop isoimmune neonatal thrombocytopenia appear normal at birth but within hours develop scattered petechiae and purpuric hemorrhages, with platelet counts below 30,000/μL. Intracranial hemorrhage is the primary cause of mortality in these infants.

Therapy is aimed at preventing intracranial hemorrhage and keeping platelet counts at hemostatically safe levels. Cesarean delivery is recommended to prevent birth trauma, thereby eliminating the potential for intracranial bleeding. Corticosteroids and IVIgG have been used as a means of antenatal treatment. Postnatal treatment is not necessary as long as the infant remains asymptomatic and the platelet count stays above 30,000/μL. Characteristically, in this disorder the platelet count begins to decrease shortly after birth, with low levels reached several hours later. When the infant manifests clinical signs of bleeding and the platelet count falls below 10,000/μL, compatible platelet transfusion utilizing maternal platelets or Pl[A1]-negative donor platelets are used. An effective hemostatic response is almost always seen when transfused platelets are compatible with maternal antibody. Table 27–11 reviews and summarizes the mechanisms of selected platelet defects previously described.

Thrombocytosis

Increases in platelet counts indicate increased platelet production or proliferation of megakaryocytes. Thrombocytosis implies a moderate increase in platelet counts; however, counts of 500,000 to 1,000,000/ μL may also be seen. Thrombocytosis may result from reactive transient stimuli to the bone marrow or may be associated with an underlying malignancy (Table 27–12).

Thrombocytosis Associated with Myeloproliferative Syndromes

The myeloproliferative syndromes, characterized by the autonomous proliferation of a pluripotent stem cell, are associated with thrombocytosis. Bleeding, thrombosis, platelet defects, and increases in platelet counts are seen in association with all the myeloproliferative syndromes. Essential thrombocythemia has platelet counts that often exceed 1 million per microliter. Polycythemia vera and agnogenic myeloid metaplasia are also associated with thrombocytosis. Based on observations of patients with reactive thrombocytosis and normal platelet function in which bleeding and thrombotic complications are uncommon, thrombocytosis alone is not the sole factor in the development of bleeding and thrombosis in the myeloproliferative syndromes. It has been suggested that these complications result from qualitative platelet defects. (The MPDs as they relate to specific platelet defects are further discussed in the section on acquired platelet defects and in Chap. 21.)

Reactive Transient Thrombocytosis

Thrombocytosis is seen following splenectomy. Within the first 2 weeks, platelet levels rise and then

TABLE 27–11	Mechanisms of Selected Platelet Defects		
Disorder	**Pathogenesis**	**Platelet Abnormality**	**Molecular Defect**
vWD	Autosomal/acquired	Adhesion	Decreased vWf multimers
Bernard-Soulier	Autosomal	Adhesion	GPIb/IX
Glanzmann's thrombasthenia	Autosomal	Aggregation/clot retraction	GPIIb/IIIa
Secretion	Congenital/acquired	Impaired release/secretion of granules	Storage pool deficiency
Uremia	Acquired	Multiple defects	Primarily mediated by uremic toxins
Paraproteinemias/ dysproteinemias	Acquired	Multiple defects	Paraproteins coat membrane
Liver disease	Acquired	Multiple defects	FDPs coat platelets; altered metabolism
Immune thrombocytopenia	Alloimmunization	Multiple defects	Pl[A1] (HPA-1a)
Heparin-induced thrombocytopenia	Alloimmunization	Aggregation/ thrombocytopenia	IgG immune complexes
HIV-related thrombocytopenia	Autoimmunization/ alloimmunization	Thrombocytopenia	Uncertain at present

TABLE 27–12   **Causes of Thrombocytosis**
Myeloproliferative Syndromes
Essential thrombocythemia
Polycythemia vera
Agnogenic myeloid metaplasia
Chronic myelocytic leukemia
Secondary (Reactive) Thrombocytosis
Postsplenectomy
Postoperative
Acute blood loss
Epinephrine
Bone marrow recovery
Vitamin B_{12} therapy
Folic acid therapy
Drug-induced thrombocytopenia
Chemotherapy
Iron-deficiency anemia
Malignancy
Hodgkin's disease
Carcinoma
Osteogenic sarcoma
Chronic infections
Osteomyelitis
Tuberculosis
Chronic inflammation
Inflammatory bowel disease
Collagen vascular disease

return to normal over a period of months after splenectomy. Platelet counts may increase as much as two to six times preoperative levels. Platelet survival has been documented to be normal. It has been suggested that the thrombocytosis seen after splenectomy is a result of increased platelet production since elimination of the splenic pool can account for no more than a 50% rise in the platelet count.[59] Regulation of thrombopoiesis is thought to be moderated by a humoral factor produced by the spleen. Thrombocytosis is also observed postoperatively. The nature of the mechanism is not clearly understood; however, hypoxia during anesthesia may be a cause.

Thrombocytosis is a common finding associated with acute hemorrhage. The platelet count is generally elevated within a day or so after hemorrhage as a result of increased marrow stimulation. Similar responses may be seen following therapeutic phlebotomy for polycythemia vera.

Iron-deficiency anemia has classically been associated with thrombocytosis. Thrombocytosis is also associated with underlying malignancy and chronic inflammatory or infectious processes. In iron-deficiency anemia, the increased platelet count is generally found in the initial stages of the disease. Iron repletion will cause the platelet count to return to normal. The process by which the platelet count increases in these disorders in poorly understood.

Patients with reactive thrombocytosis have elevated platelet counts as well. Bleeding and thrombosis are uncommon and platelet function is normal. Increased numbers of megakaryocytes are found in the marrow.

Administration of epinephrine will create a transient thrombocytosis caused by platelet release from the spleen. Chemotherapeutic agents such as vincristine and other vinca alkaloids will elevate the platelet count. Other causes of thrombocytosis are listed in Table 27–12.

The platelet count in reactive thrombocytosis may exceed 1,000,000/μL, characteristic of essential thrombocythemia (ET). Unlike the situation in ET, however, there is little tendency for hemorrhagic and thrombotic complications to occur in reactive thrombocytosis.

Hypercoagulable States

Study of qualitative and quantitative platelet disorders should include discussion of hyperactive platelets as they relate to hypercoagulable and thrombotic states. This alteration in platelet function generally represents a rather special acquired platelet defect.

Thrombotic disorders are a heterogeneous group of inherited (uncommon) or acquired (common) conditions that predispose the patient to arterial and/or venous thrombosis. Thrombosis is a pathologic process that causes disturbances in normal hemostasis resulting in thrombus formation with vaso-occlusion. Thrombus formation is thought to occur when there are changes in blood flow, vessel wall integrity, and coagulation factors and their inhibitors. Individuals susceptible to thrombi formation, or those with a history of thromboembolic events, are said to be hypercoagulable (see Chap. 30).

VASCULAR DISORDERS

The hereditary and acquired vascular disorders are quite variable, and therefore the clinical manifestations also vary. The most common clinical and diagnostic finding of vascular disorders are petechiae and purpura (Table 27–13).

Inherited Vascular Disorders

Hereditary Hemorrhagic Telangiectasia (Osler-Weber-Rendu Disease)

This rather common disorder is inherited as an autosomal-dominant trait. The classic telangiectatic lesions usually do not appear until the second or third

TABLE 27–13 **Vascular Disorders Associated with Bleeding**	
Hereditary Vascular Disorders	**Acquired Vascular Disorders**
Hereditary hemorrhagic telangiectasia	Paraproteinemias
Ehlers-Danlos syndrome	Amyloidosis
Marfan's syndrome	Autoimmune disorders
Osteogenesis imperfecta	Henoch-Schönlein syndrome
Giant hemangioma	Cushing's syndrome
	Diabetes mellitus
	Senile purpura
	Steroid purpura
	Drugs
	Psychogenic purpura

decade of life and may be pinpoint, nodular, or spider-like in appearance. They occur predominantly on the mucous membranes of the skin and the sublingual and buccal areas. Bleeding in childhood is rare; it does not appear until later in life. Hereditary hemorrhagic telangiectasia manifests as recurrent and severe epistaxis and gastrointestinal bleeds from telangiethatic lesions. The classic diagnostic triad is: (1) an inherited trait, (2) presence of telangiectasia, and (3) bleeding from telangiectatic lesions. Coagulation tests, bleeding time, and platelet counts are usually normal. Therapy is directed at controlling localized epistaxis.

Ehlers-Danlos Syndrome

This syndrome is characterized by extreme vascular fragility, skin fragility, and hyperextensible joints. It is a rare connective tissue disorder which is inherited as an autosomal dominant trait. Bleeding may clinically manifest as a result of increased fragility of subcutaneous vessels and is variable. Petechiae, purpura, and gastrointestinal and gingival bleeds are often present. Abnormal laboratory tests include prolonged bleeding time, and a positive Rumpel-Leede tourniquet test. Abnormal platelet aggregation and adhesion has been described in association with this syndrome.

Marfan's Syndrome

This disorder is an inherited autosomal dominant trait characterized by skeletal and ocular defects, and cardiovascular abnormalities such as dissecting aneurysms. This vascular disorder is associated with abnormal collagen formation. Patients exhibit easy bruising and may bleed excessively during surgical procedures. Coagulation tests are generally normal. Poorly characterized platelet defects have been reported.

Pseudoxanthoma Elasticum

This very rare disorder, inherited as an autosomal recessive trait, is characterized by significant hemorrhages in which the elastic fibers of the entire arterial system are abnormal. Patients present with easy bruising and may develop life threatening gastrointestinal bleeds. Intra-articular bleeding with hemarthrosis is common. Thrombosis affecting major arteries of the limbs may also be present.

Osteogenesis Imperfecta

This disorder is inherited as an autosomal-dominant trait in which there is defective bone matrix. Easy and spontaneous bleeding, epistaxis, hemoptysis, and intracranial hemorrhages are associated with this disorder.

Giant Hemangiomas

This syndrome, characterized by tumorous masses composed of thin-walled blood vessels commonly found in the skin and subcutaneous tissue, is generally present at birth. The hemangiomatous lesions may be widespread, involving a single organ or multiple organs. Most patients present with chronic DIC that may become acute. Treatment consists of surgical removal or radiation therapy in uncomplicated cases.

Acquired Vascular Disorders

The acquired vascular disorders are far more common than the hereditary disorders previously discussed. Hemorrhagic and thrombotic tendencies that manifest by petechiae, purpura, and thrombosis in the appropriate clinical setting characterize the acquired vascular disorders.

Paraproteinemia and Amyloidosis

Patients with paraprotein disorder and amyloidosis often develop a diffuse vascular disease with associated hemorrhage and thrombosis. It is believed that increased levels of complement-fixing immunoglobulins (IgM, IgG) cause release of histamine, platelet aggregation, and leukocyte chemotaxis, thereby increasing vascular permeability and small vein thrombosis. The associated hyperviscosity syndrome causes stasis and ischemia, thereby increasing vascular permeability resulting in epistaxis, purpura, and petechiae, as well as organ hemorrhage. Patients with malignant paraproteins often have DIC because of endothelial damage.

In primary amyloidosis, hemorrhage is the classic hallmark as a result of deposition of amyloid on the endothelium. Petechiae, purpura, ecchymosis, easy bruisability, and spontaneous hemorrhages into organs are characteristic. In secondary amyloidosis, hemorrhagic as well as thrombotic tendencies are noted as a result of amyloid deposits along the endothelium as well as perivascular infiltration. The bleeding in amyloidosis is thought to be caused by perivascular infiltration. Platelet function may be abnormal; rarely patients present with thrombocytopenia. A deficiency of factor X and other factors has been reported.[60] It is believed that factor X binds to the amyloid deposits. See Figure 27–3, which shows the characteristic periorbital distribution seen in amyloid purpura.

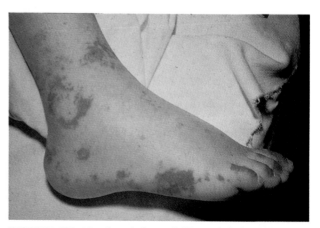

FIGURE 27–12 Anaphylactoid (Henoch-Schönlein) purpura. Purpuric lesions of the foot.

TABLE 27–14 **Common Drugs That Cause Vasculitis**		
Aspirin	Digoxin	Methyldopa
Allopurinol	Estrogens	Penicillin
Atropine	Furosemide	Phenacetin
Belladonna	Indomethacin	Quinine
Chloramphenicol	Iodine	Quinidine
Chloral hydrate	Isoniazide	Sulfonamides
Coumarin	Meprobramate	Tolbutamide

Autoimmune Disorders

Disorders involving circulating immune complexes are associated with a diffuse vasculitis and hemorrhagic and thrombotic tendencies. Most often the circulating immune complexes attach to the endothelium, whereby they fix complement, causing chemotaxis of leukocytes, increased vascular permeability, fibrin deposition, and vascular damage. A specific antibody directed against the endothelium is a rare mechanism of autoimmune-induced vasculitis and is limited to the allergic purpuras such as Henoch-Schonlein purpura. Figure 27–12 demonstrates this type of purpuric lesion located on the foot.

Infections

Many bacterial, viral, rickettsial, or protozoal infections have an associated vasculitis with hemorrhagic and thrombotic tendencies. Vascular damage occurs from the deposition of immune complexes within the vessel walls following infection or by endotoxin production. Characteristically, purpura develops symmetrically on the buttocks and posterior thighs. Diphtheria, septicemia from *Meningococcus* or *Steptococcus* species, smallpox, measles, Rocky Mountain spotted fever, and malaria are infections commonly associated with purpura.

Drugs

Drug-induced vasculitis is a common cause of acquired vascular defects. An allergic mechanism has

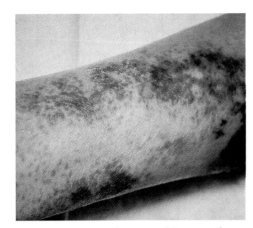

FIGURE 27–14 Steroid purpura (skin manifestations).

been described. Table 27–14 lists some of the drugs implicated in causing purpura in the face of a normal platelet count.

Psychogenic Purpura

This disorder is predominantly seen in middle-aged women with a positive history of psychiatric disorders and is manifested by spontaneous painful ecchymoses. Characteristically, the ecchymoses are confined to the limbs, rarely affecting the trunk. The purpuric lesions are believed to develop from subcutaneous extravasation of red cells as a result of injury to the skin.[61]

Miscellaneous Disorders

Malignant hypertension, diabetes mellitus, Cushing's disease, eclampsia, and senile purpura are disorders that cause vascular damage with increased vascular permeability and fibrin deposition. Ecchymoses, purpura, and a marked increase of thrombosis are common clinical manifestations seen in these disorders. In senile purpura (Fig. 27–13), in persons on prolonged corticosteroid therapy (Fig. 27–14), or in patients with Cushing's disease, purpura of the hands and forearms is common. Tables 27–11 and 27–13 summarize the various qualitative and quantitative platelet and vascular disorders discussed.

CASE STUDY

A 47-year-old African-American woman presented to the hospital with easy bruisability, petechiae, right-sided weakness, mild confusion, headaches, nausea, and vomiting.

On admission, physical examination revealed a temperature of 104°F, blood pressure of 150/70 mm Hg, pulse 80, and respirations 14 per minute. Decreased motor strength of the right extremities was noted. Examination revealed scattered petechiae over the inner thighs bilaterally with the upper extremities demonstrating petechiae and ecchymoses of the forearm.

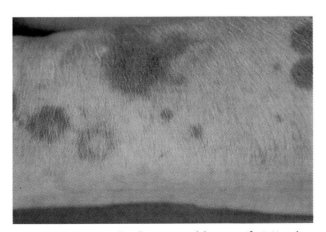

FIGURE 27–13 Senile purpura (skin manifestations).

Admission laboratory findings showed a hematocrit of 21%, white cell count of 10.0×10^9/L, platelet count of 18.0×10^9/L, and a reticulocyte count of 7.0%. PT, APTT, and fibrinogen values were normal. FDPs were positive with a titer of 1:32. The DAT and tests for circulating anticoagulants were negative. The peripheral smear showed a moderate poikilocytosis with the presence of schistocytes. Serum creatinine was 5.1 mg/dL; blood urea nitrogen, 160 mg/dL; calcium, 7.6 mg/dL; total serum protein, 4.2 mg/dL; and albumin, 2.4 g/dL. Urinalysis was remarkable with +3 proteinemia and numerous red blood cells. A bone marrow aspirate revealed moderate megakaryocytic hyperplasia with mild erythroid hyperplasia. Electrocardiogram and chest radiograph were normal.

A tentative diagnosis of thrombotic thrombocytopenic purupura was made. The patient was given 12 units of plasma over a 15-hour period without noticeable clinical change. To help correct renal function, the patient was placed on dialysis and began steroid therapy in conjunction with dipyridamole. Over the next several days of therapy, her renal, neurologic, and hematologic profile improved. She was discharged after the sixteenth day of hospitalization and maintained on prednisone and dipyridamole. One month later, all laboratory findings were normal. After 12 months, she is symptom-free and receiving no medication.

Questions

1. What other conditions would be considered in the differential diagnosis?
2. What are the characteristics of TTP?
3. What characteristics differentiate this condition from DIC?

REFERENCES

1. Ginsburg, D: Biology of inherited coagulopathies: von Willebrand factor. Hematol Oncol Clin North Am 6:1011, 1992.
2. Bloom, AL: von Willebrand factor: Clinical features of inherited and acquired disorders. Mayo Clin Proc 66:743, 1991.
3. Miller, JL, et al: Mutation in the gene encoding the alpha chain of platelet glycoprotein Ib in platelet-type von Willebrand disease. Proc Nat Acad Sci USA 88:4761, 1991.
4. Kottke-Marchand, K: Laboratory diagnosis of hemorrhagic and thrombotic disorders. Hematol Oncol Clin North Am 8:809, 1994.
5. Ruggeri, ZM: New insights into the mechanism of platelet adhesion and aggregation. Semin Hematol 31:229, 1994.
6. Nurden, AT, George, JN, and Phillips, DR: Human platelet membrane glycoproteins: Their structure, function and biological significance. In Phillips, DR and Schulman, MA (eds): The Biology of Platelets. Academic Press, New York, 1986, p 159.
7. Hourdille, P, et al: von Willebrand factor bound to glycoprotein Ib is cleared from the platelet surface after platelet activation by thrombin. Blood 79:2011, 1992.
8. Nurden, P, et al: Two-way trafficking of membrane glycoproteins on thrombin-activated human platelets. Semin Hematol 31:240, 1994.
9. Weiss, HJ, Turitto, VT, and Baumgarter, HR: Role of

shear rate and platelets in promoting fibrin formation on rabbit endothelium. Studies utilizing patients with quantitative and qualitative platelet defects. J Clin Invest 78:1072, 1986.
10. Brass, LF, et al: Structure and function of the human platelet thrombin receptor. J Biol Chem 276:13795, 1992.
11. Yamamoto, N, et al: Glycoprotein Ib-dependent and GP-Ib independent pathways of thrombin-induced platelet activation. Blood 77:1740, 1991.
12. Fox, JB et al: Identification of a membrane skeleton in platelets. J Cell Biol 106:1525, 1988.
13. White, JG and Gerrard, JM: Ultrastructure features of abnormal platelets. Am J Pathol 85:590, 1976.
14. Brown, CH, et al: Glanzmann's thrombasthenia: Assessment of the response to platelet transfusion. Transfusion 15:124, 1975.
15. White, JG: Ultrastructural studies of the gray platelet syndrome. Am J Pathol 95:445, 1979.
16. Weiss, HJ, et al: Heterogeneity in storage pool deficiencies: Studies on granule-bound substances in 18 patients including variants deficient in alpha granules, PF4, B-thromboglobulin and platelet derived growth factor. Blood 54:1296, 1979.
17. Lewis, JH, Zucker, MB, and Ferguson, JH: Bleeding tendency in uremia. Blood 11:1073, 1956.
18. Escolar, G, Casa, A, and Bastidi, E: Uremic platelets have a functional defect affecting the interaction of von Willebrand's factor with glycoprotein IIb-IIIa. Blood 76:1336, 1990.
19. Boneu, B and Fernandez, F: The role of the hematocrit in bleeding. Transfusion Med Rev 1:182, 1987.
20. Huraib, S, et al: Effect of recombinant human erythropoietin (r-HuEPO) on the hemostatic system in chronic hemodialysis patients. Clin Nephrol 36:252, 1991.
21. Taylor, JE, et al: Erythropoietin and spontaneous platelet aggregation in hemodialysis patients. Lancet 338:1361, 1991.
22. Janson, PA, et al: Treatment of the bleeding tendency in uremia with cryoprecipitate. N Engl J Med 303:7318, 1980.
23. Mannucci, PM, et al: Deamino-8-D-arginine vasopressin shortens the bleeding time in uremia. N Engl J Med 308:8, 1983.
24. Bick, RL: Alterations of hemostasis associated with malignancy. Etiology, pathophysiology, diagnosis and management. Semin Thromb Hemost 5:1, 1978.
25. Patterson, WP: Coagulation and cancer: An overview. Semin Oncol 17:137, 1990.
26. Silgals, RM and Sacher, RA: Quantitative and qualitative vascular and platelet disorders, both congenital and acquired. In Pittiglio, DH and Sacher, RA (eds): Clinical Hematology and Fundamentals of Hemostasis. FA Davis, Philadelphia, 1987, p 354.
27. Carvalho, ACA and Rao, AK: Acquired qualitative platelet defects. In Coleman, RW, Hirch, J, Marder, VJ, and Salzman, EW (eds): Hemostasis and Thrombosis: Basic Principles and Clinical Practice. JB Lippincott, Philadelphia, 1987, p 752.
28. Cortelazzo, S, Viero, P, and Barbui, T: Platelet activation in myeloproliferative disorders. Thromb Haemost 45:211, 1981.
29. Woodman, RC and Harker, LA: Bleeding complications associated with cardiopulmonary bypass. Blood 76:1980, 1990.
30. Terraris, VA, et al: Platelet aggregation abnormalities after cardiopulmonary bypass. Blood 83:299, 1994.
31. Blauhut, B, et al: Effects of high-dose aprotinin on blood loss, platelet function, fibrinolysis, complement and renal function after cardiopulmonary bypass. J Thorac Cardiovasc Surg 101:958, 1991.

32. Murano, G and Bick, RL: Basic Concepts of Hemostasis and Thrombosis. CRC Press, Boca Raton, 1980, p 188.
33. Carvalho, ACA and Rao, AK: op. cit. p 761.
34. Moschcowitz, E: Hyaline thrombosis of the terminal arterioles and capillaries: A hitherto undescribed disease. Proc NY Pathol Soc 24:21, 1924.
35. Remuzzi, GR, et al: Thrombotic thrombocytopenic purpura deficiency of plasma factors regulating platelet-vessel-wall interaction. N Engl J Med 299:311, 1978.
36. Bukowski, RM: Thrombotic thrombocytopenic purpura: A review. Prog Hemost Thromb 6:287, 1982.
37. Amorsi, EC and Ultman, JE: Thrombotic thrombocytopenic purpura. Report of 16 cases and review of the literature. Medicine 45:135, 1966.
38. Gutterman, LA and Stevenson, TD: Treatment of thrombotic thrombocytopenic purpura with vincristine. JAMA 247:1433, 1982.
39. Fitzgerald, GA, Mass, RL, and Stern, R: Intravenous prostacyclin in thrombotic thrombocytopenic purpura. Ann Intern Med 96:227, 1982.
40. Kottke-Marchant, K: Laboratory diagnosis of hemorrhagic and thrombotic disorders. In Hyun, BH (ed): Diagnostic Hematology. WB Saunders, Philadelphia, 1994, p 809.
41. Boshkov, LK, et al: Heparin-induced thrombocytopenia and thrombosis: clinical and laboratory studies. Br J Haematol 84:322, 1993.
42. Lusher, JM and Iyer, R: Idiopathic thrombocytopenic purpura in children. Semin Thromb Hemost 3:3, 1977.
43. Lightsey, AS Jr, McMillan, R, and Koenig, HM: Childhood idiopathic thrombocytopenic purpura: Aggressive management of life threatening complications. JAMA 232:734, 1975.
44. Cheung, N-KV, et al: Platelet associated immunoglobulin G in childhood idiopathic thrombocytopenic purpura. J Pediatr 102:366, 1983.
45. George, JN, El-Harake, MA, and Raskob, GE: Chronic idiopathic thrombocytopenic purpura. N Engl J Med 331:1207, 1994.
46. Snyder, HW, et al: Experience with protein A-immunoadsorption in treatment-resistant adult immune thrombocytopenic purpura. Blood 79:2237, 1992.
47. Kernoff, LM, Blake, KCH, and Shackleton, D: Influence of the amount of platelet-bound IgG on platelet survival and site of sequestration in autoimmune thrombocytopenia. Blood 55:730, 1980.
48. Baldini, M: Idiopathic thrombocytopenic purpura. N Engl J Med 274:1245, 1966.
49. Picozzi, VJ, Roeske, WR, and Creger, WP: Fate of therapy failures in adult idiopathic thrombocytopenic purpura. Am J Med 69:690, 1980.
50. Kaden, BR, Rosse, WF, and Hauch, TW: Immune thrombocytopenia in lymphoproliferative diseases. Blood 53:545, 1979.
51. Stricker, RB: Hemostatic abnormalities in HIV disease. In Mitsuyasu, RT and Golde, DW (eds): Hematologic and Oncologic Aspects of HIV Disease. WB Saunders, Philadelphia, 1991, p 249.
52. Rousselet, MC, et al: Idiopathic thrombocytopenic purpura in patients at risk for acquired immunodeficiency syndrome. Arch Pathol Lab Med 112:1242, 1988.
53. Rosenthal, N: The blood picture in purpura. J Lab Clin Med 13:303, 1928.
54. Schulman, RN and Jordan, JV, Jr: Platelet immunology. In Coleman, RW, Hirsh, J, Marder, VS, and Salzman, EW (eds): Hemostasis and Thrombosis: Basic Principles and Clinical Practice. JB Lippincott, Philadelphia, 1987, p 460.
55. Shulman, NR, et al: Immunoreaction involving platelets. V. Post-transfusion purpura due to a complement-fixing antibody against a genetically controlled platelet antigen:

A proposed mechanism for thrombocytopenia and its relevance in "autoimmunity." J Clin Invest 40:1597, 1981.
56. Morrison, FS and Mollison, PL: Post-transfusion purpura. N Engl J Med 275:243, 1966.
57. Shulman, NR and Jordan, JV, Jr: Platelet immunology. In Coleman, RW, Hirsh, J, Marder, VS and Salzman, EW (eds): Hemostasis and Thrombosis: Basic Principles and Clinical Practice. JB Lippincott, Philadelphia, 1987, p 473.
58. Bracey, AW and Shulman, NR: Effects of plasma exchange in an unusual case of post transfusion purpura. Transfusion 23:428a, 1983.
59. Shulman, NR and Jordan, JV, Jr: Platelet kinetics. In Coleman, RW, Hirsh, J, Marder, VJ, and Salzman, EW (eds): Hemostasis and Thrombosis: Basic Principles and Clinical Practice. JB Lippincott, Philadelphia, 1987, p 447.
60. Greipp, PR, Kyle, RA, and Bowie, EJW: Factor X deficiency in amyloidosis: A critical review. Am J Hematol 11:443, 1981.
61. Ratnoff, OD: The psychogenic purpuras: A review of autoerythrocyte sensitization, autosensitization to DNA, "hysterical" and factitial bleeding and religious stigma. Semin Hematol 17:192, 1980.

BIBLIOGRAPHY

Bailliere's Clinical Haematology, International Practice and Research: In Caen, JP (ed): Platelet Disorders, 2:3, July 1989.
Bick, RL: Perplexing Thrombotic and Hemorrhagic Disorders. Hematol Oncol Clin North Am 6:6, 1992.
Coleman, RW and Rao, AK: Platelets in Health and Disease. Hematol Oncol Clin North Am 4:1, 1990.
Penner, JA and Hassouna, HI: Coagulation Disorders I. Hematol Oncol Clin North Am 6:5, 1992.
Penner, JA and Hassouna, HI: Coagulation Disorders II. Hematol Oncol Clin North Am 7:6, 1993.

QUESTIONS

1. A patient presents with a platelet count of 212×10^9/L and a bleeding time of 12 minutes. These results most probably suggest:
   a. Decreased platelet production
   b. Defective platelet function
   c. Increased platelet production
   d. Increased platelet destruction

2. Which of the following clinical manifestations is most characteristic of a platelet disorder:
   a. Mucosal bleeds
   b. Hemarthrosis
   c. Retroperitoneal hemorrhage
   d. Deep muscle hematomas

3. Which of the following is not characteristic for Bernard-Soulier syndrome?
   a. Prolonged bleeding time
   b. Absent platelet aggregation in response to bovine vWf or human vWf plus ristocetin
   c. Abnormal platelet aggregation in response to ADP, collagen, and epinephrine
   d. Abnormality in platelet membrane GPIb/IX

4. Which of the following is not characteristic of Glanzmann's thrombasthenia?

a. Prolonged bleeding time
b. Giant platelets with thrombocytopenia
c. Absent platelet aggregation in response to ADP, thrombin, collagen, and epinephrine
d. Normal platelet aggregation to ristocetin and bovine vWf

5. Which of the following statements is not true regarding acute idiopathic thrombocytopenia (ITP)?
a. Thrombocytopenia occurs following a viral infection.
b. Spontaneous remissions are common.
c. Found primarily in young children.
d. Platelet counts are generally higher than in chronic ITP.

6. Thrombocytopenia, fever, renal disease, microangiopathic hemolytic anemia, and neurologic complications are hallmark characteristics of:
a. Hemolytic uremic syndrome (HUS)
b. Disseminated intravascular coagulation (DIC)
c. Thrombotic thrombocytopenic purpura (TTP)
d. Idiopathic thrombocytopenic purpura (ITP)

7. What disorders are classically associated with thrombocytosis?
a. Myeloproliferative syndromes
b. Autoimmune disorders
c. Immunodeficiency syndrome-HIV
d. Renal disease

8. Which of the following is not an inherited vascular defect?
a. Ehlers-Danlos syndrome
b. Marfan's syndrome
c. Amyloidosis
d. Giant hemangiomas

9. Which condition is classified as nonimmunologic thrombocytopenia?
a. Disseminated intravascular coagulation
b. Idiopathic thrombocytopenic purpura
c. Storage pool defects
d. Bernard-Soulier syndrome

10. Which condition is classified as immunologic thrombocytopenia?
a. Disseminated intravascular coagulation
b. Idiopathic thrombocytopenic purpura
c. Storage pool defects
d. Bernard-Soulier syndrome

ANSWERS

1. **b** (pp 509–510)
2. **a** (p 510 [Table 27–1])
3. **c** (pp 511–513)
4. **b** (p 513)
5. **d** (pp 520–522)
6. **c** (p 519)
7. **a** (p 524)
8. **c** (p 526)
9. **a** (pp 518, 520)
10. **b** (p 520)

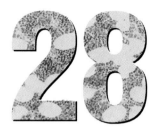

Disorders of Plasma Clotting Factors

Carol C. Caruana, H(ASCP)SH
Sharon L. Schwartz, MT(ASCP)

Objectives

At the end of this chapter, the learner should be able to:
1 List various defects that impair the coagulation system.
2 Name the vitamin K–dependent factors.
3 Describe the differences between hemophilia A and von Willebrand's disease.
4 Name the factor deficiency responsible for causing hemophilia A.
5 Name the factor deficiency responsible for causing hemophilia B.
6 Describe laboratory methods used to identify factor deficiencies.
7 Describe circulating anticoagulants and inhibitors.
8 Describe laboratory methods used to identify anticoagulants and inhibitors.
9 Discuss various etiologies and treatment modalities for various factor deficiencies.

This chapter covers disorders of plasma clotting factors and how these disorders directly affect hemostasis. Information is provided in detail on each of the coagulation factors and their deficiencies (Table 28–1 and see Table 26–19). Additionally, discussions include information on the lupus anticoagulant and specific factor inhibitors. The recommended blood component therapy for each specific plasma clotting defect is discussed. A summary of the materials presented and several case studies that illustrate the information are presented at the end of the chapter.

The transformation of liquid blood to a gel is a very complex process. The end result is the cessation of blood flow or hemostasis. Clotting factors circulate as inactive zymogens or precursors of serine proteases, which have serine as a portion of their active enzymatic site and function to cleave peptide bonds. (Chapter 27 discusses the activation of the zymogens that participate in the coagulation pathways leading to the formation of an insoluble fibrin clot. See Tables 27–8 and 28–1).

Plasma clotting deficiencies can impair hemostasis. These plasma clotting defects are a result of:
1. Decreased synthesis of the factors
2. Production of abnormal molecules that interfere with the coagulation pathways

TABLE 28-1	**Factor Deficiencies**				
Factor	Deficiency	Minimum for Hemostasis	Half-Life	Laboratory	Clinical
I	Afibrinogenemia (rare) Autosomal recessive-homozygous	50–100 mg%	120 hr	No clot formation Abnormal PT, APTT, TCT; no fibrinogen	Umbilical stump bleeding, easy bruising, ecchymosis, gingival oozing hematuria, poor wound healing
	Hypofibrinogenemia (rare) Autosomal recessive-heterozygous			Abnormal PT,APTT,TCT; low fibrinogen	Mild bleeding, thrombotic episodes
	Dysfibrinogenemia Variable inheritance Uncommon variants			Fibrinogen; qualitative: abnormal quantitative: normal	Possible hemorrhage, possible thrombosis, possible asymptomatic
II	Hypoprothrombinemia (extremely rare), autosomal recessive	30–40%	100 hr	Abnormal PT, APTT	Postoperative bleeding, epistaxis, menorrhagia, easy bruising
V	Parahemophilia Autosomal recessive 1/1,000,000-homozygote	10%	25 hr	Abnormal PT, APTT, BT	Epistaxis, menorrhagia, easy bruising
VII	Hypoproconvertinemia Incomplete autosomal recessive variable expression: 1/500,000	10%	5 hr	Abnormal PT, normal APTT	Epistaxis, menorrhagia, cerebral hemorrhage
VIII	Hemophilia A (classic hemophilia) sex-linked recessive 1/10,000	30%	8–12 hr	Abnormal APTT; normal PT, BT	May be severe, moderate, mild—spontaneous hemorrhage, hemarthroses, crippling, muscle hemorrhage, post traumatic postoperative bleeding
	von Willebrand's syndrome variable inheritance, variants: autosomal dominant variable penetrance: 1/80,000	20–40%	16–24 hr	Variable results Platelet studies, BT, APTT	Mucous membrane bleeding, superficial wound bleeding-variable depending on level of VIII:C levels
IX	Hemophilia B (Christmas disease) sex-linked recessive 1/100,000	30–50%	20 hr	Abnormal APTT; normal PT	May be severe, moderate, mild—spontaneous hemorrhage, hemarthroses, crippling, muscle hemorrhage, post traumatic postoperative bleeding, ecchymoses
X	Stuart-Prower defect Autosomal recessive <1/500,000-homozygous 1/500 heterozygous	10%	65 hr	Abnormal PT, APTT	Menorrhagia, ecchymoses, central nervous system bleeding, excessive bleeding after childbirth
XI	Hemophilia C-Incomplete autosomal recessive pseudo-dominant 1/100,000	20–30%	65 hr	Abnormal APTT; normal PT	Mild bleeding, bruising, epistaxis retinal hemorrhage, menorrhagia
XII	Hageman trait (rare) Autosomal recessive	Unknown	60 hr	Abnormal APTT Normal PT	Asymptomatic—rarely bleed, thrombosis
XIII	Factor XIII deficiency Autosomal recessive	1%	150 hr	Normal PT, APTT; clot soluble in 5 M urea	Umbilical cord bleeding, delayed wound healing, minor injuries causing prolonged bleeding, fetal wastage, excessive fibrinolysis, male sterility, intracranial hemorrhage

		TABLE 28-1 Factor Deficiencies (*Continued*)				
Factor	**Deficiency**	**Minimum for Hemostasis**	**Half-Life**	**Laboratory**	**Clinical**
PK	Prekallikrein (Fletcher factor) Autosomal recessive	Unknown	35 hr	Abnormal APTT: shortening of time after prolonged incubation with activator	Asymptomatic
HMWK	Fitzgerald deficiency (rare) Autosomal recessive	Unknown	156 hr	Abnormal APTT	Asymptomatic

Source: From Pittiglio, DH, et al: Treating hemostatic disorders. A problem oriented approach. In Pittiglio, DH: Hemostasis Overview. American Association of Blood Banks, Arlington, VA. 1984. p 28 with permission.

Abbreviations: PT = Prothrombin time; APTT = activated partial thromboplastin time; BT = bleeding time; HMWK = high-molecular-weight kininogen; TCT = thrombin clotting time

3. Loss or consumption of the coagulation factors
4. Inactivation of these factors by inhibitors or antibodies[1]

Transmission of the plasma defects may be inherited as sex-linked or autosomal disorders. These deficiencies may also be acquired as a result of vitamin K deficiency, liver disease, hemorrhage, or a consumptive coagulopathy such as disseminated intravascular coagulation (DIC), induction of anticoagulant therapy, and treatment with various drugs.

DISORDERS OF PLASMA CLOTTING FACTORS AND LABORATORY EVALUATION

Factor I (Fibrinogen)

Fibrinogen is a large glycoprotein produced in the liver with a molecular weight (M_r) of 340,000 daltons and participates in the final stages of coagulation. The fibrinogen molecule consists of two sets of three different polypeptide chains, Aα, Bβ, and γ, and has a half-life of about 3 days.[2] The interaction of these chains, combined with the activity of the enzyme thrombin, yields a network of insoluble strands called *fibrin*.[3] Fibrin monomers are produced by the cleavage of the fibrinopeptides A and B from the terminal ends of the α and β chains of the fibrinogen molecule. In the final stages these soluble monomers then polymerize to form soluble fibrin strands. In order to stabilize the soluble fibrin strands, factor XIII, which is also activated by thrombin, acts as the stabilizing factor, cross-linking the fibrin monomers to produce insoluble fibrin. This process produces a stable fibrin clot. The normal plasma concentration of fibrinogen in the circulation is 200 to 400 mg/dL.

Afibrinogenemia

Afibrinogenemia, a rare inherited autosomal recessive trait, can cause profuse bleeding after slight trauma and delay in wound healing. Initial symptoms include bleeding from the umbilical cord. Other symptoms can include intracranial bleeding, epistaxis, gastrointestinal bleeding, and menorrhagia. Hemarthrosis is uncommon for this disorder. Mild to moderate thrombocytopenia can occur, but platelet counts are rarely less than 100,000/μL.[4,5]

Treatment for this disorder includes cryoprecipitate, fresh frozen plasma (FFP), and whole blood transfusions if profuse bleeding has occurred.

The laboratory evaluation for this disorder should include: prothrombin time (PT), activated partial thromboplastin time (APTT), fibrinogen (activity and antigen), Reptilase time (RT), and thrombin time (TT) (see Table 28-2). The results of these tests will show marked abnormality: prolongation of the PT, APTT, RT, and TT, and the absence of measurable fibrinogen. Mixture with adsorbed plasma or pooled normal plasma corrects these defects. Platelet aggregation was found to be abnormal in two studies where fibrinogen was absent in platelets of patients with this disorder.[6]

Hypofibrinogenemia

Hypofibrinogenemia is an autosomal recessive disorder where the level of fibrinogen is found to be in the 20 to 100 mg/dL range. Unlike the situation in afibrinogenemia, hemorrhage after trauma is an infrequent finding. Umbilical bleeding is a common symptom, as are other hemorrhagic symptoms noted with afibrinogenemia. In hypofibrinogenemia, the degree in which laboratory tests are abnormal is dependent on the level of fibrinogen present in the plasma.

Dysfibrinogenemia

When the structure of the fibrinogen molecule is altered in either amino acid sequence or carbohydrate composition, the normal interactions of fibrinogen with its enzymes and cofactors is disrupted, leading to the formation of an abnormal protein and thereby causing defective fibrin formation.

Dysfibrinogenemia is a qualitative defect that can be either inherited, mostly as an autosomal dominant trait, or acquired as a result of some underlying disease, most often liver disease.

Polymerization of fibrin monomers, prepared by treating the abnormal molecules with large amounts of thrombin, has been found to be normal in several cases.[7] However, with lower thrombin concentrations, as in the diluted thrombin time (DTT) test, polymerization is delayed because of the lower cleavage rate of the abnormal peptide.[8] A common laboratory finding is a normal quantitative value of functional fibrinogen with a mild to markedly prolonged DTT. The level obtained by immunochemical assay of fibrinogen is very often higher than the level determined by functional assay. The anticoagulants heparin, hirudin, and the antithrombins can also prolong the DTT. To evaluate the cause of the abnormal DTT, a Reptilase time (RT) should be performed.[9,10] Reptilase, a thrombinlike enzyme extracted from the snake venom of *Bothrops atrox*, can be used to evaluate for the presence of these anticoagulants or confirmation of dysfibrinogenemia.[11] Reptilase is unaffected by heparin, hirudin, and antithrombins, and the RT will remain normal in their presence (Table 28–2).

Factor II (Prothrombin)

Prothrombin, M_r 71,600 daltons, is synthesized in the liver, is the most abundant of the vitamin K–dependent blood-clotting proteins, and circulates as a zymogen to a serine protease.[12] Prothrombin is converted to thrombin by the reactions of factor Xa in the presence of factor Va acting as a "cofactor" of phospholipid and calcium ions. Deficiencies of prothrombin delay generation of thrombin, thus contributing to hemorrhagic symptoms.

Hypoprothrombinemia

It has been suggested that the mode of inheritance of hypoprothrombinemia is autosomal recessive.[13] Patients who are either double heterozygous or homozygous with this rare condition may have symptoms with prothrombin levels from 2% to 25% of normal activity. However, the type and severity of symptoms may vary with the level of functional prothrombin available. Epistaxis, menorrhagia, postpartum hemorrhage, and

hemorrhage following surgery or trauma and broad spectrum antibiotic use are exhibited with prothrombin levels of less than 2% to less than 50%. Ingestion of aspirin has exacerbated bleeding tendencies. Prothrombin levels approaching 50% of normal activity generally do not have bleeding problems. Variable prolongation of both the PT and activated partial thromboplastin time (APTT) and a normal thrombin time (TT) are obtained in individuals with this deficiency. These screening assays are not specific for this deficiency. Diagnosis is dependent on specific assays for functional and/or immunologic prothrombin. In hypoprothrombinemia, both the levels of functional and immunologic prothrombin activity are decreased. Mixing studies with either aged serum or adsorbed plasma will show no correction of the PT or aPTT.

Dysprothrombinemia

The mode of inheritance of dysprothrombinemia is the same as in hypoprothrombinemia.[14] Bleeding manifestations may occur that are similar to those described with hypoprothrombinemia. The functional level of prothrombin is decreased and the immunologic level is normal. Vitamin K deficiency, induction and therapeutic warfarin therapy, liver disease, and the presence of antibodies to prothrombin must be distinguished from dysprothrombinemia and hypoprothrombinemia.

Treatment includes administration of FFP, prothrombin complex concentrates, and concentrates containing factors II, VII, IX and X.

Factor V (Proaccelerin)

Rapid enzymatic reactions that include protein cofactors have a vital role in normal blood coagulation. Factor V and factor VIII (antihemophilic factor) enhance these reactions. The absence of either of these factors leads to bleeding. Owren[15,16] discovered factor V deficiency in a 21-year-old woman with a lifelong bleeding history. The discovery showed that this clotting factor was not vitamin K–dependent. Factor V deficiency is inherited as an autosomal recessive trait.[17] This extremely rare condition has a probability of occurrence of 1 person per 1 million population.[18] This

TABLE 28–2	**Differential Diagnosis of Fibrinogen Disorders and Heparin**			
Test	Afibrinogenemia	Hypofibrinogenemia	Dysfibrinogenemia	Heparin
Bleeding time	P	N	N	N
Prothrombin time	P	P	P	P
APTT	P	P	P	P
Thrombin time	P	P	P	P
Reptilase time	P	P	P	N
Thrombin coagulase	P	P	N	N
Fibrinogen level (clotting assay)	10 mg/dL	20–100 mg/dL	10 mg/dL	N
Fibrinogen (immunologic assay)	Absent	20–100 mg/dL	N	N
Platelet aggregation	Abnormal	N	N	N(ABN)
Fibrinolytic test	N	N	N	N

Source: From Girolami, A, et al: Rare and quantitative and qualitative: Abnormalities of coagulation. Changes Hematol 14(2):388, 1985, with permission.

Abbreviations: N = Normal; P = Prolonged; ABN = Abnormal; APTT = activated partial thromboplastin time.

factor is synthesized by the liver and is present in the α granules of platelets.[19] Factor V has an M_r of 350,000 daltons and a short half-life, and is heat-labile. It functions as a cofactor in the conversion of prothrombin to thrombin. It is converted to its active cofactor, factor Va, by the action of thrombin or factor Xa, in the presence of calcium and phospholipids. The enzymes of Russell's viper venom can also activate factor V.

Ecchymoses, epistaxis, menorrhagia, and gingival, gastrointestinal tract, umbilical, and central nervous system bleeding are associated with deficiencies of factor V. Hemorrhagic manifestations are usually noted in individuals with less than 10% activity. Hemarthrosis seldom occurs even in severely deficient patients. Combined factors V and VIII deficiencies have been reported in several families.

Acquired factor V deficiency can be the result of the appearance of specific antibodies or associated with a variety of diseases, such as liver disease, carcinoma, tuberculosis, disseminated intravascular coagulation (DIC), and other causes.[20] The PT and APTT are prolonged and are corrected with the addition of normal plasma. Mixing studies with adsorbed plasma also show a correction of the PT and APTT. However, mixing studies with aged serum do not correct the prolongation of either the PT or the APTT. The thrombin time (TT) is normal. To avoid contamination of the plasma factor V level, plasma must yield platelet counts of less than $10,000/\mu l$. Functional factor activity is decreased or absent. Correction with the addition of normal plasma will not occur in the presence of an inhibitor. Factor V-deficient patients are often treated with fresh or fresh-frozen plasma. Cryoprecipitate does not contain adequate amounts of factor V to be used in therapy.

Factor VII (Proconvertin)

The division of the coagulation system into the intrinsic and extrinsic systems was created as a useful tool for laboratory diagnoses. It has recently been recognized that this division does not occur in vivo as tissue factor/factor VIIa complex is responsible for the activation of factor IX as well as factor X.

The initiation of the coagulation pathways in vivo begins with the extrinsic system involving components of the vascular and blood elements. A major component is tissue factor, which functions as a cofactor. Tissue factor is synthesized by macrophages and endothelial cells and is composed of a single polypeptide chain. The predominant plasma protein of the entrinsic system is factor VII, a vitamin K-dependent protein with an M_r of 50,000. It is produced in the liver and its activity is increased by factor XIIa or IXa and requires tissue factor, thrombin, and calcium ions to form VIIa.

Factor VII deficiency is a rare inherited autosomal recessive trait.[21,22] Clinically, factor VII–deficient patients have deep muscle hematomas, joint hemorrhage, epistaxis, and menorrhagia. The PT is prolonged with a normal APTT (factor VII is not measured in the APTT test system). The PT can be fully corrected with Russell's viper venom and mixing with aged serum (Table 28–3). Documentation of factor VII deficiency requires the one-stage factor assay. Patients who have less then 1% clotting activity can have severe

TABLE 28–3 Laboratory Findings for Factor VII Deficiency

Test	Results	Normal Values
PT	>20 s	10.3–14.0 s
APTT	<34.0 s	23.0–34.0 s
Factor VII assay	<1.0%	100%
Russell's viper venom	18.0 s	<25.0 s
Other factor activity	100%	100%

hemorrhagic manifestations. Factor VII deficiency can be acquired with liver disease, warfarin therapy, or vitamin K deficiency. Treatment of factor VII deficiency includes FFP, prothrombin complex concentrates, and vitamin K.

Factor VIII

Factor VIII, a large glycoprotein, is essential in the middle phase of coagulation.[23] It circulates as a complex of von Willebrand factor (FVIII:vWf) and the procoagulant, factor VIII (FVIII:C).[24] Factor VIII:C, with an M_r of 330,000 daltons, is synthesized primarily in the liver, and von Willebrand factor (FVIII:vWf), a glycoprotein, is synthesized by megakaryocytes and endothelial cells. Only 1% to 2% of the complex is the procoagulant FVIII:C and the remaining protein is FVIII:vWf, which mediates platelet adhesion. The defect in hemophilia A is not an absence of factor VIII complex but rather a molecular defect or absence of its procoagulant portion (FVIII:C).[25] The vWf:Ag of the FVIII complex is found to be normal in patients with hemophilia. When injury occurs, FVIII:vWf serves as a carrier to concentrate the FVIII:C at the site of injury. Factor VIII:C accelerates the conversion of factor X to factor Xa in the presence of factor IXa, calcium, and phospholipids (Tables 28–4, 28–5, and 28–6). (See Chap. 27 and Table 28–1.) Factor VIII:C is thermolabile and can rapidly lose activity unless the plasma is stored below $-70°C$.

Hemophilia A

Hemophilia A is the most common hereditary coagulation disorder. It is a sex-linked bleeding disorder that has been documented for centuries. The fifth-century Talmud described a bleeding episode that occurred after circumcision. Modern rabbinic command forbids the circumcision of any child in whom the diagnosis of hemophilia has been made.[26] The disorder was found in the Royal House of Stuart in Europe and Russia. Queen Victoria, a carrier, was the source of hemophilia in four subsequent generations.[27,28] The gene resides on the X chromosome, thereby producing sons with the disease and daughters who will be obligatory carriers of the trait. The female carrier does not usually exhibit clinical bleeding. She has two X chromosomes, only one of which produces functional FVIII:C. The ratio of antigenic FVIII to procoagulant FVIII (vWF:Ag/FVIII:C) should be approximately 2:1 in the carrier.[29] In approximately one-third of newly diagnosed cases of hemophilia A, there may be no pre-

TABLE 28–4   **Selected Properties of Factor VIII:C and von Willebrand Factor***

	Factor VIII:C	von Willebrand Factor
Cellular site of biosynthesis	Hepatic	Endothelial cells and megakaryocytes
Plasma concentration	50–150 U/L	50–150 U/L
Molecular weight	265,000 (plus carbohydrate)	1–2 million
Principal biologic activity	Procoagulant cofactor	Platelet adhesion to vessel wall
Assay functional	APTT factor Xa formation	Bleeding time, platelet adhesion, platelet aggultination (e.g., ristocetin-induced)
Immunologic	IRMA, ELISA, immunoblot:inhibitor neutralization	Quantitative:IRMA, ELISA, electroimmunoassay (Laurell)
Inheritance	X-linked recessive	Autosomal
Clinical disorder due to deficiency	Hemophila A	von Willebrand's disease

Source: From Marder, VJ, et al: Standard nomenclature for factor VIII and von Willebrand factor: A recommendation by the International Committee on Thrombosis and Hemostasis. Thromb Haemost 54(4):871, 1985 with permission.
*In plasma, the two proteins are present as a bimolecular complex called the factor VIII–von Willebrand factor complex.

vious family history of bleeding. This suggests that a mutation may be evident, or there could be several generations of "silent carriers" of the sex-linked recessive trait.[30,31] Patients with FVIII:C levels of less than 1% (0.01 U/mL) have severe hemorrhagic disease that requires constant transfusion therapy. These patients are classified as severe hemophiliacs. Patients with levels greater than 5% (0.05 U/mL) are considered mild hemophiliacs and have a less severe hemorrhagic disease. The moderately severe hemophiliac has levels that fall between the two ranges. Hemarthrosis is a primary symptom involving knees, elbows, ankles, shoul-

TABLE 28–5   **Proposed Abbreviations for Factor VIII and von Willebrand Factor***

Attribute	ABBREVIATION	
	Proposed	Outmoded
Factor VIII		
Protein	VIII	VIII:C
Antigen	VIII:Ag	VIIIC:Ag
Function	VIII:C	—
von Willebrand factor		
Protein	vWF	VIIIR:Ag, VIII/vWF, AHF-like protein
Antigen	vWF:Ag	VIIIR:Ag, AHF-like antigens
Function	—	VIIIR:RCo, VIIIR:vWF†

Source: From Marder, VJ, et al: Standard nomenclature for factor VIII and von Willebrand factor: A recommendation by the International Committee on Thrombosis and Haemostasis. Thromb Haemost 54(4):871, 1985, with permission.
*The two proteins form a bimolecular complex that can be abbreviated as VIII/vWF.
†These abbreviations have been used to indicate the ristocetin cofactor activity of von Willebrand factor. Because neither this test nor any other in vitro test completely reflects vWF activity, no abbreviation is recommended as representative of its function.

ders, hips, and wrists. Other symptoms include hematuria, intracranial bleeding, hematomas, and unexplained spontaneous hemorrhage.

Approximately 10% to 15% of patients with hemophilia A develop antibodies or inhibitors to FVIII:C.[32] The inhibitors are usually temperature-dependent and are immunoglobulin (IgG) in nature. These inhibitors are capable of neutralizing FVIII:C at 37°C.[33] Administration of antihemophilic factor (AHF) may lead to a rise in antibody titers in patients who have developed antibodies to AHF.[33]

Many forms of treatment are available for hemophilia A. Concentrates of human plasma such as AHF are widely used. Many hemophiliacs are treated with highly purified, heat-treated lyophilized preparations of FVIII concentrate. Although cryoprecipitate is a rich source of FVIII, it is not the product of choice because of the high incidence of parenterally transmitted hepatitis C. New technologies that produce synthetic recombinant deoxyribonucleic acid (DNA) FVIII significantly lower the incidence of viral transmission. Patients who have developed antibodies to human FVIII concentrates often respond to treatment with porcine FVIII. Factor IX concentrates of prothrombin complex have been used in severe cases. A level of 30% of normal activity is the ideal therapeutic level for maintaining hemostasis.

The laboratory findings for patients with hemophilia A are a prolongation of the APTT, normal PT, and a normal bleeding time. Mixing studies with normal or adsorbed plasma correct the prolongation of the APTT. Aged serum does not correct the prolongation of the APTT. The deficiency is further characterized by low to absent levels of FVIII:C, normal levels of vWF:Ag (Fig. 28–1), and normal platelet function assays. The presence of an inhibitor can be established when mixing studies with normal plasma do not correct the prolonged aPTT. The level of activity is measured using a modified one-stage factor assay using the aPTT test and quantitating the inhibitor in Bethesda units.[34] One Bethesda unit of inhibitor corresponds to 50% residual FVIII:C activity after incubation with normal plasma for 2 hours.

TABLE 28–6 **Comparison of Hemophilia A and Classic von Willebrand's Disease**

	Hemophilia A	von Willebrand's Disease
Deficiency	VIII:C, VIII:AHF	VIII:vWF
Inheritance	Recessive, X-linked	Dominant, autosomal
Clinical bleeding	Hemarthrosis, muscle, soft tissue, visceral	Gums, gastrointestinal tract, mucous membranes
Bleeding disorder	Moderate to severe (60% to severe)	Mild to moderate
Laboratory tests		
Bleeding time	N	A
Clot retraction	N	N
Glass bead retraction	N	A
Platelet count	N	N
Ristocetin aggregation	N	A
PT	N	N
APTT	A	A
VIII	A	A
vWF:Ag	N	A

Abbreviations: N = normal; A = abnormal.

von Willebrand's Disease

In 1926, a 5-year-old girl from the Åland Islands off the coast of Finland was evaluated by Dr. Erich von Willebrand for a severe bleeding disorder. After thoroughly investigating the family members and patient, Dr. von Willebrand concluded that this was a previously undescribed bleeding disorder. von Willebrand's disease (vWD) differs from classical hemophilia A in three cardinal manifestations: autosomal inheritance rather than sex-linked; consistently prolonged bleeding times; and mucocutaneous bleeding rather than hemarthroses and deep muscle hemorrhage. It was not until the 1970s that von Willebrand factor (vWF) and factor VIII (FVIII:C) were found to be different proteins produced by different cells under different genetic control.[35]

The vWF is composed of a series of high-molecular-weight multimers with M_r ranging from 600,000 to 20 million daltons. It circulates in the plasma as a heterogenous mixture, produced by megakaryocytes and endothelial cells. vWF is stored and secreted from granules called Weibel-Palade bodies in endothelial cells, and α granules in platelets.[36] It binds to the subendothelium because of interaction with collagen.[37] After injury, vWF interacts with the glycoprotein Ib (GPIb) receptor on platelets resulting in their activation and adhesion to the subendothelium. This action can be initiated in vitro using platelet-rich plasma and the antibiotic ristocetin, or the snake venom extract botrocetin. Ristocetin, an antibiotic similar in structure to vancomycin, was removed from clinical use when it was discovered that it caused thrombocytopenia. Shortly thereafter, ristocetin was shown to aggregate normal platelets but to cause little or no aggregation in patients with vWD.[38] Normal or hemophiliac plasma can correct this defect because of the presence of vWF. This platelet aggregation assay may not be sensitive to mild reductions of vWf and is not quantitative. A quantitative assay, using formalin-fixed normal washed platelets and serial dilutions of normal plasma and patient plasma, allows for a more sensitive measurement. This is known as the ristocetin cofactor activity

(vWFR:Co) assay. In this method, the fixed platelets are not metabolically active and the response to ristocetin is termed *ristocetin-induced platelet agglutination*. When metabolically active platelet-rich plasma is exposed to ristocetin, the response is termed *aggregation*, because once vWF binds to its receptor, it will induce glycoprotein IIb/IIIa (GPIIb/IIIa) receptor-dependent aggregation (ristocetin-induced platelet aggregation)[39] (Fig. 28–2).

As stated previously, vWF circulates as a complex with FVIII:C. Patients with vWD, who may have reduced or absent levels of vWF may also have reduced levels of FVIII:C. However, levels of FVIII:C are usually slightly greater than the level of vWF:Ag, presumably because there is a normal gene present for FVIII:C and the potential binding sites are saturated when levels of vWF:Ag are reduced.[40] The effects of the ABO blood grouping have a significant effect on the amount of vWF:Ag produced. Individuals who are type A, B, and AB have much greater mean vWF:Ag plasma concentrations than blood type O individuals.[41]

Patients with vWD present with mucocutaneous bleeding as well as frequent instances of epistaxis, ecchymosis, easy bruisability, gastrointestinal bleeding, menorrhagia, and hemorrhage following surgery. This is because of the inability of platelets to adhere to the subendothelial surface following injury to the blood vessel.[42,43] vWF is an acute-phase reactant that increases during stress or pregnancy, or after surgery. This makes diagnoses or evaluation difficult in patients suspected of having vWD. Therefore, it may be necessary to study these patients on multiple occasions to rule out vWD as the cause of mild bleeding symptoms.[44,45]

Because of the variant forms of vWD that have been described, the clinical presentation may vary. Since vWF is the carrier protein for factor VIII:C, it is not unusual for patients with vWD to have reduced concentrations. Patients who have severe forms of vWD generally present with normal PT, prolongation of the APTT that corrects with the addition of normal plasma, normal platelet counts, and abnormal bleeding time

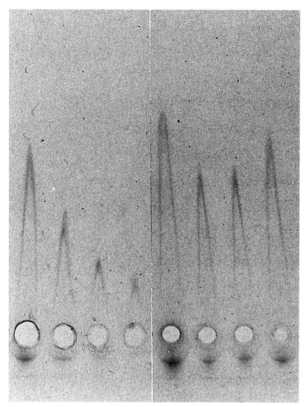

FIGURE 28–1 Quantitative immunoelectrophoresis of vWF:Ag. Laurell rockets in agarose gel. The first four peaks are the standard curve dilutions, followed by various vWF:Ag levels. Peak height is proportion to concentration.

test. The bleeding time (BT) is used to assess the function of platelets in hemostasis. Although the bleeding time is not a good screening test because of problems of standardization and interpretation, it is virtually always prolonged in patients with vWD. In milder forms of vWD, the bleeding time may be normal.[46] The most commonly used bleeding time test is known as the Ivy bleeding time. The laboratory assessment should include FVIII:C, vWF:Ag, vWFR:Co, platelet aggregation studies, and vWF multimeric analysis. Multimeric analysis will further confirm the specific variant form. Identification is essential for proper treatment. The von Willebrand variants include type I, IIa, IIb, III, and pseudo-platelet type (Table 28–7).

Type I is a partial quantitative deficiency and the most common type. Patients have a reduced to normal vWF; FVIII:C can be normal; and there are usually decreased levels of vWF:Ag and vWFR:Co. With type I there is a normal distribution of multimers. Type IIa is a qualitative defect of vWF. The absence of high-molecular-weight multimers decreases the platelet-dependent functions. The vWFR:Co is lower than the vWF:Ag. Type IIb is also a qualitative defect of vWF; the plasma shows a lack of large multimers, whereas the platelet vWF:Ag multimers are normal. A very important distinguishing feature is that patients have enhanced aggregation studies using low concentrations of ristocetin; this is the result of a plasma effect, not an intrinsic abnormality of the platelets (see Fig. 28–2). Because of this increased response, and the fact that some patients may have thrombocytopenia, treatment with desmopressin (DDAVP) is not indicated. Type III is a complete quantitative deficiency of vWF. vWF:Ag, vWFR:Co, and multimers are virtually undetectable, whereas FVIII:C is usually 2% to 5% of normal.

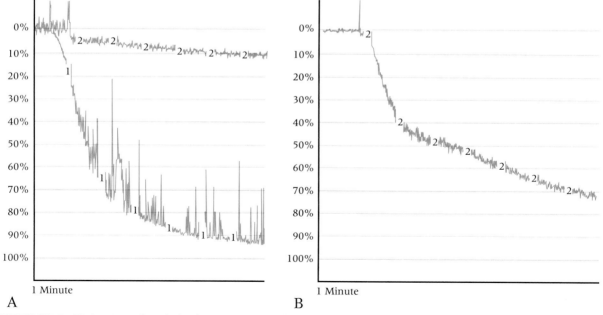

FIGURE 28–2 Ristocetin-induced platelet aggregation. (*A*) (*1*) Normal response to ristocetin 1.2 U/mL. (*2*) Normal response to ristocetin 0.6 U/mL (*B*) Abnormal response to ristocetin 0.6 U/mL characteristic of type IIb von Willebrand's.

TABLE 28–7 **Laboratory Diagnosis of Classic von Willebrand's Disease (Type IA) and Variants***

| | AUTOSOMAL DOMINANT | | | | AUTOSOMAL RECESSIVE | |
	Type IA	Type IIA	Type IIB	Platelet-type	Type IIC	Type III
Bleeding time	Increased or normal	Increased	Increased	Increased	Increased	Increased
Platelet count	Normal	Normal	Normal or decreased	Low normal or decreased	Normal	Normal
VIII:C	Normal or decreased	Normal or decreased	Normal or decreased	Normal or decreased	Normal	Markedly decreased
vWF:Ag	Decreased	Decreased or normal	Decreased or normal	Normal or decreased	Decreased or normal	Markedly decreased
Ristocetin cofactor	Decreased	Markedly decreased	Decreased or normal	Decreased or normal	Decreased	Markedly decreased
Crossed immunoelectrophoresis of plasma vWF	Normal	Abnormal	Abnormal	Abnormal	Abnormal	Variable
Multimeric structure of vWF						
Plasma	Normal	Absence of largest and intermediate multimers	Absence of largest multimers	Absence of largest multimers	Absence of largest multimers and abnormal band structure	Variable
Platelets	Normal	Absence of largest and intermediate multimers	Normal	Normal	Absence of largest multimers and abnormal band structure	Variable
Ristocetin-induced platelet aggregation in patient PRP	Decreased or normal	Markedly decreased	Increased	Increased	Decreased	Markedly decreased
Ristocetin-induced binding of vWF to platelets						
Patient plasma + normal platelets		Decreased	Increased	Normal or decreased		
Normal plasma + patient platelets		Normal	Normal	Increased		
vWF-induced aggregation of unstimulated patient platelets in PRP			Absent	Present		

Source: From Miller, JL: Blood coagulation and fibrinolysis. In Henry, JB (ed): Clinical Diagnosis and Management, 17 ed. WB Saunders, 1984, p 777, with permission.
Abbreviations: VIII:C = VIII coagulant activity; vWF:Ag = von Willebrand factor antigen; PRP = platelet-rich plasma.

Concentrates of FVIII, cryoprecipitates, and vWF have been used to treat vWD. Commercial FVIII concentrates are not useful because they lack the high-molecular-weight multimers of vWF (Fig. 28–3). Desmopressin (DDAVP) is a synthetic vasopressin used to treat patients with diabetes insipidus. This medication causes both the vWF and FVIII:C to rise. Patients with type I vWD can be treated with DDAVP before dental work or surgery and after bleeding episodes, thereby avoiding exposure to blood products. Type III vWD does not respond to DDAVP, and thrombocytopenia may occur in type IIb. The use of DDAVP as a treatment for type IIb can cause the release of abnormal vWF molecules. This abnormal molecule binds to normal platelets and thus causes accelerated clearance of normal platelets, resulting in thrombocytopenia.

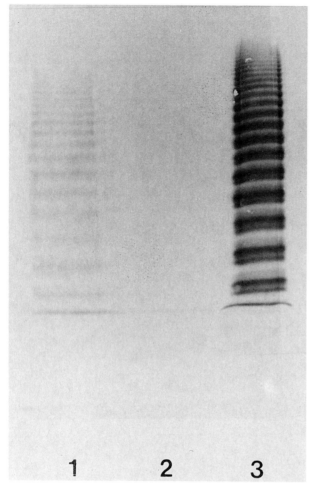

FIGURE 28–3 vWF:Ag multimers. Samples of (1) normal plasma, (2) von Willebrand plasma, and (3) cryoprecipitate underwent electrophoresis in SDS-agarose gel. A Western blotting technique was performed. The gel on nitrocellulose paper was incubated first with a rabbit antihuman vWF:Ag antibody and then with goat antirabbit IgG; then it was stained.

Factor IX (Christmas Factor)

Factor IX (FIX), a single-chain glycoprotein, is synthesized in the liver, and is vitamin K–dependent. It has a M_r of approximately 60,000 daltons. In the coagulation sequence, FIX participates in the intrinsic pathway, where it is activated by factor XIa in the presence of calcium ions to become a serine protease, factor IXa_β.[47] A second mechanism of activation, which bypasses contact activation, occurs via tissue factor and factor VIIa.[48] Additionally, FIX can be activated by a protease from Russell's viper venom,[49,50] which leads to the formation of factor IXa_α. This activated factor, in the presence of FVIIIa, calcium ions, and phospholipid, activates factor X.[51] Although FIXa alone is capable of slowly activating factor X in the presence of phospholipid and calcium ions, neither FVIII alone nor FVIII plus thrombin activates factor X in the absence of FIXa.[52]

Factor IX deficiency, also known as hemophilia B, is a sex-linked recessive bleeding disorder. Females with the deficiency are quite rare, but carrier states and spontaneous mutations do occur. Although the clinical symptoms are quite similar, blood from a patient with hemophilia A does not normalize the clotting time in blood from a patient with hemophilia B.[53,54] Hemophilia B became known as "Christmas disease" by Biggs and colleagues,[55] after their first patient with the disease. Since then FIX has also been known as Christmas factor, and plasma thromboplastin component (PTC).

The incidence of inherited FIX deficiency in the normal population is approximately 1 per 100,000.[56] The level of FIX activity determines the severity of the disorder, with the most severe deficiencies having less than 1% activity, and the milder deficiencies having 5% to 25% activity. In severe hemophilia B, there is total absence of FIX, demonstrated by the absence of clottable activity as well as antigen. Some hemophilia B patients synthesize a nonfunctional variant of the FIX molecule, whereas others do not have identifiable FIX antigen in the plasma and therefore have a true absence of synthesis of the molecule.[57] Measurement of FIX antigen and clottable activity levels greatly increases the accuracy of determining carrier status.[58] Acquired deficiency states can be seen in patients with liver disease or vitamin K deficiency and in patients on oral anticoagulant therapy.

Treatment of patients with severe to moderate FIX deficiency consists of regular infusions of fresh-frozen plasma, prothrombin-complex concentrates which contain factors II, VII, IX, and X or FIX concentrates. Mild deficiencies usually receive treatment in association with minor as well as major surgery. The most serious complication in patients with hemophilia B is the formation of antibodies to FIX. These are extremely difficult to handle, especially in life-threatening situations, and occur in approximately 10% of patients with this deficiency.[59,60]

The laboratory findings in FIX deficiency include normal values for PT, thrombin clotting time, and bleeding time. There is prolongation of the APTT, which corrects with the addition of normal plasma. Factor IX is present in serum, but not adsorbed plasma. One-stage factor assay of FIX activity will produce decreased to absent levels.

Factor X (Stuart-Prower Factor)

Factor X is a vitamin K–dependent glycoprotein with a M_r of 58,800 daltons. It is composed of a light chain and a heavy chain held together by a single disulfide bond.[61,62] The heavy chain contains the catalytic domain of the protein.[63] It is synthesized in the liver and released into the plasma as a precursor to a serine protease. The conversion of factor X to its proteolytic form, factor Xa, involves the cleavage of a peptide bond in the heavy chain. This reaction, in the intrinsic system, is catalyzed by factor IXa in the presence of factor VIIIa, calcium ions, and phospholipid. This same bond is cleaved by factor VIIa in the presence of tissue factor in the extrinsic system.[64]

Inherited factor X deficiency is extremely rare. Its

transmission is autosomal-recessive with an occurrence of less than 1 per 500,000; however, the heterozygous state can occur in approximately 1 per 500.

Deficiency of factor X may occur at any age, with the most severe hemorrhagic symptoms occurring in the very young. Bleeding sites vary according to the severity of the deficiency. Clinical symptoms range from easy bruising, epistaxis, gastrointestinal bleeding, or menorrhagia in mildly affected patients to hemarthrosis, central nervous system hemorrhage, and severe postoperative hemorrhage in the most severely affected patients.

Usually, the diagnosis of inherited factor X deficiency can be made by an appropriate family history and laboratory data. However, differentiating between inherited and acquired deficiencies should include the consideration of liver disease and vitamin K deficiency. Acquired factor X deficiencies usually coincide with other vitamin K–dependent factor disorders. Factor X deficiencies have been reported in patients with amyloidosis.[65]

Variant forms of factor X deficiency exist because of amino acid substitutions or deletions. As a result of these genetic changes, the function of the molecule is altered. This manifests itself in-vitro as variable results with standard coagulation studies (Table 28–8).[66]

The laboratory results seen in this deficiency include a prolonged PT and APTT, which corrects upon the addition of normal plasma or aged serum. Adsorbed plasma does not correct the prolongation of the PT or aPTT. Thrombin times and bleeding times are normal. The "Stypven" time or Russell's viper venom time test will be prolonged because this assay is dependent on factors II, V, and X in the presence of phospholipid. Factor activity, typically using PT methodology, will be decreased or absent (see Table 28–8). It is interesting to note, however, that factor assays based on either the PT or aPTT may be used to determine factor activity, but in variant forms of factor X deficiency discrepancies can occur in the values obtained, depending on which methodology is used.

Treatment consists of transfusions with fresh frozen plasma or prothrombin-complex concentrates. However, the need for such measures should be guided by the severity of the hemorrhagic episode. Levels of 10% are considered adequate for hemostasis. Unless the deficiency is acquired by poor diet or oral anticoagulant therapy, the disorder does not usually respond to vitamin K therapy.

TABLE 28–8 Laboratory Findings for Factor X Deficiency

Test	Results	Normal Values
PT	>30.0 s	10.3–14.0 s
APTT	>70.0 s	23.0–34.0 s
Factor X assay	<1.0%	100%
Russell's viper venom	55 s	<25.0 s
Other factor activity	100%	100%

Factor XI (Plasma Thromboplastin Antecedent)

Factor XI is a plasma glycoprotein with an M_r of 143,000 daltons and participates in the intrinsic coagulation pathway.[67] It is one of the contact factor proteins involved in early coagulation. It is synthesized by the liver and secreted into the plasma as a zymogen to a serine protease that circulates as a complex with high-molecular-weight kininogen (HMWK).[68] Structurally, it is composed of two identical polypeptide chains linked by a single disulfide bond.[69,70] After contact with a negatively charged surface, factor XI is activated by factor XIIa. The resulting serine protease is composed of two light chains containing the active sites and two heavy chains bridged by disulfide bonds.[71,72] The heavy chains of factor XIa are necessary for binding to HMWK and its substrate, factor IX.[73]

Factor XI deficiency, also once known as Rosenthal syndrome or hemophilia C, is seen predominately in the Ashkenazi Jewish population. It is inherited as an autosomal recessive trait. The incidence in the general population is approximately 1 in 100,000.[74] The heterozygous frequency within the Ashkenazi Jewish population is nearly 1 in 8.[75]

Factor XI is the only factor of the contact system (which also consists of factor XII, HMWK, and prekallikrein), in which a deficiency may lead to a bleeding diathesis. However, plasma levels do not always predict the occurrence of postoperative or post-traumatic bleeding. Symptoms can be mild, ranging from bruising, epistaxis, menorrhagia, hematuria, prolonged or delayed postpartum bleeding, and bleeding following dental extractions, to severe hemorrhage requiring massive replacement therapy. Levels of factor XI may fluctuate with time, and bleeding episodes vary in response to a variety of surgical procedures.[76] There is, however, some degree of correlation between the severity of hemostatic challenge and severe bleeding.[77] Levels of less than 15% factor activity are considered severely deficient and result in postoperative bleeding.

Replacement therapy is not needed in patients with factor XI deficiency unless they are scheduled for surgery. Preoperative infusion of fresh or fresh-frozen plasma, or the supernatant plasma after the removal of cryoprecipitate, may be required to avoid severe hemorrhage. Increase in factor activity levels to 20% to 30% of normal is adequate for hemostasis.[78] Circulating alloantibodies (inhibitors) can arise in patients with severe factor XI deficiency after exposure to plasma products. Further plasma infusions will not control bleeding, but may respond to activated prothrombin-complex concentrates, such as those used to treat patients with factor VIII or IX inhibitors.[79]

The laboratory features associated with a factor XI deficiency include a normal PT, and a prolonged aPTT, which corrects with the addition of normal plasma, adsorbed plasma, and aged serum. The bleeding time and thrombin clotting time are both normal. Specific factor XI activity assay will produce decreased or absent levels. Freezing and thawing the plasma can cause activation of the contact system and significantly shorten the aPTT in factor XI–deficient patients.

Therefore, it is advisable to perform the factor activity assay on fresh plasma drawn in plastic syringes and placed into anticoagulated siliconized or nonwettable test tubes.[80] Normal factor XI levels are considered to be 0.70 to 1.30 U/mL. Heterozygous individuals have levels ranging between 0.20 and 0.70 U/mL, whereas patients homozygous for factor XI deficiency have levels of less than 0.15 U/mL. Because of the variability in factor activity in some individuals, repeat testing is warranted in questionable cases.

Chapter 26 discussed the "cascade" theory of blood coagulation, which included the intrinsic, extrinsic, and common pathways of hemostasis. Activation of the surface-mediated pathway (contact system) can be achieved with factor XII, prekallikrein (PK), factor XI, and HMWK. With the exception of factor XI, which is associated with hemorrhagic tendencies, the remaining proteins participate in the inflammatory response, complement activation, fibrinolysis, and kinin formation.[81]

Factor XII (Hageman Factor)

Factor XII (FXII) is a single-chain β-globulin with a M_r of 76,000 daltons.[82] It is one of the members of the contact factor system, is believed to be synthesized by the liver, and circulates as an inactive zymogen. Contact with negatively charged surfaces in vitro such as glass, celite, kaolin, or ellagic acid (solid-phase activation) causes autoactivation of factor XII and its conversion to a serine protease.[83] This process initiates the intrinsic pathway of coagulation. In vivo (fluid-phase) activation occurs by contact with contents of cell membranes and components of leukocytes. In this process FXII undergoes a conformational change exposing its active site, which then converts prekallikrein to kallikrein and activates FXI.[84] Factor XIIa is formed by the enzymatic cleavage by enzymes such as trypsin, plasmin, or kallikrein, forming a two-chain molecule comprised of a heavy chain and a light chain held by a disulfide bond.[85] The presence of small amounts of FXIIa leads to activation of its substrates: prekallikrein, FXI, and HMWK.

Deficiency of factor XII, known as Hageman trait, is inherited in an autosomal recessive fashion. This disorder is not associated with clinical bleeding or hemorrhage. There may, however, be an increased incidence of thrombotic diseases, such as myocardial infarction or thromboembolism. Patients are asymptomatic and pose no hemorrhagic surgical risk. The deficiency is usually coincidentally discovered during presurgical screening. Laboratory analysis indicates a normal PT and prolonged aPTT, which corrects on the addition of normal plasma, adsorbed plasma, or aged serum. Specific factor analysis yields decreased or absent levels of functional FXII, which is required for definitive diagnosis. Care should be exercised to prevent contact activation during specimen collection by drawing into plastic syringes and placing the blood into siliconized anticoagulated test tubes. Freezing and thawing should be avoided by testing the plasma when freshly drawn. Normal FXII activity levels fall in the range of 0.70 to 1.40 U/mL, with heterozygotes having 40% to 60% of normal activity.

Factor XIII (Fibrin-Stabilizing Factor)

In the final stages of the coagulation process, there is generation of thrombin; polymerization of fibrin; and activation of factor XIII (FXIII), which is responsible for the formation of a stable fibrin clot. FXIII is a proenzyme for plasma transglutaminase, and in the presence of fibrin, thrombin converts FXIII to an enzyme called factor XIIIa.[86,87] It is the only enzyme in the coagulation system that is not a serine protease. Factor XIIIa functions as a catalyst, forming bonds between various protein substrates such as fibrin monomers, α_2-plasmin inhibitor, fibronectin, and collagen.[88] The action of this cross-linking of various plasma and extracellular matrix proteins contributes to hemostasis, wound healing, and maintenance of pregnancy.

FXIII has an M_r of 320,000 daltons and circulates with fibrinogen. Extracellular or plasma FXIII has two subunits, α_2 and β_2 chains. The α_2 chains exist in various tissues and cells such as the placenta, platelets, macrophages, and prostate, and contains the active catalytic site for transglutaminase activity. The β subunit is synthesized in the liver and circulates as a free dimer or as a complex with the α subunit. It is postulated that the β subunit contributes to the stabilization of the α subunit; however, the function of the β subunit remains unknown.

Factor XIII deficiency is inherited as an autosomal recessive trait, with a high frequency of consanguinity in families with this disorder.[89] Clinically, the homozygous deficiency has moderate to severe hemorrhagic diatheses. This is characterized by the initial stoppage of bleeding followed by recurrence of bleeding 36 hours or more after the initial traumatic event. This results from the dissolution of the fibrin clot that initially formed and was not stabilized by FXIII. These soluble fibrin clots are highly susceptible to degradation by plasmin. This disorder can be diagnosed at birth because the most common clinical symptom is bleeding from the umbilical stump. Acquired partial deficiency has been reported with several diseases, including leukemias, disseminated intravascular coagulation, and severe liver disease. Treatment includes transfusion with fresh frozen plasma or cryoprecipitate.

All routine laboratory screening tests for hemostasis will indicate normal results; PT, APTT, fibrinogen, bleeding time, and platelet count. The screening test for FXIII deficiency is based on the solubility of a recalcified plasma clot in 5 M urea solution. If the plasma is deficient in FXIII, the clot will dissolve within 24 hours. This is a qualitative test only and does not reflect the level of FXIII present, although activity of approximately 1% of normal is sufficient to prevent both an abnormal test result and symptoms in vivo.[90]

Prekallikrein (Fletcher Factor)

Prekallikrein (PK), a single-chain protein with a M_r of approximately 100,000 daltons, is synthesized in the liver.[91] Prekallikrein is the substrate for factor XII to form kallikrein and factor XIa. Approximately 75% circulates bound to HMWK,[92] and 25% circulates as free PK.

There is no ethnic or racial predilection for this disorder. It has been reported to be inherited as both an autosomal dominant and recessive trait with no apparent associated clinical bleeding disorders.[93] Patients with this deficiency have experienced thrombotic events, and vascular permeability is also defective.[94]

A marked prolongation of the APTT is characteristic of this disorder. Mixtures of patient plasma with normal plasma, adsorbed plasma, or aged serum will correct the aPTT. Interval incubations of patient's plasma with kaolinlike activators shortens the APTT.

High-Molecular-Weight Kininogen (Fitzgerald Factor)

High-molecular-weight kininogen (HMWK) has a M_r of 200,000 daltons. The deficiency has been described as autosomal recessive, and like PK shows no predilection to race. HMWK is known as the *contact activation cofactor* and is required for contact activation.[95] Its binding to endothelial cells is necessary for the binding of factor XI and its activation to factor XIa as well as for the activation of factor IX to IXa by factor XIa.[96] This deficiency presents with a markedly prolonged aPTT that corrects with the addition of normal plasma, adsorbed plasma, or aged serum. Although there is no apparent associated clinical bleeding disorder, patients have been observed with deep vein thrombosis and pulmonary embolus.[97]

Since there is no bleeding associated with factor XII, prekallikrein, or high-molecular-weight kininogen deficiencies, replacement therapy is not needed. Patients who require major surgery have had no incidence of bleeding.

CIRCULATING ANTICOAGULANTS–INHIBITORS

Circulating anticoagulants are acquired inhibitors of the coagulation mechanism. These are endogenously produced and interfere with various in vitro coagulation tests. When detected, it is important to differentiate their specificity because some are clinically significant, whereas others are inconsequential. These defects are composed of immunoglobulins directed against either specific clotting factors or components of the assay system.

Specific Factor Inhibitors

The acquired inhibitors directly inhibit clotting factor activity and are characterized as antibodies. The antibodies occur secondary to transfusion, clotting factor replacement therapy, or both. They can also occur de novo in patients with no known coagulopathy. These patients are often elderly and may have benign monoclonal gammopathies.

Factor VIII:C inhibitors can develop in patients with hemophilia A as a result of transfusion. The inhibitor has also been found in patients with rheumatoid arthritis, systemic lupus erythematosus, drug reaction, and different forms of malignancy. The mortality rate is approximately 20%. Spontaneous remission has been reported in approximately 38% of cases.[98]

Factor VIII:C inhibitors are predominately IgG antibodies and do not interfere with the function of vWF. Additionally, the antibodies do not interfere with the bleeding time. The inhibitor should be suspected in patients with hemophilia when transfused factor VIII product has a short half-life or hemostasis is difficult to achieve. A normal PT and a prolongation of the aPTT with little to no correction when mixed with normal plasma is a laboratory finding. The inhibitor can be expressed by incubating normal plasma with the patient's plasma and measuring the residual factor VIII:C activity. A test specimen having 50% residual factor VIII:C activity of normal is considered to contain 1 Bethesda unit of inhibitor. Treatment of patients with specific inhibitors can include factor VIII concentrates, immunosuppressive therapy, porcine factor VIII, and plasmapheresis for patients with very high inhibitor levels.

Spontaneously acquired inhibitors to factor II, VII, and X are very rare. Factor II inhibitors are described in association with lupus anticoagulant. There have been several reports of factors XI and XII inhibitors. Several cases were reported as factor XI deficiency with acquired inhibitors post transfusion and other cases occurring in patients with SLE.[99,100] Acquired factor V inhibitor is also rare; it has occurred in only one reported case of factor V deficiency. The remaining cases occurred in elderly patients who previously had normal levels.[101] Patients who exhibit this inhibitor vary in clinical bleeding. The laboratory findings include prolongation of both the PT and the aPTT and the addition of normal plasma does not correct the prolongations.

Nonspecific Inhibitors—Lupus Anticoagulants

Nonspecific inhibitors, as their name implies, are not directed against specific clotting factors. These are usually not associated with a bleeding risk and are not temperature-dependent, as in the case of anti-VIII:C or anti-V.[102–104] However, these inhibitors have been associated with thrombosis, fetal wastage, and thrombocytopenia, with or without autoimmune disorder.

The lupus anticoagulant was first recognized in patients with systemic lupus erythematosus (SLE).[105] This designation is a misnomer, however, because these inhibitors often occur in patients without SLE. Therefore, it is more appropriate that they be termed *lupuslike anticoagulants* (LLA). They are usually polyclonal IgG or IgM, also IgA or in combination. They occur spontaneously, or associated with autoimmune diseases such as SLE, acquired immune deficiency syndrome (AIDS), infectious diseases (bacterial, viral, protozoal), antibiotic and other drug exposure, strokes, spontaneous abortions, and lymphoproliferative disorders.[98]

Patients possessing lupuslike anticoagulants present in the laboratory with a prolonged APTT and a normal PT. In some cases both the PT and APTT are prolonged. These results give the impression that the

TABLE 28–9 Confirmatory Test for Lupus Anticoagulants: Increased Phospholipid*

Test	Nature of Phospholipid	Other Features	Sensitivity	Heparin	Oral Anticoagulant	Factor Deficiency	Specific Inhibitors	Comments
Platelet neutralization procedure (PNP)	Outdated washed platelets freeze-thawed	Use with sensitive APTT system	Sensitive in most cases with APTT 12s above upper limit of normal	False positive	False positive	—	Weak factor V inhibitor may be positive	Stored aliquots of platelets Stable-3 mo @ –20 C
High phospholipid APTT	Cephalin 1:200 1:50, 1:25 4-8× normal concentration	Kaolin activator	—	—	—	—	—	In original study, time-dependent pattern noted
Rabbit brain neutralization (RBNP)	Platelet high conc (use 4× more lipid)	Kaolin, tilt tube	Original study 30/31 patients had + test only 18/30 had + TTI	False positive	No effect	No effect	Slight shortening with factor VIII & XI inhibitors	—
Ptd-liposome APTT	PtdSer vehicle final conc (24 × 10 moles/L)	Kaolin Manchester APTT reagent	—	False positive	No effect	No effect	No effect with factor VIII & IX inhibitor	Other lipids (phosphatidylserine, no effect)
Inside-out membrane absorption test	Washed fresh human RBC-lysed with phosphate buffer	Use APTT mixture	—	No effect, ECTEOLA is used to absorb heparin	—	No effect	No effect with factor VIII inhibitor	—

Source: From Triplet, DA and Brandt, JT: Confirmatory test for lupus anticoagulant. Hematol Pathol 2(33):121, 1988, with permission.

*The confirmatory test for lupus anticoagulants may be divided into two categories. First is the use of test systems that seek to accentuate the effect of the anticoagulant by decreasing the amount of phospholipid in the test. Thus, the available phospholipid surfaces necessary for the prothrombinase complex are limited and the presence of a low titer antiphospholipid antibody will prolong the coagulation time. The TTI (tissue thromboplastin inhibitor) and the dRVVT (dilute Russell's viper venom time) are examples of this system. The second group of tests rely on increased amounts of phospholipid to either neutralize or bypass the phospholipid antibodies and shorten the prolonged coagulation time (PNP).

TABLE 28–10 Confirmatory Tests for Lupus Anticoagulants: Decreased Phospholipid

Test	Nature of Phospholipid	Other Features	Sensitivity	Heparin	Oral Anticoagulant	Factor Deficiency	Specific Inhibitors	Comment
Tissue thromboplastin inhibition (TTI)	Simplastin diluted with saline 1:50 & 1:500	—	Sensitive but not specific; positive in 10% normal subject	False positive 0.2–0.8 U/ml of heparin	False positive	False positive with factor VII, X, V, VIII, IX deficiency	False positive with factors VIII, IX, or V inhibitors	May be negative with IgM drug-induced LA
Dilute Russell viper venom test (RVVT)	Thrombofax 1.8 TBS Correction 0.1 ml Ionophore platelets	RVV diluted 1:200 TBS	Sensitive when compared with APTT & TTI	False positive	False positive corrected by mixing studies	False positive with factor V & X deficiency	False positive with factor V inhibitor	Correction studies may use ionophore* platelets or PNP
KCT	No added phospholipid; KCT very sensitive to residual platelets	May use mixture of normal & patient plasma	Presence of platelets will significantly shorten KCT in presence of LA	—	—	—	—	Use of filtered plasma will increase sensitivity
Dilute phospholipid APTT (PL-aPTT)	Thrombofax diluted 1:5,1:10; 1:20; 1:40	Mixing patient & normal 1:1 & 0.5 silica	—	No effect if protamine added	No effect	No effect	Strong inhibitor (>10 Bethesda Units) may give false positive	

Source: From Triplett, DA and Brandt, JT: Confirmatory test for lupus anticoagulants. Hematol Pathol 2(3):121, 1988, with permission.
Abbreviation: KCT = Kaolin clotting time.

patient may have a bleeding tendency. It should be noted that some patients with the lupus inhibitor have had clinically significant bleeding. The bleeding can be attributed to a depression of prothrombin activity. In these cases the factor II activity has been found to be approximately 20% of normal resulting in severe and even fatal bleeding.[106,107] However, thrombosis is the major problem in patients with LLA. A mixing study with normal plasma shows no correction of the prolonged APTT. What is occurring in vitro is a direct reaction against ionic phospholipids, which are present in the reagents used for coagulation screening assays (PT and APTT). This will also affect any factor assays based on these methodologies; however, LLAs do not inactivate the clotting factors in vitro; they inhibit the formation of the prothrombinase complex (factors Xa, Va, calcium ions, factor II, and phospholipid surfaces) causing a prolongation of the clotting time.[108–110] There is also evidence that plasma immunoglobulins are affected by nonprocoagulant phospholipid cardiolipin. There is a high incidence of thrombotic disease in patients with elevated anticardiolipin antibody.[111] This was first noted with a high prevalence of falsely positive tests for syphilis (VDRL), the reagent component of which is the antigen cardiolipin. Patients who have LLA have been found to have elevated levels of anticardiolipin antibodies in their plasma.[112]

Testing for confirmation of the LLA should include the use of test systems that have high phospholipid content that neutralizes or bypasses the inhibitor. These tests include the platelet neutralization procedure (PNP) and the high phospholipid APTT. PNP phospholipid is derived from washed, buffered, frozen platelets. This increase in phospholipid will correct the abnormal APTT. Methodologies using altered phospholipid structures (hexagonal phospholipids) have

also been used as confirmatory techniques. False-positive tests occur in heparinized patients (Table 28–9). Prolonged APTT results in patients when clotting factor deficiencies are not corrected with the PNP. An additional method using a low concentration of phospholipid is known as the dilute Russell viper venom time (dRVVT) (Table 28–10). This venom, which is an extract from the venom of *Vipera russellii*, directly activates factor X. By diluting the venom, whereby there is enough activity to activate factor X, and providing a dilute, buffered phospholipid as the cofactor for prothrombinase production, the sensitivity to inhibitors directed at phospholipid is increased and a prolonged clotting time is achieved. One-stage factor assays will show artificially decreased factor activity caused by impaired reactivity of the phospholipid reagent used in the test system. The dRVVT is also affected by the presence of heparin[113] and Coumadin.

SUMMARY

A complete personal and family history is of utmost importance in beginning a workup for a hemostatic defect. This should also include a list of any prescription or over-the-counter medications.

Tables 27–9 and 27–10, in the section titled "Quantitative Platelet Disorders," Chapter 27, should be reviewed at this time. This section of Chapter 27 gives an interpretation of screening for various coagulation abnormalities. Table 28–11 provides more reinforced information on the clotting factor defects and their laboratory diagnosis.

A battery of screening tests for coagulation abnormalities should be performed, including:

TABLE 28–11	**Factor Deficiencies and Test Results**											
Factor	BT	PT	APTT	Adsorbed Plasma	Aged Serum	TT	Fibrinogen	Urea Solubility	Platelet Count	D-Dimer	FDP
I	N	A	A	C	NC	A	A	N	N	—	—
II	N	A	A	NC	NC	N	N	N	N	—	—
V	A	A	A	C	NC	N	N	N	N	—	—
VII	N	A	N	NC	C	N	N	N	N	—	—
VIII:C	N	N	A	C	NC	N	N	N	N	—	—
VIII:VWF	A	N	A	C	C	N	N	N	N	—	—
IX	N	N	A	NC	C	N	N	N	N	—	—
X	N	A	A	NC	C	N	N	N	N	—	—
XI	N	N	A	C	C	N	N	N	N	—	—
XII	N	N	A	C	C	N	N	N	N	—	—
XIII	N	N	N	—	—	N	N	A	N	—	—
Prekallikrein	N	N	A*	C	C	N	N	N	N	—	—
HMWK	N	N	A	C	C	N	N	N	N	—	—
Plasminogen	N	N	N	—	—	N	N	N	N	—	—
DIC	—	A	A	—	—	A	A	N	A	A	A
Antithrombin III	N	N	N	—	—	N	N	N	N	—	—

Source: From Pittiglio, DH, et al: Treating hemostatic disorders. A problem-oriented approach. In Pittiglio, DH: Hemostatis Overview. American Association of Blood Banks, Arlington, VA, 1984, p 31, with permission.

Abbreviations: N = Normal; C = Correction; NC = No correction; BT = Bleeding time; PT = Prothrombin time; APTT = Activated partial thromboplastin time; DD = D-dimer; FDP = fibrin degradation products.

*The APTT will shorten after prolonged activation of the contact system.

1. Complete blood count (CBC), platelet count, and differential smear to observe platelet morphology
2. Prothrombin time (PT)
3. Activated partial thromboplastin time (APTT)
4. Fibrinogen
5. Thrombin time
6. Bleeding time

When the platelet count and morphology are normal, the results of the PT and APTT should be evaluated as follows:

1. For an abnormal PT, a mixing study using pooled normal plasma should be performed. If the PT is corrected, perform factor assays for II, V, VII, and/or X. If the deficiency is the result of fibrinogen, this will have been detected in the primary screen.
2. For abnormal PTs that do not correct with a mixing study, inhibitors to any of these factors should be considered.
3. For a prolonged PT with a normal APTT, a factor VII deficiency should be considered. Assay for factor VII activity.
4. For an abnormal APTT, a mixing study using pooled normal plasma should be performed. If the APTT is corrected, deficiency could be caused by factors VIII:C, IX, XI, XII, prekallikrein, or high-molecular-weight kininogen.
5. For abnormal APTTs that do not correct with mixing study, inhibitors to any of these factors should be considered, as well as the presence of the lupus anticoagulant or the anticoagulant heparin.
6. For specimens that have both an abnormal APTT and abnormal PT that correct with mixing studies, deficiencies of factors I (fibrinogen), II, V, and X should be considered.

When testing for individual factor deficiencies, a factor assay specific for the suspected coagulation factor defects should be performed. Mixing studies using normal pooled plasma can help laboratory workers narrow their search for the specific factor in question. When inhibitors such as the lupus anticoagulant or one that is specific for a certain factor are suspected, mixing studies and incubations should be performed. All specific factor inhibitors should be quantitated for the level of the inhibitor present. This is imperative because it lends valuable information to the physicians in their treatment plan.

The thrombin time assesses thrombin-fibrinogen interaction and may be abnormal in patients who have hypofibrinogenemia or dysfibrinogenemia, and as a result of circulation inhibitors. In these cases, the PT and APTT both may be prolonged.

Inhibitors such as fibrin-degradation products (FDPs) occurring in patients with DIC and following administration of heparin usually prolong the thrombin time. The thrombin time is the most sensitive index of heparin presence and of DIC.

ACKNOWLEDGMENTS

The authors gratefully acknowledge the contributions of Judith Brody, MD.

CASE STUDY 1

A 12-year-old boy underwent tooth extraction in preparation for orthodontia. Persistent bleeding followed. History was remarkable for bruising and frequent epistaxis. The patient's mother also experienced easy bruising and menorrhagia.

Physical examination revealed several medium-sized ecchymotic lesions on the lower extremities. Laboratory findings were as follows (reference ranges in parentheses):

PT	12.0 s	(10–14 s)
APTT	39.5 s	(23–33 s)
BT	>15 min	(2–9 min)
Platelet ct.	300,000/μL	(150–450 × 10^9/L)
FVIII:C	30 U/L	(50–150 U/L)
vWf:Ag	45 U/L	(50–150 U/L)
vWfR:Co	41%	(50–150%)
RIPA*	Depressed response	
Multimers	Normal	

The history of bruising, epistaxis, and dental bleeding with a prolonged aPTT, BT, and reduced FVIII:C, vWF:Ag, vWfR:Co, and RIPA are indicative of classic von Willebrand disease (type 1).

Questions

1. What blood product can correct the RIPA value in this case?
2. What laboratory values reflect a type 1 von Willebrand disease?
3. What form of therapy would be indicated here?

CASE STUDY 2

A full-term male infant was born by normal vaginal delivery. Thirty hours post partum there was new onset of oozing of blood at the umbilical stump. Laboratory analysis included:

CBC and platelet count	Normal
PT	14.0 sec (10–14 s)
APTT	36 sec (22–37 s)
Fibrinogen	400 mg/dL (160–450 mg/dL)

Clinical presentation did not indicate a hemorrhagic tendency. Late onset of umbilical bleeding prompted the evaluation of factor XIII. Recalcified plasma clot exposed to 5 M urea dissolved within 4 hours. This is conclusive of factor XIII deficiency.

Questions

1. Is the 5 M urea dissolution test a qualitative or quantitative determination?
2. What treatment is indicated for this patient?

CASE STUDY 3

A 5-year-old boy presented in the emergency room with a massive hemarthrosis of the right knee after falling off a playground swing. Physical examination revealed a well-nourished child with no fractures or other ecchymoses. He was afebrile. Laboratory findings were as follows:

*Ristocetin-induced platelet aggregation

CBC and platelet count	Normal
PT	13 s (10–14 s)
APTT	>100 s (23–27 s)
Fibrinogen	325 mg/dL (160–450 mg/dL)
BT	6 min (2–9 min)

Further studies included:

aPTT 1:1 mix	32 sec (control = 30 s)
FVIII:C	<1 U/L activity (50–150 U/L)
vWf:Ag	90% (50–150%)

This patient received a diagnosis of classic hemophilia A.

Questions

1. Given a FVIII deficiency, what did the technologist use when performing this mixing study?
2. What treatment is indicated for this patient?
3. Which factors are present in adsorbed plasma? In serum?

CASE STUDY 4

A 40-year-old woman was scheduled for an elective surgical procedure. Preadmission testing revealed the following results:

CBC and platelet count	Normal
PT	18.0 s (10–14 s)
APTT	30.0 s (23–33 s)

After further examination, the patient stated that she had episodes of epistaxis and easy bruising. Additional laboratory testing included:

PT 1:1 mix	13.0 s	Control = 12.0 s
FVII	30 U/L	(50–150 U/L)

This patient has factor VII deficiency. Factor VII is not measured by the aPTT and is normal, whereas the PT is sensitive to deficiencies of the extrinsic system (factors I, II, V, VII, X) and is prolonged in these cases.

Questions

1. What fluid was used to perform the mixing study and subsequent PT correction?
2. What treatment is indicated here?
3. Why was the PT prolonged and the aPTT normal in this case?

CASE STUDY 5

A 29-year-old woman was seen by her obstetrician for prenatal care. She had three previous pregnancies, two resulting in spontaneous first-trimester miscarriage and the third in fetal demise at 28 weeks' gestation. Laboratory values were as follows:

CBC and platelet count	Normal
PT	11.5 s (10–14 s)
APTT	45.0 s (23–33 s)
Fibrinogen	375 mg/dL (160–450 mg/dL)

Further studies included:

APTT 1:1 mix	43.0 s (Control = 29.5 s)
dRVVT	33 s (<25 s)
PNP	32 s; NaCl 47 s

Anticardiolipin antibodies:

IgG	55 units	(0–14 units)
IgA	5 units	(0–15 units)
IgM	12 units	(0–5 units)

This patient has a lupuslike anticoagulant with anticardiolipin–antiphospholipid antibodies. These are known to cause recurrent spontaneous abortion, as well as thrombotic events such as stroke, deep vein thromboses, and pulmonary embolism.

Questions

1. What complex is inhibited by LA causing a prolongation of the clotting time?
2. Why did the PNP correct the aPTT in this patient?
3. What form of treatment is indicated here?

CASE STUDY 6

A 25-year-old man was admitted for hernia repair. Admission laboratory data were as follows:

CBC and platelet count	Normal
PT	12.5 s (10–14 s)
APTT	74.0 s (23–33 s)

APTT 1:1 mix showed full correction of prolongation

FVIII:C	97 U/L	(50–150 U/L)
F IX	104 U/L	(50–150 U/L)
F XI	110 U/L	(70–130 U/L)
F XII	96 U/L	(70–140 U/L)

Interval incubation of the patient's plasma with the APTT reagent containing micronized silica as the activator produced the following results:

5-min incub.	74.0 s
10-min incub.	57.0 s
15-min incub.	35.0 s

Assay for prekallikrein activity (Fletcher factor) = <5% (50–150%)

This patient was deficient for Fletcher factor. Contact system deficiencies (XII, HMWK, Prekallikrein) do not pose any hemorrhagic risk.

Questions

1. Why was the aPTT affected exclusive of the PT?
2. What treatment is indicated here?
3. What fluids are appropriate ingredients for mixing studies in this deficiency?

CASE STUDY 7

A 65-year-old woman with liver disease was admitted to the medical intensive care unit. Admission laboratory data were as follows:

PT	14.5 s (10–14 s)
APTT	36.0 s (23–33 s)
Fibrinogen	175 mg/dL (160–450 mg/dL)
Thrombin time	18 s (4–12 s)

Prolongation of the APTT and thrombin time could be caused by the presence of heparin. This should be ruled out before further testing is performed.

Reptilase time	29 s (18–22 sec)

PT and APTT 1:1 mix showed full correction of the prolongations.

Factors VIII:C, IX, XI, and XII were within normal limits.

This patient was not on heparin, as evidenced by the prolonged Reptilase time. The combination of a decreased fibrinogen clottable activity, prolonged thrombin time, and Reptilase time are indicative of a dysfibrinogenemia, especially in patients with liver disease. Slight prolongation of the PT may also be noted and will not be attributable to any extrinsic factor deficiency. Immunologic assay of fibrinogen usually results in higher values than the functional (clottable) assay.

Questions

1. Given the Reptilase time, why can it be said this patient is not on heparin therapy?
2. Differentiate between the TT and RT with regard to heparin.
3. What treatment is indicated here?

CASE STUDY 8

A 60-year-old woman was admitted to the emergency room with hemorrhage into the right arm and right breast. No previous history of bleeding or medication was indicated. Laboratory data upon admission were as follows:

PT	12.0 s	(10–14 s)
APTT	58.0 s	(23–33 s)
Fibrinogen	400 mg/dL	(160–450 mg/dL)
APTT 1:1 mix	40 s	control = 29 s
dRVVT	21 s	(<25 s)
PNP	58 s	NaCl = 59 s

This patient does not have a lupuslike anticoagulant, but still does not correct on mixing with normal plasma. Further studies must be performed. Incubation of the patient's plasma with normal plasma in various dilutions for 2 hours at 37°C indicates the presence of an inhibitor by showing prolongation of the aPTT over time. Also, factor analysis indicates decreased activity for a specific factor because of the presence of an inhibitor.

FVIII:C	10 U/L	(50–150 U/L)
F IX	90 U/L	(50–150 U/L)
F XI	95 U/L	(70–130 U/L)

Specific factor inhibitor analysis for factor VIII:C resulted in 8 Bethesda units of inhibitor activity (normal = <0.5 units). One Bethesda unit of inhibitor is equivalent to 50% residual factor activity of normal after incubation at 37°C for 2 hours. This patient developed a spontaneous inhibitor to factor VIII that resulted in the massive bleeding into her arm and breast.

Questions

1. What fluid was used to perform the 1:1 ratio mixing study?
2. What test result rules out a lupus anticoagulant?
3. What treament is indicated here?

CASE STUDY 9

A 37-year-old man was seen by his physician for a routine physical examination. A full blood workup was drawn and sent to a reference laboratory for analysis. Results were as follows:

CBC and platelet count	Normal
PT	12.0 s (10–14 s)
APTT	60.0 s (23–33 s)
Thrombin time	4.5 s (4–12 s)

The patient was asymptomatic for any bleeding. Testing was continued and produced the following results:

APTT 1:1 mix	32 s (control = 29 s)
FVIII:C	90 U/L (50–150 U/L)
F IX	77 U/L (50–150 U/L)
F XI	45 U/L (70–130 U/L)

This patient was found to have factor XI deficiency. The initial history revealed that he was of eastern European–Ashkenazi Jewish background. This factor deficiency is prevalent among this population. The patient's factor level was not depressed enough to produce symptoms, but could have posed a significant surgical risk. Heterozygous factor XI deficiency has a variable presentation and bleeding risk may not correlate with factor levels.

Questions

1. Why was the aPTT affected exclusive of the PT in this case?
2. What does the mixing study aPTT result indicate?
3. What treatment is indicated here?

CASE STUDY 10

A 16-year-old boy with a diagnosis of amyloidosis was admitted to the hospital with severe gastrointestinal bleeding. Admission laboratory data included:

CBC:	Anemia due to chronic blood loss	
Platelet count:	Normal	
PT	45 s	(10–14 s)
APTT	95 s	(23–33 s)
Fibrinogen	400 mg/dL	(160–450 mg/dL)
Thrombin time	5 s	(4–12 sec)
PT 1:1 mix	13 s	control = 12 s
APTT 1:1 mix	30 s	control = 29 s
Russell's viper venom time:	55 s (14–20 s)	
F II	75 U/L	(50–150 U/L)
F V	93 U/L	(50–150 U/L)
F IX	90 U/L	(50–150 U/L)
F X	5 U/L	(50–150 U/L)

This patient was determined to have factor X deficiency secondary to amyloidosis. Other vitamin K–dependent factors were normal, as was factor V, which ruled out nutritional deficit or liver involvement.

Questions

1. Why were both the PT and aPTT prolonged in this case?
2. What test results indicate a factor deficiency as opposed to a circulating anticoagulant?
3. If adsorbed plasma were used in the mixing study, what would you expect the result to be?

REFERENCES

1. Rock, G: Defects of plasma clotting factors. In Pittiglio, DH and Sacher, RA (eds): Clinical Hematology and Fundamentals of Hemostasis, ed 1. FA Davis, Philadelphia, 1987, p 365.
2. Hantgan, RR, Francis, CW, and Marder, VJ: Fibrinogen structure and function. In Coleman, RW, et al. (eds): Hemostasis and Thrombosis: Basic Principles and Clinical Practice, ed 3. JB Lippincott, Philadelphia, 1994, p 277.
3. Ibid, p 277.
4. Bommer, W, Kunzer, W, and Schroer, H: Kongenitale Afibrinogename, Teil I. Ann Paediatr 200:46, 1963.
5. Gralnick, HR and Connaghan, DG: In Williams, WJ et al. (eds): Hematology, ed 5, McGraw-Hill, New York, 1994, p 1441.
6. Girolami, A, et al: Rarer quantitative and qualitative abnormalities of coagulation. In Clinics in Hematology: Coagulation Disorders, Vol. 14, no. 2. WB Saunders, Philadelphia, 1985, p 385.
7. Henschen, A, Kehl, M, Southan, C, et al: Genetically abnormal fibrinogens—some current characterization strategies. In Haverkate, F, Henschen, A, Nieuwenhuizen, and W, Straub, PW (eds): Fibrinogen—Structure, Functional Aspects, Metabolism. Walter de Gruyter, Berlin, 1983, p 125.
8. McDonagh, J, Carrell, N, and Lee, MH: In Colman, RW, et al (eds): Hemostasis and Thrombosis: Basic Principles and Clinical Practice, ed 3. JB Lippincott, Philadelphia, 1994, p 321.
9. Reptilase is a registered trademark of Pentapharm Ltd.
10. Latallo, ZS and Teisseyre, E: Evaluation of Reptilase-R and thrombin clotting time in the presence of fibrinogen degradation products and heparin. Scand J Haematol 13(Suppl):261, 1971.
11. Donati, MB, Vermylen, J, and Verstraete, M: Fibrinogen degradation in vivo: Effect on the reptilase time and on the thrombin time. Scand J Haematol 13(Suppl):259, 1971.
12. Davie, EW, Fujikawa, K, and Kisiel, W: The coagulation cascade: Initiation, maintenance and regulation. Biochemistry 30:10363, 1991.
13. Shapiro, SS and McCord, IS: Prothrombin. In Spaet, TH (ed): Progress in Hemostasis and Thrombosis, vol. IV. New York, Grune & Stratton, 1978.
14. Chong, L-L, Chau, W-K, and Ho, C-H: A case of "super" warfarin poisoning. Scand J Haematol 36:314, 1986.
15. Owren, PA: The coagulation of blood: Investigation on a new clotting factor. Acta Med Scand (Suppl)194:1, 1947.
16. Owren, PA and Cooper, T: Parahemophilia. Arch Intern Med 95:194, 1955.
17. Colman, RW: Factor V. Prog Hemost Thromb 3:109, 1976.
18. Jandl, JH: Blood: Textbook of Hematology. Little Brown, Boston, 1987.
19. Chiu, HC, Schick, P, and Colman, RW: Biosynthesis of coagulation Factor V by megakaryocytes. J Clin Invest 75:339, 1985.
20. Nesheim, ME, Nichols, WL, Cole, TL, et al: Isolation and study of acquired inhibitor of human coagulation factor V. J Clin Invest 77:405, 1986.
21. Hall, CA, Rapaport, SI, Ames, SB, and De Groot, JA: A clinical and family study of hereditary proconvertin (factor VII) deficiency. Am J Med 37:172, 1964.
22. Dische, FE and Benfield, V: Congenital Factor VII deficiency: Haematological and genetic aspects. Acta Haematol 21:257, 1959.
23. Davie, EW, Fujikawa, K, and Kisiel, W: The coagulation cascade: Initiation, maintenance and regulation. Biochemistry 30:10363, 1991.
24. Tuddenham, EGD, Lane, RS, Rotblat, F, et al: Response to infusion of proelectrolyte fractionated human factor VIII concentrates in human haemophilia A and von Willebrand disease. Br J Haematol 52:259, 1982.
25. Hoyer, LW and Rick, ME: Implications of immunological methods for measuring antihemophilic factor (factor VIII). Ann NY Acad Sci 240:97, 1975.
26. Miale, JB: Hemostasis and blood coagulation: Hemophilia (factor VIII deficiency). In Miale, JB (ed): Laboratory Medicine: Hematology, ed 6. CV Mosby, St. Louis, 1982, p 823.
27. Ibid.
28. McGlasson, DL: Defects of plasma clotting factors. In Harmening, DM (ed): Clinical Hematology and Fundamentals of Hemostasis, ed 2, FA Davis, Philadelphia, 1992, p 463.
29. Ratnoff, OD and Bennett, B: The genetics of hereditary disorders of blood coagulation. Science 179:1291, 1973.
30. McGlasson, DL: Defects of plasma clotting factors. In Harmening, DM (ed): Clinical Hematology and Fundamentals of Hemostasis, ed 2. FA Davis, Philadelphia, 1992, p 468.
31. Miller, JL: Blood coagulation and fibrinolysis. In Henry JB (ed): Clinical Diagnosis and Management, ed 17. WB Saunders, Philadelphia, 1984, p 765.
32. Weiss, AE: Circulating inhibitors in hemophilia A and B: Epidemiology and methods of detection. In Brinkhous, KM and Henker, HC (eds): Handbook of Hemophilia. Excerpta Medica, Amsterdam, 1975, p 29.
33. Shapiro, SS: Hemorrhagic disorders associated with circulating inhibitors. In Ratnoff, OD and Forbes, CD (eds): Disorders of Hemostasis. Grune & Stratton, Orlando, FL, 1984, p 271.
34. Kasper, CK, et al: A more uniform measurement of factor VIII inhibitors. Thromb Diath Haemorrh 34:869, 1975.
35. Bennett, B, Forman, WB, and Ratnoff, OD: Studies on the nature of antihemophilic factor (factor VIII): Further evidence relating the AHF-like antigens in normal and hemophiliac plasma. J Clin Invest 52:2191, 1973.
36. Wagner, EE, Olmstead, JB, and Marder, VJ: Immunolocalization of von Willebrand protein in Weibel-Palade bodies of human endothelial cells. J Cell Biol 95:355, 1982.
37. Enbal, A and Loscalzo, J: Glycocalicin binding to vWf adsorbed onto collagen-coated or polystyrene surfaces. Thromb Res 56:347, 1989.
38. Howard, NA and Firkin, BG: Ristocetin—a new tool in the investigation of platelet. Thromb Diath Haemorrh 26:362, 1971.
39. Montgomery, RR and Coller, BS: Von Willebrand disease. In Colman, RW, et al (eds): Hemostasis and Thrombosis: Basic Principles and Clinical Practice, ed 3. JB Lippincott, Philadelphia, 1994, p 141.
40. Montgomery, RR and Coller, BS: Von Willebrand disease. In Colman, RW, et al (eds): Hemostasis and Thrombosis: Basic Principles and Clinical Practice, ed 3. JB Lippincott, Philadelphia, 1994, p 146.
41. Montgomery, RR and Coller, BS: Von Willebrand disease. In Colman, RW, et al (eds): Hemostasis and Thrombosis: Basic Principles and Clinical Practice, ed 3. JB Lippincott, Philadelphia, 1994, p 144.
42. Coller, BS: Von Willebrand's disease. In Ratnoff, OD and Farbes, CD (eds): Disorders of Hemostasis. Grune & Stratton, Orlando, FL 1984, p 241.
43. Holmberg, L and Nelson, IM: Von Willebrand's disease. In Clinics in Hematology: Coagulation Disorders, vol 14, no 2. WB Saunders, Philadelphia, 1985, p 461.
44. Lombardi, R, Mannucci, PM, Seghatchian, MJ, et al: Alterations of factor VIII vWf in clinical conditions associated with an increase in its plasma concentration. Br J Haematol 49:61, 1981.
45. Scholtes, MC, Gerretsen, G, and Haak, HL: The factor

VIII ratio in normal and pathological pregnancies. Eur J Obstet Gynecol Reprod Biol 16:89, 1983.

46. Nilsson, IL, Magnusson, S, and Borchgrevink, C: The Duke and Ivy methods for determination of bleeding time. Thromb Diath Haemorrh 10:223, 1963.

47. Hedner, U and Davie, EW: Factor IX. In Colman, RW, et al (eds): Hemostasis and Thrombosis—Basic Principles and Clinical Practice, ed 2. JB Lippincott, Philadelphia, 1987, p 41.

48. Østerud, B and Rapaport, SI: Activation of factor IX by the reaction product of tissue factor and factor VII: Additional pathway for initiating blood coagulation. Proc Nat Acad Sci USA 74:5260, 1977.

49. DiScipio, RG, Kurachi, K, and Davie, EW: Activation of human factor IX (Christmas factor). J Clin Invest 61:1528, 1978.

50. Lindquist, PA, Fujikawa, K, and Davie, EW: Activation of bovine factor IX (Christmas factor) by factor XIa (activated plasma thromboplastin antecedent) and a protease from Russell's viper venom. J Biol Chem 253:1902, 1978.

51. Hedner, U and Davie, EW: Factor IX. In Colman RW, et al (eds): Hemostasis and Thrombosis—Basic Principles and Clinical Practice, ed 2. JB Lippincott, Philadelphia, 1987, p 43.

52. Hultin, M and Nemerson, Y: Activation of factor X by factors IXa and VIII. A specific assay for factor IXa in the presence of thrombin-activated factor VIII. Blood 52:928, 1978.

53. Biggs, R and Macfarlane, RG: The reaction of haemophilic plasma to thromboplastin. J Clin Pathol 4:445, 1951.

54. Aggeler, PM, White, SG, Glendening, MB, et al: Plasma thromboplastin component (PTC) deficiency: A new disease resembling hemophilia. Proc Soc Exp Biol Med 79:692, 1952.

55. Biggs, R, Douglas, AS, Macfarlane, RG, et al: Christmas disease: A condition previously mistaken for haemophilia. Br Med J 2:1378, 1952.

56. Biggs, R: The inheritance of defects in blood coagulation. In Biggs, R and Rizza, CR (eds): Human Blood Coagulation, Haemostasis and Thrombosis, ed 3. Blackwell Scientific, Oxford, 1984, p 92.

57. Meyer, D, Bidwell, E, and Larrieu, MJ: Cross-reacting material in genetic variants of hemophilia B. J Clin Pathol 25:443, 1972.

58. Orstavik, KH, Veltkamp, JJ, Bertina, RM, et al: Detection of carriers of hemophilia B. Br J Haematol 42:293, 1979.

59. Nilsson, IM, Hedner, U, and Ahlberg, A: Hemophilia prophylaxis in Sweden. Acta Paediatr Scand 65:129, 1976.

60. Brinkhous, KM, Roberts, HR, and Weiss, AE: Prevalence of inhibitors in hemophilias A and B. Thromb Diath Haemorrh 51(Suppl):315, 1972.

61. DiScipio, RG, Hermodson, MA, Yates, SG, and Davie, EW: A comparison of human prothrombin, Factor IX (Christmas factor), Factor X (Stuart factor), and protein S. Biochemistry 16:698, 1977.

62. DiScipio, RG, Hermodson, MA, and Davie, EW: Activation of human Factor X (Stuart factor) by a protease from Russell's viper venom. Biochemistry 16:5253, 1977.

63. Titani, K, Fujikawa, K, Enfield, DL, et al: Bovine Factor X_1 (Stuart factor): Amino acid sequence of heavy chain. Proc Nat Acad Sci USA 72:3082, 1975.

64. Ichinose, A and Davie, EW: The blood coagulation factors: Their cDNAs, genes, and expression. In Colman, RW, et al. (eds): Hemostasis and Thrombosis: Basic Principles and Clinical Practice, ed 3. JB Lippincott, Philadelphia, 1994, p 36.

65. Griep, PR, Kyle, RA, and Bowie, EJW: Factor X deficiency in amyloidosis: A critical review. Am J Hematol 11:443, 1981.

66. Roberts, HR and Lefkowitz, JB: Inherited disorders of prothrombin conversion. In Colman, RW, et al. (eds): Hemostasis and Thrombosis: Basic Principles and Clinical Practice, ed 3. JB Lippincott, Philadelphia, 1994, p 211.

67. Davie, EW, Fujikawa, K, and Kisiel, W: The coagulation cascade: Initiation, maintenance, and regulation. Biochemistry 30:10363, 1991.

68. Thompson, RE, Mandle, R, Jr, and Kaplan, AP: Association of Factor XI and high-molecular-weight kininogen in human plasma. J Clin Invest 60:1376, 1977.

69. Kurachi, K and Davie, EW: Activation of human Factor XI (plasma thromboplastin antecedent) by XIIa (activated Hageman factor). Biochemistry 16:5831, 1977.

70. Bouma, BN and Griffin, JH: Human blood coagulation Factor XI: Purification, properties, and mechanism of activation by activated Factor XII. J Biol Chem 252:6432, 1977.

71. Fair, BD, Saito, H, Ratnoff, O, and Rippon, WB: Detection by fluorescence of structural changes accompanying the activation of Hageman factor (Factor XII) (39773). Proc Soc Exp Biol Med 155:199, 1977.

72. Fujikawa, K, Chung, DW, Hendrickson, LE, and Davie, EW: Amino acid sequence of human factor XI, a blood coagulation factor with four tandem repeats that are highly homologous with plasma prekallikrein. Biochemistry 25:2417, 1986.

73. Baglia, PA, Sinha, D, and Walsh, PN: Functional domains in the heavy chain region of factor XI: A high-molecular-weight kininogen-binding site and substrate binding site for factor IX. Blood 74:244, 1989.

74. Roberts, HR and Hoffman, M: Hemophilia and related conditions—inherited deficiencies of prothrombin (factor II), factor V, and factors VII to XII. In Beutler, E, et al (eds): Williams Hematology, ed 5. McGraw-Hill, New York, 1995, p 1433.

75. Seligsohn, U: High gene frequency of factor XI (PTA) deficiency in Ashkenazi Jews. Blood 51:1223, 1978.

76. DeLa Cadena, RA, Wachtfogel, YT, and Colman, RW: Contact activation pathway: Inflammation and coagulation. In Colman, RW, et al (eds): Hemostasis and Thrombosis: Basic Principles and Clinical Practice, ed 3. JB Lippincott, Philadelphia, 1994, p 230.

77. Ibid, p 230.

78. Ibid, p 231.

79. Roberts, HR and Hofman, M: Hemophilia and related conditions—inherited deficiencies of prothrombin (factor II), factor V, and factors VII to XII. In Beutler, E, et al (eds): Williams Hematology, ed 5. McGraw-Hill, New York, 1995, p 1434.

80. Ibid, p 1434.

81. Colman, RW: Surface mediated defense reactions: The plasma contact activation system. J Clin Invest 73:1249, 1984.

82. Fujikawa, K and Davie, EW: Human factor XII (Hageman factor). Methods Enzymol 80:198, 1981.

83. Cochrane, CG, Revak, SD, and Wuepper, KD: Activation of Hageman factor in solid and fluid phases: A critical role of kallikrein. J Exp Med 138:1564, 1973.

84. Loscalzo, J: Pathogenesis of thrombosis. In Beutler E, et al. (eds): Williams Hematology, ed 5. McGraw-Hill, New York, 1995, p 1527.

85. DeLa Cadena, RA, Wachtfogel, YT, and Colman, RW: Contact activation pathway: Inflammation and coagulation. In Colman, RW, et al (eds): Hemostasis and Thrombosis: Basic Principles and Clinical Practice. JB Lippincott, Philadelphia, 1994, p 219.

86. Lorand, L and Kornishi, K: Activation of fibrin stabilizing factor of plasma by thrombin. Arch Biochem Biophys 105:58, 1964.

87. Naski, MC, Lorand, L, and Shafer, JA: Characterization of the kinetic pathway for fibrin promotion of α-throm-

bin-catalyzed activation of plasma Factor XIII. Biochemistry 30:934, 1991.

88. Folk, JE and Finlayson, JS: The epsilon gamma-glutamyl lysine crosslink and the catalytic role of transglutaminases. Adv Protein Chem 31:3, 1977.

89. Colman, RW, Hirsch, J, Marder, VJ, and Salzman, EW: Hemostastis and Thrombosis: Basic Principles and Clinical Practice, ed 3. JB Lippicott, Philadelphia, 1994, p 309.

90. Miletich, JP: Factor XIII: Laboratory analysis. In Beutler E, et al (eds): Williams Hematology, ed 5. McGraw-Hill, New York, 1995, p L91.

91. Bagdasarian, A, Lahiri, B, Talamo, RC, et al: Immuno-chemical studies of plasma kallikrein. J Clin Invest 54:1444, 1974.

92. Mandle, R, Jr, Colman, RW, and Kaplan, AP: Identification of prekallikrein and high-molecular-weight kininogen as a complex in human plasma. Proc Nat Acad Sci USA 73:4179, 1976.

93. Hattersley, PG and Hayse, D: Fletcher factor deficiency: A report of three unrelated cases. Br J Haematol 18:411, 1970.

94. Goodnough, LT, Saito, H, and Ratnoff, OD: Thrombosis or myocardial infarction in congenital clotting factor abnormalities and chronic thrombocytopenia: A report of 21 patients and a review of 50 previously reported cases. Medicine 62:248, 1983.

95. Schiffman, S and Lee, P: Preparation, characterization, and activation of a highly purified factor XI: evidence that a hitherto unrecognized plasma activity participates in the interaction of factor XI and XII. Br J Haematol 27:101, 1974.

96. Berrettini, M, Schleef, RR, Heeb, MJ, et al: Assembly and expression of an intrinsic factor IX activator complex on the surface of cultured human endothelial cells. J Biol Chem 267:19833, 1992.

97. Cheung, PP, Kunapuli, SP, Watchfogel, YT, et al: Total kininogen deficiency (Williams Trait) is due to an Arg-stop mutation in exon 5 of the human kininogen gene. Blood 78:391a, 1991.

98. Feinstein, DI: Immune coagulation disorders. In Colman, RW, et al (eds): Hemostasis and Thrombosis: Basic Principles and Clinical Practice, ed 3. JB Lippincott, Philadelphia, 1994, p 881.

99. Reece, EA, Clyne, LP, Romero, R, et al: Spontaneous factor XI inhibitors: Seven additional cases and review of the literature. Arch Intern Med 144:525, 1984.

100. Poon, MC, Saitor, H, and Koopman, WJ: A unique precipitating autoantibody against plasma thromboplastin antecedent associated with multiple apparent clotting factor deficiencies in patient with systemic lupus erythematosus. Blood 63:1309, 1984.

101. Feinstein, DI: Acquired disorders of hemostasis. In Colman RW, et al: Hemostasis and Thrombosis: Basic Principles and Clinical Practice, ed 3. JB Lippincott, Philadelphia, 1944, p 888.

102. Brandt, JT, Britton, A, and Kraut, EA: Spontaneous factor V inhibitor with unexpected laboratory features. Arch Pathol Lab Med 110:24, 1986.

103. McGlasson, DL, et al: Platelet neutralization procedure (PNP): Atypical results seen with a factor V deficiency with and without the presence of an inhibitor. Clin Lab Sci 3:2, 1990, p 119.

104. Triplett, DA and Brandt, JT: Lupus anticoagulants: Misnomer, paradox, riddle. Epiphenomenon. Hematol Pathol 2:121, 1988.

105. Conley, CL and Hartmann, RC: A hemorrhagic disorder caused by circulating anticoagulant in patients with disseminated lupus erythematosus. J Clin Invest 31:621, 1952.

106. Loeliger, A: Prothrombin as a co-factor of the circulating anticoagulant in systemic lupus erythematosus. Thromb Diath Haemorrh 3:237, 1959.

107. Bonnin, JA, Cohen, AK, and Hicks, ND: Coagulation defects in a case of systemic lupus erythematosus with thrombocytopenia. Br J Haematol 2:168, 1956.

108. Shapiro, SS and Thiagarajan, P: Lupus anticoagulants. In Spaet, T (ed): Progress in Hemostasis and Thrombosis, vol 6. Grune & Stratton, New York, 1982, p 263.

109. Shapiro, SS, Thiagarajan, P, and DeMarco, L: Mechanism of action of the lupus anticoagulant. Ann NY Acad Sci 370:359, 1981.

110. Thiagarajan, P, Shapiro, SS, and DeMarco, L: Monoclonal immunoglobulin M coagulation inhibitor with phospholipid specificity. Mechanism of a lupus anticoagulant. J Clin Invest 66:397, 1980.

111. Harris, EN, Chan, JK, Asherson, RA, et al: Thrombosis, recurrent fetal loss and thrombocytopenia: Predictive value of the anticardiolipin antibody test. Arch Intern Med 146:2153, 1986.

112. Harris EN, Boey, ML, Macworth-Young CG, et al: Anticardiolipin antibodies: Detection by radioimmunoassay and association with thrombosis in systemic lupus erythematosus. Lancet 2:1211, 1983.

113. Alving, BM, Baldwin, PE, Richards, RL, and Jackson, BJ: The dilute phospholipid APTT. A sensitive assay for verification of the lupus anticoagulants. Thromb Haemost 54:709, 1985.

QUESTIONS

1. Which of the following can produce defects that lead to impairment of the coagulation system?
   a. Decreased factor synthesis
   b. Interference of abnormal molecules
   c. Loss, consumption, or inactivation of factors
   d. All of the above

2. Which of the following diseases show decreased activity of factor VIII:C?
   a. Hemophilia A
   b. Hemophilia B
   c. Parahemophilia
   d. Hemophilia C

3. Which coagulation disorder has decreased activity of factor VIII:C, vWF:Ag, vWF R:Co and a prolonged bleeding time test?
   a. Hypoprothrombinemia
   b. von Willebrand's disease
   c. Hemophilia A
   d. Hemophilia B

4. The dissolution of a clot with 5 M urea is an indication of which factor deficiency?
   a. Factor II
   b. Factor XIII
   c. von Willebrand's disease
   d. Lupus anticoagulant

5. The factor defect that has a normal APTT and a prolonged PT is:
   a. Factor I
   b. High-molecular weight kininogen
   c. Factor VII
   d. Factor X

6. A patient with amyloidosis can have which factor deficiency?
   a. Factor V
   b. Factor X

c. Factor VIII:C
d. Factor II

7. The reptilase time will be normal with:
   a. Heparin
   b. Dysfibrinogenemia
   c. Afibrinogenemia
   d. Hypofibrinogenemia

8. Which of the following is considered a low phospholipid test for LLA identification?
   a. Platelet neutralization procedure
   b. Ionophore platelet procedure
   c. Dilute Russell's viper venom time
   d. Kaolin clotting time

ANSWERS

1. **d** (pp 531, 533)
2. **a** (p 535)
3. **b** (p 538)
4. **b** (p 542)
5. **c** (p 535)
6. **b** (pp 540–541)
7. **a** (p 534 [Table 28–2])
8. **c** (p 546)

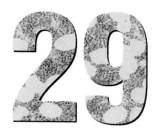

29

Interaction of the Fibrinolytic, Coagulation, and Kinin Systems and Related Pathology

John Lazarchick, MD
Joette Kizer, MT(ASCP)

Molecular Components: Physicochemical and Functional Properties
  Plasminogen
  Plasminogen Activators
  Plasminogen Activator Inhibitor 1 (PAI-1)
  Plasmin
  Plasmin Inhibitors
Congenital Abnormalities

Disseminated Intravascular Coagulation
  Triggering Mechanism: Associated
    Clinical Disorders
  Clinical Presentation
  Laboratory Diagnosis
  Therapy
Related Disorders
Case Study

Objectives

At the end of this chapter, the learner should be able to:
1 Name the components of the coagulation and fibrinolytic systems.
2 Describe the physiologic interactions of these proteolytic systems.
3 Have an understanding of the clinical and laboratory abnormalities associated with disseminated intravascular coagulation.
4 Understand the laboratory abnormalities associated with primary fibrinolysis versus disseminated intravascular coagulation.

Normal hemostasis is the result of the balanced interaction of the vascular endothelium and platelets with four biochemical systems:[1,2] the coagulation; fibrinolytic; kinin; and, to a lesser extent, complement systems. The interrelationship among these systems is illustrated in Figure 29–1. Detailed discussion of the ever-emerging central role of the vascular endothelium in hemostasis and inflammation is beyond the scope of this chapter and the reader is referred to several excellent reviews on the topic.[3,4] When a stimulus initiates activation of the coagulation system with resultant fibrin formation and the establishment of a hemostatic barrier, a series of enzymes comprising the fibrinolytic system are simultaneously activated to lyse the fibrin thrombus and re-establish vessel lumen integrity and blood flow. This chapter deals with the biochemistry of the components of this fibrinolytic system, its associated pathophysiologic disorders, and the laboratory tests available to evaluate individual components and overall function.

MOLECULAR COMPONENTS: PHYSICOCHEMICAL AND FUNCTIONAL PROPERTIES

The molecular components of the fibrinolytic system consist of: (1) the plasma protein plasminogen; (2) its active enzymatic form, plasmin; (3) a group of plasminogen activators that convert plasminogen to plasmin; (4) plasmin inhibitors, most prominently α_2-plasmin inhibitor; and (5) fibrin/fibrinogen, which serve as substrate for the active enzyme plasmin (Table 29–1).

Plasminogen

Native plasminogen is a single-chain plasma zymogen of approximately 90,000 daltons (d) that circulates in two molecular forms, which differ only in their carbohydrate content.[5] It is synthesized by the liver and

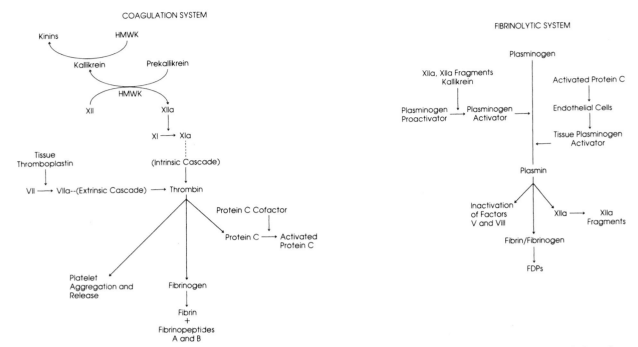

FIGURE 29–1 This schematic summarizes the interaction of the coagulation, fibrinolytic, and kinin systems. High-molecular-weight kininogen and prekallikrein catalyze the activation of factor XII to XIIa. Factor XIIa then promotes the conversion of prekallikrein to kallikrein. The latter liberates kinins from high-molecular-weight kininogen, thus completing the positive feedback loops of the contact phase of coagulation. Thrombin formed through the extrinsic or intrinsic cascade systems then converts fibrinogen to fibrin and induces platelet aggregation release. Thrombin bound to thrombomodulin on the endothelial surface activates protein C, which indirectly promotes tissue plasminogen activator release from endothelial cells in addition to direct stimulation of these cells by thrombin to release tissue plasminogen activator. A second point of interaction between these systems can also result in formation of plasminogen activator. Kallikrein, in association with factor XIIa and XIIa fragments, converts a plasmin proactivator to its activated state. Through either activating system, plasminogen can be proteolytically cleaved to form plasmin. Plasmin not only lyses fibrin and inactivates factors V and VIII but also degrades factor XIIa to inactivate fragments that are a component of the second plasminogen activator system.

has a half-life of 2 days. The plasma content is approximately 20 mg/dL. Each form of this molecule has an amino acid terminal glutamic acid (Glu-plasminogen) and is capable of undergoing limited proteolytic cleavage of this region to an incomplete molecule with lysine as the new terminal amino acid (Lys-plasminogen). This latter form is more readily converted to active plasmin by plasminogen activators than the Glu-plasminogen form and is probably of greater physiologic significance.

Plasminogen Activators

The conversion of either form to active plasmin can be initiated through a variety of direct or indirect mechanisms.[6] This group of activating proteins is collectively known as *plasminogen activators*. Regardless of the initiating mechanism, activation of plasminogen to yield plasmin proceeds through the cleavage of the same arginine 560–valine 561 bond in the Glu and Lys forms of plasminogen. These activators are either endogenous or exogenous in origin. Endogenous activators are serine proteases present in the blood and a variety of other tissues, particularly the vascular endothelium. With the initiation of the contact phase of coagulation (see Chap. 26), factor XIIa, XIIa fragments, XIa, kallikrein, and high-molecular-weight kininogen

interact to yield plasminogen-activating ability.[7] The exact biochemical steps involved in the formation of this intrinsic activator are not completely understood. The activator activity generated by this pathway slowly converts plasminogen to plasmin. The primary source of activators, however, is the vascular endothelium, the site of synthesis of both endothelial cell urokinase, which is a single-chain precursor and tissue plasminogen activator (TPA). The former probably plays a minimal role in in vivo fibrinolysis, with TPA being the main activator. Its greater efficiency in thrombolytic therapy and potential for pharmacologic manipulation has led to its widespread use as a therapeutic fibrinolytic agent. This mechanism is probably the major physiologic activator of plasminogen. TPA is an endothelial cell product with a molecular weight of approximately 68,000 d.[8] Although a number of biochemical stimuli, including histamine, vasopressin, bradykinin, and adrenaline, can induce TPA release, thrombin generated as result of activation of the coagulation system is the most important release inducer. Thrombin thus serves as a coagulant component (converting fibrinogen to fibrin, aggregating platelets); as a stimulant to dampen the coagulant process by binding to its endothelial cell receptor, thrombomodulin, thus allowing for the generation of activated protein C; and finally and paradoxically as an initiator of fibrinolysis. Acti-

TABLE 29–1	**Components of the Fibrinolytic System**
Component	**Comments**
1. Plasminogen	Circulating zymogen form with molecular weight of 90,000 daltons
2. Plasminogen activators:	
Tissue activator	Endogenous activator liberated from endothelial cells by the action of thrombin
Factor XIIa, kallikrein	Contact phase activator that generated the initiation of coagulation
Factor XIIa fragments	
Factor XIa	
Urokinase	Proteases produced in the kidney and secreted in the urine
Streptokinase	Bacterial cell product; forms complex with plasminogen that has intrinsic activating activity
3. Plasminogen activator inhibitor 1	Endogenous inhibitor of tissue plasminogen activator; synthesized and secreted by endothelial cells and platelets
4. Plasmin	Active serine protease of 70,000 to 75,000 daltons
5. α_2-Plasmin inhibitor	Primary inhibitor of plasmin; forms irreversible complex with plasmin
α_2-macroglobulin	Serves as a plasmin inhibitor only when α_2-plasmin inhibitor binding sites are saturated
6. Fibrinogen, fibrin	Plasmin substrates; proteolytic cleavage results in generation of degradation products

vated protein C exerts a negative feedback control on the coagulation process by proteolytically cleaving activated coagulant factors Va and VIIIa, thus limiting further clot formation.[9,10] This latter function of activated protein C is accelerated by its formation of a complex with protein S, which serves as a cofactor. TPA has a high affinity for fibrin and its adsorption to fibrin clots greatly enhances plasminogen conversion to plasmin. Because of a high affinity of both the plasminogen activator and plasminogen for fibrin rather than fibrinogen, the effect of this reaction is accentuated on the surface of and within the clot. Release of TPA from endothelium is also responsive to a variety of other stimuli including venous occlusion, strenuous exercise, and treatment with vasoactive drugs including the vasopressin derivative 1-desamino-8-D-arginine vasopressin (DDAVP). TPA activity is increased many times under these conditions.[11]

Exogenous activators have been available for clinical use for a number of years. One of these, urokinase, is synthesized by the kidney in addition to the vascular endothelium, as previously mentioned, and excreted in the urine.[12] It can also be identified in vitro using kidney cell cultures and is a potent direct activator of plasminogen. Its major drawbacks are its expense and its relatively lower affinity for fibrin compared to TPA. A consequence of the latter property is that the plasmin generated digests not only fibrin but also circulating fibrinogen, and therefore the development of severe hypofibrinogenemia is not uncommon with its use. The other exogenous activator, streptokinase, is a

product of beta-hemolytic streptococci. It is not a serine protease and has no intrinsic proteolytic activity, but is capable of forming a 1:1 stoichiometric complex with plasminogen. This interaction results in a conformational change of the plasminogen molecule and exposure of its active serine site.[13] The streptokinase–plasminogen complex can then undergo autocatalysis to yield other activators, namely SK-Glu-plasmin and SK-Lys-plasmin. Any of these forms will readily convert free plasminogen to plasmin. Since streptokinase is a bacterial protein, a major limitation with its use in thrombolytic therapy is the induction of an immune response with resulting antibody development and an inhibition of its activity.

Plasminogen Activator Inhibitor 1 (PAI-1)

This inhibitor is a member of the family of protease inhibitors, which includes antithrombin III, α_2-macroglobulin, α_1-antitrypsin, and α_2-antiplasmin; they are collectively referred to as *serpins* (*serine protease inhibitors*). PAI-1 is a 53,000-d glycoprotein also synthesized by vascular endothelium and released primarily in an inactive, latent state.[14] It is an acute-phase reactant and can be induced by a variety of stimuli including interleukin-1, endotoxin, and thrombin. Its primary substrate is TPA. Thus regulation of fibrinolysis is dependent upon the interaction of TPA with PAI-1. Under basal conditions, most of the TPA released is bound to PAI-1. Excessive levels of this inhibitor have been associated with thrombotic disease.

Plasmin

The pivotal serine protease generated through these complex biochemical processes is plasmin. This protein has a molecular weight of 77,000 to 85,000 d, depending on whether Lys-plasmin or Glu-plasmin is formed, and has a transient plasma half-life measured in seconds.[15] Plasmin has the ability to proteolytically degrade both fibrin in clots and native fibrinogen in the circulation into a series of well-characterized end products collectively known as fibrin/fibrinogen degradation products (FDPs). This process results in an asymmetrical, progressive breakdown of fibrin and fibrinogen.[16] The earliest recognized component is fragment X, which is still capable of clotting. A recent finding has been the identification of a small peptide fragment from the B beta chain of fibrinogen that is released simultaneously with the formation of the X fragment. Measurement by radioimmunoassay of the B beta 15-42* peptide may prove of value in the documentation of early fibrinolytic states.[17,18] The X fragment undergoes further plasmin attack to yield unclottable Y and D fragments. The Y fragment is further digested to yield an additional D fragment and a single E fragment. It is now realized that the proteolytic cleavage of cross-linked fibrin, that is, fibrin transaminated through the action of factor XIIIa and calcium, results in other intermediate degradation products, for example, D2E without the generation of fragment D or E. This proteolytic product is referred to as the D-dimer.

These breakdown products have specific inhibitory effects on the coagulation system and thereby suppress further clot formation. Fragment X is capable of clotting slowly and exerts an anticoagulant effect by competing with fibrinogen for thrombin. It also forms slowly polymerizing complexes with fibrin monomers and inhibits the polymerization step. Fragment D forms abnormal complexes with fibrin monomers as it polymerizes. Fragment E is not known to have any specific anticoagulant effect. In high concentrations (>100 μg/mL), the degradation products are capable of inhibiting platelet aggregation and release. Plasmin also exerts a direct limiting effect on the coagulation process by being able to cleave proteolytically and render factors V and VIII inactive in addition to proteolysing factor XII and platelet glycoprotein Ib, the von Willebrand factor receptor.

Plasmin Inhibitors

Although plasmin formation characteristically takes place in the area of fibrin deposition with little free plasmin circulating, this enzyme, if unchecked by the presence of specific inhibitors, would result in circulating fibrinogen being digested and the blood being rendered unclottable. The primary physiologic inhibitor of plasmin in vivo is α_2-plasmin inhibitor.[19] It rapidly binds to the lysine binding site on plasmin in a 1:1 molar ratio in an irreversible manner. Measurement of these plasmin:α_2-plasmin inhibitor complexes has been suggested as an indicator for activation of the fibrinolytic system. Plasmin adsorbed onto fibrin during

the fibrinolytic process appears to be protected from this inhibitor because it binds to fibrin through the same lysine-binding site. Since this binding site on plasmin is occupied, the inhibitor cannot bind and clot lysis can proceed. The overall effect is to ensure that plasmin activity is limited to the area of fibrin deposition and to prevent free plasmin from circulating. Other protease inhibitors in plasma include α_2-macroglobulin, C1 inactivator, and α_1-antitrypsin. Of these, only α_2-macroglobulin has a role in plasmin inhibition during normal hemostasis but participates only when α_2-plasmin-inhibitor binding sites for plasmin are saturated.

CONGENITAL ABNORMALITIES

Congenital abnormalities of the fibrinolytic system are rare.[20] Only three cases of an abnormal plasminogen have been reported. In each of these reports the patient had a history of recurrent thrombotic episodes. Low levels of TPA activity have been documented in two families and were associated with a similar thrombotic tendency. Deficiencies of α_2-plasmin inhibitor have been reported in four families to date and, in contrast, are associated with a severe hemorrhagic tendency. Acquired abnormalities of the fibrinolytic system are much more common and will be discussed in the section on disseminated intravascular coagulation and related disorders.

In summary, an integrated system of serine proteases is brought into play once the coagulation process is initiated in response to disruption of blood vessel integrity (Fig. 29–2). The response is balanced so that the same reaction that initiated thrombin formation and fibrin deposition also initiates a series of reactions to lyse the clot. Factor XIIa with other components of the contact phase of coagulation convert plasminogen to plasmin; thrombin stimulates endothelial cells to release TPA with subsequent plasmin generation. Excess TPA activity is controlled by the presence of plasminogen activator inhibitor. Because of the high affinity of plasmin for fibrin, most of these fibrinolytic processes are taking place at the site of fibrin deposition within the damaged blood vessel. The presence of plasmin inhibitors further ensures that the proteolytic process is limited to this area.

DISSEMINATED INTRAVASCULAR COAGULATION

When there is damage to a blood vessel an ordered, integrated series of reactions involving the coagulation, fibrinolytic, kinin, and complement systems occurs on endothelial cells and platelets at the site of injury as outlined in the previous chapters, with the initial formation and subsequent lysis of fibrin deposits. The initial formation of the fibrin clot prevents further hemorrhage and initiates vascular repair. The subsequent clot lysis serves to re-establish blood flow and vascular integrity. This process is normally self-limited and localized. Under certain pathologic stimuli, the coagulation response may be accentuated and the normal inhibitory mechanisms overwhelmed. Activa-

---

*Amino acid sequence numbering of this peptide.

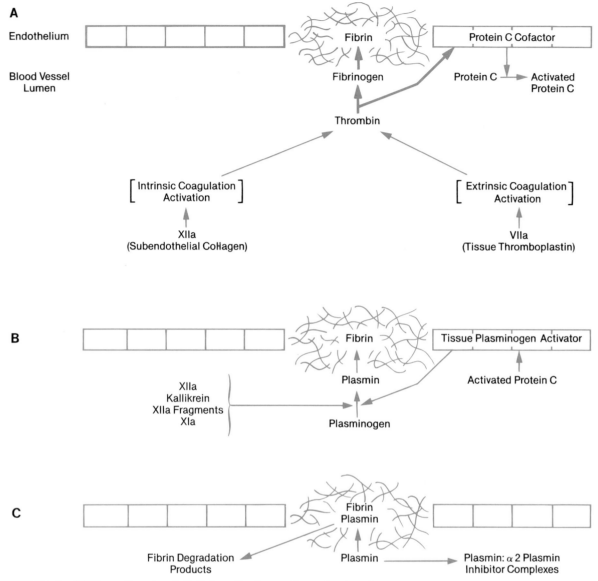

FIGURE 29-2 (*A*) Disruption of endothelial continuity results in platelet adherence, factor XIIa and VIIa formation, and the generation of thrombin to fibrin to reestablish a temporary barrier. Secondarily and simultaneously, thrombin complexes with thrombomodulin on the endothelial surface. Protein C, once bound to this complex, is rapidly converted to its activated state. (*B*) Activated protein C indirectly causes release of tissue plasminogen activator from endothelial cells in addition to direct stimulation and release of this glycoprotein by thrombin. (*C*) Plasmin-induced proteolysis of the fibrin clot results in the formation of fibrin degradation products. Reendothelialization of the damaged blood vessel begins as clot dissolution is occurring. Excess plasmin is irreversibly complexed with its inhibitor, α 2-plasmin inhibitor, preventing proteolysis of circulating fibrinogen.

tion of the coagulation system under these circumstances causes consumption of the coagulation factors and platelets with subsequent thrombus formation not only at the site of endothelial damage, but in a random manner throughout the microcirculation.[21] This hemorrhagic syndrome has been referred to as disseminated intravascular coagulation (DIC), defibrination syndrome, or consumptive coagulopathy. Simultaneous with and secondary to the activation of the coagulation cascade, the fibrinolytic system is activated.

Regardless of the nature of the inciting stimulus, the pathophysiologic effect of this process will be reflective of the balance between fibrin deposition (action of thrombin) and fibrinolysis (action of plasmin). The clinical manifestations thus can be diffuse hemorrhage (see Fig. 27–6), caused by depletion of platelets and coagulation factors, ischemic tissue damage caused by vascular occlusion, or the occurrence of both simultaneously in different areas of the microvasculature.

Triggering Mechanism: Associated Clinical Disorders

The diverse stimuli that are capable of triggering the coagulation cascade in this manner all act through one or more of three mechanisms:[22] (1) activation of the extrinsic coagulation pathway by the release of tissue thromboplastin, (2) activation of the intrinsic coagulation pathway with factor XIIa formation, and (3) direct activation of factors X or II. The exact sequence of intermediary events by which certain of the stimuli initiate coagulation is well understood, but with other stimuli this process is unknown. DIC from direct activation of factor VII seen after massive injury or in certain obstetrical complications results from release of tissue thromboplastin from the injured tissue or from amniotic fluid entering the circulation. Certain tumors, particularly mucinous adenocarcinomas, are rich in thromboplastin-like material and may act through the same mechanism. The coagulopathy seen with red cell lysis may be a result of the release of thromboplastin-like activity from the stroma of these cells. All pathologic stimuli that result in activation of the intrinsic system probably do so indirectly by first inducing endothelial cell damage with subsequent exposure of the subendothelium. Platelet adherence and aggregation and factor XII activation can then occur. This is the proposed mechanism of DIC associated with anoxia, immune complex formation, and sepsis. New experimental insight regarding sepsis now suggests that the mechanism of DIC induced by endotoxins, the lipopolysaccharide constituents of gram-negative organisms, may be more complicated with endotoxin inducing release of a number of cytokines including tissue necrosis factor α (TNF-α) and interleukin-1 (IL-1) with the primary activation of coagulation occurring through the extrinsic (tissue-factor-dependent) pathway rather than the intrinsic pathway.[23] TNF-α is capable of inducing tissue factor activity in monocytes and on both the luminal and subendothelial surfaces of endothelial cells. Tissue factor can bind and activate factor VII; the complex of TF-VIIa can then activate factor X with subsequent thrombin formation. Direct activation of coagulation factors can also occur in the presence of proteolytic enzymes. The venoms of certain snakes act through this mechanism; for example, Russell's viper venom activates factor X, whereas venom from the sand rattlesnake causes direct conversion of prothrombin to thrombin. Certain malignancies have also been reported to have direct factor X–activating capability, and this property may account from the DIC seen in these states. A list of clinical conditions associated with these triggering mechanisms is given in Table 29–2.

Clinical Presentation

The clinical presentation depends greatly on which of the proteolytic processes (coagulant or fibrinolytic) is dominant. This allows for a wide spectrum, ranging from an acute, severe hemorrhagic disorder to a low-grade disorder with predominantly thrombotic manifestations. A number of factors are important in determining the final clinical picture, including the magnitude and duration of the triggering stimulus; the functional ability of reticuloendothelial system, particularly the liver, to remove from circulation activated coagulation factors, fibrin monomers, fibrin/fibrinogen products, as well as immune complexes; the compensatory ability of the liver and the bone marrow to accelerate clotting factor and platelet production; and finally the extent to which any particular organ is involved with hemorrhage or thrombus.[19]

Laboratory Diagnosis

The laboratory findings in patients with DIC reflect the direct or indirect effects of excess thrombin and plasmin generation (Table 29–3). The constellation of laboratory abnormalities in any particular patient, however, will depend on the nature, magnitude, and duration of the triggering stimulus; the compensatory

---

TABLE 29–2 Clinical Conditions Associated with Disseminated Intravascular Coagulation

Thromboplastin Release—Factor VII Activation

Placental abruption	Promyelocytic leukemia
Trauma	Retained dead fetus syndrome
Fat emboli syndrome	Acute intravascular hemolysis*
Mucin-secreting adenocarcinoma	Amniotic fluid embolus*
Sepsis*	Cardiopulmonary bypass surgery

Endothelial Cell Damage—Factor XII Activation

Immune complex disease	Burns
Intravascular hemolysis*	Vasculitis
Liver disease*	Anoxia
Heat stroke	Acidosis
Sepsis*	

Factor X/II Activation

Snake venoms	Liver disease*
Acute pancreatitis	Fat emboli syndrome*

*More than one mechanism may be involved.

TABLE 29–3 **Laboratory Tests to Detect Excess Thrombin and/or Plasmin Activity**

Excess Protease	Effect	Laboratory Tests
Thrombin	Fibrinogen utilization	Fibrinogen concentration, thrombin/Reptilase time, prothrombin and activated partial thromboplastin times
	Utilization/degradation of other coagulation factors	Prothrombin and activated partial thromboplastin times, coagulation factor assays
	Fibrin monomer generation	Soluble fibrin monomer complexes
	Fibrinopeptide A/B release	Fibrinopeptides A and B
	Platelet aggregation/release	Platelet count, β-thromboglobulin and platelet factor 4
	AT-III complex formation	Thrombin-antithrombin III complexes, AT-III level
Thrombin/plasmin	Proteolysis of fibrinogen/fibrin	Fibrin degradation products, D-dimer concentration, B-beta 15-42 peptide assay
	Release/activate	Tissue plasminogen
	Plasminogen activators and inhibitors	Activator level, plasminogen activator inhibitor level
	Soluble fibrin monomer/fibrinogen FDP complexes	Soluble fibrin monomer complexes
Plasmin	Plasminogen utilization	Plasminogen concentration
	Proteolysis of fibrinogen/fibrin	Fibrin degradation products, thrombin/Reptilase times, platelet aggregation and release tests
	Complexes with inhibitor	α_2-Plasmin inhibitor concentration, α_2-plasmin inhibitor–plasmin complexes
	Proteolysis of factors V/VIII	Factor assays

capacity available; and the underlying disease state. Although the ultimate confirmatory test would be the direct demonstration of fibrin deposition in biopsy material from an involved blood vessel, this is not practical. As a result, a multitude of tests have been utilized by various laboratories to make this diagnosis.[18,24] It should be pointed out that no single test is diagnostic of DIC; however, in the appropriate clinical setting (patient history and type of bleeding), a battery of tests can ensure a diagnosis of DIC. Indirect tests that lack specificity for thrombin action include the prothrombin, activated partial thromboplastin, and thrombin/Reptilase clotting times. Utilization and degradation of the clotting factors in the DIC process result in prolongation of each of these global tests. Since platelets are also consumed during the coagulation process and their contents released, the finding of thrombocytopenia and elevated plasma levels of the platelet-specific proteins beta-thromboglobulin and platelet factor 4 would be expected. The plasma inhibitor antithrombin III will complex with thrombin and activated factor X and result in diminished plasma levels of antithrombin III. The presence of thrombin-antithrombin complexes formed can also be determined using an enzyme-linked immunoabsorbent assay (ELISA) system. If the fibrin deposition does not completely occlude the lumen of the damaged blood vessel, red cells may undergo a shearing effect as they traverse this area with resultant fragmentation and the development of a microangiopathic hemolytic anemia (see Fig. 27–7).

Conversion of prothrombin to thrombin is the result of cleavage from the parent molecule of a small, inactive peptide referred to as prothrombin fragment 1.2 (PF1+2). Measurement of this activation peptide has thus far been used primarily for diagnosis of a hypercoagulable state; however, it may have equal utility as a molecular marker for DIC. Specific tests for direct evidence of thrombin activity relate to the action of thrombin on fibrinogen. Other than certain snake venoms, thrombin is the only enzyme that releases the specific peptides fibrinopeptide A and B from the fibrinogen molecule. Both ELISA and radioimmunoassays are available commercially to measure each fibrinopeptide.[25] The major drawback of measuring these peptides, paradoxically, is the extreme sensitivity of the assay, which is such that elevated levels can be seen in clinical conditions in which thrombin is only transiently generated. As a consequence of fibrinopeptide release, soluble fibrin monomers are formed that are capable of forming complexes with intact fibrinogen molecules or with FDPs. The ability to precipitate these complexes from plasma is the basis for two paracoagulation assays, the ethanol gelation test and the protamine sulfate test. In our laboratory, we are currently measuring soluble fibrin monomer complex formation using a latex agglutination assay for these soluble fibrin monomer complexes. Positive tests for any of these three methods are indirect indications that thrombin was generated, therefore, the coagulation system had to have been activated.

Tests for the secondary activation of the fibrinolytic system in DIC are primarily directed at demonstrating the action of plasmin on fibrin/fibrinogen. As has already been mentioned, a series of cleavage products are formed, the FDPs. The anticoagulant action of these fragments has been noted in the previous section. A number of immunologic tests are available to measure one or more of the fibrinogen fragments and can yield quantitative information on the degree of fibrinolysis. Because of its ease of performance and specificity, that is, evidence of plasmin action on cross-linked fibrin, the D-dimer assays are gaining wide popularity as the immunologic assays of choice. A relatively recent development has been the recognition of an early cleavage product of the B-beta chain of the fibrinogen dimer, peptide B-beta 15-42.[17] Clinical assessment of the utility of the radioimmunoassay for the B-beta 15-42 peptide in diagnosing accelerated fibrinolysis has confirmed its value; however, because it is difficult to perform, it is not recommended for routine evaluation. Direct measurement of the plasminogen concentration in plasma can also be performed, and commercial assays are available. An indication of increased plasminogen activator activity seen in early stages of DIC can be obtained by performing a euglobulin lysis time.[26] The euglobulin fraction of plasma contains plasminogen, plasminogen activator, plasmin, and fibrinogen. The rapidity of lysis of the fibrin clot is directly related to plasminogen activator levels. The sensitivity of this global assay, however, is limited. As discussed, it is now possible to directly quantitate each component with commercially available kits. Assays for α_2-plasmin inhibitor levels and for circulating plasmin:α_2-plasmin inhibitor complexes are under investigation for clinical use.

Table 29–4 summarizes laboratory tests available to diagnose DIC and the constellation of results one can find in this syndrome depending on the balance between thrombin and plasmin activities and the compensatory capacity of the patient. This table describes three generalized clinical states of DIC with the typical laboratory abnormalities associated with each. The decompensated DIC state refers to a condition in which active hemorrhage is evident and in which the consumption of the coagulation factors and platelets exceeds the capacity to increase the synthesis of these components. In the compensated state, laboratory evidence of an accelerated coagulation and fibrinolytic process is apparent (increased FPA, soluble fibrin monomer complexes, increased β-thromboglobulin, increased FDPs or D-dimer levels, presence of plasmin:α_2-plasmin inhibitor complexes), but the rate of synthesis of the coagulation components is balanced with the rate of destruction. Because of this balance, the PT, APTT, thrombin time and platelet count are usually normal or only mildly abnormal. Confirmation of DIC is then based on finding evidence of coagulation activation peptides (FPA, prothrombin fragment 1.2), complexes of activated coagulant/fibrinolytic components (thrombin–antithrombin III, plasmin–α_2-antiplasmin) in addition to increased fibrin(ogen) degradation products and elevated β-thromboglobulin or platelet factor 4 levels. The hypercoagulable state is the result of excess thrombin present in the plasma with a delayed or lessened plasmin response. In this condition evidence of coagulation activation is apparent (increased levels of FPA, thrombin–antithrombin III complexes, prothrombin fragment 1.2, β-thromboglobulin), but all fibrinolytic activation markers are absent or minimally increased. A characteristic finding in this form of DIC is a shortened APTT. It should be realized that these clinical states are not static, and it is not unusual for one to evolve into one of the others, depending on the nature of the underlying disease process and the response to therapy.

Therapy

Therapy for DIC is essentially twofold: treatment or removal of the underlying pathologic stimulus and maintenance of blood volume and hemostatic function.[21,22] Dramatic improvement in the patient's clinical status with abrupt cessation of bleeding and normalization of the coagulation abnormalities can be

TABLE 29–4 **Laboratory Tests to Diagnose DIC**			
Routine Test	**Decompensated**	**Compensated**	**Hypercoagulable**
Prothrombin time	I	N	N
Activated partial thromboplastin	I	N	D
Thrombin time/Reptilase time	I	N/I	N/I
Fibrinogen	D	N	I
Platelet count	D	N/D	N
D-dimer/Fibrin(ogen) Degradation products	I	I	N/I
Euglobulin lysis test	N/I/D	N/D	N
Soluble fibrin monomer Complexes	P	P	Ng
Antithrombin III	D	N/D	N/D
Special Test	**Decompensated**	**Compensated**	**Hypercoagulable**
Coagulation factor levels	D	N/D	I
Fibrinopeptide A	I	I	I
Plasminogen	D	N/D	N
Plasmin:α_2-plasmin Inhibitor complexes	I	I	N
β-Thromboglobulin/platelet factor 4 levels	I	I	I
Thrombin–Antithrombin III complexes	I	I	I
Prothrombin fragment 1.2	I	I	I

Abbreviations: I = Increased; D = Decreased; N = Normal; P = Positive; Ng = Negative

seen in certain cases of DIC with removal of the underlying pathologic stimulus alone, for example, DIC associated with a retained dead fetus. In cases of DIC associated with septicemia, appropriate antibiotic therapy is imperative to control the pathologic process, that is, bacterial- or endotoxin-induced vascular damage. Blood component replacement therapy with transfusion of packed red blood cells, fresh frozen plasma, and platelets to maintain blood volume and to support hemostatic function is indicated in these patients with active bleeding or whose compensatory capacity is limited. In addition to fresh frozen plasma, cryoprecipitate (enriched in fibrinogen, factor VIII, and fibronectin) and prothrombin complex (enriched in vitamin K–dependent clotting factors) are often used as supplemental sources of blood component therapy. The administration of heparin in DIC has been advocated by a number of investigators, but its use is still controversial.[21,27] On the premise that the underlying pathologic basis for DIC is generation of excess thrombin, and that thrombosis, especially of small vessels, is the process that most affects morbidity and mortality, heparin should theoretically be indicated to slow or stop the coagulation process by complexing with antithrombin III to inhibit thrombin or Xa. This ameliorating effect has been noted with the use of subcutaneous low-dose heparin therapy in mild to moderate DIC.[21] Its use can result in increased bleeding, and because heparin itself affects a number of coagulation tests, it is often difficult to monitor the effect of conventional therapy. Heparin should be used and is most effective in cases of DIC that present with clinical evidence of a hypercoagulable state with evident vascular thrombosis. When major peripheral vessels are occluded as part of the hypercoagulable process, the use of fibrinolytic agents (recombinant TPA, streptokinase, or urokinase) may be indicated as an initial management choice with subsequent heparinization, but clinical experience with this form of therapy is minimal. Table 29–5 summarizes the previously described profile of DIC.

RELATED DISORDERS

Primary fibrinolysis is an unusual situation in which plasmin is formed in the absence of coagulation taking place. The clinical presentation in this disorder is similar to DIC, with diffuse hemorrhage occurring as a result of increased plasma fibrinolytic activity. Several mechanisms can initiate this process. The presence of proteolytic enzymes in plasma that are capable of either directly or indirectly converting plasminogen into plasmin can occur in certain disease states. The genitourinary system is enriched in urokinases that can enter the systemic circulation following various uro-

TABLE 29-5 Profile of DIC

Synonyms	Conditions Associated with DIC	Suggested Triggering Mechanisms	Clinical Manifestations	Clinical Laboratory Findings	Sequential Therapy

1. Consumptive coagulopathy
2. Defibrination syndrome
	Obstetric accidents
	Intravascular hemolysis
	Septicemia
	Viremia (varicella)
	Leukemias:
	  Acute
	  Promyelocytic
	  Other
	Solid malignancy
	Acidosis alkalosis
	Burns
	Crush injury and tissue necrosis
	Vascular disorders
		Amniotic fluid, which possesses thromboplastic activity
		Retained fetus, which possesses thromboplastic activity
		By-product of red cell hemolysis (phospholipid)
		Antigen/antibody complexes
		Endotoxin release
		Chronic stasis
		Complement activation
			1. *General signs:* significant hemorrhaging (usually from 3 unrelated sites: melena and hematemesis, epistaxis, or hemoptysis) fever, hypotension, acidosis, hypoxia, proteinuria, hematuria
			2. *Specific signs:* petechiae, purpura, gangrene, wound bleeding, venipuncture bleeding, subcutaneous hematomas
			3. *Microthrombi*
			4. *End-organ dysfunction*
				Hypofibrinogenemia
				Abnormal PT
				Abnormal PTT
				Abnormal thrombin time
				Abnormal platelet count
				Abnormal tourniquet test
				Abnormal clot retraction
				Abnormal factors V and VIII
				Positive fibrin(ogen)-split products
				Positive protamine sulfate test
				Positive ethanol gelatin test
				Antithrombin III consumption
				Leukocytosis
				Schistocytosis
				Thrombocytopenia
				Reticulocytosis
					1. Remove or treat triggering process
					2. Stop or slow coagulation process
					  a. Miniheparin
					  b. Heparin
					  c. Antiplatelet drugs
					  d. AT-III concentrates
					3. Blood component replacement
					  a. Platelets
					  b. Cryoprecipitate
					  c. Prothrombin complex
					  d. AHF
					4. Antifibrinolytic therapy*
					  a. Epsilon aminocaproic acid (EACA)

*Sequential therapy used only after clotting is stopped (3% of patients may require this therapy).

logic procedures. The fibrinolytic state seen with metastatic prostatic carcinoma is another example of this mechanism. The basis for the hemorrhagic state seen following cardiopulmonary bypass surgery is complex, with platelet dysfunction and hemodilution of coagulant proteins being the primary defects, but activation of the plasminogen-plasmin system with increased fibrinolytic activity is well documented. The failure of the hepatic clearance mechanism to remove plasminogen activator accounts for the increased fibrinolytic activity seen in a variety of hepatic disorders, particularly cirrhosis. Under normal circumstances, the hepatic reticuloendothelial system removes not only activated clotting proteins but plasminogen activator from the systemic circulation. When this function is impaired by hepatic disease, or in patients who have portocaval shunting procedures, the removal of plasminogen activator is less than adequate and hyperplasminemia occurs, with resultant hemorrhage. Increased fibrinolytic activity can also be seen in patients undergoing liver transplantation, especially during the reperfusion phase following reanastomosis of vessels.

The occurrence of DIC with secondary fibrinolysis is well documented in patients with acute promyelocytic leukemia. It is now recognized, however, that the coagulopathy these patients develop may also result from a primary fibrinolysis. The mechanism(s) is unsettled but may involve direct activation by the leukemic cells with release of a urokinase-type or tissue-type plasminogen activator.[28]

The coagulation abnormalities seen in these fibrinolytic disorders are similar to those in DIC with prolonged PT, APTT, and thrombin times. These defects result from the hypofibrinogenemic state induced by the proteolytic cleavage of fibrinogen by excess plasmin in addition to the catabolic effect of this enzyme on factors V and VIII. FDP concentrations are increased and, as previously noted, further interfere with coagulation by acting as antithrombins. With the excess plasmin activity the euglobulin lysis time is typically shortened. Since thrombin is not generated during this pathologic process, several laboratory tests can readily distinguish primary fibrinolysis from DIC. The platelet count is typically normal; fibrinopeptides A and B levels are not elevated, and circulating fibrin monomer complexes and elevated D-dimer levels are absent in primary fibrinolysis in contrast to the results in DIC.

Thrombotic thrombocytopenic purpura (TTP) is the syndrome of unknown etiology in which fibrin and platelet thrombi are formed diffusely throughout the microvasculature in contrast to the localized thrombus formation seen in DIC.[29] The clinical picture consists of a pentad of findings: (1) fever, (2) microangiopathic hemolytic anemia, (3) thrombocytopenia, (4) azotemia, and (5) vacillating neurologic deficits. Despite fibrin and platelet deposition, this disorder is not typically associated with excessive activation of the coagulation system. Supportive evidence that this syndrome represents an abnormality of the fibrinolytic system is suggested by the finding of diminished or absent fibrinolytic activity, particularly of TPA, in plasma and blood vessels affected with microthrombin. Therapy has not been standardized but antiplate-

let drugs, for example, aspirin or dipyridamole, plasmapheresis, and exchange transfusion have been used either singularly or in combination with variable success (see Chap. 27). Table 29–6 summarizes the other causes of fibrinolytic activation.

CASE STUDY

A 32-year-old woman, gravida 3, para 2, in her 36th week of gestation, noted the sudden onset of lower abdominal pain and profuse vaginal bleeding. She was rushed to the emergency room. On examination she was noted to be hypotensive with a blood pressure of 70/40 and had a marked tachycardia. Large ecchymoses and continuous oozing of blood from venipuncture sites were evident. A fetal heart tone was barely audible. Births of her other children were uncomplicated and the family history was negative for a hemorrhagic diathesis.

Initial coagulation studies revealed PT = 26 s (normal, 11 to 13 s); APTT = 84 s (normal, 24 to 30 s); platelet count = 20,000 (normal, 140,000–440,000/μL); fibrinogen = 85 mg/dL (normal, 145 to 350 mg/dL); FDPs >40 μg/mL (<10 ug/mL); protamine sulfate test positive (negative). Blood smear showed numerous red cell fragments present.

A diagnosis of DIC was made based on the patient's clinical presentation and the supportive laboratory data. The patient was placed on intravenous fluids to maintain her blood pressure and given 2 units of fresh-frozen plasma and 10 units of platelets. She was taken to the operating room and underwent a caesarean section. Her bleeding abated postoperatively and all coagulation parameters returned to normal within 36 hours.

This case is illustrative of an obstetric complication, placental abruption, which resulted in an acute DIC syndrome. Several triggering mechanisms have been postulated as an explanation for the underlying coagulopathy in this disorder, including the release of thromboplastin-like material from the amniotic fluid and tissue necrosis in the area of the retroperitoneal hemorrhage. The laboratory parameters are consistent with a consumptive coagulopathy and secondary fibrinolysis. With the delivery and removal of the placenta, the source of the triggering mechanism was removed and the pathologic process stopped. Restoration of normal hemostatic parameters occurs within hours postoperatively and usually no further blood component replacement therapy is required.

Questions

1. What abnormal red cell morphology represents red cell fragmentation?
2. What laboratory parameters given would you expect to correct upon transfusion of fresh frozen plasma?
3. What tests indicate that fibrinolysis is occuring?
4. Give reasons why this patient is thrombocytopenic.

TABLE 29–6   Other Causes of Fibrinolytic Activation

Clinical Condition	Mechanism	Clinical Manifestation	Other Hemostatic Alterations

1. Chronic liver disease	Abnormal fibrinolytic inhibitor (α_2-macroglobulin)
	Abnormal hepatic clearance of plasminogen activators
		Often fulminant hemorrhage with massive hemoptysis, hematachezia, melena or epistaxis
		May also demonstrate petechiae, purpura, spider telangiectasia, ecchymoses
			1. Hypofibrinogenemia (due to lysis
			2. Elevated FDP (X,Y,D, and E)
			  a. Defective fibrin monomer/polymerization
			  b. Platelet dysfunction
			3. Proteolysis of factors V, VIII, IX, XI
			4. Platelet defects
			  a. Thrombocytopenia
			  b. Platelet dysfunction (FDP, PF 3)
			5. Coagulation protein defects
			  a. Decreased synthesis of II, VII, IX and X
			  b. Decreased synthesis of Fletcher factor
			  c. Decreased or dysfunctional synthesis of AT-III

2. Cardiopulmonary bypass (CPB)	Unclear; possibly direct activation of fibrinolysis by the oxygenation system of pump-induced accelerated flow rates may alter endothelial plasminogen	Hemorrhage; hematuria, petechiae/purpura, and oozing from intravenous site in conjunction with increased chest tube loss	1. Hyperfibrinolysis results in
			  a. Elevated FDP
			  b. Hypofibrinogenemia
			  c. Low factors V and VIII
			2. Functional platelet defect
			  a. CPB-induced
			  b. Drug-induced
			3. Thrombocytopenia
			4. Hyperheparinemia-heparin rebound(?)
			5. DIC(?)

3. Malignancy	Poorly understood; in several instances tumor extracts possess the ability to activate directly or indirectly the fibrinolytic system (e.g., gastric carcinoma, sarcomas, and prostatic carcinoma)	Thrombosis/hemorrhage	1. Thrombocytopenia 2. Platelet function defects 3. Elevated FDP 4. Decreased AT-III 5. DIC(?)

4. Acute promyelocytic leukemia	Release of urokinase-type and tissue-type plasminogen activators from leukemic cells	Severe hemorrhage	1. Hypofibrinogenemia (due to fibrin(ogen) lysis
			2. Marked elevation of FDP(X, Y, D, and E)
			  a. Defective fibrin monomer/polymerization
			  b. Platelet dysfunction
			3. Proteolysis of V, VIII, XI, XII
			4. Decreased plasminogen
			5. Plasmin: α 2-antiplasmin complexes

REFERENCES

1. Kaplan, AP, et al: Interaction of the clotting, kinin forming, complement and fibrinolytic pathways. NY Acad Sci 389:25, 1982.
2. Sundsmo, JS and Fan, DS: Relationships among the complement, kinin, coagulation and fibrinolytic systems. Springer Semin Immunopathol 6:231, 1983.
3. Benedict, CR, Pakala, R, and Wilkerson, JT: Endothelial-dependent procoagulant and anticoagulant mechanism. Tex Heart Inst J 21:86, 1984.
4. Esmon, CT: Cell mediated events that control blood coagulation and vascular injury. Ann Rev Cell Biol 9:1, 1993.
5. Castellino, FJ: Recent advances in the chemistry of the fibrinolytic systems. Chem Rev 81:431, 1981.

6. Miller, JL: Normal fibrinolysis. In Henry, JB (ed): Clinical Diagnosis and Management by Laboratory Methods. 17th ed, WB Saunders, Philadelphia, 1984, p 769.
7. Mandle, RJ and Kaplan, AP: Hageman factor-dependent fibrinolysis: Generation of fibrinolytic activity by the interaction of human activated factor XI and plasminogen. Blood 54:850, 1979.
8. Bachman, F and Kruithof, IEKO: Tissue plasminogen activator: Chemical and physiological aspects. Sem Thromb Hemost 10:6, 1984.
9. Owen, WG: The control of hemostasis. Arch Pathol Lab Med 106:209, 1982.
10. Owen, WG and Esmon, CT: Functional properties of an endothelial cell cofactor for thrombin-catalyzed activation of protein C. J Biol Chem 256:5532, 1981.
11. Prowse, CV and Cash, JD: Physiologic and pharmacologic enhancement of fibrinolysis. Sem Throm Hemost 10:51, 1984.
12. Rickli, EE: The activation mechanism of human plasminogen. Thromb Diath Haemorrh 34:386, 1975.
13. Brogden, RN, Speight, TM, Avery, GS: Streptokinase: A review of its clinical pharmacology, mechanism of action and therapeutic uses. Drugs 5:357, 1973.
14. Edelberg, JM, Sane, DC, and Pizzo, SV: Vascular regulation of plasminogen activator inhibitor-1 activity. Semin Thromb Hemost 20:319, 1994.
15. Gonzalez-Gronow, M, Violand, BN, Castellino, FJ: Purification and some properties of the glu- and lys-human plasmin heavy chains. J Biol Chem 252:2175, 1977.
16. Marder, VJ, et al: High molecular weight derivatives of human fibrinogen produced by plasmin. I. Physicochemical and immunologic characterization. J Biol Chem 244:2111, 1968.
17. Kudryk, B, et al: Measurement in human blood of fibrinogen/fibrin fragments containing the B-beta 15-42 sequence. Throm Res 25:277, 1982.
18. Ockelford, A and Carter, J: DIC: Application and utility of diagnostic tests. Semin Thromb Hemost 8:198, 1982.
19. Aoki, N and Harpel, PC: Inhibitors of the fibrinolytic enzyme system. Semin Thromb Hemost 10:24, 1984.
20. Kwaan, HC: Disorders of fibrinolysis. Med Clin North Amer 56:163, 1972.
21. Bick, RL: Disseminated intravascular coagulation: Objective criteria for clinical and laboratory diagnosis and assessment of therapeutic response. Clin Appl Thromb/Hemost 1:3, 1995.
22. Muller-Berghaus, G: Pathophysiology of generalized intravascular coagulation. Semin Thromb Hemost 3:209, 1977.
23. Levi, M, et al: Pathogenesis of disseminated intravascular coagulation in sepsis. JAMA 270:975, 1993.
24. Fareed, J, et al: Impact of automation on the quantitation of low molecular weight markers of hemostatic defects. Semin Thromb Hemost 9:355, 1983.
25. Hirsh, J: Blood tests for the diagnosis of venous and arterial thrombosis. Blood 57:1, 1981.
26. Buckell, H: The effect of citrate on euglobulin methods of estimating fibrinolytic activity. J Clin Pathol 11:403, 1958.
27. Mant, MJ and King, EG: Severe, acute disseminated intravascular coagulation. A reappraisal of its pathophysiology, clinical significance and therapy based on 47 patients. Am J Med 47:557, 1979.
28. Tallman, MS, et al: New insights into the pathogenesis of coagulation dysfunction in acute promyelocytic leukemia. Leuk Lymph 11:27, 1993.
29. Bukowski, RM: Thrombotic thrombocytopenic purpura: A review. Prog Hemost Thromb 6:287, 1982.

QUESTIONS

1. D-dimer formation is the result of plasmin's action on:
   a. Fibrin monomer
   b. Fibrinogen
   c. Cross-linked fibrin
   d. Fibrin degradation products

2. Inactivation of factors Va and VIIIa is the result of:
   a. Thrombin
   b. Protein S
   c. TPA
   d. Activated protein C

3. In primary fibrinolysis, which of the following lab tests will be abnormal?
   a. Platelet count
   b. D-dimer level
   c. Fibrin peptide A level
   d. Thrombin time

4. In DIC presenting clinically as a hypercoagulable state, it is not unusual for which of the following coagulation times to be paradoxically shortened?
   a. Reptilase time
   b. Euglobulin lysis time
   c. Activated partial thromboplastin time
   d. Thrombin time

5. The primary inhibitor of the fibrinolytic system is:
   a. Antithrombin III
   b. α_2-antiplasmin
   c. Protein C
   d. α_2-macroglobulin

Answers

1. **c** (p 557)
2. **d** (p 556)
3. **d** (p 564)
4. **c** (p 561)
5. **b** (p 557)

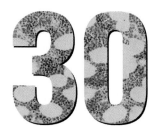

Introduction to Thrombosis and Anticoagulant Therapy

Michel M. Canton, PharmD

Regulation of Coagulation and Fibrinolysis
  Thrombotic Factors
  Antithrombotic Factors
  Regulation of Fibrinolysis
Pathophysiology of Thrombosis
  Conditions Predisposing to Recurrent
   Thrombosis

Antithrombotic Therapies and Monitoring
  Vitamin K Antagonists: Oral
   Anticoagulants
  Heparin Therapy
  Thrombolytic Therapy
Case Study

Objectives

At the end of this chapter, the learner should be able to:
1. Name natural anticoagulants and inhibitors present in plasma.
2. Name the most important serine-protease inhibitor and its cofactor.
3. Identify vitamin K–dependent inhibitors.
4. Identify components of plasminogen activation.
5. List similarities for deficiencies of antithrombin III, heparin cofactor II, protein C, and protein S.
6. Name laboratory tests for evaluation of antiphospholipid antibody syndrome.
7. Explain the action of oral anticoagulants and the mechanism of heparin.
8. Name the most common laboratory test used to monitor oral anticoagulant therapy.
9. Name laboratory tests used to monitor heparin therapy.
10. Name laboratory tests used for monitoring fibrinolytic therapy that are not affected by the presence of therapeutic heparin.

Since the first description by Egeberg[1] in 1965 of a Norwegian family with congenital deficiency of antithrombin III (AT-III) and a thrombotic diathesis, understanding of the existing connections between alteration of coagulation inhibitors and thromboembolisms progressed rapidly. Abnormalities of hemostasis, as observed in venous thrombosis, reflect disturbances in two regulatory mechanisms, the physiologic coagulation inhibitors and the fibrinolytic system. Hereditary deficiencies in AT-III, protein C, protein S, and defects of the fibrinolytic system, as well as the existence of antiphospholipid antibodies, are the abnormalities most directly associated with thromboembolic disease in patients under 40 years of age. In patients over 40, cancer is the major cause of thromboembolic disease.[2] The nonspecific binding of heparin to these plasma proteins decreases the anticoagulant effect of heparin by limiting its availability to interact with AT-III. This is particularly important in monitoring heparin's anticoagulant response in patients with thromboembolic disease, since several of these heparin-binding proteins are acute-phase reactants, the levels of which increase in ill patients. This phenomenon may also account for the resistance of some patients to the anticoagulant effect of heparin. Standard heparin inhibits platelet function and increases vascular permeability, which may account for its association with hemorrhage at concentrations that should produce antithrombotic effects.[3] The regulation of hemostasis is complex and involves interactions of many key components of the coagulation system. These components are able to bind to specific platelet receptors to form small amounts of thrombin. Natural anticoagulant mechanisms act to oppose the generation of the latter enzyme. Two types of natural anticoagulants or inhibitors are present in the plasma: (1) AT-III and heparin cofactor II (HC-II), which are serine-protease inhibitors; and (2) protein C, which, when activated in activated protein C (APC), is capable of degrading activated factors V (Va) and VIII (VIIIa) in the presence of its cofactor protein S.

If platelet activation occurs, prothrombin is brought into proximity with the prothrombinase complex, and significant amounts of thrombin can be generated. This overproduction of thrombin might overwhelm the natural anticoagulant mechanism. Therefore, the thrombotic accident can be defined as the result of an imbalance between the procoagulant and the anticoagulant systems.[4]

The fibrinolytic system is as complex as the coagulation system. The cause-and-effect relationship between the frequency of deficiencies in the physiologic fibrinolytic system and the occurrence of thromboembolism is yet to be established. However, it seems that the most common abnormality is the presence of an excess of plasminogen activator inhibitor 1 (PAI-1), leading indirectly to a decreased functional availability of the tissue plasminogen activator (TPA).[5]

REGULATION OF COAGULATION AND FIBRINOLYSIS

As mentioned before, in a normal, healthy person, procoagulant and anticoagulant systems are in equilibrium (Fig. 30–1). This balance may be tipped in either direction by a change in clinical circumstances. Because the levels of regulatory and procoagulant proteins vary, a patient may vacillate among a thrombotic, a prothrombotic, and a balanced state (Fig. 30–2).

Although the exact roles of platelets and other cells have still to be defined, blood cells, platelets, endothelial cells, subendothelial structures, and plasma components play important roles. The expression of these functions will be either a thrombotic factor or an antithrombotic reaction during the occurrence of thrombosis.

Thrombotic Factors

The Platelets

Thrombin generation in plasma is greatly accelerated by the presence of platelets. Indeed, the activated platelets have an enhanced capacity to catalyze interactions between the activated coagulation factors. This capacity is caused by a rearrangement of the phospholipid structure of the platelet membrane that accompanies the platelet shape change, which offers support for the surface-dependent activation process of coagulation. The platelet release reaction also contributes to the thrombogenesis because, when platelets are exposed to various stimuli (e.g., thrombin), the alpha granule contents are released. These granules contain the platelet-specific proteins, platelet factor (PF) 4, β-thromboglobulin, platelet-derived growth factor, and a variety of other proteins, including fibrinogen, factor V, and von Willebrand factor (vWF), which provide platelet aggregation, thrombin generation, and local platelet adhesion.

Thrombin

Thrombin is one of the most fascinating enzymes in the coagulation system (Table 30–1). First, thrombin

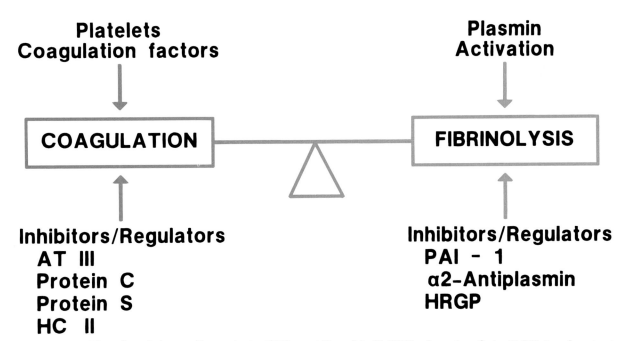

FIGURE 30–1 Physiologic balance of hemostasis. AT III = antithrombin III; HC II = heparin cofactor II; PAI-1 = plasminogen activator inhibitor-1; HRGP = histidine-rich glycoprotein.

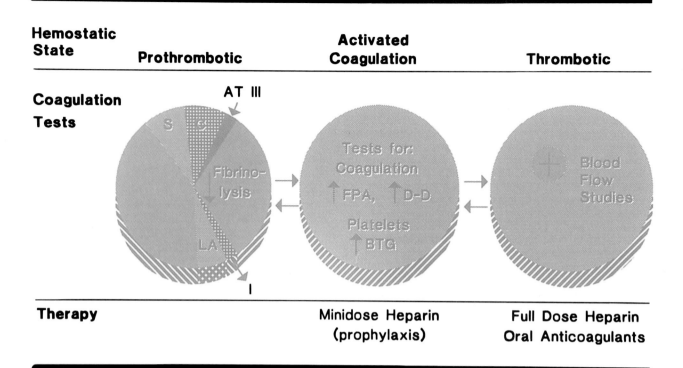

Hemostatic State	Prothrombotic	Activated Coagulation	Thrombotic

FIGURE 30–2 Continuum of hypercoagulability. With the new laboratory tests, approximately 55% of patients with recurrent thrombosis will be found to have demonstrable abnormalities. The relative proportion of each abnormality is shown in the prothrombotic category. S = protein S; C = protein C; D-D = D-dimer; βTG = beta-thromboglobulin; LA = lupus anticoagulant; I = fibrinogen; FPA = fibrinopeptide A. (From American Bioproducts Co., with permission.)

proteolytically cleaves fibrinogen to produce two molecules of fibrinopeptide A and two molecules of fibrinopeptide B from the Aα and Bβ fibrinogen chains, respectively—an event that converts fibrinogen to fibrin monomer. The released fibrin monomers may polymerize to form fibrin thrombi. Thrombin converts plasma and platelet factor XIII to an active transglutaminase, which, in turn, cross-links fibrin with covalent amide bonds that render the fibrin insoluble. Thrombin can "activate" the procoagulant factors, factors VIII and V, to participate in amplifying its own generation.

Thrombin participates in the activation of protein C, which serves as an anticoagulant to inactivate factors VIIIa and Va. Therefore, thrombin indirectly possesses some antithrombotic activities, limiting the extent of its own generation.

Thrombin also binds to platelets at low concentration and initiates shape change, aggregation, and secretion. Thrombin stimulates the platelets to make PF 3 available on the surface, which facilitates the prothrombin complex to generate more thrombin from prothrombin.

Antithrombotic Factors

The normal plasma contains a sophisticated system of serine protease inhibitors capable of inhibiting many of the activated proteases generated during coagulation (Fig. 30–3).

Antithrombin III

The most important of these inhibitors is AT-III, an α_2-glycoprotein with a molecular weight (MW) of 58,000 daltons (d). It is composed of a single chain of 432 amino acids.[6] Its in vivo half-life is about 2 to 3 days. Normally, AT-III is a relatively weak inhibitor of the serine protease, but it may be activated by various

TABLE 30–1 **Roles of Thrombin**
Cleaves fibrinogen to form fibrinopeptides A and B and fibrin monomers
Activates factors V, VIII, and XIII and protein C
Activates platelets to aggregate and secrete
Contributes to the generation of platelet procoagulant activity
Induces endothelial release of PAF,* prostacyclin, vWF, interleukin-1, thrombospondin, TPA, and PAI-1
Induces granulocyte chemotaxis and adherence to endothelial monolayers to macromolecules
Depression of reticuloendothelial clearance of activated products of coagulation

*Platelet-activating factor.

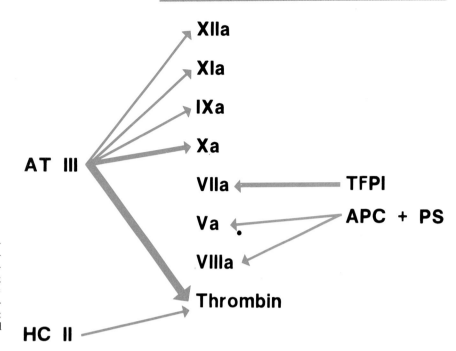

FIGURE 30-3 Physiologic inhibitors of coagulation. AT III = antithrombin III; APC = activated protein C; XIIa = activated factor XII; HC II = heparin cofactor II; PS = protein S, TFPI = tissue factor pathway inhibitor. (From Samama, MM: Hotel-Dieu Hospital, Paris, personal communication, 1983.)

glucosaminoglycans—in particular heparin and the heparin sulfates.[7] Heparin, which is highly negatively charged, interacts with a domain in the AT-III molecule containing a high density of basic amino acids, particularly lysine. As a result, conformational changes occur in AT-III, making its active center containing arginine more available to the active serine residue of thrombin and other serine proteases. A complex is formed between AT-III and the serine protease, which possesses no enzyme and no inhibitor activity. As the complex forms, the heparin molecule falls off and is ready to react on another AT-III molecule. Therefore, heparin administered even in small doses converts AT-III from a slow, relatively ineffective inhibitor to a fast, effective one.

Heparin Cofactor II

Heparin cofactor II (HC-II) was first identified by Birginshaw in 1974[8] and isolated by Tollefsen in 1981.[9] The primary amino acid structure of HC-II is quite distinct from that of AT-III. HC-II also possesses an affinity for heparin that is significantly less than that of AT-III. The specificity of HC-II is narrowly restricted to thrombin. The other mucopolysaccharides such as dermatan sulfate are able to accelerate dramatically the action of this protease inhibitor. Indeed, it appears likely that the observed anticoagulant effects of mucopolysaccharides other than heparin are primarily a result of interactions with HC-II. HC-II probably plays a minimal role when heparin is used clinically as an anticoagulant. Tollefsen has suggested that HC-II may function as a second-line inhibitor of thrombin after its activation by dermatan sulfate present on the surface of the vessel wall. Toulon and associates[10] also suggested that HC-II was present in a functional active form in human platelets and that platelet HC-II could

play a role in the regulation of thrombin generated on the platelet surface.[11]

The Protein C System

Protein C, identified in 1960, is a vitamin K–dependent zymogen that, once activated by thrombin, proteolytically degrades factors VIIIa and Va, two of the major cofactors involved in thrombin generation[12] (Fig. 30-4).

Protein C has a molecular weight of 62,000 d. It is a glycoprotein with heavy and light chains linked by a disulfide bond. Thrombin cleaves a specific ArgLeu bond at the amino terminus of the heavy chain to release a 12-amino-acid activation peptide resulting in activation of protein C.[13] A cofactor for thrombin-mediated activation of protein C was identified on the surface of the endothelial cells and designated thrombomodulin,[14] an integral membrane protein. Once thrombin binds to thrombomodulin, there appears to be a conformational change in thrombin as it loses its procoagulant activities. Thrombin bound to thrombomodulin no longer activates platelets or factors V, VIII, or XIII, nor does it cleave fibrinogen. Thrombin activation of protein C in the presence of thrombomodulin is modulated by activated factor V (Va). Low factor Va concentrations, which can be generated on and bound to endothelial cell surfaces, enhance the activation rate, whereas high concentrations of factor Va or light chain of factor V inhibit protein C activation. This mechanism provides a feedback control on the activation process of protein C. Protein C function is significantly enhanced in the presence of its cofactor protein S, and phospholipids.[15] In the absence of adequate quantities of protein S, protein C function is inadequate to control the generation of thrombin. Factors VIIIa and Va appear to be relatively resistant to

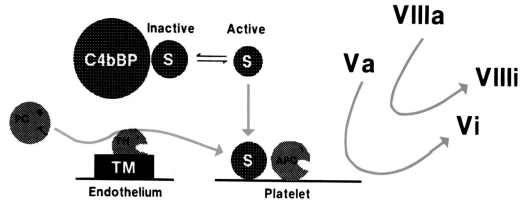

FIGURE 30–4 Activation of protein C system. In plasma protein S (S) is found both free and in complex with C4b binding protein (C4bBP). The free protein S is functionally active and serves on the membrane surface as cofactor for the degradation of factors Va and VIIIa by activated protein C (APC). The enzymatic degradation of V and VIII results in inhibition of the clotting cascade. The production of APC from protein C (PC) by the thrombin (TH)-thrombomodulin (TM) complex also occurs on the endothelial cell surface. (From Comp,[36] p 178, with permission.)

proteolysis in the presence of their associated serine proteases (factors IXa and Xa, respectively), suggesting that downward regulation of thrombin generation by protein C occurs in concert with decreasing quantities of factors IXa and Xa. Protein S is a vitamin K–dependent protein that is produced in the liver as well as in

megakaryocytes and endothelial cells.[16] Protein S is synthesized and released as a single chain with a molecular weight of 69,000 to 84,000 d. It is unique among the vitamin K–dependent coagulation proteins in that it is not the zymogen of a serine protease. Plasma protein S circulates in two forms, one bound

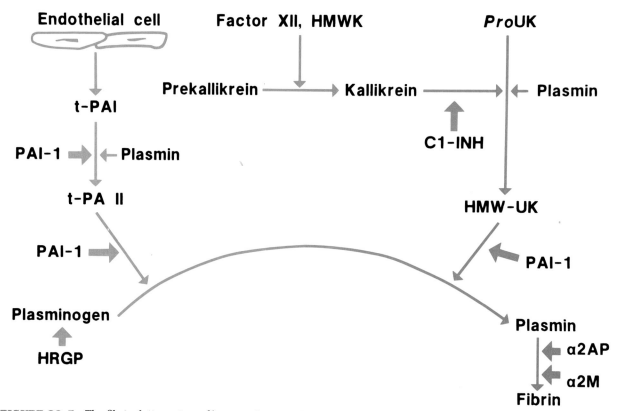

FIGURE 30–5 The fibrinolytic system of human plasma. t-PAI = single-chain tissue-type plasminogen activator, also called sct-PA; T-PA II = two-chain tPA (tct-PA); PAI-1 = plasminogen activator inhibitor-1 (endothelial type); HRGP = histidine-rich glycoprotein; HMWK = high-molecular-weight kininogen; Pro-UK = pro-urokinase, also called single-chain urinary-type PA (scu-PA); HMW-UK = high-molecular-weight urokinase, also called two-chain u-PA (tcu-PA); C'l-INH = Cl inhibitor; α2AP = Alpha-2-antiplasmin; α2-M = Alpha-2-macroglobulin. (From Bachmann,[23] p 194, with permission.)

TABLE 30–2 **Inhibitory Effect of the Serine-Protease Inhibitors**	
Serpin	**Inhibitory Effects**
α_2-Antiplasmin	Plasmin
α_2-Macroglobulin	Thrombin, plasmin, kallikrein
α_1-Antitrypsin	Thrombin, trypsin, chymotrypsin, factor XIa, elastase, activated protein C
AT-III	Thrombin; factors Xa, XIIa, IXa, and XIa; plasmin; kallikrein
C1 inhibitor	Kallikrein, plasmin, factors XIIa and XIa, C1 esterase
Antichymotrypsin	Chymotrypsin
HC-II	Thrombin
Protein C inhibitor	Activated protein C
PAI-1 and PAI-2	Plasminogen activators

to the C4b-binding protein (C4b-BP) from the complement system, the other free. Only the free form of protein S functions as protein C cofactor. Platelets contain protein S. Therefore, activation of platelets provides not only a surface for procoagulant reactions, but also a surface and a cofactor for eventual control of the thrombin generation (see Fig. 30–4). In 1983, the presence of an inhibitor of APC in human plasma was described.[17] Initially, it was hypothesized that a deficiency of the protein C inhibitor (PCI) was the cause of the combined factor VIII/V deficiency.[18] Later this theory was refuted and the original results were explained as the result of the repeated freezing and thawing of the test samples.[19] Suzuki and coworkers[20] described the purification and characterization of a plasma glycoprotein (MW 57,000 d) that neutralizes APC activity by forming a 1:1 stoichiometric complex. This inhibitor, PCI-I, was shown to be identical to the plasminogen activator inhibitor 3 (PAI-3). More recently a second inhibitor of protein C was described. Unlike PCI-I, this PCI-II is believed to be heparin-independent and has a relatively high concentration.[21] The amino acid analysis revealed that PCI-II is identical to α_1-antitrypsin. Finally, analysis of the kinetics of APC inactivation in the plasma from a patient congenitally deficient in α_1-antitrypsin showed that there is probably a third inhibitor of APC in plasma different from PCI-I and from α_1-antitrypsin.[22]

Regulation of Fibrinolysis

Physiologic fibrinolysis results in the proteolytic degradation of polymerized fibrin.[4] The central reaction in this system is the conversion of a proenzyme, plasminogen, to the proteolytic enzyme plasmin. Plasminogen is a 90,000-d glycoprotein synthesized in the liver. Its half-life is 2 to 3 days. Plasminogen circulates free or bound to histidine-rich glycoprotein (HRGP), to α_1-antiplasmin, and to fibrinogen. The physiologic activation of plasminogen is achieved by the extrinsic pathway initiated by the TPA released from the endothelial cells after stimulation, and by the intrinsic pathway consisting of a factor XIIa–dependent activator and urokinase[23] (Fig. 30–5). A specific group of inhibitors has been described that controls the fibrinolytic process in the plasma. These serine protease inhibitors are members of the protein superfamily called *serpins*. They are structurally homologous to many inhibitors of the serine proteases of the coagulation system (Table 30–2). Plasmin activity is regulated and inhibited by a number of plasma proteins such as α_2-antiplasmin, α_2-macroglobulin, α_1-antitrypsin, AT-III (especially in the presence of heparin), and C1 esterase inhibitor. Physiologically, α_2-antiplasmin is the main plasmin inhibitor. α_2-Antiplasmin is a 60,000-d glycoprotein circulating in the plasma at a concentration of 1 micromole (μM). Its properties include the immediate inhibition of plasmin, its interference with the absorption of plasminogen to fibrin, and its susceptibility to factor XIII–catalyzed cross-linking to fibrin. The combined effects of these three characteristics render α_2-antiplasmin much more specific and effective in inhibition of fibrinolysis than any of the other major inhibitors. Plasminogen activators (PAs) are inhibited by a number of specific proteins. In recent years, research has revealed the existence of at least three different inhibitors of the extrinsic system: PAI-1, PAI-2, and PAI-3, identified in plasma and urine[24] (Table 30–3). PAI-3 has also been described as one of the APC inhibitors, PCI-I. The most important inhibitor is PAI-1, a 50-kd plasma glycoprotein that is the primary fast-acting inhibitor of TPA and a member of the serpin protein superfamily. The physiologic plasma concentration of PAI-1 varies widely from 0 to 60 ng/mL with an average range of 5 to 20 ng/mL. The physiologic fibrinolytic activity seems to result primarily from the balance between TPA and its first inhibitor.

TABLE 30–3 **TPA Inhibitors**			
	PAI-1	**PAI-2**	**PAI-3**
Origin	Plasma Platelets Endothelial cell Granulocytes	Placenta Leukocytes Macrophages	Urine Plasma
MW	54,000	47,000	50,000
Inhibitory effect	TPA UK	TPA UK	UK APC
Concentration	0–1.3 nM	2 μM (3rd trimester)	—

Abbreviations: UK = urokinase; APC = activated protein C; MW = molecular weight; nM = nanomoles; μM = micromoles.

PATHOPHYSIOLOGY OF THROMBOSIS

Conditions Predisposing to Recurrent Thrombosis

Hereditary Disorders

Congenital or acquired changes in coagulation or fibrinolysis have been associated with an increased risk of thrombosis. The possibility of a hereditary defect predisposing to recurrent thrombosis should be entertained whenever a patient under the age of 40 presents with unexplained or recurrent thrombosis. The differential diagnosis includes evaluation of proteins C and S, serpin family, as well as the fibrinolytic system. Unfortunately there is no global test for these systems and each individual parameter has to be tested.

Functional assays (clotting or chromogenic assays) are always preferred because immunologic assays such as the Laurell method, enzyme-linked immunosorbent assay (ELISA), and radial immunodiffusion (RID) may miss qualitative defects. A diagnosis should never be based on a single determination, particularly if the sample is obtained at the time of the thrombotic episode.

AT-III and HC-II Congenital Deficiencies The prevalence of the AT-III deficiency is about 1 in 5000 in the normal population.[25] In patients with antecedents of venous thrombosis, the frequency of the defect is about 2% to 3%. The trait is inherited in an autosomal dominant manner. The clinical manifestations are essentially deep venous thrombosis (DVT), often complicated by pulmonary embolism. The occurrence of superficial thrombosis is relatively rare with AT-III. The AT-III deficiency seems to be also associated with arterial thrombosis.[26] It is important to mention that more than 90% of affected family members develop thrombosis episodes at some point in their lives, usually before the age of 40.[27] These thrombotic episodes often occur after a triggering event such as surgery, confinement to bed, pregnancy, or even oral contraceptive use. The variants of the disease have been classified into two types and five subtypes,[28] as shown in Table 30–4.

The AT-III deficiencies are usually heterozygous and the AT-III levels are reported at about 50% (25% to 60%) of normal. The only cases of homozygous AT-III deficiencies belonged to subtype IIc.

TABLE 30–4 Classification of AT-III Congenital Deficiencies

Type I	Quantitative Defect
Subtype Ia	Reduced synthesis or increased turnover
Subtype Ib	Reduced synthesis or increased turnover with alteration of heparin-binding site
Type II	Qualitative Defect
Subtype IIa	Abnormalities of both active and heparin-binding sites
Subtype IIb	Abnormal active site
Subtype IIc	Abnormal heparin-binding site

Autosomal-dominant hereditary deficiency of heparin cofactor II (HC-II), a hypercoagulable disorder, has been described in several kindreds. At this point, it is unclear whether heterozygous deficiency of HC-II is associated with a thrombotic tendency. Most of the affected family members described to date have been asymptomatic.

Various methods have been described for the measurement of AT-III or HC-II. Functional assays are recommended that reflect the antithrombin activity. The endpoint is measured using synthetic chromogenic substrates. These methods can be easily automated and standardized.

Protein C and Protein S Congenital Deficiencies Several hereditary disorders of the protein C system have been identified and described.[29] Hereditary deficiency of protein C, whether heterozygous or homozygous, typically has an autosomal mode of inheritance. As with AT-III deficiency, the first thrombotic episode in these individuals classically occurs before they reach 40 years of age. The heterozygous deficiency is associated with DVT or pulmonary embolism, as well as with an increased risk of warfarin-induced skin necrosis. These episodes may occur when the deficient patient is receiving large doses of warfarin. The level of protein C in the heterozygous patient is typically found between 30% and 65% of the normal level.[30] The prevalence of this defect varies widely between 1 in 16,000 and 1 in 200 to 300 individuals. Indeed, Miletich[31] has screened almost 5000 asymptomatic blood donors, of whom 79 had plasma levels of protein C under 65% of normal. None of these subjects had personal or familial thrombotic antecedents.

Thus, it is suggested that some additional risk factors besides protein C deficiency may be necessary for the development of venous thrombosis. It is estimated that heterozygous protein C deficiency may account for 8% to 10% of all cases of recurrent DVT. Homozygous protein C deficiency is rare (1 in 500,000 births). In the classic form, affected newborn infants develop purpura fulminans and an acute form of disseminated intravascular coagulation (DIC) within the first 2 days of life. As described with AT-III deficiency, several types of protein C defects have been reported.[32]

Subsequently, type I protein C deficiency is characterized by low antigenic and functional levels of the protein. In those with type II deficiency, the antigenic level of protein C is normal, and the structural abnormality of the protein is marked with a low functional activity of the molecule. Therefore protein C deficiencies should be screened by using a protein C functional assay (clot-based[33] or chromogenic assay[34]), as this will detect both types I and II. Once a low protein C activity is determined, an immunologic assay should be performed to distinguish type I from type II protein C deficiency. Recently, a low clot-based protein C level but normal chromogenic protein C level has been reported in a patient with DVT.[35]

Protein S deficiency differs significantly from deficiencies of the other vitamin K–dependent plasma proteins. Most individuals with protein S deficiency appear to have normal or moderately reduced levels of total protein S antigen, which suggests that the functional protein S deficiency involves the quantitative distribution of protein S between free and bound forms

TABLE 30–5 Proposed Classification of Hereditary Protein S Deficiency

	Free Protein S	Protein S Activity	Total Protein S
Type I	Low	Low	Low
Type IIa	Low	Low	Normal
Type IIb*	Normal	Low	Normal

*No cases reported to date.

and not an abnormality of the protein S per se. Comp[36] has proposed a classification of the congenital protein S deficiencies based on the free, total, and activity protein S levels (Table 30–5). The mode of inheritance of the type I defect is clearly autosomal-dominant. Although most of the protein S–deficient patients reported in the literature presented with DVT, most recently several cases of severe cerebral arterial thrombosis were reported associated with protein S deficiency. Immunologic assays (ELISA, Laurell) for both total and free protein S are commonly used. However, functional assays have been described[37] that will be preferable.

Fibrinolytic Defects Impaired capacity to increase the catalytic concentration of TPA in plasma after stimulation (as from the venous occlusion test) has been associated with an increased risk of thromboembolism.[23] An impaired fibrinolytic potential has also been suggested to be an important risk factor for arterial thrombosis and atherosclerosis. More recently, it has been shown that the reduced TPA activity in patients with an inherited or acquired tendency to venous thrombosis as well as in patients with coronary artery disease may be related to a deficient release of TPA from the vessel wall, an increased level of PAI-1, or both.

In support of a causative role of PAI-1 in thrombotic disease, an increased level of PAI-1 appears to constitute a risk factor for reinfarction in survivors of myocardial infarction and is the most commonly encountered abnormality in idiopathic DVT. However, it cannot be excluded that the increase in PAI-1 levels in septic shock merely reflects a nonspecific acute-phase reactant behavior without direct pathogenic consequences. The evaluation profile of the fibrinolytic system should consist of measurement of TPA and PAI-1 levels before and after venous occlusions. Plasminogen, α_2-antiplasmin, fibrinogen, and TPA–PAI-1 complex should also be determined.

Acquired Thrombotic Disorders

Hospitalized patients may also present risk factors that are difficult to sort out and quite different from those found in young adults with recurrent thrombosis. In general, hospitalized patients show an activation state, frank thrombosis, or both. A particular case is the presence of antiphospholipid antibodies that have been recently linked to a variety of clinical findings, including arterial and venous thrombosis, recurrent spontaneous abortions, and fetal loss, as well as thrombocytopenia.[38]

Primary Antiphospholipid Antibody Syndrome This syndrome is characterized by the production of antiphospholipid antibodies that leads to immune thrombocytopenia in patients with a history of arterial or venous thrombosis and/or unexplained recurrent spontaneous abortions, stillbirths, abruptio placentae, or early pre-eclampsia. The detection of the antiphospholipid antibodies (APA) is the biologic cornerstone in the diagnosis of this recently described syndrome[39] characterized by thrombotic episode or recurrent fetal loss. Beaumont[40] probably described the first case of association of recurrent pregnancy loss and a circulating anticoagulant; however, Laurell and Nilsson[41] received credit for the first report of such an association. Soulier and Boffa[42] reported a series of three women with histories of recurrent spontaneous abortion associated with previous thromboembolic events. The triad of recurrent fetal loss, thromboembolism, and lupus anticoagulant (LA) is called the Soulier-Boffa syndrome.

Finally, Hughes[43] was the first to propose the concept of an APA syndrome. The laboratory evaluation of APA is usually performed through two types of tests: (1) coagulation tests to identify a phospholipid-dependent inhibitor of fibrin formation (platelet neutralization test, dilute Russell viper venom time, tissue thromboplastin inhibition assay, kaolin clotting time, and APTT), and (2) highly specific ELISA for APA. The platelet neutralization test remains the confirmatory test for the clotting-based assays.

The criteria for diagnosis of a *primary* APA syndrome include at least two of the following clinical manifestations that have been related to high titers of APA: DVT, arterial occlusion, thrombocytopenia, hemolytic anemia, recurrent fetal loss, leg ulcers, and livedo reticularis with the systemic absence of lupus erythematosus (SLE) or other connective tissue disorders. The laboratory workup for diagnosis of APA syndrome is shown in Figure 30–6. Recently, a prospective study demonstrated an association between the presence of circulating APA and stroke.[44]

Drug-Induced Thrombotic Disorders Because the major coagulation inhibitors and regulators may be affected by commonly used antithrombotic drugs or other medications, such as L-asparaginase and oral contraceptives, it is essential to evaluate the possible effects of such medications in order to explain a low level of AT-III or protein C or protein S (Table 30–6). For its anticoagulant action, heparin requires the presence of AT-III. Heparin therapy was associated with a considerable progressive reduction in AT-III binding capacity and antigenic protein. This decrease in AT-III is usually independent of its initial concentration. Plasma AT-III level returned to normal 2 to 3 days after the patient stopped receiving heparin. This finding is very relevant to the interpretation of clinical

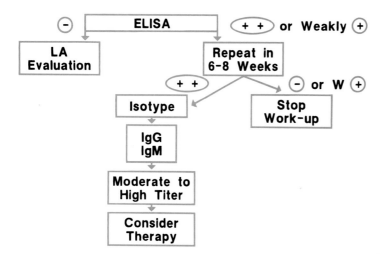

FIGURE 30-6 Antiphospholipid antibody (APA) syndrome, evaluation for APA.

data in patients treated with heparin and may suggest that the decrease of AT-III may be related to the thrombotic complications sometimes encountered during heparin therapy. The level of AT-III during heparin therapy rarely drops below 70% of normal. Therefore, a level of less than 60% may be a real defect rather than an acquired one. In this case, AT-III assay must be repeated 3 days after heparin administration was interrupted. Heparin cofactor II is not affected by anticoagulant therapies.[11]

Oral anticoagulants are known to affect the level of all vitamin K–dependent coagulation factors, including protein C and protein S. Therefore the interpretation of assays for these inhibitors may be difficult. Previously, the use of ratios of protein C antigen to factor X antigen or protein C to factor II antigen have been

recommended. However, because factor VII has a half-life similar to that of protein C (6 to 7 hours), a ratio of protein C antigen to factor VII antigen may be more appropriate. In this case, stable patients receiving oral anticoagulation yield similar values for both protein C and factor VII, provided that similar assay systems are used for determination of antigen ratios. Protein S is also depressed during oral anticoagulation. A considerable variation in plasma protein S levels is observed among individuals with similar intensity of anticoagulation. Ratios between protein S antigen and factor II antigen may be useful to assess protein S status during warfarin and treatment. Oral contraceptives (OC) have been shown to affect protein S level.[45] Because protein S is distributed in plasma in two forms (free protein S and that bound to C4b-BP), a decrease of the total protein S level as a result of OC use may result in a more significant decrease of the active form, the free protein S. In addition, the thromboembolic complications of OC use are often associated with periods of physiologic stress, such as the postoperative period and during episodes of trauma and infection. Because C4b-BP is an acute-phase reactant, an elevated level of C4b-BP could shift the protein S to the complexed inactive form. This shift in protein S could further compromise the already reduced free protein S level found in OC users and thus might be a predisposing factor to thrombosis. L-Asparaginase inhibits protein synthesis in leukemic cells. This accounts for its therapeutic effect in acute lymphoblastic leukemia but is also responsible for depression of a variety of proteins synthesized in the liver. The affected coagulation factors are fibrinogen, AT-III, protein C, and protein S.[46] These findings probably account for enhancement of thromboembolic risk in patients with predisposing factors such as immobilization, obesity, damage of vascular endothelium, or release of procoagulants from neoplastic cells.

Thrombosis and Malignancy Activation of coagulation is a fundamental event in the pathogenesis of tumor growth and metastasis.[2] Venous thrombosis may be the first indication of malignancy in an otherwise healthy individual.[47] Among the most common coagulation abnormalities reported in several large series of cancer patients are elevation of fibrin(ogen) deg-

TABLE 30–6 **Causes of Acquired Defects of Coagulation Inhibitors**	
Inhibitors	**Causes of Acquired Defects**
AT III	DIC Liver disease Nephrotic therapy Oral contraceptives L-Asparaginase
Protein C	Oral anticoagulant treatment DIC Vitamin K deficiency Newborn infants After plasma exchange Postoperative state L-Asparaginase Liver disease
Protein S	Oral anticoagulant treatment Pregnancy Oral contraceptives Vitamin K deficiency Liver disease Diabetes type I Acute inflammation Newborn infants

radation products (FDPs) and an increase or a decrease of fibrinogen, factors V and VIII, and other clotting factors. Several studies have revealed elevated levels of plasma fibrinopeptide A in almost all patients with acute leukemia.[46] It should be emphasized that none of the clotting tests currently available is specific for cancer. More recently, a study postulated the possible role of thrombospondin, a large platelet-secreted protein that promotes platelet aggregation and cell adhesion, in the mediation of tumor cell metastasis.[48] This study suggested that thrombospondin may play a role in the development of human metastatic colorectal carcinoma.

Thrombosis and Pregnancy A number of thrombogenic factors operate during normal pregnancy and delivery, including a decrease in fibrinolytic activity, an increase of plasma fibrinogen and factor VIII, and a release of tissue thromboplastin into the circulation at the time of placental separation. The hemostatic capacity appears to increase progressively during normal pregnancy. This may represent a physiologic adaptation to ensure efficient control of bleeding at the time of placental separation. A parallel reduction in TPA and increased PAI activities can be observed during normal pregnancy, with rapid return to nonpregnant levels post partum. D-dimer level is elevated during the third trimester. Although protein C and AT-III levels remain normal during pregnancy, both are decreased during pre-eclampsia. In normal pregnancy and pre-eclampsia, levels of both free and total forms of protein S are decreased[49] (see Table 30-6). A decrease in functional protein S activity during the early puerperium may be connected with the risk of developing thrombotic episodes during the postpartum period. Fibronectin may be a valuable marker for the detection of pre-eclamptic states.[50]

Thrombosis and Major Trauma Deep vein thrombosis and pulmonary embolism are common complications after major trauma. Five independent risk factors for deep vein thrombosis following major trauma have been defined.[51] These include older age, blood transfusions given, surgery, fracture of the femur or tibia, and spinal cord injury, which are associated with a higher risk of thrombosis. In one study in which prophylaxis was *not* used, 58% of patients admitted to the trauma unit developed deep vein thrombosis in their lower extremities.[51] In addition, deep vein thrombosis was found in 50% of patients with major injuries involving the face, chest, or abdomen; 54% of patients with major head injuries; 62% with spinal injuries; and 69% with lower-extremity orthopedic injuries.[51] Thrombi were detected in 80% of patients with femoral fracture, 77% with tibial fractures, and 61% with pelvic fractures.[51] As a result, safe and effective prophylactic treatment is necessary in patients with major trauma.

Disseminated Intravascular Coagulation Recognition of the simultaneous formation of thrombin and plasmin in the appropriate clinical setting is the definition of the diagnosis of DIC. The pathogenesis of DIC in most instances is the generation of procoagulant material with secondary fibrinolysis. Using a specific hemagglutination assay for fibrin monomers (FS test), results of this assay will remain positive in most cases of DIC, thus showing that thrombin is being generated

during the early activation stage of DIC. Whereas an acute DIC is usually characterized with a hemorrhagic syndrome, the diagnosis of subacute or chronic DIC is suggested by the presence of unexplained thrombosis in patients suspected or proven to have an underlying malignancy or who have mucin-producing adenocarcinomas. Chronic DIC develops in as many as 25% of pregnant women in whom a dead fetus has been retained for more than 5 weeks. Whatever the etiology and the severity of the DIC, AT-III, protein C, fibronectin, and other plasma protein levels are decreased. Although depressed levels are probably not helpful in the diagnosis of DIC, recognition of their presence may be important in the pathogenesis and may suggest modes of therapy.[52] Other laboratory findings associated with DIC include an acquired aberrant decrease of α_1-antitrypsin, perhaps reflecting the inhibition of activated protein C.

Suggested Test Panel for Recurrent Thrombosis

When a thrombotic disorder is suspected in a young patient, the coagulation laboratory can aid the clinician in (1) assessing the prothrombotic or prethrombotic state, (2) detecting an activated coagulation state, and (3) monitoring anticoagulant therapy. A particular area of concern for both clinicians and laboratories is the proper interpretation of the test results, especially when there is a familial history of thrombotic events. Labeling a patient with a hereditary disease such as protein C or S deficiency has significant ramifications. Because these disorders are autosomal-dominant, 50% of the family members may potentially be affected. Therefore the laboratory and physician must be absolutely sure that the diagnosis is correct. Two factors are critical: drawing an appropriate blood sample and doing family studies for substantiation. The laboratory studies and tests for recurrent thrombosis should follow the panel shown on Table 30-7.

TABLE 30-7 Suggested Test Panel for Recurrent Thrombosis

Test	Recommended Methodology
Protein C	Functional and antigenic assay
Protein S	Antigenic assay for total and free forms (functional assay preferable when available)
AT-III	Functional assay
Fibrinogen	Clauss method (clot-based assay)
Plasminogen	Functional assay
LA test	Increased phospholipid: PNP Decreased phospholipid: dRVVT
APA	ELISA for APA IgG and IgM
PAI-1 and TPA	Functional and antigenic assay (before and after venous occlusion)
TPA—PAI-1 complexes	Antigenic assay

Abbreviation: dRVVT = dilute Russell viper venom time.

ANTITHROMBOTIC THERAPIES AND MONITORING

Administration of intravenous heparin followed by long-term oral anticoagulants is the therapy of choice for most patients with DVT. Warfarin sodium, a dicumarol derivative, is now the most popular vitamin K antagonist used in the United States. Low-molecular-weight heparin (LMWH) preparations are commercially available and may well replace standard heparin because it is easier to administer and does not require laboratory monitoring. LMWHs have been reported to be safe and effective for the prevention and treatment of venous thromboembolism. Finally, AT-III concentrates are available commercially and there is still controversy on their use in prophylaxis and treatment of venous thromboembolism. In addition, protein C concentrates are available commercially but are not FDA-approved and can be used only for compassionate use (when no other treatment is available).

Vitamin K Antagonists: Oral Anticoagulants

Mechanism of Action

All the vitamin K–dependent coagulation proteins, factors II, VII, IX, and X, protein C, and protein S, are characterized in their structure by a specific chain where some glutamic acid residues undergo a gamma-carboxylation. This gamma-carboxylation is vitamin K–dependent. The presence of these carboxylated groups is necessary for the binding of calcium ions required for the formation of the various activation complexes during the activation of the coagulation. The classic oral anticoagulants present a structural similarity with vitamin K. Therefore these anticoagulants are able to inhibit the regeneration step of reduced vitamin K (Fig. 30–7). Because the reduced vitamin K, together with a carboxylase activity, is needed to convert the precursors of the vitamin K–dependent coagulation factors into the zymogens that are further activated to form the active coagulation enzymes, the inhibition of the reduced vitamin K by dicumarol-type anticoagulants blocks the final synthesis step of these vitamin K–dependent proteins. The peak effect of the vitamin K antagonists does not occur until 36 to 72 hours after drug administration. Indeed, the effect of the drug is delayed until the normal clotting factors are cleared from the circulation. The rate of disappearance of the coagulation factors depends on their in vivo half-life (Fig. 30–8). Factor VII and protein C have similar half-lives (6 to 7 hours). Their respective levels fall during the initiation of the therapy, whereas the levels of functionally active factors II, IX, X, and protein S remain normal. That explains why, during the initiation of oral anticoagulation, the drug has the potential to be thrombogenic. This is because the low level of factor VII is counteracted by the low level of protein C, with

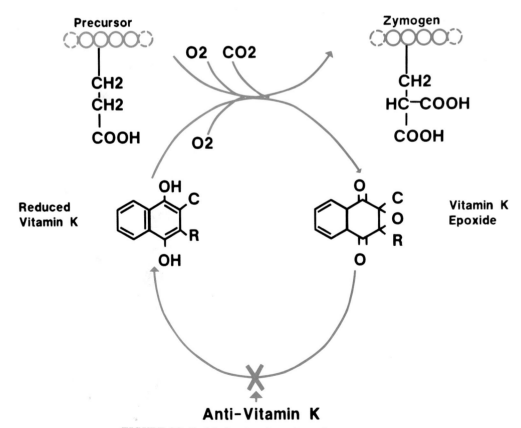

FIGURE 30–7   Mechanism for action of anti-vitamin K.

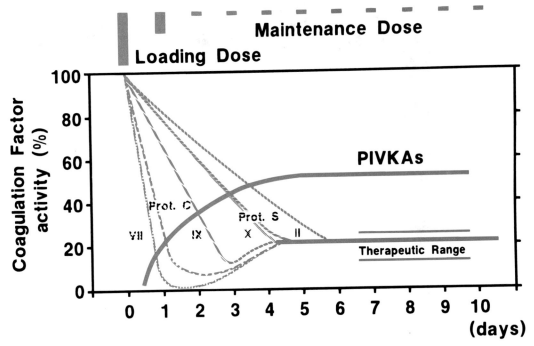

Maintenance Dose

Loading Dose

PIVKAs = Proteins Induced by Vitamin K Antagonist or Absence

FIGURE 30-8 PIVKAs = Proteins induced by vitamin K antagonist or absense: Effect of oral anticoagulants on plasma activity of vitamin K-dependent coagulation factors. (From Loeliger, EA: In AMHP van der Besselaar et al., (eds): Thromboplastin Calibration and Oral Anticoagulant Control, Martinus Nijhoff, Boston, 1984. p 2, with permission.)

almost normal levels of procoagulant factors II, IX, and X. These factors drop after 72 to 96 hours and then the anticoagulant properties of the anticoagulant drug can be expressed. This justifies the need for an overlapping of oral anticoagulant therapy with heparin therapy for 3 to 4 days.

Clinical Applications

The clinical use of warfarin has been established in: (1) prevention of DVT (warfarin is effective for DVT prophylaxis following hip fractures, hip surgery, and possibly other forms of general abdominal surgery); (2) long-term use following pulmonary embolism and DVT; (3) prevention of arterial emboli originating from the heart; and (4) acute myocardial infarction.

Laboratory Monitoring

The most common laboratory test used to monitor oral anticoagulant therapy is the conventional prothrombin time (PT). The PT evaluates the extrinsic pathway of the coagulation. Therefore it is sensitive to the decrease of factors II, VII, and X. However, the PT does not reflect the effect of the drug on factor IX.

Further confusion about the appropriate therapeutic range has occurred because the available reagents used for the determination of the PT may vary in sensitivity to the vitamin K–dependent factors and in response to the drug. Numerous international trials have shown that considerable differences may exist in the

same plasma, depending not only on the origin of the reagent but also on the method used to read the test. Therefore, each reagent should have its own therapeutic range defined, using the World Health Organization (WHO)–recommended standardization protocol. The target value corresponding to the best balance between the prevention of thrombosis and the hemorrhagic risk is a function of the therapeutic indication and the clinical context. The desired anticoagulation required, usually low in presurgical situations or for prophylaxis of thrombosis, is expected to be higher in the prevention or the treatment of recurrent venous thrombosis, and even more so in arterial thrombosis or after implant of heart valves (Table 30–8).

To promote standardization of the PT for monitoring oral anticoagulant therapy, the WHO has developed an international reference thromboplastin from human brain tissue and has recommended that the PT ratio be expressed as the international normalized ratio (INR).[53] The INR value for a plasma depends on the international sensitivity index (ISI) of the reagent used. To determine the sensitivity of a given reagent, PTs obtained with it are graphed against values obtained on the same specimens using the WHO standard. A linear plot is usually obtained, the slope of which is defined as the ISI. The INR is calculated from the following formula:

$$INR = \left(\frac{\text{Patient value, in seconds}}{\text{Control value, in seconds}}\right)^{ISI}$$

TABLE 30–8 Recommended Therapeutic Range for Oral Anticoagulant Treatment		
Condition	**INR**	**Patient/Control PT Ratio**
Prophylaxis of deep venous thrombosis in high-risk medical or surgical patients	2.0–3.0	1.2–1.5
Treatment of deep venous thrombosis	2.0–3.0	1.2–1.5
Prevention of embolism	2.0–3.0	1.2–1.5
Prevention of recurrent embolism, or patients with mechanical prosthetic intravascular valves	3.0–4.5	1.5–2.0

Heparin Therapy

Structure and Heterogeneity of Standard Heparin

Heparin consists of unbranched oligosaccharide chains of varying lengths (and thus molecular weights). This natural oligosaccharide is present in mastocytes and is industrially extracted from ox lung and pork intestine. Heparin is composed of alternating units of D-glucosamine and either D-glucuronic acid or L-iduronic acid (Fig. 30–9). A variety of substitutions may occur at various sites on these basic sugars. These substitutions include the following:

For R1: —H or —OSO3
For R2: —S03 or —COCH3

The molecular weight of heparin varies from 3000 to 30,000 d with a distribution peak of about 13,000 to 15,000 d. Although the length of polysaccharide chains varies, a pentasaccharide structure that is randomly distributed along the polysaccharide chains of heparin has been identified and then synthesized.[54] In the heparins used in therapy, only one third of the polysaccharide chains carries the pentasaccharide sequence responsible for the binding to AT-III. This fraction of high affinity for AT-III is responsible for most of the anticoagulant and antithrombotic functions of heparin.

Anticoagulant Activity of Heparin

Classically, the coagulation factors are bound on the phospholipid surface of platelets or tissue. The enzymatic cascade leads to the generation of thrombin, which is then released from the phospholipid environment. In this environment, the other coagulation factors are protected from the inhibition by heparin–

AT-III complex. Therefore, thrombin, the only free coagulation enzyme, is preferentially inhibited by the heparin–AT-III complex, whereas the phospholipid-bound factors IXa and Xa are little inhibited.

Thrombin participates in its own formation by activating the platelets and the cofactors V and VIII. Any inhibition of thrombin has an impact on these feedback mechanisms and leads to more thrombin inhibition. However, during the platelet activation by thrombin, the PF 4 is released from the granules of platelets and inhibits heparin.

Thus, the complexity of the anticoagulant mechanism of heparin is related to its initial target, which is thrombin inhibition. At low doses, heparin inhibits the first traces of thrombin generated, then slows down the thrombin generation. At high doses, heparin inhibits the thrombin entirely, making the blood uncoagulable.

In addition, many other actions of heparin are known, apart from its effects on the blood coagulation, such as enzyme inhibition, tumor growth inhibition, and antibacterial activity.

Pharmacokinetics of Heparin

After intravenous (IV) administration, heparin is cleared from the blood through two distinct mechanisms. The first system is composed of the reticuloendothelial cells that bind heparin with a high affinity, then internalize before degrading heparin by desulfatation and depolymerization. The second mechanism is renal filtration. If used at therapeutic doses, heparin is principally cleared through the cellular system, which is extremely effective. At higher doses, the clearance capacity of the reticuloendothelial system (RES) mechanism is saturated, and the excess of heparin

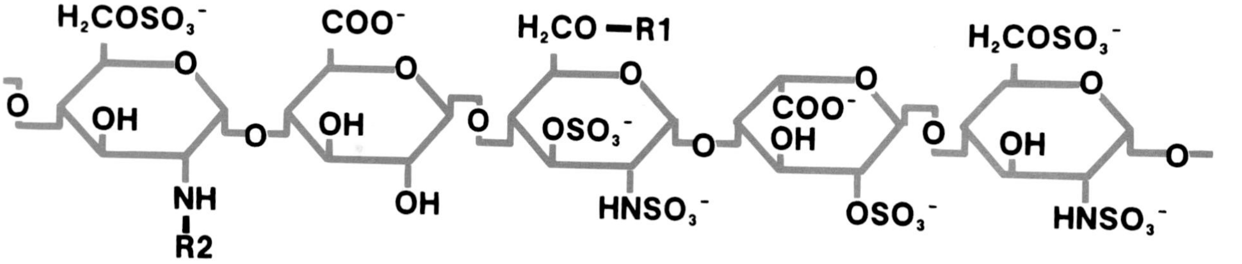

FIGURE 30–9 Heparin structure.

present in the blood is passively filtrated by the kidney. These features explain why the half-life of heparin increases with the dose administered and why, above a certain dose, the clearance curve of heparin loses its linearity and becomes concavoconvex. As an indication, the half-life of heparin after an IV injection of 60 IU/kg is about 1 h with a wide intersubject variability (30 to 90 min).[55] Standard heparin can be administered subcutaneously (SC). In this case the activity peak is obtained 2 to 4 hours after the time of the injection. The half-life depends on the level of the peak. It is classically admitted that the bioavailability of SC heparin is 30% of what is obtained with IV heparin. However, it has been shown that during curative heparinotherapy of DVT, the total heparin levels required to treat the patients are equivalent, whatever the route of drug administration. Thus, the bioavailability of the SC heparin increases with the dose administered and can reach 100% with the doses used for a curative therapy.

In 1982, Bjornsson and Wolfrom[56] showed the intersubject variability in the anticoagulant response to heparin in vitro. Several other authors have described the in vivo intersubject and circadian variability in heparin sensitivity with obvious implications in the method of choice for the monitoring of heparin.

Clinical Applications

Although the use of long-term warfarin therapy for the treatment of venous thromboembolism is well established, heparin has been proposed as the therapy of choice in treatment of DVT[57] 30 years after its discovery. Later it was suggested that it might be of use in prevention of thrombotic complications following vascular surgery,[58] myocardial infarction,[59] and extracorporeal circulation.[60] It must be emphasized that all treatment with heparin is prophylactic—either primary (to prevent thromboembolism) or secondary (to limit previous thromboembolism). The administration of heparin postoperatively in full therapeutic dose is often accompanied by bleeding complications. Subsequently, administration of small doses of heparin has been shown to prevent venous thrombosis and pulmonary embolism. A large number of clinical trials have been conducted to establish the efficacy of low-dose heparin therapy. Further studies suggested that the combined administration of low-dose heparin with dihydroergotamine may have greater efficacy than low-dose heparin alone.

In regard to the prevention of arterial thromboembolism, a renewed interest in heparin came from the observation that arterial thrombosis is not totally a platelet-driven event but is also coagulation factor–dependent. This concept was emphasized after the results of treating coronary thrombosis with thrombolytic agents.

Other studies have examined the use of heparin in patients with unstable angina. When used to treat patients with active thrombosis, heparin should be administered in doses large enough to prolong results of an appropriate coagulation test to within a defined anticoagulant level. The anticoagulant effect is usually achieved by an initial IV bolus injection of heparin, which is then followed by continuous infusion, inter-

mittent IV injection, or SC injection. The efficiency and safety of heparin given by either one or the other administration route have been compared in various prospective, randomized studies. It is possible that the incidence of bleeding during heparin therapy is related more to the total daily dose of heparin given than to its method of administration. The indications for heparin therapy are summarized in Table 30–9.

Limitations of Standard Heparin

Several limitations have been well documented for the use of standard heparin, even though it is effective in the prevention and treatment of thrombotic disorders. These include: (1) the unpredictable anticoagulant response in patients, (2) the requirement for careful laboratory monitoring, (3) the narrow benefit-to-risk ratio, and (4) the limited activity of heparin against clot-bound thrombin.[3] The narrow benefit-to-risk ratio may be defined by the fact that patients given subtherapeutic doses have a high risk of recurrent thrombotic events and overly aggressive high doses can be associated with hemorrhage.

The complicated clearance mechanism of heparin is responsible for its variable anticoagulant response. As a result, standard heparin binds to endothelial cells, matrix proteins, and macrophages, which are rapidly cleared through a saturable, dose-dependent mechanism.[3] In addition, standard heparin also binds to a variety of plasma proteins (Table 30–10).

TABLE 30–9   Indications for Heparin Therapy

Heparin Regimens	Clinical Use
Full therapeutic dose	Treatment of acute thromboembolism DVT Pulmonary embolism Acute myocardial infarction Arterial thrombosis
Low-dose	Prophylaxis of venous thromboembolism Postsurgery Stroke, acute myocardial infarction Pregnancy Thrombotic tendency
Adjusted dose	DIC Extracorporeal circulation Hemodialysis Pregnancy Prosthetic heart valves

---

TABLE 30–10   Plasma Proteins to Which Standard Heparin Binds Nonspecifically

Fibronectin
Histidine-rich glycoprotein
Vitronectin
Platelet factor 4
Von Willebrand factor

Low-Molecular-Weight Heparins

The low-molecular-weight heparins (LMWHs) are defined as products that have been developed from standard heparin by extraction processes or by controlled chemical or enzymatic depolymerization. The molecular weight of these fragments ranges from 1000 to 10,000 d, with a mean of 5000 d, approximately one third the size of standard heparin.[61] The LMWHs have antithrombin (anti-IIa) activity that is low compared with their anti-Xa activities. They are very efficiently absorbed from subcutaneous injection and have a longer half-life than standard heparins. The LMWHs act as anticoagulants by catalyzing the inactivation of thrombin and factor Xa by antithrombin III, similar to standard heparin.[61] In contrast to heparin, however, only 25% to 50% of the LMWH chains are of sufficient length to bind to both thrombin and AT-III.[3] As a result, unlike standard heparin, which has equivalent inhibitory activity against thrombin and Xa, the LMWH preparations have an anti-factor Xa-to-anti-thrombin ratio of 4:1 to 2:1, depending on their molecular weight distributions.[62] The LMWHs bind to AT-III and do not interact with platelets to the same degree as standard heparin. Therefore they may be less likely to cause bleeding in the treated patients. The LMWHs are effective as antithrombotic agents, particularly in prevention of DVT.

Currently a number of LMWH preparations have been approved by the FDA and are commercially available (Fragmin, Lovenox). These products have been proven safe and effective for the prevention and treatment of venous thromboembolism[63-65] (Table 30–11).

Advantages of LMWH

One of the major advantages of LMWHs is that these preparations produce a more predictable anticoagulant response in comparison to standard heparin.[3] This is because of the properties of the LMWH chains, which show little or no nonspecific binding to plasma proteins; therefore, the clearance of LMWH is dose-independent. As a result, laboratory monitoring is unnecessary. In addition, LMWH produces less bleeding than standard heparin in therapeutic doses. Table 30–12 summarizes and lists all the currently reported advantages of LMWHs over standard heparin.[3]

Antithrombin III Concentrates

AT-III (human) is licensed for use in the United States to treat and prevent thrombotic episodes in patients with hereditary AT-III deficiency. It has been used more extensively for over a decade in Europe to treat patients with a variety of conditions that lead to the development of venous thromboses associated with an acquired AT-III deficiency.[62]

Hereditary AT-III deficiency is associated with a high frequency of multiple venous thrombosis and pulmonary embolism because of low levels of AT-III.[66] Traditionally, replacement therapy using AT-III concentrate (with and without heparin) has been effective in treating and preventing thrombosis in the patients.[67]

Several pathologic conditions, including acute venous thrombosis, liver disease, general and orthopedic surgery, and disseminated intravascular coagulation (DIC) have been reported to be associated with acquired AT-III deficiency. AT-III concentrates have been used in a variety of these conditions to increase AT-III levels. The administration of AT-III concentrates together with heparin have been reported to be more effective than Dextran in preventing thrombotic complications following hip and knee arthroplasty.[68-70]

However, the effectiveness of AT-III concentrates in other conditions associated with thrombosis caused

TABLE 30–11 **Prophylaxis of Venous Thromboembolism**		
Category	**Complication**	**Treatment**
Orthopedic Surgery	Deep vein thrombosis (DVT)	LMWH, low-intensity warfarin Low-dose heparin or dextran
Total hip replacement (THR)	DVT	LMWH > Low-dose heparin or dextran LMWH = Low-intensity warfarin*
Total knee replacement (TKR)	DVT	LMWH > Low-intensity warfarin*
Hip fracture	DVT	LMWH > dextran LMWH = Low-intensity warfarin*
Medical and Surgery Patients	Venous thromboembolism (VT)	LMWH, Low-dose heparin Organon heparinoid
Medical patients (i.e., myocardial infarction)	VT	*LMWH = Low-dose heparin†
General surgery	VT	*LMWH = Low-dose heparin‡
Acute stroke	VT	LMWH = Organon heparinoid (organan)
Spinal cord injury	VT	LMWH > heparin

*Warfarin is cheaper but requires careful laboratory monitoring.
†Requires fewer injections and produces fewer hematomas at injection sites.
‡LMWH reduces the risk of thrombosis and pulmonary embolism to a greater extent than standard heparin.
= Similar in efficacies
> more effective

TABLE 30–12 **Advantages of LMWH**
Predictable anticoagulant response
No need for laboratory monitoring
Longer half-life when given in fixed doses (allows dosing once per day)
Greater bioavailability at low doses
Less bleeding when given in therapeutic doses
Lower incidence of heparin-induced thrombocytopenia

TABLE 30–13 **Assays for Monitoring Heparin**	
Test	**Comment**
APTT	Most commonly used test
	Inaccurate at fibrinogen level <75 mg/dL
Thrombin time	Evaluates anti-IIa* effect of heparin
	Extremely sensitive to heparin, but also to elevated FDPs and to hypofibrinogenemia
	Not commonly used in US for heparin monitoring
Heparin assays	Residual added Xa or IIa is measured by clotting assay or by cleavage of chromogenic substrate; clotting time or color development is inversely proportional to heparin concentration
Anti-Xa† clotting assay	
Anti-IIa or anti-Xa chromogenic assay	Easy to automate or standardize
	Anti-Xa chromogenic or clotting assay may be monitoring assays of choice for LMWH

Source: Courtesy of American Bioproducts Co.
*IIa = thrombin.
†Xa = activated factor X.

by an acquired AT-III deficiency is still controversial and requires additional studies.[71]

Monitoring of Heparin Therapy

Because of the potent in vivo anticoagulant activity of heparin, monitoring is justified to improve the antithrombotic efficacy of heparin and to reduce the risk of bleeding. Adjustment of dosage is another implication of the laboratory monitoring required to achieve effective heparin treatment.

Influence of Sample Collection and Storage However accurate may be the assay of heparin in plasma, its partial inactivation during the time lapse between blood collection and laboratory assay decreases the reliability of the methods for monitoring heparin therapy. This inactivation of heparin is mainly because of PF 4 or to other heparin-binding proteins. Various options have been proposed for preventing heparin inactivation during blood centrifugation and storage. Current recommendation refutes chilling the specimen after the plasma is separated because PF 4 released by platelets will cause agglutination when exposed to colder temperatures. Blood collected in combinations of citric acid, theophylline, adenosine, and dipyridamole—CTAD mixture—was found to greatly reduce the heparin loss during blood centrifugation and storage.[72]

Laboratory Tests for Heparin Monitoring The development of new heparins by manufacturers, as well as the need for more clinical trials, led to a dramatic evolution of the methods used by the control authorities and subsequently by the clinical laboratories for assessment of the heparinization level in patients.

The most popular test remains the activated partial thromboplastin time (APTT). In 1973, specific methods based on the heparin ability to neutralize factor Xa (anti-Xa assay) or factor IIa (anti-IIa assay) in plasma were developed. The introduction of chromogenic substrates methodology then paved the way for standardization of the methods and use of pharmacologic approach of monitoring heparin therapy (Table 30–13). In a limited number of laboratories protamine sulfate titrations are performed for heparin monitoring, although this procedure is tedious and very time-consuming. In addition, some reference laboratories perform direct measurement of heparin by radioimmunoassay.

Activated Partial Thromboplastin Time The sensitivity of heparin by the various commercially available APTT reagents shows considerable variation. The logic of the APTT system and its simplicity all contribute to its popularity. However, for heparin monitoring, the response of the particular APTT reagent used must be known. Individual variation in the APTT response to heparin may reflect variation in coagulation factor levels. Classically high factor VIII levels in an acute phase reaction is the main cause of a shortened APTT. This short APTT may be misinterpreted as a low response to heparin. Presence of abnormal inhibitors such as lupus anticoagulant (LA) may lead to prolonged baseline APTT.

Thrombin Time Heparin prolongs the coagulation of plasma in the presence of thrombin. Modified thrombin times have been used for heparin monitoring. However, this test may also respond to the existence of low fibrinogen and the presence of FDPs. One may note that the antithrombin level influences the thrombin clotting time, particularly at low heparin concentration.

Anti-Xa Assay: Clot-Based Method The assessment of the anti-Xa effect of heparin by this method gives a high sensitivity in detecting low heparin levels. This assay is influenced by the level of AT-III and FDPs. However, this method is less sensitive to individual variation than is the popular APTT. This assay is easily automated. It is standardized and may also be used to monitor LMWH therapy or low-dose heparin therapy.

Anti-Xa Assay: Chromogenic Substrates The introduction of synthetic substrates in the evaluation of coagulation began a new era in monitoring of heparin. The endpoint is read by an instrument, and the precision is higher than for clotting assays. The assay that follows is a modification of the original amidolytic assay:

1. Heparin + AT-III Heparin-AT-III complex
2. Heparin-AT-III + Xa Heparin-AT-III-Xa + residual Xa
3. R-pNA + residual Xa R—COOH + pNA* (yellow)

---

*Denotes chromogen.

If the test plasma is the only source of AT-III, a combined heparin–AT-III activity is measured. It would be reasonable to monitor heparin therapy in venous thrombosis by either the heparin level or global tests such as the APTT. If the heparin level is used, it should be maintained above 0.2 to 0.3 IU/mL at all times, with an upper limit of 0.5 IU/mL. If the APTT is used, it should be adjusted to 1.5 to 2 times the mean of the normal laboratory control subject.

Thrombolytic Therapy

In recent years, thrombolytic therapy has become the treatment of choice for eligible patients with acute myocardial infarction. As a consequence, the clinical use of thrombolytic therapy has increased rapidly from the small number of patients treated with these agents for DVT, pulmonary embolism, and blocked arteriovenous shunts. Monitoring of effectiveness and of bleeding complications has been the primary focus of most of the studies related to thrombolytic therapy. Several thrombolytic agents have been made available for clinical use. The aim of these drugs is to activate plasminogen into the active form plasmin. The exact mechanism of activation of plasminogen differs according to the thrombolytic agent.

Thrombolytic Agents

These agents may be classified into two groups according to their mechanism of action: (1) nonfibrin-specific plasminogen activators, which cause the conversion of plasminogen to plasmin (in this group, streptokinase and urokinase are the most widely used); and (2) fibrin-specific agents such as tissue plasminogen activator (TPA), prourokinase, and acylated plasminogen streptokinase activated complex (APSAC).

Streptokinase forms a stoichiometric complex with plasminogen leading to a modification of plasminogen, allowing the complex to activate plasminogen to plasmin. Therefore, streptokinase infusion to patients is usually associated with a systemic fibrinolytic state characterized by a plasminogen activation, a depletion of α_1-antiplasmin (the circulating physiologic inhibitor of plasmin), and fibrinogen breakdown. This mechanism implies that the streptokinase-plasminogen complex activates circulating plasminogen and fibrin-associated plasminogen equally and thus lacks significant fibrin specificity. Streptokinase is antigenic for humans and the in vivo half-life is less than 10 minutes. In contrast, urokinase is a human protein and is therefore nonantigenic. Like streptokinase, urokinase also has a minimal fibrin specificity. Its mode of action is a direct activation of plasminogen.

TPA is a fibrin-specific lytic agent. It forms a ternary complex with plasminogen on the fibrin surface. Thus, plasmin is generated directly on the surface of the fibrin clot to be lysed. Basically, fibrin increases the local plasminogen concentration by creating the interaction between TPA and plasminogen. The plasmin produced on the fibrin surface is protected from its inhibitor, α_2-antiplasmin. The in vivo half-life of TPA is less than 10 minutes.

APSAC is prepared by acylation of the plasminogen molecule's serine active site, which temporarily inac-

---

TABLE 30–14 Baseline Studies for Monitoring of Fibrinolytic Therapy

- All patients
  PT
  APTT
  CBC (with platelet count)
- Patients receiving non-fibrin-specific agents
  Thrombin time or fibrinogen assay

Source: Courtesy of American Bioproducts Co.

---

tivates it. In vivo, the APSAC binds to both fibrin and fibrinogen and the deacylation occurs relatively quickly at sites of fibrin formation but more slowly in plasma. As a result, a more sustained fibrinolytic effect occurs and the in vivo half-life of APSAC is approximately 90 minutes.

Laboratory Monitoring During Fibrinolytic Therapy

The goal for monitoring of thrombolytic therapy is twofold:

1. To predict which patients are at greatest risk for bleeding and to guide therapy
2. To assess the status of the hemostatic system before coronary artery bypass grafting in the patient who has recently received fibrinolytic therapy

A baseline study of the hemostatic functions is always indicated regardless of the underlying clinical condition being treated and the lytic agent of choice (Table 30–14). Classically, this baseline study consists of the evaluation of PT, APTT, complete blood count (CBC) in all patients, and fibrinogen assay, using the Clauss method (clotting method) or thrombin time. Then, during the therapy, it is useful to determine the extent of the coagulopathy for patients who are demonstrating significant hemorrhage. This information may guide the clinician in deciding whether or not to transfuse with substitutive products. Thrombin time and APTT show a prolongation in these patients with persistent lytic state. However, because thrombin time, as well as APTT, is affected by the presence of therapeutic heparin in these patients, it has been recently emphasized that the Reptilase time may be a more adequate method to evaluate the patients at risk of hemorrhagic complication. The Clauss fibrinogen assay is also preferred because heparin levels in the therapeutic range do not affect the test.

In summary, the only useful routine monitoring of thrombolytic therapy consists of pretreatment baseline studies and evaluation of the presence of a lytic state in patients treated with more or less nonfibrin-specific agents.[73]

CASE STUDY

A 53-year-old woman visited her doctor complaining of pain and swelling in her right calf. Physical examination revealed cyanotic coloration around her ankle, absence of pedal pulse, and sluggish capillary return in the skin. Her temperature was elevated. Previous medical history included a fractured femur and spinal cord injuries just 1 year before, caused by an automobile accident.

Laboratory studies are as follows:

PT	30 s (12–14 s)
INR	3.5
APTT	40 s (<35 s)
TT	28 s (15 s)
Fibrinogen	100 mg/dL (200–450 mg/dL)
FDP	>40 μg/mL (4.9 +/− 2.8 μg/mL)

This patient was started on heparin therapy, followed by Coumadin at 5 mg a day. Heparin was stopped in 2 weeks. Long-term oral anticoagulant therapy continued for 5 months and the prothrombin time was maintained at 20 to 22 seconds, with an average INR of 2.5. All other coagulation studies remained normal. This is a case of DVT resulting from previous trauma.

Questions

1. Why were fibrinogen degradation products increased in this patient?
2. Why was this patient initially treated with heparin?
3. What coagulation factors are affected by warfarin drugs?

REFERENCES

1. Egeberg, O: Inherited antithrombin deficiency causing thrombophilia. Thromb Diath Hemorrh 13:516, 1965.
2. Nordstrom, M, et al: Deep venous thrombosis and occult malignancy: An epidemiological study. Br Med J 308:891, 1994.
3. Bauer, K, et al: Coagulation/Hemostasis. ASH Educational Program Book. American Society of Hematology Annual Meeting, Nashville, TN, 1994.
4. Stump, D and Mann, KG: Mechanisms of thrombus formation. Ann Emerg Med 17:1138, 1988.
5. Almer, LO and Ohlin, H: Elevated levels of the rapid inhibitor of plasminogen activator (t-PAI) in acute myocardial infarction. Thromb Res 47:335, 1987.
6. Rosenberg, RD and Bauer, KA: Prothrombinase generation and the regulation of coagulation. In Loscalzo, J (ed): Thrombosis and Hemorrhage. Blackwell Scientific, Boston, 1994, p 21.
7. Bauer, K: Natural Anticoagulants and the Prethrombotic State. In Handin RI (ed): Blood: Principles and Practice of Hematology. JB Lippincott, Philadelphia, 1995, p 1320.
8. Birginshaw, GF and Shanberg, JN: Identification of two distinct cofactors in human plasma. Inhibition of thrombin and activated factor X. Thromb Res 4:463, 1974.
9. Tollefsen, DM, Majerus, DW, and Blank, MK: Heparin cofactor II: Purification and properties of a heparin-dependent inhibitor of thrombin in human plasma. J Biol Chem 257:2161, 1982.
10. Toulon, P, Aiach, M, and Gianese, F: In vitro study of a new potential antithrombotic drug MF 701 (dermatan sulfate). Ann NY Acad Sci 556:486, 1989.
11. Toulon, P, et al: Heparin cofactor II in patients with deep venous thrombosis under heparin and oral anticoagulant therapy. Thromb Res 49:497, 1988.
12. Neumann, CB, Wolf, M, and Larrieu, MJ: Protein C and Protein S: Methodological and Clinical Aspects. In Shearer, MJ, Vitamin K Dependent Protein: Analytical, Physiological, and Clinical Aspects, CRC Press, Boca Raton, FL, 1993, p 144.
13. Ibid. p 144.
14. Walker, FJ: Structural and Functional Properties of Protein C. In Hoyer, LW and Drohan, WN (eds): Recombinant Technology in Hemostasis and Thrombosis. Plenum Press, New York, 1991, p 81.
15. Bauer, K: Natural Anticoagulants and the Prethrombotic State. In Handlin, RI (ed): Blood: Principles and Practice. JB Lippincott, Philadelphia 1995, p 1321.
16. Bauer, K and Rosenberg, RD: Prothrombinase generation and the regulation of coagulation. In Loscalzo, J and Schafer, AI (eds): Thrombosis and Hemorrhage. Blackwell Scientific, Boston, 1994, p 17.
17. Suzuki, K, Nishioka, J, and Hashimoto, S: Protein C Inhibitor: Purification from human plasma and characterization. J Biol Chem 258:163, 1983.
18. Marlar, RA and Griffin, JH: Deficiency of protein C in combined factor V/VIII deficiency disease. J Clin Invest 66:1186, 1980.
19. Canfield, WM and Kiesel, W: Evidence of normal functional levels of activated protein C inhibitor in combined V/VIII deficiency disease. J Clin Invest 70:1260, 1982.
20. Suzuki, K, et al: Protein C inhibitor: Structure and function. Thromb Haemost 61:337, 1989.
21. Hieb, MJ, Bischool, R, Courtney, M, and Griffin, JH: Inhibition of activated protein C by recombinant alpha-1 antitrypsin variant with substitution of arginine for leucine for methionine. J Biol Chem 265:2365, 1990.
22. Van der Meer, FJM, et al: A second plasma inhibitor of activated protein C: Alpha 1-antitrypsin. Thromb Haemost 62:763, 1989.
23. Bachmann, F: Laboratory diagnosis of impairment of fibrinolysis in patients with thromboembolic disease. Semin Thromb Hemost 16:193, 1990.
24. Ouimet, H and Loscalzo, J: Fibrinolysis. In Loscalzo, J and Schafer, AI (eds): Thrombosis and Hemorrhage. Blackwell Scientific, Boston, 1994, p 134.
25. Ibid. p 811.
26. Johnson, EJ, Prentic, CRM, Parapia, LA: Premature arterial disease associated with familial antithrombin III deficiency. Thromb Haemost 63:13, 1990.
27. Tollefsen, DM: Laboratory diagnosis of antithrombin and heparin cofactor II deficiency. Semin Thromb Haemost 16:162, 1990.
28. Finazzi, F, Caccia, R, Burbui, T: Different prevalence of thromboembolism in the subtypes of congenital antithrombin III deficiency: Review of 404 cases. Thromb Haemost 58:1090, 1987.
29. Rick, ME: Protein C and Protein S: Vitamin K dependent inhibitors of blood coagulation. JAMA 263:701, 1990.
30. Neumann, CB, Wolf, M, and Larrieu, MJ: Op. cit. CRC Press, Boca Raton, FL, 1993, p 147.
31. Miletich, JP: Laboratory diagnosis of Protein C deficiency. Semin Thromb Haemost 16:169, 1990.
32. Berina, RM, et al: Hereditary heparin cofactor II deficiency and the risk of development of thrombosis. Thromb Haemost 57:196, 1987.
33. Martinolli, JL, Stocker, K: Fast functional protein C assay using PROTAC, a novel protein C activator. Thromb Res 43:253, 1986.
34. Waller, PA, Bauer, KA, McDonagh, J: A simple automated functional assay for protein C. Am J Clin Pathol 92:210, 1989.
35. Vasse, M, Borg, JY, Monconduitt, M: Protein C abnormality with low anticoagulant but normal amidolytic activity. Thromb Res 56:387, 1989.
36. Comp, P: Laboratory evaluation of Protein S status. Semin Thromb Haemost 16(2):178, 1990.
37. Poda, L, et al: A prothrombin time-based functional assay of Protein S. Thromb Res 60:19, 1990.
38. McNiel, HP, Chesterman, CN, Krilis, SA: Immunology and clinical importance of antiphospholipid antibodies. Adv Immunol 49:193, 1991.
39. Harris, EN: Antiphospholipid antibodies (annotation). Br J Haematol 74:1, 1990.
40. Beaumont, JL: Syndrome hémorragique acquis du à un anticorps circulant. Sangr 25:1, 1954.
41. Laurell, AB and Nilsson, IM: Hypergamma-globulinemia circulating anticoagulant and biologic false positive Was-

seman reaction: A study of 2 cases. J Lab Clin Med 49:694, 1957.

42. Soulier, JP and Boffa, MC: Avortemets a repetition, thromboses et anticoagulat circulant anti-prothrombinase. Nouv Presse Med 9:859, 1980.

43. Hughes, GVR: Thrombosis, abortion, cerebral disease and the lupus anticoagulant. Br Med J 287:1088, 1983.

44. Kushner, MJ: Prospective study of anticardiolipin antibodies in stroke. Stroke 21:295, 1990.

45. Bauer, KA: The biologic impact of hereditary defects that cause thrombosis. In Hoyer, LW and Drohan, WN (eds): Recombinant Technology in Hemostasis and Thrombosis. Plenum Press, New York, 1991, p 157.

46. Rodeghiero, F, Castaman, G and Dini, E: Fibrinopeptide A changes during remission induction treatment with L-Asparaginase in acute lymphoblastic leukemia: Evidence for blood activation. Thromb Res 57:31, 1990.

47. Donati, MB: Cancer and Thrombosis. Haemostasis 24:128, 1994.

48. Tuszinki, GP, et al: Thrombospondin mediates tumor cell metastasis (abstr). Thromb Haemost 62:22, 1989.

49. Nucei, MR and Bell, WR: Acquired hypercoagulable states. In Loscalzo, J and Schager, AI (eds): Thrombosis and Hemorrhage. Blackwell Scientific, Boston, 1994, p 845.

50. Mombaerts, P, et al: Fibrinolytic response to venous occlusion and fibrin fragment D-Dimer and fibronectin levels in normal and complicated pregnancy (abstr). Thromb Haemost 58:98, 1987.

51. Geerts, WH, Code, KI, Jay, RM, et al: A prospective study of venous thromboembolism after major trauma. N Engl J Med 331:1601, 1994.

52. Bick, RL: Disseminated Intravascular Coagulation: Objective criteria for diagnosis and treatment. Med Clin North Am 78:511, 1994.

53. Hirsh, J: Oral anticoagulant drugs. N Engl J Med 324:1865, 1991.

54. Freedman, JE and Adelman, N: Pharmacology of heparin and oral anticoagulants. In Loscalzo, J and Schafer, AI: Thrombosis and Hemorrhage, Blackwell Scientific, Boston, 1994, p 1157.

55. Ibid. p 1158.

56. Bjornsson, TD and Walfrom, KM: Intersubject variability in the anticoagulant response to heparin in vitro. Eur J Clin Pharmacol 21:491, 1982.

57. Murray, G: Heparin in surgical treatment of blood vessels. Arch Surg 40:307, 1940.

58. Jaques, LB: Heparins-anionic polyelectrolyte drugs. Pharmacol Rev 31:99, 1980.

59. Wright, IS, Marple, CD and Beck, DF: Report of the committee for the evaluation of heparin in the treatment of coronary thrombosis with myocardial infarction: A progress report on the statistical analysis of the first 800 cases by this committee. Am Heart J 36:801, 1948.

60. Best, CH, Cowan, C and MacLean, DL: Heparin and the formation of white thrombi. J Physiol 92:20, 1938.

61. Hirsh, J and Levine, MN: Low-molecular weight heparins. Blood 79:1, 1992.

62. Handlin, RI, Lux, SE, and Stossel, TP: Blood: Principles and Practice of Hematology. JB Lippincott, Philadelphia, 1995.

63. Green, D, et al: Low molecular weight heparin: A critical analysis of clinical trials. Pharmacol Rev 46:89, 1994.

64. Colwell, CW, et al for the Enoxaparin Clinical Trial Group: Use of enoxaparin, a low-molecular-weight heparin for the prevention of deep venous thrombosis after elective hip replacement. J Bone Joint Surg 76A:3, 1994.

65. Mensin, J, et al: Prevention of deep vein thrombosis following total hip replacement surgery with enoxaparin versus unfractionated heparin: A pharmacoeconomic evaluation. Ann Pharmacother 28:271, 1994.

66. Menache, D: Antithrombin III concentrates. Coagulation Disorders I. Hematol Oncol Clin North Am 6:1115, 1992.

67. Ibid.

68. Francis, CW, Pelligrini, VD, Jr, Marder, VJ, et al: Prevention of venous thrombosis after total hip arthroplasy: Antithrombin III and lost dose heparin compared with Dextrin 40. J Bone Joint Surg 71A:327, 1989.

69. Francis, CW, Pelligrini, VD Jr, Stulberg, BN, et al: Prevention of venous thrombosis after total hip arthroplasy: Comparison of antithrombin III to dextran. Bone Joint Surg 72A: 976, 1990.

70. Francis, CW, Pellegrini, VD Jr., Harris, CM, et al: Prophylaxis of venous thrombosis following total hip and total knee replacement using antithrombin III and heparin. Semin Hematol 28:39, 1991.

71. Diaz-Cremades, JM, Lorenzo, R, Sanchez, M, et al: Use of antithrombin III in critical patients. Intensive Care Med 20:577, 1994.

72. Contant, G, Goulult-Heilmann, M, and Martinoli, JL: Heparin inactivation during blood storage: Its prevention by blood collection in citric acid, theophylline, adenosine, dipyridamole-CTAD mixture. Thromb Res 31:365, 1983.

73. Bouman, CS, Ypma, ST, and Sybesma, JP: Comparison of the efficacy of D-dimer, fibrin degradation products and prothrombin fragment 1 + 2 in clinically suspected deep venous thrombosis. Thromb Res: 77:225, 1995.

QUESTIONS

1. Which of the following is not a natural anticoagulant/inhibitor?
   a. Antithrombin III
   b. Heparin cofactor II
   c. Factor Va
   d. Protein C
   e. Protein S

2. What is the most important serine-protease inhibitor?
   a. Antithrombin III
   b. Protein C and protein S
   c. Facors IXa and Xa
   d. PCI-I and α_1-antitrypsin

3. Which inhibitors are vitamin K–dependent? (Use answer choices for question 2.)

4. Which of the following characteristics are similar for deficiencies of antithrombin III, heparin cofactor II, protein C, and protein S?
   a. Onset before age 40
   b. Deep venous thrombosis
   c. Pulmonary embolism
   d. All of the above

5. What laboratory tests are performed for evaluation of primary APA syndrome?
   a. Platelet neutralization test
   b. Coagulation tests such as dilute Russell viper venom time
   c. ELISA for APA
   d. All of the above

6. What is the action of oral anticoagulants?
   a. Degrade clotting factors
   b. Block vitamin K
   c. Inhibit binding of calcium
   d. Replace activated zymogens

7. What laboratory test is most commonly used to monitor oral anticoagulant therapy?
   a. PT
   b. APTT
   c. Platelet count
   d. Protein C and protein S levels

8. What is the anticoagulant mechanism of heparin?
   a. Inhibits PF4
   b. Inhibits thrombin by complexing with AT-III
   c. Degrades AT-III
   d. Complexes with HC-II

9. Which laboratory tests are used to monitor heparin therapy?
   a. APTT
   b. Anti-Xa heparin assay
   c. Thrombin time
   d. All of the above

10. What laboratory test(s) is/are not affected by the presence of therapeutic heparin?
   a. PT and APTT
   b. Thrombin time
   c. Reptilase time
   d. Whole blood clotting time and heparin assay

ANSWERS

1. **c** (p 567)
2. **a** (p 568)
3. **b** (pp 569, 570)
4. **d** (p 572)
5. **d** (p 573)
6. **b** (p 576)
7. **a** (p 577)
8. **b** (p 578)
9. **d** (p 581)
10. **c** (p 582)

Part V

LABORATORY METHODS

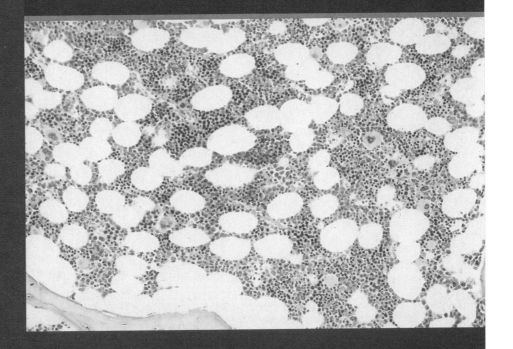

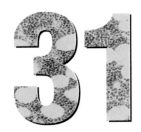

Routine Hematology Methods

Janis Wyrick-Glatzel, MS, MT(ASCP)
Virginia Hughes, BS, MT(ASCP)

Objectives

At the end of this chapter, the learner should be able to:
1 Calculate a manual white blood cell count, red blood cell count, and platelet count.
2 Calculate a percentage of reticulocytes and an absolute/corrected reticulocyte count.
3 Calculate a reticulocyte production index.
4 List errors in the performance of a centrifugal microhematocrit determination.
5 Calculate mean corpuscular volume, mean corpuscular hemoglobin, and mean corpuscular hemoglobin concentration.
6 Identify factors that affect the erythrocyte sedimentation rate.
7 Identify hemoglobins separated at alkaline and acid pH in hemoglobin electrophoresis.
8 Name a method for quantitating hemoglobin A_2 and hemoglobin F.
9 Describe the differential solubility test for hemoglobin S.
10 Describe a procedure for detecting Heinz bodies.

11 Identify conditions that show increased and decreased osmotic fragility.
12 Describe the basic principle for the Ham test and the sugar water test for paroxysmal nocturnal hemoglobinuria.
13 Explain the basic principle of the cyanmethemoglobin method for hemoglobin determination.
14 Describe the effects of a lipemic specimen on hemoglobin determinations.
15 Calculate a corrected white blood cell count for a peripheral blood smear containing more than 10 nucleated red blood cells per 100 white blood cells.

Our goal in this chapter is to present the student with basic hematologic procedures. Emphasis is placed on interpretation as well as on procedure. At the end of some of the procedures we have included a comment section that serves as a potpourri highlighting general points of information concerning the procedure, its limitations, and its interpretation.

As technology and automation have expanded, some procedures have become antiquated. We believe, however, that an understanding of the basic procedures will serve as a sound building block for the application of more advanced technology.

COLLECTION OF BLOOD SPECIMENS

Blood collection for hematologic studies can be performed via venipuncture (blood collected from a vein) or by capillary puncture (blood collected from the finger, heel, earlobe, or toe). The anticoagulant used most often in routine hematology methods excluding coagulation analyses is ethylenediamine tetra-acetic acid (EDTA).

There are many preanalytical steps to follow in the process of blood collection such as patient identification, requisition verification of laboratory orders, and biohazard safety, to name a few. These items, as well as venipuncture and capillary puncture methodology, will be discussed.

Patient Identification

Hospitalized Patients

Hospitalized patients wear a wristband with the following information: (1) patient's first and last name, and middle initial; (2) hospital number; (3) date of birth or age; (4) gender; (5) name of physician; and (6) location or room number. All of this information should be checked with the laboratory requisition form or laboratory orders for each patient. If the patient is not wearing a wristband, a nurse should be notified to verify patient identification.

Outpatients

For outpatients who have blood collected, the phlebotomist should ask the patient to recite his or her full name, address, social security number, and date of birth. The phlebotomist must check this information with the laboratory requisition form or physician's record of laboratory orders.

Safety

Universal precautions should be in practice at all times when collecting blood specimens. This means that all specimens should be handled as if they were infected with the hepatitis B virus or human immunodeficiency virus (HIV). Such safety precautions include wearing a new pair of latex gloves for each patient, washing hands between patients, and disposing of needles and contaminated supplies in a puncture-resistant biohazard container (sharps).

Verification of Laboratory Requisitions

With each request for blood collection and laboratory analysis there must be a laboratory requisition that is either written or contained in the laboratory information system (LIS). This requisition contains the following patient information:

Patient's full name
Age of patient
Social security number
Hospital number
Date and time specimen is to be collected
Physician's name
Accession or specimen number
Location where order was placed
Ordered tests

The phlebotomist needs to verify that the patient information on the requisition form or specimen label is

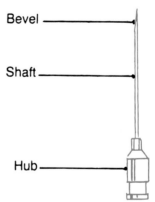

FIGURE 31-1 The hypodermic needle consisting of the bevel, shaft, and hub. The hub attaches to the syringe. (From Wedding, ME and Toenjes, SA: Medical Laboratory Procedures. FA Davis, Philadelpha, 1992, p 144, with permission.)

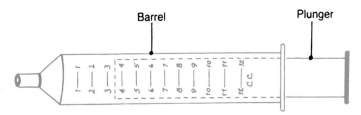

FIGURE 31-2 The syringe consisting of a barrel and plunger. (From Wedding, ME and Toenjes, SA: Medical Laboratory Procedures. FA Davis, Philadelphia, 1992, p 145, with permission.)

correct before blood is collected. He or she should be aware of the appropriate anticoagulants for the tests being performed as well as the volume of blood required.

Labeling the Blood Specimen

A properly labeled specimen is essential to patient care. The consequences of a patient being treated based on another patient's results can be detrimental and sometimes fatal, depending on the situation. Many hospitals and laboratories have implemented preprinted patient labels that contain the following information: (1) patient's first and last name, (2) age, (3) gender, (4) hospital number, (4) test ordered, (5) type of tube required, (6) social security number, (7) patient location, and (8) name of physician.

The tubes in which blood is collected should be labeled after the blood is collected and not before; this alleviates labeling another tube if blood cannot be collected successfully on the first venipuncture. If preprinted labels are not available, the patient's first and last name and social security number should be on the tube of blood.

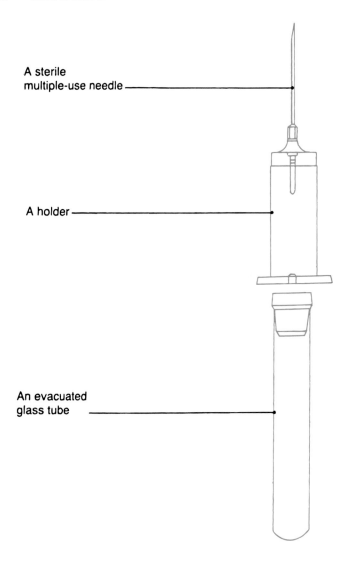

FIGURE 31-3 The evacuated tube system consisting of a double-pointed needle, a plastic holder, and a vacuum tube with rubber stopper. (From Wedding, ME and Toenjes, SA: Medical Laboratory Procedures. FA Davis, Philadelphia, 1992, p 142, with permission.)

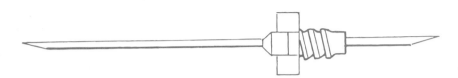

FIGURE 31-4 The multisample needle, pointed at both ends with one end insulated in a rubber sheath. (From Wedding, ME and Toenjes, SA: Medical Laboratory Procedures. FA Davis, Philadelphia, 1992, p 143, with permission.)

Venipuncture Methodology

Principle

Venipuncture can be performed via syringe or by using the more popular evacuated tube system.[1] Syringes have become somewhat antiquated in the blood collection scenario because of multisample availability with the evacuated tube system. However, this technique is still available and used on patients with small veins, in blood culture collection, and in arterial blood gas collection. Briefly, once the needle (attached to the syringe) enters the vein, blood will appear in the hub of the syringe (Fig. 31-1). The phlebotomist or person performing the blood collection controls the volume of blood being collected by pulling up on the plunger (Fig. 31-2). Once the syringe is filled, the phlebotomist releases the tourniquet and withdraws the needle. The blood collected must be placed into the correct tubes as soon as possible to avoid coagulation (clotting) of the specimen.

The evacuated tube system offers the benefit of multisample blood collection. This means that more than one tube of blood can be collected with one needlestick. An evacuated tube system usually consists of a disposable sterile needle, a needle holder, and an evacuated tube (Fig. 31-3). Briefly, the multisample needle is pointed at both ends (Fig. 31-4). The end covered with a rubber sheath is screwed into the needle holder; the other gets inserted into the vein. Once the vein is entered (Figs. 31-5 and 31-6), tubes can be inserted into the body of the needle holder, puncturing the rubber sheath to withdraw the blood. Additional tubes can be filled in this manner. This apparatus alleviates the transfer of blood from the syringe to appropriate collection vials, which subjects the specimen to hemolysis because of the speed at which blood from the syringe is ejected. The reader should refer to any phlebotomy textbook for the actual procedure.

Capillary Puncture Methodology

In hematologic studies, blood collected by capillary puncture is most often performed on the pediatric population and to a lesser extent on elderly patients and

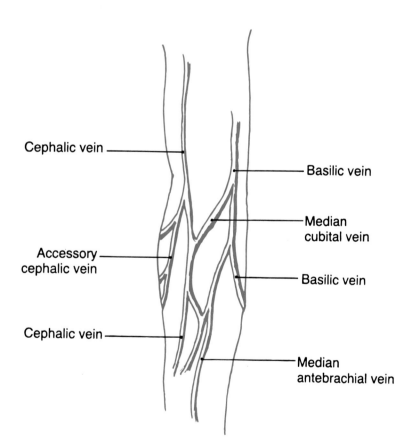

Cephalic vein

Accessory cephalic vein

Cephalic vein

Basilic vein

Median cubital vein

Basilic vein

Median antebrachial vein

FIGURE 31-5 The path of veins of the arm. (From Wedding, ME and Toenjes, SA: Medical Laboratory Procedures. FA Davis, Philadelphia, 1992, p 148, with permission.)

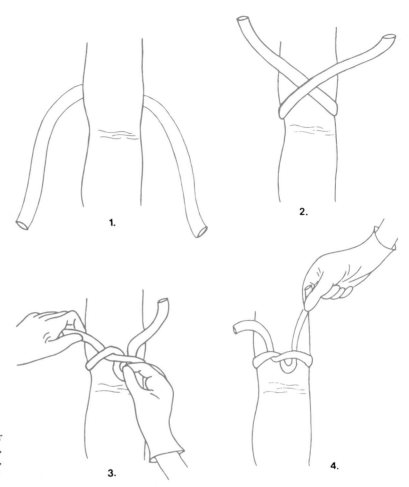

FIGURE 31-6 Application of the rubber tourniquet. (From Wedding, ME and Toenjes, SA: Medical Laboratory Procedures. FA Davis, Philadelphia, 1992, p 147, with permission.)

those whose veins are collapsed or indiscriminate to the phlebotomist. The most common site for a capillary stick in infants is the plantar surface of the heel perpendicular to the big toe or perpendicular to the fourth or fifth toe on the opposite side of the foot. In older infants and the elderly population, the palmar (fleshy) surface of the distal phalanx of the second, third, or fourth fingers may be punctured, with the middle finger being the first choice.[2] Briefly, the site of puncture is warmed to enhance blood flow, cleansed with isopropyl alcohol, and punctured with a sterile lancet. The first drop is wiped away and the appropriate volume of blood is collected into either microhematocrit tubes (heparinized) or microcontainers that contain EDTA. (Refer to any phlebotomy textbook for the actual procedure.)

MANUAL BLOOD CELL COUNTS

Hemacytometer

The *hemacytometer* counting chamber is used for cell counting. It is constructed so that the distance between the bottom of the *coverslip* and the surface of the counting area of the chamber is 0.1 mm (Fig. 31–7).

The surface of the chamber contains two square ruled areas separated by an H-shaped moat. These two squares are identical, allowing the technologist to duplicate the cell count. Each has a total area of 9 mm² (3 mm on each side). These squares are divided into nine primary squares (Fig. 31–8), each with an area of 1 mm² (1 mm on each side). The four corner primary squares are used when counting leukocytes. These four corner primary squares are further divided into 16 smaller secondary squares, each with an area of 0.04 mm². The four corner and center secondary squares of the center primary square (see Fig. 31–8) are used to count erythrocytes. All 25 secondary squares of the center primary square are used to count

HEMACYTOMETER

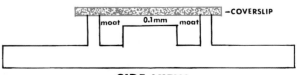

SIDE VIEW

FIGURE 31-7 Hemacytometer, side view.

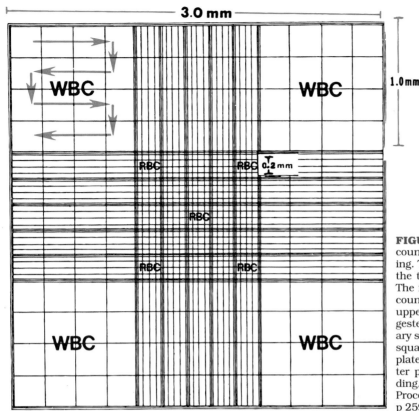

FIGURE 31–8 Spencer Bright-Line double counting system with improved Neubauer ruling. This represents an enlarged view of one of the two ruled squares of the hemacytometer. The four corner primary squares are used for counting white blood cells. The arrows in the upper left corner square represent the suggested counting pathway of cells. Five secondary squares (labeled RBC) of the center primary square are used for counting red blood cells. In platelet enumeration, all 25 squares of the center primary square are counted. (From Wedding, ME and Toenjes, SA: Medical Laboratory Procedures. FA Davis, Philadelphia, 1992, p 259, with permission.)

platelets, and each of these 25 squares is further divided into 16 smaller tertiary squares (see Fig. 31–8).

The boundary lines of the central primary square are either double or triple. When the boundary line is double, all the cells within the square and those touching the innermost line are counted. If the boundary line is triple, all of the cells within the squares and those touching the middle line inward are counted.

Hemacytometers and coverslips should meet the specifications of the National Bureau of Standards and are so marked by the manufacturer. A standardized coverslip should be used that has been ground to fit the specifics of the hemacytometer, ensuring a uniform depth and therefore a constant volume (see Fig. 31–7). A regular coverslip cannot be used.

Manual Cell Counting

With the introduction of sophisticated electronic equipment such as the Coulter Counter into the field of hematology, there is a diminished need for manual cell counting. However, a knowledge of this method is still important. Manual cell counts are often performed in patients with extreme cases of thrombocytosis, thrombocytopenia, leukocytosis, and leukopenia. Perhaps the most clear-cut use for manual cell counts is for measuring body fluids such as cerebral spinal fluid (CSF) and pleural fluid, since these can be counted only by manual methods.

Blood Dilution Vials

Dilution of blood samples may be performed by using prepackaged blood dilution vials available from manufacturers, such as the Unopette kit by Becton-Dickinson Vacutainer System (Fig. 31–9). Each vial is

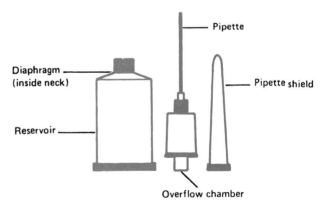

FIGURE 31–9 Unopette system, consisting of a reservoir containing a diluent, a pipet used to deliver specimen into reservoir, and a pipet shield used to puncture plastic seal of reservoir and as a cap for the pipet to prevent evaporation. (From Wedding, ME and Toenjes, SA: Medical Laboratory Procedures. FA Davis, Philadelphia, 1992, p 255, with permission.)

filled with premeasured diluent and capillary pipets appropriate for the necessary dilutions. A wide variety of test vials are available including those for white blood cells (WBCs), platelets, red blood cells (RBCs), eosinophils, and hemoglobin. With the implication of infectious disease such as hepatitis and acquired immunodeficiency syndrome (AIDS), mouth suctioning pipets are no longer advocated as proper procedure for making dilutions with micropipet. Any changes in dilution factors that may vary with the manufacturer must be kept under consideration. Once the dilutions are made, the manual counts may be performed as described below.

Red Blood Cell Count Using the Unopette System (Fig. 31–9)

The Unopette system of red cell enumeration is an easier and less tedious procedure than the Thoma diluting pipet. The correct volume of diluent is contained in the Unopette reservoir, which eliminates "overshooting" the diluent with a manual diluting pipet.

Specimen Freeflowing capillary or well-mixed anticoagulated venous blood. EDTA is the anticoagulant of choice.

Principle Venous or capillary blood samples are drawn by capillary action at a specific volume into the

Unopette reservoir containing RBC diluent. The reservoir is then mixed by inversion several times and charged onto the hemacytometer to be counted microscopically.

Equipment

Unopette reservoir No. 5851 containing 1.99-mL diluting fluid

Sodium chloride	8.5 g
Sodium azide	0.1 g
Distilled water	1000 mL

Capillary pipet (10 μL)
Hemacytometer and coverslip
Microscope
Hand counter
Petri dish lined with moist filter paper

Procedure

1. Using the protective shield on the capillary pipette, puncture the diaphragm of the reservoir (Fig. 31–10A).
2. Remove shield from pipette assembly by twisting.
3. Holding pipet almost horizontally, touch tip of pipet to blood. Pipet will fill by capillary action (see Fig. 31–10B). Filling will cease automati-

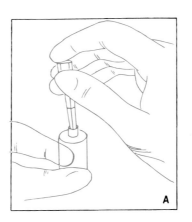
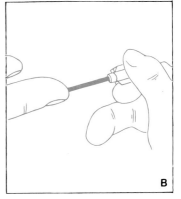
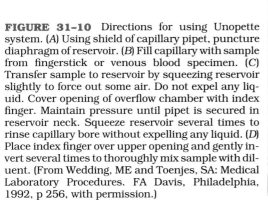
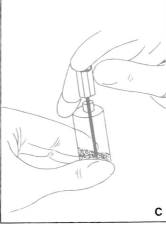
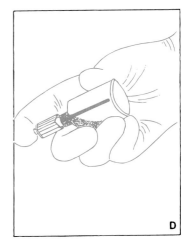

FIGURE 31–10 Directions for using Unopette system. (*A*) Using shield of capillary pipet, puncture diaphragm of reservoir. (*B*) Fill capillary with sample from fingerstick or venous blood specimen. (*C*) Transfer sample to reservoir by squeezing reservoir slightly to force out some air. Do not expel any liquid. Cover opening of overflow chamber with index finger. Maintain pressure until pipet is secured in reservoir neck. Squeeze reservoir several times to rinse capillary bore without expelling any liquid. (*D*) Place index finger over upper opening and gently invert several times to thoroughly mix sample with diluent. (From Wedding, ME and Toenjes, SA: Medical Laboratory Procedures. FA Davis, Philadelphia, 1992, p 256, with permission.)

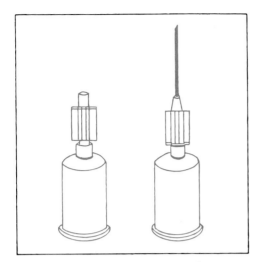

FIGURE 31–11 Unopette conversion to dropper assembly by withdrawing pipet from reservoir and securing it in reverse position. (From Wedding, ME and Toenjes, SA: Medical Laboratory Procedures. FA Davis, Philadelphia, 1992, p 258, with permission.)

cally when the blood reaches the end of the capillary bore in the neck of the pipet.[3]

4. Wipe the outside of the capillary pipet to remove excess blood that would interfere with the dilution factor.
5. Squeeze reservoir slightly to force out some air while simultaneously maintaining pressure on reservoir.
6. Cover opening of overflow chamber of pipet with index finger and seat pipet securely in reservoir neck (see Fig. 31–10C).
7. Release pressure on reservoir. Then remove finger from pipet opening. At this time negative pressure will draw blood into reservoir.
8. Squeeze reservoir gently two or three times to rinse capillary bore forcing diluent up into, but not out of, overflow chamber, releasing pressure each time to return mixture to reservoir.
9. Place index finger over upper opening and gently invert several times to thoroughly mix blood with diluent (see Fig. 31–10D).

10. Let mixture stand 10 minutes before charging hemacytometer.
11. To charge hemacytometer, convert to dropper assembly by withdrawing pipet from reservoir and reseating securely in reverse position (Fig. 31–11).
12. Invert reservoir and discard the first 3 or 4 drops of mixture.
13. Clean the hemacytometer and its coverslip with an alcohol pad and then dry with a wipe.
14. Carefully charge hemacytometer with diluted blood by gently squeezing sides of reservoir to expel contents until chamber is properly filled (Fig. 31–12).
15. Place hemacytometer in moist Petri dish for 10 minutes to allow red cells to settle. (Moistened filter paper retains evaporation of diluted specimen while standing)
16. Mount the hemacytometer on the microscope and lower its condenser.
17. Procedure for counting RBCs:
    a. Cells are scanned under a 10× objective to ensure even distribution.
    b. Use a 40X objective (high-dry) to count the erythrocytes in the 5 squares labeled RBC of the center primary square (see Fig. 31–8). This counting procedure is repeated on the opposite side of the hemacytometer.
    c. To count the cells in the tertiary squares, use the following pattern:
       1. Count cells starting in the upper left corner square, continue counting to the right hand square, drop down to the next row; continue counting from the right hand square to the left square (see Fig. 31–8). Continue counting in this fashion until the total area in that secondary square has been counted.
       2. Count all cells that touch any of the upper and left lines, do not count any cell that touches a lower or right line (Fig. 31–13).
    d. The difference between the highest and lowest number of cells of the 10 squares should be no greater than 25.

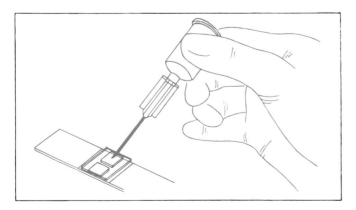

FIGURE 31–12 Charging of hemacytometer by Unopette inversion of reservoir dropper assembly. The first three or four drops are discarded before hemacytometer is loaded. (From Wedding, ME and Toenjes, SA: Medical Laboratory Procedures. FA Davis, Philadelphia, 1992, p 258, with permission.)

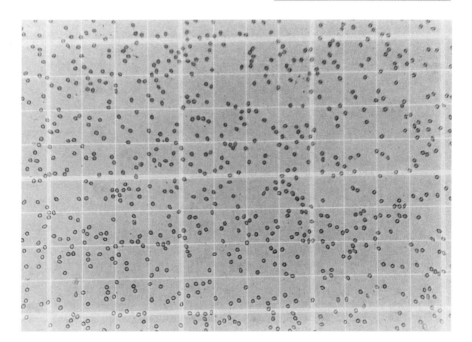

FIGURE 31–13 Photography of erythrocytes loaded onto a Neubauer hemacytometer at ×100 magnification. These squares represent 6 of 25 secondary squares of the center primary square.

Note: Diluted blood samples must be examined within 2 hours and must be thoroughly mixed just before their admission onto the hemacytometer.[4]

Calculations The basic formula for the calculation of the number of RBCs per cubic millimeter of diluted blood is as follows:

$$\text{No. of cells/mm}^3 = \frac{\text{No. of cells} \times \text{Depth factor} \times \text{Diluting factor}}{\text{Area}}$$

$$= \frac{\text{No. of cells} \times 10 \times 200}{0.2 \times 0.2 \times 5}$$

Note: Depth factor equals depth of chamber, which is 0.1 mm. This must be multiplied by 10 to get 1 mm³.

A factor of 10,000 may be employed for simplification, which is the result of:

$$\frac{\text{Depth factor} \times \text{Dilution factor}}{\text{Area}} \quad \text{or} \quad \frac{10 \times 200}{0.2} = 10,000$$

Conversion to SI Units To convert this number to SI units (system of internationalized units) or 10^{12} RBCs/L, a factor of 10^6 is used, so that 5.0×10^6 RBCs/mm³ $\times 10^6 = 5.0 \times 10^{12}$/L. This factor of 10^6 represents a conversion in the total volume of the 5 squares counted, which is 1.00 uL converted to liters.

Interpretation

Normal Values

Newborn	$4.4–5.8 \times 10^{12}$/L
Infant/child	$3.8–5.5 \times 10^{12}$/L
Adult male	$4.7–6.1 \times 10^{12}$/L
Adult female	$4.2–5.4 \times 10^{12}$/L

Errors in RBC Enumeration Erroneous results in RBC counting may be the result of an incorrect dilution, faulty equipment, technique, or nature of the sample.

The blood sample must be free of clots and thoroughly mixed. The technologist must pay close attention when filling the chamber because overfilling would change the depth factor while raising the coverslip and underfilling would produce falsely decreased red cell counts.

White Blood Cell and Platelet Counts Using the Unopette System

Principle Free-flowing capillary or well-mixed anticoagulated venous blood is added to a diluent at a specific volume in the Unopette reservoir. The diluent lyses the erythrocytes but preserves leukocytes and platelets. The diluted blood is added to the hemacytometer chamber. Cells are allowed to settle for 10 minutes before leukocytes and platelets are counted. (Refer to manufacturer's instructions for the procedure.)

Equipment

Unopette reservoir no. 5854/5855 (1.98 mL of diluent)

Ammonium oxalate	11.45 g
Sorensen's phosphate buffer	1.0 g
Thimerosal	0.1 g
Purified water	qs to 1000 mL

Unopette capillary pipet, 20-μL capacity
Hemacytometer and coverslip
Microscope
Lint-free wipe
Alcohol pads
Hand counter
Petri dish lined with moist filter paper

Specimen Free-flowing capillary or well-mixed anticoagulated venous blood. EDTA is the anticoagulant of choice.

Procedure

1. Puncture diaphragm of Unopette reservoir and add sample using a 20-μL capillary pipette as described in RBC count using the Unopette system.
2. Let diluent-blood mixture stand 10 minutes to allow RBCs to hemolyze. This mixture can stand for up to 3 h.
3. Charge the hemacytometer as described in RBC counts using the Unopette system.
4. Place hemacytometer in a Petri dish lined with moist filter paper and let sit for 10 minutes to allow cells to settle.

Count and Calculations A *leukocyte count* is performed with a Neubauer hemacytometer as follows:

1. Under 10× magnification, leukocytes are counted in all nine large squares of counting chamber.
2. Total WBC/mm^3 = (No. of cells × 10 × 100)/9
3. Or one can more easily determine the total cell count by adding 10% of count to total number of cells counted, and then multiplying this figure by 100 to get total leukocyte count. This is a simplification of the general formula described in other sections, which involves multiplying the cells counted by 10 to correct the depth of chamber and dividing by the number of squares enumerated.[5]

Example If an average of 60 cells is counted on both sides of chamber, add 10%, or 6, to 60 and multiply by 100 to get 6600 leukocytes/mm^3. This number can then be multiplied by a factor of 10^6 to derive SI units or 6.6×10^9/L.

A *platelet count* is performed with a Neubauer hemacytometer as follows:

1. Under 40× magnification using bright-light or phase microscopy, platelets are counted in all 25 small squares within the large center square (see Fig. 31–8). Duplicate counts on a sample (e.g., both sides of a hemacytometer) should agree within 10% for counts to be acceptable.
2. Multiply the average number of platelets counted on both sides of chamber by 1000 to get total platelet count/mm^3. Multiply this number by a factor of 10^6 to have the platelet count in SI units or 10^9/L. This step of multiplying by 1000 simplifies multiplication of dilution factor (100) and depth (10) which is equal to 1000.[6]

Example An average of 230 platelets were enumerated on both sides of the hemacytometer using the Unopette system for platelet determinations.

$$\text{Platelets/mm}^3 = 230 \times 1000 = 230{,}000/\text{mm}^3 \times 10^6 = 230 \times 10^9/\text{L}.$$

Note: If another hemacytometer is used, calculations appropriate to the particular type should be employed.

Comments

1. Diluent and blood should be properly mixed before filling the hemacytometer.
2. The hemacytometer must be properly filled to avoid erroneous results in manual cell counting.
3. If the chamber is overfilled, as indicated by the presence of excess fluid in the moat of hemacytometer, clean hemacytometer and recharge chamber. As with all manual counts, the diluent sample must be thoroughly mixed before charging the hemacytometer, which must be properly filled.
4. A highly elevated leukocyte or platelet count may make accurate counting difficult. In either instance, a secondary dilution should be made. When calculating the total count, adjust the formula to allow for secondary dilution. There are physiologic variations to consider when performing WBC counts. Higher counts are seen following exercise, emotional stress, anxiety, and food intake. Blacks generally show slightly lower WBC counts than whites.
5. Platelets appear as dense, dark bodies and can be round, oval, or rodlike, sometimes showing dendritic processes (Fig. 31–14). Their internal granular structure and pearlescent sheen allow the platelets to be distinguished from debris, which is often refractile. RBCs appear as ghost cells. Use caution when RBCs have inclusions present, so as not to confuse the inclusion with platelets.
6. If platelet clumping is observed, redilute count. If clumping is still present, obtain a fresh specimen. Because of the adhesive quality of platelets, fingerstick specimens are least desirable.
7. The phase platelet determination should be compared with a review of the blood film for correction of count and morphology.

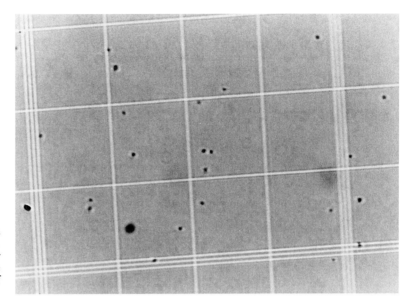

FIGURE 31–14 Photograph of platelets loaded onto a hemacytometer using a ×40 objective (phase contrast). The platelets appear as dense, refractile, dark bodies that can be round, oval, or rod-shaped with a diameter of approximately 2–4 um.

8. EDTA is the anticoagulant of choice when performing phase platelet counts. The student should be aware of "platelet satellitosis" when using this anticoagulant.[7] Platelet satellitosis appears as neutrophils ringed with adhesive platelets. Obtain correct platelet counts by collecting a fresh specimen with sodium citrate as the anticoagulant. When sodium citrate is used as an anticoagulant, make the correction for the dilution by multiplying by 1.1.
9. Ordinary light microscopy may be used; however, in this method differentiation and enumeration are more difficult.

Interpretation
Normal values (WBC)

Newborn	$9.0{-}30.0 \times 10^9/L$
1 week	$5.0{-}21.0 \times 10^9/L$
1 month	$5.0{-}19.5 \times 10^9/L$
6–12 months	$6.0{-}17.5 \times 10^9/L$
2 years	$6.2{-}17.0 \times 10^9/L$
Child/adult	$4.8{-}10.8 \times 10^9/L$

Normal values (Platelets)

$130{-}400 \times 10^9/L$

Reticulocyte Count Using the Miller Disc

Principle Reticulocytes are immature RBCs that contain remnant cytoplasmic ribonucleic acid (RNA) and organelles such as mitochondria and ribosomes. Reticulocytes are visualized by staining with vital dyes (such as new methylene blue) that precipitate the RNA and organelles, forming a filamentous network of reticulum. The reticulocyte count is a means of assessing the erythropoietic activity of the bone marrow.

Reagents New methylene blue. Dissolve 10.0 g of new methylene blue (NMB) and 8.9 of NaCl (0.152 mol/L) in 1000 mL of distilled water. Filter through What-

man #1 filter paper before use. Store at room temperature.

Equipment

Miller ocular disc
Whole blood anticoagulated with EDTA
Microscope slides
10 × 75 mm test tubes
6-inch capillary tubes
Hand counter

Procedure

1. Add an equal number of drops of thoroughly mixed EDTA anticoagulated blood and NMB mixture to a glass 10 × 75-mm tube.
2. Make a conventional wedge smear and let air dry. Do not counterstain with Wright's stain.
3. Use a 100× objective and a 10× ocular secured with a Miller disc (Fig. 31–15) or similar apparatus and count the reticulocytes and RBCs on the smear. As in differential enumeration of WBCs, choose a section of the smear where cells are close to each other but not touching or overlapping. Count a total of 20 fields.

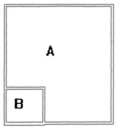

FIGURE 31–15 The visible field of the Miller ocular disc. In each field reticulocytes are counted in the larger square (A) and red blood cells are counted in the smaller square (B). The area of square B is one-ninth of square A.

4. In each field count RBCs in the smaller square and reticulocytes in the larger square (see Fig. 31–15).

Calculations   Calculate the percentage of reticulocytes per the following formula:

$$\% \text{ Reticulocytes} = \frac{\text{Total reticulocytes in larger square}}{\text{Total RBC in smaller square} \times 9} \times 100$$

This calculation is usually based on a total of 1000 erythrocytes counted. (*Example:* 10 reticulocytes and 900 RBCs)

$$\% \text{ Reticulocytes} = \frac{10}{900 \times 9} \times 100 = 0.12\%$$

Interpretation
Normal values

Newborn (0–2 weeks)	2.5–6.0%
Adult	0.5–2.0%

The absolute reticulocyte count is calculated per the following formula:

$$\text{Absolute reticulocyte count} = \frac{\% \text{ Reticulocyte count} \times (\text{RBC count}) (10^{12}/\text{L})}{100}$$

The absolute reticulocyte count expresses the number of reticulocytes in 1 mm³ of whole blood; it is not a percentage of RBCs. The normal value is $60 \times 10^9/\text{L}$ or 60,000/mm³. Higher reticulocyte counts have been reported in normal persons living at an altitude greater than 60,000 feet above sea level, with significantly higher values in women than in men.[8]

The reticulocyte count is most often expressed as a percentage of total red cells. In states of anemia, the reticulocyte percentage is not a true reflection of reticulocyte production. A correction factor must be used so as not to overestimate marrow production, because each reticulocyte is released into whole blood containing few RBCs—a low hematocrit (Hct)—thus relatively increasing the percentage. The corrected reticulocyte count may be calculated by the following formula:

$$\text{Corrected reticulocyte count} = \frac{\text{Reticulocyte (\%)} \times \text{Patient Hct\%}}{45 \text{ (avg. normal Hct)}}$$

For example, if a patient presenting with a reticulocyte count of 12% and a hematocrit of 24%, the corrected reticulocyte count would be 12% times (24/45) or 6.4%. In other words, the patient who presents with a reticulocyte count of 12% and a hematocrit of 24% would have the equivalent of a reticulocyte count of 6.4% in a patient with a hematocrit of 45%.

Estimating RBC production by using the corrected reticulocyte count may yield erroneously high values in patients when there is a premature release of younger reticulocytes from the marrow (owing to increased erythropoietin stimulation). The premature reticulocytes are called "stress or shift" reticulocytes. These result when the reticulocytes of the bone marrow pool are shifted to the circulation pool to compensate for anemia. The younger stress reticulocytes present with more filamentous reticulum. The mature reticulocyte may present with granular dots representing reticulum. Normally, reticulocytes lose their reticulum within 24 to 27 hours after entering the peripheral circulation. The premature stress reticulocytes have increased reticulum and require 2 to 2.5 days to lose their reticulum, resulting in a longer peripheral blood maturation time (Table 31–1).

The peripheral smear should be carefully reviewed for the presence of many polychromatophilic macrocytes, thus indicating stress reticulocytes and the need for a correction for both the RBC count and the presence of stress reticulocytes. The value obtained is called the reticulocyte production index (RPI). To calculate the RPI, the following formula is used:

$$\text{RPI} = \frac{\text{Reticulocyte count \%} \times \text{Patient's Hct}/45 \text{ (normal Hct)}}{2 \text{ (Stress reticulocyte maturation time at 25\% Hct)}}$$

so that if a patient has a *corrected* reticulocyte of 12% and a hematocrit of 25%, the RPI is 12/2 or 6. An RPI equal to or greater than 3 represents an adequate response to anemia by the bone marrow, whereas an RPI of less than 2 is considered an inadequate response of erythropoiesis by the bone marrow to a state of anemia (Fig. 31–16).

TABLE 31–1 **The Maturation Time for Reticulocytes**	
Maturation Time	**Hematocrit (%)**
1 day	45
1.5 days	35
2 days	25
3 days	15

According to the pattern of reticulum and the degree of maturation, reticulocytes can be divided into four categories from the youngest to the most mature.

There is a high degree of inaccuracy in the manual reticulocyte count owing to error ($+/-2\%$ in low counts and $+/-7\%$ in high counts) and lack of reproducibility because of the inaccuracy of the blood film. However, these inaccuracies have been overcome with the application of reticulocyte enumeration by flow cytometry. This procedure is described in the section on automated reticulocyte counts.

Comments

The reticulocyte count is elevated: (1) in patients with hemolytic anemia, (2) in those with hemorrhage (acute and chronic), (3) following treatment of iron-deficiency anemia and the megaloblastic anemias, and (4) in patients with uremia (see Fig. 31–16).

The reticulocyte count is decreased in cases of: (1) aplastic anemia; (2) aplastic crises of hemolytic anemias; and (3) ineffective erythropoiesis as seen in thalassemia, pernicious anemia, and sideroblastic anemia.

Reticulocytopenia in the presence of a suggested hemolytic anemia may often make diagnosis difficult. The diagnosis of a hemolytic anemia can be made because the combination of both hemolysis and reticulocytopenia results in a rapidly falling hemoglobin and hematocrit.

By convention, singly dotted reticulocytes are not counted. A reticulocyte must contain two or more discrete blue granules. The granular reticulum of the reticulocyte may be confused with Heinz bodies. Heinz bodies stain as light blue-green granules present at the periphery of the red cell.

Manual Reticulocyte Count without the Miller Disc

Procedure

1. Mix equal amounts of blood and new methylene blue staining solution in a test tube.
2. Draw the blood-dye mixture up into a capillary pipet. Allow the mixture to stand for 10 minutes at room temperature.
3. Prepare thin wedge smears of blood-dye mixture using 1 small drop. Air-dry. Do not fix or counterstain slides with Wright's stain.
4. Under oil immersion, count all red cells in each field where the cells do not overlap, inclusive of reticulocytes.
5. Count 1000 red cells in consecutive oil immersion fields. Record the number of reticulocytes seen.

Calculations

1. Calculate the percent of reticulocytes as follows:

$$\% \text{ Reticulocytes} = \frac{\text{Reticulocyte count}/1000 \text{ RBCs}}{10}$$

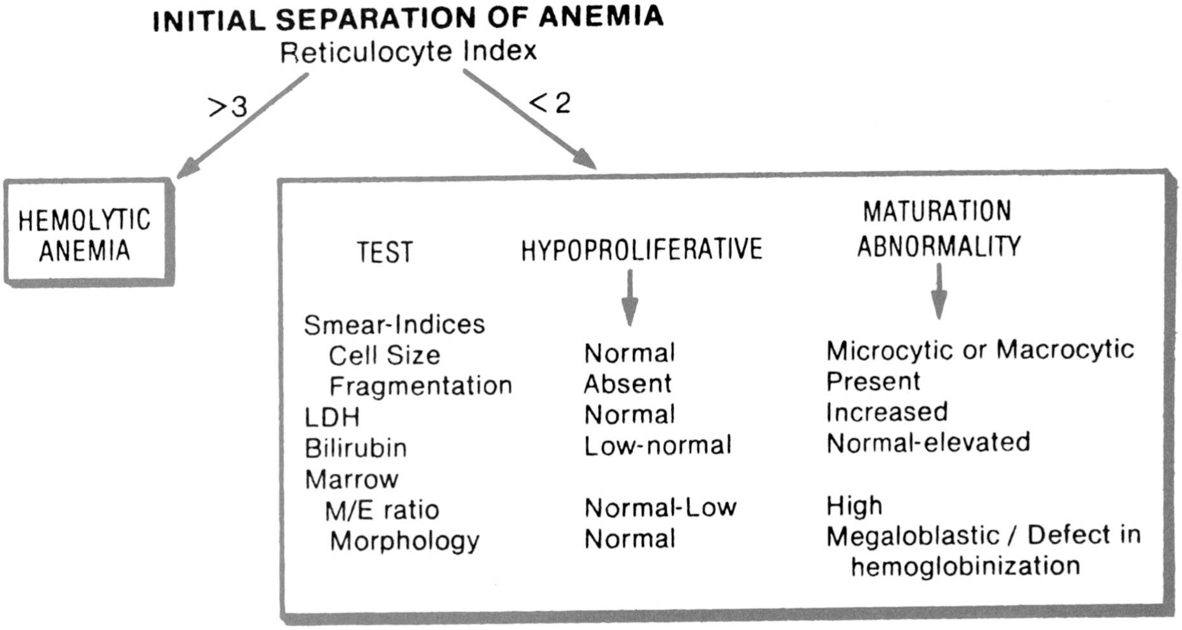

INITIAL SEPARATION OF ANEMIA
Reticulocyte Index

	TEST	HYPOPROLIFERATIVE	MATURATION ABNORMALITY
Smear-Indices			
	Cell Size	Normal	Microcytic or Macrocytic
	Fragmentation	Absent	Present
LDH		Normal	Increased
Bilirubin		Low-normal	Normal-elevated
Marrow			
	M/E ratio	Normal-Low	High
	Morphology	Normal	Megaloblastic / Defect in hemoglobinization

>3 → HEMOLYTIC ANEMIA

<2

FIGURE 31–16 The initial separation of anemia. Anemia may be broadly classified on the basis of the reticulocyte index as hemolytic (index >3) or impaired production, either a hypoproliferative or maturation abnormality (index <2). Further tests are required to separate the latter two functional defects as shown.

Note: Counting 1000 red cells is sufficient for normal or increased reticulocyte counts. However, for decreased reticulocyte counts, 2000 or more red cells should be counted. A proper quality control sample should be run in parallel to verify accurate reporting; such samples are available through manufacturers and contain known reticulocyte values.

AUTOMATED RETICULOCYTE COUNTS

Reticulocyte Count by Flow Cytometry

The reticulocyte count is one of the most important diagnostic indicators of erythropoietic activity. Its usage in the clinical laboratory is paramount to the diagnosis and monitoring of the hemolytic anemias, blood loss, and inherent erythropoietic response of the bone marrow. The measurement of reticulocytes by flow cytometry has alleviated many of the inaccuracies associated with manual methods, such as standard error with low and high counts, lack of reproducibility among technologists, and inconsistent use of the Miller disc. Figure 31–17 illustrates "gating" of RBCs in a flow cytometry analysis of reticulocyte enumeration. Refer to Chapter 24 for a detailed description of flow cytometry and its applications.

Reticulocyte Count Using Coulter Instrumentation (see Chap. 32)

Principle

Retic prep[9] reagent contains two solutions that effectively precipitate basophilic RNA from red blood cells and remove hemoglobin from the erythrocyte, leaving the precipitate complex intact. The total RBC population is then measured using the VCS concept of volume, conductivity, and light scatter on Coulter reticulocyte instrumentation.

Reagents and Equipment

Coulter Retic Prep reagent kit:
Reagent A
New methylene blue in buffered solution 0.06%
Reagent B
Sulfuric acid with stabilizers store at 0.08%
room temperature

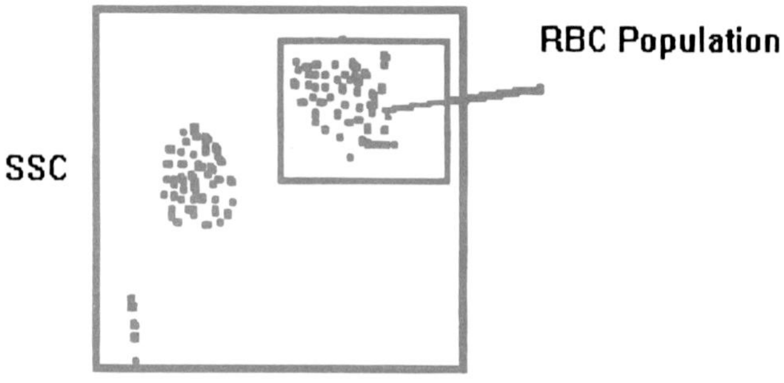

FIGURE 31–17 "Gating" of RBCs in a flow cytometry analysis of reticulocyte enumeration. Platelets, noise, and other debris are excluded from count. FSC = forward scatter; SSC = side scatter.

Coulter instrumentation with reticulocyte capability
2-μL and 50-μL air displacement pipettes
Pipette tips
12×75 mm disposable test tubes
STAT-MATIC Repetitive Dispenser, Model 5819 or equivalent timer
Note: Refer to specific instrument protocol for sampling procedures.

Specimen

Whole blood collected by venipuncture or fingerstick methodology and placed into EDTA collection tubes.

Procedure

1. Collect blood as described above.
2. Prime STAT-MATIC dispenser to fill outlet and inlet tubing of reagent B, making sure no bubbles are present in tubing.
3. Label two 12×75 test tubes. Mark one A and one B.
4. Dispense 4 drops of reagent A into tube labeled A while positioning bottle in a vertical direction (angled position will change prepared dilution).
5. Into the tube marked A, dispense 50 μL of thoroughly mixed whole blood or quality control specimen. Be careful not to let blood adhere to side of tube. Gently mix by inversion and allow to stand for 5 minutes at room temperature, but no longer than 60 minutes.
6. Transfer 2 μL of blood-stain mixture from tube A into the bottom of tube B.
7. Position tube marked B containing the blood-stain mixture at a 30° angle under the tip of the reagent B dispenser. Press down on the STAT-MATIC dispenser plunger releasing 2 mL of reagent B into tube B. Do not mix; wait 30 seconds before aspirating sample into instrument.

Note: To ensure that no bubbles occur when dispensing reagent B, let it run down the side of tube at a rapid speed to ensure mixing with blood-stain solution.

Comments

1. Sample preparation should be carried out at room temperature.
2. The accuracy of reticulocyte enumeration might be compromised if RBC inclusions, stained by new methylene blue, are present in increased numbers.[10]

RED BLOOD CELL INDICES

Principle

The values obtained for the erythrocyte count, hematocrit, and hemoglobin concentration can be further used to calculate RBC indices, which define the size and hemoglobin content of the average RBC in a given specimen of blood. The values for the RBC indices are useful tools in the classification of anemias.

The three most commonly used RBC indices are: (1) mean corpuscular volume (MCV), (2) mean corpuscular hemoglobin (MCH), and (3) mean corpuscular hemoglobin concentration (MCHC).

Definitions

Mean Corpuscular Volume

This is the average volume of the RBC, in cubic microns (μ^3) or femtoliters (fL). Normal erythrocytes have an MCV of 80 to 98 fL (replaces old units, μ^3). Results below 80 fL indicate a smaller than normal MCV; that is, the cells are on the average microcytic. Similarly, an MCV of greater than 100 fL indicates the cells are macrocytic.

It is imperative to interpret the value for MCV along with a careful inspection of the peripheral blood smear, because the MCV is only a mean volume measurement. It is possible, for example, to have a wide variation in cell size—from cells that are microcytic to some that are macrocytic—and still have an MCV within the normal range. This may be true if there is a large number of reticulocytes in the peripheral blood because reticulocytes usually have a larger volume than adult cells have.

$$MCV = \frac{\text{Hematocrit (\%)} \times 10}{\text{RBC count (in millions/mm}^3)}$$

or

$$MCV = \frac{\text{Hematocrit (L/L)} \times 10^{15}\ \text{fL/L}}{\text{RBC count } (\times 10^{12}/\text{L})}$$

or

$$MCV = \frac{\text{Hct (L/L)} \times 10^3\ \text{fL}}{\text{RBC/L}}$$

where 1 fL = 10^{15}/L

This value is reported in fL(μ^3) to the nearest whole number. Normal values for MCV are 80 to 94 fL for males and 81 to 99 fL for females.

Example: Hematocrit = 42% or .42 L/L, RBC = 5.7×10^{12} L/L

$$MCV = \frac{.42 \times 10^3\ \text{fL}}{5.7/\text{L}}$$

$$= 74\ \text{fL}$$

Mean Corpuscular Hemoglobin

This is the average weight of hemoglobin, in absolute units, in the RBC. The result gives the average content of hemoglobin per erythrocyte in picograms (pg) or micromicrograms ($\mu\mu$g). The MCH value is usually higher in newborns and infants because their MCV is higher than that of adults.

$$MCH = \frac{\text{Hemoglobin (g/100 mL)} \times 10}{\text{RBC count (millions/mm}^3)}$$

or

$$MCH = \frac{\text{Hemoglobin (g/100 mL)} \times 10^{13}\ \text{pg/L}}{\text{RBC count } (\times 10^{12}/\text{L})}$$

or

$$MCH = \frac{\text{Hemoglobin g/L pg}}{\text{RBC/L}}$$

Note: Multiplying by 10^{13} is a conversion to picograms (Hgb g/100 mL $\times$ 10 $\times$ 10^{12}). 1 g = 10^{12} pg

Example: Hemoglobin = 14.0 g/100 mL, RBC count = 5.2×10^{12}/L

$$MCH = \frac{14.0\ \text{(g/100 mL)} \times 10^{13}\ \text{pg/L}}{5.2 \times 10^{12}/\text{L}}$$

$$= 27\ \text{pg}$$

Normal values for MCH = 27 to 31 pg

Mean Corpuscular Hemoglobin Concentration

This is the average concentrations of hemoglobin in each individual RBC. It is a ratio of the weight of hemoglobin to the volume of the RBC.

$$MCHC = \frac{\text{Hemoglobin (g/100 mL)} \times 100}{\text{Hematocrit (\%)}}$$

or

$$MCHC = \frac{\text{Hemoglobin (g/100 mL)}}{\text{Hematocrit (L/L)}}$$

Example: Hemoglobin = 15 g/100 mL, Hematocrit = 45%. The MCHC is calculated as:

$$MCHC = \frac{15\ \text{g/100 mL} \times 100}{45\%}$$

$$= 33.3\%$$

This value is reported to the nearest 10th of a percent. Normal values for MCHC = 32.0 – 36.0% (Fig. 31–18).

RBC Distribution Width (RDW)

This is the coefficient of variation of the red cell volume distribution. It is provided by automated hematology instruments and is used as an indication of anisocytosis. An elevated RDW may be seen on blood smears with varying degrees of anisocytosis. This parameter is useful in distinguishing iron-deficiency anemia (increased) from thalassemia (normal).[11]

$$RDW = \frac{\text{Standard deviation of RBC volume} \times 100}{\text{Mean MCV}}$$

Normal values for RDW = 11.5% to 14.5%

Comments

Determination of the MCV, MCH, and MCHC gives valuable information that helps to characterize RBCs. According to the MCV, erythrocytes may be classified as normocytic, microcytic, or macrocytic. Based on the MCHC, erythrocytes may be classified as normochromic or hypochromic (Table 31–2). The MCH only expresses the mean weight of hemoglobin per erythrocyte.

OTHER ROUTINE HEMATOLOGY METHODS

Erythrocyte Sedimentation Rate (ESR)

Definition

The ESR test measures the settling of erythrocytes in diluted human plasma over a specified time period.[12] This numeric value is determined (in millimeters) by measuring the distance from the bottom of the surface meniscus to the top of erythrocyte sedimen-

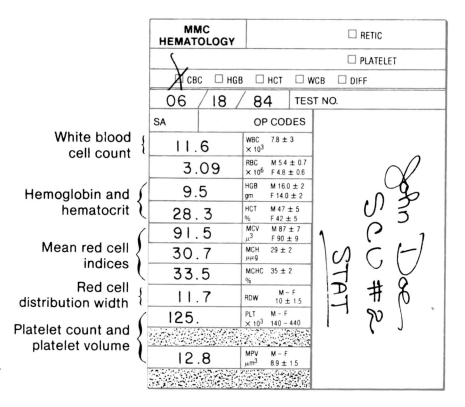

White blood cell count {

Hemoglobin and hematocrit {

Mean red cell indices {

Red cell distribution width {

Platelet count and platelet volume {

MMC HEMATOLOGY		☐ RETIC	
		☐ PLATELET	
☒ CBC ☐ HGB ☐ HCT ☐ WCB ☐ DIFF			
06 / 18 / 84	TEST NO.		

SA		OP CODES	
11.6	WBC × 10³	7.8 ± 3	
3.09	RBC × 10⁶	M 5.4 ± 0.7 F 4.8 ± 0.6	
9.5	HGB gm	M 16.0 ± 2 F 14.0 ± 2	
28.3	HCT %	M 47 ± 5 F 42 ± 5	
91.5	MCV μ³	M 87 ± 7 F 90 ± 9	
30.7	MCH μμg	29 ± 2	
33.5	MCHC %	35 ± 2	
11.7	RDW	M − F 10 ± 1.5	
125.	PLT × 10³	M − F 140 − 440	
12.8	MPV μm³	M − F 8.9 ± 1.5	

FIGURE 31-18 The results of blood cell counts and indices.

tation in an vertical column containing diluted whole blood that has remained perpendicular to its base for 60 minutes. Various factors affect the ESR, such as RBC size and shape, plasma fibrinogen, and globulin levels, as well as mechanical and technical factors.

The ESR is directly proportional to the RBC mass and inversely proportional to plasma viscosity. In normal whole blood, RBCs do not form rouleaux; the RBC mass is small and therefore the ESR is decreased (cells settle out slowly). In abnormal conditions when RBCs can form rouleaux, the RBC mass is greater, thus increasing the ESR (cells settle out faster).

Historically, there have been two methods of performing an ESR—the Westergren method[13] and the Wintrobe and Landsberg method.[14]

Westergren ESR Determination

This method is preferred by NCCLS standards because of its simplicity and greater distance of sedimentation measured in the longer Westergren tube. The straight tube is 30 cm long, 2.5 mm in internal diameter, and calibrated in millimeters from 0 to 200. Approximately 1 mL of blood is required.[15] In addition, the tubes negate the process of pipetting whole blood

directly into the tube with a glass Pasteur pipet; instead, a solution of sodium citrate is mixed with 1 mL of blood. The Westergren tube is then plunged vertically into the blood mixture and blood fills by capillary action to the top of the tube. A Westergren rack is also provided.

Reagents and Equipment

Westergren tubes
Westergren rack
Disposable pipets
0.5 mL sodium citrate or sodium chloride in puncture ready vials
EDTA anticoagulated whole blood

Procedure

1. Collect whole blood anticoagulated with EDTA.
2. Dilute whole blood with 0.5 mL of 3.8% sodium citrate or 0.85% sodium chloride.
3. Mix blood-diluent solution.
4. Insert Westergren tube into plungable vial cap of diluent mixture. Let blood draw to top of tube by capillary action. Place tube in Westergren rack in an vertical position and leave undisturbed for 1 hour.
5. After 1 hour has passed, record the distance in millimeters from the top of the column of red cells to the plasma-red cell interface. Again, the buffy coat should not be included in this measurement.

Normal Values

Adult men   0–15 mm/h
Adult women   0–20 mm/h

Comments   The ESR is not a very specific or diagnostic test. Despite the time constraints and the lack

TABLE 31–2	**Classification of Anemia**		
MCV (fL)	**MCHC %**	**Classification**	
80–100	32–36	Normocytic, normochromic	
<80	<32	Microcytic, hypochromic	
>100	32–36	Macrocytic, normochromic	

of specificity among disorders that can cause an abnormal ESR, however, the test is still used in many institutions as a screening test.

Perhaps the usefulness of this test lies in its ability to differentiate among diseases with similar symptoms or to monitor the course of an existing disease. For example, early in the course of an uncomplicated viral infection, the ESR is usually normal, but it may rise later with a superimposed bacterial infection. Within the first 24 hours of acute appendicitis, the ESR is not elevated, but in the early stage of acute pelvic inflammatory disease or ruptured ectopic pregnancy, it is elevated. The ESR is elevated in established myocardial infarction but normal in angina pectoris. It is elevated in rheumatic fever, rheumatoid arthritis, and pyogenic arthritis, but not in osteoarthritis. The ESR can be an index to disease severity. In many cases it can be an index of the activity of pulmonary tuberculosis. In general, there is no direct correlation between fever and the ESR.

Factors that Affect the ESR

Plasma Factors   Increased plasma concentration of fibrinogen, along with immunoglobulin, will result in rouleaux formation and an increased ESR. It can therefore be expected that disease states that are characterized by hyperfibrinogenemia or elevated immunoglobulin levels will result in an increased ESR.

Extreme increases in plasma viscosity slow down the ESR, thus resulting in a decreased ESR.

RBC Factors   When rouleaux formation cannot occur, owing to the shape or size of the RBC, a decreased or low ESR is expected. This is observed with sickle cells and spherocytes. The ESR is of little diagnostic value in severe anemia or in hematologic states evidenced by poikilocytosis. Table 31–3 lists factors that influence the ESR.

Anticoagulants   Sodium citrate or EDTA can be used without an effect on the ESR. Sodium or potassium oxalate can cause RBC shrinkage. Heparin causes only a slight amount of shrinkage, but a falsely elevated ESR. Our anticoagulant of choice is EDTA because of its routine use in the hematology laboratory.

Mechanical Factors   Different normal values are given for various methods owing to variations in the caliber of the tube and height of the column of blood.

A number of years ago, Wintrobe and Landsberg[12] proposed a method of correcting the ESR for anemia, based on the patient's hematocrit level. The significance of a corrected ESR is still debatable because the hematocrit can vary according to the type and severity of anemia present and therefore may influence the corrected ESR. As a result, we do not correct the ESR for anemia in our laboratory.

TABLE 31–3 **Factors Affecting the ESR**	
Increase	**Decrease**
Rouleaux formation	Microcytes
Fibrinogen (elevated)	Sickle cells
Immunoglobulin (excess)	Spherocytes

Hematocrit

Principle (Centrifugal Microhematocrit Method)

Hematocrit is defined as the volume occupied by erythrocytes (RBCs) in a given volume of blood and is usually expressed as a percentage of the volume of the whole blood sample.

The hematocrit is usually determined by spinning a blood-filled capillary tube in a centrifuge. The Coulter Counter series of analyzers provides an indirect measurement of hematocrit (see section on automated cell counting).

Reagents and Equipment

Capillary tubes, heparinized or plain (75 mm)
Microhematocrit centrifuge
Microhematocrit reader (needed only if centrifuge does not have one incorporated in the tube holder)

Procedure

1. Draw venous blood from an antecubital vein and into potassium EDTA. Take care to avoid tourniquet stasis, as this can elevate venous hematocrit results. Carefully mix the blood, preferably on a mechanical rotator. Blood specimen may also be obtained through capillary puncture using a heaparinized capillary tube to collect the specimen.
2. Once adequately mixed, place the unmarked end of a plain capillary tube in the blood and let it fill rapidly to approximately three quarters of its length. Tipping the tube horizontally will speed filling. Then remove the tube from the blood and wipe it clean of excess blood.
3. Seal the capillary tubes by placing the dry end into the tray with sealing compound at a 90° angle. Rotate the capillary tube slightly and remove it from the tray. The sealant plug should be from 4 to 6 mm long. Inspect the seal carefully for a perfectly flat bottom, perpendicular to the length axis.[16]
4. Secure the filled capillary tubes in the microhematocrit centrifuge with the sealed end toward the periphery. This should be done in duplicate at end-to-end positions. Make sure to record the numbers where tubes are seated in the centrifuge.
5. Centrifuge for 5 minutes at a set speed (force is approximately 14,500 rpm). This separates RBCs from plasma and leaves a band of buffy coat consisting of WBCs and platelets at the interface.
6. Allow the centrifuge to stop on its own; *do not hand brake.*
7. Read the hematocrit as the percent of whole venous blood occupied by RBCs. Using a constant-bore capillary tube, obtain a distance ratio on a microhematocrit reader. Set the reader first with the clay-red cell interface at 0%. Next, shift the ruled scale or etched line to 100% and align it with the plasma meniscus. Read down to the percent spiral line that intersects with the RBC–WBC interface. This percent is the hematocrit value. Do

not include the buffy coat layer in this value. If it exceeds 2%, it should be recorded and noted as volume of packed WBCs.

8. Results should duplicate within 1%.

Interpretation Normal values:

	Percent	SI Units (L/L)
Newborn	53–65	0.53–0.65
Infant/child	30–43	0.30–0.43
Man	42–52	0.42–0.52
Woman	37–47	0.37–0.47

Comments

1. Incomplete sealing of the capillary tubes will give falsely low results because, in the process of spinning, RBCs and a small amount of plasma will be forced from the tube.
2. If the buffy coat is included in the RBCs when reading the result, the hematocrit will be falsely elevated.
3. The microhematocrit centrifuge should never be forced to stop by applying pressure to the metal coverplate. This will cause the RBC layer to "sling" forward and results in a falsely elevated value.
4. The hematocrit is usually three times the hemoglobin value.
5. The Standard International (SI) unit (L/L) of reporting expresses the hematocrit as the volume of packed RBCs in relation to volume of whole blood.

PREPARATION OF BLOOD SMEARS AND GROSS EXAMINATION

Preparation of the Peripheral Blood Smear

The preparation and examination of a peripheral blood smear is one of the most frequently requested tests in the hematology laboratory. This procedure is requested not only for the diagnosis of hematologic disorders but also to provide information for diagnosis of nonhematologic diseases, for indicating side effects in chemotherapy, and for monitoring patient therapy. Reasons such as these make it essential that a blood smear be prepared correctly and examined in such a way as to provide the physician with an accurate interpretation.[17]

Two methods are routinely used to prepare blood smears:

1. Slide-to-slide or "push" smears
2. Automatic spinner

Blood smears are prepared with EDTA-anticoagulated blood to minimize degenerative changes in the blood cells. The collection tube must be completely filled with the appropriate amount of blood so that it can mix with the anticoagulant. If there is an excess of anticoagulant, artifacts will occur. To ensure good preservation of cellular morphology, differential smears should be made as soon as possible and no later than 3 h after collection.[18]

Slide-to-Slide Method

Principle A small drop of blood is placed near the frosted end of a clean glass slide. A second slide is used as a spreader. The blood is streaked in a thin film over the slide (Fig. 31–19). The slide is allowed to air-dry and is then stained.

Equipment

1. Glass slides, 3 × 1 inch (precleaned with frosted edge)
2. Capillary tubes, plain

Procedure

1. Fill a capillary tube three-quarters full with the anticoagulated specimen.
2. Place a drop of blood, about 2 mm in diameter, approximately 1/3 inch from the frosted area of the slide.
3. Place the slide on a flat surface, and hold the narrow side of the nonfrosted edge between your left thumb and forefinger.
4. With your right hand, place the smooth clean edge of a second (spreader) slide on the specimen slide, just in front of the blood drop.
5. Hold the spreader slide at a 30° angle, and draw it back against the drop of blood.
6. Allow the blood to spread almost to the edges of the slide.
7. Push the spreader forward with one light, smooth, and fluid motion. A thin film of blood in the shape of a bullet with a feathered edge will remain on the slide.
8. Allow the blood film to air-dry completely before staining.

Comments

1. A good blood film preparation will be thick at the drop end and thin at the opposite end.

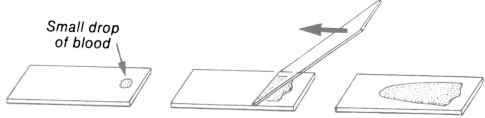

FIGURE 31–19 Preparation of a peripheral blood smear, slide-to-slide technique.

2. The blood smear should occupy the central portion of the slide and should not touch the edges.
3. The thickness of the spread when pulling the smear is determined by the (1) angle of the spreader slide (the greater the angle, the thicker and shorter the smear),[15] (2) size of the blood drop; and (3) speed of spreading.
4. This is one of the easiest and most popular methods for producing a blood smear, but it does not produce quality smears. The WBCs are unevenly distributed and RBC distortion is seen at the edges. Smaller WBCs such as lymphocytes tend to reside in the middle of the feathered edge. Large cells such as monocytes, immature cells, and abnormal cells can be found in the outer limits of this area.

Automatic Spinner Technique

Principle Although there are several automatic slide spinners on the market, their basic principle remains the same. A small quantity of patient blood is placed in the middle of a 3 × 1 inch glass slide. The slide is held in a horizontal position by a platen. The motor of the spinner is activated and accelerates rapidly to a predetermined speed. When the slide has spun for its predetermined time, the motor quickly stops.

A slide with a monolayer of cells is produced, suitable for evaluation. An even distribution of cells over the entire slide makes this preparation ideal for performing differentials on samples with low WBC counts, as well as normal and abnormal specimens. One disadvantage is that the slides must be extremely clean to prevent the shearing and spreading of cells as they are spun. The main disadvantage to this method is the hazard of blood aerosols from the spinner. Unfortunately, this disadvantage has led to the decline in the use of this method.

Staining of the Peripheral Blood Smear by Romanowsky Methods

Principle A Romanowsky stain is any stain combination consisting of eosin Y or eosin B with methylene blue and/or any of its oxidation products. Such stains produce the typical purple coloration of leukocyte nuclei and neutrophilic granules as well as the numerous blues and pinks found in other cell types.[19] Methyl alcohol is used as both a solvent and fixative in this procedure.

Reagents and Equipment

1. Stain
   a. Powdered commercial Wright stain   9 g
   b. Powdered commercial Giemsa stain   1.0 g
   c. Glycerin   90 mL
   d. Absolute anhydrous methyl alcohol
       2910 mL
   Ingredients are mixed in a brown bottle 1 month before use. Mixture should be thoroughly shaken and filtered before staining smears.
2. 15 M phosphate buffer, pH 6.4.

Procedure

1. Align blood smeared slides on horizontal rack so that smears are facing upward.
2. Cover the entire smear for 1 minute with prepared stain.
3. Carefully add buffer in same quantity as stain and mix by maneuvering slide. Do not let stain mixture spill off slides.
4. Rinse stain with neutral distilled water until stained area appears pink.
5. Allow slide to air-dry.

Comments

1. Insufficient washing, alkaline stain, or prolonged staining may lead to bluish-red cells and dark blue nuclei.
2. Inadequate staining, prolonged washing, or stain that is too acidic may lead to red cells that have stained too red and pale-grey-blue nuclei.
3. Precipitates present on slides may be caused by insufficient washing, allowing stain to dry on slides, or by using dirty slides.[20] Only precleaned slides should be used for staining blood smears.
4. Table 31–4 describes the characteristic staining patterns of Romanowsky-like stains on the cellular components of hematologic cells.

The Hema-Tek Automated Slide Stainer

Principle The Hema-Tek slide stainer (Fig. 31–20) is a fully automated benchtop instrument capable of housing up to 25 slides. These slides are pulled along a metal platen and stained at a rate of one slide per minute. This instrument has delivered uniform reproducibility and is nearly maintenance-free. The stain is contained in a "stain-pak" that sits within the instrument connected by stylets and tubing and consists of Wright-Giemsa stain, buffer, and rinse. These stains are triggered to pump and deliver a certain amount of

TABLE 31–4 **Romanowsky Staining Patterns of Hematologic Cells**	
Cellular Constituent	**Color**
Nuclei	Purple
Myeloblast cytoplasm	Blue
Promyelocyte cytoplasm	Blue
Myelocyte cytoplasm	Pink
Metamyelocyte cytoplasm	Pink
Neutrophil cytoplasm	Pink
Lymphocyte cytoplasm	Blue
Monocyte cytoplasm	Gray-blue
Erythroblast cytoplasm	Dark blue
Erythrocyte	Pink
Basophilic granules	Purple-black
Eosinophilic granules	Reddish orange
Neutrophilic granules	Pink-purple
Platelet granules	Pink-purple
Azurophilic granules	Red or purple
Auer body inclusions	Purple
Dohle body inclusions	Blue
Howell-Jolly bodies	Purple
Cabot rings	Pink-purple

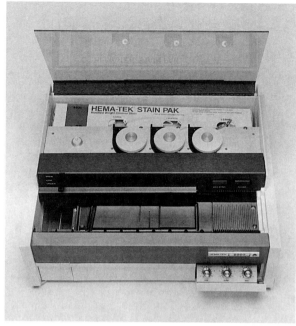

FIGURE 31–20 THe Hema-Tek Slide Stainer and Stain-Pak. (Courtesy of the Bayer Corporation, Tarrytown, NY.)

TABLE 31–5 **Estimation of Total WBC Count from the Peripheral Blood Smear**	
No./High Power Field	**Estimated Total WBC Count/cu mm**
2–4	4000–7000
4–6	7000–10,000
6–10	10,000–13,000
10–20	13,000–18,000

cu mm = cubic millimeters

solution to the slide via capillary space on the instrument.

Once the slide has been stained and rinsed, it will then pass through a final panel on the metal platen to be air-dried. The slides then drop into a separate compartment where they can sit until the differential is performed. For further inquiries, the reader is referred to the Ames Hema-Tek operation manual.[21]

Examination of the Peripheral Blood Smear

There are several necessary steps in the examination of a peripheral blood smear.

Low-Power (×10) Scan

1. Determine the overall staining quality of the blood smear.
2. Determine if there is a good distribution of the cells on the smear.
   a. Scan the edges and center of the slide to be sure there are no clumps of RBCs, WBCs, or platelets.
   b. Scan the edges for abnormal cells.
3. Find an optimal area for the detailed examination and enumeration of cells.

   a. The RBCs should not quite touch each other.
   b. There should not be areas containing large amounts of broken cells or precipitated stain.
   c. The RBCs should have a graduated central pallor.

High-Power (×40) Examination

1. Determine the WBC estimate.
   a. The WBC estimate is performed under high power (400×) according to the values given in Table 31–5.
2. Correlate the WBC estimate with the WBC counts per mm^3.
3. Evaluate the morphology of the WBCs and record any abnormalities such as toxic granulation or Dohle bodies.

Oil Immersion (×100) Examination

1. Perform a 100 WBC differential count.
   a. All WBCs are to be included.
2. Evaluate RBC anisocytosis, poikilocytosis, hypochromasia, polychromasia, and inclusions.
3. Perform a platelet estimate and evaluate platelet morphology.
   a. Count the number of platelets in 10 oil immersion fields.
   b. Divide by 10.
   c. Multiply by $15,000/mm^3$ if slide was prepared by an automatic slide spinner; multiply by $20,000/mm^3$ for all other blood smear preparations.
4. Correct any total WBC count per mm^3 that has greater than 10 nucleated red blood cells (NRBCs) per 100 WBCs.
   a. When performing the WBC differential, do not include NRBCs in your count, but report them as the number of NRBCs per 100 WBCs.
   b. Use the following formula to correct a WBC count:

$$\text{Corrected WBCs/mm}^3 = \frac{\text{WBC/mm}^3 \times 100}{100 + \text{no. of NRBCs/100 WBCs}}$$

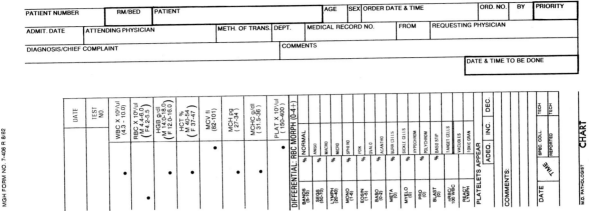

FIGURE 31–21 Hematology laboratory report sample form illustrating the complete blood count (CBC).

The examination of the peripheral blood smear is performed as part of the hematologic laboratory workup called the complete blood count (Fig. 31–21).

Buffy Coat Preparation for Decreased WBC Counts

Principle The WBC:RBC ratio contained with an EDTA tube is increased by centrifugation and removal of the top layer of cells. Albumin and normal saline are added to the tube to prevent cell overcrowding. Aliquots of the cell suspension are cytocentrifuged onto slides and stained with Wright-Giemsa stain for WBC classification.[22]

Specimen EDTA anticoagulated venous blood is the specimen of choice.

Procedure

1. Centrifuge the blood sample for 5 minutes at 2000 rpm.
2. Transfer the top layer of cells (approx. 0.5 mL) to a Wintrobe hematocrit tube. This layer will contain red cells.
3. Centrifuge the Wintrobe tube for 5 minutes at 2000 rpm.
4. Carefully remove the plasma without disturbing the cells.
5. Transfer the top layer of cells (approximately 0.03 mL) to a 20-mL plastic vial.
6. Prepare a 1% to 2% RBC suspension with normal saline in the plastic vial.
7. Add 3 drops of 22% bovine albumin/10 mL to RBC suspension.
8. Add 6 drops of the suspension to the cytocentrifuge holders attached to slides.
9. Centrifuge the specimen for 5 minutes at 1400 rpm.
10. Allow the slides to air-dry before staining with Wright-Giemsa stain.

Comments

1. This method of buffy coat preparation alleviates the tedious counting of a low number of WBCs on the peripheral blood smear and misrepresentation of a 100 white cell differential.
2. The amount of albumin added may vary depending on the presence of artifacts on the blood smear. If there is an excess of albumin, the cells will appear too dark.

TESTS FOR HEMOGLOBINS

Hemoglobinometry

Principle

Hemoglobin, the main component of the RBC, transports oxygen to and CO_2 from the body's tissues. Hemoglobin in circulating blood is a mixture of hemoglobin, oxyhemoglobin, carboxyhemoglobin, and minor amounts of other forms of this pigment. It is necessary to prepare a stable derivative involving all forms of hemoglobin in the blood in order to measure this compound accurately. The cyanmethemoglobin (HiCN) derivative can be conveniently and reproducibly prepared and is widely used for hemoglobin determination. All forms of circulating hemoglobin are readily converted to HiCN except for sulfhemoglobin, which is rarely present in significant amounts. Cyanmethemoglobin can be measured accurately by its absorbance in a colorimeter.

The basic principle of the cyanmethemoglobin (HiCN, hemoglobin-cyanide method) is that blood diluted in a solution of potassium ferricyanide yields oxidation to the ferric state (Fe^{3+}) to form methemeglobin (Hi-hemoglobin). This solution reacts with potassium cyanide to form stable cyanmethemoglobin, which is read on a spectrophotometer at 540 nm.

Procedure

Automated hematology analyzers routinely perform hemoglobin determinations. The reader is referred to manufacturer instructions for specific methodology.

Interpretation

Normal values (g/100 mL)

Man	14–17
Woman	12.5–15
Newborn	17–23
3-month-old	9–14
10-year-old	12–14.5

Hemoglobin Electrophoresis

Principle

Electrophoresis is defined as the movement of charged particles in an electric field. The different normal and abnormal hemoglobins show different mobilities of migration patterns in an electric field at a fixed pH. The usual support medium is cellulose acetate at an alkaline pH of 8.5. The procedure that follows is from Helena Laboratories, and all reagents and apparatus are available through their organization.[23]

Reagents

1. Hemolysate reagent
2. Controls A_1FSC; normal A_1A_2 patient
3. Buffer: Supre-Heme buffer (one envelope is dissolved in distilled water and diluted to 980 ml *tris*-EDTA-boric acid buffer, pH 8.4)
4. Ponceau S stain
5. Destain: 5-mL glacial acetic acid per 100 mL distilled water, a 5% solution
6. Dehydrating agent: Absolute methanol
7. Clearing solution: 150-mL glacial acetic acid, 350 mL absolute methanol, and 20 mL Clear Aid
8. Titan III-H cellulose acetate plates.

Equipment

1. Cliniscan
2. Helena Titan power supply
3. Incubator-oven-dryer
4. Electrophoresis chamber
5. Super Z sample well plate
6. Super Z aligning base
7. Applicator
8. Zip-zone chamber wicks

Procedure

1. Preparation of hemolysate: Spin EDTA blood for 20 minutes at 3000 rpm to pack the RBCs. Remove the plasma and buffy coat. Add 6 drops of hemolysate reagent to 1 drop of packed RBCs. Let stand for 1 minute; then vortex for 1 minute. Hemolysate may be frozen and then thawed to ensure complete hemolysis.
2. Preparation of electrophoretic chamber: Pour 100 mL of buffer into each outer compartment. Soak a wick in each compartment, and then drape it over the bridge, making sure it contacts the buffer. Cover the chamber.
3. Preparation of cellulose acetate plates: Number the plates on the bottom right of the glossy side. Wet the plates by slowly lowering the rack into a container of buffer. Allow to soak for at least 5 minutes.
4. Preparation of sample well plates: Clean with distilled water and dry each well with a cotton swab. Prepare two rinse plates by filling the wells with distilled water. Prepare the patient samples by using a 5-lambda microdispenser to fill the wells on clean dry plates. Patient samples should be run in duplicate, and a normal A_1A_2 and A_1FSC control should be run on each plate. Cover with glass slide to prevent evaporation.
5. Loading of cellulose acetate plates:
   a. Prime the applicator by depressing several times into the same well plate and then depressing once on a blotter.
   b. Remove the cellulose acetate plate from the buffer; blot once firmly; and place on the aligning base with the number at the bottom left.
   c. Load the applicator by depressing three times into the sample well plate; then transfer the applicator to the aligning base, and depress the bar firmly for 5 seconds.
   d. Place the plate, glossy side up, across the bridge in the electrophoresis chamber.
6. Electrophoresis at 350 volts for 25 minutes.
7. Staining:
   a. Apply Ponceau S for 5 minutes. Drain for 5 to 10 seconds.
   b. Four successive washes of 5% glacial acetic acid are used to destain. Leave in each for 2 minutes, draining for 5 seconds between each wash.
   c. Use two successive washes of absolute methanol to dehydrate. Leave for 2 minutes in each, draining for 5 seconds between each wash.
   d. Apply clearing solution for 5 minutes.
   e. Dry vertically for 1 to 2 minutes.
   f. Dry in the oven for 3 to 4 minutes, acetate side up.
8. Scan the plate with the Cliniscan using a 525-nm filter, slit size 5, and optics filter wheel V-2 O.D.
9. Label the plate and store in a plastic envelope as a permanent record.

Results

Variant hemoglobins are reported in relative percentages.

Hemoglobin A_1 (HbA$_1$)	96.0–98.6%
Hemoglobin A_2 (HbA$_2$)	1.5–4.0%
Hemoglobin F (HbF)	
At birth	60.0–90.0%
After 1 yr of age	1.0–2.0%

Comments

At an alkaline pH, hemoglobins S and D have the same mobility, as do hemogobins A_2, C, E, and O_{Arab}. These hemoglobins may be separated by electrophoresing on citrate agar at an acid pH (Fig. 31–22). Hemoglobin A_2 may also be quantitated by column. HbF separates from HbA in this system and migrates slightly closer to the origin. However, cellulose acetate electrophoresis is not recommended as an initial screening test during the neonatal period because

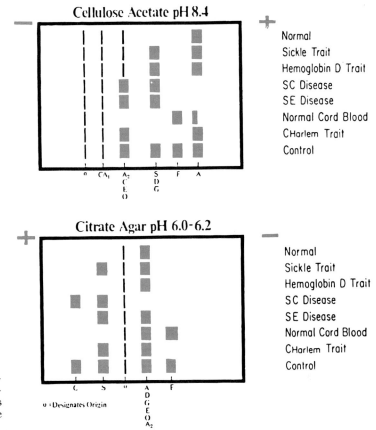

FIGURE 31-22 Comparative hemoglobin electrophoresis. Hemoglobin electrophoresis on cellulose acetate and citrate agar indicating patterns of mobility. The width of the band is not indicative of hemoglobin concentration.

large amounts of HbF form a heavy band overlapping the adjacent bands of HbA or HbS.[24] The procedure for separation and quantitation of HbF is based on acid and/or alkali resistance (see HbF denaturation).

Citrate Agar Hemoglobin Electrophoresis

Principle

As mentioned earlier, electrophoresis is the movement of charged particles in an electric field. Using citrate agar at an acid pH facilitates the separation of hemoglobins that migrate together on other media (cellulose acetate) at a different pH (alkaline). The following procedure is that of Helena Laboratories, and all reagents and apparatus are available from their organization.

Reagents

1. Hemolysate reagent
2. Controls A_1FSC; normal A_1A_2
3. Buffer: Citrate buffer. Dissolve one package in distilled water and dilute to 1 L.
4. Stain:
   a. 10 mL of 5% glacial acetic acid
   b. 5 mL of toluidine in methanol
   c. 1 mL of sodium nitroferricyanide in water
   d. 1 mL of 3% hydrogen peroxide
   e. Prepare fresh on day of use.
5. Titan IV citrate agar plates

Equipment

1. Helena Titan power supply
2. Electrophoresis chamber
3. Sample well plate
4. Aligning base
5. Applicator
6. Sponge wicks

Procedure

1. Preparation of hemolysate: Spin EDTA blood for 20 minutes at 3000 rpm to pack the red cells. Remove the plasma and buffy coat. Add 10 drops of hemolysate reagent to 1 drop of packed RBCs. Let stand for 1 minute, then vortex for 1 minute. Hemolysate may be frozen and then thawed to ensure complete hemolysis.
2. Preparation of electrophoresis chamber: Pour 100 mL of buffer into each outer compartment. Soak a sponge wick in each compartment, then place it so that the top of the sponge protrudes over the inner ridge of the compartment. Cover the chamber.
3. Preparation of sample well plates: Clean all wells with distiled water and dry with cotton swabs. Prepare the patient samples by using a 5-lambda microdispenser to fill the wells. Patient hemolysates should be run in duplicate, plus an A_1FSC and an A_1A_2 control should be run on each plate. Cover the plate with a glass slide to prevent evaporation.

4. Loading of citrate agar plates:
   a. Prime the applicator by pressing several times into the sample well plate, and then dispensing once on a blotter.
   b. Place the Titan IV citrate agar plate on the aligning base.
   c. Load the applicator by pressing three times into the sample well plate; then transfer applicator to the aligning base.
   d. Depress the applicator onto the gel surface using no pressure, and allow hemolysate to absorb for 1 minute.
5. Place the plate gel side down across the inner ridges of the electrophoresis chamber with the application point near the anode.
6. Electrophorese for 40 minutes, at 40 mA per plate and 50 V per plate.
7. Staining:
   a. Place the plate in a staining dish and puddle the stain over the surface. Let stand for 5 to 10 minutes.
   b. Rinse with distilled water for 10 minutes.
   c. Cover with another gel plate and seal with tape to store.

Results

With this procedure, hemoglobin S and D can be separated. Hemoglobin D, instead of migrating with HbS as in an alkaline buffer, will migrate with HbA. This procedure also separates hemoglobins A_2 and E from HbC, as hemoglobins A_2 and E will migrate with HbA, leaving HbC by itself. The pattern distributes thus from cathode to anode: hemoglobins C, S, A_1, A_2, D, E, and F (see Fig. 31–22).

Hemoglobin A_2 by Column
Principle

This is an anion-exchange chromatography method. The anion exchange resin is a preparation of cellulose covalently coupled to small positively changed molecules, which will attract negatively charged molecules. Hemoglobins have positive or negative charges, owing to properties of their component amino acids. Here buffer and pH favor net negatively charged hemoglobins, which are attracted and bound to the resin. Once bound, the hemoglobins can be selectively eluted and measured on a spectrophotometer. This procedure (the Sickle-Thal column method) is that of Helena Laboratories.

Reagents

1. Control: Quik column control
2. Sickle-Thal Quik Column
3. Hemoglobin A_2 developer
4. Hemoglobin S developer
5. Hemolysate reagent C

All are available from various manufacturers

Equipment

1. Column rack and collection tubes
2. Spectrophotometer

Procedure

1. Preparation of hemolysate: Add 50-lambda EDTA blood plus 200-lambda hemolysate reagent C to a small test tube. Vortex vigorously and allow to stand 5 minutes before use.
2. Preparation of columns:
   a. Allow to come to room temperature.
   b. Turn each column upside down twice, place it in the rack, remove top cap, and resuspend with a pipet.
   c. Remove the bottom cap and allow the buffer to drain out.
   d. After the resin repacks, remove any buffer remaining at the top, being careful not to disturb the resin.
3. Slowly apply 100 lambda of patient hemolysate to the column and allow to absorb into the resin.
4. Put 100 lambda of patient hemolysate in a large collection tube and Q.S. to 15 ml with distilled water. Label this tube "total fraction."
5. Elution of HbA_2:
   a. Slowly apply 3 mL of HbA_2 developer and allow to pass through the column into the small collection tube (approximately 30 minutes).
   b. Q.S. the tube to 3 mL with distilled water.
6. Elution of HbS (optional):
   a. Slowly add 10 mL of HbS developer to the column in aliquots of 3 mL, 3 mL, and 4 mL.
   b. Allow it to pass through the column into a large collection tube (approximately 1.5 to 2 hours).
   c. Q.S. the tube to 15 mL with distilled water.
7. Using the spectrophotometer at 415 nm, record the absorbance of the HbA_2 eluate, the HbS eluate, and the total fraction.

Results

$$\% \ HbA_2 = \frac{OD \ HbA_2 \ eluate \times 100}{5 \times OD \ total \ fraction}$$

$$\% \ HbS = \frac{OD \ HbS \ eluate \times 100}{OD \ total \ fraction}$$

where OD = optical density

The HbS eluate is optional, as it can be picked up on alkaline electrophoresis.

The normal range for HbA_2 is 1.5 to 4.0%. This can be used to separate HbA_2 and HbC or HbE. Elevated levels of HbA_2 may be useful in diagnosing a β-thalassemia. Be careful not to underload or overload the column with the hemolysate. Overloading the column may cause incomplete separation of the HbA_2. Underloading the column may make visual collection of the HbA_2 fraction impossible.[25]

Solubility Test for Hemoglobin S
Principle

Sickling hemoglobin, which is defined as any hemoglobin that causes erythrocytes to sickle under conditions of low oxygen tension, in a deoxygenated state will form a precipitate when exposed to a high molarity phosphate buffer solution.[26] This precipitation is the result of tactoids forming from deoxygenated hemoglobin molecules producing a turbid solution. This turbidity is qualitatively determined from the inability to visualize black type lines on a white background. This procedure utilizes packed red blood cells.

4. Stock solution:

Dibasic potassium phosphate, anhydrous (1.24 mol), K_2HPO_4	216 g
Monobasic potassium phosphate, crystals (1.24 mol), KH_2PO_4	169 g
Saponin	10 g
Distilled water	to 1 L

Note: Reagent should be stored at 4°C for approximately 1 month and should be checked against a known positive and negative control. There are many commercial kits available that mimic this procedure, (i.e., Sickle-quik, General Diagnostics), and each new reagent should be checked with known positive and negative controls.

Working Solution Sodium hydrosulfite (dithionite) $Na_2S_2O_4$ (5 mg/mL of stock reagent) is added on the day of testing.

Procedure

1. Pipet 2 mL of working solution into a labeled 12 mm × 75 mm test tube.
2. Allow working solution to warm to room temperature.
3. Centrifuge whole blood (EDTA) at 1500 to 2000 g for 5 minutes to remove buffy coat and plasma.
4. Add 10 μL of packed erythrocytes.
5. Mix and wait 5 minutes.
6. Hold tube approximately 2.5 cm in front of white card with black lines.
7. Read for qualitative determination of turbidity.

Results

A negative result (indicating no sickling hemoglobins) occurs when the black lines are visible through the test solution.

A positive result (indicating the presence of a sickling hemoglobin) is indicated by a very turbid solution in which the black lines cannot be seen through the test solution) (see Fig. 11–11). Other sickling hemoglobins may be present; therefore, this test is not specific for hemoglobin S. Table 31–6 depicts hemoglobins that can be present from negative and positive results of this test. Both positive and negative controls must be run for each solubility test performed.

Comments

1. Erroneous results may be seen in normal blood transfused to an anemic patient whose native blood contains a sickling hemoglobin, or blood transfused that contained a sickling hemoglobin.
2. Cold reagent may cause inaccurate results as well as whole blood used instead of packed cells,

Reagents and Equipment

1. 12 × 75 mm disposable glass or plastic test tubes.
2. Reading card with 14-point or 18-point black type in straight lines on a white background, approximately 0.5 cm apart (see Fig. 11–11).
3. Centrifuge (1500–2000 g)

the latter because of excess gamma globulins, extreme leukocytosis, or hyperlipidemia.[24]

Acid Elution for Hemoglobin F

Principle

Hemoglobin F in RBCs is resistant to acid elution; therefore, it can be precipitated and stained. Hemoglobin A will be eluted from the RBCs. This is a modification of the original Kleihauer stain.

Reagents

1. Fetal cell fixing solution: 80% reagent alcohol
2. Fetal cell buffer solution: citrate buffer 0.027 M
3. Fetal cell stain: erythrosin B
4. Control: 0.1 mL of cord blood plus 0.9 mL of normal adult blood

Procedure

1. Add 2 drops of EDTA blood to 3 drops of 0.85% saline.
2. Prepare a monolayer film of this suspension. Allow to air-dry.
3. Immerse film in fixing solution for 5 minutes at room temperature.
4. Rinse in distilled water and allow to air-dry.
5. Immerse in buffer solution for 8 to 10 minutes at room temperature.
6. Immediately immerse in staining solution for 3 minutes at room temperature.

TABLE 31–6 **Hemoglobins Present in Positive/Negative Solubility Tests**	
Positive	**Negative**
Hb C$_{Harlem}$	Hb A
HbS	Hb F
Hb S$_{Travis}$	Hb C
Hb C$_{Ziguinchor}$	Hb D
	Hb G
	Hb E
	Lepore
	Hb A$_2$

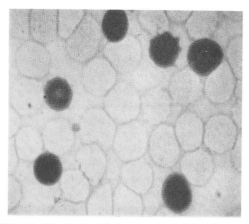

FIGURE 31–23 Betke-Kleihauer stain of blood from a newborn. Red-staining cells contain hemoglobin F; clear staining cells contain hemoglobin A. (From Diggs, LW: Hematology. In Listen, Look and Learn. Health and Education Resources, Inc., Bethesda, MD, with permission.)

7. Rinse in distilled water and allow to air-dry.
8. Examine for the presence of cells staining for fetal hemoglobin.

Results

Cells containing HbF will stain bright pink-red. Those containing only HbA will be very light pink (Fig. 31–23). The stain may be useful in distinguishing hereditary persistence of fetal hemoglobin (HPFH), in which most RBCs show an even distribution of HbF, from a high level of HbF in a patient with thalassemia minor (in which the distribution of HbF is uneven). The percentage of fetal cells may be calculated if this stain is to be used to assess fetal cells in maternal circulation.[27]

Staining for Heinz Bodies

Principle

Heinz bodies are denatured hemoglobulin precipitated in the RBC and attached to the RBC membrane. They are not visible with Wright's stain but show up with supravital staining (crystal violet) and phase microscopy (see Fig. 4–1).

Reagents and Equipment

1. Crystal violet solution: 1.0 g of crystal violet dissolved in 50 mL of a 0.85% saline solution, which is shaken for 5 minutes and filtered before storage.
2. Methyl violet solution: 0.5 g of methyl violet dissolved in 100 mL of a 0.85% saline solution, which is shaken for 5 minutes and filtered before storage.
   Note: A 0.75% saline solution may be used. This slightly hypotonic solution may swell the cells.
3. Glass slides and coverslip
4. Microscope

Procedure

1. Mix equal volumes of EDTA blood and stain in a small test tube. Either stain may be used.
2. Incubate for 20 minutes at room temperature.
3. Remix the blood-stain solution and transfer 1 drop to a slide.
4. Place a coverslip on the slide and examine for Heinz bodies under oil immersion.

Results

Heinz bodies appear as irregular, refractile, purple inclusions, 1 to 3 μm in diameter, located on the periphery of the cell. They may even seem to be outside the cell. Reticulocytes are not stained by this technique.[28]

TESTS FOR HEMOLYTIC ANEMIAS

Osmotic Fragility

Principle

Whole blood is added to a series of saline dilutions. Exposure to hypotonic solution causes water to be drawn into the erythrocyte through osmosis. This eventually leads to swelling of the erythrocyte, leaking, and bursting of the cell. Once the cell bursts, hemoglobin is released and can be measured with a spectrophotometer. The presence or absence of hemolysis is an effective measure of erythrocyte susceptibility to hypotonic damage. This test is more than just an index of cell shape; it is also a measure of the surface-to-volume ratio. When an RBC's membrane surface decreases and its volume remains the same or increases, the cell becomes more turgid and less deformable. This is because the RBC membrane is flexible but not elastic. The result of this loss of surface-to-volume ratio is similar to what happens to a small plastic bag that is filled with more and more water.

Spherocytes, which have a decreased surface-to-volume ratio, demonstrate an increased osmotic fragility. This is because of their inability to swell in a hypotonic medium before leaking hemoglobin. Sickle cells, target cells, and other poikilocytes are relatively resistant to osmotic change and therefore demonstrate a decreased fragility.

Reagents and Equipment

1. Twenty-four 12 × 75 mm test tubes
2. Two 5-mL serologic pipet (TD); one 3-mL pipet
3. Parafilm squares
4. One heparinized normal control sample
5. One heparinized patient sample
6. Linear graph paper
7. 1% NaCl solution: Weight 1.0 g NaCl crystals on an analytical balance. Place crystals in a 100-mL volumetric flask and fill to the mark with distilled water. Stir to completely dissolve NaCl.
8. Spectrophotometer
Note: Procedure can also be performed using Unopette Erythrocyte Fragility Test Kit by Becton Dickinson Vacutainer Systems. When using this kit, note

that saline dilutions are prepackaged in individual reservoirs.

Procedure

1. Arrange two series of 12 tubes in the rack. Label both sets of tubes 1 through 12. The first series of tubes 1 through 12 is for the patient and the second series is for the control.
2. With a 5-mL pipet and 1% NaCl solution, and with the other 5-mL pipet, add distilled water into the series of patient tubes according to the following schedule:

Tube	1% NaCl (mL)	Distilled Water (mL)	NaCl% Final Concentration
1	4.25	0.75	0.85
2	3.50	1.50	0.70
3	3.25	1.75	0.65
4	3.00	2.00	0.60
5	2.75	2.25	0.55
6	2.50	2.50	0.50
7	2.25	2.75	0.45
8	2.00	3.00	0.40
9	1.75	3.25	0.35
10	1.50	3.50	0.30
11	1.25	3.75	0.25
12	0.75	4.25	0.15

3. Thoroughly mix the contents of each tube by covering with parafilm and inverting several times.
4. With a 3-mL pipette, transfer 2.5 mL of solution from the first set of tubes to the corresponding second set. Only one pipette is necessary if you start to transfer with the most dilute solution.
5. Draw blood into a tube containing heparin. Immediately add 50 μL of blood into each tube of the first set. The blood should drop directly into the solution. Do not allow the blood to drop onto the sides of the tube.
6. Add 50 μL of known normal blood, collected in the same manner, to each tube in the second set.
7. Let the tubes sit at room temperature for half an hour.
8. Mix gently and centrifuge at 2000 rpm for 5 minutes.
9. When interpreting results, note which tubes show initial and complete hemolysis. Initial hemolysis is recognized by a faintly pink supernatant and a cell button at the bottom of the tube. Complete hemolysis is seen as a red supernatant with possibly a button of cell stroma at the bottom of the tube.
10. This test may be quantitated by measuring each tube on the spectrophotometer. To do this, two additional tubes are necessary. The first is a blank containing 50 μL of blood to which 2.5 mL of 0.9% NaCl is added, which will result in no hemolysis. The second blank is complete (100%) hemolysis and is obtained by adding 50 μL of blood to 2.5 mL of distilled water.

11. These blanks are run in parallel with the other tubes.
12. After centrifugation, the supernatant of each tube is removed, and its optical density (OD) is read in a spectrophotometer using a 540-nm filter.[29] The percentage of hemolysis in each tube is calculated using the following equation:

$$\% \text{ Hemolysis} = \frac{\text{OD }(x) - \text{OD } 0.85\%}{\text{OD }(o) - \text{OD } 0.85\%} \times 100$$

where OD(x) represents absorbance of sample solution of NaCl concentration and OD(o) represents a sample blank, NaCl concentration (0.00%). An osmotic fragility curve may be drawn by plotting the percentage of hemolysis in each tube against the corresponding concentration of NaCl solution, as shown (Fig. 31–24). It is helpful to plot the normal control with the patient so that any difference can be seen more clearly.

Interpretation

1. Patient values are always reported with the value of the control. With the normal samples, initial hemoysis is generally around 0.45%, with complete hemolysis occurring at 0.30% or 0.35%.
2. Examples of initial and complete hemolysis in various conditions follow:

	Initial Hemolysis (%NaCl)	Complete Hemolysis (%NaCl)
Normal	0.45	0.35
Hereditary spherocytosis	0.65	0.45
Acquired hemolytic anemia	0.50	0.40
Hemolytic disease of the newborn	0.55	0.40
Thalassemia	0.35	0.20
Sickle-cell anemia	0.35	0.20

It may be necessary in some cases to incubate the patient's heparinized blood for 24 hours at 37°C. This will enhance increased osmotic fragility, which may reveal a subtle but abnormal osmotic fragility not apparent upon initial testing.

Comments

1. Fresh heparinized blood is recommended, but defibrinated blood may be used. Oxalate, EDTA, or citrate should not be used because of the additional salts present.
2. Perform this test immediately because cell shape and osmotic conditions change with time.
3. Osmotic fragility can be altered by pH and temperature.
4. If the plasma is significantly jaundiced, replace the plasma with isotonic saline before testing to prevent interference.
5. Hemolytic organisms in a blood specimen can cause erroneous results owing to hemolysis, which is not attributed to test conditions.

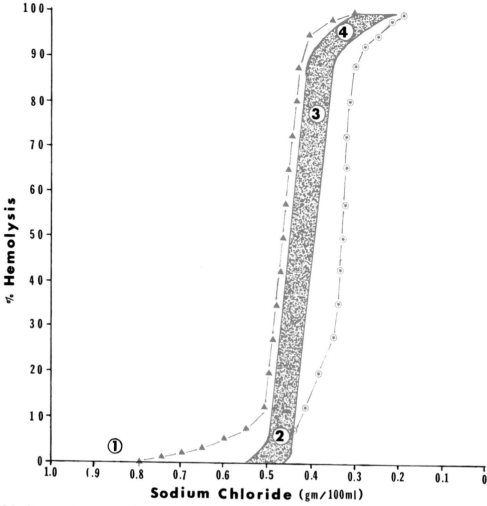

FIGURE 31–24 Comparative osmotic fragility curve (*sickle-cell anemia; hereditary spherocytosis). Normal range is indicated by shaded area. 1 = normal biconcave disc; 2 = disc-to-sphere transformation; 3 = disc-to-sphere transformation; 4 = lysis.

6. If the patient has a low hemoglobin level, wash patient and control cells once with isotonic saline and resuspend with equal volumes of RBCs and saline for both specimens. This will correct for the anemia.

7. In some anemias, when poikilocytosis accompanies a low hemoglobin level, decreased osmotic fragility may be seen. This may be partly the result of decreased hemoglobin concentration and not of the presence of poikilocytes.

Acidified Serum Test (Ham Test) for Paroxysmal Nocturnal Hemoglobinuria

Principle

Confirmation of diagnosis of paroxysmal nocturnal hemoglobinuria (PNH) is dependent on a positive acidified serum test result. The RBCs of patients with PNH are complement-sensitive. In this test, complement will affix to the RBCs at a slightly acidic pH, become activated by the alternative pathway, and result in lysis of the RBCs.[30]

Reagents and Equipment

1. Venous patient specimen
2. Venous normal control (ABO compatible)
3. Five 12 mm × 75 mm test tubes
4. 0.2 N HCL
5. 1-mL serologic pipets
6. Two Erlenmeyer flasks
7. Glass beads

Procedure

1. Collect venous specimens from patient and control in a plastic syringe and defibrinate by swirling in an Erlenmeyer flask that contains glass beads.
2. Centrifuge the defibrinated blood and separate serum from cells. Save the normal control serum, the patient's serum, and RBCs.

3. Wash the RBCs from the patient and control three times with isotonic saline, and dilute to a 50% cell suspension.

4. Label test tubes 1 through 5.
5. Add the reagents to the five tubes in numerical order, as shown in the accompanying table.

Reagents	Tubes 1	2	3	4	5
Patient serum	0.5 mL	0.5 mL			
Normal serum			0.5 mL	0.5 mL	0.5 mL
0.2 N HCl		0.5 mL	0.5 mL		0.05 mL
Patient's RBCs (50%)	1 drop	1 drop	1 drop	1 drop	
Normal RBCs (50%)					1 drop

6. Cover with parafilm and incubate all tubes for 1 hour at 37°C.
7. Centrifuge and examine supernatant for hemolysis.

Interpretation

1. Patients with PNH will demonstrate hemolysis in tubes 2 and 3. Tube 3 was run in the event that the patient had decreased complement levels.
2. Little or no hemolysis will be seen in tubes 1 and 4.
3. No hemolysis should be seen in the control, tube 5.

Comments

1. The optimum pH for this test is 6.5 to 6.7.
2. Blood containing a large number of spherocytes, as seen in hereditary spherocytosis (HS), may result in a false-positive result.
3. The test result may be positive also in hereditary erythroblastic multinuclearity with positive acidified serum (HEMPAS) test. There are, however, two differentiating features; in HEMPAS the RBCs are not lysed by the patient's own acidified serum, and the sugar water test result is negative for patients with this condition.

Sugar Water Test for Paroxysmal Nocturnal Hemoglobinuria

Principle

In patients with PNH, the sucrose solution provides a low ionic strength environment that allows complement proteins to bind to the RBCs. These abnormal cells are extremely complement sensitive, which results in complement-mediated lysis.

Reagents and Equipment

1. Stock sucrose solution: Dissolve 486 g sucrose and 5.1 g sodium barbital in 500 mL distilled water. Adjust the pH to 7.3 to 7.4 with HCl and water to reach 1 L. Store at 4°C.
2. Working sucrose solution: Mix 20 mL stock solution with 80 mL water.
3. Test tubes, 12 mm × 75 mm
4. 1 mL serologic pipets
5. Spectrophotometer

Procedure

1. Prepare a 50% blood suspension from EDTA-anticoagulated whole blood. Determine the ABO blood group.
2. Access type-compatible fresh normal serum or serum from an AB donor. Serum can be stored at −20°C for up to one week.
3. Prepare the following mixtures using 12 mm × 75 mm test tubes:

Test Tube	1	2	3	4
Sucrose, mL	0.90	0.95	0.95	
Cells, mL	0.05	0.05		0.05
Serum, mL	0.05		0.05	
0.01 M NH₄OH, mL				0.95

4. Incubate mixtures for 60 minutes at room temperature.
5. After incubation add 4 mL of 0.15 M NaCl and centrifuge to remove residual cells for 1 to 2 minutes at 3400 rpm.
6. Take absorbance readings of the supernatant against a water blank at 540 nm.

Calculations

The percent lysis is calculated by the following formula:

$$\% \text{ lysis} = \frac{\text{OD tube 1} - (\text{OD tube 2} + \text{OD tube 3}) \times 100}{(\text{OD tube 4} - \text{OD tube 2})}$$

Comments

1. Though this test does not always accurately reflect complement-sensitive cells, a percent lysis value of greater than 5 ascertains a diagnosis of PNH.[31]
2. Other disease states may yield less than 5% lysis such as megaloblastic anemia and autoimmune hemolytic anemia causing false-positive results.
3. Fresh samples should be used to retain potent complement activity on PNH cells.

Autohemolysis Test

Principle

When defibrinated blood is incubated at 37°C for 48 hours, only minimal hemolysis will occur. In patients with hereditary spherocytosis (HS), autohemolysis is increased. The addition of glucose or adenosine triphosphate (ATP) to the incubation state will decrease the percentage of the abnormal hemoysis seen in the spherocytes of HS patients.

Reagents and Equipment

1. Ammonia water: Add 0.4 mL concentrated ammonium hydroxide to 1 L of deionized water.
2. 0.239 M ATP: Weigh out 121 mg of ATP, dilute with 1 mL saline, and carefully neutralize to pH 7.5 to 8.0 with 1 M NaOH. This solution must be sterilized through a 0.45-μm pore filter unit syringe.
3. Sterile 10% dextrose in 0.85% NaCl solution.
4. Sterile 125-mL Erlenmeyer flasks with approximately 25 glass beads (4 mm)
5. Sterile polypropylene tubes with caps (12 × 75 mm)
6. Sterile 5-mL pipets
7. Sterile 3-mL syringes
8. Spectrophotometer set to read at 540 nm
9. Assorted volumetric flasks, test tubes, and Pasteur pipets

Procedure

Day 1

1. Draw 25 mL of blood from the patient, and carefully defibrinate by swirling blood in a sterile 125-mL Erlenmeyer flask with glass beads. Repeat the same procedure for a control sample.
2. Prelabel six sterile 12 mm × 75 mm polypropylene tubes for each patient, and control and dispense the appropriate reagents as follows:

	Tubes					
	1*	2*	3	4	5	6
10% dextrose in saline (ml)			0.1	0.1		
0.239 M ATP (ml)					0.1	0.1

*Tubes 1 and 2 remain plain.

3. Add 2 mL of the appropriate defibrinated blood to each tube and gently rotate to mix.
4. Incubate for 24 hours in a 37°C incubator.
5. Prepare a 1:100 dilution of defibrinated blood by pipetting 0.5 mL of whole blood into a 50-mL volumetric flask, and bring it to volume with ammonia water. This is done for both the control and the patient blood.
6. Centrifuge remaining defibrinated blood, and remove serum.
7. Prepare a reagent blank by making a 1:10 dilution of serum with 4.5 mL ammonia water. This is done for both the control and the patient serum.
8. Refrigerate serum for use on day 3.
9. Read the OD of the whole blood dilutions against the serum blanks at 540 nm. Record these results.

Day 2

1. Rotate incubated samples gently, and reincubate for an additional 24 hours.

Day 3

1. Gently mix incubated samples, and pool pairs.
2. Perform a spun hematocrit on each sample (total three hematocrits per patient and control). Record results.
3. Pour each sample into a tube, and centrifuge for 5 minutes at 2500 rpm.
4. Remove the serum from each tube, and prepare a 1:10 dilution of each serum with ammonia water (0.5 mL serum with 4.5 mL ammonia water).
5. Make a 1:10 dilution of original serum saved from day 1. This will be your serum blank.
6. Read the OD of the serum samples made in step 4 at 540 nm using the sample prepared in step 5 as the reagent blank.

Calculations

The percentage of hemolysis for each tube is calculated as shown here:

$$\% \text{ Hemolysis} = \frac{(100 - \text{Hct of tube}) \times \text{OD of serum sample}}{\text{OD of whole blood} \times 10}$$

Normal Values	Lysis at 48 h
Without added dextrose	0.2–2.0%
With added dextrose	0–0.9%
With added ATP	0–0.8%

Comments

When normal blood is incubated for 48 h under sterile conditions, the amount of hemolysis is relatively small. If dextrose or ATP is added, hemolysis is further slowed.

INCUBATION HEMOLYSIS

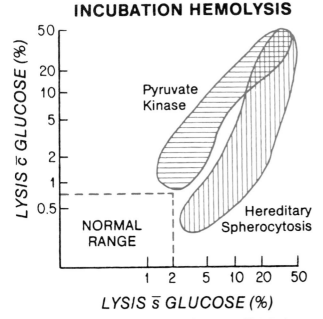

FIGURE 31-25 Incubation hemolysis test. This test provides a further measure of cell resistance to hemolysis. Pyruvate-kinase-deficient blood demonstrates an abnormal rate of hemolysis that is independent of the presence or absence of glucose in the incubation media. In contrast, the blood from a patient with hereditary spherocytosis shows more marked hemolysis when glucose is absent ($\bar{s}$). (From Hillman, RS and Finch, CA: Red Cell Manual, ed. 7. FA Davis, Philadelphia, 1996, p 124, with permission.)

Increased autohemolysis occurs in many types of hemolytic anemia. The patterns that may be observed, according to Dacie and Lewis,[32] are as follows:

1. Type I: Patients whose red cells show slight autohemolysis, corrected by dextrose, as seen in G6PD deficiency, hexokinase deficiency, and acquired nonspherocytic hemolytic anemia.
2. Type II: Patients with moderate autohemolysis without dextrose and in whom correction with dextrose does not take place, as seen in pyruvate kinase deficiency and acquired spherocytic hemolytic anemia.
3. Type III: Patients with marked autohemolysis without dextrose correction, seen in HS and triose phosphate isomerase deficiency (Fig. 31–25).

The autohemolysis test is no longer used in the differential diagnosis of nonspherocytic congenital hemolytic anemia, because specific enzymatic assays are now available that are considerably more accurate. It is, however, a useful screening test for some RBC enzyme deficiencies in the detection of hemolysis.

REFERENCES

1. Stockbower, JM, et al: Procedures for the Collection of Diagnostic Blood Specimens by Venipuncture, ed. 3. NCCLS H3-A3, Villanova, PA, July 1991, p 13.
2. Levitt, MJ, et al: Skin puncture and blood-collecting techniques for infants. Clin Chem 25:183, 1979.
3. The Unopette System for RBC Determinations, Becton-Dickinson, Rutherford, NJ, 1991.
4. Sonnenwirth, AC and Jarett, L: Gradwohl's Clinical Laboratory Methods and Diagnosis, ed 8, vol 1. CV Mosby, St Louis, 1980, p 795.
5. The Unopette System for WBC/Platelet Determinations. Becton-Dickinson, Rutherford, NJ, 1991, p 8.
6. Sonnenwirth, AC and Jarett, L: Gradwohl's Clinical Laboratory Methods and Diagnosis, ed. 8 vol 1, CV Mosby, St Louis, 1980, p 800.
7. Dale, NL and Schumacher, HR: Platelet satellitism—new spurious results with automated instruments. Lab Med 13:5, 1982.
8. Finch, CA, et al: Method for Reticulocyte Counting. NCCLS H16-P, vol 5, no 10, Villanova, PA, 1985, p 226.
9. Coulter Retic-Prep. Coulter Corporation, Miami, FL PN 7507938-C, 10/93.
10. Lee, LG, Chen, CH, and Chin, LA: Thiazole orange: A new dye for reticulocyte analysis. Cytometry 7:508, 1986.
11. Williams, WJ, Beutler, E, Erslev, AJ, and Lichtman, MA: Hematology, ed 4 McGraw-Hill, New York, p 15.
12. Koepke, JA, Bull, BS, and van Assendelft OW: Reference Procedure for the Erythrocyte Sedimentation Rate (ESR) Test, NCCLS H2-A2, ISSN 3099-0273, vol 8, no 3, Villanova, PA, 1988.
13. Westergren, A: Die Senkungsreaction. Ergeb Inn Med Kinderheilkd 5:531, 1924.
14. Wintrobe, MM and Landsberg, JW: A Standardized technique for blood sedimentation test. Am J Med Sci 189:102, 1935.
15. Henry, JB: Clinical Diagnosis and Management by Laboratory Methods, ed 18. WB Saunders, Philadelphia 1991, p 599.
16. van Assendelft, OW, et al: Procedure for Determining Packed Cell Volume by the Microhematocrit Method, NCCLS, H7-A, vol 5, no 5, Villanova, PA, 1985, p 107.
17. O'Connor, BH: A Color Atlas and Instruction Manual of Peripheral Blood Cell Morphology. Williams & Wilkins, Baltimore, 1984.
18. Dacie, JV and Lewis, SM: Practical Hematology, ed 4. Grune & Stratton, New York, 1968.
19. Marshall, PN, Bentley, SA, and Green, FJ: Romanowsky Blood Stains, NCCLS H32-P, vol 6, no 2, 1986, p 65.
20. Sonnenwirth, AC and Jarett, L: Gradwohls Clinical Laboratory Methods and Diagnosis, ed 8, vol 1, CV Mosby, St Louis, 1980, p 763.
21. Ames Hema-Tek Operational Manual. Miles Laboratories, ed 2. Elkhart, IN, 1980.
22. DeNunzio, J: Buffy coat preparation for leukopenic specimens. Lab Med, 16:497, 1985.
23. Helena Laboratories, Method for Hemoglobin Electrophoresis, Beaumont, TX, 1985.
24. Kim, HC, Adachi, K, and Schwartz, E: Separation of hemoglobins. In Williams, WJ, et al (eds): Hematology, ed 4, McGraw-Hill, New York, 1990, p 1711.
25. Schneider, RG: Chromatographic (Microcolumn) Determination of Hemoglobin A_2, NCCLS H9-A, vol 9, no 17, Villanova, PA, 1989, p 935.
26. Schneider, RG, et al: Solubility Test for Confirming the Presence of Sickling Hemoglobins, NCCLS H10-A, vol 6, no 10, Villanova, PA, 1986, p 209.
27. Screening Test for the Detection of Erythrocyte Containing Fetal Hemoglobin in Maternal Blood. Simmler Inc, St Louis, MO.
28. Beutler, E: Heinz body staining. In Williams, WJ, et al (eds): Hematology, ed 4. McGraw-Hill, New York, 1990, p 1701.
29. Beutler, E: Osmotic fragility. In Williams, WJ, et al (eds): Hematology, ed 4. McGraw-Hill, New York, 1990, p 1727.
30. Bauer, JD, Ackermann, PG, and Toro, G: Clinical Laboratory Methods, ed 8. CV Mosby, St Louis, 1974, p 220.
31. Beutler, E: Sucrose hemolysis and acidified serum lysis tests. In Williams, WJ, et al (eds): Hematology, ed 4, McGraw-Hill, New York, 1990, p 1729.
32. Dacie, JV and Lewis, SM: Practical Hematology, ed 4. Grune & Stratton, New York, 1968.

QUESTIONS

1. Twenty microliters of blood are drawn into a Unopette system for a WBC count. Fifty cells are counted on one side and 52 on the other side of a hemocytometer (4 large squares). Calculate the WBC count.
   a. 12.5×10^9/L
   b. 12.7×10^9/L
   c. 12.0×10^9/L
   d. 13.0×10^9/L

2. If a patient has a reticulocyte count of 8% with a hematocrit of 18%, what is the corrected reticulocyte count?
   a. 20%
   b. 2.3%
   c. 3.2%
   d. 8%

3. Which of the following errors will cause falsely elevated results for a centrifugal microhematocrit?
   a. Reading of buffy coat with red cells
   b. Incomplete sealing of capillary tubes
   c. Allowing the centrifuge to stop without braking
   d. All of the above

4. Which of the following factors affect(s) the ESR?
   a. Increased fibrinogen
   b. Extreme poikilocytosis
   c. Use of heparin as an anticoagulant
   d. All of the above

5. What type of hemoglobin electrophoresis would be best to separate hemoglobins S and D?
   a. Cellulose acetate at alkaline pH.
   b. Citrate agar at acid pH.
   c. Either cellulose acetate or citrate agar may be used.

6. What is the principle for the acid elution test for HbF?
   a. HbF is resistant to acid elution; it can be precipitated and stained.
   b. HbF is susceptible to acid elution; it can be dissolved and measured photometrically.
   c. HbF is resistant to acid elution; it can be separated by aspirating the acid from the remaining hemoglobin.
   d. HbF is susceptible to acid elution; it can be destroyed and the denatured hemoglobin can be detected by a color reaction

7. Which condition shows increased osmotic fragility?
   a. Hereditary spherocytosis
   b. Sickle-cell anemia

c. Acquired hemolytic anemia
   d. Hemolytic disease of the newborn

8. What is the basic principle of both the Ham test and the sugar water test for PNH?
   a. Complement-mediated RBC lysis
   b. Precipitation of abnormal RBCs
   c. Vital staining of affected RBCs
   d. Differential agglutination of RBCs

9. Calculate the corrected WBC count for a smear containing 20 NRBCs (WBC count = 4500/μL).
   a. 4500/μL; no need to correct
   b. 375/μL
   c. 4480/μL
   d. 3750/μ

10. What is the principle of the cyanmethemoglobin method in the colorimetric determination of hemoglobin?
    a. Potassium ferricyanide oxidizes hemoglobin to methemoglobin; potassium cyanide converts methemoglobin to cyanmethemoglobin.
    b. Potassium cyanide oxidizes hemoglobin to methemoglobin: potassium ferricyanide converts methemoglobin to cyanmethemoglobin.
    c. Potassium ferricyanide oxidizes hemoglobin to cyanmethemoglobin: cyanmethemoglobin degenerates to form potassium cyanide.
    d. Potassium cyanide reduces hemoglobin to cyanmethemoglobin.

ANSWERS

1. **b** (pp 598–599)
2. **c** (p 600)
3. **a** (p 606)
4. **d** (p 605)
5. **b** (p 612)
6. **a** (p 613)
7. **a** (p 614)
8. **a** (pp 616, 617)
9. **d** (p 608)
10. **a** (p 609)

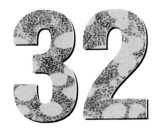

Principles of Automated Differential Analysis

Ellen Hope, MS, SH(ASCP)H
Ellinor I.B. Peerschke, PhD

Objectives

At the end of this section, the learner should be able to:

1 Explain the main use of the leukocyte histogram/scattergram differential.
2 Decide when to accept an automated leukocyte histogram/scattergram differential or perform a conventional manual differential.
3 Determine the correct action to be taken when a result is flagged.
4 Interpret patient data generated by both Coulter and Technicon instruments, including the hemogram parameters, red blood cell histograms, platelet histograms, and white cell histograms/scattergrams.

The differential analysis of peripheral blood smears consists of the examination and identification of leukocyte subpopulations, an evaluation of red blood cell (RBC) morphology, and an estimation of platelet sufficiency. It represents one of the most frequently ordered and most time-consuming hematology test procedures. Differential analysis of peripheral blood has been considered the single laboratory test from which the most information regarding patient disease status can be derived.[1] Examination of peripheral blood smears, for example, can reveal hematologic abnormalities such as anemia and leukemia, aid in the identification of infectious conditions including infectious mononucleosis and parasitemia, monitor the progress of disease, and follow a patient's response to therapy.[2]

In the past decade, reliable automated methods for analyzing peripheral blood cell populations have emerged.[3-7] In addition to providing complete blood count (CBC) parameters such as white blood cells (WBC), red blood cells (RBC), hemoglobin (Hgb), hematocrit (Hct), platelets (PLT), and RBC indices, current instruments also quantify WBC subpopulations, and identify samples with abnormalities for further review. Many instruments also determine parameters such as red cell and platelet distribution widths (RDW and PDW) and mean platelet volume (MPV).

The automated leukocyte analysis eliminates statistical variations associated with 100- or 200-cell manual differential counts based on the increased number of cells (several thousand) that are analyzed. This has also contributed to the increased sensitivity of automated leukocyte differentials to abnormalities such as the clumping of platelets and the presence of nucleated red blood cells (nRBCs) and leukemic blasts.[8,9] Moreover, a number of studies suggest that the automated differential is more efficient and cost-effective than the manual procedure.[10,11]

Despite the advantages of using the automated differential to evaluate hematologically normal patients, further studies are required before automated methods replace the manual procedure,[5] particularly in evaluating blood samples from oncology patients,[12,13] and neonatal intensive care populations.[14]

Automated differential analysis is currently based on the quantitation and evaluation of cell volume, cell light scattering, and cytochemistry, used alone or in combination. Applications of cell volume analysis are illustrated by the Coulter (Model S Plus IV) three-part screening differential, which provides information about granulocytes, lymphocytes, and mononuclear

cell fractions.[15,16] Coulter's newer VCS technology (Models STKS and MAXM) combines volume, conductivity, and light scatter in a single integrated system that enumerates neutrophils, eosinophils, basophils, monocytes, and lymphocytes illustrated in a three-dimensional scatterplot of cell populations and subpopulations.[17] Applications of VCS technology are illustrated by the Coulter Model STKS. The leukocyte differential, available from Technicon systems, demonstrates cell analysis based on light-scattering events and cytochemistry.[18] The Sysmex (NE-Series) hematology analyzers from TOA Medical Electronics Co. Ltd. use a combination of technologies for identifying and separating leukocyte cell populations and subpopulations, including the electronic resistance detection principle with radiofrequency signals for recognizing cell density characteristics of leukocyte populations. These instruments generate a WBC scattergram and red cell and platelet histograms.[19]

EVALUATION OF BLOOD SPECIMENS BY CELL VOLUME ANALYSIS: THE COULTER DIFFERENTIAL

The third-generation Coulter Model S Plus Series (S Plus II, S Plus III, S Plus IV, S Plus V, S Plus VI, and the STKR [pronounced "stacker"]) instruments generate three histograms representing WBC, RBC, and platelet volume distributions, expressed in femtoliters (fL). Histograms of WBCs, RBCs, and platelets are displayed simultaneously with CBC information.

Leukocyte Histogram Analysis

Leukocytes in ethylenediaminetetra-acetic acid (EDTA)–anticoagulated peripheral blood are separated into three major cell fractions by cell volume analysis (Fig. 32–1). Using an isotonic saline solution and lysing reagent to dilute and differentially shrink WBCs, the instruments differentiate between lymphocytes (lymphocytes and atypical lymphocytes), granulocytes (segmented neutrophils, bands, metamyelocytes, eosinophils, and basophils), and mononuclear cells (monocytes, promyelocytes, myelocytes, plasma cells, and blasts) based on differences in nuclear size and cytoplasmic complexity. Cells with a volume of approximately 35 to 90 fL are defined as lymphocytes. Those with volumes ranging from 160 to 450 fL are

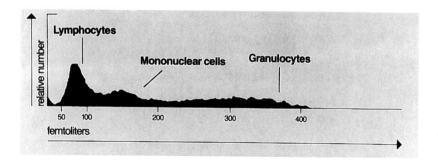

FIGURE 32–1 Coulter leukocyte histogram differential. (From Significant Advances in Hematology, Coulter Electronics, Hialeah, FL, 1983, p 8, with permission.)

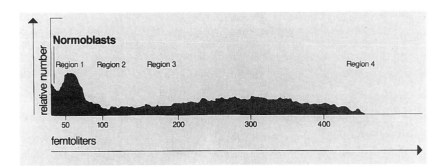

FIGURE 32-2 Region flags (*R flags*) superimposed on Coulter WBC histogram. (From Significant Advances in Hematology, Coulter Electronics, Hialeah, FL, 1983, p 9, with permission.)

classified as granulocytes, and those ranging from 90 to 160 fL are identified as mononuclear cells. Results are expressed in absolute and relative numbers for each cell category.[5]

To highlight results that are out of range, the Coulter instrument backlights the offending number. Backlighting occurs in the presence of abnormal cells or interferences to alert the operator to the possibility of erroneous or abnormal results. Region flag indicators or R flags (R1, R2, R3, R4) indicate the specific location(s) of abnormalities in the WBC size distribution (Fig. 32-2). They may also denote overlapping of two or more of the cell populations at the four designated threshold/valley regions (35, 90, 160, and 450 fL) of the WBC size distribution histogram. Common abnormalities associated with each flag[20] are listed in Table 32-1.

The presence of backlighting and/or flagging of the results suggests that a manual differential count or careful microscopic scanning of a stained peripheral blood smear is indicated. The decision to perform a manual differential should be based on the individual laboratory's established criteria for manual review of automated histogram differential analysis. Examples

of criteria for manual review and reference values for the automated histogram differential, established at a tertiary-care hospital, appear in Tables 32-2 and 32-3.

Red Cell Histogram Analysis

Particles with a volume of greater than 36 fL and less than or equal to 360 fL are identified as RBCs. The RBC histogram displays particles with a volume greater than 24 fL, but the mean corpuscular volume (MCV) is calculated from the area under the curve of the RBC histogram, depicted in Figure 32-3. Deviations in the shape and position of the RBC histogram indicate changes in RBC size and/or shape.

The availability of red cell parameters such as RBC, Hgb, Hct, MCV, mean corpuscular hemoglobin (MCH), and mean corpuscular hemoglobin concentration (MCHC), in conjunction with information derived from RBC histograms, may provide valuable information for assessing erythrocytic disorders. The RDW represents a parameter that quantifies relative anisocytosis. It is calculated as the coefficient of variation (CV) of the

TABLE 32-1 **Abnormalities Associated with Specific Flagging Regions of the Coulter Model S Plus Series WBC Histogram**		
R Flag	**Region**	**Abnormality**
R1	Far left	Erythrocyte precursors Cryoglobulins Nonlysed erythrocytes Giant and/or clumped platelets
R2	Between lymphocytes and monocytes	Blasts Basophilia Eosinophilia Plasma cells Abnormal/variant lymphocytes
R3	Between monocytes and granulocytes	Abnormal cell populations Eosinophilia Immature granulocytes
R4	Far right	Increased absolute granulocytes
RM		Multiple flags

Source: From Pierre, RV: Seminar and Case Studies: The Automated Differential. Coulter Electronics, Hialeah, FL, 1985, p 9, with permission.

TABLE 32–2 Criteria for Manual Review of the Coulter Histogram Differential Established at a Tertiary Care Hospital

WBC count	$<4.0 \times 10^9/L$
	$>15.0 \times 10^9/L$
Monocytes	$>15.0\%$
Lymphocytes	$>50\%$
Granulocytes	$<50\%$
All backlighting	
All R flags	
All incomplete computations	

TABLE 32–3 Reference Values for Selected Blood Cell Parameters Established at a Tertiary Care Hospital

Granulocytes	50–75%
Lymphocytes	25–40%
Monocytes	4–10%

TABLE 32–4 Calculation of the RDW as Determined by Coulter

$$RDW = \frac{SD}{Mean} \times 100$$

Normal range = 11.5–14.5%

Source: From Pierre, RV: Seminar and Case Studies: The Automated Differential. Coulter Electronics, Hialeah, FL, 1985, p 38, with permission.

MCV (Table 32–4). Its usefulness in the early detection of iron deficiency (increased RDW) and in distinguishing between iron deficiency and β-thalassemia (normal RDW) has been suggested.[21]

Platelet Histogram Analysis

The PLT histogram displays native platelet size. Particles with volumes ranging from 2 to 20 fL are counted. The raw data are fitted to a log-normal distribution (Fig. 32–4), from which the reported platelet count is calculated.

The MPV and PDW are additional parameters describing platelet size. The MPV is equivalent to the MCV and is inversely proportional to the platelet count (Fig. 32–5).[22] The PDW measures uniformity of platelet size and is equivalent to the RDW. In combination with the platelet histogram, the MPV and PDW provide greater distinction between normal and abnormal platelet populations.

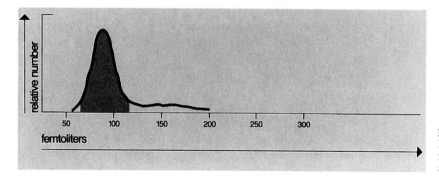

FIGURE 32–3 Normal Coulter RBC histogram. (From Significant Advances in Hematology, Coulter Electronics, Hialeah, FL, 1983, p 11, with permission.)

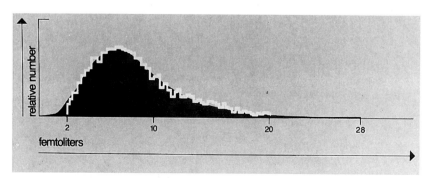

FIGURE 32–4 Normal Coulter platelet histogram. (From Significant Advances in Hematology, Coulter Electronics, Hialeah, FL, 1983, p 13, with permission.)

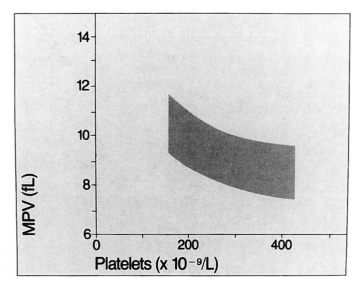

FIGURE 32–5   Coulter MPV normogram. (From Significant Advances in Hematology, Coulter Electronics, Hialeah, FL, 1983, p 14, with permission.)

ADVANCES IN COULTER LEUKOCYTE DIFFERENTIAL ANALYSIS: VCS TECHNOLOGY

Coulter Models STKS and MAXM

The Coulter WBC differential has been expanded to include enumeration of eosinophils and basophils, by combining measurements of cell volume with conductivity and light-scatter data. Light-scattering characteristics provide additional information about cell structure and shape. This technology is particularly useful for identifying eosinophils. Conductivity measurements are made using a high-frequency electromagnetic probe and reflect the nuclear, granular, and chemical properties of cells. Conductivity measurements aid in differentiating among cells of similar size, such as lymphocytes and basophils that differ in internal structure.

An example of WBC analysis by the Coulter Model STKS (pronounced "stack-S," Fig. 32–6) is provided in Figure 32–7. Individual cells are depicted as points on a scatterplot, reflecting cell volume and light-scatter-

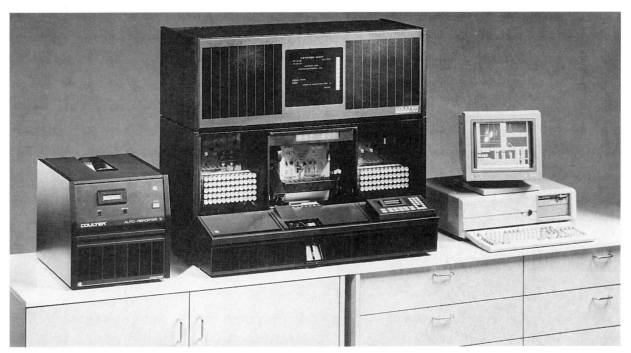

FIGURE 32–6   Coulter STKS Hematology System. (Courtesy of Coulter Corp., Miami, FL.)

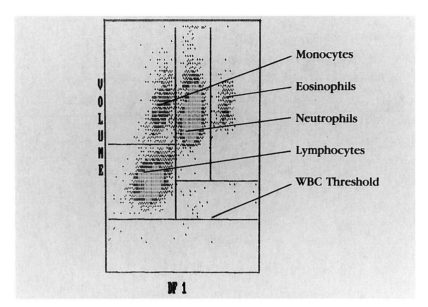

FIGURE 32–7 White blood cell analysis by Coulter VCS technology. (From Coulter VCS Technology Casebook, Coulter Electronics, Hialeah, FL, 1989, p 62, with permission.)

ing characteristics. Clusters of cells are identified as monocytes, eosinophils, lymphocytes, and neutrophils based on their relative position on the scatterplot. Separate scatterplots comparing cell volume and conductivity properties are generated to quantify basophils.

Floating discriminators examine areas between different cell populations. Abnormalities are identified by specific region flags. The STKS flagging system is enhanced by providing specific alphanumeric codes and three types of messages including suspect, definitive,

and condition messages. Common abnormalities associated with each flagging message appear in Table 32–5. Suspect messages flag abnormal cell populations or distributions such as certain red cell abnormalities, platelet clumping, variant lymphocytes, and immature granulocytes. These messages appear in the cell classification window on the sample analysis display and abnormalities should be confirmed by a microscopic review. Definitive messages flag decreases and increases for all test parameters

	TABLE 32–5 **Summary of Flagging Messages Generated by the Coulter VCS Differential**		
Population	**Suspect**	**Condition**	**Definitive**
White Cells	Immature grans Variant lymphs Blasts Review slide	Normal WBC pop. Abnormal WBC pop. No message Edited data Full clog Partial clog 1 Partial clog 2	Leukocytosis Leukopenia Neutrophilia Neutropenia Monocytosis Lymphocytosis Lymphopenia Basophilia Eosinophilia
Red Cells	Dimorphic RBC pop. Microcytic RBCs/RBC fragments RBC agglutination	Normal RBC pop. Abnormal RBC pop. No message Edited data	Anemia Microcytosis Macrocytosis Anisocytosis Poikilocytosis Hypochromia Pancytopenia Erythrocytosis
Platelets	Giant platelets Platelet clumping	Normal Plt pop. Abnormal Plt. pop. No message	Thrombocytosis Thrombocytopenia Large platelets Small platelets

Source: Adapted from Pierre, R: Seminar and Case Studies: The Automated Differential. Coulter Electronics, Inc, Hialeah, FL, July 1991, p 75.

based on numeric limits set by the laboratory. A message appears in the cell classification window on the sample analysis display if the results of the sample exceed preset limits. Condition messages indicate whether the white cell, red cell, and platelet populations are abnormal or normal. In addition to flagging messages, data from cell counts, white cell scatter plots, and size-distribution histograms are sent to a data management system (DMS). As much as 1000 sets of results may be stored by this system.

EVALUATION OF BLOOD SPECIMENS BY LIGHT SCATTERING AND CYTOCHEMICAL ANALYSIS: THE TECHNICON DIFFERENTIAL

Enumeration and identification of blood cells by the Technicon automated blood analyzer (Fig. 32–8) is based on optical flow cytometry, cytochemistry, and light scattering. The instrument's sampling mechanism divides blood samples into aliquots that are treated in four separate reaction chambers; the red cell and platelet reaction chamber, hemoglobin reaction chamber, basophil/lobularity reaction chamber, and perioxidase reaction chamber. Cells are counted as they pass through a flow cell. A laser beam is located on one side of the flow cell. As the cells pass in front of the beam, they are counted by a light-scatter detector.

Red Cell and Platelet Histogram Analysis

Red cells and platelets are identified on the basis of their light-scattering properties. A buffered reagent isovolumetrically fixes and spheres platelets and red cells while light scattered at high and low angles concurrently measures cell volume and optical density. Red cell and platelet histograms are generated based on light-scatter measurements translated into cell volume. Additional parameters such as RDW and platelet cell volume (PCV) are derived from these histograms. The instrument's interpretive report identifies and grades (1+ to 4+) various RBC abnormalities including microcytosis, macrocytosis, hypochromia, hyperchromia, and anisocytosis.

Technicon's RDW reference range of 10.2% to 11.8% is different from the Coulter range of 11.5% to 14.5%.[23] The difference is likely because of each instrument's individualized mathematical trimming of the data. Because the absolute value reported for the CV of RBC size is variable based on the program of each standardized analyzer, each laboratory should determine its own normal ranges.[21]

Leukocyte Analysis

WBCs are fixed with formaldehyde and stained with peroxidase in the peroxidase reaction chamber. The chamber is heated to a relatively high temperature that lyses PLTs and RBCs and causes the WBCs to be fixed and dehydrated. Narrow forward-angle light scatter and tungsten light optics are used to measure WBC size and peroxidase activity, respectively. Myeloperoxidase is a granulocyte enzyme marker that is present to varying degrees in neutrophils, eosinophils, and monocytes but absent from basophils, lymphocytes, and blasts.[24]

A peroxidase scattergram depicting peroxidase staining intensity on the abscissa and cell size on the ordinate is generated (Fig. 32–9). Each point in the scattergram characterizes the peroxidase activity and size of a single cell. Clusters of points represent distinct leukocyte subpopulations.

A specific basophil count is determined separately in the basophil/lobularity chamber. Whole blood is exposed to an acid buffer that selectively lyses all cells

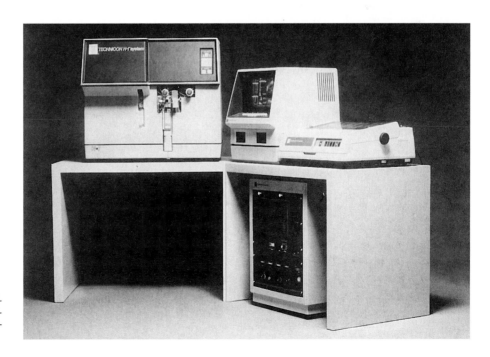

FIGURE 32-8 Technicon H-1 System. (Courtesy Bayer Diagnostic Division, Bayer Corporation, Tarrytown, NY.)

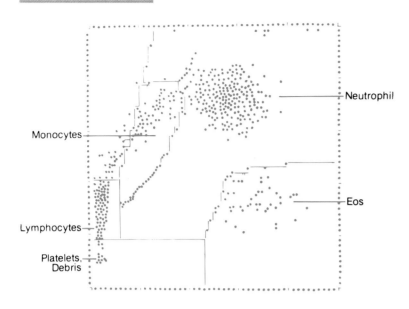

FIGURE 32–9 Technicon WBC/peroxidase scattergram. Cell size is indicated on the ordinate axis, peroxidase activity on the abscissa. (From Brown, BA: Special hematology procedures. In Brown, BA: Hematology: Principles and Procedures, ed 5. Lea & Febiger, Philadelphia, 1988, p 388, with permission.)

except basophils. The resulting particles are subsequently sorted, and their forward angle and light-scattering properties quantified. Because basophils are resistant to lysis, they appear larger than the bare nuclei of other leukocytes, scatter more light, and appear higher on the vertical axis of the scattergram (Fig. 32–10). A fixed horizontal threshold separates the nuclei of other WBCs from basophils.

The WBC differential report generated by Technicon instruments not only includes the relative percentages and absolute values for neutrophils, lymphocytes, monocytes, eosinophils, and basophils but also provides additional interpretive data to signal the presence of abnormalities. The differential report defines the proportion of leukocytes with high myeloperoxidase content, designated the HPX fraction, and the percentage of large unstained cells (LUC). Increased myeloperoxidase activity may be associated with reactive states, megaloblastic anemia, or hyperprolifer-

ative granulopoiesis,[18] whereas increased numbers of LUCs may reflect the presence of atypical lymphocytes or blasts.[25] Normal ranges of 0% to 3.7% for LUCs and 0% to 5.4% for HPX have been established.[26]

EVALUATION OF BLOOD SPECIMENS BY ELECTRONIC RESISTANCE DETECTION WITH HYDRODYNAMIC FOCUSING TECHNIQUE: THE SYSMEX DIFFERENTIAL

Sysmex is the brand name of hematology analyzers manufactured by TOA Medical Electronics Company, Limited, Kobe, Japan (TOA). TOA has manufactured hematology products since 1961 and developed a comprehensive series of hematology analyzers that includes: NE-Alpha Integrated System, NE-Series systems (NE-8000/7000/6000/5500/4500), an au-

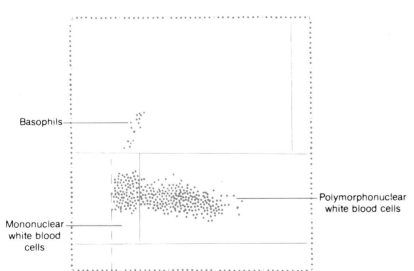

FIGURE 32–10 Technicon cytogram for basophil/lobularity. (From Brown, BA: Special hematology procedures. In Brown, BA: Hematology: Principles and Procedures, ed 5. Lea & Febiger, Philadelphia, 1988, p 389, with permission.)

tomated reticulocyte analyzer (R-3000), and the HS Series (SE-9000) Hematology workstation.[27] The following is an overview of the Sysmex NE-Series systems.

The NE-Series hematology analyzers provide test results for 23 parameters comprised of 8 CBC parameters, 5 analytical platelet and red cell parameters, 10 WBC differential parameters, 1 WBC scattergram, and 5 histograms. Relative percentages and absolute values for neutrophils, monocytes, lymphocytes, basophils, and eosinophils are reported and additional interpretive reports provide comprehensive information for each test sample. Interpretive comments are very useful in assessment of data analysis and identification of abnormal samples.[19]

Red Cell and Platelet Histogram Analysis

The NE-Series systems generate RBC and PLT histograms along with the following associated parameters: RBC distribution width by standard deviation (RDW-SD), RBC distribution width by coefficient of variation (RDW-CV), PLT distribution width (PDW), and PLT large cell ratio (P-LCR). Red cell histograms are generated in a manner similar to that used for platelets. The principal differences occur in the methods used to eliminate interferences of small red cells on the platelet count and histogram and in the particle selection for generating the histogram.

In order to size and count the red cells and platelets, the direct current (DC) detection method is enhanced by hydrodynamic focusing with sheath flow technology. The hydrodynamic focusing technique is a modification of the electronic resistance detection method. The DC method enhanced by hydrodynamic focusing eliminates problems known to be associated with the DC detection method such as inconsistent sizing, coincidence, and recirculating cells.[19]

Leukocyte Analysis

The principles used in generating the WBC histograms and scattergram include simultaneous measurements of blood cells by radiofrequency (RF) and DC detection methods for identifying and delineating WBC populations. There are separate detector blocks for the determination of cell populations. The RF method detects and sizes lyse-treated cells based on density and nuclear size, whereas the DC method sizes the entire cell, nucleus, and cytoplasm. Cell pulses detected by RF and DC methods are then displayed as a three-dimensional WBC scattergram. The WBC scattergram contains information about the distribution of lymphocytes, monocytes, and granulocytes. Normal cells appear in areas different from the area in which abnormal cells appear. Abnormal WBCs, such as immature granulocytes, shift to the left; blasts, atypical lymphocytes, nucleated RBCs, and platelet clumping are detected in cell distribution on the WBC scattergram. The number of cells in each size position rises from the plane of the matrix, creating peaks in the various size positions and separating the different populations of cells by the use of eight floating discriminators. The WBC trimodal histogram demonstrates the separation of particle populations into regions of gran-

ulocytes, monocytes, and lymphocytes. Separate histograms are also generated for basophil and eosinophil populations utilizing the DC detection method and cell-specific lyse reagents. The basophil histogram provides useful information about the appearance of immature granulocytes because immature granulocytes are least likely to be lysed by the lysing reagent that measures basophils.[28]

QUALITY CONTROL AND QUALITY ASSURANCE

Quality control measures for the automated screening differential consist of performing daily, monthly, and annual instrument maintenance procedures as specified by the manufacturer and evaluating instrument accuracy and precision on a daily or per-shift basis with stabilized controls for which target values— mean ± standard deviation (SD) have been established.[29] Usually three levels of control material are analyzed to evaluate instrument performance over the spectrum of clinically relevant values. In addition, establishing action limits for manual review of automated results is essential. Separate criteria for review of automated results should be established for adult and pediatric patient populations, as well as for oncology, acquired immunodeficiency syndrome (AIDS), and transplant patients. Action limits on RDW, Hgb, and RBC count and indices may be included to trigger a morphological evaluation of blood films for RBC abnormalities. Similarly, action limits on platelet counts should be established to verify manually low automated platelet counts.

Participation in external quality assurance programs provided by manufacturers of quality control materials and the American Society of Clinical Pathologists should be included in a comprehensive quality control program.[30] Comparison of laboratory performance with that of other laboratories evaluating aliquots of the same specimen by the same method (intralaboratory quality control) provides an independent assessment of instrument accuracy. Comparison of laboratory values with those reported by other institutions should include not only a comparison of the test results but also, when applicable, a comparison of the standard deviation. An increased standard deviation may indicate problems in instrument performance, comprehensive instrument control, and maintenance; and problem logs can provide valuable information.

CASE STUDIES: LEUKOCYTE HISTOGRAM/SCATTERGRAM ANALYSIS

The following cases illustrate automated differential analysis of whole blood by Coulter (S Plus IV and STKS) and Technicon (H-6000 and H-1) instruments.

Case 1: Granulocytosis/Neutrophilia

The Coulter WBC histogram (Fig. 32–11) depicts a large granulocyte population spanning the region be-

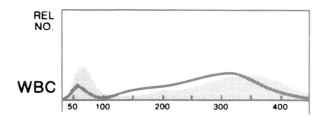

WBC	16.8
LY %	8.2
MO%	7.2
GR %	84.6
LY #	1.4
MO #	1.2
GR #	14.2

FIGURE 32–11 Coulter S Plus IV histogram depicting granulocytosis and neutrophilia. The shaded area represents the normal WBC distribution. (From Pierre,[20] p 23, with permission.)

tween 200 and 400 fL, a small lymphocyte population, and few mononuclear cells. The shaded area represents the normal WBC distribution. An elevated WBC count is consistent with a shift to the left. Manual differential analysis revealed 56% bands, 35% neutrophils, 8% lymphocytes, and 1% monocytes.

Neutrophilia

Coulter STKS WBC scatterplot depicts neutrophilia (Fig. 32–12). WBC, 30.5×10^9/L; 91% neutrophils. Manual differential analysis revealed 48% neutrophils, 24% bands, 10% metamyelocytes, 6% myelocytes, and 12% lymphocytes.

Case 2: Acute Lymphoblastic Leukemia

Examination of Coulter WBC histogram (Fig. 32–13) reveals a single WBC peak spanning the region between 50 and 150 fL. The shaded area represents the normal WBC distribution. An R2 flag alerts the operator to the skewed patient WBC distribution to the right of the normal lymphocyte peak. The R3 flag reflects the absence of a normal granulocyte peak. Manual differential analysis revealed the presence of 11% lymphoblasts, 50% lymphocytes, 32% neutrophils, 1% metamyelocytes, and 6% myelocytes.

Acute Lymphoblastic Leukemia

Coulter STKS WBC scatterplot (Fig. 32–14) demonstrates the presence of lymphoblasts at the top of the scatterplot, overlapping areas that would contain normal monocytes and neutrophils. A suspect blast flag was generated by the instrument. Manual differential showed 18% lymphocytes, 49% blasts, 23% neutrophils, and 10% monocytes.

Case 3: Acute Lymphoblastic Leukemia

Examination of the Technicon WBC/peroxidase scattergram (Fig. 32–15) reveals a marked increase in LUCs (66%). Note the vertical band of lymphoid blasts extending upward from the lymphocytic region.

Case 4: Chronic Lymphocytic Leukemia

The Coulter WBC histogram (Fig. 32–16) reveals abnormal cell populations to both left and right of the normal lymphocyte peak, indicated by the shaded region between 50 and 100 fL. The peak to the right represents lymphocyte doublets that were counted coincidentally owing to the extremely elevated WBC count (more than 99×10^9/L). Dilution of the blood sample to achieve a WBC count of less than 50×10^9/L eliminated this peak. The abnormal cell population on the

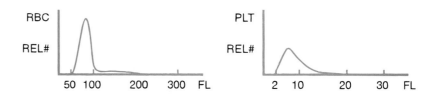

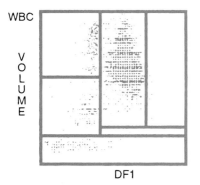

FIGURE 32–12 Coulter STKS WBC scatterplot depicting neutrophilia. WBC 30.5×10^9/L, 91% neutrophils.

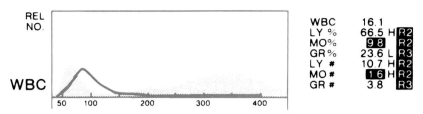

FIGURE 32-13 Coulter S Plus IV histogram depicting acute lymphoblastic leukemia. The shaded area represents the normal WBC distribution. (From Pierre,[20] p. 16, with permission.)

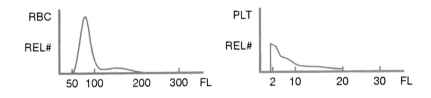

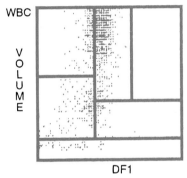

FIGURE 32-14 Coulter STKS WBC scatterplot demonstrating the presence of lymphoblasts at the top of the scatterplot overlaping areas that would contain normal monocytes and neutrophils. A suspect blast flag was generated by the instrument.

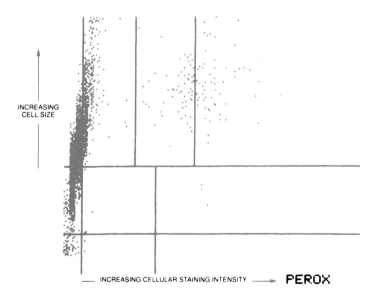

FIGURE 32-15 Technicon WBC/peroxidase scattergram illustrating a case of acute lymphoblastic leukemia. (From Simmons, A: Apparatus and automation. In Simmons, A: Hematology: A Combined Theoretical and Technical Approach. WB Saunders, Philadelphia, 1989, p 370, with permission.)

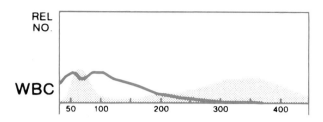
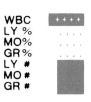

FIGURE 32–16 Coulter S Plus IV histogram illustrating a case of chronic lymphocytic leukemia. The shaded area represents the normal WBC distribution. (From Pierre,[20] p 32, with permission.)

left side of the normal lymphcyte peak is consistent with a pattern of B-cell chronic lymphocytic leukemia.

Chronic Lymphocytic Leukemia

Coulter STKS WBC scatterplot (Fig. 32–17) illustrates a case of chronic lymphocytic leukemia. Note the predominance of a lymphocytic population. Manual differential revealed 72% lymphocytes, 12% atypical lymphs, and 16% neutrophils.

Case 5: Chronic Lymphocytic Leukemia

Technicon scattergram (Fig. 32–18) reveals a major concentration of cells in the lymphocyte region and a small granulocyte component.

Case 6: Acute Myeloblastic Leukemia

Examination of the Coulter WBC histogram (Fig. 32–19) shows a broadening and shift to the right of the lymphocyte peak. An R2 flag suggests an increased mononuclear cell population. Examination of the blood film indicated the presence of 82% blasts, 12% lymphocytes, and 6% monocytes.

Case 7: Acute Myeloblastic Leukemia

Examination of the Technicon WBC/peroxidase scattergram (Fig. 32–20) reveals a large cluster of LUCs representing blasts.

Case 8: Chronic Myelocytic Leukemia

The Coulter WBC histogram (Fig. 32–21) demonstrates a broadened curve extending through the mononuclear and immature granulocyte regions, and an elevation at the right of the normal lymphocyte peak. This irregularity is characteristic of the lymphopenia and granulocytosis associated with granulocytic immaturity, often seen in chronic myeloproliferative disorders. An R1 flag suggests the presence of nucleated RBCs and/or clumped platelets.

Case 9: Chronic Myelocytic Leukemia in Blast Crisis

Coulter STKS WBC scattergram (Fig. 32–22) illustrates a case of chronic myelogenous leukemia in blast crisis. A suspect blast flag was generated by the instrument. A manual differential showed 35% blasts, 1% promyelocytes, 4% myelocytes, 1% metamyelo-

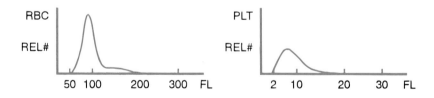

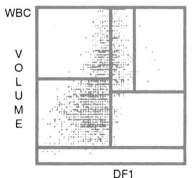

FIGURE 32–17 Coulter STKS WBC scatterplot illustrating a case of chronic lymphocytic leukemia. Note the predominance of a lymphocytic population.

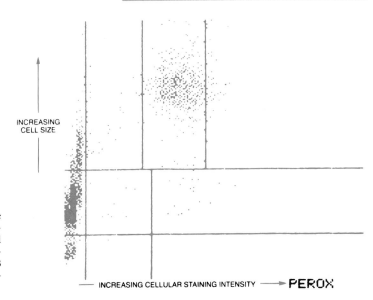

FIGURE 32-18 Technicon WBC/peroxidase scattergram illustrating a case of chronic lymphocytic leukemia. (From Simmons, A: Apparatus and automation. In Simmons, A: Hematology: A Combined Theoretical and Technical Approach. WB Saunders, Philadelphia, 1989, p 371, with permission.)

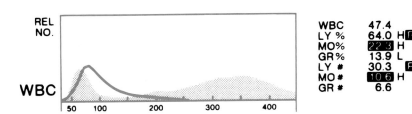

WBC	47.4	
LY %	64.0	H R2
MO%	22.3	H
GR %	13.9	L
LY #	30.3	R2
MO #	10.6	H
GR #	6.6	

FIGURE 32-19 Coulter S Plus IV depicting acute myeloblastic leukemia. The shaded area represents the normal WBC distribution. (From Pierre,[20] p 27, with permission.)

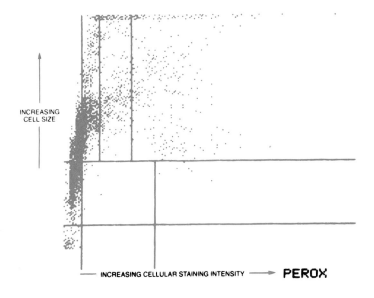

FIGURE 32-20 Technicon WBC/peroxidase scattergram depicting acute myeloblastic leukemia. (From Simmons, A: Apparatus and automation. In Simmons, A: Hematology: A Combined Theoretical and Technical Approach. WB Saunders, Philadelphia, 1989, p 367, with permission.)

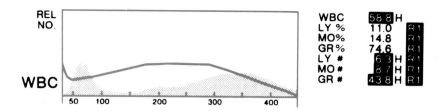

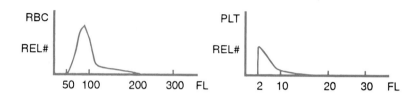

FIGURE 32–21 Coulter S Plus IV histogram illustrating a case of chronic myelocytic leukemia. The normal WBC distribution is depicted by the shaded area. (From Pierre,[20] p 25, with permission.)

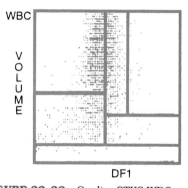

FIGURE 32–22 Coulter STKS WBC scattergram illustrating a case of chronic myelocytic leukemia in blast crisis. A suspect flag was generated by the instrument. Note the presence of cells with increased volume overlapping regions normally containing monocytes and neutrophils.

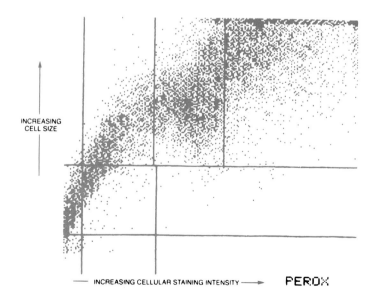

FIGURE 32–23 Technicon WBC/peroxidase scattergram depicting chronic myelocytic leukemia. (From Simmons, A: Apparatus and automation. In Simmons, A: Hematology: A Combined Theoretical and Technical Approach. WB Saunders, Philadelphia, 1989, p 367, with permission.)

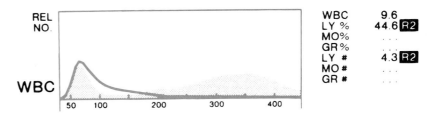

FIGURE 32-24 Coulter S Plus IV histogram depicting infectious mononucleosis. The shaded area represents the normal WBC distribution. (From Pierre,[20] p 12, with permission.)

cytes, 5% bands, 36% neutrophils, 10% basophils, 5% monocytes, and 3% lymphocytes. Note the presence of cells with increased volume overlapping regions normally containing monocytes and neutrophils.

Case 10: Chronic Myelocytic Leukemia

Cells are spread diagonally across the Technicon WBC/peroxidase scattergram (Fig. 32–23). An increase in the number of cells with high peroxidase activity is depicted in the upper right section of the scattergram. This pattern is typical of the increased numbers of immature granulocytes seen in this malignancy.

Case 11: Infectious Mononucleosis

The Coulter WBC histogram (Fig. 32–24) reveals an abnormal WBC distribution with a lymphocyte peak that was shifted to the right of normal, suggesting the presence of an abnormal lymphocyte/mononuclear population. The R2 flag is consistent with the presence of large atypical lymphocytes. Note the similar WBC distribution in Case 6, acute nonlymphocytic leukemia, emphasizing the impotance of manual review of automated differential results.

Case 12: Monocytosis

Coulter STKS WBC scatterplot (Fig. 32–25) depicts monocytosis. Note the increased concentration of cells in the monocyte region. Scan of the corresponding stained peripheral blood smear confirmed the presence of 24% monocytes.

Case 13: Eosinophilia

Coulter STKS WBC scatterplot (Fig. 32–26). Note the increased number of cells in the eosinophil region. Manual differential analysis confirmed the presence of 10% eosinophils.

Case 14: Nucleated Red Blood Cells

The Coulter WBC, RBC, and PLT histograms (Fig. 32–27) all show abnormal cell distributions. The RBC histogram shows a left-shifted curve with interference below 35 fL. The WBC histogram depicts an extremely high peak to the left of the normal lymphocyte region, accompanied by an R1 flag. The platelet histogram failed to return to baseline near 20 fL. These patterns are consistent with the presence of nRBCs (affecting the WBC histograms) and RBC fragments (affecting RBC and PLT histograms).

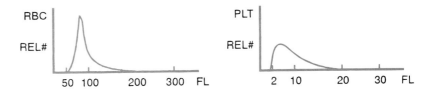

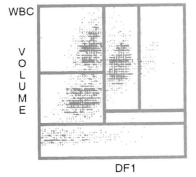

FIGURE 32-25 Coulter STKS WBC scatterplot depicting monocytosis. Note the increased concentration of cells in the monocyte region.

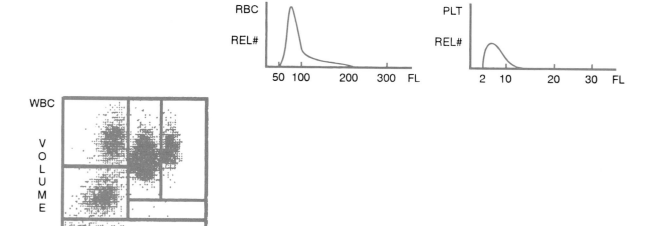

FIGURE 32–26 Coulter STKS WBC scatterplot. Note the increased number of cells in the eosinophil region.

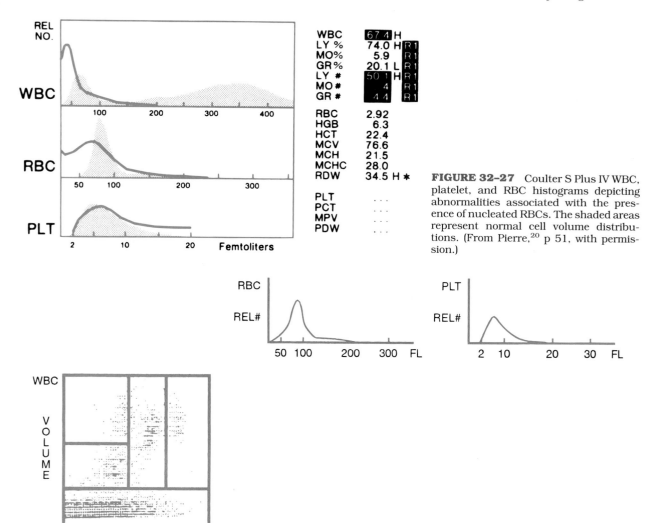

WBC	67.4	H
LY %	74.0	H R1
MO%	5.9	R1
GR%	20.1	L R1
LY #	50.1	H R1
MO #	4	R1
GR #	4.4	R1
RBC	2.92	
HGB	6.3	
HCT	22.4	
MCV	76.6	
MCH	21.5	
MCHC	28.0	
RDW	34.5	H *
PLT	. . .	
PCT	. . .	
MPV	. . .	
PDW	. . .	

FIGURE 32–27 Coulter S Plus IV WBC, platelet, and RBC histograms depicting abnormalities associated with the presence of nucleated RBCs. The shaded areas represent normal cell volume distributions. (From Pierre,[20] p 51, with permission.)

FIGURE 32–28 Coulter STKS WBC scatterplot depicting an increase in particles appearing below the WBC threshold in a specimen containing nucleated red blood cells and Howell-Jolly bodies.

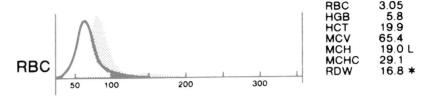

RBC	3.05
HGB	5.8
HCT	19.9
MCV	65.4
MCH	19.0 L
MCHC	29.1
RDW	16.8 ∗

FIGURE 32-29 Coulter S Plus IV RBC histogram illustrating a case of iron-deficiency anemia. The shaded area represents normal RBC volume distribution. (From Pierre,[20] p 43, with permission.)

Nucleated Red Blood Cells

Coulter STKS WBC scatterplot (Fig. 32–28) depicts an increase in particles appearing below the WBC threshold in a specimen containing nucleated red blood cells and Howell-Jolly bodies. Manual differential revealed 2% nRBCs, and occasional Howell-Jolly Bodies.

CASE STUDIES: RED CELL AND PLATELET ANALYSIS

Because RBC and PLT histograms generated by Coulter and Technicon instruments are not significantly different, Coulter case studies are provided to depict some of the more frequently encountered abnormalities.

Case 15: Iron-Deficiency Anemia

The RBC histogram (Fig. 32–29) shows an RBC distribution curve that is shifted to the left, which is characteristic of microcytosis. The slightly elevated RDW is consistent with iron deficiency and is flagged for review.

Case 16: Folic Acid Deficiency

The RBC histogram (Fig. 32–30) demonstrates an abnormal shift to the right, suggesting macrocytosis. Note the extremely elevated MCV and RDW, reflecting marked macrocytosis and anisocytosis, respectively.

Case 17: Cold Agglutinins

The Coulter RBC histogram (Fig. 32–31) appears relatively normal except for a slight elevation at the far right of the curve. Red cell indices, however, are flagged with the letter "H," emphasizing marked elevations in the MCH and MCHC. In addition, RBC parameters show discrepancies among the RBC count, Hgb, and Hct, which normally differ by a factor of 3.[27] The Hct and the RBC count are disproportionately low, which is characteristic of cold agglutinins.

Case 18: Sickle-Thalassemia

The Coulter RBC histogram (Fig. 32–32) demonstrates an abnormal shift to the left of the RBC volume distribution representing a moderate microcytosis. The RBC parameters are consistent with microcytic anemia (decreased MCV) and anisocytosis (increased RDW). In addition to iron deficiency, an increased RDW has been reported in patients with hemoglobin SS, hemoglobin SC, and S-beta-thalassemia.[30]

Case 19: Post-RBC Transfusion

The Coulter STKS RBC histogram (Fig. 32–33) depicts a dimorphic RBC population in a patient who had received a RBC transfusion. Distinct microcytic and normocytic RBC populations are apparent.

Case 20: Platelet Clumping

The Coulter PLT histogram (Fig. 32–34) appears normal. A PLT count, however, is not computed, based on disagreement among simultaneous independent automated PLT count determinations. The WBC histogram depicts interference of approximately 35 fL. This is confirmed by an R1 flag. Careful examination of the peripheral blood smear reveals the presence of PLT clumps. The RBC histogram is unremarkable.

Case 21: Giant Platelets

The Coulter PLT histogram (Fig. 32–35) is grossly abnormal and fails to return to baseline near 20 fL. The R1 flag reflects the high left shoulder of the WBC histogram. Examination of a stained peripheral blood film reveals the presence of giant platelets. The RBC histogram is unremarkable.

Although examples in the case studies section have focused only on Coulter and Technicon analyzers, a number of other automated hematology analyzers perform CBCs and histogram/scattergram differentials. Some of these include CELL-DYN systems (Abbott Diagnostics, Mountain View, CA); HC-1020 (Danam, Dallas, TX); and ABX series (ABX, Horsham, PA). We do not endorse any particular model. Owing to the abundance of hematology analyzers and publication

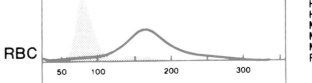

RBC	1.05 L
HGB	5.9
HCT	16.7
MCV	158.7 H
MCH	56.2 H
MCHC	35.4
RDW	31.5 H∗

FIGURE 32-30 Coulter S Plus IV RBC histogram depicting folic acid deficiency. The shaded area represents normal RBC volume distribution. (From Pierre,[20] p 45, with permission.)

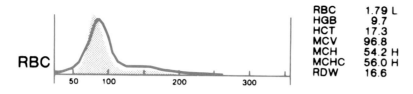

RBC	1.79 L
HGB	9.7
HCT	17.3
MCV	96.8
MCH	54.2 H
MCHC	56.0 H
RDW	16.6

FIGURE 32–31   Coulter S Plus IV RBC histogram depicting abnormalities associated with the presence of cold agglutinins. The shaded area represents normal RBC volume distribution. (From Pierre,[20] p 55, with permission.)

FIGURE 32–32   Coulter S Plus IV RBC histogram depicting a case of sickle thalassemia. The shaded area represents normal RBC volume distribution. (From Pierre,[20] p 50, with permission.)

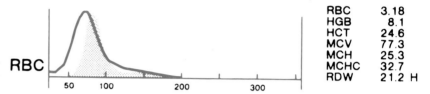

RBC	3.18
HGB	8.1
HCT	24.6
MCV	77.3
MCH	25.3
MCHC	32.7
RDW	21.2 H

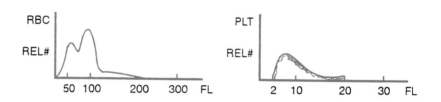

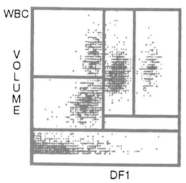

FIGURE 32–33   Coulter STKS RBC histogram depicting a dimorphic RBC population.

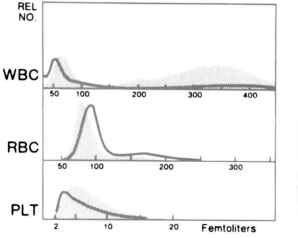

WBC	7.1
LY %	41.6 R1
MO%	10.4 R1
GR%	48.0 R1
LY #	3.0 R1
MO #	.7 R1
GR #	3.4 R1
RBC	4.64
HGB	15.9
HCT	46.1
MCV	99.3
MCH	34.3
MCHC	34.5
RDW	12.3

PLT	. . .
PCT	. . .
MPV	. . .
PDW	. . .

FIGURE 32–34   Coulter S Plus IV RBC histogram depicting abnormalities associated with platelet clumping. The shaded area represents normal platelet volume distribution. (From Pierre,[20] p 71, with permission.)

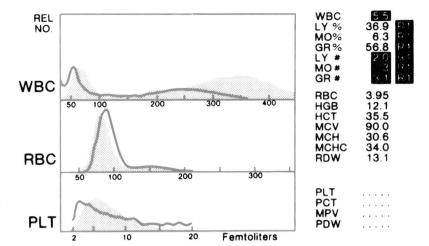

FIGURE 32–35 Coulter S Plus IV RBC histogram reflecting the presence of giant platelets. The shaded area represents normal platelet volume distribution. (From Pierre,[20] p 73, with permission.)

CONCLUSION

Future trends point to increased hematology testing, requiring automated specimen processing, multitest analysis, and advances in data processing. Thus, in addition to the improved accuracy and precision of automated whole blood differential analysis, new advances in hematology analyzers are directed at improving laboratory safety, productivity, efficiency, and work flow. Because current automated analyzers with histogram differential capabilities generate comprehensive interpretive reports containing detailed information about abnormalities, careful evaluation of the data can provide an efficient screening tool.

A review of the literature, however, underscores the importance of the smear differential for confirming and reviewing automated results.[3–5,29] Confirmatory evaluation of blood smears to identify abnormalities can be considerably more efficient and less labor-intensive with the help of automated differential results. Automated results can direct the technologist to focus on specific problems.

Improved features such as user-friendly software, bar code sample identification, closed tube sampling, and greater sample throughput enhance overall laboratory safety, efficiency, and productivity. Moreover, these advanced features contribute to cost-effective laboratory operations and efforts to preserve quality patient care despite the current shortages in qualified laboratory personnel.

In the past, automated hematologic analysis of bone marrow aspirates and body fluids has not been feasible because of limitations associated with samples, very low cell counts, the presence of microclots and extraneous debris, decreased sample volume, and interferences by heparin anticoagulants. Recent advances in instrumentation have overcome such obstacles, and automated procedures for analyzing body fluids and bone marrow specimens are being investigated.

REFERENCES

1. Hyun, BH, Ashton, JK, and Dolan, K: Practical Hematology. WB Saunders, Philadelphia, 1975, p 193.
2. O'Connor, BH: A Color Atlas and Instruction Manual of Peripheral Blood Cell Morphology. Williams & Wilkins, Baltimore, 1984, p 1.
3. Watson, JS and Davis, RA: Evaluation of the Technicon H-1 hematology system. Lab Med 18:316, 1987.
4. Miers, MK, et al: Evaluation of the Coulter S Plus IV three-part differential as a screening tool in a tertiary care hospital. Am J Clin Pathol 87:745, 1987.
5. Griswold, DJ and Champagne, VD: Evaluation of the Coulter S-Plus IV three-part differential in an acute care hospital. Am J Clin Pathol 84:49, 1985.
6. Greendyke, RM, et al: A comparison of differential white blood cell counts using manual technic and the Coulter S-Plus IV. Am J Clin Pathol 84:348, 1985.
7. Rumpke, CL: Statistical reflections on finding atypical cells. Blood Cells 11:141, 1985.
8. Cox, CJ, et al: Evaluation of the Coulter Counter Model S Plus IV. Am J Clin Pathol 84:297, 1985.
9. Bollinger, P: The Technicon H-1 hematology analyzer: Sensitivity and specificity of blast identification in peripheral blood. In Simson, E, et al (eds): Proceedings of the Technicon H-1 Hematology Symposium. Technicon Instruments Corp, New York, 1985, p 39.
10. Kalish, RJ and Becker, K: Evaluation of the Coulter S-Plus IV three-part differential in a community hospital, including criteria for its use. Am J Clin Pathol 86:751, 1986.
11. Gauvin, GP, et al: Evaluation of the SYSMEX CC-800/PDA-410 system with trimodal histogram for white cell differential analysis. Lab Med 18:373, 1987.
12. Lai, AP, et al: Automated leucocyte differential counts in acute leukemia: A comparison of the Hemalog D, H600 and Coulter S-Plus IV, Clin Lab Haematol 8:33, 1986.
13. Drewinko, B: Utility of the Technicon H-1 system in malignant disease. In Simson, E, et al (eds): Proceedings of the Technicon H-1 Hematology Symposium, Technicon Instrument Corporation, New York, 1985, p 23.
14. Nelson, L, et al: Laboratory evaluation of differential white blood cell count information from the Coulter S-

Plus IV and Technicon H-1 in patient populations requiring rapid "turnaround" time. Am J Clin Pathol 91:563, 1989.

15. Payne, BA and Pierre, RV: Using the three-part differential: Part I. Investigating the possibilities. Lab Med 17:459, 1986.
16. Payne, BA and Pierre, RV: Using the three-part differential: Part II. Implementation of the system. Lab Med 17:517, 1986.
17. Coulter Electronics, Inc: Multidimensional leukocyte differential analysis. Coulter Hematology Analyzer. II, 1:1–6, June 1989.
18. Ross, DW and Bentley, SA: Evaluation of an automated hematology system (Technicon H-1). Arch Pathol Lab Med 110:803, 1986.
19. Howen, B, Walters, J, and Broden, P (eds): In NE-Series User's Guide: A Practical Approach to Interpreting NE-Series Scattergrams and Histograms. Toa Medical Electronics Co., Ltd., Kobe, Japan, 1991, p 2–6.
20. Pierre, RV: Section One: WBC case studies. In Pierre, RV: Seminar and Case Studies: The Automated Differential. Coulter Electronics, Hialeah, FL, 1985, p 7.
21. Bessman, JD: Red cells. In Bessman, JD: Automated Blood Counts and Differentials. John Hopkins University Press, Baltimore, 1988, p 5.
22. Bessman, JD: Platelets. In Bessman, JD: Automated Blood Counts and Differentials. John Hopkins University Press, Baltimore, 1986, p 57.
23. Tatsumi, N, Tsuda, I, Yokomatsu, Y, et al: Development of an Hematology Analyzer. Sysmex J 13:21, 1990.
24. Lamb, AA, Ansell, B, and Garvey, MB: Performance Characteristics of the Sysmex NE-8000 Automated Hematology Analyzer. A Hematology Monograph. Baxter Diagnostics, McGaw Park, IL, 1990, p 1–14.
25. Rickets, C: Intralaboratory quality control using control samples. In Cavill, I (ed): Methods in Hematology Quality Control. Churchill-Livingstone, New York, 1982, p 151.
26. Ward, PG, Warlo, F, and Lewis, SM: Standardization for routine blood counting—the role of interlaboratory trials. In Cavill, I (ed): Methods in Hematology Quality Control. Churchill-Livingstone, New York, 1982, p 102.
27. Cornbleet, PJ and Kessinger, S: Evaluation of Coulter S-Plus three-part differential in population with a high prevalence of abnormalities. Am J Clin Pathol 84:620, 1985.

BIBLIOGRAPHY

Bessman, JD, Gilmore, PR, Jr, and Gardner, FH: Improved classification of anemias by MCV and RDW. Am J Clin Pathol 80:322, 1983.
Burns, ER and Wenz, HB: Quantitative evaluation of the hematopoietic system. In Tilton, RC, Balows, A, Hohnadel, DC, and Reiss, RF (eds): Clinical Laboratory Medicine, Mosby–Year Book, St Louis, 1992, p 859.
Coulter Hematology Education Series: Significant Advances in Hematology. Coulter Electronics, Hialeah, FL, 1983.
Coulter Hematology Education Series: Coulter VCS Technology Casebook. Coulter Electronics, Hialeah, FL, 1989.
Dotson, M: Automation in Hematology. In Schoeff, LE and Williams, RH (eds): Principles of Laboratory Instruments. CV Mosby, St Louis, 1993, p 361.
Turgeon, ML: Clinical Hematology: Theory and Procedures, ed 2. Little, Brown, Boston, 1993.
Watson, JS and Dotson, M: Multiparameter hematology instruments. In Lotspeich-Steininger, CA, Stiene-Martin, EA, and Koepke, JA (eds): Clinical Hematology: Principles, Procedures, and Correlations. JB Lippincott, Philadelphia, 1992, p 496.

QUESTIONS

1. What is the main use of the leukocyte histogram differential?
   a. Diagnostic laboratory test for hematologic diseases
   b. Research tool for the routine hematology laboratory
   c. Replacement for the conventional manual differential
   d. Screening tool for hematologic diseases

2. What should be the basis for the decision to accept an automated leukocyte histogram differential or to perform a conventional manual differential?
   a. Each individual laboratory's established criteria for manual review of automated differential analysis
   b. Availability of qualified technologists
   c. Laboratory workload
   d. Manufacturer's recommendation

3. A 47-year-old woman was admitted to the hospital for elective surgery. Her bleeding history was unremarkable. Results from her admission CBC revealed normal RBC parameters, an increased WBC count, and a decreased PLT count. The Coulter WBC histogram revealed a large shoulder to the left of the lymphocyte region accompanied by an R1 flag. The letter "H" appeared next to the WBC count. What should be done first to verify these results?
   a. Examine the patient's blood smear for the presence of blasts and immature granulocytes, shift to the left.
   b. Request another sample from the patient and repeat the automated CBC and differential on the new sample.
   c. Notify the hematologist.
   d. Examine the patient's stained peripheral blood smear for platelet clumps and/or nRBCs.

4. An RBC histogram that shows an RBC distribution curve that is shifted to the left is characteristic of:
   a. Macrocytosis
   b. Anisocytosis
   c. Microcytosis
   d. Spherocytosis

5. Which of the following best describes the principle of the Coulter Model STKS?
   a. Laser and light scatter
   b. Volume, cell size and cytochemistry
   c. Volume, conductivity and light scatter
   d. Laser and immunofluorescence

6. The RDW represents a parameter that quantifies relative:
   a. Macrocytosis
   b. Anisocytosis
   c. Platelet size
   d. Microcytosis

7. The MPV and PDW are parameters describing:
   a. White cell size
   b. Red cell size
   c. Platelet size
   d. Multiple cell size

8. The Coulter Model S Plus IV differentiates lymphocytes, granulocytes, and mononuclear cells based on differences in:
   a. Overall cell size
   b. Cytoplasmic size
   c. Nuclear size and cytoplasmic complexity
   d. Nuclear size

9. Which area of the cell size distribution WBC histogram from a Coulter analyzer illustrated below is appropriate for a mononuclear population curve?
    a. a
    b. b
    c. c
    d. d

10. Region flags or R flags indicate which of the following?
    1. A decreased RBC count
    2. Specific locations of abnormalities in the WBC size distribution
    3. Erroneous results
    4. Overlapping of two or more of the cell populations at the four threshold areas of the WBC size distribution histogram
        a. 1, 2, 3
        b. 1, 3
        c. 2, 4
        d. 4 only

ANSWERS

1. **d** (p 622)
2. **a** (p 623)
3. **d** (p 623)
4. **c** (pp 623, 624)
5. **c** (p 626)
6. **b** (p 627)
7. **c** (p 624)
8. **c** (p 622)
9. **c** (pp 622–623)
10. **c** (p 623)

a.   a
b.   b
c.   c
d.   d

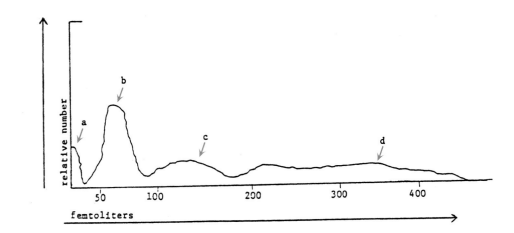

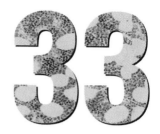

Special Stains and Cytochemistry

Mary Loring Perkins, MS, MT(ASCP)SH*
Deirdre E. DeSantis, MS, MT(ASCP)SBB*

Cytochemical Stains
   Leukocyte Alkaline Phosphatase Stain
   Myeloperoxidase Stain
   Alternative Method–Myeloperoxidase
     Stain
   Sudan Black B Stain

Cytochemical Esterases
   Specific Esterase (Naphthol AS-D
     Chloroacetate)
   Nonspecific Esterase (Alpha-Naphthol
     Butyrate)
   Combined Esterase

Other Stains
   Acid Phosphatase Stain/Tartrate-Resistant
     Acid Phosphatase
   Periodic Acid-Schiff Reaction
   Terminal Deoxynucleotidyl Transferase
     Test

Objectives

At the end of this chapter, the learner should be able to:
1. Interpret the score of leukocyte alkaline phosphatase staining and formulate a probable clinical diagnosis.
2. Discuss the clinical applications of myeloperoxidase staining methods.
3. Compare and contrast myeloperoxidase methods and Sudan black B methods in regard to cells identified and diagnostic applications.
4. Identify the types of cells that are stained by the specific esterase stain.
5. Discuss nonspecific esterase staining in regard to cells identified and the diagnostic value of sodium fluoride inhibition studies.
6. Discuss the diagnostic value of the acid phosphatase tartrate-resistant acid phosphatase stain.
7. Describe the clinical applications of Periodic acid-Schiff staining.
8. Discuss the clinical applications of terminal deoxynucleotidyl transferase methods.

Wright-stained peripheral blood smears and bone marrow preparations are routinely evaluated to identify and characterize erythrocytes, leukocytes, and platelets for the diagnosis of hematologic disorders. The presence of early precursor cells in particular blast cells may present a challenge to the technologist be-

cause the routine evaluation of morphological features may not always reveal evidence for classifying the cell line. Approximately 10% of all acute leukemias are reported to be undifferentiated by examination of morphological criteria alone. Cytochemical and immunocytochemical methods apply biochemical techniques for the identification of cellular elements such as enzymes or lipids to differentiate hematopoietic cell lines and aid in the diagnosis and classification of the acute leukemias and other hematologic conditions (see Chap. 18). Routine cytochemical stains, their proce-

*The coauthors acknowledge Milka Montiel, MD, for the staining of bone marrow preparations.

TABLE 33–1   **Cytochemical Reactions**

	Px	SBB	PAS	"Specific" Esterase (NCA)	"Nonspecific" Esterase (NA or NB)	αNA with NaF	αNA or αNB with NaF
Normal Cells							
Granulocytes	4+	4+	4+*	4+	(+/−)	(+/−)	
Monocytes	2+	2+	2+*	−	4+	−	
Lymphocytes	−	−	−/+	−	−/+("dot")	−/+("dot")	
Platelets or megakaryocytes	−	−	2+	−	+/−		
Erythroid cells	−	−	−	−		−	
Leukemic Blasts and Immature Cells							
ALL	−	−	−/+*	−	−/+("dot")		−/+("dot")
AML	+	+	+*	+	(+/−)		(+/−)
AMML	+	+	+*	+	+		(+/−)
AMoL	+	+	+*	−	+		−(+/−)
EL	−	−	+	−	−		−

Source: Mary Jo Fackler, B.Sc., M.T.(ASCP), S.H., with permission.
Abbreviations: Px = peroxidase; SBB = Sudan black B; PAS = periodic acid-Schiff; NCA = naphthol AS-D chloroacetate; NA = α naphthol acetate; NB = α-naphthol butyrate; NaF = sodium fluoride; ALL = acute lymphoblastic leukemia; AML = acute myelogenous leukemia; AMML = acute myelomonocytic leukemia; AMoL = acute monocytic leukemia; El = erythroleukemia.
*Diffuse background staining of cytoplasm and fine PAS granulation.
"dot" = staining reaction confined to small circular area of cytoplasm.

dures, and their applications will be presented in this chapter. Table 33–1 describes the expected reactions of normal cells, leukemic blasts, and immature cells to cytochemical stains.

CYTOCHEMICAL STAINS

Leukocyte Alkaline Phosphatase Stain

Purpose

The leukocyte alkaline phosphatase (LAP) enzyme is located in the tertiary or microvesicular granules of segmented neutrophils, bands, and some metamyelocytes. LAP activity increases with stages of neutrophil maturity. The enzyme is combined with a substrate at an alkaline pH to form a colored precipitate at sites of hydrolysis.

This cytochemical procedure is primarily relied on to distinguish chronic myelogenous leukemia (CML) from leukemoid reactions and myeloproliferative disorders such as polycythemia vera or myelofibrosis. One hundred *mature* neutrophils and bands are counted on an LAP-stained blood smear and are visually evaluated and scored according to the staining characteristics listed in Table 33–2.

Scoring should be performed on an area of the slide where the cell distribution is most suitable for differential counting. The edges of the smear or areas of cell overlapping should be avoided. Counts should be performed by two technologists since the scoring method is somewhat subjective. The two counts should match by approximately 10%. Because score values vary for different disease states as well as with technical bias, each laboratory must establish its own normal values.

Principle

The LAP within the neutrophil hydrolyzes the substrate naphthol AS-BI phosphate. The hydrolyzed substrate then couples with the dye (fast red-violet salt LB) and precipitates out at the site of enzyme activity. The degree of staining noted is proportional to enzymatic activity.

Specimen

Fingerstick specimens are acceptable; however, fresh heparinized samples of whole blood are routinely used. The use of ethylenediaminetetraacetic acid (EDTA)-anticoagulated blood is not recommended because it inhibits LAP activity. If staining is to be delayed, fix slides and store at −20°C within 2 hours of specimen collection. Optimally, smears should be thin.

TABLE 33–2   **Leukocyte Alkaline Phosphatase Scoring**

LAP Scoring Scale and Characteristics		
Grade	**Stain Intensity**	**Granulation**
0	None	None
1+	Fine/diffuse	Occasional
2+	Moderate	Moderate
3+	Strong	Many
4+	Brilliant	Nucleus obscured

TABLE 33–3 **LAP Score Calculation**

Grade	Number of Cells Counted	Calculation	LAP Score
0	60	$0 \times 60 = 0$	0
1+	20	$1 \times 20 = 20$	20
2+	14	$2 \times 14 = 28$	28
3+	5	$3 \times 5 = 15$	15
4+	1	$4 \times 1 = 4$	4
Total	100		67

LAP Control

Establishing limits for LAP control:
1. Obtain fresh heparinized sample from an individual with an elevated LAP score. Samples from a pregnant woman in the last trimester or a woman on oral contraceptives are suitable. The control is usually stable for 12 months.
2. Prepare smears, allow to dry, fix with LAP fixative, and rinse. Allow fixed smears to air-dry, then store at −20°C.
3. Prepare and read a series of slides from the new control and the old control. A minimum of five slides for each control is recommended. Calculate the mean LAP score with a control range of ±15.

Reagents

Control: Heparinized blood with score of approximately 200. Fix and store at −20°C.
1. Fixative: Store at room temperature. Reagent expires in 90 days, pH 4.2 to 4.5.
   Sodium citrate (formula weight (FW) 294.10) 0.282 g
   Citric acid (FW 210.14) 1058 g
   Deionized water 200 mL
   Acetone 300 mL
   Allow dry reagents to dissolve in water before adding acetone.
2. Substrate solution: Aliquots of 45 mL are stored at −20°C. Reagent expires in 8 months.
   2-amino-2-methyl-1,3-propanediol 13.15 g 0.1 N HCl 125 mL
   Check the pH (9.5 to 9.7) before adding 0.2 g naphthol AS-BI phosphate dissolved in 10 mL N,N-dimethylformamide. Add sufficient quantity (QS) with deionized water to 2500 mL.
3. Dye: 40 mg aliquots of fast red-violet salt LB are stored at −20°C.
4. Mayer's hematoxylin counterstain

Procedure

1. Allow smears to dry for 30 minutes. (This helps to keep the cells from washing off slides when rinsing after fixation.)
2. Fix smears in fixative for 30 seconds at room temperature.
3. Rinse with distilled water.
4. Thaw substrate solution to room temperature (22°C to 24°C); check with thermometer.
5. Add dye to substrate solution, gently agitate, filter, and use immediately.
6. Place slides, including control, in mixture for 15 minutes at room temperature.
7. Rinse slides in distilled water.
8. Counterstain with Mayer's hematoxylin for 2 minutes.
9. Rinse slides in distilled water.
10. Air-dry and mount with synthetic medium.

Interpretation

One hundred *mature* neutrophils and bands are counted and graded according to the scale 0 to 4+ presented in Table 33–2. To calculate the LAP score, the grade of staining is multiplied by the number of neutrophils counted for that grading. The final LAP score is obtained by adding together the value of each grade score. An example of LAP score calculation is provided in Table 33–3.

Report patient score if control is within established limits. Each laboratory must establish its own normal values. The normal LAP scores recommended for this method range between 11 and 95.

LAP activity is decreased in patients with CML, paroxysmal nocturnal hematuria (PNH), sickle cell anemia, sideroblastic anemia, and hereditary hypophosphatasia. Increased activity is seen in leukemoid reactions, myeloproliferative disorders such as polycythemia vera, and myelofibrosis (Table 33–4). As

TABLE 33–4 **LAP Reactivity in Various Disorders**

	Leukemoid Reaction	Chronic Granulocytic Leukemia	Acute Granulocytic Leukemia	Polycythemia Rubra Vera (PRV)	Myelofibrosis	Paroxysmal Nocturnal Hematuria	Pregnancy
Leukocyte alkaline phosphatase score	↑	↓	Varies	↑	Varies	↓	↑

Source: From procedures by Mary Loring Perkins, M.T.(ASCP), S.H., and Joe Marty, M.S., M.T.(ASCP).

previously noted, increased LAP values are also noted during the third trimester of pregnancy.

Comments

1. *Thin* blood smears should be prepared so that the white blood cells (WBCs) do not touch erythrocytes. Thick smears may falsely elevate results.
2. Only segmented and bandform neutrophils are scored. Do not include other cells. Monocytes and eosinophils do not stain.
3. Leukocyte alkaline phosphatase slides need to be scored as quickly as possible. The dye tends to fade.

Myeloperoxidase Stain

Purpose

Peroxidase enzyme is present in the primary (or azurophilic) granules of cells in the myeloid lineage and plays a central role in effective microbial killing during phagocytosis. The peroxidase in these granules is referred to as myeloperoxidase (MPO), which distinguishes it from other peroxidases such as eosinophilic peroxidase and platelet peroxidase. Myeloperoxidase is valued as a marker for myeloid cells since it is almost exclusive to primary granules in the neutrophil. Primary granules are present from the promyelocyte stage (late blast) to the neutrophilic stage of maturation. Accordingly, promyelocyte, myelocytes, metamyelocytes, bands, and segmented neutrophils are strongly positive for MPO. These granules are described to be absent in myeloblast; however, limited MPO activity is demonstrated at the sites of future primary granule synthesis with staining methods. This characteristic of myeloblasts is most useful for differentiating blast cells in acute myelogenous leukemias such as FAB subclasses M1, M2, and M3 from blast cells in acute lymphocytic leukemia (ALL).

Principle

Peroxidase enzymes are known to catalyze the oxidation of certain substances by hydrogen peroxide. Accordingly, in the presence of MPO, hydrogen peroxide oxidizes the substrate, 3-amino-9-ethylcarbazole (AEC), which will form a blue/black precipitate that may be easily identified as coarse granulation under light microscopy (Fig. 33–1).

Specimen

Smears or bone marrow touch preparations may be used. A fresh capillary sample is preferred for smears, however, EDTA, heparinized, or oxalated specimens are acceptable. Fresh samples are required since peroxidase activity decreases with exposure to light and heat or on prolonged storage.

Reagents

1. Fixative (buffered formalin acetone pH 6.6). Stored at 4° to 10°C, reagent has a shelf-life of 90 days.

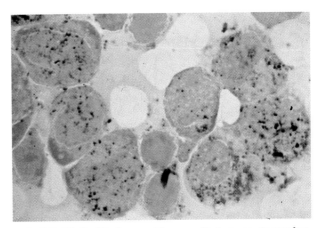

FIGURE 33–1 Myeloperoxidase positivity in acute myelogenous leukemia (M2).

    a. Na_2HPO_4 anhydrous (FW 141.96) 0.2 g
       KH_2PO_4 anhydrous (FW 136.09) 1.0 g
       Deionized water 300 mL
    b. Add 250-mL reagent-grade formalin 37%.
    c. Add 450-mL reagent-grade acetone.
    d. The pH should be 6.6. If necessary, adjust the pH with appropriate buffer salt.
2. 0.02 M acetate buffer pH 5.2. Stored at 4° to 10°C, reagent has a shelf-life of 90 days.
    a. 900 mL distilled water
    b. 2.72 g sodium acetate (FW 136.08)
    c. Adjust the pH to 5.2 with dilute acetic acid.
    d. Bring the volume to 1000 mL with distilled water.
3. Hydrogen peroxide 30%
4. 3-amino-9-ethylcarbazole (AEC substrate)
5. Dimethylsulfoxide (DMSO)
6. Mayer's hematoxylin

Procedures

1. Fix smears or bone marrow touch preparations for 15 seconds.
2. Rinse with deionized water.
3. Incubate smears for 8 minutes at room temperature in a freshly made filtered mixture containing the following:
    AEC 10 mg
    DMSO 6 mL
    Acetate buffer 50 mL
    Hydrogen peroxide 30% 0.005 mL
4. Rinse with deionized water.
5. Stain with Mayer's hematoxylin for 2 minutes.
6. Rinse in deionized water.
7. Air dry and mount with coverslip.

Interpretation

1. Positive staining for MPO is indicated by the presence of blue-black granules. Most cells in the myelocytic series demonstrate strongly positive peroxidase activity indicated by coarse blue-black granulation (see Fig. 33–1). Positive activity of blasts should be evaluated because reactivity in

mature granulocytes is not of diagnostic importance.

2. Positive staining is also noted in eosinophils and monocytes. Monocytes demonstrate weakly positive or diffuse staining with only a few peroxidase-positive granules present. Monoblasts noted in acute monocytic leukemia are usually negative, whereas monoblasts in acute myelomonocytic leukemia may demonstrate weak reactivity. Eosinophils reveal strong peroxidase activity.

3. Because Auer rods are strongly peroxidase-positive, MPO staining is useful for demonstrating their presence.

4. Early myeloblasts, erythroblasts, lymphocytes, mature basophils, and plasma cells are generally negative for myeloperoxidase.

Comments

1. Because peroxidase enzymes are sensitive to light, smears should be stained immediately and stored in the dark. Smears that are older than 2 weeks or that have been exposed to excessive light should not be reported as peroxidase-negative. If smears are to be stained at a later date, they should be fixed, air-dried, and stored in an envelope in the freezer.

2. Permount should not be used for mounting. Color usually fades before microscopic observation can be made. In addition, xylene should not be used to clean unmounted slides.

3. A positive control may be obtained from healthy individuals.

4. One indicator of overincubation is positive peroxidase activity in red blood cells.

Alternative Method—Myeloperoxidase Stain

Purpose

MPO staining methods are useful for identifying myelocytic leukemias because granulocytes and their precursors stain positive, whereas cells of the lymphoid and erythroid lineage stain negative. If the standard MPO methods do not stain blasts that are still suspected to be of myeloid origin, an alternative method can be used. As noted, the myeloperoxidase enzyme is present in the primary granules of myeloid cells. They first appear in the early promyelocyte stage and persist through subsequent stages of maturation. Limited MPO activity is noted in myeloblasts. This method is particularly useful for identifying blasts in poorly differentiated forms of AML such as FAB subclass M1.

Principle

In the presence of MPO, hydrogen peroxide oxidizes the substrate, benzidine dihydrochloride, which forms a black precipitate. The oxidized substrate essentially appears at the site of the enzyme activity and is interpreted as a positive marker for the presence of myeloperoxidase.

Specimen

Smears or bone marrow touch preparations can be used. A fresh capillary sample is preferred for smears; however, EDTA, heparinized, or oxalated specimens are acceptable. Fresh samples are required, since peroxidase activity decreases with exposure to light and heat or on prolonged storage.

Reagents

1. Fixative (stored at room temperature, reagent has a shelf life of 90 days).
   Formaldehyde (37%) 10 mL
   Absolute ethyl alcohol 190 mL
2. Zinc sulfate solution
   Zinc sulfate ($ZnSO_4$, $7H_2O$) 0.38 g
   Deionized water 10 mL
3. Substrate solution: Filtered and stored at room temperature, reagent expires in 6 months.
   Add reagents in order, mixing well after each addition.
   Ethyl alcohol (30%) 100 mL
   Benzidine dihydrochloride 0.3 g
   Zinc sulfate solution 1.0 mL
   Sodium acetate (F.W. 136.1) 1.0 g
   Hydrogen peroxide (30%) 0.005 mL
   Sodium hydroxide (1.0 N) 1.5 mL
   Safranin O 0.2 g
   Note: Benzidine is a potential carcinogen, and the following precautions should be taken when handling the reagent or its solutions.
   a. Wear protective clothing including gloves, laboratory coat, and mask when weighing out powders.
   b. Use mechanical aids for all pipetting.
   c. Clean up spills immediately.
   d. Wash hands after completion.
   e. Weigh benzidine in hood.
   f. The 30% alcohol may be warmed with hot tap water to facilitate dissolving of the benzidine.

Procedure

1. Fix smears or bone marrow touch preparations for 60 seconds.
2. Rinse with deionized water.
3. Incubate for 30 seconds in substrate solution at room temperature.
4. Rinse with deionized water.
5. Air-dry and mount with a coverslip.

Interpretation

Positive staining for peroxidase activity is indicated by the presence of black granulation. Enzyme activity noted in blasts is of the most diagnostic importance while positive reactions in mature granulocytes provide limited diagnostic value.

Sudan Black B Stain

Purpose

Sudan black B (SBB) is a fat-soluble dye. SBB staining patterns correlate closely with the patterns ob-

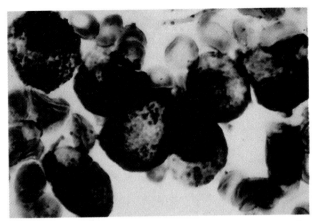

FIGURE 33-2 Sudan black positivity in acute promyelocytic leukemia (M3).

served with MPO methods. Accordingly, neutrophils are strongly positive with SBB staining (Fig. 33–2). The intensity and coarseness of staining increases with the stages of myelocytic maturation. The term *sudanophilic* has been applied as a characteristic of cellular structures that are stained by Sudan black. In comparison with MPO reactions, all cellular structures that demonstrate MPO activity also demonstrate sudanophilia. One advantage of SBB methods over MPO methods is the increased stability of SBB-stained smears when exposed to sunlight or heat and when stored for prolonged periods.

Although SBB methods have largely been replaced by myeloperoxidase methods, SBB staining has been described to be reliable in identifying cells of myeloid lineage and for distinguishing the blast cells in acute myelogenous leukemia (FAB subclasses M1, M2, and M3) from the blast cells in acute lymphocytic leukemia (ALL).

Principle

SBB stains phospholipids, neutral fats, and sterols. The mechanism by which the SBB reaction demonstrates the presence of phospholipid is not clearly understood, but is believed to be based on the ability of fat-soluble dye to disassociate from its solvent and penetrate lipoprotein complexes. Phospholipids are concentrated in the primary, secondary, and tertiary granules of neutrophils and, to a lesser extent, in the lysosomal granules of monocytes and macrophages. Lymphocyte and lymphocyte precursors are generally negative with SBB; however, rare exceptions of SBB positivity have been noted in Burkitt's lymphoma and in the blast crisis associated with chronic lymphocytic leukemia (CLL).

Specimen

Smears or bone marrow touch preparations may be used. A fresh capillary sample is preferred for smears; however, EDTA, heparinized, or oxalated specimens are acceptable.

Reagents

1. Polyvinyl pyrrolidone (K-29-33)
2. Phosphate buffer, pH 7.2
   0.15 M Na_2HPO_4, (21 g/L) 7.0 mL
   0.15 M $Na_2H_2PO_4$ H_2O (20.7 g/L) 3.0 mL
   Distilled water 30.0 mL
3. Fixative, pH 5.5; store at room temperature in amber bottle; expires in 90 days.
   a. Dissolve 10 g of Plasdone in 400 mL of absolute ethanol.
   b. Add 75 mL of 37% formaldehyde.
   c. Add 10 mL phosphate buffer pH 7.2.
   d. Add 15 mL liquefied phenol.
4. SBB solution expires in 1 year.
   a. Dissolve 1.5 g of SBB in 500 mL of absolute ethanol.
   b. Stir with a magnetic stirrer for 60 minutes; filter before use.
5. Phosphate: Phenol buffer expires in 6 months.
   a. Dissolve 0.48 g anhydrous Na_2HPO_4 (FW 141.96) in 400 mL of distilled water.
   b. Dissolve 64 g of crystalline phenol (or 72.8 mL of liquified phenol) in 120 mL of absolute ethanol and mix with the phosphate.
6. Nuclear counterstain expires in 1 year.
   a. 1% aqueous cresol violet
7. Background stain expires in 1 year.
   a. 0.2% aqueous light green to which 2 drops of glacial acetic acid have been added

Procedure

1. Fix smears or touch preparations for 60 seconds.
2. Rinse three times with tap water.
3. Incubate slides in the following mixture for 60 minutes (prepare daily):
   a. 20 mL phosphate-phenol buffer
   b. 30 mL Sudan black B solution
   c. Filtering solution is not necessary.
4. Rinse in 70% ethanol.
5. Air-dry.
6. Counterstain for 10 seconds in 1% violet. Wash three times in tap water. Air-dry.
7. Counterstain for 10 seconds in 0.2% light green. Wash three times in tap water. Air-dry and mount with coverslip.

Interpretation

1. Positive staining for SBB is indicated by the presence of brown-black cytoplasmic granules. Most cells in the myelocytic series demonstrate a strongly positive SBB reaction (see Fig. 33–2).
2. Positive staining is also noted in eosinophils and monocytes. Monocytes demonstrate weakly positive or diffuse staining. Eosinophils reveal strong SBB reactivity that is described by distinct staining of an outer shell with a clear or unstained center.
3. Early myeloblasts, lymphocytes, erythroblasts, mature basophils, megakaryocytes, and platelets are generally negative for SBB staining.

Comments

1. Mayer's hematoxylin or Giemsa stain may be used as counterstains.
2. Normal blood smears should always be run as a positive control.

CYTOCHEMICAL ESTERASES

Esterases are enzymes that are found in a variety of tissues and hematopoietic cell lines. Esterases are known to hydrolyze aliphatic and aromatic ester bonds. In regard to hematopoietic cells, they are capable of splitting naphthol and naphthol derivatives from their esters.

Certain esterases have been demonstrated in leukocytes that have been separated into nine subtypes or isoenzymes. These isoenzymes may be classified as either *specific* or *nonspecific*, depending on the particular substrate hydrolyzed and the optimum pH for enzyme activity.

Isoenzymes 1, 2, 7, 8, and 9 are referred to as specific (or chloroacetate) esterases (SE) because they are found in all stages of myelocytic maturation and mast cells. Accordingly, specific esterases are valued as a marker for early cells of myeloid lineage. The SE enzymes hydrolyze the substrate, naphthol AS-D chloroacetate (NASDA), at a neutral or slightly alkaline pH and are resistant to sodium fluoride treatment.

Nonspecific esterases (NSE) comprise isoenzymes 3, 4, 5, and 6, which are found in a variety of cell types such as monocytes, plasma cells, megakaryocytes and certain T-lymphocyte subsets. Depending on the nonspecific esterase, either alpha-naphthol butyrate or alpha-naphthol acetate is hydrolyzed at a slightly acid pH. The nonspecific esterase activity of monocytes and monoblasts may be distinguished from the nonspecific esterase activity of other cells with the addition of an inhibitor such as sodium fluoride to the incubation medium. The NSE activity of monocytes and macrophages is inhibited or abolished, whereas the activity of other cells remains unaffected (Figs. 33–3 and 33–4). The NSE reaction is often used as a specific marker for early monocytes and macrophages.

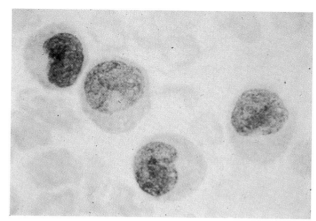

FIGURE 33–4 Nonspecific esterase stain with sodium fluoride inhibition in acute monocytic leukemia (M5b).

Cytochemical esterase staining is used as a tool for differentiating cells in the myeloid series from cells in the monocytic series. The results of staining have been relied on to distinguish precursor cells in acute myelogenous leukemia (FAB subclasses M2 and M3) from precursor cells in acute myelomonocytic leukemia (FAB subclass M4) and acute monocytic leukemia (FAB subclass M5).

Specific Esterase (Naphthol AS-D Chloroacetate)

Purpose

Specific esterase staining is valued as a marker for early cells of myeloid lineage and is used most often to identify precursor cells in acute myelogenous leukemias. Specific esterase is present in the primary granules of myeloid cells.

Principle

The specific esterase enzyme within granulocytes hydrolyzes the substrate naphthol chloroacetate. The hydrolyzed substrate then couples with the diazo salt (hexazotized pararosaniline). The diazo dye precipitates out at the site of enzymatic activity. Positive activity is easily identified under light microscopy by the presence of granulation.

Specimen

Paraffin sections, smears, and bone marrow touch preparations are used. Fresh capillary samples are preferred for smears; however, anticoagulated blood is acceptable.

Reagents

1. Esterase fixative, pH 6.6; stored at 4°C, reagent expires in 90 days.
   a. In 120 ml of deionized water dissolve:
   Na_2HPO_4 (F.W. 141.96) 0.08 g
   KH_2PO_4 (F.W. 136.09) 0.40 g

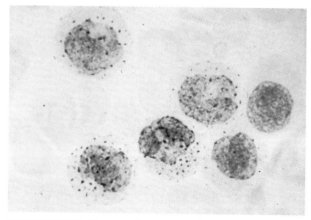

FIGURE 33–3 Nonspecific esterase alpha naphthol acetate positivity in acute monocytic leukemia (M5b).

Formaldehyde 37% 100 mL
Acetone 180 mL

b. Adjust pH to 6.6 if necessary with appropriate buffer salt.

2. Phosphate buffer, 0.1 M pH 6.5; stored at 4°C, reagent expires in 90 days. Discard if mold develops.
NaH_2PO_4 H_2O (FW 137–99) 9.45 g
Na_2HPO_4 (FW 141.96) 4.47 g
Deionized water 1000 mL
Check pH and adjust to 6.5 if necessary with appropriate buffer salt solution.

3. Substrate solution. Store in glass (not plastic) stoppered bottle at 4°C. Reagent expires in 30 days.
a. Dissolve 100 mg of naphthol AS-D chloroacetate in 10 ml of N,N-dimethylformamide (FW 73.1).

4. Pararosaniline solution: Store in brown bottle at 4 to 10°C. Expires in 3 months. Caution: Pararosaniline is a potential carcinogen.
a. Dissolve 1.0 g pararosaniline HCl (FW 323.8) in 20 mL distilled water plus 5 mL concentrated HCl. Solution may be gently heated to dissolve pararosaniline.
b. Filter.

5. Sodium nitrite solution. *Must be prepared daily.*
a. Dissolve 1.0 g $NaNO_2$ (FW 69.0) in distilled water to a volume of 25 mL.

6. Mayer's hematoxylin

7. Acid alcohol working solution
70% ethanol 5 mL
Deionized water 995 mL
Concentrated HCl 0.05 mL

8. Bluing agent
$NaHCO_3$ 1 g
Deionized water 100 mL

Procedure

1. Deparaffinize and hydrate sections. The fixative B5 may be used if the fixation time is short and if the mercury precipitate is not removed with iodine.

2. For blood smears and imprints, fix in esterase fixative and wash well with deionized water at 4°C for 30 seconds.

3. Incubate slides in the "incubation mixture" for 30 minutes. The incubation mixture is prepared as follows:
a. To 40 mL of buffer add 1.0 mL of substrate solution.
b. In a separate test tube, add 0.1 mL of sodium nitrite solution to 0.1 mL of pararosaniline solution. Wait 1 minute and add buffer substrate solution.
c. Filter.

4. After 30 minutes at room temperature, check control slide microscopically. If the reacting cells are not red enough, refilter the solution and replace slides for 15 to 30 minutes.

5. Wash slides in running tap water for 5 minutes.

6. Counterstain for 2 minutes in Mayer's hematoxylin.

7. Rinse well with deionized water.

8. Dip in bluing solution until counterstain turns from purple to blue (approximately 10 dips).

9. Wash, dry, and mount smears with Permount. Tissue sections must be rehydrated and cleared in xylene before mounting.

Interpretation

The cytoplasm of granulocytes and tissue mast cells appears red. Nuclei are counterstained blue in cells of the granulocytic series (Fig. 33–5).

Comments

Esterase activity is inhibited to varying degrees by mercury, acid solutions, heat, and iodine. False-negative reactions may occur under the following conditions:

1. Slides overheated during the drying process.
2. Mercury crystals removed from tissues with an iodine solution.
3. Tissues fixed in an acid fixative such as Zenker's (formalin or acetic) or Bouin's fixative.
4. Tissues decalcified in an acid solution.
5. Solutions used that are too old.

Nonspecific Esterase (Alpha-Naphthol Butyrate)

Purpose

Nonspecific esterase (NSE) activity is valued as a marker for early monocytes and macrophages when used in conjunction with sodium fluoride inhibition studies. Because a number of cells express activity with NSE staining, the incubation medium may be modified by the addition of sodium fluoride. The NSE activity of monocytes and macrophages is inhibited or abolished, whereas the activity of other cells remains unaffected. NSE is used most often to identify precursor cells in the acute myelomonocytic (FAB subclass M4) and acute monocytic leukemias (FAB subclass M5).

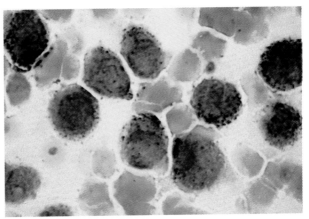

FIGURE 33–5 Specific esterase naphthol-AS-D chloroacetate positivity in acute promyelocytic leukemia (M3).

Principle

The nonspecific esterase enzyme within cells hydrolyzes the substrate alpha-naphthol butyrate. The hydrolyzed substrate then couples with the diazo salt (hexazotized pararosaniline). The diazo dye forms a precipitate at the site of enzymatic activity. Positive activity is easily identified under light microscopy by the presence of granulation.

Specimen

Smears or bone marrow preparations may be used. A fresh capillary sample is preferred; however, EDTA, heparinized, or oxalated specimens are acceptable.

Reagents

1. Esterase fixative, pH 6.6; stored at 4°C, reagent expires in 90 days.
   a. In 300 mL of deionized water dissolve:
      Na_2HPO_4 (FW 141.96) 0.2 g
      KH_2PO_4 (FW 136.09) 1.0 g
      Formaldehyde 37% 250 mL
      Acetone 450 mL
   b. Adjust pH to 6.5 if necessary with appropriate buffer salt. (*Note:* pH has tendency to increase if allowed to sit. If pH is near 6.5, allow to stand overnight, and then test new fixative on known positive.)
2. Phosphate buffer 0.15 M, pH 6.3; stored at 4°C, reagent expires in 90 days. Discard if mold growth is observed.
   NaH_2PO_4, H_2O (FW 137.99) 8.02 g
   Na_2HPO_4 (FW 141.96) 2.4 g
   Deionized water 1000 mL
   Check the pH and adjust to 6.3 if necessary with appropriate buffer salt.
3. Substrate solution: Store in glass stoppered bottle at 4°C to 10°C. Good for 1 month. Dissolve 250 mg alpha-naphthol butyrate in 12.5 mL ethylene glycol monomethyl ether (Eastman Kodak). If alpha-naphthol butyrate is in liquid form, then use 0.225 mL/12.5 mL of solvent.
4. Sodium nitrite solution. Prepare daily.
   a. Dissolve 1.0 g $NaNO_2$ (FW 69.0) in distilled water to a volume of 25 mL.
5. Pararosaniline solution (possible carcinogen; see under comments). Stored in brown bottle at 4°C to 10°C, reagent has a shelf life of 90 days.
   a. Dissolve 1.0 g pararosaniline HCl (FW 323.8) in 20 mL distilled water plus 5 mL concentrated HCl. Solution may be gently heated to dissolve pararosaniline.
6. Mayer's hematoxylin
7. Acid alcohol working solution
   70% ethanol 15 mL
   Deionized water 995 mL
   Concentrated HCl 10.05 mL
8. Bluing agent
   $NaHCO_3$ 1 g
   Deionized water 100 mL

Procedure

1. Fix smears for 30 seconds at 4°C to 10°C in esterase fixative.

2. Wash three times with deionized water.
3. Air-dry smears and place in Coplin jar.
4. Incubate smears for 45 minutes at room temperature in the following mixture:
   a. To 40 mL of buffer (pH 6.3) add 2 mL of substrate solution.
   b. In a separate container, add 0.2 mL sodium nitrite solution to 0.2 mL pararosaniline solution. Wait 1 minute and add to buffer substrate solution.
   c. Filter into Coplin jar.
5. Wash well with deionized water.
6. Counterstain with hematoxylin for 2 minutes.
7. Wash well with deionized water.
8. Place slides in bluing reagent for 30 seconds.
9. Wash well with deionized water.
10. Air-dry and mount with Permount.

Interpretation

Megakaryocytes, macrophages, plasma cells, and monocytes demonstrate positive reactivity by the presence of brick-red precipitate. Certain subsets of T lymphocytes demonstrate punctate staining. Granulocytes are generally negative. With the addition of sodium fluoride to the incubation medium, NSE activity in monocytes is reduced or abolished, whereas the NSE activity of others cells remains unchanged (see Figs. 33–3 and 33–4).

Comments

1. Pararosaniline is a possible carcinogen and the following precautions should be taken when handling the reagent or its solutions.
   a. Wear protective clothing: gloves, laboratory coat, smock. Wear a mask when weighing out powders.
   b. Use mechanical pipetting aids for all pipetting.
   c. Immediately clean up all spills.
   d. Wash hands after completion.
2. A control must be run to be sure reagents are working.
3. Hexazotized reagents are unstable and must be used immediately.
4. Fixation keeps the enzyme from washing out of the cell during staining and improves the morphological preservation of the cells.
5. Smears should be fixed after drying, even if staining is to be performed at a later date.
6. Since this method depends on an enzymatic reaction, care must be taken to preserve enzyme activity by avoiding exposure to light and heat as well as prolonged storage. Store fixed smears in freezer.
7. *For sodium fluoride inhibition studies, add NaFl 1.5 mg/mL to incubation mixture.*

Combined Esterase

Purpose

Combined esterase studies are used to evaluate the ratio of myelocytic and monocytic cells on a smear. This staining method is most often relied upon to differentiate acute myelomonocytic leukemia (FAB subclass M4) from acute monocytic leukemia (FAB subclasses M5a and M5b). The combined esterase approach is especially valuable when a limited number of smears are available.

Principle

The esterase enzymes within cells hydrolyze the substrate alpha-naphthol butyrate and naphthol AS-D chloroacetate. The hydrolyzed substrate then couples with the dye, fast-blue BB, or pararosaniline, and the colored complex formed precipitates out at the site of enzymatic activity.

Specimen

This may be a fresh smear or a bone marrow touch preparation. For smears, fresh capillary samples are preferred; however, anticoagulated specimens are acceptable.

Reagents

1. Esterase fixative pH 6.6. Stores at 4°C, reagent expires in 3 months.
   a. In 120 mL of deionized water dissolve:
      Na_2HPO_4 (FW 141.96) 0.08 g
      KH_2PO_4 (FW 136.09) 0.40 g
   b. Formaldehyde 37% 100 mL
   c. Acetone 180 mL
   d. Adjust pH to 6.6 if necessary with appropriate buffer salt.
2. Phosphate buffer pH 7.4. Stored at 4°C, reagent expires in 90 days. Discard if any mold is observed.
   a. NaH_2PO_4 H_2O (FW 137.99) 1.67 g
   b. Na_2HPO_4 (FW 141.96) 7.74 g
   c. Deionized water 1000 mL
   d. Adjust pH to 7.4 if necessary with appropriate buffer salt solution.
3. Naphthol AS-D chloroacetate. Store at 0°C.
4. Substrate solution. Stored at 4°C in glass-stoppered bottle, reagent expires in 30 days.
   a. Naphthol AS-D chloroacetate 20 mg
   b. N,N-dimethylformamide (FW 73.1) 10 mL
5. Fast blue BB salt. Store at 0°C.
6. Mayer's hematoxylin
7. Bluing agent
   $NaHCO_3$ 1 g
   Deionized water 100 mL
8. Refer to nonspecific esterase procedure for reagents needed for step 1 of this combined esterase procedure.

Procedure

1. Perform as for a nonspecific esterase procedure, but do not counterstain.
2. Incubate slides in the following filtered mixture for 20 minutes at room temperature:
   Buffer 38 mL
   Substrate solution 2mL
   Fast-blue BB 20 mg
3. Wash well with deionized water.
4. Counterstain with hematoxylin for 2 minutes.
5. Wash well with deionized water.
6. Place slides in bluing reagent for 30 seconds.
7. Wash, air-dry, and mount with coverslip.

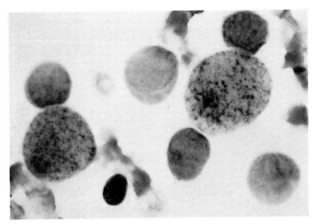

FIGURE 33–6   Combined esterase positivity in acute myelomonocytic leukemia (M4).

Interpretation

Monocytes and macrophages demonstrate diffusely brown/red staining. T lymphocytes usually stain with punctate red granules. Mast cells, early promyelocytes, and later granulocytes demonstrate a granular blue staining (Fig. 33–6).

OTHER STAINS

Acid Phosphatase Stain/Tartrate-Resistant Acid Phosphatase

Purpose

Acid phosphatase is a lysosomal enzyme that is present in many tissues and hematopoietic cells. Numerous isoenzymes have been identified, with several appearing to be cell-specific. Seven isoenzymes have been classified as nonerythrocytic with isoenzymes 2 and 4 being noted in neutrophils and monocytes; isoenzyme 3 in lymphocytes and platelets and isoenzyme 5 in the hairy cells seen in leukemic reticuloendotheliosis (hairy cell leukemia). The findings of alkaline phosphatase staining alone are of limited diagnostic value unless run in conjunction with tartrate inhibition studies. With the addition of tartrate to the incubation medium, the acid phosphatase activity of all isoenzymes is abolished with the exception of isoenzyme 5. Because isoenzyme 5 is specific to hairy cells, the finding of *tartrate resistance* on a smear supports the diagnosis of leukemic reticuloendotheliosis (Fig. 33–7).

Acid phosphatase activity has been shown to be higher in T lymphocytes than in B lymphocytes and is therefore useful for identifying lymphoblasts in many cases of acute T-lymphocytic leukemia. T lymphocytes demonstrate focal speckled staining wherever Golgi bodies are found. This presentation is not specific to T lymphocytes and may be noted in other cells such as myeloblasts and erythroblasts. Additional cytochemical markers should be evaluated before making a diagnosis of acute T-lymphocytic leukemia.

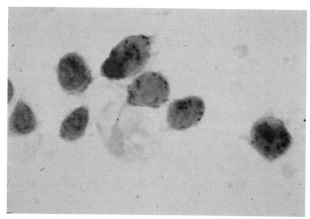

FIGURE 33–7 Tartrate-resistant acid phosphatase (TRAP) stain of peripheral blood showing positivity in hairy cells and no staining in neutrophils.

Principle

The acid phosphatase within the white cell hydrolyzes the substrate naphthol AS-BI phosphoric acid. The hydrolyzed substrate then couples with the dye (hexazotized pararosaniline) and precipitates out at the site of enzymatic activity. The addition of tartrate to the incubation medium inhibits all acid phosphatase isoenzyme activity with the exception of the enzyme fraction found in hairy cell leukemia (isoenzyme 5).

Specimen

Smears, bone marrow touch preparations, or frozen sections may be used. Fresh capillary samples are preferred; however, EDTA or heparinized specimens are acceptable.

Reagents

1. Acid phosphatase fixative, pH 5.4; stored at 4°C to 10°C, reagent expires in 90 days. Discard if RBC morphology is poor.
   a. Dissolve 0.63 g citrate acid (FW 210.14) in 30 mL of deionized water.
   b. Add 10 mL of methanol and 60 mL of acetone.
   c. Mix and adjust the pH to 5.4 with concentrated NaOH solution.
2. 0.1 N acetate buffer, pH a.2; stored at 4°C, reagent expires in 90 days.
   a. 600 mL distilled water
   b. 13.6 g sodium acetate (FW 136.1)
   c. Adjust the pH to 5.2 with 1.0 M acetic acid. Bring the volume to 1000 mL with distilled water.
3. Tartrate sodium acetate buffer, pH 5.2; stored at 4 to 10°C, reagent expires in 3 months.
   a. Dissolve 3.75 g of L-(+)-tartaric acid in 490 mL of 0.1 N acetate buffer.
   b. Adjust the pH to 5.2 with concentrated NaOH.

   c. Bring the volume to 500 mL with distilled water.
4. 0.1 M acetic acid
   a. 200 mL distilled water
   b. 1.25 mL glacial acetic acid (F.W. 60.05, 16N)
5. L-(+)-Tartaric acid
6. Substrate solution: Stored in glass-stoppered bottle at 4° to 10°C, reagent has a shelf-life of 30 days. Discard if it turns pink.
   a. Dissolve 100 mg naphthol AS-BI phosphoric acid in 10.0 ml N,N-dimethylformamide.
   b. When used infrequently, make up fresh by adding 10 mg naphthol AS-BI phosphoric acid in 1.0 ml N,N-dimethylformamide.
7. 4% sodium nitrate solution; prepare daily.
   a. Dissolve 1.0 g $NaNO_2$ (FW 69.0) in distilled water to a volume of 25 mL.
8. 4% pararosaniline solution (possible carcinogen; see comments under nonspecific esterase). Stored in brown bottles at 4 to 10°C, reagent has a shelf-life of 90 days.
   a. Dissolve 1.0 g pararosaniline HCl (FW 323.8) in 20 mL distilled water plus 5 mL concentrated HCl. Solution may be gently heated to dissolve pararosaniline. Filter.
9. Mayer's hematoxylin
10. Acid alcohol solution
    Concentrated HCl 0.05 mL
    100% ethanol 3.5 mL
    Deionized water 996.5 mL
11. Bluing reagent
    $NaHCO_3$ 1 g
    Deionized water 100 mL

Procedure

1. Fix smears, touch preparations, or frozen section for 30 seconds with cold fixative.
2. Wash three times with deionized water. Air-dry.
3. Incubate smears or imprints at 37°C in the appropriate filtered mixture:
   a. Acid phosphatase stain
      Acetate buffer 50 mL
      Stock substrate solution 2 mL
   In a separate container, add 0.2 mL of 4% sodium nitrate solution to 0.2 ml of 4% pararosaniline solution. Wait 1 minute, and then add to buffer substrate solution.
   b. Tartrate-resistant acid phosphatase (TRAP) stain
      Acetate-tartrate buffer 50 mL
      Stock substrate solution 2 mL
   In a separate container, add 0.2 mL of 4% sodium nitrate solution to 0.2 mL of 4% pararosaniline solution. Wait 1 minute and then add to buffer substrate solution.
4. Incubate for 60 minutes at 37°C.
5. Wash three times in tap water.
6. Counterstain with hematoxylin for 2 minutes.
7. Rinse well with deionized water.
8. Place in bluing solution for 30 seconds.
9. Wash, dry, and mount with Permount. Frozen tissue sections must be dehydrated and cleared in xylene before mounting.

Interpretation

Acid phosphatase activity is demonstrated by the presence of an orange-red precipitate with pararosaniline. The test result is considered positive when two or more cells exhibit strong (4+) activity. The presence of lymphoblasts may be indicated if acid phosphatase staining is present in a focal speckled pattern at the sites of Golgi bodies. Increased activity has occasionally been observed in myeloma cells.

Comments

1. A control must be run along with patient samples to ensure that reagents are working properly.
2. As hexazotized reagents are unstable, they must be used immediately.
3. Fixation prevents the enzyme from washing out of the cell during staining and improves the morphological preservation of the cells.
4. Enzyme activity may be extended by avoiding exposure to light and heat as well as prolonged storage.
5. Smears may be kept at room temperature for at least 2 weeks without apparent loss of enzymatic activity.
6. After a few weeks, reaction products may precipitate out (salting-out phenomenon) and be confused with true positive staining.
7. Controls should be fixed, air-dried, and stored at −20°C.
8. Increasing the temperature beyond 37°C causes inactivation of the enzyme and decomposition of the azo dye, resulting in nonspecific precipitation.
9. Mayer's hematoxylin as a counterstain gives a light gray tint to the cytoplasm of the leukocytes which may mask weak enzymatic activity. In contrast, methyl green may give poor nuclear detail, but weak enzymatic activity in the cytoplasm is not masked.

Periodic Acid-Schiff Reaction

Purpose

Periodic acid-Schiff (PAS) stains cytoplasmic glycogen, which is present in a variety of hematopoietic cells. As many cell lines exhibit PAS positivity, evaluation of the pattern and intensity of staining may be useful for differentiating cell lines. Lymphocytes, granulocytes, monocytes, and megakaryocytes all demonstrate positive reactivity with varying intensity and pattern. Generally, early granulocytes stain in a light, diffuse pattern, with increasing intensity and coarseness noted with stages of maturation. Lymphocyte staining is more granular and coarse. Lymphoblasts in ALL (FAB subclasses L1 and L2) have been known to exhibit "block" staining. One important clinical application of PAS staining is for supporting the diagnosis of erythroleukemia (FAB subclass M6). Normal erythrocytes and erythrocyte precursors will present with negative reactivity, whereas erythrocyte precursors in erythroleukemia demonstrate intense PAS positivity. Occasionally, positive PAS reactions have been noted in refractory anemias and thalassemia. Lymphocytes

in Burkitt's type ALL (FAB subclass L3) stain negative with PAS. Although still popular in many clinical laboratories, PAS methods have largely been replaced by more specific cytochemical markers that are capable of establishing more definitive diagnoses.

Principle

PAS oxidizes complex carbohydrates such as glycogen to aldehydes. The aldehydes react with Schiff's reagent to release a colored product. Basic fuchsin is a frequently used dye that imparts a magenta color (Fig. 33–8).

Specimen

Smears or bone marrow touch preparations may be used. Anticoagulants do not inhibit activity. Paraffin tissue sections may also be used, but sections must first be hydrated.

Reagents

1. Fixative: Stored at room temperature, reagent has a shelf-life of 1 year.
   37% reagent-grade formalin 50 mL
   Absolute ethanol 450 mL
2. 1% Periodic acid: Stored at room temperature, reagent has a shelf-life of 3 months.
   Periodic acid 5 g
   Deionized water 500 mL
3. Schiff's reagent: Stored at 4°C, reagent has a shelf-life of 3 months.
   Basic fuchsin Cl 42500 2.5 g
   Deionized water 500 mL
   Sodium metabisulfite 5 g
   1 N HCl 50 mL
   Stir all ingredients for 2 h, or until solution turns yellow (light amber). Add 4.0 g of activated charcoal. Filter until all charcoal is removed from solution. Do not use solution if it turns pink.
4. 0.5% sodium metabisulfite ($Na_2S_2O_5$): Stored at room temperature, reagent has a shelf-life of 3 months.

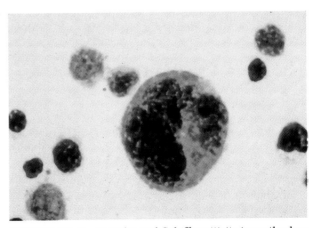

FIGURE 33-8   Periodic acid-Schiff positivity in erythroleukemia (M6).

Sodium metabisulfite 2.5 g
Deionized water 500 ml
5. Hematoxylin (see hematoxylin counterstain)
6. Acid alcohol solution: Stored at room temperature, reagent expires in 6 months.
1% HCl in 70% ethanol 2.5 mL
Deionized water 497.5 mL
7. 1% sodium bicarbonate solution. At room temperature, reagent has a shelf-life of 6 months.
Sodium bicarbonate 5 g
Deionized water 500 mL

Procedure

1. Fix smears for 15 minutes. Paraffin tissue sections must be hydrated if they have already been fixed.
2. Rinse *gently* in deionized water. Vigorous rinsing may lead to the loss of cells/tissue from the slides.
3. Place in periodic acid for 10 minutes.
4. Rinse in deionized water and dry.
5. Place dried smears in Schiff's reagent for 30 minutes.
6. Place in three 10-minute changes of metabisulfite solution.
7. Wash in deionized water for 10 minutes.
8. Counterstain with hematoxylin for 2 minutes.
9. Rinse in deionized water.
10. Place in sodium bicarbonate (bluing) solution for 30 seconds.
11. Rinse in deionized water, dry (tissue needs to be dehydrated), and mount with Permount.

Interpretation

Cellular structures that stain positive for PAS appear bright magenta. Lymphocytes, granulocytes, monocytes, and megakaryocytes may demonstrate positive reactivity with varying intensity and pattern. Neutrophils present on the smear may serve as a suitable positive control. Normal erythrocytes and erythrocyte precursors are negative. In erythroleukemia (FAB subclass M6), the erythrocyte precursors usually stain intensely positive; however, early red cells may occasionally be positive in sideroblastic anemia, iron deficiency, and thalassemia. Lymphoblasts in Burkitt's type ALL stain PAS-negative. The findings of PAS staining should not be used to distinguish the leukemias because staining patterns are variable.

Terminal Deoxynucleotidyl Transferase Test

Purpose

Terminal deoxynucleotidyl transferase (TdT) is valued as a marker for primitive lymphoid populations. This nucleus derived enzyme is observed in pre-B cells and T lymphoblasts, but is absent in B lymphocytes. TdT activity is elevated in FAB classes L1 and L2, which include T-cell, null cell and sometimes pre-B-cell leukemias. Furthermore, 90% of acute lymphocytic leukemia and lymphoblastic lymphoma patients demonstrate strong TdT activity. TdT is regarded as specific for primitive cells of lymphoid lineage; however, exceptions have been noted in a significant number of patients presenting with acute undifferentiated leukemia and CML blast crisis. TdT methods are generally relied on to differentiate acute lymphocytic leukemia from acute myelogenous leukemia when morphologic classification is uncertain. TdT may be assayed by immunofluorescence and immunoperoxidase techniques as well as by radioimmunoassay.

Principle

TdT is classified as a deoxyribonucleic acid (DNA) polymerase that is present in lymphocytic cells. Fluorescein isothiocyanate (FITC)–labeled goat anti-rabbit antibody is incubated with the sample. TdT activity in the nucleus is indicated by the presence of fluorescence in cells.

Specimen

A nonheparinized bone marrow aspirate or one in which the cells have been separated and washed three times with culture media (RPMI-1640) and 2% fetal calf serum may be used. Peripheral blood samples may be used; however, special specimen collection is required. Slides should be stored at 4°C in the dark and stained within a few days of preparation.

Reagents

1. Antiserum, Kit No. 9311 SB (Bethesda Research Laboratories)
2. Rabbit anticalf TdT, affinity-purified IgG
3. Goat antirabbit IgG, FITC conjugated
   a. The endpoint of antibody activity should be determined each time a new batch of antiserum is received.
   b. Dilute antiserum to optimum ratio using diluting media. An eight- to tenfold dilution is recommended for the rabbit anticalf TdT, and a 70- to 100-fold dilution for the goat anti-rabbit TdT.
   c. Store anti-TdT at 4°C. Aliquot antirabbit antiserum (20 lambda) and store at −20°C.
4. Diluting media: RPMI with 2% fetal calf serum and 0.1% sodium azide.
5. Phosphate buffered solution (PBS), pH 7.4
   $NaH_2PO_4 \cdot H_2O$ 0.4 g
   Na_2HPO_4 1.6 g
   NaCl 8.0 g
6. Controls
   a. Prepare cytopreps from a known ALL patient with a positive TdT.
   b. Air-dry cytopreps.
   c. Wrap with plastic wrap.
   d. Freeze and store at −70°C.
   e. Bring to room temperature before unwrapping.
   f. Follow test procedure and treat as an unknown sample.
   g. A negative control may be prepared from mouse serum and a phosphate buffer solution.

Procedure

1. Circle an area rich in nucleated cells on the side with a diamond scribe. Fix slides in methanol at 4°C for 30 minutes.
2. Rinse well in PBS to remove all fixative. Do not air-dry.
3. Hydrate the fixed slides in PBS for 5 minutes at room temperature.
4. Carefully wipe off all the sample on the slide outside the circle. Apply 10 μL of primary antibody (anticalf TdT) onto this area and distribute it over the circle. Incubate for 30 minutes at room temperature in a humid chamber. It is very important that the slide does not dry out.
5. Wash slides with three changes of PBS over a period of 15 minutes to remove excess antibody. Wipe off all the excess PBS around the circle, being especially careful not to let the sample dry out.
6. Apply 15 μL of secondary antibody [FITC F(ab')$_2$ goat, antirabbit IgG] to the circled area of the slide and incubate for 30 minutes at room temperature in a humid chamber.
7. Repeat wash procedure as in step 5.
8. Apply a small drop of mounting medium and cover with a coverslip.
9. Examine the nuclei for fluorescence at 495 nm excitation with a barrier filter. Record the intensity of fluorescence, 0 to 4+, and the percentage of cells that are positive. The preparation can be stored in the dark in the refrigerator for several days.

Interpretation

Most patients with T-cell and precursor B-cell ALL and lymphoma have positive TdT activity. In addition, 50% of patients with acute undifferentiated leukemia and 30% of patients in CML blast crisis also exhibit TdT activity. Approximately 5% of patients with AML exhibit TdT activity. In summary, TdT is valued as a marker for identifying primitive lymphoid cells.

Comments

1. Peripheral blood, bone marrow aspirate smears, or touch preps may be examined for TdT activity. The slides should be stored for no longer than 7 days at room temperature. Optimally, staining should be carried out as soon as possible.
2. A control slide should be run with patient samples as well as with each new lot number of reagents.

BIBLIOGRAPHY

Abramson, JS and Wheeler, JG: The Neutrophil. Oxford Press, Oxford, 1993.

Bell, A, Hippel, T, and Goodman, H: Use of cytochemical and FAB classification in leukemias and other pathologic stages. Am J Med Technol 47:6, 1981.

Brownman, GP, Neame, PB, and Soamboonsrup, P: The contribution of cytochemistry and immunophenotyping to the reproducibility of the FAB classification in acute leukemia. Blood 68:134, 1986.

Catovsky, D and Foa, R: The Lymphoid Leukaemias. Butterworth, London, 1990.

Elghetany, M, MacCallum, JM, and Davey, FR: The use of cytochemical procedures in the diagnosis of acute and chronic myeloid leukemia. Clin Lab Med 10:4, 1990.

Ellas, JM: A rapid sensitive myeloperoxidase stain using 4-chloro-1-naphthol. Brief scientific reports. Am J Clin Pathol 73:797, 1980.

Handin, RI, Lux, SE, and Stossel, TP: Blood: Principles and Practice of Hematology. JB Lippincott, Philadelphia, 1995.

Heckner, F, Lehmann, HP, and Kao, YS: Practical Microscopic Hematology, ed 4. Lea & Febiger, Philadelphia, 1994.

Kaplow, LS: Simplified myeloperoxidase stain using benzidine dihydrochloride. Blood 26:215, 1965.

Kaplow, LS: Substitute for benzidine in myeloperoxidase stains. Am J Clin Pathol 63:451, 1974.

Kass, L: Esterase activity in erythroleukemia. Am J Clin Pathol 67:368, 1977.

Kass, L and Peters, CL: Esterases in acute leukemias. Am J Clin Pathol 69:273, 1978.

Kjedsberg, C, et al: Practical Diagnosis of Hematologic Disorders. ASCP Press, Chicago, 1989.

Kung, PC, et al: Terminal deoxynucleotidyl transferase in the diagnosis of leukemia and malignant lymphoma. Am J Med 64:788, 1978.

Janckila, AJ, Li, CY, Lam, KW, et al: The cytochemistry of tartrate-resistant acid phosphatase. Am J Clin Pathol 70:45, 1978.

Li, CY, Yam, KW, and Yam, LT: Esterases in human leukocytes. J Histochem Cytochem 21:1, 1973.

Li, CY, Yam, KW, and Yam, KW: Acid phosphatase isoenzyme in human leukocytes in normal and pathologic conditions. J Histochem Cytochem 18:473, 1970.

Lotspeich-Steininger, CA, Stiene-Martin, EA, and Koepke, JA: Clinical Hematology: Principles, Procedures and Correlations. JB Lippincott, Philadelphia, 1992.

Melvin, L: Comparison of techniques for detecting T-cell acute lymphocytic leukemia. Blood, 54:1, 1979.

Miale, JB: Laboratory Medicine: Hematology, ed 6. CV Mosby, St Louis, 1982.

Nadjii, M, and Morales, AR: Immunoperoxidase: II. Practical applications. Lab Med 15:33, 1984.

Naeim, F, Gatti, RA, and Yunis, JJ: Recent advances in diagnosis and classification of leukemias and lymphomas. Disease Markers 8:231, 1990.

Nathan, DG and Oski, FA: Hematology of Infancy and Childhood. WB Saunders, Philadelphia, 1993.

Sheehan, HL, and Storey, GW: An improved method of staining leukocyte granules with Sudan black B. J Pathogen Bacteriol 59:336, 1947.

Sun, T, Li, CY, and Yam, LT: Atlas of Cytochemistry & Immunochemistry of Hematologic Neoplasms. ASCP Press, Chicago, 1985.

Rodak, BF: Diagnostic Hematology. WB Saunders, Philadelphia, 1995.

Rozenszajin, L, et al: The esterase activity in megaloblasts, leukaemic and normal haemotopoietic cells. Br J Haematol 14:605, 1968.

Rutenberg, AM, Rosales, CL, and Bennett, JM: An improved histochemical method for the demonstration of leukocyte alkaline phosphatase activity: Clinical application. J Clin Lab Med 65, 1965.

William, WJ, Beutler, E, Erslev, AJ, and Lichtman, MA: Hematology, ed 5. McGraw-Hill, New York, 1995.

Wislocki, GB, Rheingold, JJ, and Dempsey, EW: The occurrence of the Periodic acid-Schiff reaction in various normal cells of blood and connective tissue. Blood 4:562, 1949.

Yam, LT, Li, CY, and Crosby, W: Cytochemical identification of monocytes and granulocytes. Am J Clin Pathol 55:283, 1971.

QUESTIONS

1. A 66-year-old woman presents with an LAP score of 22. What is a possible clinical correlation for this score?
a. Normal
b. Leukemoid reaction
c. Chronic granulocytic leukemia
d. Pregnancy

2. In which condition would the majority of cells stain positive with myeloperoxidase and Sudan Black B?
a. Acute lymphocytic leukemia
b. Acute myelogenous leukemia
c. Chronic lymphocytic leukemia
d. Erythroleukemia

3. Which of the following cells would demonstrate positive staining with Sudan black B?
a. Lymphocyte
b. Basophil
c. Promyelocyte
d. Erythroblast

4. Which of the following cells would stain positive using the specific esterase stain?
a. Megakaryocytes
b. Macrophages
c. Neutrophils
d. Lymphocytes

5. Staining of which of the following cell lines would be inhibited by the addition of sodium fluoride to nonspecific esterase methods?
a. Megakaryocyte
b. Plasma cell
c. Lymphocyte
d. Monocyte

6. For which of the following disease states would the acid phosphatase/TRAP stain have diagnostic value?
a. Erythroleukemia
b. Hairy cell leukemia
c. Chronic lymphocytic leukemia
d. Burkitt's lymphoma

7. For which of the following disease states would Periodic acid-Schiff staining have diagnostic value?
a. Erythroleukemia
b. Hairy cell leukemia
c. Chronic lymphocytic leukemia
d. Myelomonocytic leukemia

8. Which condition(s) demonstrate(s) positive TdT activity?
a. T-cell ALL
b. Null cell ALL
c. Pre-B ALL
d. All of the above

ANSWERS

1. **a** (p 644)
2. **b** (pp 645, 647)
3. **c** (p 647)
4. **c** (p 649)
5. **d** (p 650)
6. **b** (p 651)
7. **a** (p 653)
8. **d** (p 654)

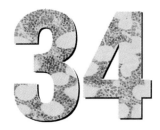

34

Coagulation

Gordon E. Ens, MT(ASCP)
Janis Wyrick-Glatzel, MS, MT(ASCP)

Objectives

At the end of this chapter, the learner should be able to:
1 Explain the diagnostic use of a bleeding time.
2 Correlate platelet aggregation results with clinical conditions.
3 Explain the use of the activated partial thromboplastin time and prothrombin time.
4 Explain the use of the thrombin time and Reptilase time.
5 List conditions having low and high fibrinogen levels.
6 Relate clinical conditions to measurements of factor VIII–related antigen.
7 Identify methods for laboratory diagnosis of protein C deficiency and protein S deficiency.
8 Identify an activated partial thromboplastin time result that indicates presence of circulating anticoagulants.
9 List criteria for the laboratory detection of lupus inhibitors.
10 Explain the use of the latex agglutination test in the diagnosis of disseminated intravascular coagulation.

GENERAL POINTS REGARDING COAGULATION PROCEDURES

1. Most coagulation procedures are performed on plasma, thereby requiring the addition of calcium in order to perform the tests because the anticoagulant used, sodium citrate, binds free calcium.
2. Testing is performed at 37°C ± 1°.
3. Each laboratory should develop its own normal values reflecting the methodology, reagents, instrumentation, and patient population.
4. The technique used in obtaining and processing the patient's blood sample and the conditions under which samples are stored or transported determine the integrity of the final test result. Traumatic venipuncture may result in activation of coagulation factors, and improper storage conditions may result in the deterioration or (in the case of factor VII) activation of coagulation factors.
5. Sodium citrate (3.2% or 3.8%) is the anticoagulant used for routine clot-based procedures. Other anticoagulants such as ethylenediaminetetraacetic acid (EDTA), heparin, and oxalate are unacceptable.
6. The ratio of blood to anticoagulant should be 9:1. This may vary as long as the final concentration of sodium citrate remains 3.2% or 3.8% of the final blood mixture. A disproportion of anticoagulant to blood is seen in patients with polycythemia and those with moderate to severe anemia.
7. Immunologic assays are currently available for a number of coagulation factors, inhibitors, and proteins involved in fibrinolysis. Because these assays determine the presence or absence of these proteins and not their biologic activity, functional testing should be performed in addition when possible.
8. Enzyme-specific synthetic substrates: In the past, evaluation of hemostasis has relied on traditional procedures based on the detection of clot formation. The innovation of enzyme-specific synthetic substrates has had a great impact on the field of hemostasis. The knowledge of molecular structures for different enzymes and the cleavage points of their corresponding substrate factors has led to the development of synthetic substrates that are cleaved by a single factor enzyme. Synthesis of synthetic substrates occurs when the amino acids of the substrate on the molecule fit into the active sites and the binding sites of the enzyme. All synthetic substrates rely on cleavage of the peptide by their specific enzymes, releasing a chromogenic complex such as paranitroaniline or a fluorogenic complex such as aminoisophthalic acid dimethyl ester (AIE), which may be detected and measured by means of a spectrophotometer or fluorimeter. Various synthetic chromogenic and fluorogenic assays exist for the evaluation of plasmin, plasminogen activator, α_2-antiplasmin, kallikrein, antithrombin III (AT-III), factor Xa, thrombin, and several other serine proteases, making these assays applicable for routine laboratory testing. Procedures using synthetic substrates have certain advantages over the traditional clot formation techniques. They are rapid to perform, sensitive, allow a greater degree of standardization, require smaller sample volumes, and are well suited for automation. Synthetic substrates facilitate measuring the activity of the clotting factor and their inhibitors. Often individual stages of a reaction can be assayed without having to observe the entire cascade of the clotting process. As the field of blood coagulation continues to undergo major technical advancement, the use of synthetic substrates will gain increasing significance and may replace some of the time-honored clotting tests currently used in the routine clinical laboratory.

PLATELET FUNCTION TESTS

Bleeding Time

Principle

Bleeding time is defined as the time taken for a standardized skin wound to stop bleeding. On vessel injury, platelets adhere and form a hemostatic platelet plug. Bleeding time measures the ability of these platelets to arrest bleeding and, therefore, measures platelet number and function. Capillary contractility and both the intrinsic and extrinsic systems of coagulation function in a minor capacity in the bleeding time. Bleeding time is measured as a screening procedure used to detect both congenital and acquired disorders of platelet function. The bleeding time assesses in vivo platelet function.

Several devices are available for making standardized incisions when performing a bleeding time.

Method

Caution: Each patient should be informed that, with any bleeding time procedure, the possibility of faint scarring exists. Keloid formation, although rare, may occur in certain patients.

Reagents and Equipment

Sterile bleeding time device
Stopwatch, with seconds available
Sphygmomanometer
Filter paper disc (Whatman No. 11)
Alcohol swab
Butterfly bandage and covering bandage

Procedure

Before a bleeding time is measured, it is important that a platelet count from within the past 24 hours be available. The bleeding time is directly influenced by platelet number if the patient's platelet count is less than 100,000 per mm[1].

1. Place the patient's arm on a steady support with the muscular area over the lateral aspect of the forearm exposed. The preferred site for the procedure is 5 cm below the antecubital crease. Take care to avoid surface veins, scars, and

bruises. If the patient has a notable amount of hair, lightly shave the area first.

2. Place the sphygmomanometer at 40 mmHg. The time between the inflation of the cuff and the incision should be between 30 and 60 s. Hold at this pressure for the duration of the test.
3. Cleanse the arm with an alcohol swab and allow it to air-dry.
4. Remove the device from the package, being careful not to contaminate the instrument by touching or resting the blade-slot end on any unsterile surface.
5. Remove the safety clip.
6. Hold the device securely between thumb and middle finger.
7. Gently rest the device on the patient's forearm and apply minimal pressure so that both ends of the instrument are lightly touching the skin.
8. Push the trigger and start the stopwatch simultaneously. The blade will make an incision 5 mm long by 1 mm deep.
9. Remove the device from the patient's forearm immediately after making the incision.
10. After 30 s, blot the flow of blood with filter paper. Bring the filter paper close to the incision, but do not touch the paper directly to the incision so as not to disturb the formation of a platelet plug.
11. Blot the blood every 30 s thereafter until blood no longer stains the paper. Stop the timer. Bleeding time is determined to the nearest 30 s. If the bleeding continues after 15 minutes, terminate the test and apply pressure to the incision site. Report the bleeding time as greater than 15 minutes.
12. Remove the blood pressure cuff and carefully cleanse around the incision site with alcohol. Apply butterfly bandage across the cut and keep in place for 24 hours to prevent scarring.

Interpretation

Normal values are from 2.5 to 9.5 minutes. Owing to variations in technique and patient population, it is recommended that each laboratory establish its own "normal" values. Prolonged bleeding times are found in the following situations: thrombocytopenia, platelet count less than 100,000 per mm^3, platelet dysfunction, after the administration of aspirin or aspirin-containing drugs, and after the administration of other drugs that inhibit platelet function such as antihistamines.

Comment

If the incision fails to bleed or if a small vein is cut, disregard the bleeding time of the incision and repeat test.

The bleeding time should be measured in the diagnostic workup of a qualitative platelet disorder, not for the evaluation of a coagulation factor deficiency.

The bleeding time increases in proportion to the decrease in platelet count. The use of aspirin, aspirin-containing drugs, and antihistamines causes a prolonged bleeding time. The patient should be instructed not to take any aspirin or drugs containing aspirin for 1 week before the test. The bleeding time should be measured in the diagnostic workup of a qualitative platelet disorder.

Platelet Aggregation

Principle

Platelets function in primary hemostasis by forming an initial platelet plug at the site of vascular injury. The phenomenon occurs partly through the ability of platelets to adhere to one another, a process known as *aggregation*. Substances that can induce platelet aggregation include collagen, adenosine diphosphate (ADP), epinephrine, thrombin, serotonin, arachidonic acid, the antibiotic ristocetin, snake venoms, antigen-antibody complexes, soluble fibrin monomer complexes, and fibrin(ogen)olytic degradation products (FDPs). These aggregating agents induce platelet aggregation or cause platelets to release endogenous ADP, or both. Platelet aggregation is an essential part of the investigation of any patient with a suspected platelet dysfunction.

Platelet aggregation is studied by means of a platelet aggregometer, a photo-optical instrument connected to a chart recorder. Platelet-rich plasma, which is turbid in appearance, is placed in a cuvette, warmed to 37°C in the heating block of the instrument, and stirred by a small magnetic bar. Light transmittance through the platelet-rich plasma is recorded. The addition of an aggregating agent causes the formation of larger platelet aggregates with a corresponding increase in light transmittance, owing to a clearing in the platelet-rich plasma. The change in light transmittance is converted to electronic signals and recorded as a tracing by the chart recorder.

Note: There are some basic requirements for platelet aggregation as an in vitro means of evaluating platelet function:

1. In performing platelet aggregation studies, a clean venipuncture is crucial. Hemolyzed samples should not be studied because RBCs contain ADP.
2. Plasma from fasting patients is preferred for testing. Lipemic samples may obscure changes in optical density owing to platelet aggregation.
3. Sodium citrate is the anticoagulant used in aggregation studies. Keep in mind that in vitro aggregation is dependent on the presence of calcium ions. The concentration of calcium even after anticoagulation may be sufficient for aggregation to occur.
4. Fibrinogen must be present in the test sample for aggregation to occur.
5. The plasma sample should not come in contact with a glass surface unless the surface is siliconized. Platelets adhere to glass.
6. Aggregation studies should be performed at 37°C at a pH of 6.5 to 8.5. To help maintain pH values, all samples, once collected, should be capped to prevent CO_2 loss.
7. Test samples should be maintained at room temperature during processing. Cooling inhibits the platelet aggregating response. Just before per-

forming the test, the plasma is incubated at 37°C in the heat block of the aggregometer.

8. Stirring is necessary to bring the platelets in close contact with one another to allow aggregation to occur.

9. All aggregation studies should be performed within 3 hours of sample collection.

10. It is essential that the patient refrain from taking any anti-inflammatory drugs 1 week before the test. These drugs inhibit the platelets' release reaction.

11. Thrombocytopenia makes evaluation of the aggregation responses difficult.

12. Aggregating agents should be prepared fresh daily and brought to room temperature before use. They must have known potency and be added in small volumes.

13. Control tests using platelet-rich plasma from a known donor must be performed with the test samples.

Reagents and Equipment

Control and test platelet-rich plasma
Aggregometer and cuvettes
Magnetic stirring bar
Pipets
Normal saline
Aggregating agents
Adenosine-5'-phosphate (ADP)   Prepare 100 μmol/L, 50 μmol/L, 25 μmol/L, and 10 μmol/L solutions in saline.
Collagen   Prepare a 40 μg/mL and a 20 μg/mL working concentration.
Ristocetin   Prepare 15 mg/mL, 12 mg/mL, and 10 mg/mL working solutions.
Arachidonic acid   Prepare a 0.50 mmol/L solution.
Epinephrine   Prepare 20 μmol/L and 200 μmol/L solutions in 0.1% sodium metabisulphite.

Procedure

1. Centrifuge the citrated venous blood sample at room temperature (18°C to 25°C) at 150 to 200 g for 10 to 15 minutes. Dilute the platelet-rich plasma with platelet-poor plasma to obtain a platelet count of 250×10^9/L. Plasma may be left at room temperature in capped plastic tubes for up to 2 hours before testing. Repeat procedure for control sample.

2. Turn on heating block of the aggregometer 30 minutes before tests are to be run.

3. Pipet the appropriate volume of plasma into a cuvette and place into the 37°C heat block for 1 minute to warm the test plasma.

4. Place a magnetic stirring bar into the cuvette and turn on the motor. Adjust the speed of the stirring bar to between 800 and 1100 rpm (the speed that yields optimal platelet aggregation when strong concentrations of ADP are added to normal plasma). Adjust the absorbance of the plasma to 0.40, and adjust the chart recorder so that the difference in absorbance between platelet-rich and platelet-poor plasma causes the pen to cover the width of the paper.

5. Pipet 0.1 mL of aggregating agent to the plasma. Observe the aggregation curve for 3 minutes.

6. Tests are usually performed with three dilutions of ADP, collagen, ristocetin, and epinephrine for patient and normal plasma samples.

Interpretation

Low concentrations of ADP induce biphasic aggregation (i.e., both a primary and a secondary wave of aggregation); very low concentration of ADP induce a primary wave followed by disaggregation; and high concentrations of ADP induce a single, broad wave of aggregation.[2] A biphasic aggregation response to ADP is not seen in patients with platelet release disorders. Patients with Glanzmann's thrombasthenia show incomplete aggregation with ADP regardless of the final concentration. Platelet aggregation induced by collagen is characterized by a lag period before aggregation, followed by only a single wave of aggregation.[3] A biphasic aggregation response is seen with the antibiotic ristocetin; however, often only a single broad wave of aggregation will occur. In patients with severe von Willebrand's disease, aggregation to ristocetin is characteristically absent. Decreased to normal aggregation to ristocetin can be seen in patients with mild von Willebrand's disease. Correction of the abnormal ristocetin aggregation curves can be seen by the addition of normal, platelet-poor plasma to the patient's platelet-rich plasma.

Abnormal ristocetin-induced platelet aggregation may occur in patients with Bernard-Soulier syndrome, platelet storage pool defects, and idiopathic thrombocytopenia purpura. Platelet aggregation induced with arachidonic acid causes a rapid secondary wave of aggregation. Biphasic aggregation is observed with epinephrine. One-third to one-half of normal, healthy patients produce a primary wave of aggregation with epinephrine.[4] The aggregating agent thrombin induces a biphasic wave of aggregation. Platelet aggregation induced by serotonin normally produces a wave of aggregation with a maximum of 10% to 30% transmittance followed by disaggregation (Figs. 34–1 and 34–2).[4]

Comment

In evaluating patients with suspected platelet disorders, the aggregating agents most commonly used are ADP in various concentrations, collagen, epinephrine, and ristocetin.

Aspirin, aspirin compounds, and anti-inflammatory drugs inhibit the secondary wave of aggregation by inhibiting the release reaction of the platelet. Reduced or absent aggregation as well as disaggregation curves may be observed in patients taking medication containing aspirin. The intensity of platelet aggregation may be estimated by recording the change in absorbance as a percentage of the difference in absorbance between platelet-rich and platelet-poor plasma. This has limited usefulness because absorbance is dependent on the size and density of platelet clumping and the number of platelets that aggregate. A more complex analysis of aggregation related to the rate of ag-

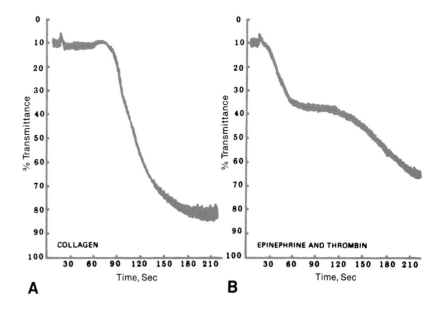

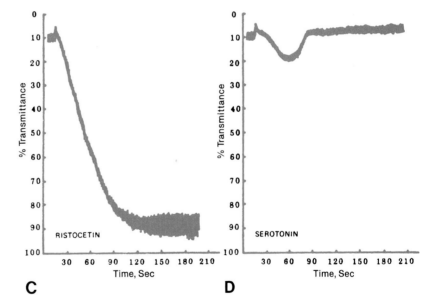

FIGURE 34-1 Aggregation curves with various aggregating agents. (*A*) Aggregation curve induced by collagen. Note the lag time before aggregation followed by a single wave of aggregation. (*B*) Aggregation curve induced with epinephrine and thrombin. Note the biphasic wave of aggregation. (*C*) Aggregation curve induced by ristocetin. A biphasic wave of aggregation as well as a single wave of aggregation may be seen. (*D*) Aggregation curve induced by serotonin. Generally a single wave of aggregation followed by disaggregation is seen.

gregation may also be obtained. However, visual interpretation of the aggregation curves suffices and can establish whether aggregation is abnormal or normal.

Platelet Factor 3 Availability

Principle

Platelets serve as templates on which activation of coagulation proteins can occur by releasing a phospholipid (platelet factor 3) that acts as a partial thromboplastin, which is necessary for the intrinsic conversion of prothrombin to thrombin. Platelet factor 3 (PF 3) is not available in normal intact circulating platelets. It is released when platelets are activated by a stimulus such as celite or kaolin, which are contact activators. The recalcification time of platelet-rich plasma (PRP) is shortened when plasma is incubated with celite before the addition of calcium. Celite causes the release of PF 3 from the patient's platelets and activation of intrinsic coagulation. Platelet-rich plasma, a source of PF 3, and platelet-poor plasma (PPP), which is low in PF 3 activity, are compared with an activated partial thromboplastin reagent for activity.

Reagents and Equipment

Celite 505, 1% suspension in 0.85% NaCl
0.025 M CaCl$_2$
Platelin plus activator
Activated partial thromboplastin time (APTT) assay equipment
Plastic tubes and pipettes

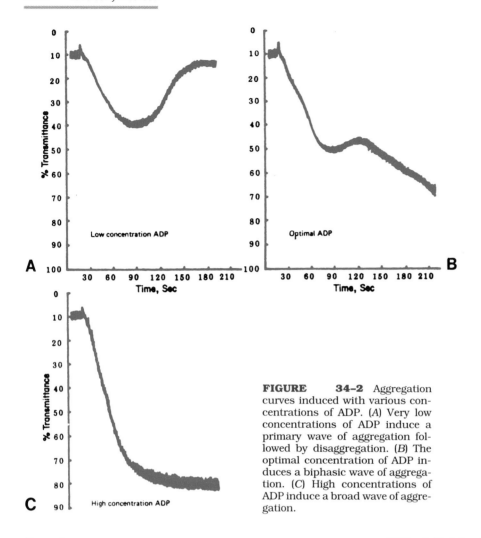

FIGURE 34–2 Aggregation curves induced with various concentrations of ADP. (A) Very low concentrations of ADP induce a primary wave of aggregation followed by disaggregation. (B) The optimal concentration of ADP induces a biphasic wave of aggregation. (C) High concentrations of ADP induce a broad wave of aggregation.

Procedure

1. Obtain 9.0 mL of blood with a plastic syringe and place in a plastic tube containing 1.0 mL of 3.8% sodium citrate and mix thoroughly. Generally, hemolyzed samples are not satisfactory. The phospholipid in the membrane of the red cells may act like PF3 and yield questionable results.
2. Platelet-rich plasma   Spin the citrated sample at 1500 rpm for 5 minutes. Do not use the centrifuge brake; gently remove sample from the centrifuge. Remove as much of the plasma as possible using a plastic pipet and place in a plastic tube labeled PRP.
3. Platelet-poor plasma   Respin the blood sample for 10 to 15 minutes at 1500 rpm. Remove as much plasma as possible with a plastic pipet and place in a plastic tube labeled "PPP."
4. Determine the clotting time for the following three assays:
   a. Control   Add 0.1 mL platelin plus activator to 0.1 mL PPP and incubate for 5 minutes at 37°C. Add 0.1 mL of 0.025 M CaCl$_2$. Obtain clotting time.
   b. PRP   Add 0.1 mL of 1% celite suspension to 0.1 mL PRP and incubate for 5 minutes at 37°C. Add 0.1 mL of 0.025 M CaCl$_2$. Obtain clotting time.
   c. PPP   Add 0.1 mL 1% celite suspension to 0.1 mL PPP and incubate for 5 minutes at 37°C. Add 0.1 mL of 0.025 M CaCl$_2$. Obtain clotting time.

Interpretation

The PRP and celite should have a clotting time close to that of the control. In vitro platelin acts like PF 3, so recalcifying the PRP and control produces similar test systems and results.

The PPP has a prolonged clotting time because of a lack of platelets and PF 3. If the PRP clotting time is prolonged, close to the PPP time, PF 3 activity is reduced in the patient sample.

TEST TO MEASURE THE INTRINSIC SYSTEM

Activated Partial Thromboplastin Time

Principle

The APTT is a screening test used to measure the intrinsic pathway of coagulation, or more precisely, to assay all the plasma coagulation factors with the exception of factors VII and XIII and PF 3. The formation of fibrin occurs at a normal rate only if the factors involved in the intrinsic pathway (factors XII, XI, IX, and

VIII) and the common pathway (factors I, II, V, and X) are present in normal concentrations. Optimal activation is achieved by the addition of a platelet phospholipid substitute, which eliminates the test's sensitivity to platelet number and function, as well as the addition of activators such as kaolin, celite, and ellagic acid, which eliminates the variability of activation by glass contact. The APTT is also used to monitor heparin therapy.

Reagents and Equipment

Coagulation analyzer
Commercial activated thromboplastin

Procedure

1. Obtain 4.5 mL of blood by means of clean venipuncture. Mix by gentle inversion with 0.5 mL of 0.109 M sodium citrate.
2. Centrifuge for 10 minutes at 1500 rpm. Collect plasma and store in plastic tubes at 4°C until use. Testing should be performed within 4 h.
3. Reconstitute activated thromboplastin reagent according to directions.
4. Perform APTT according to manufacturer's package insert.
5. Record time for fibrin formation.
6. All testing on both control and test plasma should be performed in duplicate. (Normal duplicate results should be within ± 0.5 seconds of each other; therapeutic results within ±1.0 second.) Calculate the mean clotting time and report results in seconds to the nearest 10th. Note: the exact procedure varies according to the methodology used to measure fibrin formation.

Interpretation

Each laboratory should develop its own normal range; however, the normal range used in this text is <35 sec. The test result is abnormal in patients with deficiencies of all factors involved in the intrinsic pathway. The APTT is prolonged with levels of factors 30 to 40 percent of normal, depending on reagent sensitivity. Hypofibrinogenemia (levels less than 100 mg/dl) will prolong the APTT. When the APTT is used to monitor heparin therapy, it is typically prolonged 1.5 to 2.5 times the control level.

Comment

Both the APTT and the prothrombin times (PT) should be performed as screening procedures, since together the tests evaluate the intrinsic, extrinsic, and common pathways of coagulation.

TESTS TO MEASURE THE EXTRINSIC SYSTEM

One-Stage Prothrombin Time (Quick)[5]
Principle

The prothrombin time (PT) is the time required to form a fibrin clot when plasma is added to a thromboplastin-calcium mixture. The test is a measure of the extrinsic pathway of coagulation involving factors II, V, VII, and X (as well as fibrinogen). Tissue thromboplastin activates factor VII, which proceeds through the cascade, ultimately generating thrombin. The thrombin thus formed converts fibrinogen to fibrin. The rate of fibrin formation therefore depends on the level of factors II, V, VII, and X and fibrinogen, and thus measures the overall activity of these factors.

The test is a valuable screening procedure used to indicate possible factor deficiencies of the extrinsic pathway. The PT test is sensitive to the vitamin K-dependent factors of the extrinsic pathway (factors II, VII, and X) and is therefore used as a means of monitoring oral anticoagulant therapy. (The fourth vitamin K–dependent factor, factor IX, is measured by the APTT.)

Reagents and Equipment

Coagulation analyzer
Commercial thromboplastin

Procedure

1. Obtain 4.5 mL of blood by means of a clean venipuncture. Mix by gentle inversion with 0.5 mL of 0.109 M sodium citrate. (Blood collection vacutainer tubes containing sodium citrate may be used.)
2. Centrifuge for 10 minutes at 1500 rpm. Collect plasma and store at 4°C until use. Testing should be performed within 4 hours.
3. Reconstitute thromboplastin-$CaCl_2$ reagent according to directions.
4. Perform PT procedure according to the manufacturer's package insert.
5. Record time for fibrin formation.
6. All testing on both control and test plasma must be performed in duplicate. (Normal duplicate results should be within ± 0.5 s of each other; therapeutic results within ± 1.0 s.) Calculate the mean clotting time and report results in seconds to the nearest tenth of a second when monitoring oral anticoagulant therapy. The International Normalized Ratio (INR) should be reported, using the International Sensitivity Index (ISI) of the thromboplastin.

$$INR = \frac{(Patient\ PT)}{(Mean\ of\ normal\ range)} \times ISI$$

Interpretation

Normal PT is approximately 11 to 13 s. Each laboratory must develop its own "normal" range.

The PT is prolonged in individuals with a factor deficiency involving a single factor (as in patients with a congenital deficiency) or involving multiple factors (as in patients with acquired deficiencies, e.g., those with liver disease receiving coumarin therapy or those with vitamin K deficiency) and in the presence of circulating anticoagulants such as FDPs and heparin.

In patients with polycythemia, the PT is prolonged as a result of a change in the ratio of anticoagulant to plasma. PT also yields shortened results when stored for longer than 3 h.

Coagulation Factor Assays

One-Stage Quantitative Assay Method for Factors II, V, VII, and X

Principle The PT is the basis of this test system, with specific factor-deficient plasmas being used instead of a correction plasma or serum. The percentage of factor activity is determined by the amount of correction detected when specific dilutions of patient plasma are added to a factor-deficient plasma. These results are obtained from an activity curve made from dilutions of normal reference plasma and specific factor-deficient plasma.

Reagents and Equipment

Thromboplastin
Specific factor-deficient plasma (II, V, VII, X)
Imidazole buffered saline, pH 7.3 ± 0.1
Normal reference plasma (commercial reference plasma with known factor levels)
Equipment—same as that used for PT assay

Procedure

1. Preparation of activity curve
   a. Prepare 1:10, 1:20, 1:40, 1:80, 1:160, 1:320, 1:640, and 1:1280 serial dilutions of the normal reference plasma with imidazole-buffered saline. The 1:10 dilution is considered 100% factor activity.
   b. Warm thromboplastin to 37°C (Table 34–1).
   c. Perform the following test procedure on each dilution:
      (1) Add 0.1 mL of specific factor-deficient plasma to 0.1 of diluted normal reference plasma and warm to 37°C for allotted time.
      (2) Add 0.2 mL thromboplastin to the sample and determine the clotting time.
      (3) Repeat procedure on duplicate sample and average results.
   d. Plot results on 2 × 3 cycle log graph paper, with percent factor activity on the X axis and seconds on the Y axis. Draw a best-fit line. The curve will demonstrate a plateau at the least concentrated dilutions and should be plotted as such, demonstrating the end of sensitivity for the assay.
2. Procedure for testing patient plasma
   a. Prewarm thromboplastin to 37°C.
   b. Prepare a 1:10 dilution of citrated patient plasma with imidazole-buffered saline. It is im-

portant to keep samples and dilutions refrigerated until they are to be tested.
   c. Add 0.1 mL of specific factor-deficient plasma to 0.1 mL of diluted patient plasma.
   d. Add 0.2 ml thromboplastin to sample and determine the clotting time.
   e. Repeat procedure on a duplicate sample and average results.
   f. Read the percent activity directly from the activity curve (Fig. 34–3). A 35-s result on a 1:10 dilution of plasma would be interpreted as 8.3% activity.

Interpretation

A range of 50% to 150% is considered normal. Each laboratory should define its own range.

Comment

1. If the result is greater than 100%, dilute the test sample with buffered saline until results fall within the sensitivity range of the curve.
2. Calculate the percent activity of the dilution tested and multiply by the dilution factor for the percent activity of the patient sample.
3. These tests require the same considerations as the APTT and PT assay in regard to quality control, specimen handling, reagent preparation, and points of procedural importance. The assay should be performed on the same equipment and in the same manner as all other coagulation assays in the laboratory.

One-Stage Quantitative Assay Method for Factors VIII, IX, XI, and XII

Principle The APTT is the basis of this test system. This method is also based on the ability of patient plasma to correct specific factor-deficient plasma. Results in percent activity are obtained from an activity curve.

Reagents and Equipment

APTT reagent
0.025 M $CaCl_2$
Specific factor-deficient plasma (VIII, IX, XI, and XII)
Normal reference plasma (with known factor levels)
Imidazole-buffered saline, pH 7.3 ± 0.1
Equipment for APTT assay

TABLE 34–1 **Preparation of Test Dilutions for Reference Plasma in the One-Stage Assay for Factors**

Tube No.	Amount of Plasma	Imidazole Buffered Saline	Dilution	% of Factor
1	0.1 mL	0.9 mL	1:10	100.00
2	0.5 mL of 1	0.5 mL	1:20	50.00
3	0.5 mL of 2	0.5 mL	1:40	25.00
4	0.5 mL of 3	0.5 mL	1:80	12.50
5	0.5 mL of 4	0.5 mL	1:160	6.25
6	0.5 mL of 5	0.5 mL	1:320	3.13
7	0.5 mL of 6	0.5 mL	1:640	1.56
8	0.5 mL of 7	0.5 mL	1:1280	0.78

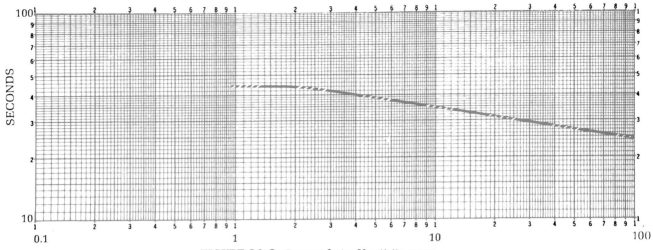

FIGURE 34–3 Percent factor V activity curve.

Procedure

1. Preparation of activity curve:
   a. Prepare a 1:10, 1:20, 1:40, 1:80, 1:160, 1:320, 1:640, 1:1280 serial dilution of the normal reference plasma with imidazole-buffered saline (see Table 34–1). The 1:10 dilution is considered 100% factor activity.
   b. Prewarm the CaCl$_2$ and APTT reagent to 37°C.
   c. Perform the following test procedure on each dilution.
      (1) Add 0.1 mL of specific factor-deficient plasma and 0.1 mL of diluted normal reference plasma to 0.1 mL APTT reagent. Mix well and incubate for the specified time.
      (2) Add 0.1 mL CaCl$_2$ into the mixture at the specified time and determine the clotting time.
      (3) Repeat the procedure on a duplicate sample and average results.
   d. Plot results on 2 × 3 cycle log graph paper, with percent factor on the X axis and seconds on the Y axis. Draw a best-fit line. The curve will demonstrate a plateau at the least concentrated dilutions and should be plotted as such, demonstrating the end of sensitivity for the assay.
2. Procedure for testing patient plasma:
   a. Prewarm CaCl$_2$ and APTT reagent to 37°C.
   b. Prepare a 1:10 dilution of citrated patient plasma with imidazole-buffered saline. It is important to keep samples and dilutions refrigerated until they are to be tested.
   c. Add 0.1 ml of specific factor-deficient plasma and 0.1 mL of diluted patient plasma to 0.1 mL APTT reagent. Mix well and incubate for the allotted time.
   d. Add 0.1 ml CaCl$_2$ into the mixture at the specified time and determine the clotting time.
   e. Repeat the procedure on a duplicate sample and average the results.
   f. Read the percentage of activity directly from activity curve (see Fig. 30–3).

Results A range of 50% to 150% is considered normal. Each laboratory must define its own range.

TESTS TO MEASURE FIBRIN FORMATION

Thrombin Time

Principle

The thrombin time (TT) is the time required for thrombin to convert fibrinogen to an insoluble fibrin clot. Fibrin formation is triggered by the addition of thrombin to the specimen and therefore bypasses prior steps in the coagulation cascade. The TT does not measure defects in the intrinsic or extrinsic pathways. The test is affected by the levels of fibrinogen, dysfibrinogenemia, and the presence of circulating anticoagulants (antithrombins) such as heparin, plasmin, and FDPs.

Reagents and Equipment

Coagulation analyzer
Commercial thrombin reagent
Normal control plasma

Procedure

1. Prepare platelet-poor plasma. Separate plasma and immediately refrigerate at 4°C or store on ice. Test should be performed as soon as possible; however, stoppered refrigerated plasmas are stable for 4 hours.
2. Perform all tests in duplicate according to manufacturer's instructions.
3. Measure the clotting time.

4. If the patient's average clotting time greatly exceeds the average control time, the test should be repeated using a 1:1 mixture of patient's plasma and normal or control plasma (see Interpretation).

Interpretation

Normal value is approximately 15 seconds. The TT is prolonged in patients with hypofibrinogenemia (usually less than 100 mg/dl), in those with dysfibrinogenemia, and in the presence of circulating anticoagulants (heparin, FDP).

If the mixing test results in a clotting time that approximates that of the control plasma, a deficiency or a molecular abnormality of fibrinogen is most likely indicated. If the mixing tests fail to correct the TT, the presence of a circulating inhibitor is indicated.

The thrombin time does not differentiate a state of DIC from primary fibrinolysis; however, it is a sensitive test for determining the process of DIC.

Reptilase Time

Principle

The Reptilase time is similar to the TT except that, with the former, clotting technique is initiated with the snake venom enzyme, reptilase. Reptilase, thrombin-like in nature, hydrolyzes fibrinopeptide A from the intact fibrinogen molecule, in contrast to thrombin, which hydrolyzes fibrinopeptide A and B from fibrinogen. The clot that forms by the action of reptilase on fibrinogen is more fragile than that formed by thrombin's action on fibrinogen. The reptilase time is not inhibited by heparin. There is only a minimum effect on the reptilase time by FDPs.

Reagents and Equipment

Coagulation analyzer
Reptilase-R
Platelet-poor citrated plasma (control and test plasma)

Procedure

1. Obtain 4.5 mL of blood by means of a clean venipuncture. Mix by gentle inversion with 0.5 mL of 0.109 M sodium citrate. Reject any specimens that are hemolyzed.

2. Prepare platelet-poor plasma by centrifugation at 1500 rpm for 10 to 15 minutes.
3. Perform all tests according to manufacturer's instructions.
4. Measure the clotting time. Calculate the average clotting time and report results in seconds.
5. All testing, on both control and test plasma, must be performed in duplicate. (Duplicate results should agree within ± 0.5 s.) Calculate the average clotting time and report results in seconds.

Interpretation

Normal values are 18 to 22 s. Except for fibrinogen Oklahoma and fibrinogen Oslow, all the congenital dysfibrinogenemias have an infinite Reptilase time. The Reptilase time is also infinitely prolonged in cases of congenital afibrinogenemia. In states of hypofibrinogenemia, the Reptilase time may be variable, dependent on the levels of fibrinogen present. The Reptilase time is moderately prolonged in the presence of FDPs and is unaffected by heparin (see test comparison below).

Comment

In the presence of heparin, thrombin is inhibited by way of AT-III. However, heparin does not interfere with reptilase's ability to cleave fibrinopeptide A from fibrinogen. A comparison of both TT and reptilase time will aid in detecting the presence of thrombin inhibitors such as heparin (Table 34–2).

Fibrinogen

Principle

Fibrinogen can be quantitatively measured by a modification of the TT because the thrombin clotting time of dilute plasma is inversely proportional to the concentration of fibrinogen. This method involves clotting dilutions of both patient's test plasma and control plasma with an excess of thrombin. Results are calculated from a calibration curve.

Reagents and Equipment

Coagulation analyzer
12 × 75 test tubes
Commercial fibrinogen determination kit
1. Thrombin, 100 NIH units per mL, bovine lyophilized. Reconstitute with 1.0 mL distilled water.

TABLE 34–2 **Test Comparison**		
Thrombin Time	**Reptilase Time**	**Defect**
Infinitely prolonged	Infinitely prolonged	Dysfibrinogenemia
Infinitely prolonged	Infinitely prolonged	Afibrinogenemia
Prolonged	Equally prolonged	Hypofibrinogenemia
Prolonged	Normal	Heparin
Prolonged	Slight to moderately prolonged	FDPs

2. Fibrinogen standard   Fibrinogen concentration is standardized by the macro-Kjeldahl method. Reconstitute with 1.0 mL distilled water. Mix by gentle inversion; do not shake.
3. Owren's Veronal buffer, pH 7.35.
4. Control (with a known fibrinogen concentration).

Procedure

1. Mix nine parts of freshly collected blood to one part 3.8% sodium citrate.
2. Centrifuge for 15 minutes at 1500 *g*. Collect plasma.

Preparation of Calibration Curve

3. Make dilutions of the fibrinogen standard with Owren's Veronal buffer as follows: 1:5, 1:15, and 1:40. Make all transfers from the first test tube.
   a. 1:5 dilution (first tube): 1.6 mL buffer to 0.4 mL fibrinogen standard.
   b. 1:15 dilution (second tube): 0.8 mL buffer to 0.4 mL mixture from the first test tube
   c. 1:40 dilution (third tube): 2.8 mL buffer to 0.4 mL mixture from the first test tube
4. Perform duplicate determinations on each dilution of fibrinogen standard as follows:
   a. Incubate 0.2 mL fibrinogen standard dilution at 37°C for at least 2 minutes but no more than 5 minutes.
   b. Add 0.1 mL thrombin reagent.
   c. Measure the clotting time. Average the values.

Calibration Curve   Using the graph paper furnished, plot the clotting time in seconds on the vertical axis versus the concentration of fibrinogen standard dilutions on the horizontal axis. Depending on the known concentration of fibrinogen in the standard, the points on the horizontal axis will approximate the three vertical lines marked 1:5, 1:15, and 1:40. Connecting the plotted points usually approximates a straight line. The calibration curve may be extended to a minimum of 50 mg/mL and a maximum of 800 mg/mL.

Sample Assay

1. Make a 1:10 dilution of test plasmas and control using Owren's Veronal buffer as follows: 0.1 mL plasma to 0.9 mL buffer.
2. Perform duplicate determinations on each dilution of test sample.
   a. Incubate 0.2 mL sample dilution at 37°C for at least 2 minutes but no more than 5 minutes.
   b. Add 0.1 mL thrombin reagent.
   c. Measure the clotting time. Average the values.
3. Read results from calibration curve and record in mg/dL (Fig. 34–4).

Interpretation

Normal values range from 200 to 400 mg/dL. Prolonged clotting times may indicate either a low fibrinogen concentration or the presence of inhibitors such as heparin or circulating FDPs. The effect of heparin may be excluded by performing the TT using reptilase in place of thrombin because reptilase is unaffected by heparin. A comparison of clotting times using both TT and reptilase may help to distinguish a fibrinogen deficiency from a dysfibrinogenemia.

Low fibrinogen levels are seen in infants and children and in those with congenital afibrinogenemia or hypofibrinogenemia. Acquired deficiencies are seen in states of liver disease, DIC, and fibrinolysis.

High fibrinogen levels are seen in pregnancy and in women taking oral contraceptives. Fibrinogen is considered an acute-phase reactant, and therefore high levels may be seen in states of acute infection, neoplasms, collagen disorders, nephrosis, and hepatitis.

Comment

If a prolonged clotting time is obtained using a 1:10 dilution of patient plasma, this may indicate low fibrinogen levels of 50 mg/dL or less. Retest sample using a 1:20 dilution. If a short clotting time is obtained using a 1:10 dilution of patient plasma, this may indicate high fibrinogen levels of 800 mg/dL or more.

A number of automated instruments are available that measure fibrinogen concentrations based on change in optical density as part of the prothrombin time determination.

Fibrinogen antigen levels may also be assayed by means of radial immunodiffusion (RID).

Factor XIII Screening Test

Principle

Stabilization of the fibrin clot depends on plasma factor XIII, which converts hydrogen bonds to covalent bonds by transamination. In the absence of factor XIII, the hydrogen-bonded fibrin polymers are soluble in 5 M urea or 1% monochloroacetic acid.

Reagents and Equipment

5 M urea or 1% monochloroacetic acid
Bovine thrombin (200 NIH units/mL)
0.15 NaCl
Patient plasma
37°C water bath

Procedure

1. Add 0.5 mL of patient plasma and 0.1 mL thrombin solution to a 12 × 75 mm test tube.
2. Incubate at 37°C for 30 minutes.
3. Remove the clot from the test tube with a glass rod.
4. Wash the clot with cold saline.
5. Place the clot in a clean 12 × 75 mm test tube containing 1 mL of 5 M urea or 1 mL of 1% monochloroacetic acid.
6. Incubate the tube at room temperature for 24 hours.

Interpretation

After 24 hours, the presence of a formed clot indicates a plasma factor XIII concentration of greater than 1% of normal.

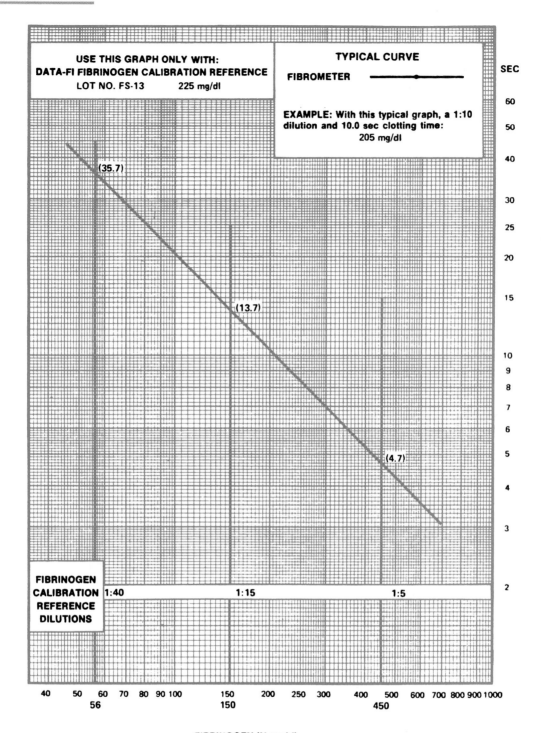

USE THIS GRAPH ONLY WITH:
DATA-FI FIBRINOGEN CALIBRATION REFERENCE
LOT NO. FS-13   225 mg/dl

TYPICAL CURVE
FIBROMETER ————•————

SEC

EXAMPLE: With this typical graph, a 1:10
dilution and 10.0 sec clotting time:
205 mg/dl

(35.7)

(13.7)

(4.7)

FIBRINOGEN
CALIBRATION   1:40   1:15   1:5
REFERENCE
DILUTIONS

40   50   60   70   80 90 100   150   200   250   300   400   500   600 700 800 900 1000
56   150   450

FIBRINOGEN IN mg/dl

FIGURE 34-4   Fibrinogen calibration curve.

Comment

A deficiency of factor XIII is not detected by other coagulation tests; therefore, hemostatic evaluation is not complete without a factor XIII assay. Because the minimum level of factor XIII is about 5%, this assay will reliably detect those individuals with a rare factor XIII deficiency.[6]

Patients who present with a homozygous deficiency of factor XIII show dissolution of a fibrin clot, usually within 1 h.

TESTS FOR VON WILLEBRAND'S DISEASE

Measurement of von Willebrand Factor Antigen

Principle

Von Willebrand factor antigen (vWF:Ag) can be quantitated using enzyme-linked immunosorbent assay (ELISA), radioimmunoassay (RIA), or Laurell rocket electrophoresis. These methods measure total von Willebrand factor protein, independent of its ability to function. An enzyme immunoassay is most frequently used for the quantitative determination of von Willebrand factor (vWF) and is frequently assayed by the sandwich technique, also known as ELISA (Fig. 34–5).

A microtiter plate coated with specific rabbit anti-human vWF antibodies captures the vWF to be measured. Rabbit anti-vWF antibody coupled with peroxidase then binds to the remaining free antigenic determinants of vWF, forming the "sandwich." The bound enzyme peroxidase is then detected by its activity on the substrate ortho-phenylenediamine in the presence of hydrogen peroxide. The reaction is stopped with a strong acid. The intensity of the color produced is directly related to the vWF concentration present in the plasma sample.

The vWF of low molecular weight is responsible for the procoagulant activity, and reacts with homologous antibodies that appear in certain polytransfused type A hemophiliacs. The other entity is of high molecular weight, composed of monomers, each of molecular weight 850,000 d, which aggregate to form polymers of molecular weight as high as 20 million. This structure is the support of the "Willebrand activity" and the "ristocetin cofactor." The monomer itself is composed of subunits, each of molecular weight about 200,000, linked with one another by disulfide bridges and composing a carbohydrate portion. This entity is synthesized by the endothelial cells. The von Willebrand factor is present in platelets.

Reagents and Equipment:

Optical density reader with 492-nm filter
Vortex
Multiple adjustable pipet and tips
12 × 75 plastic tubes
3 M H_2SO_4
Hydrogen peroxide (H_2O_2): 30%
Calibrator
Normal and abnormal controls
Commercial ELISA vWF kit

Procedure

1. Collect blood by double-syringe technique with one part of buffered sodium citrate plus nine parts of whole blood. Blue-top vacutainer tube with buffered sodium citrate may be used if a discard tube is drawn first and then the blue top is filled to the proper amount.
2. Centrifuge blood as soon as possible for 10 minutes at 3000 rpm.
3. Remove plasma immediately and put into a plastic tube. Cap and refrigerate for no more than 4 h before testing.
4. Freeze plasma at −20°C if unable to perform test.
5. Immediately before testing the plasma, rapid thawing in a 37°C water bath is recommended to prevent denaturation of fibrinogen.
6. Perform assay according to manufacturer's package insert.

Interpretation

The vWF level increases above normal during pregnancy, use of birth control pills, physical exercise, and stress. It also rises with age.

The vWF level is decreased in von Willebrand diease. Elevated vWF levels are observed when there is injury to the vascular endothelium, such as in cancer, fever, or hepatic or renal disorder, during the postoperative period, thrombosis, and myocardial infarction.

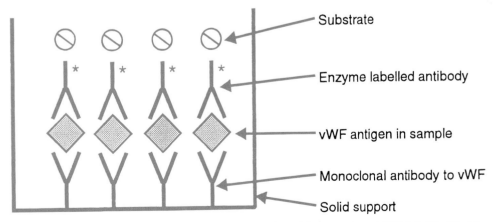

FIGURE 34–5 Principle of the sandwich ELISA test for von Willebrand factor antigen (vWF:Ag). (Modified from Constantine, N, et. al.: Retroviral Testing, Essentials for Quality Control and Laboratory Diagnosis. CRC Press, Inc., Boca Raton, 1992, p 71, with permission.)

von Willebrand Factor Function Assay

von Willebrand factor (vWF:RCo, ristocetin cofactor) is produced in the endothelial cells and is composed of large and small multimers. It is the property of the factor VIII/vWF complex that is responsible for agglutination of platelets in the presence of ristocetin. Decreased and/or increased amounts of agglutination are becoming very important in diagnosis and prognosis of several disease states. In von Willebrand disease, it is usually decreased with the exception of type IIB and "pseudo" or "platelet type." Levels of von Willebrand factor are determined by the ability of a test plasma and ristocetin to induce agglutination of a standardized platelet suspension.

Principle

In this test, normal reconstituted lyophilized platelets are mixed with dilutions of plasma. Ristocetin is added and the rate of aggregation is quantitated. The rate of aggregation is proportional to vWF factor activity.[7] The activity of unknown test samples is extrapolated from a reference graph obtained by testing dilutions of normal pooled plasma.

Reagents and Equipment

Platelet aggregometer
Aggregometer cuvettes
12 × 75 mm plastic screw-cap test tubes
Plastic centrifuge tubes
Micropipets
Lyophilized platelets
Ristocetin reagent
Normal pooled plasma
Calibrator

Procedure

1. Collect blood by double-syringe technique with one part of buffered sodium citrate plus nine parts of whole blood. A blue-top Vacutainer tube with buffered sodium citrate may be used if a discard tube is drawn first and then the blue top is filled to the proper amount.
2. Centrifuge blood as soon as possible for 10 minutes at 3000 rpm.
3. Remove plasma immediately into a plastic tube and refrigerate for no more than 4 h before testing.
4. Freeze plasma at −20°C if unable to perform test.
5. Prepare dilutions of reference pooled plasma in normal saline as follows: 1:2, 1:4, 1:8, and 1:16. The dilution of 1:2 represents 100%.
6. Prepare dilutions of patient's test plasma in normal saline as follows: 1:2 and 1:4.
7. Prepare the reference blank as follows: 0.25 mL reconstituted platelets are added to 0.25 mL of normal saline in an aggregometer cuvette and mix.
8. To a second aggregometer cuvette, pipet 0.4 mL reconstituted platelets. Add 0.05 mL of 1:2 reference-pool dilution to the cuvette. Incubate at 37°C for 2 minutes in aggregometer.

9. Add a magnetic stirring bar to the cuvette.
10. Set the baselines for 0% and 100% on the aggregometer.
11. When the 0% baseline has stabilized, add 0.05 mL of ristocetin. Note the point of ristocetin addition to the chart paper.
12. Observe aggregation until point of completion.
13. Repeat steps 4 through 10 on each serial dilution of reference plasma.
14. Repeat steps 4 through 10 on each serial dilution of patient's test plasma.

Calculation

1. Draw a slope along the steepest linear portion of the agglutination curve, being sure the line intersects the chart baseline.
2. From the point of intersection at the baseline, measure over 2 cm. At the 2-cm point, draw a perpendicular line that intersects the slope line.
3. Read the slope value off the chart paper.
4. Preparation for the standard curve: Plot the slope value of each dilution of Cryocal on semi-log graph paper, with the percentages on the abscissa and the slope value on the ordinate.
5. Controls and Patients: Read the slope value of each control and test plasma off the standard curve. Multiply by the appropriate dilution factor. Report in percentage of normal.

Interpretation

Normal values are 50% to 150% activity (compared with normal pooled plasma as reference). Patients with vWD range from 0% to 50% activity. There is a high degree of correlation between the activity of vWF in vitro and its activity in vivo, as assayed by means of the bleeding time.[7] The results typically correlate well with factor VIII:Ag. vWF activity may become normal in individuals with vWD and during inflammation or pregnancy, or following transfusion with components rich in factor VIII despite the prolonged bleeding times.[8,9] Patients who present with a variant form of vWD may show prolonged bleeding times in the face of decreased to normal vWF levels but increased activity to ristocetin.[10,11]

Normal or increased levels of vWF are found in patients with hemophilia A and in those with Bernard-Soulier syndrome.

Certain disease states such as diabetes mellitus, hyperthyroidism, liver disease, chronic renal failure, pregnancy, endothelial cell damage, and disorders of the myeloproliferative syndrome may cause an increase in the level of vWF activity. Because of these variations, it is suggested that two or three separate assays be performed before making a diagnosis.

TESTS FOR NATURAL AND PATHOLOGIC CIRCULATING ANTICOAGULANTS

AT-III Assay

Antithrombin III (AT-III) is a naturally occurring inhibitor of blood coagulation and plays an important role in maintaining blood in the fluid state. It is an α_2-globulin synthesized in the liver, circulating in the plasma, and is the major plasma inhibitor responsible for neutralizing the activity of thrombin, factors IXa and Xa, and plasmin. AT-III slowly, progressively, and irreversibly inhibits the action of thrombin by forming a 1:1 stoichiometric complex with thrombin. This complex forms when the active serine site of thrombin binds with the arginine site of antithrombin. The inhibition of thrombin by AT-III is greatly accelerated by heparin.

AT-III can be measured by a variety of techniques.[12] The most frequently used assays are: (1) chromogenic substrate assays, (2) Laurell rocket electroimmunoassay, (3) Mancini radial immunodiffusion, and (4) microlatex particle immunologic assay.

AT-III Synthetic Substrate Assay

Principle

Chromogenic AT-III assays measure the functional levels of AT-III in plasma by an amidolytic method using a synthetic substrate. Plasma containing AT-III is diluted in the presence of heparin and incubated with excess thrombin, forming an AT-III–thrombin–heparin complex. The remaining thrombin catalyzes the release of p-nitroaniline (pNA) from the chromogenic substrate. The release of pNA is measured by either an endpoint or kinetic method at 405 nm. The absorbance obtained is inversely proportional to the concentration of AT-III in the sample and may be quantitated by interpolation from a calibration curve.

Reagents and Equipment

Instrument reader at 405 nm
Chromogenic substrate kit
Multiple pipets and tips
Calibrator
Normal and abnormal controls
Buffered saline

Procedure

1. Collect blood by double-syringe technique with one part of buffered sodium citrate plus nine parts of whole blood. Blue-top Vacutainer tube with buffered sodium citrate may be used if a discard tube is drawn first and then the blue top is filled to the proper amount.
2. Centrifuge blood as soon as possible for 10 minutes at 3000 rpm.
3. Remove plasma immediately into a plastic tube and refrigerate for no more than 4 h before testing.
4. Freeze plasma at $-20°C$ if unable to perform test.
5. Immediately before testing the plasma, rapid thawing in a 37°C water bath is recommended to prevent denaturation of fibrinogen.
6. Perform testing according to manufacturer's package insert.

Radial Immunodiffusion

Reagents and Equipment

Phosphate buffer   pH 6.5
K_2HPO_4 0.56 g
KH_2PO_4 0.93 g
Na_2EDTA 1.0 g
Mix salts with 1000 mL of distilled H_2O
$3\frac{1}{4} \times 4$ inch Kodak glass slides precoated with 0.1% agarose
5-μL pipet
Well cutter
Template
Agarose, stain, destaining solution, AT-III antiserum, control serum and patient serum (all the same as for AT-III electroimmunoassay)

Procedure

1. Prepare precoated glass slides with 1% agarose in phosphate buffer pH 6.5. Add 0.25 mL of AT-III antiserum to agar.
2. Make a template with 20 wells 3 mm in diameter.
3. By following the pattern of the template, cut 20 wells 3 mm in diameter in the agar. Lift the agar from the wells with suction.
4. Prepare dilutions of control serum: undiluted (100%), 1:2 (50%). Dilutions are made with phosphate buffer.
5. Place 5 μL of each dilution in each well. The 200% reference well receives 10 μL of serum.
6. Place the slide in a moist chamber and incubate at 37°C for 18 hours.
7. Dry and stain, as described for AT-III rocket assay.

Calculation

1. Measure the diameter of the circles in two directions that are perpendicular to one another.
2. Use the mean diameter of each control sera to make a standard curve. Plot on log-log paper.
3. Determine the percent AT-III in each patient sample from the standard curve.

Microlatex Particle Immunologic Assay

Principle

When a beam of monochromatic light is allowed to traverse a suspension of microlatex particles to which specific antibodies have been attached by covalent bonding, and if the light is of a wavelength that is much greater than the diameter of the latex particles, it can pass through the latex suspension unabsorbed. However, in the presence of the antigen being tested, the antibody-coated particles agglutinate to form aggregates of diameters greater than the wavelength of the light and the latter is absorbed. There is a direct relationship between the observed absorbance value and the concentration of the antigen being measured.

Reagents and Equipment

Instrument
Commercial microlatex kit

Multiple adjustable pipet and tips
Normal saline
Normal and abnormal control

Procedure

1. Collect blood by double-syringe technique with one part of buffered sodium citrate plus nine parts whole blood. Blue-top Vacutainer with buffered sodium citrate may be used if a discard tube is drawn first and then the blue top is filled to the proper amount.
2. Centrifuge blood as soon as possible for 10 minutes at approximately 3000 rpm.
3. Remove plasma immediately into a plastic tube and refrigerate for no more than 4 h before testing.
4. Freeze plasma at $-20°C$ if unable to perform test. Plasma is stable for 1 month.
5. Immediately before testing the plasma, rapid thawing in a 37°C water bath is recommended to prevent denaturation of fibrinogen.
6. Perform assay according to manufacturer's package insert.

Interpretation

Since 1965, AT-III has been considered important as a result of the description of the first known hereditary deficiency and its consequences: the congenital decrease of the AT-III level is accompanied by a high frequency in spontaneous thromboembolic disorders.

Hereditary qualitative deficiencies are less frequent: these are identified by their antigenic AT-III levels being normal, while their AT-III activity levels are depressed.

Quantitative AT-III deficiencies are more frequent: They are identified by both of the AT-III antigenic and activity levels being depressed. In addition to these deficiencies, a number of acquired deficiencies have been described, including DIC, nephrotic syndrome, liver diseases, oral contraceptives, postsurgical state, and following prolonged heparin therapy.

Protein C Assays

Protein C is a vitamin K–dependent serine protease that functions as a major regulatory protein in the control of coagulation. Activated protein C is a potent anticoagulant and mediates this activity by proteolytically inactivating cofactor Va and factor VIIIa, and also enhances fibrinolytic activity in plasma. Cofactors Va and VIIIa are important in accelerating the activation of prothrombin and factor X.

Components of the protein C system include proteins C and S, C4b-binding protein, thrombomodulin, activated protein C inhibitor (plasminogen activator inhibitor 3), and factor V. Protein S, a second vitamin K–dependent factor, is a necessary cofactor in the reaction in which factor Va is inactivated by protein C. Activated protein C resistance, typically the result of a mutation on the factor V gene, has also recently been described.[13,14]

Laboratory diagnosis of a protein C deficiency is by means of antigenic or functional assays. Antigenic assays use RIAs, Laurell rocket immunoelectrophoresis, and an ELISA method. Functional assays detect activated protein C by clot-based or synthetic chromogenic substrate methods. The APTT and the PT are not sensitive to decreases in protein C levels.

Protein C Enzyme Immunologic Assay

Principle A microtiter plate coated with specific rabbit antihuman protein C antibodies captures the protein C to be measured. Rabbit antiprotein C antibody coupled with peroxidase then binds to the remaining free antigenic determinants of protein C, forming the "sandwich." The bound enzyme peroxidase is then detected by its activity on the substrate orthophenylendiamine in the presence of hydrogen peroxide. The reaction is stopped with a strong acid. The intensity of the color produced is directly related to the protein C concentration present in the plasma sample.

Reagents and Equipment

Optical density reader with 490-mm filter
Microtiter plate rocker
Vortex for mixing dilutions
Commercial synthetic substrate kit
Multiple adjustable pipet and tips
12×75 plastic tubes
1 N HCL
Hydrogen peroxide (H_2O_2) 30%
Normal and abnormal controls

Procedure

1. Collect blood by double-syringe technique with one part of buffered sodium citrate plus nine parts of whole blood. Blue-top Vacutainer tube with buffered sodium citrate may be used if a discard tube is drawn first and then the blue top is filled to the proper amount.
2. Centrifuge blood as soon as possible for 10 minutes at 3000 rpm.
3. Remove plasma immediately and put into a plastic tube. Cap and refrigerate for no more than 4 h before testing.
4. Freeze plasma at $-20°C$ if unable to perform test.
5. Immediately before testing the plasma, rapid thawing in a 37°C water bath is recommended to prevent denaturation of fibrinogen.
6. Perform assay according to manufacturer's package insert.

Protein C Functional Assay (Synthetic Substrate Assay)

Principle Protein C in plasma is activated by a specific enzyme from southern copperhead snake venom. The amount of activated protein C is determined by the rate of hydrolysis of the synthetic substrate S-2366. The amount of pNA release measured at 405 nm is proportional to the protein C level.

Reagents and Equipment

Instrument
Multiple adjustable pipet and tips

Calibrator
Normal and abnormal control

Procedure

1. Collect blood by double-syringe technique with one part of buffered sodium citrate plus nine parts of whole blood. Blue-top Vacutainer tube with buffered sodium citrate may be used if a discard tube is drawn first and then the blue top is filled to the proper amount.
2. Centrifuge blood as soon as possible for 10 minutes at 3000 rpm.
3. Remove plasma immediately into a plastic tube and refrigerate for no more than 4 h before testing.
4. Freeze plasma at $-20°C$ if unable to perform test.
5. Immediately before testing the plasma, rapid thawing in a 37°C water bath is recommended to prevent denaturation of fibrinogen.
6. Perform assay according to manufacturer's package insert.

Comment

Heparin levels up to 3 IU/mL do not interfere in the assay. Sample blank should be determined and subtracted in plasmas from patients with a variety of conditions such as streptokinase therapy, where contact factor activation is suspected; DIC, and in women on oral contraceptives.

Clot-Based Assay

Principle   Protein C is activated in the presence of a specific antigen, snake venom.[13] The resulting activated protein C inhibits factors V and VIII, and thus prolongs the APTT of a system in which all the factors are present, in excess except for protein C, which is in the sample.

Reagents and Equipment

$CaCl_2$ 0.025 M
Owren-Koller buffer
Coagulation analyzer
Normal and abnormal controls

Procedure

1. Collect blood by double-syringe technique with one part of buffered sodium citrate plus nine parts of whole blood. Blue-top Vacutainer tube with buffered sodium citrate may be used if a discard tube is drawn first and then the blue top is filled to the proper amount.
2. Centrifuge blood as soon as possible for 10 minutes at 3000 rpm.
3. Remove plasma immediately and put into a plastic tube. Cap and refrigerate for no more than 4 h before testing.
4. Freeze plasma at $-20°C$ if unable to perform test.
5. Immediately before testing the plasma, rapid thawing in a 37°C water bath is recommended to prevent denaturation of fibrinogen.
6. Perform assay according to manufacturer's package insert.

Comment

Heparin does not affect test results when present at a concentration less than 1 U/mL of plasma. Higher levels of heparin may lead to an overestimation of the protein C level.

Interpretation

Low levels of protein C are observed at birth as a result of liver immaturity. In adults, the protein C level appears to be independent of age and sex. Acquired deficiencies of protein C are observed in the following cases: hepatic disorders such as hepatitis and cirrhosis, DIC, and oral anticoagulant therapies. In these cases the interpretation of test results is difficult if the patient has had a history of thromboses and is receiving anticoagulant treatments.

Protein S Functional Assay

Protein S, a second vitamin K–dependent factor, is required for activated protein C anticoagulant activity. Both functional and antigenic assays for protein S exist. Because protein S exists in two states, bound and free, interpretation of laboratory tests is more complex than for protein C. Protein S bound to C4b-binding protein (C4b-BP) has little or no cofactor activity; free protein S is functional. It is recommended that both free protein S and total protein S be determined. Total protein S can be determined by means of Laurell rocket electrophoresis performed at 25°C. Higher temperatures dissociate the complex, whereas reduced temperatures make interpretation difficult. Distribution of free and bound protein S is determined by crossed immunoelectrophoresis in which free protein S migrates faster than C4b-BP-bound protein S. Semiquantitative information about protein S distribution is obtained by comparing normal plasma patterns with those in the patients. The functional protein S assay is based on the observation that activated protein C will not anticoagulate plasma in the absence of protein S. Protein S–deficient plasma is clotted by factor Xa in a one-stage assay that uses cephalin. Activated protein C is then added. A linear relationship exists between the concentration of protein S and the prolonged clotting time. Normal plasma added to protein S–deficient plasma causes a prolonged clotting time proportional to the amount of normal plasma added. Functional protein S determinations are obtained by comparing the clotting time response of normal plasma with that of the patient. The presence of heparin and factor Va interferes with this assay, as do oral anticoagulants.

Principle

Protein S is a vitamin K–dependent cofactor for the anticoagulant and the profibrinolytic effects of activated protein C. In normal plasma, about 60% of protein S is in complex with C4b binding protein, whereas the other 40% is in free form. Only free protein S has functional cofactor activity.[15]

Protein S activity is determined by measuring the clotting time in a system that includes bovine thromboplastin, activated protein C and calcium. Activated protein C is generated in vitro by activation of protein S–deficient plasma.

Reagents and Equipment

Coagulation analyzer
Commercial kit
Multiple adjustable pipet and tips
Calibrator
Normal and abnormal controls

Procedure

1. Collect blood by double-syringe technique with one part of buffered sodium citrate plus nine parts of whole blood. Blue-top Vacutainer tube with buffered sodium citrate may be used if a discard tube is drawn first and then the blue top is filled to the proper amount.
2. Centrifuge blood as soon as possible for 10 minutes at 3000 rpm.
3. Remove plasma immediately into a plastic tube and refrigerate for no more than 4 h before testing.
4. Freeze plasma at −20°C if unable to perform test.
5. Immediately before testing the plasma, rapid thawing in a 37°C water bath is recommended to prevent denaturation of fibrinogen.
6. Perform assay according to manufacturer's package insert.

Comment

Protein S values may be underestimated in test samples with elevated factor VIIa levels.[16] Factor VIIa may be elevated because of a clinical condition, inappropriate venipuncture, and cold activation[17] on storage. Perform additional tests when elevated factor VIIa levels are suspected by testing samples diluted 1:40 (25 μL + 975 μL) and 1:80 (25 μL + 1975 μL) using protein S–deficient plasma.

Screening Test for the Detection of Circulating Anticoagulants

Circulating anticoagulants are acquired pathologic plasma proteins that inhibit normal coagulation. Circulating anticoagulants differ from naturally occurring inhibitors such as AT-III, α_2-macroglobulin, α_2-antitrypsin, and C1 esterase and must be differentiated from anticoagulants such as heparin and coumarin analogues. Most of these pathologic anticoagulants are inhibitors or autoantibodies of the IgG class whose inhibitory effects are directed against certain coagulation factors or demonstrate specific activity against phospholipids (such as factor VIII and the prothrombin complex).

Some of the circulating anticoagulants that have been detected thus far have been encountered in patients with the following conditions: hemophilia A, Christmas disease, DIC, pregnancy, systemic lupus erythematosus (SLE), the plasma cell dyscrasias, Waldenstrom's macroglobulinemia, advanced age, and others.

The circulating anticoagulant directed against the factor VIII molecule is the most common specific factor inhibitor. It is seen in patients with hemophilia A and may be related to repeated therapeutic transfusions of antihemophilic factor (AHF), but is also seen in non-hemophiliac patients (e.g., women after childbirth or abortion, elderly individuals, and those with immunologic disorders such as rheumatoid arthritis). Antibodies to factor VIII may also be seen in patients known to have the severe form of von Willebrand's disease.

Other specific inhbiitors have been reported against factor IX, factor XI, factor XII, factor V, factor XIII, and inhibitors of fibrin formation.

Some patients with SLE develop an acquired circulating anticoagulant. This inhibitor demonstrates specific activity against phospholipids and thus interferes with phospholipid-dependent complexes that involve factors V and VIII.[18]

The Activated Partial Thromboplastin Time (APTT)—Mixing Studies

Principle The APTT is useful as a screening test for all types of circulating anticoagulants. The test is based on the ability of normal plasma to correct an abnormal clotting time with a factor deficiency. The addition of normal plasma will not correct the clotting time in the presence of a circulating anticoagulant.

Reagents and Equipment

APTT reagent
CaCl$_2$ (0.025 M)
Normal control plasma

Procedure

1. Collect citrated plasma from patient.
2. Mix patient's plasma with normal control plasma in a series of six 12 × 75 test tubes as follows (Table 34–3):
   Tube 6 is the control; tube 1 is 100% patient's plasma; tube 2 is 75% patient's plasma; tube 3 is 50% patient's plasma; tube 4 is 25% patient's plasma; and tube 5 is 10% patient's plasma.
3. Incubate each tube for 1 hour at 37°C.
4. Measure the APTT for each tube.

Interpretation

If the APTT is corrected by normal plasma, a factor deficiency is indicated. The addition of normal plasma supplies the coagulation factor or factors that are deficient, and thus corrects the APTT. When a factor de-

TABLE 34–3 **Dilution for APTT Mixing Studies**		
Tube No.	Patient's Plasma	Normal Control Plasma
1	0.20 mL	—
2	0.15 mL	0.05 mL
3	0.10 mL	0.10 mL
4	0.05 mL	0.15 mL
5	0.02 mL	0.18 mL
6	—	0.20 mL

ficiency is present, there should be correction of the abnormal APTT by only 10% to 25% normal plasma[19] (tubes 5 and 4).

If the APTT is not corrected by the addition of normal plasma in most of the mixtures, a strong circulating anticoagulant is indicated.

A weak circulating anticoagulant is indicated by a prolonged APTT following incubation at 37°C for 1 hour. On incubation, a weak inhibitor progressively inactivates the coagulation factor, thus prolonging the APTT. This pattern is most typical of a factor VIII inhibitor.

Comment

The circulating anticoagulant that inhibits factor VIII is a specific IgG antibody.[19] These antibodies are often present as weak circulating anticoagulants but are temperature- and time-dependent, thus causing only a slightly prolonged clotting time on fresh patient plasma. Mixing tests may yield APTT results intermediate between the clotting times of patient and normal control. On incubation at 37°C, both the patient plasma and mixing plasmas show prolonged times, but the normal control plasma shows no change. Owing to the nature of the factor VIII inhibitor, the mixture of test plasma and normal control plasma must be incubated for a period of 30 to 120 minutes to allow for the inhibitor's progressive activity.

If a factor VIII inhibitor is present, it is important to determine the level of activity periodically because the development of an inhibitor complicates the management of a patient with hemophilia when therapy involves AHF concentrates.

The thrombin time is also of value in the detection of circulating anticoagulants.

Screening Tests for the Detection of Lupus Anticoagulants

Lupus anticoagulants (LA) are antibodies (IgG, IgM, IgA, or a mixture) reactive against phospholipids, thereby prolonging in vitro phospholipid-dependent coagulation tests. First recognized in patients with systemic lupus erythematosus (SLE), lupus anticoagulants have been identified in a variety of disorders including malignancies, infections, and autoimmune disorders, as well as following drug therapy. The presence of an LA is usually not associated with a bleeding problem unless accompanied by thrombocytopenia, platelet dysfunction, or drug administration (aspirin, etc.). The LA, however, has been associated with a risk factor for venous and arterial thrombosis and recurrent spontaneous abortions.[20]

The laboratory diagnosis of a lupus inhibitor is critical in terms of distinguishing it from other specific factor inhibitors and to identify patients at potential risk for thrombotic problems. The Scientific and Standardization Committee (SSC) Sub-Committee for the Standardization of Lupus Anticoagulants of the International Society of Thrombosis and Hemostasis (ISTH) has defined the following criteria for lupus:

1. An abnormal in vitro phospholipid dependent coagulation assay.

2. Demonstration that the abnormal test is caused by an inhibitor.
3. Demonstration that the inhibitor is directed against a phospholipid and not at a specific coagulation factor.

Suspicion of an LA is most often aroused by an unexplained prolongation of the APTT that is not corrected by the addition of an equal volume of normal plasma. Confirmatory tests to identify an LA include those that decrease the phospholipid in the test system, thereby increasing the LA effect, such as the tissue thromboplastin inhibition (TTI) test, dilute Russell's viper venom time (DRVVT), and the kaolin clotting time (KCT), or those that increase the phospholipid, thereby neutralizing the LA effect, such as the platelet neutralization procedure (PNP).

Confirmatory Tests for Lupus Anticoagulants

There are several confirmatory tests for lupus, including: platelet neutralization procedure, anticardiolipin assay, kaolin clotting time, tissue thromboplastin inhibition test, and dilute Russell's viper venom test. The first two are described in this section.

Platelet Neutralization Procedure

Principle The platelet neutralization procedure (PNP) is based on the ability of platelets to correct significantly in vitro coagulation abnormalities.[21] The disrupted platelet membranes present in the freeze-thawed platelet suspension neutralize phospholipid antibodies present in the plasma of patients with LA. After the patient plasma is mixed with the freeze-thawed platelet suspension, the APTT will be "corrected" when compared with the original baseline APTT.

Interpretation

A correction of the baseline APTT of 5 s or more by the platelet suspension as compared with the control is indicative of the presence of an LA.

Comment

Specimen collection, centrifugation, and processing are critical when testing for the presence of an LA. Coagulation assays that have a phospholipid-dependent reaction are affected by the presence of platelets in platelet-poor plasma. Lupus anticoagulants are directed against phospholipids, and therefore the relative concentration of the phospholipid affects the sensitivity of the assay for detection of the LA.

Previously considered indicative of factor VIII inhibitors, time-dependent inhibition has been seen in lupus anticoagulants and factor V inhibitors.

Lupus anticoagulants demonstrate considerable heterogeneity and show variable differences in sensitivity and responsiveness of the reagent, as well as on the selection of an appropriate confirmatory test. Despite the differences in testing methodology and reagents currently available, most of these anticoagulants can be detected and identified.

Anticardiolipin Assay

Principle   Anticardiolipin antibodies (ACAs) and LAs are antiphospholipid immunoglobulins (IgG, IgM, IgA, or a combination). Several studies have shown that patients with the LA and the closely related ACA are prone to recurrent venous and arterial thrombosis, recurrent spontaneous abortions, and thrombocytopenia.[22] Some patients with anticardiolipin antibodies have been reported to show an LA. The concept of an antiphospholipid antibody syndrome has been proposed. This includes patients with antiphospholipid antibodies (APAs), whether or not an LA is present; those who have a confirmed LA only; and those who show evidence of both APA and an LA.

ELISA assays for anticardiolipin antibodies have been developed. The commercial kits use cardiolipin or a mixture of negatively charged phospholipids such as antigen (see Chap. 30).

TESTS FOR FIBRIN/FIBRINOGEN DEGRADATION PRODUCTS

Plasmin proteolytically cleaves fibrin(ogen) into fragments X and Y, known as early degradation products, and fragments D and E, known as late degradation products. These FDPs share antigenic determinants with both fibrin and fibrinogen, thus allowing for detection by immunologic methods by the use of antisera to highly purified preparations of human fibrinogen fragments D and E. Measurement of FDPs provides an indirect assay of fibrinolysis.

Thrombo-Wellcotest: Latex Agglutination Test

Principle

This test is a direct latex agglutination slide test for the detection and semiquantitation of FDPs. Latex particles in glycine buffer are coated with specific antibodies to human fibrinogen fragments D and E. The presence of FDPs in either the serum or the urine causes the latex particles to clump, yielding macroscopic agglutination. An approximate concentration of FDPs in the sample can be determined by testing the sample at different dilutions. Thrombin is added to the test sample to ensure complete clotting and complete removal of fibrinogen. The addition of a proteolytic inhibitor—soybean trypsin—prevents in vitro activation of the fibrinolytic system.

Reagents and Equipment

Commercial kit.

Procedure

1. Collect 2 mL of venous blood in a special FDP sample Vacutainer tube (provided with test kit). Mix immediately by gentle inversion several times.
2. Ring the clot to allow retraction to occur. Keep the sample tube at room temperature or 37°C for 30 minutes and centrifuge to separate serum.

TABLE 34–4 **Dilutions for FDP**		
	Tube 1	**Tube 2**
Glycine buffer	0.75 mL	0.75 mL
Serum	5 drops	1 drop
Final dilution	1:5	1:20

3. If the sample is obtained from a heparinized patient, reptilase (Abbott Laboratories, North Chicago, IL) should be added to the blood. Reptilase-R and enzyme isolated from snake venom clot fibrinogen in the presence of heparin and other such antithrombins. Reptilase-R 0.1 mL will clot 1.0 mL of blood.
4. Label two 12 × 75 test tubes. Prepare dilutions of the serum (see Table 34–4): To aliquot the buffer, use the graduated dropper provided. To deliver the sample, use the disposable pipet and bulb provided in the kit. Mix well.
5. Label two rings on the glass slide provided as 1 and 2.
6. Transfer 1 drop of the dilution from test tube 2 to position 2 on the glass slide and 1 drop from test tube 1 to position 1. Deliver the dilutions in this order.
7. Thoroughly mix the latex suspension. Add 1 drop to each position on the slide.
8. Stir the latex-serum mixture. Start with position 2 on the slide, then mix position 1. When stirring the mixture, spread to fill the circles.
9. Gently rotate the slide for no longer than 2 minutes. Observe the slide for macroscopic agglutination by viewing against a dark background.

Controls

1. Label two of the rings on the glass test slide (+) and (−) for positive and negative controls.
2. Place one drop of the appropriate control and one drop of latex suspension on the slide and mix as described earlier.
3. Read results. Failure of the controls to react as described indicates deterioration of at least one of the reagents or an improperly performed test.

Interpretation

The test is sensitive to values of 2 μg of FDP per milliliter. The presence of agglutination in position 1 indicates the presence of FDPs in a final concentration greater than 10 μg/mL. The presence of agglutination in position 2 indicates the presence of FDPs in a final concentration of greater than 40 μg/mL. For the test to be valid, if agglutination is present in position 2, it must also be present in position 1 on the slide. Agglutination in tube 1 and lack of agglutination in tube 2 indicate FDPs greater than 10 μg/mL but less than 40 μg/mL.

Lack of agglutination indicates an FDP concentration of less than 2 μg/mL. The mean normal level of serum is 4.9 ± 2.8 μg FDP per milliliter. The normal value may be elevated during exercise and stress.

The latex agglutination assay has been documented to give false-positive results with sera from patients with rheumatoid arthritis. Trace amounts of FDPs occur in the blood of normal healthy adults and children as a result of physiologic fibrinolysis.

Comment

Generally, elevated levels of FDP are associated with thrombotic episodes such as myocardial infarction, pulmonary emboli, and deep vein thrombosis, as well as with certain complications of pregnancy.

The assay is of value in the differential diagnosis of patients with certain kidney diseases. Quantitation of urine FDP levels provides a useful clinical means of monitoring glomerulonephritis and kidney rejection following transplantation.

The detection of FDPs is of great clinical value in assessing patients with DIC. A positive test result, accompanied by an elevated PT and APTT and a decrease in platelet count and fibrinogen concentration, is suggestive of DIC.

D-Dimer (D-Di) Test

Principle

Under the action of thrombin, fibrinogen is cleaved to give rise to fibrin monomers. These monomers form polymers, which are stabilized by factor XIII, forming covalent crosslinkages in the D domain to produce an insoluble fibrin clot. Plasmin, a potent clot-lysing enzyme, attacks fibrin clots as well as fibrinogen in the body. Unlike plasmin's action on fibrinogen, which produces FDPs, its action on the fibrin clot leads to the generation of cross-linked fibrin containing D-dimer. The latex particles provided in the D-DI test are coated with mouse antihuman D-dimer monoclonal antibodies. Test samples containing D-dimers when mixed with the latex particle suspension make the particles agglutinate. Other laboratory tests that may be useful in evaluation of the fibrinolytic system include fibrin monomers, ethanol gelation test, protamine sulfate test, and euglobulin lysis time.

MARKERS OF THROMBIN ACTIVATION

New assays have been developed that allow detection of molecular markers of thrombosis.[23] These molecular markers can provide specific and pertinent data for early diagnosis and management of coagulation disorders.

Before thrombin becomes biologically available, there is generation of biochemical markers in the blood. These markers of thrombosis can be employed in basically three diagnostic applications: (1) diagnosis of spontaneous thrombosis, (2) prognosis and follow-up of thrombotic disease, and (3) monitoring of anticoagulant therapies.

Under normal conditions, all individuals produce measurable quantities of molecular markers; however, significantly increased levels have been observed in persons with deep venous thrombosis, pulmonary emboli, disseminated intravascular coagulation, and

other thrombotic phenomena. Because of their short half-lives, activation peptides demonstrate blood activation only as long as the thrombotic process is ongoing.

Molecular markers offer several advantages as compared with the conventional coagulation tests. First, molecular markers are specific indicators of the activation of coagulation and fibrinolysis while conventional assays measure deficiencies of the clotting mechanism. Additionally, markers are ultrasensitive and are able to detect minute changes in the components of hemostasis.

The disadvantages of marker testing include the requirement of special anticoagulants for collection and the necessity of rapid sample processing.

Fibrinopeptide A, prothrombin fragment 1 + 2, and thrombin-antithrombin complex are the markers measured most frequently to determine the generation of thrombin. ELISA assays are currently available to test for these thrombotic markers.

ACL 3000 (AUTOMATED COAGULATION LABORATORY)

The ACL 3000 manufactured by Instrumentation Laboratory (IL) is a fully automated lab top microcentrifugal coagulation analyzer (Fig. 34–6). This technologically advanced instrument houses a microcomputer-controlled system that computes calibration data and test results to the video display unit. In operating this instrument, the technologist transfers plasma to the appropriate sample cups, which can be either 0.5 or 2.0 mL. The desired tests are then keyed into the video display unit (VDU). The analyzer, using centrifugal force, detects the samples to be run and recognizes available space on the 20-place rotor. A mechanical sampling arm automatically pipets the plasma sample and reagents into the 20-place acrylic rotor. These are mixed by a centrifugal force and parameters are measured in spinning cycles of rotation based on principles of light scatter. Results are displayed on the video display unit and printed on thermal paper.

Routine coagulation analyses, as well as factor assays and chromogenic assays, are performed on this instrument. The routine analyses include the prothrombin time (PT), the activated partial thromboplastin time (APTT), thrombin time (TT), and fibrinogen. The factor assays are grouped into the extrinsic factors (VII, X, V, and II) intrinsic factors (XII, XI, IX, and VIII), and single factors (VII, X, V, II, XII, XI, IX, and VIII). In addition, the ACL 3000 performs clottable protein C and protein S assays. These can be analyzed via pathways (extrinsic and intrinsic) or as single factors. The chromogenic assays performed on the ACL 3000 consist of AT-III, heparin, α_2-antiplasmin, plasminogen, and protein C.

Some of the more exclusive features offered by this instrument as compared to other coagulation analyzers are a bar code reader that serves to electronically identify patient specimens, a dual testing option that pairs the TT/APTT and PT-fibrinogen/APTT parameters as opposed to running these tests separately, and

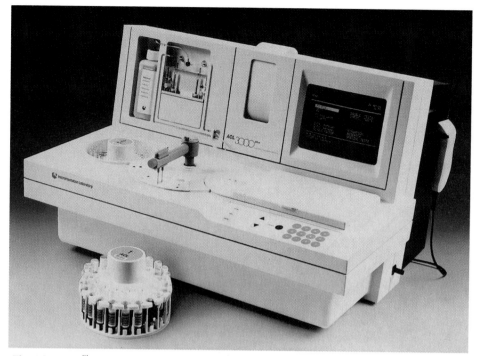

FIGURE 34–6   The ACL 3000^Plus, combining the features of the ACL 3000 with specialized software to accommodate a choice of user programmable test cycles. Loading and timing conditions may vary, and the data are sent to an external PC (not shown) for data manipulation and hemostatic imaging. Courtesy of Instrumentation Laboratory.

computer interfacing capabilities in which results can be transmitted directly to the laboratory information system (LIS). In addition, the sample carousel that holds the specimens and controls accommodates 5-mL or 3.5-mL Vacutainer tubes, alleviating transfer of plasma to specimen cups, which is economically appealing.

With minimal maintenance, the ACL delivers quality testing and versatility to coagulation studies in hospital, private, and physician office laboratories.

REFERENCES

1. Lenahan, JG and Smith, K: Hemostasis, ed 16. General Diagnostics, Division of Warner-Lambert Co, Morris Plains, NJ, 1982.
2. Born, GVR: Aggregation of blood platelets by adenosine diphosphate and its reversal. Nature 194:927, 1962.
3. Wilner, AD, Nossel, HL, and LeRoy, EC: Aggregation of platelets by collagen. J Clin Invest 47:2616, 1968.
4. Triplett, DA, et al: Platelet Function: Laboratory Evaluation and Clinical Application. American Society of Clinical Pathologists, Chicago, 1978.
5. Quick, AJ, Stanley-Brown, M, and Bancroft, FW: A study of the coagulation defect in hemophilia and jaundice. Am Med Sci 190:501, 1935.
6. Kitchens, CS and Newcomb, TF: Factor XIII. Medicine 58:413, 1979.
7. Weiss, HJ, et al: Quantitative assay of a plasma factor, deficient in von Willebrand's disease, that is necessary for platelet aggregation. Relationship to factor VIII procoagulant activity and antigen content. J Clin Invest 52:2708, 1973.
8. Ratnoff, OD and Saito, H: Bleeding in von Willebrand's disease. N Engl J Med 290:420, 1974.
9. Weiss, HJ: Relation of von Willebrand's factor to bleeding time. N Engl J Med 291:420, 1974.
10. Ruggeri, ZM, et al: Heightened interaction between platelets and factor VII/von Willebrand's factor in a new subtype of von Willebrand's disease. N Engl J Med 302:1047, 1980.
11. Ruggeri, ZM and Zimmerman, TS: Variant von Willebrand's disease. Characterization of two subtypes by analysis of multimeric composition of factor VIII/von Willebrand's factor in plasma and platelets. J Clin Invest 65:131a, 1980.
12. Miale, JB: Laboratory Medicine: Hematology, ed 6. CV Mosby, St Louis, 1982.
13. Klein, J, et al: Purification of a Protein C Activator from the venom of the Southern Copperhead snake. Biochemistry 25:4175, 1986.
14. Dahlback, B, Carlson, M, and Swensson, PJ: Familial Thrombophilia due to a Previously Unrecognized Mechanism Characterized by Poor Anticoagulant Response to Activated Protein C: Prediction of a Cofactor to Activated Protein C. Proc Natl Acad Sci 90:1004, 1993.
15. Suzuki, K and Nishoika, J: Plasma protein S activity using Protac, a snake venom derived activator of protein C. Thromb Res 49:241, 1988.
16. Preda, L, Tripodi, A, Valsechi, C, et al: A prothrombin time-based functional assay of protein S. Thromb Res 60:19, 1990.
17. Ens, GE and Newlin, F: Spurious Protein S Deficiency as a Result of Elevated Factor VII Levels. Clin Hemost Rev 9:18, 1995.
18. Schleider, MA, Nachman, RL, Jaffe, EA, et al: A clinical study of the lupus anticoagulant. Blood 48:499, 1976.
19. Sirridge, MS and Shannon, R: Laboratory Evaluation of Hemostasis and Thrombosis, ed 3. Lea & Feibger, Philadelphia, 1983, p 124.
20. Carreras, LO, et al: Arterial thrombosis, intrauterine death, and "lupus anticoagulant": Detection of immu-

noglobulin interfering with prostacyclin formation. Lancet 1:244, 1981.

21. Triplett, DA, et al: Laboratory diagnosis of lupus inhibitors: A comparison of the tissue thromboplastin inhibition procedure with a new platelet neutralization procedure. Am J Clin Pathol 79:678, 1983.
22. Harris, NE, et al: Thrombosis, recurrent fetal loss and thrombocytopenia. Predictive value of the anticardiolipin antibody test. Arch Intern Med 146:2153, 1986.
23. Jensen, R and Ens, GE: Markers of thrombin activation. Clin Hemost Rev 8:1, 1994.

BIBLIOGRAPHY

Abildgard, CF, et al. Serial studies in von Willebrand's disease: Variability versus "variants." Blood 56:4, 1980.
Alami, SY, et al. Fibrin stabilizing factor (factor XIII). Am J Med 44:1, 1968.
Ambruso, DR, et al. Antithrombin III deficiency: Decreased synthesis of a biochemically normal molecule. Blood 60:1, 1982.
Automated APTT (package insert). General Diagnostics, Morris Plains, NJ, 1977.
Bertina, RM, et al: Mutation in blood coagulation factor V associated with resistance to activated protein C. Nature 369:64, 1994.
Comp, PC, et al: An abnormal plasma distribution of protein S occurs in functional protein s deficiency. Blood 67:504, 1986.
Bauer, JD: Clinical Laboratory Methods, ed 9. CV Mosby, St Louis, 1982.
Biggs, R and Rizza, CR: Human Blood Coagulation: Hemostasis and Thrombosis, ed 3. Blackwell Scientific, Boston, 1984.
Bloom, AL: The von Willebrand syndrome. Semin Hematol 27:4, 1980.
Bockenstedt, PL: Laboratory methods in hemostasis. Thromb Hemorrhage 26:455, 1994.
Bowie, EJW, et al. Platelet adhesiveness in von Willebrand's disease. Am J Clin Pathol 52:69, 1969.
Comp, PC, Nixon, RR, and Esmon, CT: Determination of functional protein C, and antithrombotic protein, using thrombin thrombomodulin complex. Blood 63:15, 1984.
Comp, PC: Laboratory evaluation of protein S status. Semin Thromb Hemost 16:177, 1990.
Dahlback, B, et al: Familial thrombophilia due to a previously unrecognized mechanism characterized by poor anticoagulant response to activated protein C: Prediction of a cofactor to activated protein C. Proc Natl Acad Sci 90:1004, 1993.
Dahlback, B and Hildebrand, B: Inherited resistance to activated protein C is corrected by anticoagulation cofactor activity found to be a property of factor V. Proc Natl Acad Sci 91:1396, 1994.
Data-Fi Fibrinogen Determination Kit (package insert): American Dade, Division of American Hospital Supply Corporation, Miami, FL, 1978.
de Ronde, H and Bertina, RM. Laboratory Diagnosis of APC-Resistance: A Critical Evaluation of the Test and the Development of Diagnostic Criteria. Thromb Haemost 72:880, 1994.
Ebert, R: PTs, PRs, ISIs, and INRs: A primer on prothrombin time reporting. Part I: Calibration of thromboplastin reagents and principles of prothrombin time reporting. Clin Hemost Rev 7:1, 1993.
Ebert, R: PTs, PRs, ISIs, and INRs: A primer on prothrombin time reporting. Part II: Limitations of INR reporting. Clin Hemost Rev 7:1, 1993.
Eliman, L, et al: The Thrombo-Wellcotest as a screening test for disseminated intravascular coagulation. N Engl J Med 288:633, 1973.
Ens, G and Jensen, R: Coagulation instrumentation review. Clin Hemost Rev 7:1, 1993.
Ens, G and Jensen, R: Diagnosis and management of acquired bleeding disorders. Clin Hemost Rev 7:1, 1993.
Ens, G: Disorders leading to thrombosis. Clin Hematol 56:639, 1992.
Epstein, DJ, et al: Radioimmunoassay for Protein C and Factor X. Am J Clin Pathol 82:573, 1983.
Ewing, NP and Kasper, CK: In Vitro Detection of Mild Inhibitors to Factor VII in Hemophilia. Am J Clin Pathol 77:6, 1982.
Exner, T, et al: Comparison of Test Methods for the Lupus Anticoagulant: International Survey on Lupus Anticoagulants-I (ISLA-1). Thromb Haemost 64:478, 1990.
Fischbach, DP and Fogdall, RP: Coagulation: The Essentials. Williams & Wilkins, Baltimore, 1981.
Francis, RB and Thomas, W: Behavior of Protein C Inhibitor in Intravascular Coagulation and Liver Disease. Thromb Haemost 52:71, 1984.
Godal, H and Abildgaard, U. Gelation of soluble fibrin in plasma by ethanol. Scand J Haematol 3:432, 1966.
Guglielmone, HA and Vides, MA: A novel functional assay of protein C in human plasma and its comparison with amidolytic and anticoagulant assays. Thromb Haemost 67:46, 1992.
Harker, L and Thompson, AR: Manual of Hemostasis and Thrombosis, ed 3. FA DAvis, Philadelphia, 1983.
Hemostasis Committee of the "Societe Francaise De Biologie Clinique": Laboratory heterogeneity of the lupus anticoagulant: A multicentre study using different clotting assays on a panel of 78 samples. Thromb Res 66:349, 1992.
Henry, JB: Clinical Diagnosis and Management by Laboratory Methods, ed 17. WB Saunders, Philadelphia, 1984.
Hoyer, LW: The factor VIII complex: Structure and function. Blood 58:1, 1981.
Jensen, R: Activated protein C resistance. Clin Hemost Rev 9:1, 1995.
Jensen, R and Ens, G: Advances in the Diagnosis of Lupus Anticoagulant. Clin Hemost Rev 7:1, 1993.
Jensen, R and Ens, G: Components of the protein C anticoagulant system Part I. Clin Hemost Rev 6:1, 1992.
Jensen, R and Ens, G: Components of the protein C anticoagulant system Part II. Clin Hemost Rev 6:1, 1992.
Jensen, R and Ens, G: ELISA application in hemostasis. Clin Hemost Rev 7:1, 1993.
Jensen, R and Ens, G: Serine protease inhibitors. Clin Hemost Rev 7:1, 1993.
Kennedy, J: Fibrinogen, fibrin, and fibrinolysis. Dade, Division of American Hospital Supply Corporation, Miami, FL, 1974.
Koepke, JA, et al: The prediction of prothrombin time system using secondary standards. Am J Clin Pathol 68:191, 1977.
Kowalski, E: Fibrinogen derivatives and their biologic activity. Semin Hematol 5:45, 1968.
Laroche, P, et al: Rapid quantitative latex immuno assays for diagnosis of thrombotic disorders. Thromb Haemost 62:379, 1989.
Latallo, ZS and Teisseyre, E: Evaluation of reptilase-R and thrombin clotting time in the presence of fibrinogen degradation products and heparin. Scand J Haematol 4:261, 1971.
Laurell, CB: Quantitative estimation of proteins by electrophoresis in agarose gel containing antibodies. Ann Biochem 15:45, 1966.
Laurell, CB: Electroimmunoassay. Scand J Clin Lab Invest 124:21, 1972.
Lee, RL and White, PD: A clinical study of the coagulation time of blood. Am J Med Sci 145:495, 1913.
Lenahan, JG and Smith, K: Hemostasis, ed 16. General Diagnostics Division of Warner-Lambert Company, NJ, 1982.
Losowsky, MA, Hall, R, and Goldie, W: Congenital deficiency of fibrin stabilizing factor. Lancet 2:156, 1965.

Macfarlane, RG: A simple method for measuring clot retraction. Lancet 1:1199, 1939.

Mammen, EF: Congenital abnormalities of the fibrinogen molecule. Semin Thromb Hemost 1:184, 1974.

Mannucci, PM, et al: Familial dysfunction of protein S. Thromb Haemost 62:763, 1989.

Martinoli, JL, and Stocker, K: Fast functional protein C assay using Protac, a novel protein C activator. Thromb Res 43:253, 1986.

McGann, MA and Triplett, DA: Interpretation of antithrombin III activity. Lab Med 13:12, 1982.

Miale, JB: Laboratory Medicine: Hematology, ed 6. CV Mosby, St Louis, 1982.

Mielke, CH, et al: The standardized normal ivy bleeding time and its prolongation by aspirin. Blood 34:204, 1969.

Murano, G and Bick, RL: Basic Concepts of Hemostasis and Thrombosis. CRC Press, Boca Raton, FL, 1980.

National Committee for Clinical Laboratory Standards: Collection transport and preparation of blood specimens for coagulation testing and performance of coagulation assays. NCCLS Document H21-A, vol 6, no 20, 1986.

National Committee for Clinical Laboratory Standards: Tentative guidelines for the standardized collection, transport and preparation of blood specimens for coagulation testing and performance of coagulation assays; vol 2, p 4, Villanova, PA, 1982.

Nor-Partien Fibrinogen Kit (package insert): Behring Diagnostics, La Jolla, CA, 1988.

Olson, JD, et al. Evaluation of ristocetin-Willebrand's factor assay and ristocetin-induced platelet aggregation. Am J Clin Pathol 63:210, 1975.

Pabinger, I: Clinical relevance of protein C. Blut 53:65, 1986.

Patterson, BB: Clot observation—A review of an important but neglected coagulation test. Lab Med 7:12, 1976.

Platelet Neutralization Procedure. Department of Air Force, Lackland AFB, TX, 1980.

Preda, L, et al: A prothrombin time–based functional assay of protein S. Thromb Res 60:19, 1990.

Protein C Antigen Rocket EID Method (package insert): Helena Laboratories, Beaumont, TX, 1989.

Protopath Proteolytic Enzyme Detection System: Antithrombin III Synthetic Substrate Assay for Determination of AT-III Activity in Plasma (package insert). American Dade, Division of American Hospital Supply Corp, Miami, FL 1986.

Ramsey, R and Evatt, BL: Rapid assay for von Willebrand's factor activity using formalin-fixed platelets and microtitration technique. Am J Clin Pathol 72:996, 1979.

Reptilase-R (package insert): Abbott Laboratories, Diagnostics Division, IL, 93-4260, 1974.

Russell's Viper Venom Reagent for Factor X Assays (package insert): General Diagnostics, Morris Plains, NJ, 1976.

Sadler, JE: A revised classification of von Willebrand disease: For the subcomitee on von Willebrand factor of the Scientific and Standardization Committee of the International Society on Thrombosis and Haemostasis. Thromb Haemost 71:520, 1994.

Sala, N, Owen, WG, and Collen, D: A functional assay of protein C in human plasma. Blood 63:671, 1984.

Seaman, AJ: The recognition of intravascular clotting: The plasma protamine paracoagulation tests. Arch Intern Med 125:1016, 1970.

Shapiro, SS and Hultin, M: Acquired inhibitors to the blood coagulation factors. Semin Thromb Hemost 1:366, 1975.

Shitamoto, BS, Leslie, KO, and Galloway, WB: Postpartum hemophilia. Am J Clin Pathol 78:5, 1982.

Sirridge, MS and Shannon, R: Laboratory Evaluation of Hemostasis and Thrombosis, ed 3. Lea & Febiger, Philadelphia, 1983.

Spero, JA, Lewis, JH, and Hasiba, V: Disseminated intravascular coagulation: Findings in 346 patients. Thromb Haemost 43:28, 1980.

Stenflo, J and Jonsson, M: Protein S, a new vitamin K–dependent protein from bovine plasma. FEBS Lett 101:37, 1979.

Sussman, LN: The clotting time—an enigma. Am J Clin Pathol 60:5, 1973.

Thrombo-Wellcotest (package insert): Wellcome Research Laboratories, Brekenham, England, 1974.

Triplett, DA, et al: Platelet Function: Laboratory Evaluation and Clinical Application. American Society of Clinical Pathologists, Chicago, 1978.

Triplett, DA and Harms, CS: Procedures for the Coagulation Laboratory. American Society of Clinical Pathologists, Chicago, 1981.

Triplett, DA: The laboratory diagnosis of lupus anticoagulants. Presented at the Fifth International Symposium of Antiphospholipid Antibodies. San Antonio, TX, September, 1992.

Vinazzer, H, et al: Protein C: Comparison of different assays in normal and abnormal plasma samples. Thromb Res 46:1, 1987.

von Kaulla, F and von Kaulla, N: Deficiency of antithrombin III activity associated with hereditary thrombosis tendency. J Med 3:349, 1972.

Walker, FJ: Regulation of activated protein C by a new protein—A possible function for bovine protein S. J Biol Chem 255:5521, 1980.

QUESTIONS

1. What is measured by a bleeding time?
   a. Platelet number
   b. Platelet function
   c. Intrinsic and extrinsic coagulation systems
   d. Two of the above

2. Which platelet aggregation result would be characteristic for patients with Bernard-Soulier syndrome?
   a. Incomplete aggregation with ADP
   b. Primary wave of aggregation in response to collagen
   c. Abnormal ristocetin-induced platelet aggregation
   d. Primary wave of aggregation with epinephrine

3. Which of the following tests measures the intrinsic pathway of coagulation and is used to detect factor deficiencies and hypofibrinogenemia and to monitor heparin therapy?
   a. Activated partial thromboplastin time
   b. Prothrombin time
   c. Quantitative factor assay
   d. Stypven time test (Russell's viper venom time test)

4. Which test measures the extrinsic pathway of coagulation and is used to measure factor deficiencies and monitor oral coagulation therapy?
   a. Activated partial thromboplastin time
   b. Prothrombin time
   c. Quantitative factor assay
   d. Stypven time test (Russell's viper venom time test)

5. Which test does not measure defects in intrinsic or extrinsic pathways and is affected by the levels of fibrinogen and dysfibrinogenemia, as well as the presence of circulating anticoagulants?
   a. Thrombin time
   b. Prothrombin consumption test
   c. Reptilase time
   d. Fibrinogen

6. Which of the following conditions would show a short clotting time, indicating high fibrinogen levels?
   a. Disseminated intravascular coagulation
   b. Liver disease
   c. Pregnancy
   d. Fibrinolysis

7. Which condition would most likely show a decrease in factor VIII antigen?
   a. Hemophilia
   b. Female carriers of hemophilia A
   c. Myeloproliferative syndrome
   d. von Willebrand's disease

8. Which APTT result would indicate the presence of a strong circulating anticoagulant?
   a. APTT not corrected by the addition of normal plasma
   b. Prolonged APTT (more than 1 h)
   c. APTT corrected by the addition of normal plasma
   d. Any of the above results

9. Which of the following are criteria for the laboratory detection of lupus inhibitors?
   a. Abnormal APTT and/or PT
   b. Demonstration that an abnormal APTT/PT is due to inhibitors
   c. Proof that the inhibitor is directed against phospholipids
   d. All of the above

10. Which test result, using the FDPs test, would be indicative of a patient having DIC? (Assume fibrinogen concentration is indicative of DIC.)
   a. Positive FDP test result; increased PT and APTT; decreased platelet count
   b. Positive FDP test result; decreased PT and APTT; increased platelet count
   c. Negative FDP test result; increased PT, decreased APTT; decreased platelet count
   d. Negative FDP test result; decreased PT, increased APTT; increased platelet count

ANSWERS

1. **d** (p 658)
2. **c** (p 660)
3. **a** (pp 662–663)
4. **b** (p 663)
5. **a** (p 665)
6. **c** (p 667)
7. **d** (p 670)
8. **a** (p 675)
9. **d** (p 675)
10. **a** (p 677)

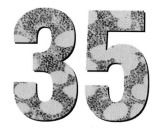

Molecular Diagnostic Techniques in Hematopathology

Margaret L. Gulley, MD

Objectives

At the end of this chapter, the learner should be able to:
1 Describe the fundamental structure of DNA.
2 Define *nucleic acid probe.*
3 List the most commonly used molecular diagnostic assays and state the purpose of each assay.
4 Describe a potential clinical application of each diagnostic test.
5 Interpret a Southern blot result.

Deoxyribonucleic acid (DNA) is the inherited substance that encodes all the information needed for cell structure and function. For this information to be expressed, it must be transmitted through an intermediary substance called ribonucleic acid (RNA). DNA and RNA are collectively called *nucleic acid.* Analysis of nucleic acid in patient samples forms the foundation for a new field of laboratory medicine called *molecular diagnostics.* In no other discipline of laboratory medicine has this technology had a greater impact than in hematology, where it is used to assist in the diagnosis of certain inherited, infectious, and malignant forms of hematologic diseases.

The laboratory methods most commonly implemented in clinical settings are Southern blot analysis,

polymerase chain reaction (PCR), and in situ hybridization. To understand how each of these methods is used, we must first review the structure of DNA and RNA. A glossary at the end of this textbook provides definitions of the new terms.

STRUCTURE OF DNA

Human DNA is packaged into 46 chromosomes, each of which is an exceptionally large molecule formed from two very long strands of nucleotides. If all 46 chromosomes were aligned end to end, they would be 3 billion nucleotide pairs long and would stretch for over 2 meters. Inside each nucleus, the DNA strands

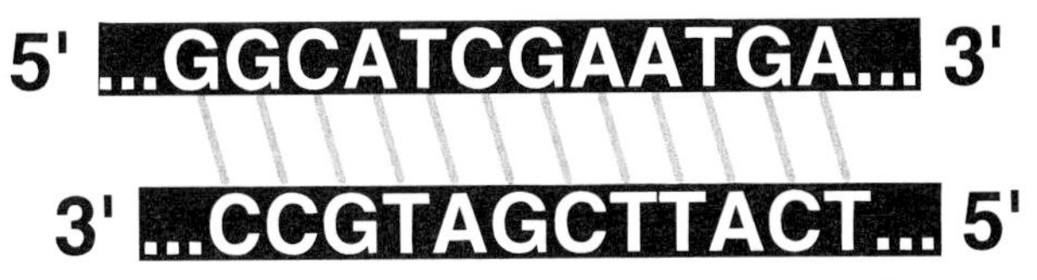

5' ▮▮...GGCATCGAATGA...▮▮ 3'

3' ▮▮...CCGTAGCTTACT...▮▮ 5'

FIGURE 35–1   DNA is composed of two strands of nucleotides that are bound to each other through hydrogen bonds (depicted as diagonal bridges). Only four types of nucleotides are present, adenine (A), thymine (T), guanine (G), and cytosine (C). Because of the characteristic biochemical structure of each nucleotide, and A on one strand can bond only to T on the other strand, and G can bond only to C. Therefore, the two strands of DNA are said to be "complementary" to each other. The strands are oriented in opposite directions with respect to the sugar and phosphate groups that link adjacent nucleotides; thus each strand has a 5' and a 3' end.

are tightly coiled around histone proteins to form chromatin. Within these long strands of nucleotides is encoded all of the information necessary for life.

Nucleotides are the basic building blocks of DNA, and they are composed of one of four different types of nitrogenous bases—adenine, guanine, thymine, or cytosine—attached to a deoxyribose sugar and phosphate moiety. The two strands of nucleotides that combine to form DNA are bound together by hydrogen bonds that form between the nucleotides on one strand and those on the opposite strand. According to the rules of complementary nucleotide pairing, an adenine in one strand can bond only with a thymine in the other strand, and guanine can bond only with cytosine. For this reason, the two strands of DNA are said to complement each other (Fig. 35–1).

Encoded within the nucleotide sequences of DNA are functional units called *genes* that serve as templates for RNA transcription and ultimately protein translation. Although all nucleated cells contain a full complement of DNA constituting that person's genome, each cell expresses only a fraction of the estimated 100,000 different genes, depending on its cell type and stage of differentiation. Gene expression results in the production of RNA, a molecule that resembles DNA except that it is single-stranded, contains ribose instead of deoxyribose, and substitutes uracil for thymine.

Recent advances in our understanding of the genetic basis of disease have led to the development of laboratory tests targeting DNA or RNA in patient samples. All current molecular diagnostic tests are based on our ability to identify a specific nucleotide sequence in DNA or RNA by using a "probe" that targets that sequence. A probe is simply a single-stranded segment of nucleic acid (either DNA or RNA) whose nucleotide sequence is complementary to the target sequence (either DNA or RNA). A probe binds to its target through a process called *hybridization*. Hybridization is usually accomplished by combining probe and target in a small tube (liquid phase) or on a membrane or glass slide (solid phase). In either case, the probe has usually been prelabeled so that it can be subsequently detected and used as a marker for the target sequence (Fig. 35–2).

APPLICATIONS OF DNA TECHNOLOGY TO DIAGNOSTIC MEDICINE

DNA technology is potentially useful in diagnosing all diseases resulting from altered DNA. These include inherited diseases, which by definition have a genetic basis, and infectious diseases in which the identification of foreign DNA or RNA indicates that a pathogen is present. Table 35–1 provides a list of inherited and infectious diseases that commonly affect the hematopoietic system and for which probe assays have been developed.

DNA technology can also be used to help diagnose and classify various types of cancer. This is because virtually all cancers harbor genetic defects that are responsible for malignant transformation. A gene whose alteration is responsible for cancer formation is called on *oncogene*. Table 35–2 lists the known oncogenes related to hematopoietic cancers. Laboratory detection of cancer-associated genetic defects not only contributes to improved diagnosis of affected patients, but in some cases may also help determine the most appropriate treatment or help monitor the response to treatment.

Each of the diagnostic applications mentioned above relies on prior basic and clinical research that has de-

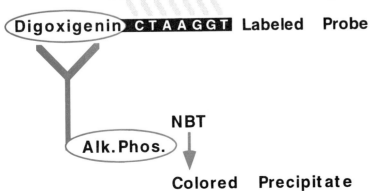

...G A T T C C A G A T G... **Target   Sequence**

Digoxigenin C T A A G G T **Labeled   Probe**

NBT

Alk. Phos.

Colored   Precipitate

FIGURE 35–2   In the laboratory, the two strands of DNA may be dissociated from one another by heating them to 95°C or treating them with a strong alkaline solution (high pH). Once separated, a strand can then bind (or "hybridize") to a probe of complementary nucleotide sequence. In the example depicted here, the probe was labeled with digoxigenin so that it could be subsequently detected by a colorimetric reaction involving alkaline phosphatase and 4-nitroblue tetrazolium chloride (NBT).

TABLE 35-1 Hematologic Diseases Amenable to Molecular Assays

Genetic Diseases

Gaucher disease

Hemoglobinopathies (sickle cell anemia, α and β thalassemias)[1-3]

Glucose-6-phosphate dehydrogenase deficiency

Bleeding and thrombotic disorders (various factor deficiencies, Bernard-Soulier syndrome, platelet storage pool deficiency, von Willebrand disease, and APC resistance)[4]

Immunodeficiency states (deficiencies of adenosine deaminase, purine nucleoside phosphorylase, and leukocyte adhesion, DiGeorge and Wiskott-Aldrich syndromes, chronic granulomatous disease)

Porphyrias

Red cell membrane defects including hereditary spherocytosis and elliptocytosis, and paroxysmal nocturnal hemoglobinuria

Infectious Diseases

Epstein-Barr virus (EBV)[5]

Cytomegalovirus (CMV)

Human immunodeficiency virus (HIV)

Human T-lymphotropic virus type 1 (HTLV1)[6]

Malaria

Mycobacteria

Mycoplasma

Parvovirus B19

Toxoplasma

APC = activated protein C

fined disease-specific genetic alterations and established molecular probe assays to detect those alterations. In the remainder of this chapter, we will review each of the most commonly used molecular diagnostic procedures. Readers desiring further information on the equipment, reagents, or step-by-step procedures are referred to one of several detailed protocol manuals.[7-10] Examples of applications of these methods are found throughout this text and in several excellent references.[8,9,11-17]

SAMPLE SOURCES FOR MOLECULAR PROCEDURES

Intact DNA is usually well preserved in tissues that are frozen within an hour of collection, and in blood samples that are less than 2 days old. One of the best tissue fixatives for preserving intact DNA is ethanol. Unfortunately, the more commonly used formalin fixation causes strand breakage that interferes with certain molecular assays. The optimal specimen for each type of molecular assay is listed under the description of each assay below.

Fortunately, DNA is a very stable molecule. For example, fragments of DNA have been recovered from fossils, skeletal remains, and bodies that were mummified thousands of years ago. Nevertheless, specimens submitted to clinical laboratories for molecular genetic assays should be handled with care to preserve intact DNA. This is particularly true for samples to be

analyzed by the Southern blot technique in which prior "degradation" (i.e., nonspecific fragmentation) of the DNA invalidates the results.

Unlike DNA, RNA is unstable because it is so easily degraded by ubiquitous natural enzymes collectively termed *RNase*. Therefore, special handling (described below) is required to preserve RNA in clinical samples.

NUCLEIC ACID EXTRACTION

Preparation of Samples

DNA or RNA is readily extracted from blood, marrow, body fluid cells, and tissue samples. In preparation for extraction of DNA from blood samples, nucleated blood cells are separated from the more abundant red cells by centrifugation in a ficoll gradient. Only the nucleated cells are retained for subsequent DNA extraction, whereas the red cells and platelets are discarded because they have no nucleus and hence contain no DNA.

In contrast to blood specimens, solid tissue specimens contain relatively few red cells, so enrichment procedures are not required. Instead, frozen tissues are finely minced, whereas paraffin-embedded tissues are sliced with an instrument called a microtome before nucleic acid extraction.

DNA Extraction from Fresh Cells or Frozen Tissue

DNA can be separated from all of the protein and lipids that compose cells by an organic chemical extraction procedure. This procedure is based on the fact that DNA is soluble in water, whereas lipids and protein are not easily dissolved in water. First, however, the patient cells are treated with detergent and proteinase enzymes to lyse their membranes and degrade their proteins. Then the organic chemical phenol is added to the cellular lysate. On centrifugation, lipids migrate to the phenol fraction at the bottom of the tube, while DNA remains in the aqueous fraction on top and protein byproducts collect at the interface between the two layers. The DNA that is preferentially isolated to the upper aqueous layer is simply pipetted into a fresh tube, where it is subsequently concentrated and further purified by precipitating it in a cold mixture of salt and ethanol. The DNA is then recovered by either spooling the long strands onto a stick or centrifuging the precipitated DNA and pouring off the supernatant. Finally, the DNA is resuspended in water and stored at 4°C for up to 1 month or at −20°C indefinitely.

Commercial kits and semiautomated instruments are now available to facilitate extraction of DNA from blood or other tissues. The resultant DNA can then be quantitated (see below) and analyzed by various molecular laboratory assays. Some assays, such as Southern blot analyses, require relatively pure and intact DNA that is largely free of protein contaminants, since such contaminants tend to inhibit restriction enzyme digestion. Other assays such as PCR can be performed on DNA that is only crudely purified or even partially degraded.

TABLE 35–2	**Genetic Abnormalities in Hematopoietic Cancers**	
Tumor Type	**Karyotype**	**Genes***
Myeloid leukemias		
Chronic myelogenous leukemia[18–22]	t(9;22)	ABL/BCR
Acute non-lymphocytic (ANLL)	t(6;9)	DEK or SET/CAN
ANLL-M1 or M2	t(8;21)	ETO/AML1
ANLL-M4eo	inv(16)	MYH11/CBFβ
ANLL-M3[23,24]	t(15;17)	PML/RARα
ANLL	t(16;21)	FUS/ERG
Chronic myelomonocytic leukemia	t(5;12)	PDGFRβ/TEL
B-cell leukemias		
Acute lymphoblastic leukemia (ALL)[25]	t(9;22)	ABL/BCR
Pre-B ALL	t(1;19)	PBX1/E2A
Pre-B ALL	t(17;19)	HLF/E2A
Pre-B ALL	t(5;14)	IL3/IgH
ALL or mixed lineage leukemia	t(various;11)	various/MLL=ALL1
Chronic lymphocytic leukemia	t(14;19)	IgH/bcl3
B-cell lymphomas[26]		
Burkitt's lymphoma[27]	t(8;14,2 or 22)	myc/IgH, Igκ, or Igλ
Mantle cell lymphoma[28,29]	t(11;14)	bcl1/IgH
Follicular lymphoma[30–32]	t(14;18)	IgH/bcl2
Diffuse large cell lymphoma	t(3;14)	bcl6/IgH
Lymphoma	t(11;14)	RCK/IgH
Lymphoma	t(10;14)	LYT-10/IgH
T-cell leukemias/lymphomas[26]		
	t(8;14)	myc/TCRαδ
	t(1;7 or 14)	SCL=TAL1 or LCK/TCRαδ or β
	(7;9)	TCRβ/TAL2
	t(7;19)	TCRβ/LYL1
	t(7;14)	TCRβ/tcl1
	t(7;9)	TCRβ/TAN1
	inv(7)	TCRβ/TCRγ
	t(11;14)	RBTN1=TTG1/TCRαδ
	t(11;7 or 14)	RBTN2=TTG2/TCRαδ or β
	t(10;7 or 14)	HOX11/TCRαδ or β
Anaplastic large cell lymphoma	t(2;5)	NPM/ALK

*In each case, the order of the genes corresponds to the order of the karyotype.

DNA Extraction from Paraffin-Embedded Tissue

First, a single 10-μm paraffin section is cut on a microtome and stuffed into a microfuge tube. Since paraffin can inhibit subsequent enzymatic reactions, some users trim excess paraffin from the block before sectioning. The resultant tissue section is typically submerged in octane to dissolve the paraffin, then washed with ethanol, dried, and incubated in a proteinase enzyme solution that degrades cellular proteins. The proteinase is subsequently heat-inactivated so that it will not interfere with future enzymatic reactions.

In nearly all cases, the DNA extracted from paraffin tissues will subsequently be used in an amplification assay such as PCR, and therefore precautions are needed to avoid contamination of the section with extraneous DNA during the histologic sectioning process. These precautions include:

1. Wear gloves. Before beginning, wipe down all work surfaces with 10% bleach to destroy any extraneous nucleic acid.

2. Change the microtome blade between cases so that minute amounts of tissue are not carried over to the next case.

3. Use a smooth-edged forceps to transfer the section into the microfuge tube. Between cases, wipe the forceps with 10% bleach, then rinse and dry it with clean absorbent gauze.

4. Do not allow bleach to contact the tissue to be analyzed since it could destroy the nucleic acid.

5. Consider interspersing "control" blocks among the cases to evaluate for contamination by extraneous DNA.

RNA Extraction

RNA can be extracted from cells by treating them with guanidine thiocyanate, a chemical that disrupts cellular membranes and also inhibits endogenous RNase activity. RNA is separated from cellular lipids and proteins by the same organic extraction technique described to isolate DNA. RNA is then further purified and concentrated by precipitation in isopropanol followed by centrifugation. The final product is resuspended in water and stored at −70°C pending further analysis.

Because RNase enzymes are ubiquitous, special precautions are required to diminish RNA degradation by such enzymes before probe analysis. In particular, gloves should be worn and all solutions and plasticware should be RNase-free. Dedicated laboratory areas and reagents are recommended.

NUCLEIC ACID QUANTITATION

DNA and RNA are quantitated by spectrophotometry, which relies on the fact that nucleic acids absorb ultraviolet light of optical density (OD) 260 nm, whereas proteins absorb at OD280. Quantity is estimated using the following formulas, which are based on the concept that an OD260 of 1 corresponds to 50 μg/mL of DNA, 40 μg/mL of RNA, or 20 μg/mL of a single stranded oligonucleotide:

$$\text{Double-stranded DNA concentration } (\mu\text{g/uL}) = \text{OD260} \times 0.05$$

$$\text{RNA concentration } (\mu\text{g/uL}) = \text{OD260} \times 0.04$$

$$\text{Single-stranded oligonucleotide concentration } (\mu\text{g/uL}) = \text{OD260} \times 0.02$$

Most commonly, a small aliquot of the unknown sample is diluted with water before spectrophotometry, so the dilution factor must be taken into account to arrive at the concentration in the original sample.

Protein contamination of a DNA sample is assessed by calculating a ratio of OD260/OD280. The expected ratio is between 1.7 and 1.8 for DNA, and 1.9 to 2.0 for RNA. A ratio below 1.7 suggests the need for repeated organic extraction to remove impurities (usually proteins) that may interfere with restriction enzyme digestion of DNA.

Alternatively, DNA can be quantitated using either (1) a fluorometer instrument that relies on the binding of Hoechst 33258 dye, or (2) electrophoresis and staining of a "yield gel" whereby lanes containing sample DNA are compared with lanes containing standard amounts of DNA. The DNA in these gels is visualized by staining with ethidium bromide, a chemical that intercalates into the DNA strands and fluoresces when exposed to ultraviolet light. Each of these techniques is suitable for quantitating very small volumes of DNA but, unlike in the spectrophotometric method, protein contamination is not assessed.

SEQUENCE-SPECIFIC FRAGMENTATION OF DNA BY RESTRICTION ENDONUCLEASES

One of the most important breakthroughs in our ability to manipulate DNA in the laboratory came with the discovery of naturally occurring enzymes that chop DNA into small fragments. An important feature of these enzymes is that they cut only at specific sequence-recognition sites. These enzymes are normally produced by bacteria as a means of defending the bacteria from foreign pathogens like bacteriophages. The ability to reproducibly cleave DNA into smaller fragments simplifies laboratory handling of an otherwise excessively large molecule.

In clinical laboratories, the enzymes most commonly used for sequence-specific cleavage of DNA are EcoR1 derived from *Escherichia coli* and recognizing 5'-GAATTC-3', BamH1 derived from *Bacillus amyloliquifaciens* and recognizing 5'-GGATCC-3', and HindIII derived from *Hemophilus influenzae* and recognizing 5'-AAGCTT-3'. Each of these enzymes cuts human DNA into thousands of smaller fragments that can subsequently be separated by size in the Southern blot procedure, or captured in vectors to produce recombinant DNA. (See "Probe Production" below.)

DIAGNOSTIC PROCEDURES FOR ANALYZING DNA

Southern Blot Analysis

Purpose To analyze the molecular structure of DNA so that disease-specific genetic alterations can be identified.

Procedure DNA is extracted from the tissue sample, cut with restriction endonucleases to produce "restriction fragments," separated by size using gel electrophoresis, and detected with probes complementary to the particular region of interest. If DNA is altered by mutation, translocation, or any other structural change, then the number and/or size of the resulting restriction fragments is altered accordingly (Fig. 35–3). Note that some people use the term *restriction fragment length polymorphism*, or RFLP, as a synonym for the Southern blot method of detecting genetic alterations.

Sample Requirements Frozen tissue, fresh body fluid or frozen cell pellet, blood or marrow. Sufficient DNA is usually obtained from a single tube of blood (7 mL) if the white count is normal or proportionally less blood if the white count is elevated, 1 to 2 mL of marrow, or 2 mm^3 of tissue or pelleted cells from a body fluid. Ethylenediaminetetraacetic acid (EDTA) anticoagulant is preferred over heparin because heparin inhibits the action of restriction endonucleases.

Assay Time Approximately 1 week

Sensitivity Moderate (about 1 target per 20 cells, or 5%)

Specificity High

Cost per Test Approximately $300 if only one sample is analyzed, less for batched samples

Clinical Applications

1. To detect any disease-specific genetic abnormality that consistently alters the size of a particular restriction fragment. Examples include certain inherited diseases, such as sickle cell anemia, and many types of cancer including hematopoietic neoplasms.[17] A list of cancer-related genetic defects is provided in Table 35–2. Note that B-cell tumors tend to have genetic defects involving

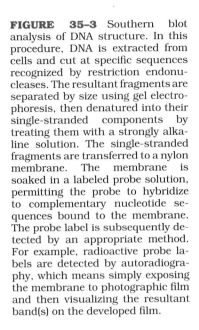

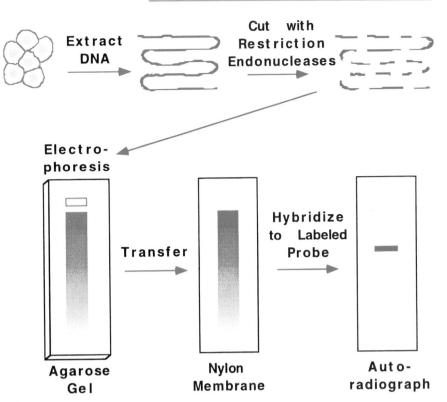

FIGURE 35-3 Southern blot analysis of DNA structure. In this procedure, DNA is extracted from cells and cut at specific sequences recognized by restriction endonucleases. The resultant fragments are separated by size using gel electrophoresis, then denatured into their single-stranded components by treating them with a strongly alkaline solution. The single-stranded fragments are transferred to a nylon membrane. The membrane is soaked in a labeled probe solution, permitting the probe to hybridize to complementary nucleotide sequences bound to the membrane. The probe label is subsequently detected by an appropriate method. For example, radioactive probe labels are detected by autoradiography, which means simply exposing the membrane to photographic film and then visualizing the resultant band(s) on the developed film.

their immunoglobulin genes, whereas T-cell tumors have defects of their T-cell receptor genes. Lymphoid tumors are thought to arise as a result of errors occurring during physiologic rearrangement of these antigen receptor genes.

2. To detect clonal rearrangement of immunoglobulin or T-cell receptor gene rearrangements in lymphoid leukemias and lymphomas.[26,33-38] This helps distinguish lymphoid neoplasms from reactive lymphoid hyperplasia, and can also be used to determine the B- versus T-cell lineage of lymphoid tumors. As a rule, B-cell tumors, including leukemias and lymphomas, exhibit clonal rearrangement of the immunoglobulin heavy-chain gene. In most cases, these B-cell tumors also exhibit coexistent clonal rearrangement of the kappa light-chain gene regardless of whether they express kappa or lambda light-chain protein. T-cell tumors usually exhibit clonal rearrangement of the T-cell receptor beta gene. In contrast, no clonal gene rearrangement is found in reactive lymphoid hyperplasia[35] (Fig. 35-4).

3. To quantitate gene amplifications associated with certain tumors, such as n-myc gene amplification associated with neuroblastoma.

4. To detect foreign DNA associated with infectious diseases, so long as the foreign DNA is relatively abundant (at least 1 target per 20 cells).

5. To detect DNA polymorphisms in forensic or paternity assays.[39]

6. To confirm the size or origin of PCR products, or to detect disease-specific genetic alterations in those products. For example, the point mutation

responsible for sickle cell anemia may be detected by a Southern blot assay or by Southern blot analysis of a PCR product.

Major Advantage   It is the most accurate method for detecting gene rearrangements in lymphoid leukemias and lymphomas.

Major Disadvantages

1. Sensitivity is relatively low. For example, tumors composing less than 5% of a tissue sample are frequently undetectable. (Controls run simultaneously with patient samples can be used to evaluate the sensitivity of each Southern blot assay.)

2. Labor-intensive and therefore costly.

3. Relatively long turn-around time.

4. Requires fresh or frozen tissue, and is not amenable to formalin-fixed tissue.

Potential Pitfalls

1. Sample DNA must be intact before beginning the Southern blot procedure. Intact DNA is characterized by very long strands of clear gel-like material that can be spooled onto a collection stick. In contrast, degraded DNA does not spool well because it is already fragmented, which confounds our ability to visualize and interpret bands on Southern blots. It should also be noted that intact DNA is difficult to pipet, whereas degraded DNA pipets easily. Nevertheless, pipetting of genomic DNA should be kept to a minimum because the shear stresses generated by pipetting contribute to fragmentation.

2. In the next step of Southern analysis, it is essential that restriction endonuclease digestion be al-

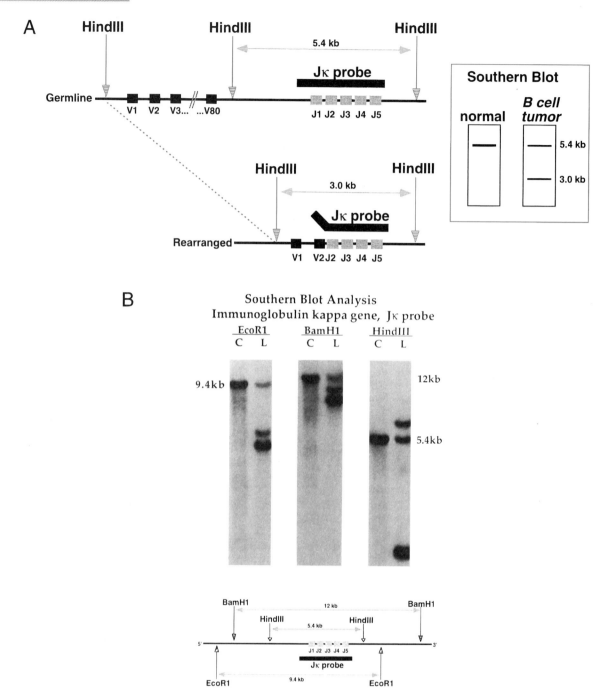

FIGURE 35–4 (A) Southern blot analysis can be used to identify B-cell tumors based on their characteristic clonal immunoglobulin gene rearrangements. Normally, during B-cell differentiation, the immunoglobulin kappa light-chain gene (Igκ) rearranges to produce a unique coding sequence that determines antibody specificity. This occurs through a process of splicing and deletion whereby 1 of 80 variable (V) regions is juxtaposed with 1 of 5 joining (J) regions. These rearrangements alter the size of the DNA fragments produced by the HindIII restriction endonuclease and recognized by hybridization to a probe (shown as a bar) spanning the Jκ region. Whereas each benign B cell rearranges its kappa gene differently, malignant B cells contain exactly the same rearrangement that was present in the B cell from which the tumor arose. This clonal gene rearrangement alters the band pattern on the Southern blot. In addition to the 3.0kb rearranged band that characterizes the particular rearrangement depicted here, there is also partial retention of the 5.4kb unrearranged (germline) Igκ gene originating from residual normal cells in the sample or from the other Igκ allele in tumor cells. (B) In the actual Southern blot autoradiograph shown here, the Jκ probe was used to detect clonal Igκ gene rearrangement in a case of chronic lymphocytic leukemia (L). In each of three different restriction endonuclease digests, the presence of two extra bands suggests that both Igκ alleles are clonally rearranged in the tumor cells or, less likely, that the tumor is biclonal. Normal control (C) tissue analyzed simultaneously identifies the position of the germline bands. A map of the Jκ region depicts the expected size of the germline bands for each restriction endonuclease.

lowed to proceed to completion. A reasonable way to evaluate the completeness of enzymatic digestion (and the degree of DNA degradation) is to examine the size distribution of DNA fragments in the agarose gel that is prepared during Southern analysis. These fragments may be visualized and photographed after staining them with ethidium bromide. Good-quality digestions are characterized by a graded distribution of fragment sizes as depicted in Figure 35–3. In contrast, incomplete digestions exhibit an excess of large fragments, whereas degraded DNA exhibits an excess of small fragments.

3. Beware of "polymorphisms." Users should be aware that DNA polymorphisms can confound the proper interpretation of Southern blot results. We define polymorphisms as natural differences in nucleotide sequence that distinguish one person's DNA from another's. In fact, every person's DNA is unique, except for that of identical twins. On average, polymorphisms occur at a rate of about 1 in every 500 nucleotide pairs. Polymorphisms can be exploited as a means of establishing identity for forensic purposes, so-called DNA fingerprinting.[39] On the other hand, polymorphisms can also interfere with molecular tests for disease-associated genetic defects. For example, a polymorphism occurring at the site where a restriction enzyme normally cleaves DNA could result in altered band sizes on the resultant Southern blot that might mimic a disease-specific structural abnormality. To overcome this pitfall, it is prudent to confirm the low polymorphism rate at the disease-related locus being examined and to design additional confirmatory tests when feasible. For example, multiple separate restriction enzyme digestions are often used to establish the likelihood that an altered band pattern on a Southern blot results from a tumor-associated genetic alteration as opposed to a simple base substitution at one restriction enzyme recognition site.[34] Alternatively, a tumor sample could be compared to normal tissue from the same patient to identify tumor-specific genetic defects.

Polymerase Chain Reaction

Introduction Polymerase chain reaction (PCR) is one of several methods for amplifying (i.e., copying) particular segments of DNA.[40] Since PCR was the first amplification method to be invented and the first to be introduced into clinical laboratories, it will be described in detail. A review article by Weidbrauk describes several other related methods of DNA amplification.[41]

Purpose To amplify target DNA a billionfold so that it may be more easily detected or further analyzed for disease-specific genetic alterations. PCR works by enzymatically replicating one particular segment of DNA from amidst all the DNA in a patient's sample. Segments as long as 40,000 base pairs (bp) have been amplified in research laboratories, but a more realistic limit in clinical samples is about 5000 bp, or even less (about 500 bp) if the DNA was extracted from fixed paraffin-embedded tissue.

Procedure DNA is isolated from the sample and mixed with: (1) an enzyme called DNA polymerase that copies DNA by converting single-stranded into double-stranded DNA; (2) short probes that flank the target sequence and serve as primers for the initiation of DNA replication by the polymerase; and (3) the building blocks (dATP, dGTP, dCTP and dTTP) needed for generating new DNA strands. The enzymatic reaction takes place in a thermocycler instrument programmed to sequentially vary the temperature of the reaction mixture so that progressive cycles of DNA replication can occur. After about 30 cycles, which takes only a few hours, about a billion copies of the target DNA are generated (Fig. 35–5). The reaction product is easily identified as a band on gel electrophoresis. Hybridization to an internal probe is an alternate method of detecting the product and moreover confirming its origin. The PCR product can then be further tested for a disease-specific genetic alteration, if appropriate.

Note: The DNA polymerase used in PCR reactions is "thermostable." This means that, unlike DNA polymerases found in mammalian cells, the polymerase used in PCR reactions can sustain near-boiling temperatures and still remain active. It is this feature that allows the PCR reaction to continue through multiple heat cycles without loss of enzyme function. Thermostable polymerase is derived from bacterial species such as *Thermus aquaticus* ("Taq") that have adapted to survive in geysers or hot pools.

Sample Requirements Fresh, frozen, fixed, or paraffin-embedded tissue, blood, marrow, or body fluid. Although several investigators have reported performing successful PCR reactions on single cells, most clinical assays rely on sample sizes of at least a million cells. Recommended minimum sample volumes are 1 mL of blood, 0.5 mL of marrow, or 0.5 mm^3 of tissue. PCR has been successfully applied to needle biopsy specimens and even cerebrospinal fluid. Although formalin fixation results in strand breakage, PCR frequently succeeds in amplifying DNA segments up to several hundred base pairs in length from formalin-fixed, paraffin-embedded tissue because only one intact target sequence is required for the reaction to proceed.

Assay Time Approximately 1 day to generate and detect reaction product; further testing of the reaction product requires additional time.

Sensitivity High. Theoretically, one target is sufficient. In practice, amplification of one target per 10^5 cells is typically achieved.

Specificity High.

Cost per Test Approximately $100 if only one sample is analyzed, less if samples are batched, more if further testing of the PCR product is required.

Clinical Applications

1. Detect foreign nucleic acid characteristic of infectious diseases. In some cases, further epidemiologic or drug susceptibility studies can be done to characterize the pathogen.
2. Selectively amplify DNA that has a particular disease-associated defect, such as the point mutation characteristic of sickle cell anemia, or the bcl2/JH translocation characteristic of follicular lymphoma, among others.

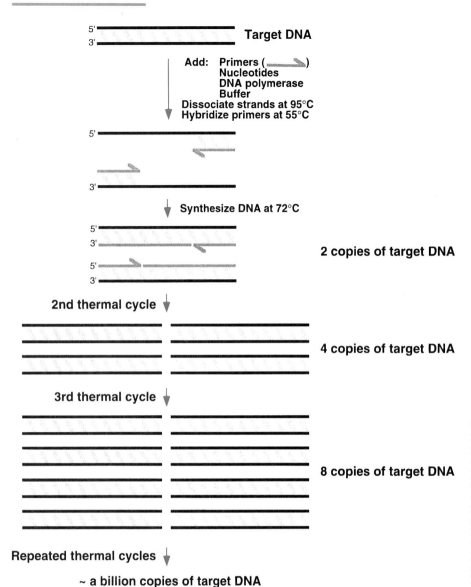

5' ▬▬▬▬▬▬▬▬▬▬▬▬
3' ▬▬▬▬▬▬▬▬▬▬▬▬ **Target DNA**

Add: Primers (▬▬▷)
Nucleotides
DNA polymerase
Buffer
Dissociate strands at 95°C
Hybridize primers at 55°C

Synthesize DNA at 72°C

2 copies of target DNA

2nd thermal cycle

4 copies of target DNA

3rd thermal cycle

8 copies of target DNA

Repeated thermal cycles

~ a billion copies of target DNA

FIGURE 35–5 Polymerase chain reaction is a method of copying a particular segment of DNA numerous times through a process of repeated cycles of heating, cooling, and DNA synthesis. To accomplish this, the target DNA is mixed with two short DNA probes called primers (shown as half-arrows) that are designed to span the segment of DNA to be amplified. Also added to the sample is an enzyme called DNA polymerase, which converts single-stranded DNA into double-stranded DNA by incorporating nucleotides starting at the 3′ end of each primer. A thermocycler instrument is programmed to sequentially heat and cool the sample. In each heat/cool cycle, the sample is first heated to 95°C to dissociate the two strands of DNA, and then cooled to 55°C to permit binding of the primers, then warmed to 72°C for enzymatic DNA replication. After the first cycle, an exact copy of the original target DNA has been produced. Then, in subsequent cycles, the products of previous cycles can serve as templates for DNA replication, permitting an exponential accumulation of DNA copies. After 30 cycles, which takes only a couple of hours, approximately a billion copies of the target DNA have been synthesized.

3. Detect minimal residual disease in cancer patients following therapy by using PCR to amplify the tumor-specific molecular defect. Such an approach has been used to predict relapse of follicular lymphoma before there is clinical or morphological evidence that residual tumor is still present.[31]
4. Detect clonal immunoglobulin or T-cell receptor gene rearrangements by using primer sets that span rearranged gene segments.[42–46] Current protocols detect clonality in about 80% of B-cell neoplasms (compared to 100% by Southern analysis). A substantial fraction of clonal T-cell receptor gene rearrangements can also be detected by PCR, but further studies are needed to confirm clinical utility in comparison with Southern analysis.

Major Advantages

1. Extremely sensitive to low numbers of target sequences.
2. Small sample size requirements.
3. Relatively fast and inexpensive unless extensive postamplification analysis is required.
4. Permits analysis of formalin-fixed, paraffin-embedded tissue that is not suitable for Southern blot analysis.

Major Disadvantage

1. Extreme precautions required to avoid contamination of samples or reagents by extraneous DNA.[47,48] Contamination by the abundant products generated from previous PCR reactions is a worrisome problem.

Reverse Transcriptase Polymerase Chain Reaction

Purpose The purpose of reverse transcriptase polymerase chain reaction (rtPCR) is to detect RNA in patient specimens (1) so that expression of a particular

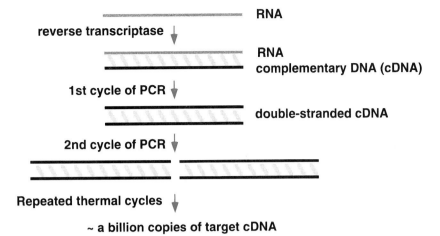

reverse transcriptase — RNA

RNA
complementary DNA (cDNA)

1st cycle of PCR — double-stranded cDNA

2nd cycle of PCR

Repeated thermal cycles

~ a billion copies of target cDNA

FIGURE 35–6   The rtPCR procedure is a method for detecting a particular RNA transcript. First, RNA serves as a template for construction of complementary DNA (cDNA) by the enzyme reverse transcriptase. Then routine PCR is done to convert the cDNA of interest to a double-stranded sequence and to amplify that sequence so that it may be readily detected or further analyzed. This procedure is a sensitive, specific, and rapid means of amplifying disease-associated RNA in a patient sample.

gene can be monitored, (2) so that an RNA virus can be identified, or (3) because RNA presents a better target for the detection of a particular disease-related sequence than does the DNA from which it was encoded.

Procedure   RNA is extracted from tissue and converted to complementary DNA (cDNA) using the enzyme reverse transcriptase in the presence of deoxyribonucleotides and primers. After cDNA production, conventional PCR is carried out to amplify the cDNA sequence of interest (Fig. 35–6).

The primers used in the reverse transcriptase step function to initiate enzymatic production of cDNA from an RNA template. If these primers are random hexamers, the resultant cDNA represents all of the various RNAs in the sample, whereas a sequence-specific primer can be used to target the RNA species of interest.

Sample Requirements   Fresh blood, marrow, body fluid, or solid tissue. Because RNA is easily degraded, samples should be processed as soon as possible after collection. If RNA extraction cannot be performed immediately, the tissue or nucleated cell pellets should be stored in a sterile, sealed container at −70°C until analysis. Some laboratories have reported successful rtPCR of fixed, paraffin-embedded tissue. Serum and plasma samples have been used in rtPCR detection of RNA viruses such as hepatitis C virus.

Assay Time   Approximately 2 days.

Sensitivity   High. (Theoretically, one target is sufficient.)

Specificity   High.

Cost per Test   Approximately $150 if only one sample is analyzed, less for batched samples.

Clinical Applications

1. Determine expression of selected genes by targeting their corresponding RNA transcripts, for example, oncogenes overexpressed in tumor samples. When used to evaluate gene expression, it is wise to design PCR primers that flank transcript splice sites and thus permit distinction of cDNA from native DNA.
2. Detect certain disease-specific chromosomal translocations where RNA is transcribed across the translocation breakpoint. In many instances, breakpoint cluster regions identified at the DNA level are further clustered by the natural process of RNA splicing, thus simplifying detection of the translocation event. Examples of fusion transcripts that are amenable to rtPCR analysis include PML/RARα, t(15;17); bcr/abl, t(9;22); AML1/ETO t(8;21); NPM/ALK, t(2;5); MLL/AF-4, t(4;11); and CBFβ/MYH11, inv16.
3. Detect minimal residual disease in cancer patients following therapy by using rtPCR to amplify tumor-specific fusion transcripts. Such an approach has been used to predict relapse of chronic myelogenous leukemia or acute promyelocytic leukemia (ANLL-M3).[22,24]
4. Detect foreign organisms using probes targeting abundantly transcribed sequences or targeting viruses having RNA genomes. Examples of RNA viruses include human immunodeficiency virus (HIV), human T-lymphotropic virus type 1 (HTLV1), and hepatitis C virus (HCV).

Major Advantages

1. Sensitive to low numbers of target sequences.
2. Small sample size requirements compared to Northern blot analysis. (Northern blot analysis is an old and laborious technique for characterizing specific RNA molecules. In the Northern procedure, cellular RNA is electrophoresed, transferred to a membrane, and then hybridized to a complementary probe. This process is analogous to Southern blotting except that restriction enzyme digestion is not necessary since RNA is much smaller than genomic DNA. The Southern technique was first described by Dr. Edwin Southern,[49] and the term "Northern" is a pun on his name.)

Major Disadvantages

1. RNA is labile and therefore all RNA-based testing requires meticulous care to avoid degradation by RNases.
2. Extreme precautions are required to avoid contamination of samples or reagents by extraneous RNA, cDNA, or products of previous reactions.

In Situ Hybridization to Cells or Tissues Immobilized on Glass Slides

Purpose To localize DNA or RNA to particular cells in a tissue section immobilized on a glass slide.

Procedure Cells or tissue sections are immobilized on glass slides that have been treated to promote adherence, for example, Silane-coated slides. Fresh cells or frozen sections are then fixed by immersion in 95% ethanol, whereas paraffin sections are immersed in xylene to diminish the amount of paraffin. Next, protease treatment permeabilizes cell membranes, allowing the target DNA or RNA to be more accessible for hybridization. A hybridization mixture is applied that contains labeled probes (20 to 2000 bases in length) complementary to the sequence of interest. The slides are incubated for several hours at a temperature that optimizes specific hybridization of probe to target. Bound probe is then detected using an appropriate signal detection method. Counterstaining permits microscopic visualization of the target nucleic acid in the context of histologic features and cytologic detail (Fig. 35–7).

Sample Requirements Fresh blood, marrow, or body fluid from which nucleated cells have been isolated; frozen tissue; or fixed paraffin-embedded tissue.

Method Variation for Flow Cytometric Analysis In a variation of this technique, fresh cells in suspension are made permeable and then hybridized to a probe complementary to the target sequence. The probe is directly or secondarily labeled with a fluorochrome that fluoresces in response to an input light. The signal can be detected and quantitated by flow cytometry.

Assay Time Approximately 2 days.

Sensitivity Moderate. (Theoretically, one target is sufficient, but in practice most users report difficulty detecting single-copy targets.)

Specificity: High.

Cost per test: Approximately $100 if only one sample is analyzed, less for batched samples.

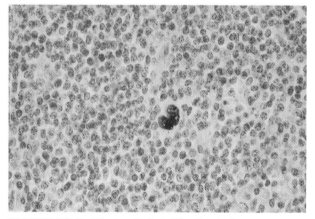

FIGURE 35–7 The in situ hybridization technique permits visualization of nucleic acid in tissue sections on glass slides. In this example, hybridization to Epstein-Barr virus EBER transcripts reveals that the viral gene product is localized to the nucleus of a Reed-Sternberg cell in a case of Hodgkin's disease. In contrast, the background lymphocytes stain only with the methyl green counterstain.

Clinical Applications

1. Determine the disease-related location of foreign organisms. This is especially important for pathogens that might also exist as "normal flora," such as cytomegalovirus or Epstein-Barr virus.
2. Detect and localize gene expression by targeting RNA transcripts.

Major Advantages

1. Permits the visualization of target nucleic acid in the context of cytologic and morphological features.
2. Sensitive to low numbers of affected cells in the sample.
3. Relatively fast results (about 2 days).

Major Disadvantage

1. Difficult to obtain adequate sensitivity for detecting rare targets. The assay works best for high copy number targets such as abundant RNA transcripts (e.g., EBER transcripts of Epstein-Barr virus) or abundant viral genomes (e.g., human papillomavirus in cervical carcinomas).

Fluorescence In Situ Hybridization

Purpose The purpose of fluorescence in situ hybridization (FISH) is to detect and localize specific DNA sequences in G-banded metaphase chromosomes using a probe labeled in such a way that it fluoresces in response to an input light. One option is a double hybridization in which one probe fluoresces green and another probe fluoresces red, thus allowing definitive identification of a particular cytogenetic alteration. Another option is hybridization to multiple probes targeting various loci along a certain chromosome (so-called chromosome painting) to permit evaluation of complex karyotypic alterations involving that chromosome.

Procedure Metaphase spreads of chromosomes are prepared on glass slides using the same methods that are employed in routine karyotyping. The chromosomal DNA is denatured and allowed to hybridize to a labeled probe complementary to the sequence of interest. Unbound probe is washed away, and the bound probe targeting the sequence of interest is visualized under a fluorescence microscope. Counterstaining with 4,6-diamidino-2-phenylindole (DAPI) permits visualization of the chromosomes (Figure 35–8).

Sample Requirements Fresh cells capable of mitosis.

Assay Time Approximately 1 to 2 days.

Sensitivity High (1 target is sufficient).

Specificity High.

Cost per Test Approximately $100 if only one sample is analyzed, less for batched samples. This cost does not include culture, preparation of the metaphase spreads, or karyotyping.

Major Advantage

1. Permits visualization of target DNA in the context of karyotypic visualization of metaphase chromosomes. This is helpful in identifying gross structural alterations that may be difficult to de-

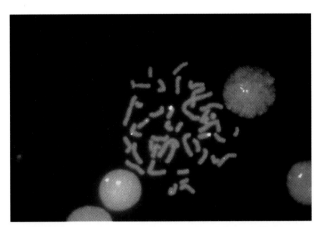

FIGURE 35-8 FISH probe detects the alpha satellite region near the centromere of chromosome 15. Two bright fluorescent signals are seen in the metaphase spread of chromosomes identifying the two number 15 chromosomes. Note that additional fluorescent signals are seen in the three nonmitotic nuclei in this photomicrograph, representing probe that is bound to chromosome 15 inside these intact nuclei. (Photomicrograph courtesy of Charleen Moore, PhD, University of Texas Health Science Center at San Antonio.)

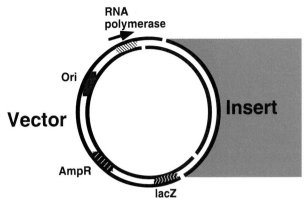

FIGURE 35-9 Vectors are vehicles for capturing and replicating specific DNA sequences. The process of using a vector to capture and manipulate a particular DNA segment is called "recombinant DNA technology." The recombined vector/insert DNA can then be replicated inside bacterial hosts using natural cellular machinery. Specialized features built into the vector assist in tracking and controlling the vector and insert. Examples of vectors include plasmids, bacteriophages, cosmids, and yeast artificial chromosomes, the latter of which can hold extremely large segments of DNA, i.e., 300kb. These vectors permit production of abundant, homogeneous probes.

fine by standard chromosomal G-banding techniques. As an example, DiGeorge syndrome is usually characterized by small deletions of chromosome 22 that can be detected with molecular probes but are difficult to visualize on routinely prepared karyotypes.

Major Disadvantages

1. Metaphase analysis requires live cells capable of entering mitosis.
2. Visualization of fluorochromes requires input light source, and the fluorochrome fades with time.

PROBE PRODUCTION

Where do DNA probes come from? Short DNA probes (less than 40 base pairs) can be synthesized in vitro, and are readily available at reasonable prices from commercial suppliers. Longer probes are usually derived from "cloned" genomic DNA. Cloning is the process by which segments of human DNA are recombined with foreign "vector" DNA to produce "recombinant DNA." Vectors are capable of self-replicating inside bacteria. By culturing bacteria containing vector DNA hitched to a particular DNA segment of interest, one can generate millions of copies of that segment. The DNA segments can then be isolated, labeled, and dissociated into their single-stranded components to form a probe (Fig. 35-9).

An alternate process of generating probes is by amplification strategies such as PCR. In this way, multiple copies of the desired DNA sequence can be generated. These copies can be labeled and dissociated into their single-stranded components to form usable probes.

RNA probes (also known as Riboprobes) are generated from DNA templates in specialized recombinant vectors. These vectors contain transcription initiation start sites that are recognized by RNA polymerase, the enzyme that is responsible for transcribing DNA to RNA. Thousands of RNA probes can be made from a single DNA template. RNA probes can be labeled during their synthesis by incorporating labeled ribonucleotides.

The optimum conditions for specific hybridization of probe to target depend on several factors including the reaction temperature, the concentration of salt and formamide in the hybridization solution, the length of the probe and its proportion of G-C versus A-T bases, and the DNA versus RNA nature of the probe and target. For each hybridization assay, reaction conditions should be optimized so that the probe preferentially binds to its intended target rather than "cross-hybridizing" with partially matched sequences.

PROBE LABELS

To be useful as probes, nucleic acid fragments must be labeled in a way that is detectable following hybridization. Probes can be labeled either during their synthesis by incorporating labeled nucleotides, or at a later time by attaching labels to existing probes. The labels that are most commonly used in clinical laboratories include biotin, digoxigenin, and radioisotopes such as ^{32}P.

Radioisotopes are famous for their remarkable sensitivity. They are detected by either autoradiography or a scintillation counter. Major disadvantages include their short shelf-life, high disposal costs, and the need for strict radiation safety precautions. Nevertheless, many diagnostic laboratories still use radioisotopes,

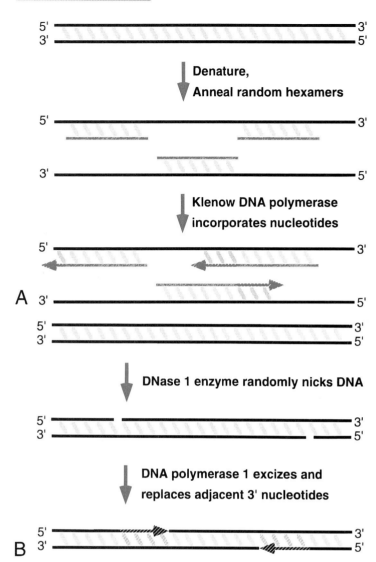

5' ━━━━━━━━━━━━━━━━━━━━━━━ **3'**
3' ━━━━━━━━━━━━━━━━━━━━━━━ **5'**

↓ **Denature,**
Anneal random hexamers

5' ━━━━━━━━━━━━━━━━━━━━━━━ **3'**

3' ━━━━━━━━━━━━━━━━━━━━━━━ **5'**

↓ **Klenow DNA polymerase**
incorporates nucleotides

5' ━━━━━━━━━━━━━━━━━━━━━━━ **3'**

A **3'** ━━━━━━━━━━━━━━━━━━━━━━━ **5'**

5' ━━━━━━━━━━━━━━━━━━━━━━━ **3'**
3' ━━━━━━━━━━━━━━━━━━━━━━━ **5'**

↓ **DNase 1 enzyme randomly nicks DNA**

5' ━━━━━━━━━━━━━━━━━━━━━━━ **3'**
3' ━━━━━━━━━━━━━━━━━━━━━━━ **5'**

↓ **DNA polymerase 1 excizes and**
replaces adjacent 3' nucleotides

5' ━━━━━━━━━━━━━━━━━━━━━━━ **3'**
B **3'** ━━━━━━━━━━━━━━━━━━━━━━━ **5'**

FIGURE 35–10   DNA probes are labeled by incorporating radioisotopes or non-isotopic markers into their nucleotide strands. (*A*) The "random primer" method capitalizes on the ability of Klenow DNA polymerase to synthesize new complementary strands of DNA starting at the free 3' ends where "hexamers" (6 base probes of random sequence) have bound to the probe template. Addition of labeled nucleotides to the reaction mixture results in a marker being incorporated into the newly synthesized DNA. (*B*) The "nick translation" method of probe labeling relies on the ability of the enzyme DNase 1 to randomly nick the backbone of DNA. Then the enzyme DNA polymerase 1 recognizes and repairs each nick, and subsequently proceeds to replace adjacent 3' nucleotides with new ones. In this way, labeled nucleotides can be incorporated into the probe.

particularly when sensitivity is critical to assay performance.

Biotin and digoxigenin are practical alternatives to radioisotopes. Biotin labels are recognized by avidin conjugates in an analogous fashion to the immunochemical use of avidin-biotin conjugates. The conjugate most commonly used is alkaline phosphatase enzyme that is subsequently detected by adding a colorimetric substrate. Unlike biotin, which is a natural substance, digoxigenin is a synthetic chemical, so it is not prone to the background problems that sometimes hamper biotin reactions. Digoxigenin labels are recognized by a specific antibody carrying an alkaline phosphatase conjugate. Alkaline phosphatase catalyzes a colorimetric or chemiluminescent reaction that signals its location (see Fig. 35–2).

There are several methods for incorporating labels into existing probes, and commercial kits are available for each of the methods described below. The most popular method of labeling a DNA probe is called *random priming*. Another is *nick translation*. Both of these procedures are suitable for labeling large DNA probes (Fig. 35–10). In contrast, short DNA probes (i.e., oligonucleotides) are efficiently labeled by a method called *end labeling*, which uses the enzyme T4 polynucleotide kinase to add labeled nucleotides to the 5' end of the probe.

FUTURE PROSPECTS OF MOLECULAR ASSAYS

DNA technology is a powerful new tool for laboratory diagnosis, and tremendous growth of this discipline is expected in the coming decades. Indeed, increasing numbers of probe-based kits are being approved by the Food and Drug Administration (FDA) for use in clinical laboratories. Among these are Southern blot kits for evaluating bcr translocations and lymphoid gene rearrangements, PCR kits to detect chlamydia and HIV, and kits for detecting ribosomal RNA of cultured organisms including mycobacteria and fungi (histoplasma, coccidioides, blastomycosis, candida, and cryptococcus). Also available are probe kits that directly detect ribosomal RNA of sexually transmitted pathogens (*Neisseria gonorrhoeae* and *Chlamydia trachomatis*) in urethral or cervical swabs.

Technological improvements will undoubtedly result in faster and less expensive methods of probe analysis. At the same time, new discoveries related to the genetic basis of human disease are fostering development of even more probe tests for various disease states. It seems likely that this technology will revolutionize laboratory diagnosis of many diseases.

ACKNOWLEDGMENTS

Polymerase chain reaction patents are owned and licensed by Hoffmann-LaRoche Molecular Systems, Inc. Riboprobe is a registered trademark of the Promega Corporation.

REFERENCES

1. Saiki, RK, et al: Enzymatic amplification of β globin genomic sequences and restriction site analysis for diagnosis of sickle cell anaemia. Science 230:1350, 1985.
2. Anonymous: Guidelines for the fetal diagnosis of globin gene disorders. J Clin Pathol, 47:199, 1994.
3. Camaschella, C, and Saglio, G: Recent advances in diagnosis of hemoglobinopathies. Crit Rev Oncol Hematol 14:89, 1993.
4. Sommer, SS, and Sobell, JL: Application of DNA-based diagnosis to patient care: The example of hemophilia A. Mayo Clin Proc 62:387, 1987.
5. Gulley, ML, and Raab-Traub, N: Detection of Epstein-Barr virus in human tissues by molecular genetic techniques. Arch Pathol Lab Med 117:1115, 1993.
6. Takemoto, S, et al: A novel diagnostic method of adult T-cell leukemia: Monoclonal integration of human T-cell lymphotropic virus type I provirus DNA detected by inverse polymerase chain reaction. Blood 84:3080, 1994.
7. Ausubel, FM, et al: Current Protocols in Molecular Biology. John Wiley Sons, New York, 1995.
8. Farkas, DH (ed): Molecular Biology and Pathology: A Guidebook for Quality Control. Academic Press, San Diego, 1993.
9. Herrington, CS and McGee, JO'D (eds): Diagnostic Molecular Pathology: A Practical Approach, vol 2. IRL Press, Oxford, 1993.
10. Sambrook, J, Fritsch, EF, and Maniatis, T: Molecular Cloning: A Laboratory Manual, ed 2. Cold Spring Harbor Laboratory Press, Cold Spring Harbor, NY, 1989.
11. Ross, DW: Introduction to Molecular Medicine, ed. 2. Springer-Verlag, New York, 1996.
12. Trent, RJ: Molecular Medicine: An Introductory Text for Students. Churchill Livingstone, Edinburgh, 1993.
13. McClatchey, KD: Clinical Laboratory Medicine. Williams and Wilkins, Baltimore, 1994, pp 117–209.
14. Fenoglio-Preiser, CM, and Willman, CL: Molecular Diagnostics in Pathology. Williams & Wilkins, Baltimore, 1991.
15. Bernstam, VA: Handbook of Gene Level Diagnostics in Clinical Practice. CRC Press, Ann Arbor, 1992.
16. Persing, DH, et al: Diagnostic Molecular Microbiology: Principles and Applications. American Society of Microbiology. Washington, DC, 1993.
17. Hanson, CA: Clinical applications of molecular biology in diagnostic hematopathology. Lab Med 24:562, 1993.
18. Blennerhassett, GT, et al: Clinical evaluation of a DNA probe assay for the Philadelphia (Ph') translocation in chronic myelogenous leukemia. Leukemia 2:648, 1988.
19. Kurzrock, R, Gutterman, JU, and Talpaz, M: The molecular genetics of Philadelphia chromosome-positive leukemias. N Engl J Med 319:990, 1988.
20. Kawasaki, ES, et al: Diagnosis of chronic myeloid and acute lymphocytic leukemias by detection of leukemia-specific mRNA sequences amplified in vitro. Proc Nat Acad Sci USA 85:5698, 1988.
21. McClure, JS and Litz, CE: Chronic myelogenous leukemia: Molecular diagnostic considerations. Hum Pathol 25:594, 1994.
22. Radich, JP, et al: Polymerase chain reaction detection of the bcr-abl fusion transcript after allogeneic marrow transplantation for chronic myeloid leukemia: Results and implications in 346 patients. Blood 85:2632, 1995.
23. Grignani, F, et al: Acute promyelocytic leukemia: From genetics to treatment. Blood 83:10, 1994.
24. Miller, WH, et al: Detection of minimal residual disease in acute promyelocytic leukemia by a reverse transcription polymerase chain reaction assay for the PML/RAR-α fusion mRNA. Blood 82:1689, 1993.
25. Westbrook, CA, et al: Clinical significance of the bcr-abl fusion gene in adult acute lymphoblastic leukemia: A Cancer and Leukemia Group B study (8762). Blood 80:2983, 1992.
26. Harris, NL, et al: A revised European-American Classification of lymphoid neoplasms: A proposal from the International Lymphoma Study Group. Blood 84:1361, 1994.
27. Shiramizu, B, and Magrath, I: Localization of breakpoints by polymerase chain reaction in Burkitt's lymphoma with 8;14 translocation. Blood 75:1848, 1990.
28. Williams, M, Meeker, T, and Swerdlow, S: Rearrangement of the chromosome 11 bcl-1 locus in centrocytic lymphoma: Analysis with multiple breakpoint probes. Blood 78:493, 1991.
29. Rimokh, R, et al: Detection of the chromosomal translocation t(11;14) by polymerase chain reaction in mantle cell lymphomas. Blood 83:1871, 1994.
30. Crisan, D, and Anstett, M: Bcl-2 gene rearrangements in follicular lymphomas. Lab Med 24:579, 1993.
31. Gribben, JG, et al: Detection by polymerase chain reaction of residual cells with the bcl-2 translocation is associated with increased risk of relapse after autologous bone marrow transplantation for B-cell lymphoma. Blood 81:3449, 1993.
32. Korsmeyer, SL: Bcl-2 initiates a new category of oncogenes: Regulators of cell death. Blood 80:879, 1992.
33. Cossman, J, et al: Molecular genetics and the diagnosis of lymphoma. Arch Pathol Lab Med, 112:117, 1988.
34. Cossman, J, et al: Gene rearrangements in the diagnosis of lymphoma/leukemia: Guidelines for use based on a multiinstitutional study. Am J Clin Pathol 95:347, 1991.
35. Gill, JI and Gulley, ML: Immunoglobulin and T-cell receptor gene rearrangement. Hematol Oncol Clin North Am 8:751, 1994.
36. Greisser, H, et al: Gene rearrangements and translocations in lymphoproliferative disease. Blood 73:1402, 1989.
37. Kamat, D, et al: The diagnostic utility of immunophenotyping and immunogenotyping in the pathologic evaluation of lymphoid proliferations. Mod Pathol 3:105, 1990.
38. Davis, RE, et al: Utility of molecular genetic analysis for the diagnosis of neoplasia in morphologically and immunophenotypically equivocal hematolymphoid lesions. Cancer 67:2890, 1991.
39. Weedn, VW, and Roby, RK: Forensic DNA testing. Arch Pathol Lab Med 117:486, 1993.
40. Faloona, FA: Specific synthesis of DNA in vitro via a poly-

merase catalyzed chain reaction. Methods Enzymol 155:335, 1987.

41. Wiedbrauk, DL: Molecular methods for virus detection. Lab Med 23:737, 1992.

42. Medeiros, L, and Weiss, L: The utility of the polymerase chain reaction as a screening method for the detection of antigen receptor gene rearrangements. Hum Pathol 25:1261, 1994.

43. Trainor, KJ, et al: Gene rearrangement in B and T-lymphoproliferative disease detected by the polymerase chain reaction. Blood 78:192, 1991.

44. Segal, GH, et al: Optimal primer selection for clonality assessment by polymerase chain reaction analysis: I. Low grade B-cell lymphoproliferative disorders of nonfollicular center cell type. Hum Pathol 25:1269, 1994.

45. Segal, GH, et al: Optimal primer selection for clonality assessment by polymerase chain reaction analysis: II. Follicular lymphomas. Hum Pathol 25:1269, 1994.

46. Chan, WC, and Greiner, TC: Diagnosis of lymphomas by the polymerase chain reaction. Am J Clin Pathol 101:273, 1994.

47. Kwok, S, and Higuchi, R: Avoiding false positives with PCR. Nature 239:237, 1989.

48. Erlich, HA, Gelfand, DH, and Saiki, RK: Specific DNA amplification. Nature 331:461, 1988.

49. Southern, EM: Detection of specific sequences among DNA fragments separated by gel electrophoresis. J Mol Biol 98:503, 1975.

QUESTIONS

1. To convert double-stranded DNA into its single-stranded components, which of the following procedures may be used?
   a. Heat DNA to 95°C
   b. Expose the DNA to a strong alkaline solution
   c. Either of the above
   d. Neither of the above

2. Which of the following assays is most appropriate for routine clinical detection of the point mutation responsible for sickle cell anemia?
   a. *In situ* hybridization
   b. Fluorescence *in situ* hybridization
   c. Cloning
   d. Southern blot analysis

3. Which statement is true about the polymerase chain reaction (PCR)?
   a. It is a method for amplifying a particular segment of DNA.
   b. The DNA polymerase enzyme that is used as a reagent in this assay is derived from tree bark.
   c. It is labor-intensive and expensive compared with Southern blot analysis.
   d. The assay does not require any probes, and therefore you need not know anything about the sequence of the target DNA.

4. Which of the following are reasonable probe labels?
   a. Digoxigenin
   b. Biotin
   c. ^{32}P radioisotope
   d. All of the above

5. Which of the following tumor types is most likely to exhibit clonal immunoglobulin gene rearrangement?
   a. Acute nonlymphocytic leukemia.
   b. B-cell lymphoma.
   c. Human T-cell lymphotropic virus type 1 (HTLV1)-related leukemia.
   d. Chronic myelogenous leukemia.

6. The following are steps in the Southern blot procedure *except*:
   a. Agarose gel electrophoresis
   b. Cut DNA with restriction endonuclease
   c. Synthesize DNA at 72°C
   d. DNA extraction

7. Which of the following chemicals is used to stain DNA in agarose gels?
   a. EcoR1
   b. Ethidium bromide
   c. Ethanol
   d. Formalin

8. Which of the following is true about restriction endonucleases?
   a. They function to replicate DNA in the polymerase chain reaction.
   b. In the "nick translation" procedure, they are used to incorporate labeled nucleotides into DNA probes.
   c. They are enzymes that cut DNA at specific recognition sequences.
   d. They function as protease enzymes to permeabilize cell membranes.

9. Which is true of the in situ hybridization procedure for analyzing paraffin tissue sections that are immobilized on glass slides?
   a. It can be used to localize DNA or RNA in the context of histologic and cytologic features.
   b. It is a means of determining DNA structure so that disease-specific gene translocations can be identified.
   c. It can amplify sequences up to 5000 nucleotides in length.
   d. All of the above.

10. Which of the following probes would be most appropriate for an assay in which you want to target the following DNA sequence, 5′-AAAGGGTCTCTCTTTTGGG-3′?
    a. 3′-GGGAAACTCTCTCCCCAAA-5′
    b. 5′-TTTCCCAGAGAGAAAACCC-3′
    c. 3′-TTTCCCAGAGAGAAAACCC-5′
    d. 3′-AAAGGGTCTCTCTTTTGGG-5′

ANSWERS

1. **c** (p 683 [Fig. 35–2])
2. **d** (p 686)
3. **a** (p 689)
4. **d** (p 693)
5. **b** (p 687)
6. **c** (p 686)
7. **b** (p 689)
8. **c** (p 686)
9. **a** (p 692)
10. **c** (p 683, also Figure 35–1)

Glossary

A

Abetalipoproteinemia: A disorder in which the absence of beta lipoproteins manifests itself in mental retardation and impaired food absorption. Clinical manifestations include acanthocytes, retinitis pigmentosa, and excess fat in the stool.

Abruptio placenta: Premature detachment of normally situated placenta.

Acanthocyte: An abnormal red cell that is slightly reduced in size and that possesses 3 to 12 spicules of uneven length distributed along the periphery of the cell membrane.

Achlorhydria: Absence of free hydrochloric acid in the stomach.

Acholuria: Absence of bile pigments in urine, occurring when unconjugated bilirubin does not pass through the glomerular filter.

Acrocyanosis: Bluish tinge to the extremities.

Actin: A muscle protein that, in conjunction with myosin particles, facilitates expansion and contraction.

Activated partial thromboplastin time (APTT): A test to evaluate the overall integrity of the clotting system that involves factors XII, XI, IX, VIII, X, V, II, and I. Usually a means of evaluating the intrinsic system of coagulation.

Acute phase reactant: Plasma protein, the concentration of which increases in response to a variety of stimuli.

Adenopathy: Swelling and morbid change in lymph nodes; glandular disease.

Adenosine diphosphate (ADP): A substance used to induce platelet aggregation that may be derived from injured tissues, erythrocytes, or platelets.

Adhesion: The molecular attraction exerted between the surfaces of bodies in contact (for example, platelets to connection tissue structures).

Afibrinogenemia: A rare blood disease characterized by the absence of fibrinogen in the plasma; may be congenital or acquired.

Agammaglobulinemia: A rare disorder in which there is a virtual absence of gamma globulins.

Agglutination: The clumping together of red blood cells or any particulate matter resulting from interaction of antibody and its corresponding antigen.

Aggregation: A clustering or clumping together (for example, platelet aggregation, which plays a critical role in hemostasis).

Agnogenic dyspoiesis: Preleukemic disorder of unknown origin, characterized by hypercellular marrow and abnormal cell maturation.

Agranulocytosis: An acute disease in which the white cell count is markedly reduced and neutropenia becomes pronounced.

Alkaline phosphatase: An enzyme that is found in a number of tissues but is chiefly used in connection with diagnosis of bone and liver disease. The granules of normal granulocytic cells contain alkaline phosphatase; patients with chronic myelogenous leukemia (CML) have decreased phosphatase activity.

Alkalosis: Excessive alkalinity of body fluids, owing to accumulation of alkalies or reduction of acids.

Allele: One of several alternate forms of a gene. In a particular person's genome, there are usually two alleles for each gene, one inherited from the mother and the other from the father. Any differences between alleles of the same gene may be referred to as polymorphisms.

Alloantibody: An antibody produced by an immune response that was stimulated by a foreign antigen.

Allograft: A tissue transplant between individuals of the same species.

Alloimmunization: The process in which a patient develops antibodies to foreign and/or white blood cell antigen(s) through transfusion or pregnancy.

Alopecia: Baldness.

Alpha chain: A type of globin chain found in hemoglobin and coded for by the alpha gene.

Alpha methyldopa (Aldomet): A common drug used to treat hypertension; frequently the cause of a positive direct Coombs' test result.

Amaurotic: Caused by the atrophying of optic nerve or vision centers.

Ameliorate: Moderate, improve.

Amniocentesis: Transabdominal puncture of the amniotic sac, using a needle and syringe, to remove amniotic fluid. The material may then be studied to detect genetic disorders or maternal-fetal blood incompatibility.

Amphophilic: Having an affinity for acid and/or basic dyes.

Amyloidosis: A metabolic disorder marked by extracellular deposition of amyloid (an abnormal protein) in the tissues; this usually leads to loss of function and organ enlargement.

Anamnestic (response): An accentuated antibody response following a secondary exposure to an antigen. Antibody levels from the initial exposure are not detectable in the patient's serum until the secondary exposure, when a rapid rise in antibody titer is observed.

Anaphylaxis: An allergic hypersensitivity reaction of the body to a foreign protein or drug.

Ancillary: Auxiliary, supplementary.

Androgenic: Causing masculinization.

Anemia: A condition in which there is reduced oxygen delivery to the tissues. It may result from increased destruction of red cells, excessive blood loss, or decreased production of red cells.

Aplastic a.: Anemia caused by aplasia of bone marrow or its destruction by chemical agents or physical factors.

Autoimmune hemolytic a.: Acquired disorder characterized by premature erythrocyte destruction owing to abnormalities in the individual's own immune system.

Diamond-Blackfan a.: A congenital pure RBC aplasia characterized by severe chronic anemia which manifests early in infancy and is associated with normal white cells and platelets.

Fanconi's a.: A congenital aplastic anemia associated with genetic anomalies. Untreated patients with Fanconi's anemia usually die of secondary infections or hemorrhage.

Hemolytic a.: Anemia caused by hemolysis of red blood cells resulting in reduction of normal red cell lifespan.

Hypoplastic a.: An normochromic, normocytic anemia of bone marrow failure that may be idiopathic, congenital, or caused by chemical agents.

Iron-deficiency a.: Anemia resulting from a greater demand on stored iron than can be met.

Megaloblastic a.: Anemia in which megaloblasts are found in the blood; usually caused by a deficiency of folic acid or vitamin B_{12}.

Microangiopathic hemolytic a.: A hemolytic process associated with thrombotic thrombocytopenic purpura (TTP), prosthetic heart valve, and burns. It is visualized in the peripheral blood smear by fragmentation of the red cells and other bizarre morphology.

Pernicious a.: A type of megaloblastic anemia caused by a deficiency of vitamin B_{12} that is directly linked to absence of intrinsic factor (IF).

Sickle-cell a.: See **Sickle-cell anemia.**

Sideroblastic a.: A disorder in which iron is not being incorporated into heme and serum iron levels are elevated. The bone marrow is hyperplastic and contains iron-laden sideroblasts.

Aneuploidy: Having an abnormal number of chromosomes.

Angina pectoris: Severe pain and constriction about the heart caused by insufficient supply of blood to the heart.

Anisochromia: The state of being not of uniform color.

Anisocytosis: Variation in the size of erythrocytes when observed on a peripheral blood smear.

Ankyrin: A pyramid-shaped protein that is a major component of the red cell cytoskeleton.

Annealing: The process by which a probe (or oligonucleotide primer in PCR reactions) binds to its complementary single-stranded target sequence.

Anoxia: The state of being without oxygen.

Antenatal: Occurring before birth.

Antibody: A protein substance developed in response to, and interacting specifically with, an antigen. In blood banking, it is found in serum, from either a commercial manufacturer or a patient. It is secreted by plasma cells.

Cross-reacting a.: An antibody that reacts with antigens functionally similar to its specific antigen.

Maternal a.: An antibody produced in the mother and transferred to the fetus in utero.

Naturally occurring a.: An antibody present in a patient without known prior exposure to the corresponding red cell antigen.

Antibody screen: Testing the patient's serum with group O reagent red cells in an effort to detect atypical antibodies.

Anticoagulant: An agent that delays or prevents blood coagulation.

Antigen: A substance that is recognized by the body as being foreign and that therefore can elicit an immune response.

Antiglobulin test (AGT) or antihuman globulin (AHG) test: Test to ascertain the presence or absence of red cell coating by immunoglobulin (IgG) and/or complement.

Direct AGT (DAT): Used to detect in vivo cell sensitization.

Indirect AGT (IAT): Used to detect antigen-antibody reactions that occur in vitro.

Antihemophilic factor (AHF): A commercially prepared source of factor VIII. (See also **Hemophilia A.)**

Antihuman serum: An antibody prepared in rabbits or other suitable animals that is directed against human immunoglobulin or complement or both. It is used to perform the AGT or Coombs' test. The serum may be either polyspecific (anti-IgG plus anticomplement) or monospecific (angi-IgG or anticomplement).

Antiplasmin: Plasma proteins that are known to neutralize free plasmin: α_2-antiplasmin, α_2-macroglobulin.

α_2-a.: The major inhibitor of plasmin.

Antipyretic: An agent that reduces fever.

Antiseptic: Preventing decay, putrefaction, or sepsis.

Antithrombin: A substance that opposes the action of thrombin and thus prevents or inhibits coagulation of blood.

Antithrombin III (AT-III): A naturally occurring inhibitor of coagulation responsible for neutralizing the activity of thrombin; factors IXa, Xa, XIa, XIIa; and plasmin. (Also known as the heparin cofactor.)

Anuria: Absence of urine formation.

Apheresis: A method of blood collection in which whole blood is withdrawn, a desired component separated and retained, and the remainder of the blood returned to the donor. (See also **Plateletpheresis; Plasmapheresis.)**

Aplasia: Failure of an organ or tissue to develop normally.

Ascites: The accumulation of serous fluid in the peritoneal cavity.

Asphyxia: Condition caused by insufficient intake of oxygen.

Asplenism: The state of being without a spleen.

Asthenic: Weak, caused by a muscular or cerebellar disease.

Asynchrony: The failure of events to occur in time with each other as they usually do. In hematology, nuclear and cytoplasmic development are mismatched.

Atypical lymphocyte: A benign reactive change in the morphologic appearance of the lymphocyte, which is frequently secondary to a viral disease (for example, infectious mononucleosis).

Auer's rod: Rod-shaped alignment of primary granules that are present only in the cytoplasm of myeloblasts and monoblasts in leukemic states.

Autohemolysis: Hemolysis of an individual's blood corpuscles by his or her own serum.

Autoimmune: Referring to the production of antibodies directed against one's own tissues, usually in association with a disease state.

Autoimmune hemolytic anemia (AIHA): Abnormality of the immune system resulting in production of antibodies against self, which occurs because of failure of the mechanism regulating the immune response.

Autologous: Of the self.

Autosomal: Relating to any of the chromosomes other than the sex (X and Y) chromosomes.

Autosplenectomy: Formation of a fibrotic, nonfunctioning spleen caused by restrictive blood flow to the organ; often seen in sickle-cell anemia.

Azotemia: Presence of increased amounts of urea in the blood.

Azurophilic granules: Primary granules.

B

Babesiosis: A rare, often severe, and sometimes fatal disease of humans caused by the protozoal parasite of the red blood cells, *Babesia microti*, and perhaps other *Babesia* species.

Band: An immature neutrophilic granulocyte with a horseshoe- or sausage-shaped nucleus (also called a stab). Makes up 2% to 6% of the normal differential count.

Base pair: A nucleotide pair of A and T, or G and C, in double-stranded DNA. The length of a DNA sequence is measured in base pairs (bp), or in thousands of base pairs = kilobases (kb).

Basophil: A mature white blood cell whose cytoplasmic granules stain deep blue-purple with basic dyes like methylene blue. Makes up 0% to 2% of the normal differential count.

Basophilia: An absolute increase in basophils.

Basophilic normoblast: An immature red cell precursor found only in the bone marrow that is characterized by a vivid blue cytoplasm and a high nuclear-to-cytoplasmic ratio. (Synonym: **Prorubricyte.**)

Basophilic stippling: Red blood cell inclusion that consists of precipitated ribonucleoprotein and mitochrondial remnants. Stippling may be fine, coarse, or punctate and is seen in toxic states such as lead poisoning, severe bacterial infection, and drug exposure.

B-cell: Named for the site of lymphopoiesis in the chicken (the bursa of Fabricius). In humans, B cells differentiate into plasma cells from lymphoid stem cells of the marrow.

Bernard-Soulier syndrome: A congenital bleeding disorder characterized by the presence of large platelets, thrombocytopenia of varying degrees, and a prolonged bleeding time.

Beta chain: A type of globin chain found in hemoglobin that is coded for by the beta gene.

Betke-Kleihauer technique: An acid elution test used to quantitate the amount of fetal hemoglobin present. Fetal hemoglobin is more resistant than adult hemoglobin to elution at acid pH during this procedure, and stains red.

Bilirubin: The orange or yellowish pigment in bile, which is carried to the liver by the blood. It is produced from hemoglobin of red blood cells by reticuloendothelial cells in the bone marrow, spleen, and elsewhere.

  Direct b.: The conjugated water-soluble form of bilirubin.

  Indirect b.: The unconjugated water-insoluble form of bilirubin.

Bilirubinemia: Pathologic condition in which excessive destruction of red blood cells occurs, increasing the amount of bilirubin found in the blood.

Bite cell: Cell in which the removal of a portion of membrane has left a permanent indentation in the remaining cell membrane.

Blackwater fever: Hemoglobinuria following chronic falciparum malaria infection.

Bleeding time: A test used to evaluate the hemostatic role of platelets in vivo.

Bradykinin: A plasma kinin.

Buffy coat: The layer of leukocytes and platelets lying directly on top of the red cell layer seen after sedimentation or centrifugation.

Burr cells (echinocytes): Red cells with approximately 10 to 30 spicules evenly distributed over the surface of the cell.

Burst-forming unit committed to erythropoiesis (BFU-E): A primitive stem cell committed to erythropoiesis and thought to be a precursor to the CFU-E.

C

C1 esterase inhibitor: A protein in the blood that inhibits the activity of plasmin as well as the activity of C1 esterase in the complement pathway.

C3a: A biologically active fragment of the C3 molecule, which demonstrates anaphylactic capabilities on liberation.

C3b: A biologically active fragment of the complement C3 molecule, which is an opsonin and promotes immune adherence.

C3d: A biologically inactive fragment of the C3b complement component formed by inactivation by the C3b inactivator substance present in serum.

C4: A component of complement present in serum, which participates in the classic pathway of complement activation.

C5a: A biologically active fragment of the C5 molecule, which demonstrates anaphylactic capabilities as well as chemotactic properties on liberation. This fragment has also been reported to be a potent aggregator of platelets.

Cabot's rings: A red blood cell inclusion resembling a figure 8. It is usually found in heavily stippled cells.

Cachexia: A condition that may result from chronic disease or certain malignancies whereby a state of malnutrition, weakness, and muscle wasting exists.

Calmodulin: A cytoplasmic calcium-binding protein.

Carcinoma: A neoplasm (new growth) or malignant tumor that occurs in epithelial tissue. A neoplasm can infiltrate or metastasize to any tissue or organ of the body.

Cardiac output: The amount of blood discharged from the left or right ventricle per minute.

Catecholamines: Biologically active amines, epinephrine and norepinephrine, derived from the amino acid tyrosine. They have a marked effect on nervous and cardiovascular systems, metabolic rate, temperature, and smooth muscle.

cDNA (complementary DNA): Synthetic DNA produced from an mRNA template by the enzyme reverse transcriptase.

Celiac: Related to the abdominal regions.

Celite: A substance that acts as a contact activator causing the release of PF 3 and the activation of the intrinsic system.

Central venous pressure: The pressure within the superior vena cava reflecting the pressure under which the blood is returned to the right atrium.

Centripetal: Moving toward the center.

Cerebriform: A word that is used to describe the brainlike convolutions of some nuclear chromatin material.

Chédiak-Higashi inclusions: Gigantic, fused lysosomal deposits seen in the cytoplasm of leukocytes.

Chelation: Combining of metallic ions with certain heterocyclic ring structures so that the ion is held by chemical bonds from each of the participating rings.

Chemokinesis: Increased activity of cells in the presence of a chemical attractant.

Chemotactic: Referring to the ability of white cells to move nondirectionally toward an attractant.

Chemotaxis: Describes movement toward a stimulus, particularly that displayed by phagocytic cells toward bacteria and sites of cell injury.

Cholecystectomy: Excision of a gallbladder.

Cholecystitis: Acute or chronic inflammation of the gallbladder.

Christmas factor: Plasma thromboplastin component (PTC); factor IX. Functions in the intrinsic system of coagulation.

Chromatin: A dark-staining substance located in the nucleus of the cell that contains the genetic material composed of deoxyribonucleic acid (DNA) attached to a protein structure.

Chromogenic: Pigment-producing.

Circulating anticoagulants: Acquired pathologic plasma proteins that inhibit normal coagulation. The majority of these pathologic anticoagulants are inhibitors or autoantibodies of the IgG class whose inhibitory effects are directed against a specific factor or a complex of coagulation factors.

Coagulation: The process of stopping blood flow from a wound. This process involves the harmonious relationship of the blood-clotting factors, the blood vessels, and the fibrin-forming and fibrin-lysing system.

Coagulopathy: A disease affecting the blood-clotting process.

Collagen: A fibrous insoluble protein found in the connective tissue, including skin, bone, ligaments, and cartilage; represents about 30% of the total body protein.

Colony-forming unit committed to erythropoiesis (CFU-E): A stem cell that is committed to forming cells of the red blood cell series.

Colony-forming unit—culture (CFU-C): Generation of stem cells using tissue culture methods. Current synonym is CFU-GM, which is a colony-forming unit committed to the production of myeloid cells (granulocytes and monocytes).

Complement: A series of proteins in the circulation that, when sequentially activated, cause disruption of bacterial and other cell membranes. Activation occurs via one of two pathways, and once activated, the components are involved in a great number of immune defense mechanisms including anaphylaxis, chemotaxis, and phagocytosis. Red cell antibodies that activate complement may be capable of causing hemolysis.

Complement fixation (CF): An immunologic test involving antigen combining with antibody and complement causing inactivation of complement.

Congenital: Present at birth.

Consanguinous: Relationship by blood (that is, being descended from a common ancestor).

Contiguous: In contact or closely associated with.

Convulsion: Involuntary muscle contraction and relaxation.

Cord cells: Fetal cells obtained from the umbilical cord at birth. They may be contaminated with Wharton's jelly.

Corticosteroid: Any of a number of hormonal steroid substances obtained from the cortex of the adrenal gland.

Coumarin drugs (Warfarin, Coumadin, Dicumarol): Oral anticoagulants that act as vitamin K antagonists and result in depression of the concentration of prothrombin and factors VII, IX, and X.

Counterelectrophoresis (CEP): An immunologic procedure involving electrophoretic movement of antigen and antibody resulting in formation of a precipitin line.

Cryoglobulin: An abnormal protein in the blood that forms gels at low temperatures.

Cryoglobulinemia: An increase in the concentration of cryoglobulins in the blood.

Cryoprecipitate: A concentrated source of coagulation factor VIII that has been prepared from a single unit of donor blood. The product also contains fibrinogen, factor XIII, and von Willebrand factor.

Cryoprotein: A protein circulating in the plasma or demonstrable in serum testing that precipitates on exposure to cold temperature.

Cryptococcosis: An infection caused by *Cryptococcus neoformans* that may affect the central nervous system with respect to the brain and meninges or the skin. It may also affect the spleen, liver, joints, and lungs.

Cyanosis: Slightly bluish or grayish discoloration of the skin caused by accumulation of reduced hemoglobin or deoxyhemoglobin in the blood as a result of oxygen deficiency or carbon dioxide buildup.

Cytochemistry: The microscopic study of the chemical constituents in cells, the purpose of which includes differentiation of cell types and assistance in the diagnosis of hematologic diseases.

Cytogenetics: The study of cytology in relation to genetics, especially the chromosomal behavior in mitosis and meiosis.

Cytokines: Growth factors, such as colony-stimulating factors and interleukins.

Cytomegalovirus (CMV): One of a group of species-specific herpes viruses.

Cytopenia: Abnormalities or deficiencies in blood cell elements.

Cytopheresis: A procedure using a machine by which one can selectively remove a particular cell type normally found in peripheral blood of a patient or donor.

Cytotoxicity: Ability to destroy.

D

Dacrocyte: See **Teardrop cell.**

Dactylitis: Painful swelling of the feet and hands.

Defibrinated: Deprived of fibrin (the conversation of fibrinogen into fibrin is the basis for the clotting of blood).

Delayed hemolytic transfusion reaction (DHTR): A hemolytic reaction that occurs when previously sensitized individuals have antibody levels that are undetectable and are once again exposed to the offending antigen(s). In most cases of DHTR the antibodies implicated are IgG.

Delta: A type of globin chain found in hemoglobin coded for by the delta gene.

Desferrioxamine: Substance obtained from certain bacteria that is used to chelate iron. This substance is used orally or parenterally in treating iron poisoning.

Diagnosis: The use of scientific and skillful methods to establish the cause and nature of a disease process.

Diapedesis: The journey of the blood cells (that is, leukocytes) through the unruptured walls of a capillary.

Diaphoresis: Profuse sweating.

Differential: Microscopic examination of a stained blood smear to determine the relative number of each type of white blood cell; an estimate of white cell, red cell, and platelet counts; and an inspection of the morphology of red cells, white cells, and platelets.

Dimer: A compound formed by the combination of two identical molecules.

Dimorphism: Existence of a two-cell population in the peripheral blood smear (for example, few microcytes, few macrocytes; few hypochromic, few normochromic).

2,3-Diphosphoglycerate (2,3-DPG): An organic phosphate in red blood cells that alters the affinity of hemoglobin for oxygen. Blood cells stored in a blood bank lose 2,3-DPG, but once infused the substance is resynthesized or reactivated.

Discocyte: See **Erythrocyte.**

Disseminated intravascular coagulation (DIC): A pathologic form of coagulation that is diffuse rather than localized, and is characterized by generalized bleeding and shock.

Diuresis: Secretion and passage of large amounts of urine.

Diuretic: An agent that increases the secretion of urine. Action is in one of two ways: by increasing glomerular filtration or by decreasing reabsorption from the tubules.

Diurnal: Occurring during the daytime.

Diverticulosis: Outpouching of the colon without inflammation or symptoms. There are many locations of diverticula but all are saccular dilatations protruding from the wall of a tubular organ.

DNA (deoxyribonucleic acid): The inherited substance that cells use to catalog, express, and propagate information. DNA is composed of two strands of nucleotides that wind around each other to form a double-stranded helix. The two nucleotide strands are held together by hydrogen bonds formed according to the following rules of complementary nucleotide pairing: G bonds with C, A bonds with T, and other combinations cannot bond. When cells divide, DNA is replicated and equally partitioned among the progeny such that each daughter cell contains a full complement of DNA known as the genome.

Dohle bodies: Single or multiple, round or oval, blue cytoplasmic inclusions (with Romanowsky stain) seen in neutrophils, usually associated with toxicity.

Donath-Landsteiner antibody test: A test usually performed in the blood bank to detect the presence of the Donath-Landstein antibody, which is a biphasic IgG antibody with anti-P specificity found in patients suffering from paroxysmal cold hemoglobinuria.

Drepanocytes: Red cells that have been transformed by hemoglobin polymerization into rigid, inflexible cells with at least one pointed projection.

Dyscrasia: An old term now used as a synonym for disease.

Dyserythropoiesis: Changes in erythroid cell nuclear chromatin pattern; some of these changes are bizarre.

Dysfibrinogenemia: A congenital disorder characterized by the synthesis of abnormal fibrinogen molecules with different functional characteristics.

Dyshematopoiesis: Abnormalities in the maturation, division, or production of blood cells.

Dyskeratosis: Any alteration in the keratinization of the epithelial cells of the epidermis.

Dysostosis: Defective ossification.

Dysplasia: Conditions or diseases characterized by developmental abnormalities or deficiencies.

Dyspnea: Labored or difficult breathing.

Dyspoiesis: Nuclear-cytoplasmic dissociation, especially in red cells.

E

Early degradation products: The large fragments X and Y that result from the proteolytic action of plasmin on fibrin or fibrinogen. Fragments X and Y have antithrombin activity.

Ecchymosis: A form of macula appearing in large, irregularly formed hemorrhagic areas of the skin, originally blue-black and changing to greenish brown or yellow.

Echinocyte: See **Burr cell.**

Eclampsia: An acute disorder of pregnant and puerperal women, associated with convulsions and coma.

Edema: A local or generalized condition in which the body tissues contain an excessive amount of tissue fluid.

Edematous: Pertaining to swelling of body tissues.

Electrophoresis: The movement of charged particles through a medium (paper, agar, gel) in the presence of an electrical field. Useful in the separation and analysis of proteins.

Elliptocyte: Pencil-shaped cells, invariably not hypochromic.

Elution: A process whereby cells that are coated with antibody are treated in such a manner as to disrupt the bonds between the antigen and the antibody. The freed antibody is collected in an inept diluent such as saline or 6% albumin. This serum can then be tested to identify its specificity using routine methods. The mechanism to free the antibody may be physical (heat, shaking) or chemical (ether, acid), and the harvested antibody-containing fluid is called an eluate.

Embolism: Obstruction of a blood vessel by foreign substances or by a blood clot.

Embolus: A mass of undissolved matter present in a blood or lymphatic vessel brought there by the blood or lymph circulation.

Endemic: Term used to describe a disease that occurs continuously in a particular population but has a low mortality rate, such as measles; used in contrast to epidemic.

Endocarditis: Inflammation of the lining membrane of the heart. May be caused by invasion of microorganisms or an abnormal immunologic reaction.

Endogenous: Produced or arising from within a cell or organism.

Endoplasmic reticulum: A connecting network of microcanals or tubules running through the cytoplasm of a cell that serves in intracellular transport.

Endothelium: A form of squamous epithelium consisting of flat cells that line the blood and lymphatic vessels, the heart, and various other body cavities. It is derived from the mesoderm.

Endotoxemia: The presence of endotoxin in the blood (endotoxin is present in the cells of certain bacteria, such as gram-negative organisms).

Eosinophil: A mature type of granulocyte in which cytoplasmic granules are large, round, and refractile and stain orange or red with Wright's stain. Composes 0% to 4% of the normal differential count.

Epistaxis: Hemorrhage from the nose; nosebleed.

Epsilon: A type of globin chain found in embryonic hemoglobins.

Epsilon aminocaproic acid (EACA): A synthetic inhibitor of plasminogen activation.

Erythroblast: A nucleated cell from which red blood cells are developed. These cells are found in the bone marrow and seen in circulatory blood in the presence of disease.

Erythroblastosis fetalis: See **Hemolytic disease of the newborn (HDN).**

Erythrocyte: A mature red blood cell or corpuscle.

Erythrocyte sedimentation rate (ESR): The rate at which red blood cells settle per hour; affected by three factors: erythrocytes, plasma, and mechanical factors.

Erythrocytosis: Abnormal increase in the number of red blood cells in circulation, secondary to many disorders.

Erythroid hyperplasia: As seen in the bone marrow, an increase in the number of immature red cell forms; usually a response to anemic stress.

Erythropoiesis: The production and maturation of erythrocytes.

Erythropoietin: A hormone that regulates red blood cell production.

Etiology: The study of the causes of disease.

Euglobulin: The fraction of plasma containing fibrinogen, plasminogen, and plasminogen activators with only trace amounts of antiplasmins.

Euglobulin lysis time: Coagulation procedure testing for fibrinolysins.

Exocytosis: Secretion of the contents of cytoplasmic granules.

Exogenous: Originating outside an organ or part.

Extracorporeal: Existing outside of the body.

Extramedullary hematopoiesis: Formation of blood cells in sites other than the bone marrow (that is, liver, spleen).

Extravascular: Outside of the blood vessel.

　E. hemolysis: Hemolysis occurring within the cells of the reticuloendothelial system.

F

Factor assay: Coagulation procedure to assay the concentration of specific plasma coagulation factors.

Factor VIII antigen: The high molecular weight component of the factor VIII molecule.

Factor VIII concentrate: A commercially prepared source of coagulation factor VIII.

Favism: An inherited condition resulting from sensitivity to the fava bean, usually seen in people of Mediterranean origin who have a deficiency in the enzyme glucose-6-phosphate dehydrogenase, which may result in a severe hemolytic episode.

Femto-: A prefix used in the metric system to signify 10^{-15} of any unit. Femtoliter (fL) is used in reporting mean corpuscular volume (MCV) of erythrocytes.

Ferritin: The storage form of iron in the tissues, found principally in the reticuloendothelial cells of the liver, spleen, and bone marrow.

Fibrin: A whitish filamentous protein or clot formed by the action of thrombin on fibrinogen, converting it to fibrin.

Fibrin monomer: The altered molecule that results from thrombin splitting fibrinopeptides A and B from two of the three paired chains of the fibrinogen molecule.

Fibrinogen: A protein produced in the liver that circulates in plasma. In the presence of thrombin, an enzyme produced by the activation of the clotting mechanism, fibrinogen is cleaved into fibrin, which is insoluble protein that is responsible for clot formation.

Fibrinogen-degradation products (FDPs): The polypeptide fragments X, Y, D, and E that result from the proteolytic action of plasmin on fibrinogen or fibrin.

Fibrinolysin: The substance, also called plasmin, that has the ability to dissolve fibrin.

Fibrinolysis: Dissolution of fibrin by fibrinolysin caused by the action of proteolytic enzyme system that is continually active in the body but increased greatly by various stress stimuli.

Fibrinopeptides: Peptides released when fibrinogen is converted to fibrin by thrombin. The fibrinopeptides released by thrombin are designated A and B.

Fibrin-split products: Products that result from fibrin digestion.

Fibrin-stabilizing factor (FSF): Factor XIII.

Fibrosis: Excessive formation of fibrous tissue.

Fitzgerald factor: High molecular weight kininogen (HMWK).

Fletcher factor: Prekallikrein.

Fractures: The sudden breaking of bones.

Fragility: Liability to break, burst, or disintegrate, as erythrocytes are prone to do when exposed to varying concentrations of hypotonic salt solutions.

Fresh frozen plasma (FFP): A frozen plasma product (from a single donor) that contains all clotting factors, especially the labile factors V and VIII. Useful for clotting factor deficiencies other than hemophilia A, von Willebrand's disease, and hypofibrinogenemia.

Friable: Easily broken or pulverized.

G

Gallops: Relating to cardiac rhythms, an abnormal third or fourth heart sound in a patient experiencing tachycardia. Gallops are indicative of a serious heart condition.

Gamma: A type of globin chain found in fetal hemoglobin. Two types exist: G gamma contains glycine at position 13 of the amino acid sequence, and A gamma contains alanine at the same position.

Gamma globulin: A protein found in plasma and known to be involved in immunity.

Gammopathy: Abnormalities of the immune or gamma system arising in a single disordered clone of cells that is able to synthesize immunoglobulin.

Gastrectomy: Surgical removal of part or all of the stomach.

Gastritis: Inflammation of the stomach, characterized by epigastric pain or tenderness, nausea, vomiting, and systemic electrolyte changes if vomiting persists. The mucosa may be atrophic or hypertrophic.

Gaucher's disease: A familial, lysosomal disorder caused by a deficiency in the enzyme betaglucocerebrosidase. Three types are identified; all three have in common the triad of hepatosplenomegaly, Gaucher's cells in the bone marrow, and an increase in serum acid phosphatase.

Gene: A functional segment of DNA that serves as a template for RNA transcription and protein translation. Regulatory sequences control gene expression, so that only a small fraction of the estimated 100,000 genes are ever transcribed in any one cell. The spectrum of gene expression in a given cell depends on the cell type and stage of differentiation, and on external signals that it receives from its environment.

Gene rearrangement: A process by which segments of DNA are cut and spliced to produce new DNA sequences. The only genes known to undergo physiologic rearrangement are the immunoglobulin genes and the T cell receptor genes that encode antigen recognition proteins expressed by B and T lymphocytes, respectively.

Genome: The total aggregate of inherited genetic material. In humans, the genome consists of 3 billion base pairs of DNA divided among 46 chromosomes (22 pairs of autosomes and two sex chromosomes).

Genotype: The genetic constitution of a particular person. Every person's genotype is unique unless he or she has an identical twin.

Gestation: In mammals, the length of time from conception to birth.

Gigantism: Excessive development of part or all of the body.

Glanzmann's thrombasthenia: A congenital bleeding disorder characterized by impaired or absent clot retraction and a failure of the platelets to aggregate with most aggregating agents, particularly ADP.

Globin: A protein constituent of hemoglobin. There are four globin chains in the hemoglobin molecule.

Glossitis: Inflammation of the tongue.

Glucose-6-phosphate dehydrogenase (G6PD): An intracellular red cell enzyme important in the hexose monophosphate pathway.

Glycolysis: Hydrolysis of sugar by an enzyme in the body.

Glycophorin: The principal integral blood cell protein, containing 60% carbohydrate and giving the red cell its negative charge. It appears on the external surface of the red cell.

Glycoprotein: A group of compounds characterized by the combination of a protein with a carbohydrate group.

Golgi apparatus: A lamellar membranous structure near the nucleus of almost all cells. The structure is best seen by electron microscopy. It contains enzymes that add terminal sugar sequences to protein moieties.

Gout: Hereditary metabolic disease that is a form of acute arthritis and is marked by inflammation of the joints. The affected joint may be at any location, but gout usually begins in the knee or foot.

Graft-versus-host (GVH) disease: A disorder in which the grafted tissue attacks the host tissue.

Granulocyte: A mature granular leukocyte; refers to band or polymorphonuclear neutrophil, eosinophil, or basophil.

Granulocytopenia: Abnormal reduction of granulocytes in the blood.

Granulomas: A granular tumor or growth usually of lymphoid and epithelial cells. It occurs in various infectious diseases such as leprosy, cutaneous leishmaniosis, yaws, and syphilis.

Granulopoiesis: The production and maturation of granulocytes.

H

Hageman factor: Synonym for coagulation factor XII.

Haplotypes: A term used in human leukocyte antigen (HLA) testing to denote the five genes (HLA-A, B, C, D, and DR) on the same chromosome.

Hapten: The portion of an antigen containing the grouping on which the specificity is dependent.

Haptoglobin: An α_2-glycoprotein produced in the liver, having three phenotypes with differing abilities to bind hemoglobin.

Heinz bodies: Large red blood cell inclusions that are formed as a result of denatured or precipitated hemoglobin. May be seen in the thalassemia syndromes, G6PD deficiency, or any of the unstable hemoglobin conditions.

Helmet cell: See **Bite cell.**

Hemagglutination: The clumping together of erythrocytes.

Hemangioma: A benign tumor of dilated blood vessels.

Hemarthrosis: Bloody effusion into the cavity of a joint.

Hematemesis: Vomiting of blood.

Hematocrit: The proportion of red blood cells in whole blood expressed as a percentage.

Hematoma: A swelling or mass of blood confined to an organ, tissue, or space and caused by a break in a blood vessel.

Hematopoiesis: Formation and development of blood cells, normally in the bone marrow. (Synonym: **Hemopoiesis.**)

Hematuria: Blood in the urine.

Heme: The iron-containing protoporphyrin portion of the hemoglobin wherein the iron is in the ferrous (Fe^{2+}) state.

Hemochromatosis: A disease of iron metabolism in which iron accumulates in body tissues, causing complications and tissue damage.

Hemoconcentration: An increase in the number of red cells, resulting from a decrease in the volume of plasma.

Hemodialysis: Removal of chemical substances from the blood by passing it through tubes made of semipermeable membranes. This procedure is used to cleanse the blood of patients in whom one or both kidneys are defective or absent and to remove excess accumulation of drugs or toxic chemicals in the blood.

Hemoglobin: The iron-containing pigment of the red blood cells that functions to carry oxygen from the lungs to the tissues. Consists of approximately 6% heme and 94% globin.

H. A.: The major portion of adult hemoglobin (95%), composed of two alpha and two beta chains.

H. A₂: A small portion of adult hemoglobin (2% to 4%), composed of two alpha and two delta chains.

H. Bart's: An abnormal hemoglobin composed of four gamma chains. Formed in α-thalassemia major, the most severe form of thalassemia occurring in anemic, edematous stillborn infants whose hemoglobin composition is almost all hemoglobin Bart's.

H. F: The major fetal hemoglobin, composed of two alpha and two gamma chains.

H. Gower 1: A type of hemoglobin found in the embryo, composed of two zeta and two epsilon chains.

H. Gower 2:   A type of hemoglobin found in the embryo, composed of two alpha and two epsilon chains.

H. H. inclusions: Red cell inclusions that are formed in the α-thalassemia in which hemoglobin (four beta chains) is in high concentration.

H. Lepore: A type of abnormal hemoglobin that is the product of a fused delta and beta gene, formed by an unequal crossing over resulting in a hemoglobin with fused delta/beta chains; a form of thalassemia.

H. Portland: A type of hemoglobin found in the embryo, composed of two zeta and two gamma chains.

Hemoglobinemia: Presence of hemoglobin in the blood plasma.

Hemoglobinopathies: The group of diseases caused by or associated with the presence of one of several forms of abnormal hemoglobin in the blood.

Hemoglobin-oxygen dissociation curve: The relationship between the percent saturation of the hemoglobin molecule with oxygen and the environmental oxygen tension.

Hemoglobinuria: The presence of free hemoglobin in the urine.

Hemolysin: An antibody that activates complement, leading to cell lysis.

Hemolysis: The destruction of red blood cells.

Intravascular h.:   The disruption of the red cell membrane and release of hemoglobin into the surrounding fluid within the vasculature.

Extravascular h: The phagocytosis of erythrocytes by the reticuloendothelial system, primarily in the spleen and liver.

Hemolytic: Pertaining to, characterized by, or producing hemolysis.

H. anemia: Anemia caused by increased destruction of erythrocytes.

H. disease of the newborn (HDN):   A disease characterized by anemia, jaundice, enlargement of the liver and spleen, and generalized edema (hydrops fetalis), owing to the maternal IgG antibodies that cross the placenta and attack fetal red cells when there is a feto-maternal blood group incompatibility. Usually caused by ABO or Rh antibodies. (Synonym: **Erythroblastosis fetalis.**)

Hemolytic uremic syndrome (HUS):   A disorder that usually affects young children and is characterized by the combination of severe hemolytic anemia and renal failure. Reticulocytosis and schistocytes are the morphologic findings of this microangiopathic hemolytic anemia.

Hemopexin: A β-globulin that has the capacity to bind hemoglobin when haptoglobin has been depleted.

Hemophilia: A hereditary blood disease characterized by impaired coagulability of the blood and a strong tendency to bleed.

H. A: A sex-linked hereditary bleeding disorder characterized by greatly prolonged coagulation time owing to a deficiency of factor VIII.

H. B: Christmas disease, a hereditary bleeding disorder caused by a deficiency of factor IX.

H. C: A hereditary bleeding disorder caused by a deficiency of factor XI.

Hemoptysis: Coughing and spitting up of blood as a result of bleeding from any part of the respiratory tract.

Hemorrhage: Abnormal internal or external bleeding. May be venous, arterial, or capillary from blood vessels into the tissues, or into or from the body.

Hemorrhagic diathesis: Predisposition to spontaneous bleeding from a trivial trauma caused by a defect in clotting or in the structure or function of blood vessels.

Hemosiderin: An iron-containing pigment derived from hemoglobin on disintegration of red cells; one method whereby iron is stored until needed for making hemoglobin.

Hemosiderinuria: The excretion of hemosiderin from disintegrated red blood cells into the urine.

Hemosiderosis: A condition in which the iron content of blood is increased.

Hemostasis: The process in which the blood clots and bleeding is arrested.

Hemotherapy: Blood transfusion as a therapeutic measure.

Heparin: A sulfonated mucopolysaccharide that acts as a powerful anticoagulant at several sites in the coagulation sequence: (1) inhibition of thrombin, (2) inhibition of factor Xa, (3) inhibition of factor IXa, and (4) inhibition of factor XIIa. Used therapeutically in the treatment of thromboembolic disease.

Hepatitis: Inflammation of the liver.

Hepatocyte: A liver cell.

Hepatomegaly: A condition characterized by enlargement of the liver.

Hepatosplenomegaly: Enlargement of the liver and the spleen.

Hereditary: Transmitted from parent to offspring.

Hereditary angioneurotic edema: A disease state in which there is no inhibition of C1 enzyme activity. There are increased levels of plasmin and complement activator.

Hereditary elliptocytosis (HE):   An inherited (autosomal dominant) intracorpuscular defect of the red cell membrane that is characterized by the presence of greater than 40% elliptical red cells on the peripheral blood smear. The condition is generally asymptomatic. There is a biochemical and genetic relationship to hereditary pyropoikilocytosis (HPP).

Hereditary erythroblastic multinuclearity with a positive acid serum (HEMPAS):   A type II congenital dyserythropoietic anemia (CDA), also known as Ham's test.

Hereditary hemorrhagic telangiectasia: A congenital hemorrhagic abnormality of the vascular system characterized by localized dilation and convolution of capillaries and venules giving rise to the characteristic telangiectases.

Hereditary persistence of fetal hemoglobin (HPFH):   A group of conditions characterized by the persistence of fetal hemoglobin synthesis into adult life.

Hereditary pyropoikilocytosis (HPP):   A relatively rare and severe autosomal recessive hemolytic anemia characterized by striking bizarre micropoikilocytosis in which the red cells bud, fragment, and form microspherocytes. In addition, the red cells are thermally unstable when heated to 45°C and strikingly fragmented in comparison to normal red cells which fragment only at 49°C.

Hereditary spherocytosis (HS):   An inherited (autosomal dominant) intracorpuscular defect of the red cell membrane (altered spectrin) that results in the most common hereditary hemolytic anemia found in whites. The morphologic hallmark of hereditary spherocytosis is the presence of spherocytes on the peripheral blood smear.

Hereditary stomatocytosis (hereditary hydrocytosis):   A heterogenous group of rare red cell membrane disorders inherited in an autosomal dominant fashion that are characterized by the presence of stomatocytes on the peripheral blood smear and alterations in the permeability of the red cell membrane to cations.

Hereditary thrombophilia: Antithrombin III deficiency; an autosomal dominant disorder in which there is an increased tendency toward thrombosis.

Heterozygous: Possessing different alleles in regard to a given characteristic.

Histamine: A substance normally present in the body that is released by the mast cells and basophils. It exerts a pharmacologic action when released from injured cells.

Histoplasmosis: An infection caused by *Histoplasma capsulatum* with clinical manifestations of anemia and leukopenia, enlargement of the spleen and liver, and fever.

Hodgkin's disease: A disease of unknown etiology producing enlargement of lymphoid tissue, spleen, and liver, with invasion of other tissues.

Homozygous: Possessing identical alleles in regard to a given characteristic.

Howell-Jolly bodies: Red cell inclusions that develop in periods of accelerated or abnormal erythropoiesis. They represent nuclear remnants containing DNA.

Human immunodeficiency virus (HIV): A lymphotropic (Ribonucleic acid—RNA) retrovirus that directly infects T helper cells (CD 4 cells) causing cell lysis, loss of cellular immunity, and the acquired immunodeficiency syndrome (AIDS).

Human leukocyte antigen (HLA): Antigens found in white blood cells that are part of the major histocompatibility complex.

Humoral: Pertaining to body fluids or substances contained in them.

Hybridization: The process in which one nucleotide strand binds to its counterpart strand by forming hydrogen bonds between long stretches of complementary nucleotides.

Hybridoma: A neoplastic cell.

Hydrophilic: Having an affinity for or readily absorbing fluid.

Hydrophobic: Having an aversion to or not readily absorbing fluid.

Hydrops fetalis: Erythroblastosis fetalis. A hemolytic disease of the newborn characterized by anemia, jaundice, enlargement of the liver and spleen, and generalized edema.

Hyperbilirubinemia: A condition characterized by an excessive amount of bilirubin in the blood.

Hypercoagulability: A condition in which activated coagulation factors are found intravascularly; may or may not be associated with increased incidence of thromboembolism.

Hyperkalemia: Excessive amounts of potassium in the blood.

Hyperlipidemia: A condition characterized by excessive amounts of lipids in the blood.

Hyperplasia: Excessive proliferation of normal cells in the normal tissue arrangement of an organ.

Hypersegmentation: An increase in the number of nuclear lobes or segments (more than 6) in segmented neutrophils; especially characteristic in vitamin B_{12} or folate deficiencies.

Hypersplenism: A condition arising as a result of an enlarged spleen. Red cell survival is significantly shortened.

Hypertension: Increase in blood pressure to above normal.

Hyperviscosity: Excessive viscosity or exaggeration of adhesive properties seen in anemias and inflammatory disease.

Hypocalcemia: Pertaining to a deficient level of calcium in the blood.

Hypochromia: Increased area of central pallor in red cells.

Hypoferremia: Pertaining to a deficient level of iron in the blood.

Hypofibrinogenemia: A congenital disorder characterized by low levels of fibrinogen, usually without any bleeding tendencies.

Hypogammaglobulinemia: Decreased blood levels of gamma globulins seen in some disease states.

Hypogonadism: Defective internal secretion of the gonads.

Hypokalemia: Pertaining to a deficient level of potassium in the blood.

Hypopituitarism: A condition caused by deficient functioning of the hypophysis cerebri, or pituitary organ, which secretes several important hormones.

Hypoplasia: Abnormal, deficient, or defective development.

Hyposplenism: Decreased or improper splenic function. A variety of conditions and splenic sizes are associated with hyposplenism; however, all have in common hematologic manifestations that suggest loss of many or all of the vital splenic functions (for example, Howell-Jolly bodies, Pappenheimer's bodies, poikilocytes, increased platelet count).

Hypotension: Decrease in blood pressure to below normal.

Hypothermia: Having a body temperature below normal.

Hypothyroidism: A condition caused by a deficiency of thyroid secretion, resulting in a lowered basal metabolism.

Hypovolemia: Diminished blood volume.

Hypoxemia: A condition characterized by insufficient oxygenation of the blood.

Hypoxia: Deficiency of oxygen.

I

Icterus: A condition characterized by yellowish skin, eyes, mucous membranes, and body fluids owing to deposition of excess bilirubin.

Idiopathic: Pertaining to conditions without clear pathogenesis or disease without recognizable cause, as of spontaneous origin.

Idiopathic thrombocytopenic purpura (ITP): Bleeding caused by a decreased number of platelets. The etiology is unknown, with most evidence pointing to platelet autoantibodies.

Idiothrombocythemia: An increase in blood platelets with unknown etiology.

Immune response: The reaction of the body to substances that are foreign or are interpreted as foreign. Cell-mediated or cellular immunity pertains to tissue destruction mediated by T cells such as graft rejection and hypersensitivity reactions. Humoral immunity pertains to cell destruction caused by antibody production.

Immune serum globulin: Gamma globulin protein fraction of serum containing antibodies.

Immunoblast: A mitotically active T or B cell.

Immunodeficiency: A decrease in the normal concentration of immunoglobulins in serum.

Immunogenicity: The ability of an antigen to stimulate an antibody response.

Immunoglobulin (Ig): One of a family of closely related, yet not identical, proteins that are capable of acting as antibodies: IgA, IgD, IgE, IgG, and IgM. The principal immunoglobulin in exocrine secretions such as saliva and tears is IgA. Immunoglobulin D may play a role in antigen recognition and the initiation of antibody synthesis. Immunoglobulin E is produced by the cells lining the intestinal and respiratory tracts and is important in forming reagin. The main immunoglobulin in human serum is IgG. A globulin formed in almost every immune response during the early period of the reaction is IgM.

Immunologic memory: The development of T and B memory cells that have been sensitized by exposure to an antigen and respond rapidly under subsequent encounters with the antigen.

Immunologic unresponsiveness: Development of a tolerance to certain antigens that would otherwise evoke an immune response.

Immunoprecipitin: An antigen-antibody reaction that results in precipitation.

Inflammation: Tissue reaction to injury. The succession of changes that occurs in living tissue when it is injured.

Inhibitor: A chemical substance that stops enzyme activity.

Insidious: Without warning.

***In situ* hybridization:** Detection of DNA or RNA within native cells by hybridization to a complementary probe. This permits microscopic visualization of the target sequence in the context of cytologic or morphologic features of the tissue or glass slides. In a variation of this procedure called fluorescence *in situ* hybridization (FISH), the target is usually a karyotypic preparation of chromosomes, and the probe is labeled in such a way that it fluoresces in response to an input light signal.

Insomnia: Inability to sleep, or sleep prematurely ended or interrupted by periods of wakefulness.

Interferon: A protein or proteins formed when cells are exposed to viruses. Noninfected cells exposed to interferon are protected against viral infection.

Interleukin (IL): A family of polypeptide products (proteins) produced by many cell types that are involved in lymphocyte recruitment, lymphocyte proliferation, and cellular responses in immunology.

Intravascular hemolysis: Hemolysis occurring within the blood vessels. (See **Hemolysis.**)

Intrinsic factor (IF): A protein secreted by the parietal cells of the stomach that is necessary for vitamin B_{12} absorption.

Intrinsic system: Initiation of blood clotting that occurs through a surface-mediated pathway.

In utero: Within the uterus.

In vitro: In glass, as in a test tube.

In vivo: In the living body or organism.

Ischemia: Local and temporary deficiency of blood supply to the tissues.

Isoagglutinins: A term used to denote the ABO antibodies anti-A, anti-B, and Anti-A,B.

Isoimmune: An antibody produced against a foreign antigen in the same species.

J

Jaundice: A condition characterized by yellowing of the skin and the whites of the eyes. One cause is excess hemolysis, which results in increased circulating bilirubin. Another cause is liver damage caused by hepatitis.

Juvenile: A common-usage term that is a synonym for neutrophilic metamyelocyte.

K

Kaolin: A surface-activated substance.

Karyorrhexis: A necrotic stage with fragmentation of the nucleus whereby chromatin is distributed irregularly throughout the cytoplasm.

Karyotype: A photomicrograph of a single cell in the metaphase stage of mitosis that is arranged to show the chromosomes in descending order of size.

Kernicterus: A form of icterus neonatorum occurring in infants. Develops at 2 to 8 days of age. Prognosis is poor if untreated.

Ketosis: The accumulation in the body of the ketone bodies: acetone, beta hydroxybutyric acid, and acetoacetic acid.

Kinin: A general term for a group of polypeptides that have considerable biologic activity (for example, vasoactivity).

Koilonychia: A disorder of the nails, which are abnormally thin and concave from side to side, with the edges turned up.

L

Late degradation products: The terminal fragments D and E that result from the proteolytic action of plasmin on fibrin or fibrinogen. Fragments D and E are known to inhibit fibrin polymerization.

Lepore: See **Hemoglobin Lepore.**

Leptocyte: Synonymous with **Target cell.**

Lethargic: Sluggish; having a lack of energy.

Leukemia: A chronic or acute disease of unknown etiologic factors characterized by unrestrained growth of leukocytes and their precursors in the tissues.

Leukemic hiatus: A phase of leukemia in which the normal maturation series of white cells is not seen because blast cells crowd out normal cells.

Leukemoid reaction: A moderate or advanced degree of leukocytes in the blood that is not a result of a leukemic disease. These reactions are frequently observed as a feature of infectious disease, drug and chemical intoxication, or secondary to nonhematopoietic carcinoma.

Leukoagglutinins: Antibodies to white blood cells.

Leukocyte: Colorless cell in blood, lymph and tissue; important to the immune system.

Leukocytosis: Increase in number of leukocytes (more than 10,000 cells/mm³) in the blood.

Leukoerythroblastosis: The presence of immature white cells and nucleated red cells on the blood smear; frequently denotes a malignant or myeloproliferative process.

Leukopenia: An abnormal decrease in the number of leukocytes in the blood.

Leukopheresis: Withdrawal of leukocytes from the circulation; may be used to obtain leukocytes for administration to patients with severe granulocytopenia.

Linkage analysis: The process of following the inheritance pattern of a particular gene in a family based on its tendency to be inherited together with another locus on the same chromosome.

Littoral cells: Cells located in the walls of blood sinuses or lymph, characterized by their flattened appearance.

Locus: A specific position along the DNA sequence composing a particular chromosome, analogous to a street address.

Lymphadenitis: Inflammation of the lymph nodes.

Lymphadenopathy: Disease of the lymph nodes.

Lymphocyte: A white blood cell formed in lymphoid tissue throughout the body, generally described as nongranular and including small and large varieties. Makes up approximately 20% to 45% of the total leukocyte count.

Lymphocytosis: An increase in lymphocytes within the blood.

Lymphoma: Asymmetrical enlargement of a group of lymph nodes, which destroys the normal histologic lymph node architecture.

Lymphopoiesis: Refers to the growth or development of lymphocytes.

Lysosomes: Part of an intracellular digestive system that exists as separate particles in the cell. Even though their importance in health and disease is certain, all the precise ways in which lysosomes affect changes are not understood.

Lysozyme (muramidase): A hydrolytic enzyme destructive to cell walls of certain bacteria. It is present in body fluids and found in high concentration within granulocytes.

M

Macrocephaly: Enlargement of the head.

Macrocyte: A red cell 9 μm in diameter or larger.

Macrocytosis: Refers to a condition in which erythrocytes are abnormally large.

Macroglobulin: A protease inhibitor present in the blood that inhibits the activity of plasmin.

Macroglobulinemia: Abnormal presence of high molecular weight immunoglobulins (IgM) in the blood.

Macroovalocytes: Refers to a condition in which ovalocytes are abnormally large.

Macrophage: Cells of the reticuloendothelial system having the ability to phagocytose particulate substances and to store vital dyes and other colloidal substances. They are found in loose connective tissues and various organs of the body.

Major histocompatibility complex (MHC): Present in all mammalian and ovarian species (analogous to human HLA complex); HLA antigens are within the MHC at a locus on chromosome 6.

Malabsorption syndrome: Disordered or inadequate absorption of nutrients from the intestinal tract. May be caused by disease that affects the intestinal mucosa such as infections, tropical sprue, gluten enteropathy, or pancreatic insufficiency, or by antibiotic therapy.

Malaria: An acute and sometimes chronic infectious disease caused by the presence of protozoan plasmodium parasites within red blood cells.

Mast cell: A tissue basophil. (See **Basophil.**)

Mastocytosis: An increase in the number of mast cells.

Mastoiditis: Inflammation of the air cells of the mastoid process.

May-Hegglin anomaly: Inclusions found in the hereditary leukocyte and platelet disorder, similar but not identical to Dohle bodies.

Mean corpuscular hemoglobin (MCH): A measure of the hemoglobin content of red corpuscles. It is reported in picograms.

$$MCH = \frac{\text{Hemoglobin in g/100 ml} \times 10}{\text{RBC count, millions of cells}/\mu l}$$

Mean corpuscular hemoglobin concentration (MCHC): A measure of concentration of hemoglobin in the average red cell.

$$MCHC = \frac{\text{Hemoglobin in g/100 ml} \times 100}{\text{Hematocrit, \%}}$$

Mean corpuscular volume (MCV): A measure of the volume of red corpuscles expressed in cubic micrometers or femtoliters.

$$MCV = \frac{\text{Hematocrit, \%} \times 10}{\text{RBC count, millions of cells}/\mu l}$$

Mediastinal: Related to the mediastinum.

Mediastinum: A septum or cavity between two principal portions of an organ.

Medullary: Concerning marrow or medulla.

Megakaryocyte: The intermediate platelet precursor cell in the bone marrow, not normally present in peripheral blood. It is a large cell, usually having a multilobed nucleus, that gives rise to blood platelets owing to a pinching off of the cytoplasm.

Megakaryopoiesis: The development of megakaryocytes in the blood.

Megaloblast: A large, nucleated, abnormal red cell precursor, 11 to 20 μm in diameter, oval and slightly irregular, resulting from a nuclear/cytoplasmic maturation asynchrony characteristic of vitamin B_{12} or folate deficiency.

Megaloblastoid: Term used to describe changes in the bone marrow that are morphologically similar to, yet etiologically different from, megaloblastic change.

Meiosis: Type of cell division of germ cells in which two successive divisions of the nucleus produce cells that contain half the number of chromosomes present in somatic cells.

Melena: Black, tarry feces caused by the action of intestinal juices on free blood.

Melanocyte: A pigment-producing cell.

Menorrhagia: Menstrual bleeding that is excessive in number of days, amount of blood, or both.

Menstruation: The periodic discharge of a bloody fluid from the uterus, occurring at more or less regular intervals during the life of a woman from puberty to menopause.

Metamyelocyte: An immature neutrophilic granulocyte with a kidney-bean-shaped nucleus or an indent, with the presence of specific granules (neutrophilic, eosinophilic, or basophilic) in the cytoplasm (such as neutrophilic metamyelocyte, eosinophilic metamyelocyte, basophilic metamyelocyte).

Metaphyseal dysostosis: Defective bone formation in the metaphysis (the portion of a developing long bone between diaphysis or shaft and epiphysis).

Metaplasia: Conversion of one kind of tissue into a form that is not normal for that tissue.

Metarubricyte: Synonymous with **Orthochromic (orthochromatophilic) normoblast.**

Metastatic: Pertaining to metastasis. (See below.)

Metastasis: Movement of bacteria or body cells, especially cancer cells, from one part of the body to another. Change in location of a disease or of its manifestation or transfer from one organ or part to another not directly connected. Spread is by the lymphatics or bloodstream.

Methemoglobin: A form of hemoglobin wherein the ferrous ion (Fe^{2+}) has been oxidized to ferric ion (Fe^{3+}), possibly owing to toxic substances such as aniline dyes, potassium chlorate, or nitrate-contaminated water.

Microaggregates: Aggregates of platelets and leukocytes that accumulate in stored blood.

Microcephaly: Abnormal smallness of the head, often seen in mental retardation. This condition is congenital.

Microcyte: An abnormally small red cell with a diameter of less than 6 μm.

Microcytosis: Refers to a condition in which the erythrocytes are abnormally small.

Microspherocytes: Small, sphere-shaped red blood cells seen in certain kinds of anemia.

Mitochondria: Slender microscopic filaments or rods 0.5 μm in diameter that can be seen in cells by using phase contrast microscopy or electron microscopy. They are a source of energy in the cell and are involved in protein synthesis and lipid metabolism.

Mitosis: Type of cell division in which each daughter cell contains the same number of chromosomes as the parent cell. All cells except sex cells undergo mitosis.

Mixed field: A type of agglutination pattern in which there are numerous small clumps of cells amid a sea of free cells.

Mixed lymphocyte culture (MLC): A technique for typing cells in which lymphocytes of different individuals are cocultured.

Mixed lymphocyte reaction (MLR): A method of tissue typing that exploits the fact that T lymphocytes are stimulated to grow in the presence of cells carrying foreign histocompatibility class II antigens.

Monoclonal: Antibody derived from a single ancestral antibody-producing parent cell.

Monocyte: A white blood cell that normally constitutes 2% to 10% of the total leukocyte differential count. This cell is 9 to 12 μm in diameter and has an indented nucleus and an abundant pale blue-gray cytoplasm containing many fine red-staining granules.

Morbidity: The number of sick persons or cases of disease in relationship to a specific population.

Mortality: The death rate; ratio of number of deaths to a given population.

Mucopolysaccharidoses: A group of hexosamine-containing polysaccharides that are the major constituent of mucus.

Multiparous: Having borne more than one child.

Multiple myeloma: A neoplastic proliferation of plasma cells, characterized by very high immunoglobulin levels of monoclonal origin.

Mutant: A variation of genetic structure.

Mutation: A change in a gene potentially capable of being transmitted to offspring.

    Frameshift m.: A change in which a message is read incorrectly because either a base is missing or an extra base is added. This results in an entirely new polypeptide because the triplet sequence has been shifted one base.

    Point m.: A change in a base in DNA that can lead to a change in the amino acid incorporated into the polypeptide. The change is identifiable by analyzing the amino acid sequences of the original protein and its mutant offspring.

Myalgia: Muscle pain.

Myeloblast: The first recognizable "mother cell" (precursor) of the granulocytic cell line.

Myelocyte: An immature granulocyte characterized by an eccentrically located round nucleus and specific granules—neutrophilic, eosinophilic, or basophilic (such as a neutrophilic myelocyte, eosinophilic myelocyte, or basophilic myelocyte).

Myelodysplasia: Abnormal division; maturation and production of erythrocytes, granulocytes, monocytes, and platelets.

Myelodysplastic syndrome (MDS): A group of primary hematologic disorders associated with abnormal division, maturation, and production of erythrocytes, granulocytes, monocytes, and platelets; also referred to as preleukemic myelodysplastic syndrome.

Myelofibrosis: Replacement of the bone marrow by fibrous tissue.

Myeloid-to-erythroid (M:E) ratio: Differential count of bone marrow obtained by dividing the number of granulocytes and their precursor cells by the number of nucleated red cells.

Myelokathexis: A moderate neutropenia related to defective release of mature granulocytes into peripheral circulation.

Myeloperoxidase: An enzyme that is present in the primary (azurophilic) granules of polymorphonuclear neutrophils, eosinophils, and monocytes-macrophages.

Myelophthisic: The process that occurs primarily in the bone marrow as a result of the crowding out of normal elements by malignant cells. A consequential reduction in normal marrow cells and release of immature hematopoietic cells (especially nucleated red cells) into the blood occur.

Myelopoiesis: The growth or development of myeloid cells in the bone marrow.

Myeloproliferative: Referring to a group of disorders characterized by autonomous proliferation of one or more hematopoietic elements in the bone marrow. In many cases, the liver and spleen are enlarged.

Myoglobin: Muscle hemoglobin.

N

Necrosis: The pathologic death of one or more cells of a portion of tissue or organ.

Neonatal: Pertaining to the first 6 weeks after birth.

Neoplasm: A new and abnormal formation of tissue such as a tumor or growth.

Neuraminidase: An enzyme that cleaves sialic acid from the red cell membrane.

Neutralization: Inactivating an antibody by reacting it with an antigen against which it is directed.

Neutropenia: The presence of abnormally small numbers of neutrophils in the circulating blood.

Neutrophil: A medium-sized mature leukocyte with a three- to five-lobed nucleus and cytoplasm containing small lilac-staining granules. Neutrophils normally constitute 50% to 70% of leukocytes in the blood.

Neutrophilia: An abnormal increase in neutrophil leukocytes.

Niemann-Pick disease: An infant disease characterized by a deficiency of sphingomyelinase, fatal within the first two years of life. It is characterized by anemia, enlargement of the liver and spleen, and leukocytosis.

Nondisjunction: Failure of a pair of chromosomes to separate during meiosis.

Nonresponder: An individual whose immune system does not respond well in antibody formation to antigenic stimulation.

Normocyte: A normal erythrocyte.

Normovolemic: Having a normal blood volume.

Nuclear-to-cytoplasmic (N:C) ratio: The proportion of nucleus to cytoplasm found in nucleated cells; often used in identification of cell maturity.

Nucleotide: The basic building block of DNA, composed of a nitrogenous base (A=adenine, T=thymine, G=guanine, or C=cytosine) attached to a sugar (deoxyribose) and a triphosphate moiety. RNA is similarly composed except that the sugar is ribose and T is replaced by U=uracil.

O

Obstetric: Referring to the branch of medicine that concerns itself with the management of women during pregnancy, childbirth, and puerperium.

Oculocutaneous: Relating to the eyes and the skin.

Oliguria: Diminished amount of urine formation.

Oncogene: A gene that contributes to the development of cancer. Most oncogenes are altered forms of normal genes (called proto-oncogenes) that function in key biochemical pathways related to cell growth or differentiation.

Opisthotonos: Extreme arching of the spine.

Opsonin: Substance in the blood serum that acts on microorganisms and other cells, facilitating phagocytosis.

Organomegaly: Enlargement of any of the specific organs of the body.

Orthochromic (orthochromatophilic) normoblast: An immature red cell precursor characterized by pink cytoplasm and a small round pyknotic nucleus. This stage of maturation is normally found only in the bone marrow.

Orthodontic: Referring to the branch of dentistry that deals with the prevention and correction of irregularities of the teeth.

Orthostatic hypotension: Decreased blood pressure with the body in an erect position.

Osmolality: The osmotic concentration of a solution determined by the ionic concentration of dissolved substances per unit of solvent.

Osmotic fragility: The ability of the red cells to withstand different salt concentrations; this is dependent on the volume, surface area, and functional state of the red blood cell membrane.

Osteoblast: An immature bone marrow cell responsible for the formation of osteocytes.

Osteoclast: Giant multinuclear cell formed in the marrow of growing bones.

Osteomyelitis: Inflammation of the bone, especially the marrow, caused by a pathogenic organism.

Osteoporosis: Increased porosity of the bone, seen most often in elderly women.

Ovalocyte: An abnormal red cell that is egg-shaped or elliptical. (Synonym: **Elliptocyte.**)

Oxyhemoglobin: The combined form of hemoglobin and oxygen.

P

P$_{50}$: The partial pressure of oxygen or oxygen tension at which the hemoglobin molecule is 50% saturated with oxygen.

Pagophagia: A craving to eat ice.

Pallor: Paleness; lack of color.

Panagglutinin: An antibody capable of agglutinating all red blood cells tested, including the patient's own cells.

Pancytopenia: A depression of each of the normal bone marrow elements: white cells, red cells, and platelets in the peripheral blood.

Panel: A large number of group O reagent red cells that are of known antigenic characterization and are used for antibody identification.

Panhyperplasia: An abnormal increase in all affected cells.

Panmyelosis: Increase in all the elements of the bone marrow.

Papilledema: Edema and inflammation of the optic nerve at its point of entrance into the eyeball.

Pappenheimer's bodies: Basophilic inclusions in the red blood cell that are clusterlike. They are believed to be iron particles; confirmation is made by Prussian blue stain.

Parachromatin: The portions of the nuclear chromatin that are nonstained or lightly stained.

Paracoagulants: A variety of substances capable of converting soluble fibrin monomer complexes into insoluble fibrin. These include protamine sulfate, ethanol, and material from staphylococci.

Paracoagulation tests: Coagulation procedures used to indicate the presence of soluble fibrin monomer complexes, which is indirect evidence of the action of thrombin on fibrinogen.

Paraproteinemia: A general term for abnormalities of the immunoglobulins, associated with one of several disease states.

Parenchymal: Relating to parenchyma, the essential parts of an organ that are concerned with its function in contradistinction to its framework.

Parenteral: Entry into the body through the intravenous (IV) or intramuscular (IM) route rather than the alimentary route.

Paresis: Partial or incomplete paralysis.

Paresthesia: Numbness.

Paroxysm: A sudden, periodic attack or recurrence of symptoms of a disease.

Paroxysmal cold hemoglobinuria (PCH): A type of cold autoimmune hemolytic anemia usually found in children suffering from viral infections in which a biphasic IgG antibody can be demonstrated with anti-P specificity. (See also **Donath-Landsteiner antibody test.**)

Paroxysmal nocturnal hemoglobinuria (PNH): An uncommon acquired form of hemolysis caused by an intrinsic defect in the red blood cell membrane, rendering it more susceptible to hemolysins in an acid environment, and characterized by hemoglobin in the urine following periods of sleep.

Pathogenesis: Origination and development of a disease.

Pathognomonic: Specifically distinctive or characteristic of a disease or pathologic condition.

Perfusion: Supplying an organ or tissue with nutrients and oxygen by passing blood or other suitable fluid through it.

Perioral paresthesia: Tingling around the mouth, occasionally experienced by apheresis donors, resulting from the rapid return of citrated plasma that contains citrate-bound calcium and free citrate.

Peroxidase: An enzyme that hastens the transfer of oxygen from peroxide to a tissue that requires oxygen; essential to intracellular respiration.

Petechiae: Pinpoint hemorrhages from arterioles or venules.

Phagocyte: Cells that ingest foreign particles, microorganisms, or other cells.

Phagocytosis: Ingestion and digestion of bacteria and particles by phagocytes.

Pharmacologic: Relating to the study of drugs and their origin, natural properties, and effects on living organisms.

Phlebotomy: Surgical opening of a vein to withdraw blood.

Phosphoglyceromutase (PGM): A red cell enzyme involved in the glycolytic pathway.

Phospholipid: A lipid containing phosphorus groups, found in the Rbc membrane.

Photodermatitis: Lesion development on exposure to sunlight.

Phototherapy: Exposure to sunlight or artificial light for therapeutic purposes.

Phox: Phagocyte oxidase subunits whose interaction results in the formation of active oxygen metabolites during the respiratory burst.

Pica: A perversion of appetite associated with ingestion of material not fit for food, such as starch, clay, ashes, or plaster, associated with severe iron-deficiency anemia.

Pico-: A prefix used in the metric system to signify 10^{-12}. A picogram is used in reporting the mean corpuscular hemoglobin.

Pinguecula: A yellowish discoloration near the corneal-scleral junction of the eye.

Pinocytosis: Process by which cells absorb or ingest nutrients and fluid.

Plaques: Small, flat growths.

Plasma: The liquid portion of whole blood containing water, electrolytes, glucose, fats, proteins, and gases. Contains all the clotting factors necessary for coagulation but in an inactive form. Once coagulation occurs, the fluid is converted to serum.

Plasma cell: A B lymphocyte-derived cell that secretes immunoglobulins or antibodies.

Plasmacyte: A plasma cell.

Plasmacytosis: The presence of plasma cells in blood.

Plasma protein fraction (PPF): Also known as Plasmanate. Sterile pooled plasma stored as a fluid or freeze-dried. Used for volume replacement.

Plasma thromboplastin antecedent (PTA): Factor XI involved in the intrinsic coagulation pathway.

Plasmacytomas: Localized or generalized tumor masses of plasma cells.

Plasmapheresis: Removal of blood, separation of plasma by centrifugation, and reinjection of the cells into the body. Used as a means of obtaining plasma and in the treatment of certain pathologic conditions.

Plasmin: Fibrinolytic enzyme derived from its precursor, plasminogen.

Plasminogen: A protein found in many tissues and body fluids. It is important in preventing fibrin clot formation.

Plasmodium: See **Malaria.**

Platelet: A round or oval disc, 2 to 4 μm in diameter, de-

rived from the cytoplasm of the megakaryocyte, a large cell in the bone marrow. Plays an important role in blood coagulation, hemostasis, and blood thrombus formation.

Platelet adhesion: The interaction of platelet surface glycoproteins with connective tissue elements of the subendothelium, requiring von Willebrand factor as a plasma cofactor.

Platelet aggregation: Platelet-to-platelet interaction dependent on calcium.

Platelet concentrate: Platelets prepared from a single unit of whole blood or plasma and suspended in a specific volume of the original plasma. Also known as random donor platelets.

Platelet factor (PF) 3: A phospholipid found within the platelet membrane required for coagulation. Platelet factor 3 assays are used to evaluate platelet disorders.

Platelet plug: Platelets that function in arresting bleeding by "plugging" any damage in the vessel wall and providing phospholipids essential for blood coagulation. The development of a hemostatic platelet plug depends on adhesion, aggregation, and consolidation.

Plateletpheresis: A procedure using a machine by which one can selectively remove platelets from a donor or patient.

Platelet-rich plasma (PRP): Plasma that is derived from a citrated blood sample spun at 1500 rpm for 5 minutes.

Platelin: A substance that acts in vitro like PF3.

Plethora: Congestion causing distention of the blood vessels.

Pleural effusion: Fluid in the pleural space.

Pluripotential stem cell: A generalized parent cell that gives rise to a common lymphoid stem cell, which differentiates into T or B cell ontogeny or a colony-forming unit (CFU).

Pneumonitis: Inflammation of the lung.

Poikilocytosis: Variation in shape of red cells.

Polyacrylamide gel: A type of matrix used in electrophoresis upon which substances are separated.

Polyagglutination: A state in which an individual's red cells are agglutinated by all sera regardless of blood type.

Polychromasia: Describes the blue-gray color of some younger red cells in evaluation of red blood cell morphology. Increased polychromasia is a sign of a very active bone marrow.

Polychromatophilic normoblast: An immature red cell precursor characterized by blue-gray cytoplasm and round, eccentrically located nucleus with a distinct chromatin/parachromatin pattern of staining, and normally only found in the bone marrow. (Synonym: **Rubricyte.**)

Polyclonal: Antibodies derived from more than one antibody-producing parent cell.

Polycythemia: An excess of red blood cells in the peripheral blood.

P. vera: A chronic life-shortening myeloproliferative disorder involving all bone marrow elements, characterized by an increase in red blood cell mass and hemoglobin concentration.

Polymerase chain reaction (PCR): A procedure for copying a specific DNA sequence a billion times. To accomplish this, short DNA probes are designed to flank the target sequence. These probes serve as primers to initiate synthesis of new complementary nucleotide strands by the enzyme DNA polymerase. The whole process takes place in a thermocycling instrument that sequentially varies the reaction temperature to optimize probe binding, DNA synthesis, and denaturation before the next cycle of synthesis. In this way, target sequences up to several thousand base pairs in length may be replicated many times.

Polymorphism: A genetic system that possesses numerous allelic forms, such as a blood group system.

Polymorphonuclear neutrophil (PMN): A mature granulocyte with neutrophilic granules and a segmented nucleus (also called segmented neutrophil). (See **Neutrophil**.)

Polyspecific Coombs' sera: A reagent that contains antihuman globulin sera against IgG and C3d.

Porphobilinogen: A precursor of porphobilin that is a dark-pigmented nonporphyrin.

Porphyria: A group of inherited disorders caused by excessive production of porphyrins in the bone marrow or the liver. Two types are recognized: erythropoietic and hepatic.

Portal hypertension: Increased pressure in the portal vein as a result of obstruction of the flow of blood through the liver.

Postpartum: Occurring after childbirth.

Precipitation: The formation of a visible complex (precipitate) in a medium containing soluble antigen (precipitinogen) and the corresponding antibody (precipitin).

Precipitin: An antibody formed in the blood serum of an animal by the presence of a soluble antigen, usually a protein. When added to a solution of the antigen, it brings about precipitation. The injected protein is called the antigen and the antibody produced is the precipitin.

Preleukemia (myelodysplastic syndrome): A clinical syndrome in which the bone marrow shows marked hypocellularity with clusters of immature cells that in many cases evolve into true nonlymphocytic leukemia.

Priapism: Abnormal, painful, and continued erection of the penis caused by disease, accompanied by loss of sexual desire.

Primary fibrinolysis: Activation of the fibrinolytic system that is not secondary to coagulation.

Primary hemostasis: The interaction of platelets and the vascular endothelium to stop bleeding following vascular injury.

Proaccelerin: Factor V; functions in the common pathway of coagulation as a cofactor.

Proband: The initial subject presenting a mental or physical disorder; the heredity of this individual is studied to determine if other members of the family have had the same disease or carry it. (Synonym: **Propositus/proposita.**)

Probe: A tool for identifying a particular nucleotide sequence. A probe is a strand of nucleotides whose sequence is complementary to the target sequence and is thus capable of hybridizing to it. Probes are usually labeled in a way that permits their detection, so that the probe serves as a marker for the target sequence. Probes and their targets may be composed of either deoxyribonucleotides (DNA) or ribonucleotides (RNA). For probe binding to be effective, both the probe and target must be single-stranded. Double-stranded nucleic acid can be converted to its single-stranded components by the application of heat or a strong alkaline solution.

Proconvertin: Factor VII; functions in the extrinsic system of coagulation.

Prodrome: A symptom indicative of an approaching disease.

Progranulocyte: An immature white blood cell precursor found only in the bone marrow that is the characteristic stage of maturation at which azurophilic nonspecific granules first appear in the cytoplasm of the granulocytic cell line.

Pronormoblast: The first recognizable "mother cell" (precursor) of the erythrocytic cell line. (Synonym: Rubriblast.)

Prophylaxis: Any agent or regimen that contributes to the prevention of infection and disease.

Propositus/Proposita: The initial individual whose condition led to investigation of a hereditary disorder or to a serologic evaluation of family members. (Synonym: **Proband.**)

Proprioception: The awareness of posture movement and change in equilibrium and the knowledge of position, weight, and resistance of objects in relation to the body.

Prorubicyte: See **Basophilic normoblast.**

Prostaglandins: A group of fatty acid derivatives present in many tissues, including prostate gland, menstrual fluid, brain, lung, kidney, thymus, seminal fluid, and pancreas.

Prosthesis: Replacement of a missing part by an artificial substitute, such as an artificial extremity.

Prostration: Absolute exhaustion.

Protamine sulfate: A substance used to detect the presence of soluble fibrin monomer complexes. It is also used to neutralize the effects of heparin. (See also **Paracoagulants.**)

Prothrombin: Factor II; functions in the common pathway of coagulation.

Prothrombin complex: A commercially prepared concentrate of the vitamin K-dependent factors, prothrombin, and factors VII, IX, and X in lypholized form. Preparations of prothrombin complex are used therapeutically to treat acquired and congenital hemorrhagic disorders.

Prothrombin consumption test (PCT): A test that measures prothrombin activity in serum after coagulation has taken place.

Prothrombin time (PT): A test to evaluate the overall integrity of the clotting system that involves factors VII, X, V, II, and I. Commonly referred to as a means of evaluating the extrinsic system of coagulation.

Protoporphyrin: A porphyrin whose iron complex forms the heme of hemoglobin and the prosthetic groups of myoglobin and certain respiratory pigments.

Pulmonary artery wedge pressure: Pressure measured in the pulmonary artery at its capillary end.

Pulse pressure: The difference between the systolic and diastolic blood pressures.

Punctate: Having pinpoint punctures or depressions on the surface; marked with dots.

Purpura: A condition with various manifestations and diverse causes, characterized by hemorrhages into the skin, mucous membranes, internal organs, and other tissues.

Pyelogram: A radiograph of the ureter and renal pelvis.

Pyknosis (pyknotic): Condensation and shrinkage of cells through degeneration.

Pyoderma: Any acute inflammatory skin disease of unknown origin. Bacteria may be cultured from the lesions, but there are normal resident flora.

Pyogenic: Producing pus (for example, pyogenic infection).

Pyropoikilocytosis: See **Hereditary pyropoikilocytosis.**

Pyroprotein: A serum protein that precipitates on exposure to hot temperatures.

Pyruvate kinase deficiency: An enzymatic disorder in the Embden-Meyerhof Pathway caused by a deficiency in prruvate kinase. Hemolysis and anemia persist after splenectomy. The trait is autosomal-recessive.

R

Raynaud's disease: A peripheral vascular disorder characterized by abnormal vasoconstriction of the extremities on exposure to cold or during emotional stress. A history of symptoms for at least 2 years is necessary for diagnosis.

Recessive: In genetics, incapable of expression unless carried by both members of a set of homologous chromosomes; not dominant.

Recipient: A patient who is receiving a transfusion of blood or a blood product.

Recombinant human erythropoietin (rHuEpo): A genetically engineered erythropoietin.

Red cell distribution width (RDW): This measurement is included on some instruments as part of the complete blood count. It measures the distribution of red blood cell volume and is equivalent to anisocytosis on the peripheral blood smear. It is calculated as the coefficient of variation of the red cell volume and is expressed as a percentage (normal 11.5% to 14.5%).

Refractory: Not responsive to therapy.

Reniform—kidney bean shape: Characteristic shape of the nucleus of metamyelocytes; often used to distinguish metamyelocytes from myelocytes and neutrophilic bands; may also be used to characterize the appearance of reactive lymphocytes.

Replication: The process by which DNA is copied during cell division. Replication is carried out by the enzyme DNA polymerase, which recognizes single-stranded DNA and fills in the appropriate complementary nucleotides to produce double-stranded DNA. Synthesis usually begins at a junction where double-stranded DNA lies next to single-stranded DNA, and synthesis proceeds in a 5' to 3' direction. In the laboratory, replication of specific DNA sequences can be artificially induced. This permits us to produce and label DNA probes, determine the sequence of target DNA, and amplify DNA sequences as exploited by polymerase chain reaction.

Reptilase: An enzyme, thrombinlike in nature, derived from the venom of *Bothrops atrox*. Predominantly hydrolyzes fibrinopeptide A from the fibrinogen molecule, in contrast to thrombin, which hydrolyzes fibrinopeptides A and B.

R. time: A coagulation procedure similar to thrombin time except that clotting is initiated with the snake venom enzyme reptilase.

Respiratory distress syndrome (RDS): A condition, formerly known as hyaline membrane disease, accounting for more than 25,000 infant deaths per year in the United States. Clinical signs, including delayed onset of respiration and low Apgar score, are usually present at birth.

Respiratory syncytial virus (RSV): A common viral cause of acquired neutropenia in children.

Restriction endonuclease: An enzyme that cleaves double-stranded DNA at a specific nucleotide sequence. For example, EcoR1 cleaves DNA only where the sequence 5'-GAATTC-3' is present. A variety of other endonucleases have different sequence recognition sites. The ability to reproducibly cleave DNA into smaller fragments simplifies molecular analysis of an otherwise quite long molecule. (Human chromosomes exceed 10^7 nucleotides in length.)

Reticular dysgenesis: A disorder characterized by a combined deficiency of antibody production and cellular immunity; reported to be a selective failure of stem cells committed to the myeloid and lymphoid cell lines. Death occurs shortly after birth.

Reticulocyte: A red blood cell containing a network of granules or filaments representing an immature stage in development. Reticulocytes normally make up about 1% of circulating red blood cells.

Reticulocytopenia: A condition characterized by decreased erythrocytes.

Reticuloendothelial system (RES): Term applied to those cells scattered throughout the body that have the power to ingest particulate matter. Includes histiocytes of loose connective tissue; reticular cells of lymphatic organs; Kupffer's cells of the liver; cells lining blood sinuses of the spleen, bone marrow, adrenal cortex, and hypophysis; and other cells.

Retinopathy: Any disorder of the retina.

Rh immune globulin (Rhlg): A passive form of anti-D given within 72 hours of delivery to all Rh-negative mothers delivering an Rh-positive fetus.

Ribonucleic acid (RNA): A nucleic acid that controls protein synthesis in all living cells. There are three different types, and all are derived from the information encoded in the DNA of the cell. Messenger RNA (mRNA) carries the code for specific amino acid sequences from the DNA to the cytoplasm for protein synthesis. Transfer RNA (tRNA) carries the amino acid groups to the ribosome for protein synthesis. Ribosomal RNA (rRNA) exists within the ribosomes and is thought to assist in protein synthesis.

Ribosome: A cellular organelle that contains ribonucleoprotein and functions to synthesize protein. Ribosomes may be single units or clusters called polyribosomes or polysomes.

Rickettsia: Any of the microorganisms belonging to the genus *Rickettsia*.

Ristocetin: Drug used in platelet aggregation studies.

Rouleaux: A group of red blood corpuscles arranged like a roll of coins, owing to an abnormal protein coating on the cells' surfaces; seen in multiple myeloma and Waldenstrom's macroglobulinemia.

Rubriblast: See **Pronormoblast.**

Rubricyte: See **Polychromatophilic normoblast.**

Russell's viper venom (Stypven): Snake venom with thromboplastic activity.

S

Sarcoidosis: A disease of unknown etiology characterized by widespread granulomatous lesions that may affect any organ or tissue of the body.

Sarcoma: Cancer arising from connective tissue such as muscle or bone. It may affect the bones, bladder, kidneys, liver, lungs, parotids, and spleen.

Schistocyte: An abnormal red cell that is formed when pieces of the red cell membrane become fragmented. Whole pieces of the red cell membrane appear to be missing, causing bizarre-looking red cells.

Sclera: A tough, white fibrous tissue that covers the so-called white of the eye. It extends from the optic nerve to the cornea.

Scleroderma: A chronic disease of unknown etiology that causes sclerosis of the skin and certain organs, including the gastrointestinal tract, lungs, heart, and kidneys. The skin feels tough and leathery, may itch, and later becomes hyperpigmented.

Screening cells: Group O reagent red cells that are used in antibody detection or screening tests.

Scurvy: A deficiency of vitamin C characterized by hemorrhagic manifestations and abnormal formation of bones and teeth.

Senescence: The aging process of the red cells.

Sensitization: A condition of being made sensitive to a specific substance (such as an antigen) after the initial exposure to that substance. Results in the development of immunologic memory that evokes an accentuated immune response with subsequent exposure to the substance.

Sepsis: A pathologic state, usually febrile, resulting from the presence of microorganisms or their poisonous products in the bloodstream.

Septicemia: Presence of bacteria in the blood. The microorganisms may multiply and cause overwhelming infection and death.

Sequestration: An increase in the quantity of blood within the blood vessels, occurring physiologically or produced artificially.

Serine protease inhibitors: Plasma proteins such as antithrombin III. The activity of the various enzymes (serine proteases) involved in the coagulation sequence is controlled to a variable extent primarily by these plasma proteins, generally known as inhibitors.

Serine proteases: A family of proteolytic enzymes with the amino acid serine at the active site.

Serositis: Inflamed condition of a serous membrane.

Serotonin: A chemical present in platelets that is a potent vasoconstrictor.

Serum: The fluid that remains after blood has clotted.

Sex linkage: A genetic characteristic located on the X or Y chromosome.

Sézary syndrome: A skin disease characterized by infiltration with atypical Sezary cells. This exfoliative dermatitis is considered a variant form of mycosis fungoides.

Shift to the left: An abnormal cell maturation situation that occurs when increased bands, less mature neutrophils, and smaller average number of lobes are found in segmented cells; may be caused by infection, hematologic disorders, or physiologic factors.

Shift to the right: An abnormal cell maturation situation that occurs when more than one hypersegmented cell is seen; indicative of vitamin B_{12} or folate deficiency.

Shock: A clinical syndrome in which the peripheral blood is inadequate to return sufficient blood to the heart for normal function, particularly transport of oxygen to all organs and tissues.

Sickle cell: An abnormal red cell seen in patients who possess high quantities of hemoglobin S, an abnormal hemoglobin. The red cell is crescent- or sickle-shaped.

S.-c. anemia: Hereditary, chronic anemia in which abnormal sickle- or crescent-shaped erythrocytes are present. It is caused by the presence of hemoglobin S in the red blood cells. The gene that causes this disease occurs with high frequency in African and Mediterranean populations.

Sickle trait: Blood that is heterozygous for the gene coding for the abnormal hemoglobin of sickle-cell anemia.

Sideroblast: A ferritin-containing normoblast in the bone marrow. Makes up from 20% to 90% of normoblasts in the marrow.

Siderocyte: A non-nucleated red blood cell containing iron in a form other than hematin and confirmed by a specific iron stain such as the Prussian blue reaction.

Siderosis: A form of pneumoconiosis resulting from inhalation of dust or fumes containing iron particles.

Sodium dodecyl sulfate (SDS): An anionic detergent that renders a net negative charge to substances it solubilizes.

Somatic: Pertaining to nonreproductive cells or tissues.

Southern blot: A procedure to evaluate the structure of DNA, named after its inventor, Dr. Edwin Southern. First, DNA is cleaved at a specific nucleotide sequence by the action of restriction endonucleases. The resulting DNA fragments are separated by size using agarose gel electrophoresis, and then denatured using a strongly basic solution that converts double-stranded DNA into its single-stranded components. The fragments are transferred to a membrane, where they are immobilized and then hybridized to a complementary labeled probe. Detection of the probe label permits identification of the DNA fragments containing the sequence of interest. Genetic defects often result in alteration of the size and/or number of the target fragments.

Specificity: The affinity of an antibody and the antigen against which it is directed.

Spectrin: A large molecule, found on the inner surface of red blood cell membrane, that is responsible for the biconcave shape of the red cell as well as for its deformability.

Spectrophotometer: Device for measuring the amount of color in a solution by comparison with the spectrum.

Spherocyte: An abnormal red blood cell shape: Spherocytes are smaller than normal red cells, have a concentrated hemoglobin content, and have a decreased surface-to-volume ratio.

Spherocytosis: See **Hereditary spherocytosis.**

Splenomegaly: Enlargement of the spleen seen in several blood disorders.

Sprue: A disease endemic in many tropical regions and occurring sporadically in temperate countries, characterized by weakness, loss of weight, steatorrhea, and various digestive disorders.

Spurious: Not true or genuine; adulterated; false.

Stab: See **Band.**

Staphylococcal clumping test: A coagulation procedure used to detect the presence of fibrin-fibrinogen degradation products. The test uses a strain of staphylococcus that clumps in the presence of fibrinogen, fibrin monomers, or X and Y fragments.

Steatorrhea: Increased secretion of sebaceous glands, fatty stools.

Stenosis: Constriction or narrowing of a passage or orifice.

Steroid hormones: Hormones of the adrenal cortex and the sex hormones.

Stertorous: Pertaining to laborious breathing.

Stomatocyte: An abnormal red cell shape; this shape appears as having a slitlike area of central pallor.

Strabismus: Disorder of the eye in which optic axes cannot be directed to the same object. Strabismus can result from reduced visual activity, unequal ocular muscle tone, or an oculomotor nerve lesion.

Streptokinase: A product of beta-hemolytic streptococci capable of liquefying fibrin.

Stroma: The red cell membrane that is left after hemolysis.

Stuart-Prower factor: Factor X; functions in the common pathway of coagulation.

Stypven time test: A coagulation procedure used to distinguish between a deficiency of factor VIII and a deficiency of factor X.

Supernatant: Floating on surface, as oil on water.

Supervention: The development of an additional condition as a complication to an existing disease.

Syncytial: Of the nature of a syncytium, which is a group of cells in which the protoplasm of one cell is continuous with that of adjoining cells, such as the mesenchyme cells of the embryo.

Systemic: Pertaining to a whole body rather than to one of its parts.

Systemic lupus erythematosus (SLE): A disseminated autoimmune disease characterized by anemia, thrombocytopenia, increase IgG levels, and the presence of four IgG antibodies: antinuclear antibody, antinucleoprotein antibody, anti-DNA antibody, and antihistone antibody. Believed to be caused by suppressor T-cell dysfunction.

Systolic pressure: Maximum blood pressure that occurs at ventricular concentration. The upper value of a blood pressure reading.

T

Tachycardia: Abnormal rapidity of heart action, usually defined as a heart rate greater than 100 beats per minute.

Tachypnea: Abnormal rapidity of respiration.

Tanned red cell hemagglutination inhibition immunoassay (TRCHII): A test that is the reference method for the assay of fibrinogen degradation products.

Target cell: This abnormal red cell looks like a "bull's eye" with hemoglobin concentrated in the center and on the rim of the cell.

Tay-Sachs disease: Originally termed amaurotic infantile idiocy, this disorder is an autosomal recessive gangliosidoses caused by a deficiency of the enzyme hexosaminidase A. Its incidence in the Ashkenazi Jewish population is 100 times greater than that in the non-Jewish population.

T-cell: One of the cells derived from lymphoid stem cells.

Teardrop cell: An abnormal red cell, shaped like a tear, seen frequently in the myeloproliferative disorders. (Synonym: **Dacrocyte.**)

Telangiectasia: The presence of small, red focal lesions, usually in the skin or mucous membrane, caused by dilation of capillaries, arterioles, or venules.

Template bleeding time: The elapsed time it takes for a uniform incision made by a template and blade to stop bleeding; a test of platelet function in vivo assuming a normal platelet count.

Tertian malaria: Malaria in which sporulation occurs every 48 hours. Symptoms are more common during the day;

paroxysms divided into chills, fever, and sweating stages. Benign tertian malaria is caused by *Plasmodium vivax*, malignant tertian malaria by *Plasmodium falciparum.*

Tetany: A nervous affliction characterized by intermitent spasms of the muscles of the extremities.

Thalassemia: A group of hereditary anemias produced by either a defective production rate of alpha or the beta hemoglobin polypeptide. This disorder is inherited in the homozygous or heterozygous state.

   T. major: The homozygous form of deficient beta chain synthesis, which is very severe and presents itself during childhood. Prognosis varies, however; the younger the child when the disease appears, the more unfavorable the outcome.

Thermal amplitude: The range of temperature over which an antibody demonstrates serologic or in vitro activity or both.

Thrombin: An enzyme that converts fibrinogen to fibrin so that a soluble clot can be formed.

Thrombin time (TT): A coagulation procedure that measures the time required for thrombin to convert fibrinogen to an insoluble fibrin clot.

Thrombocytopathies: Inherited disorders of platelets.

Thrombocytopenia: Decreased numbers of platelets.

Thrombocythemia: A condition marked by increased platelets in the blood.

Thrombocytosis: Increased numbers of platelets.

Thromboembolism: An embolism; the blocking of a blood vessel by a thrombus (blood clot) that has become detached from the site of formation.

Thrombopoiesis: The formation of platelets.

Thrombosis: The formation or development of a blood clot or thrombus.

Thrombotic thrombocytopenic purpura (TTP): A severe condition characterized by thrombocytopenia, microangiopathic hemolytic anemia, renal dysfunction, neurologic abnormalities, and fever.

Thymidine: An essential ingredient used in DNA synthesis and incorporated by T lymphocytes undergoing blast transformation in response to foreign HLA-D antigens in the mixed lymphocyte culture test.

Thymoma: A disorder of the thymus marked by anemia as a result of selective hypoplasia of RBC precursors in bone marrow.

Thyromegaly: Enlargement of the thyroid gland.

Tinnitus: Buzzing in the ears.

Tissue plasminogen activator (TPA): A clotting factor produced by vascular endothelial cells that selectively binds to fibrin as it activates fibrin-bound plasminogen.

Tissue thromboplastin: Factor III; functions in the extrinsic system of coagulation.

Titer score: A method used to evaluate more precisely than simple dilution by comparing the titers of an antibody. Agglutination at each higher dilution is graded on a continuous scale; the total is the titer score.

Total iron-binding capacity (TIBC): The amount of iron that transferrin can bind; normal range is 250 to 360 μg/dl. TIBC = unsaturated iron-binding capacity (UIBC) or amount of additional iron that transferrin can bind above that which is already complexed + serum Fe.

Toxic granulation: Medium to large metachromatic granules that are evenly distributed throughout the cytoplasm. May be seen in severe bacterial infections, severe burns, and other conditions.

Trabeculae: Bands or bundles of connective tissue.

Trait: A characteristic that is inherited.

Transcription: The process of RNA production from DNA, which requires the enzyme RNA polymerase.

Transferase: An enzyme that catalyzes the transfer of atoms or groups of atoms from one chemical compound to another.

Transferrin: A glycoprotein synthesized in the liver, with the primary function of iron transport.

Transfuse: To perform a transfusion.

Transfusion: The injection of blood, a blood component, saline, or other fluids into the bloodstream.

T. reaction: An adverse response to a transfusion.

Translation: The production of protein from the interactions of the RNAs.

Translocation: Transfer of a portion of one chromosome to its allele.

Transplacental: Through the placenta.

Transposition: The location of two genes on opposite chromosomes of a homologous pair.

U

Ubiquitous: Existing everywhere at the same time.

Uremia: The presence of urine or urine components in the blood.

Urokinase: A trypsinlike protease, found in the urine and synthesized by the kidney, that activates plasminogen by proteolytic cleavage. Differs from tissue plasminogen activators in that urokinase reacts with plasminogen in the fluid phase of blood.

Urticaria: A vascular reaction of the skin similar to hives.

V

Vaccine: A suspension of infectious organisms or components of them that is given as a form of immunization to establish resistance to the infectious disease caused by the same organism.

Vacuolization: The presence of cavity in a cell's protoplasm.

Valvular: Relating to or having a valve.

Variable region: Portion of the immunoglobulin light and heavy chains in which amino acid sequences vary tremendously. These amino acid variations permit the different immunoglobulin molecules to recognize different antigenic determinants. In other words, the variable region determines the antigen against which the antibody will react, thus providing each antibody molecule with its unique specificity. The variable region is located at the amino terminal region of the molecule.

Vascular: Pertaining to or composed of blood vessels.

Vasculitis: Inflammation of a blood or lymph vessel.

Vasoconstriction: Constriction of blood vessels.

Vasodilatation: Dilatation of blood vessels, especially small arteries and arterioles.

Vaso-occlusive: Obstruction of the vasculature by some pathologic process that seriously impedes blood flow.

Vasovagal syncope: Syncope resulting from hypotension caused by emotional stress, pain, acute blood loss, fear, or rapidly rising from a recumbent position.

Venipuncture: Puncture of a vein for any purpose.

Venom: A poison excreted by some animals such as insects or snakes and transmitted by bites or stings.

Venule: A tiny vein continuous with a capillary.

Verrucous: Wartlike, with raised portions.

Vertigo: Dizziness.

Viremia: Refers to the presence of a virus in the blood.

Viscosity: Having sticky or glutinous attributes.

Vitamin K: A fat-soluble vitamin required for maintenance of normal blood levels of the vitamin K-dependent factors: prothrombin and factors VII, IX, and X. Vitamin K is necessary for carboxylation of specific glutamic acid residues in the postprotein synthesis of the vitamin K-dependent factors.

von Willebrand's disease (vWD): A congenital bleeding disorder inherited as an autosomal dominant trait and characterized by a decreased level of factor VIII:C and a prolonged bleeding time.

von Willebrand factor (vWF): A component of the factor VIII molecule that mediates platelet interaction with subendothelium.

W

WAIHA: Warm autoimmune hemolytic anemia.

Whole blood clotting time: A test that evaluates the overall activity of the intrinsic system of coagulation.

Wiskott-Aldrich syndrome: A congenital platelet storage pool defect characterized by immunologic alteration, recurrent pyogenic infection, and eczema.

X

Xerocyte: A dehydrated red blood cell having a peculiar morphologic appearance (that is, hemoglobin concentration at one pole of the red cell).

Z

Zeta: A type of globin chain found in embryonic hemoglobin.

Zymogen: A substance that, when paired with its zymase, becomes an enzyme.

Index

A number in *italics* indicates a figure; a number followed by a "t" indicates a table.